Electronic Study Tools At Your Fingertips!

This new edition of **Clinically Oriented Anatomy** now includes two free CD's containing many powerful study tools for students. Case studies, 3-D anatomical images, and USMLE-style questions will help you review course material and study for course and board exams.

- The *Clinically Oriented Anatomy Student CD* contains interactive case studies that highlight the application of anatomy to clinical practice and 135 all-new USMLE-style review questions.

- The second CD contains a 45-day free trial to *Interactive Functional Anatomy*, produced by Primal Pictures. *Interactive Functional Anatomy* uses three-dimensional models of MRI images to generate a unique body of layered, rotatable anatomical illustrations. Annotations accompany the images to provide information about the anatomy being viewed. The program is delivered on CD and access is for 45 days only.

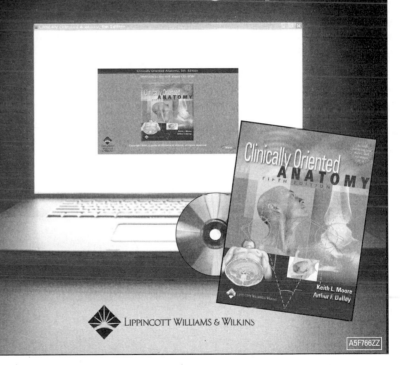

LIPPINCOTT WILLIAMS & WILKINS

A5F766ZZ

Clinically ▶Oriented Anatomy

FIFTH EDITION

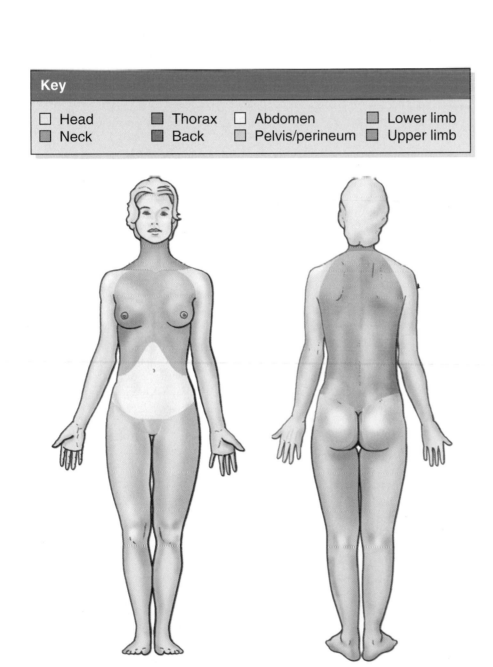

Key			
☐ Head	■ Thorax	☐ Abdomen	■ Lower limb
■ Neck	■ Back	■ Pelvis/perineum	■ Upper limb

Anterior view   **Posterior view**

Clinically ▶Oriented Anatomy

FIFTH EDITION

Keith L. Moore, Ph.D., F.I.A.C., F.R.S.M.

Professor Emeritus in Division of Anatomy, Department of Surgery
Former Chair of Anatomy and Associate Dean for Basic Medical Sciences
Faculty of Medicine, University of Toronto
Toronto, Ontario, Canada

Arthur F. Dalley II, Ph.D.

Professor of Cell and Developmental Biology
Director, Medical Gross Anatomy and Anatomical Donations Program
Department of Cell and Developmental Biology
Vanderbilt University School of Medicine
Nashville, Tennessee, U.S.A.

In collaboration with, and with content provided by,
Anne M. R. Agur, B.Sc. (OT), M.Sc., Ph.D.

Associate Professor in Division of Anatomy, Department of Surgery
Department of Physical Therapy and Department of Occupational Therapy
Division of Biomedical Communications, Department of Surgery
Institute of Medical Science
Faculty of Medicine, University of Toronto
Toronto, Ontario, Canada

With the developmental assistance and dedication of
Marion E. Moore, B.A.

LIPPINCOTT WILLIAMS & WILKINS
A **Wolters Kluwer** Company

Philadelphia • Baltimore • New York • London
Buenos Aires • Hong Kong • Sydney • Tokyo

Acquisitions Editor: Betty Sun
Developmental Editor: Kathleen H. Scogna
Marketing Manager: Joe Schott
Production Editors: Jennifer Glazer and Christiane Odyniec
Designer: Doug Smock
Compositor: Maryland Composition Company, Inc.
Printer: R. R. Donnelly & Sons—Willard

351 West Camden Street
Baltimore, MD 21201

530 Walnut Street
Philadelphia, PA 19106

Printed in the United States of America

First Edition, 1980
Second Edition, 1985
Third Edition, 1992
Fourth Edition, 1999
Spanish Translation, 2002, published by Editorial Médica Panamericana, S.A.
Complex Chinese Translation, 2003, published by The Leader Book Company
Simplified Chinese Translation, 2004, published by Henan Scientific and Technical Publishing House
French Translation, 2001, published by DeBoeck Universite
Italian Translation, 2001, published by Casa Editrice Ambrosiana
Japanese Translation, 2004, published by Igaku Shuppan
Portuguese Translation, 2001, published by Editora Guanabara Koogan

Library of Congress Cataloging-in-Publication Data

Moore, Keith L.
  Clinically oriented anatomy / Keith L. Moore, Arthur F. Dalley II ; in collaboration with, and with content provided by Anne M.R. Agur ; with the developmental assistance and dedication of Marion E. Moore.–5th ed.

    p. ; cm.
  ISBN 0-7817-3639-0
  1. Human anatomy. 2. Anatomy, Pathological. I. Dalley, Arthur F. II. Agur, A. M. R. III. Title.
  [DNLM: 1. Anatomy. QS 4 M822c 2006]
  QM23.2.M67 2006
  611–dc22

                    2004028886

To purchase additional copies of this book, call our customer service department at **(800) 638-3030** or fax orders to **(301) 824-7390.** International customers should call **(301) 714-2324.**

Visit Lippincott Williams & Wilkins on the Internet: http://www.LWW.com. Lippincott Williams & Wilkins customer service representatives are available from 8:30 am to 6:00 P.M., EST.

05 06 07 08 09
2 3 4 5 6 7 8 9 10

To Marion

My best friend, wife, colleague, and mother of our five children for her love,

unconditional support, and understanding, and in loving memory

of our son Warren, who is sadly missed. • (KLM)

To Muriel

My bride, best friend, counselor, and mother of our boys; and to our

family—Tristan, Lana, and Elijah Grey, Denver, and Skyler—with love

and great appreciation for their support, understanding, good humor,

and—most of all—patience • (AFD)

To Our Students

You will remember some of what you hear, much of what you read,

more of what you see, and almost all of what you experience and understand fully.

Preface

A quarter century has passed since the first edition of *Clinically Oriented Anatomy* appeared on bookstore shelves; six years have passed since the fourth edition was published. The relatively long interval between editions results from efforts to continue to make this book even more student friendly and authoritative. This fifth edition has therefore been *thoroughly revised* with significant new changes and updates.

Key Features

Clinically Oriented Anatomy has been widely acclaimed for the relevance of its clinical correlations. As in previous editions, the fifth edition places clinical emphasis on anatomy that is important in general practice, diagnostic radiology, emergency medicine, and general surgery. Special attention has been directed toward assisting students in learning the anatomy they will need to know in the twenty-first century, and to this end new features have been added and existing features updated.

Clinical correlations. Popularly known as "blue boxes," the clinical information sections have grown, and many of them are now supported by photographs and/or dynamic color illustrations to help with understanding the practical value of anatomy.

"Bottom Line" summaries. A new feature in this edition, frequent Bottom Line boxes summarize the preceding information, ensuring that primary concepts do not become lost in the many details necessary for thorough understanding. These summaries provide a convenient means of ongoing review.

Anatomy described in a practical, functional context. A more realistic approach to the musculoskeletal system emphasizes the action and use of muscles and muscle groups in daily activities. New material has been added to address gait and grip. The eccentric contraction of muscles, which accounts for much of their activity, is now discussed along with the concentric contraction that is typically the sole focus in anatomy texts. This perspective is important to most health professionals, including the growing number of physical and occupational therapy students using this book.

Surface anatomy. Surface anatomy sections, identified by their yellow-screened background, feature all-new color photographs, clearly demonstrating anatomy's relationship to physical examination and diagnosis. Both natural views of unobstructed surface anatomy and illustrations superimposing anatomical structures on surface anatomy photographs are components of each regional chapter.

Medical imaging. Each regional chapter ends with sections on medical imaging, identified by their green-screened backgrounds. These sections provide various combinations of plain and contrast radiographic, MRI, CT, and ultrasonography studies, often with correlative line art as well as explanatory text, to help prepare future professionals who need to be familiar with diagnostic images.

Case studies, accompanied by clinicoanatomical problems and 105 new USMLE-style multiple-choice questions. These interactive case studies and multiple-choice questions are included on an accompanying CD, providing a convenient and comprehensive means of self-testing and review.

Extensive new art program. The extensive new art program implemented in the fourth edition has been extended and revised. An effort has been made to ensure that all the anatomy presented and covered in the text is also illustrated. The text and illustrations have been developed to work together for optimum pedagogical effect, aiding the learning process and reducing the amount of searching required to find structures. The great majority of the clinical conditions are now supported by photographs and/or color illustrations; multipart illustrations often combine dissections, line art, and medical images; most tables appear in color and are illustrated to aid the student's understanding of the structures described.

Terminology. The terminology fully adheres to the new *Terminologia Anatomica* (1998), approved by the International Federation of Associations of Anatomists (IFAA). Although the official English-equivalent terms are used throughout the book, when new terms are introduced, the Latin form, used in Europe, Asia, and other parts of the world, is also provided. The roots and derivations of terms are provided to help students understand meaning and increase retention. Eponyms, although not endorsed by the IFAA, appear in parentheses in this edition—for example, sternal angle (angle of Louis)—to assist students who will hear eponymous terms during their clinical studies.

Retained and Improved Features

Students and faculty have told us what they want and expect from *Clinically Oriented Anatomy,* and we listened:

- A *comprehensive text* enabling students to fill in the blanks, as time allotted for lectures continues to decrease, laboratory guides become exclusively instructional, and multiauthored lecture notes develop inconsistencies in comprehension, fact, and format.

- A *resource capable of supporting areas of special interest and emphasis* within specific anatomy courses that *serves the anatomy needs of students during both the basic science and the clinical phases of their studies.*

- A *thorough Introduction* that covers important systemic information and concepts basic to the understanding of the anatomy presented in the subsequent regional chapters. Students from many countries and backgrounds have written to express their views of this book— gratifyingly, most are congratulatory. Health professional students have more diverse backgrounds and experiences than ever before. Curricular constraints often result in unjustified assumptions concerning the prerequisite information necessary for many students to understand the presented material. The Introduction includes efficient summaries of functional systemic anatomy. Student comments specifically emphasized the need for a systemic description of the nervous system and the peripheral autonomic nervous system (ANS) in particular. The increased coverage of the ANS implemented in the fourth edition has been strengthened and further supported with new illustrations in this edition.

- Routine facts (such as muscle attachments, innervations, and actions) presented in *tables organized to demonstrate shared qualities and illustrated to demonstrate the provided information. Clinically Oriented Anatomy* provides more tables than any other anatomy textbook.

- *Illustrated clinical correlations* that not only describe but also *show anatomy as it is applied clinically* .

- *Illustrations that facilitate orientation.* Many orientation figures have been added, along with arrows to indicate the locations of the inset figures (areas shown in close-up views) and viewing sequences. Almost all illustrations have been completely relabeled, moving the viewpoint out of the legend and next to each part of every illustration. Labels have been placed to minimize the distance between label and object, with leader lines running the most direct course possible.

- *Case studies with practice questions* that review and underscore important aspects of clinically applied anatomy are useful in preparation for internal and external examinations, such as the USMLE.

Additional Features

- More than 130 new full-color illustrations, including many multipart illustrations combining dissections, line art, and medical images such as CTs and MRIs have been added to this edition.

- Boldface type indicates the main entries of anatomical terms when they are introduced and defined; italic type indicates anatomical terms important to the topic and region of study. Boldface is also used in the surface anatomy (yellow) boxes to indicate visible or palpable features and to introduce clinical terms in the clinical correlation (blue) boxes.

- Useful content outlines appear at the beginning of every chapter.

- Instructor's resources and supplemental materials, including images exportable for *Power Point* presentation, are available—both specific to COA and through the institutional version of Dynamic Human Anatomy, which includes many resources from the LWW portfolio of anatomy products.

Commitment to Educating Students

This book is written for health science students, keeping in mind those who may not have had a previous acquaintance with anatomy. We have tried to present the material in an interesting way so that it can be easily integrated with what will be taught in more detail in other disciplines such as physical diagnosis, medical rehabilitation, and surgery. We hope this text will serve two purposes: to educate and to excite. If students develop enthusiasm for clinical anatomy, the goals of this book will have been fulfilled.

Keith L. Moore
University of Toronto
Faculty of Medicine

Arthur F. Dalley, II
Vanderbilt University
School of Medicine

Acknowledgments

We wish to thank the following colleagues who were invited by the publisher to assist with the development of this fifth edition through their critical analysis and review of an initial draft of the manuscript.

- Patricia A. Brewer, Ph.D., Assistant Professor, Department of Physical Therapy, University of Texas Health Science Center at San Antonio, San Antonio, Texas.

- Matthew Davey, M.D., Registrar, Intensive Care Unit, The Canberra Hospital, Canberra, ACT, Australia.

- Duane E. Haines, Ph.D., Professor and Chairman, Department of Anatomy, The University of Mississippi Medical Center, Jackson, Mississippi.

- Kenneth H. Jones, Ph.D., Assistant Professor, Department of Anatomy and Medical Education, Ohio State University, College of Medicine and Public Health, Columbus, Ohio.

- William A. Roy, Ph.D., Associate Professor of Anatomy, The University of Mississippi Medical Center, Jackson, Mississippi.

- Joel A. Vilensky, Ph.D., Professor of Anatomy, Department of Anatomy and Cell Biology, Indiana University School of Medicine, Fort Wayne, Indiana.

- Michael P. Zumpano, Ph.D., Associate Professor, Department of Anatomy, New York Chiropractic College, Seneca Falls, New York.

Several students, who have since graduated, were also invited by the publisher to review an initial draft of the manuscript:

- Renee Hsia, M.D., M.Sc., Emergency Medicine Resident, Stanford University Hospital, Stanford, California.

- *John C. Teeters*, M.D., Resident, University of Rochester Medical Center, Rochester, New York.

In addition to reviewers, many people—some of them unknowingly—helped us by perusing, discussing, or contributing to parts of the manuscript and/or providing constructive criticism of the text and illustrations in this and previous editions:

- Dr. Peter Abrahams, Consultant Clinical Anatomist, University of Cambridge and examiner to the Royal College of Surgeons of Edinburgh, Cambridge, United Kingdom.

- Dr. Robert D. Acland, Professor of Surgery/Microsurgery, Division of Plastic and Reconstructive Surgery, University of Louisville, Louisville, Kentucky.

- Dr. Oloruntosin Akindele, Tofunmi Medical Center, Igbogbo, Lagos State, Nigeria.

- Dr. Julian J. Baumel, Professor Emeritus of Biomedical Sciences, Creighton University School of Medicine, Omaha, Nebraska.

- Dr. Edna Becker, Associate Professor of Medical Imaging, University of Toronto Faculty of Medicine, Toronto, Ontario, Canada.

- Dr. Donald R. Cahill, Professor of Anatomy (retired; former Chair), Mayo Medical School; former Editor-in-Chief of *Clinical Anatomy,* Rochester, Minnesota.

- Dr. Joan Campbell, Assistant Professor of Medical Imaging, University of Toronto Faculty of Medicine, Toronto, Ontario, Canada.

- Dr. Stephen W. Carmichael, Professor and Chair of Anatomy, Mayo Medical School, Editor-in-Chief of *Clinical Anatomy*, Rochester, Minnesota.

- Dr. Carmine D. Clemente, Professor of Anatomy and Orthopedic Surgery, University of California, Los Angeles School of Medicine, Los Angeles, California.

- Dr. James D. Collins, Professor of Radiological Sciences, University of California, Los Angeles School of Medicine/Center for Health Sciences, Los Angeles, California.

- Dr. Raymond F. Gasser, Professor of Anatomy, Louisiana State University School of Medicine, New Orleans, Louisiana.

- Dr. Ralph Ger, Professor of Anatomy and Structural Biology, Albert Einstein College of Medicine, Bronx, New York; Associate Chairman, Department of Surgery, Nassau County Medical Center, East Meadow, New York.

- Dr. Douglas J. Gould, Associate Professor, University of Kentucky, Lexington, Kentucky.

- Dr. Daniel O. Graney, Professor of Biological Structure, University of Washington School of Medicine, Seattle, Washington.

- Dr. David G. Greathouse, Professor and Chair, Belmont University School of Physical Therapy, Nashville, Tennessee.

- Dr. Masoom Haider, Assistant Professor of Medical Imaging, University of Toronto Faculty of Medicine, Toronto, Ontario, Canada.

- Dr. John S. Halle, Professor, Belmont University School of Physical Therapy, Nashville, Tennessee.

- Dr. Jennifer L. Halpern, Resident in Orthopedic Surgery and Rehabilitation, Vanderbilt University School of Medicine, Nashville, Tennessee.

- Dr. Walter Kuchareczyk, Professor and Chair of Medical Imaging, University of Toronto Faculty of Medicine; Clinical Director of Tri-Hospital Magnetic Resonance Centre, Toronto, Ontario, Canada.

- Dr. Nirusha Lachman, Program Chair, Anatomy, Durban Institute of Technology, Durban, South Africa.

- Dr. H. Wayne Lambert, Instructor, Cell and Developmental Biology and Cancer Biology, Vanderbilt University School of Medicine, Nashville, Tennessee.

- Dr. Michael von Lüdinghausen, University Professor, Anatomy Institute, University of Würzburg, Würzburg, Germany.

- Dr. Shirley McCarthy, Director of MRI, Department of Diagnostic Radiology, Yale University School of Medicine, New Haven, Connecticut.

- Dr. Lillian Nanney, Professor of Plastic Surgery, Vanderbilt University School of Medicine, Nashville, Tennessee.

- Dr. Todd R. Olson, Professor of Anatomy and Structural Biology, Albert Einstein College of Medicine, Bronx, New York.

- Dr. Wojciech Pawlina, Professor of Anatomy, Mayo Medical School, Rochester, Minnesota.

- Dr. David Peck, Associate Professor of Anatomy and Neurobiology (retired), University of Kentucky School of Medicine, Lexington, Kentucky.

- Dr. T. V. N. Persaud, Professor of Human Anatomy and Cell Science Faculties of Medicine and Dentistry, University of Manitoba, Winnipeg, Manitoba, Canada.

- Dr. Cathleen C. Pettepher, Associate Professor of Cancer Biology, Vanderbilt University School of Medicine, Nashville, Tennessee.

- Dr. Thomas H. Quinn, Professor of Biomedical Sciences, Creighton University School of Medicine, Omaha, Nebraska.

- Dr. George E. Salter, Professor of Anatomy, Department of Cell Biology, University of Alabama at Birmingham, Birmingham, Alabama.

- Dr. Tatsuo Sato, Professor and Head (retired), Second Department of Anatomy, Tokyo Medical and Dental University Faculty of Medicine, Tokyo, Japan.

- Professor Colin P. Wendell-Smith, Department of Anatomy and Physiology, University of Tasmania, Hobart, Tasmania, Australia.

- Dr. Andreas H. Weiglein, Associate Professor, Institut fur Anatomie, Medical University Graz, Graz, Austria.

- Dr. David G. Whitlock, Professor of Anatomy, University of Colorado Medical School, Denver, Colorado.

Our grateful appreciation is extended to Marion Moore, the senior author's wife (of 55 years), for her friendly help and patience with the preparation of the manuscript. She prepared many drafts of each chapter and provided tactful, constructive criticism as the "polishing" process progressed. We also wish to acknowledge the excellent work of Kathleen Scogna, the Senior Developmental Editor. Her great efforts cannot be overstated. The quality of this edition is the result in no small part of her critical perspective, keen observations and insights, encouragement, advocacy, great attention to detail, and detailed text–art coordination.

Art plays a major role in facilitating learning. We extend our sincere gratitude and appreciation for the skills, talents, and timely work of our medical illustrators for this edition, Rob Duckwall of Dragonfly Media Group and Valerie Oxorn, who contributed many new and modified illustrations. David Rini also contributed to the art program in this edition. Wayne Hubble at LWW did a masterful job of labeling, relabeling, and resizing artwork. E. Anne Rayner, Senior Photographer, Vanderbilt Medical Art Group did an excellent job photographing the surface anatomy models, working in association with Dr. Anne Agur and the junior author (AFD). We greatly appreciate the contribution our models made to the quality of this edition. Much of the art was originally prepared for the fourth edition by Craig Durant and colleagues at J/B Woolsey Associates, Elkins Park, Pennsylvania. Although the number of illustrations from *Grant's Atlas of Anatomy* continues to be reduced and replaced by new art, we gratefully acknowledge the excellent art done by the following: Dorothy Foster Chubb, Elizabeth Blackstock, Nancy Joy, Nina Kilpatrick, David Mazierski, Stephen Mader, Bart Vallecoccia, Sari O'Sullivan, Kam Yu, and Caitlin Duckwall.

Many thanks also to those at Lippincott Williams & Wilkins who participated in the development of this edition: Betty Sun, Executive Editor; Crystal Taylor, Acquisitions Editor; and Jennifer Glazer and Christiane Odyniec, Production Editors. We would like to thank Joe Schott and his marketing colleagues for their imaginative and informative marketing and promotion of the previous and current editions. Finally, thanks is due to the sales division at LWW, which has played a key role in the continued success of this book.

Keith L. Moore
Arthur F. Dalley II

Abbreviations

a., aa.	arteries		lev.	levator
ant.	anterior		lit.	literally
B.C.E	before the Common (Christian) era		M	male
C	cervical		m., mm.	muscles
C.E.	Common (Christian) era		Mediev.	medieval
Co	coccygeal		Mod.	modern
dim.	diminutive		post.	posterior
e.g.	for example		S	sacral
et al.	and others		sup.	superior
F	female		sup.	superioris
Fr.	French		supf.	superficial
G.	Greek		T	thoracic
i.e.	that is		TA	*Terminologia Anatomica,* tibialis anterior
inf.	inferior		T. major	teres major
L	liter, lumbar		v., vv.	veins
L.	Latin		vs.	versus

Figure Credits

Introduction

Agur AMR: *Grant's Atlas of Anatomy*, 9th ed. Baltimore: Williams & Wilkins, 1991. BI.5.

Agur AMR, Dalley AF: *Grant's Atlas of Anatomy*, 11th ed. Baltimore: Lippincott Williams & Wilkins, 2004. I.47.

Daffner RH: *Clinical Radiology: The Essentials*, 2nd ed. Baltimore: Williams & Wilkins, 1998. I.45.

Hamill JH, Knutzan K: *Biochemical Basis of Human Movement*, 2nd ed. Baltimore: Lippincott Williams & Wilkins, 2003. I.20.

Rassner G: *Atlas of Dermatology*, 3rd ed. Trans: Burgdorf WHC. Philadelphia: Lea & Febiger, 1994. BI.2 (photograph).

Roche Lexikon Medizin, 4th ed. Munich: Urban & Schwarzenberg, 1998. BI 8.

Stedman's Medical Dictionary, 27th ed. Baltimore: Lippincott Williams & Wilkins, 2000. BI.2 (artist: Neil O. Hardy, Westport, CT), BI.3, BI.4 (artist: Neil O. Hardy, Westport, CT).

van de Graaff K: *Human Anatomy*, 4th ed. Dubuque, IA: WC Brown, 1995. BI.1.

Wicke L: *Atlas of Radiologic Anatomy*, 6th English ed. Ed and Trans: Taylor AN. Baltimore: Williams & Wilkins, 1998. [Wicke L: *Roentgen-Anatomie Normalbefunde*, 5th ed. Munich: Urban & Schwarzenberg, 1995.] I.48, I.49, I.50, I.51.

Willis MC: *Medical Terminology: The Language of Health Care*. Baltimore: Lippincott Williams & Wilkins, 1995. BI.7.

Chapter 1

Acuson Computed Sonography Corporation. Mountain View, CA. 1.70.

Agur AMR: *Grant's Atlas of Anatomy*, 9th ed. Baltimore: Williams & Wilkins, 1991. 1.1, 1.11, 1.12, 1.14, 1.15, 1.26A & B, 1.37, 1.43, 1.44, 1.47B, 1.53, 1.55A & B, 1.59, 1.60A & B, 1.66D.

Agur AMR, Dalley AF: *Grant's Atlas of Anatomy*, 11th ed. Baltimore: Lippincott Williams & Wilkins, 2004. 1.4 (modified), 1.5 (modified), 1.7, 1.8A & B (modified), 1.19 (modified), 1.24A, 1.25, 1.27A & B, 1.28A, 1.41, 1.46, 1.47A, 1.52 (modified), 1.66B, 1.68A & B, 1.69, 1.72, B1.25A & B.

Agur AMR, Ming JL: *Grant's Atlas of Anatomy*, 10th ed. Baltimore: Williams & Wilkins, 1999. 1.64, 1.71A, B1.12B, B1.17.

Bickley LS, Szilagyi PG: *Bates' Guide to Physical Examination*, 8th ed. Baltimore: Lippincott Williams & Wilkins, 2002. B1.6A.

Brant WE, Helms CA: *Fundamentals of Diagnostic Radiology*, 2nd ed. Baltimore: Williams & Wilkins, 1999. B1.6B.

Clay JH, Pounds DM: *Basic Clinical Massage Therapy: Integrating Anatomy and Treatment*. Baltimore: Lippincott Williams & Wilkins, 2002. Table 1.2A & B.

Dean D, Herbener TE: *Cross-Sectional Anatomy*. Baltimore: Lippincott Williams & Wilkins, 2000. 1.23.

Hall-Craggs ECB: *Anatomy as the Basis of Clinical Medicine*, 3rd ed. Baltimore: Williams & Wilkins, 1995. B1.7.

Madden ME. *Introduction to Sectional Anatomy*. Baltimore: Lippincott Williams & Wilkins, 2000. 1.71B.

Stedman's Medical Dictionary, 27th ed. Baltimore: Lippincott Williams & Wilkins, 2000. 1.22C (artist: Michael Schenk, Jackson, MS), B1.9 (artist: Neil O. Hardy, Westport, CT), B1.11

(artist: Mikki Senkarik, San Antonio, TX; photograph courtesy of Olympus America, Inc., Melville, NY), B1.12*A* (artist: Neil O. Hardy, Westport, CT), B1.13 (artist: Neil O. Hardy, Westport, CT; photographs of bronchus, carina, and trachea from Feinsilver SH, Fein A: *Textbook of Bronchoscopy.* Baltimore: Williams & Wilkins, 1995; photograph of bronchoscopy procedure courtesy of Temple University Hospital, Philadelphia, PA), B1.16 (artist: Neil O. Hardy, Westport, CT), B1.18 (artist: Neil O. Hardy, Westport, CT), B1.21 (artist: Neil O. Hardy, Westport, CT), B1.22 (photograph courtesy of the Burdick Corporation; artist: Neil O. Hardy, Westport, CT).

Torrent-Guasp F, Buckberg GD, Clemente C, et al.: The structure and function of the helical heart and its buttress wrapping. I. The normal macroscopic structure of the heart. *Semin Thoracic Cardiovasc Surg* 13:30, 2001. 1.40*A.*

Chapter 2

Agur AMR: *Grant's Method of Anatomy,* 9th ed. Baltimore: Williams & Wilkins, 1975. 2.29*A,* 2.44*A* & *B.*

Agur AMR: *Grant's Atlas of Anatomy,* 9th ed. Baltimore: Williams & Wilkins, 1991. 2.17, 2.25*A,* 2.31*B,* 2.34*D,* 2.35*B* & *C,* 2.44*B,* 2.49*C* & *D,* 2.53*B,* 2.60, 2.61, 2.64*A–D,* 2.76*A,* 2.81*C,* 2.86 (modified), 2.87*A* & *B,* B2.7.

Agur AMR, Dalley AF: *Grant's Atlas of Anatomy,* 11th ed. Baltimore: Lippincott Williams & Wilkins, 2004. 2.1, 2.6*A,* 2.8*A,* 2.10, 2.24, 2.30*A* & *B,* 2.31*A,* 2.33*A,* 2.34*A,* 2.42*A* (modified), 2.46*C,* 2.48*A,* 2.49*B,* 2.52, 2.58, 2.63, 2.67*A–C,* 2.71*A* (modified), 2.76*B,* 2.77, 2.81*A* & *B,* 2.82*A–C,* 2.83*B* & *C,* 2.85, 2.88*A,* B2.15*A,* B2.20, Table 2.7, Table 2.9*C–E,* Table 2.11, Table 2.12 (modified), Table 2.15*A* & *B.*

Agur AMR, Ming JL: *Grant's Atlas of Anatomy,* 10th ed. Baltimore: Williams & Wilkins, 1999. 2.57.

Bickley LS, Szilagyi PG: *Bates' Guide to Physical Examination,* 8th ed. Baltimore: Lippincott Williams & Wilkins, 2002. SA2.4 (modified).

Brant WE, Helms CA: *Fundamentals of Diagnostic Radiology,* 2nd ed. Baltimore: Williams & Wilkins, 1999. B2.9.

Clay JH, Pounds DM: *Basic Clinical Massage Therapy: Integrating Anatomy and Treatment.* Baltimore: Lippincott Williams & Wilkins, 2002. Table 2.2.

Dean D, Herbener TE: *Cross-Sectional Anatomy.* Baltimore: Lippincott Williams & Wilkins, 2000. 2.88*B* & *C.*

Gartner LP, Hiatt JL: *Color Atlas of Histology,* 3rd ed. Baltimore: Lippincott Williams & Wilkins, 2001. 2.46*D.*

Haines DE: *Neuroanatomy: An Atlas of Structures, Sections, and Systems.* Baltimore: Williams & Wilkins, 1994. 2.41 (inset).

Lockhart RD, Hamilton GF, Fyfe FW: *Anatomy of the Human Body.* Philadelphia: Lippincott, 1959. B2.2.

Moore KL, Agur AMR: *Essential Clinical Anatomy,* 2nd ed. Baltimore: Lippincott Williams & Wilkins, 2000. Table 2.4.

Olympus America, Inc. B2.17 (photograph of colonoscope).

Roche Lexikon Medizin, 3rd ed. Munich: Urban & Schwarzenberg, 1993. B2.17 (photograph of diverticulosis), B2.28*B.*

Rosse C, Gaddum-Rosse P: *Hollinshead's Textbook of Anatomy,* 5th ed. Philadelphia, Lippincott-Raven, 1997. 2.70.

Sauerland EK: *Grant's Dissector,* 12th ed. Baltimore: Lippincott Williams & Wilkins, 1999. 2.12*C,* 2.49*E,* B2.23, Table 2.9*B,* Table 2.15*C* (modified).

Stedman's Medical Dictionary, 27th ed. Baltimore: Lippincott Williams & Wilkins, 2000. 2.25*B* (artist: Neil O. Hardy, Westport, CT), 2.34*C* (artist: Neil O. Hardy, Westport, CT), 2.45*C* (artist: Neil O. Hardy, Westport, CT), B2.5, B2.8 (photograph courtesy of Mission Hospital Regional Medical Center, Mission Viejo, CA), B2.10 (artist: Neil O. Hardy, Westport, CT), B2.11 (artist: Neil O. Hardy, Westport, CT), B2.15*B* (part *D:* artist: Neil O. Hardy, Westport, CT), B2.16*A* & *B* (artist: Neil O. Hardy, Westport, CT), B2.17 (diverticulosis: artist: Neil O. Hardy, Westport, CT; colonoscopy: artist: Mikki Senkarik, San Antonio, TX), B2.18.

Chapter 3

Agur AMR: *Grant's Atlas of Anatomy,* 9th ed. Baltimore: Williams & Wilkins, 1991. 3.4*A* & *B,* 3.11*A–C,* 3.14*B,* 3.20*A,* 3.21, 3.24, 3.27*A,* 3.31*A* & *B,* 3.42*A* & *B,* 3.48*D,* 3.49*A,* 3.53*A* & *B,* 3.54, 3.55, 3.58, 3.59*B.*

Agur AMR, Dalley AF: *Grant's Atlas of Anatomy,* 11th ed. Baltimore: Lippincott Williams & Wilkins, 2004. 3.2 (modified), 3.3*B* & *C,* 3.6*B–D,* 3.10*A,* 3.19 (modified), 3.30 (modified), 3.33, 3.35 (modified), 3.37, 3.47 (modified), 3.49*B,* 3.50, 3.51, 3.56, 3.57, 3.59*A,* 3.63, Table 3.1*A* & *B,* Table 3.6.

Agur AMR, Ming JL: *Grant's Atlas of Anatomy,* 10th ed. Baltimore: Williams & Wilkins, 1999. 3.25 (modified).

Bassett, DL: *A Steroscopic Atlas of Anatomy. Section VI: The Pelvis, 153-4 and 154-1.* Portland, OR: Sawyers, 1961. 3.38*B* & *C.*

Beckman CR: *Obstetrics and Gynecology,* 4th ed. Baltimore: Lippincott Williams & Wilkins, 2002. B3.2*A,* B3.10, B3.20, B3.23.

Berek JS: *Novak's Gynecology,* 13th ed. Baltimore: Lippincott Williams & Wilkins, 2002. Table 3.5 (modified).

Bristow RE: Johns Hopkins School of Medicine, Baltimore, MD. B3.22.

Das Lexicon der Gesundheit. Munich: Urban & Schwarzenberg Verlag, 1996. 3.48*E* (artist: Jonathan Dimes).

Fuller J, Schaller-Ayers J: *A Nursing Approach, 2nd ed.* Philadelphia: Lippincott, 1994. B3.11 (artist: Larry Ward, Salt Lake City, UT), B3.15*A* & *B* (artist: Larry Ward, Salt Lake City, UT).

Hall-Craggs ECB: *Anatomy as the Basis of Clinical Medicine,* 3rd ed. Baltimore: Williams & Wilkins, 1995. B3.2*B.*

Lee JKT, Sagel SS, Stanley RJ, et al.: *Computed Body Tomography with MRI Correlation,* 3rd ed. Baltimore: Lippincott Williams & Wilkins, 1998. 3.62*A–C.*

Stedman's Medical Dictionary, 27th ed. Baltimore: Lippincott Williams & Wilkins, 2000. B3.6*D* (modified), B3.8, B3.12, B3.14*A, C–F,* B3.17*A–D,* B3.21, B3.24*A,* B3.27, B3.28 (artist: Neil O. Hardy, Westport, CT).

Chapter 4

Agur AMR: *Grant's Atlas of Anatomy,* 9th ed. Baltimore: Williams & Wilkins, 1991. 4.32*A* & *B,* Table 4.13.

Agur AMR, Dalley AF: *Grant's Atlas of Anatomy,* 11th ed. Baltimore: Lippincott Williams & Wilkins, 2004. 4.2*A–D* (modified), 4.4*A–C* (modified), 4.5*A* & *B,* 4.5*C,* 4.8, 4.14*C,* 4.15*A* & *B,* 4.20, 4.23, 4.25, 4.26, 4.30*A,* 4.31, 4.33, 4.38, B4.1, Table 4.1*A,* Table 4.2.

Agur AMR, Ming JL: *Grant's Atlas of Anatomy,* 10th ed. Baltimore: Williams & Wilkins, 1999. 4.3.

Becker RF, Wilson JW, Gehweiler JA: *Anatomical Basic of Medical Practice.* Baltimore: Williams & Wilkins, 1974. 4.35, B4.16*F.*

Clark CR: *The Cervical Spine,* 3rd ed. Philadelphia: Lippincott Willliams & Wilkins, 1998. 4.2*A–E,* B4.3*D* & *E,* B4.14*C.*

Lee JKT, Sagel SS, Stanley RJ, et al.: *Computed Body Tomography with MRI Correlation,* 3rd ed. Baltimore: Lippincott Williams & Wilkins, 1998. B4.2*F* & *G,* B4.12*C–E.*

Lockhart RD, Hamilton GF, Fyfe FW: *Anatomy of the Human Body.* Philadelphia: Lippincott, 1959. B4.4*A* & *B.*

MacKinnon PCB, Morris JF: *Oxford Textbook of Functional Anatomy, Vol. 1. Musculoskeletal System.* Oxford, UK: Oxford University Press, 1986. 4.5*C* (orientation figure).

Olson TR: *Student Atlas of Anatomy.* Baltimore: Williams & Wilkins, 1996. 4.1*C,* Table 4.5, Table 4.6.

Roland LP. *Merritt's Textbook of Neurology,* 9th ed. Baltimore: Williams & Wilkins, 1995. 4.41, B4.5*B.*

Wicke L: *Atlas of Radiologic Anatomy,* 6th English ed. Ed and Trans: Taylor AN. Baltimore: Williams & Wilkins, 1998. [Wicke L: *Roentgen-Anatomie Normalbefunde,* 5th ed. Munich: Urban & Schwarzenberg, 1995.] 4.40, 4.41.

Yochum TR, Rowe LJ: *Essentials of Skeletal Radiology, Vol. 2,* 2nd ed. Baltimore: Lippincott, Williams & Wilkins, 1996. 4.37, B4.4*C* & *D,* B4.12*A* & *B,* B4.13*A–D,* B4.27*B* & *C.*

Chapter 5

Agur AMR: *Grant's Atlas of Anatomy,* 9th ed. Baltimore: Williams & Wilkins, 1991. 5.5*B,* 5.28.

Agur AMR, Dalley AF: *Grant's Atlas of Anatomy,* 11th ed. Baltimore: Lippincott Williams & Wilkins, 2005. 5.9, 5.10, 5.13*A* & *B,* 5.14*B,* 5.17*A* & *B,* 5.18, 5.22, 5.23*A–C,* 5.27*D,* 5.30*A* & *B,* 5.31 (modified), 5.32, 5.33, 5.34, 5.35, 5.36, 5.37, 5.38*A,* 5.39, 5.40, 5.43*B,* 5.44, 5.46, 5.50, 5.53, 5.56*A* & *B,* 5.58*A* & *B,* 5.59, 5.60, 5.61*B* & *D,* 5.62*B* & *D,* 5.65, 5.66*B,* 5.67*A* & *B,* 5.70, 5.76*A* & *B,* 5.78, B5.9, B5.13*B,* SA5.4*C,* Table 5.1, Table 5.2, Table 5.3*B–F* & *H,* Table 5.4*A,* Table 5.6*C–J,* Table 5.7*B* & *C* (modified), Table 5.10*A,* Table 5.10 *B* (inset), Table 5.13*A,* Table 5.14*A* (right), Table 5.14*B* (right), Table 5.14*C* (right).

Agur AMR, Ming JL: *Grant's Atlas of Anatomy,* 10th ed. Baltimore: Williams & Wilkins, 1999. Table 5.4*A,* Table 5.4*B–H.*

Basmajian JV, Slonecker CE: *Grant's Method of Anatomy: A Clinical Problem-Solving Approach,* 11 ed. Baltimore: Williams & Wilkins, 1989. 5.47*A* & *B.*

Bickley LS, Szilagyi PG: *Bates' Guide to Physical Examination,* 8th ed. Baltimore: Lippincott Williams & Wilkins, 2002. SA5.2*E.*

Clay JH, Pounds DM: *Basic Clinical Massage Therapy: Integrating Anatomy and Treatment.* Baltimore: Lippincott Williams & Wilkins, 2002. 5.16*C,* 5.24*A,* 5.52*C,* SA5.4*A,* Table 5.3*G,* Table 5.6*A* & *B,* Table 5.7*A,* Table 5.8, Table 5.10*C–F,* Table 5.12, Table 5.13*B,* Table 5.14*A* (left), Table 5.14*B* (left), Table 5.14*C* (left).

Daffner RH: *Clinical Radiology—The Essentials.* Baltimore: Williams & Wilkins, 1993. B5.23 (radiograph), B5.25*D.*

Frick, Leonhardt, Starck: *Human Anatomy 1: General Anatomy.* Stuttgart: Thieme Verlag, 1991. 5.15*B* & *C* (modified).

Olson TR: *Student Atlas of Anatomy.* Baltimore: Williams & Wilkins, 1996. 5.63*B* & *D* (modified).

Palastanga NP, Field DG, Soames R: *Anatomy and Human Movement,* 4th ed. Oxford, UK: Butterworth-Heinemann, 2002. B5.25 (modified).

Roche Lexikon Medizin, 4th ed. Munich: Urban & Schwarzenberg, 1998. B5.27, B5.28.

Rose J, Gamble JG. *Human Walking,* 2nd ed. Baltimore: Williams & Wilkins, 1994. Table 5.3*A.*

Wicke L: *Atlas of Radiologic Anatomy,* 6th English ed. Ed and Trans: Taylor AN. Baltimore: Williams & Wilkins, 1998. [Wicke L: *Roentgen-Anatomie Normalbefunde,* 5th ed. Munich: Urban & Schwarzenberg, 1995.] 5.5*A,* 5.71*B,* 5.72, 5.73*A* & *B,* 5.73*C* (orientation figure), 5.75.

Willis MC: *Medical Terminology: A Programmed Learning Approach to the Language of Health Care.* Baltimore: Lippincott Williams & Wilkins, 2002. B5.23 (drawings)

Yochum TR, Rowe LJ: *Essentials of Skeletal Radiology, Vol. 2,* 2nd ed. Baltimore: Lippincott, Williams & Wilkins, 1996. B5.21.

Chapter 6

Agur AMR: *Grant's Atlas of Anatomy,* 9th ed. Baltimore: Williams & Wilkins, 1991. 6.55*B,* 6.61*C,* 6.78*A–C,* 6.80.

Agur AMR, Dalley AF: *Grant's Atlas of Anatomy,* 11th ed. Baltimore: Lippincott Williams & Wilkins, 2004. 6.1, 6.7*D,* 6.11*A–D,* 6.14, 6.23*D* (modified), 6.25, 6.26, 6.30*D,* 6.32*B,* 6.34, 6.37*B* & *C,* 6.37*E* (modified), 6.40*A* & *B,* 6.41 (modified), 6.42*A–C,* 6.45, 6.49*B,* 6.50 (modified), 6.52*A* & *B,* 6.55*A,* 6.56, 6.60*B,* 6.62*B* & *D,* 6.63*B,* 6.69, 6.71*B* & *C,* 6.72*A* & *B,* 6.74*B,* 6.76*B,* 6.77*B,* 6.79, B6.29*C,* SA6.11*A* & *B,* SA6.17, Table 6.1*E,* Table 6.2*A–E,* Table 6.5 (bottom left), Table 6.6I (far left), Table 6.6II (far left), Table 6.7*A–E,* Table 6.8 (left), Table 6.9 (left; modified), Table 6.9 (right), Table 6.11 (top left and right), Table 6.12.

Agur AMR, Ming JL: *Grant's Atlas of Anatomy,* 10th ed. Baltimore: Williams & Wilkins, 1999. 6.2*A* & *B,* 6.24*B,* 6.28, 6.29, 6.30*A–C,* 6.31, 6.32*A,* 6.33*A* & *B,* 6.59, B6.7, B6.25, B6.31.

Anderson JE: *Grant's Altas of Anatomy,* 7th ed. Baltimore: Williams & Wilkins, 1978. 6.38*A* & *B* (modified).

Anderson MK, Hall SJ, Martin M: *Foundations of Athletic Training,* 3rd ed. Baltimore: Lippincott Williams & Wilkins, 1995. B6.14.

Basmajian JV, Slonecker CE: *Grant's Method of Anatomy: A Clinical Problem-Solving Approach,* 11 ed. Baltimore: Williams & Wilkins, 1989. 6.73*B.*

Clay JH, Pounds DM: *Basic Clinical Massage Therapy: Integrating Anatomy and Treatment.* Baltimore: Lippincott Williams & Wilkins, 2002. Table 6.1*A–D.*

Hall-Craggs ECB: *Anatomy as the Basis of Clinical Medicine,* 3rd ed. Baltimore: Williams & Wilkins, 1995. 6.68 (modified), B6.13.

Meschan I. *An Atlas of Anatomy Basic to Radiology.* Philadelphia: Saunders, 1975. B6.9 (left).

Moore KL, Agur AMR: *Essential Clinical Anatomy,* 2nd ed. Baltimore: Lippincott Williams & Wilkins, 2000. 6.8*A* & *B.*

Rowland LP: *Merritt's Textbook of Neurology,* 9th ed. Baltimore: Williams & Wilkins, 1995. B6.5.

Salter RB. *Textbook of Disorders and Injuries of the Musculoskeletal System,* 3rd ed. Baltimore: Williams & Wilkins, 1998. B6.9 (right), B6.35.

Chapter 7

Agur AMR: *Grant's Atlas of Anatomy,* 9th ed. Baltimore: Williams & Wilkins, 1991. 7.14, 7.41*A,* 7.52*A* & *B,* 7.59*A.*

Agur AMR, Dalley AF: *Grant's Atlas of Anatomy,* 11th ed. Baltimore: Lippincott Williams & Wilkins, 2004. 7.1*A,* 7.1*D,* 7.2*A* & *B,* 7.3*A* & *B,* 7.5*A–C,* 7.9, 7.10*A,* 7.11, 7.12*C,* 7.16, 7.20, 7.21, 7.23, 7.27*C,* 7.32, 7.34, 7.36A. 7.39, 7.40*A* & *B,* 7.41*C,* 7.43*E,* 7.47*C,* 7.48, 7.50, 7.53, 7.55, 7.60, 7.63*B,* 7.65*B,* 7.69*A* & *C,* 7.73, 7.75*A,* 7.77 (modified), 7.78*B,* 7.83, B7.5, B7.6*A* & *B,* Table 7.2, Table 7.8*B.*

Agur AMR, Ming JL: *Grant's Atlas of Anatomy,* 10th ed. Baltimore: Williams & Wilkins, 1999. 7.13, 7.25, 7.30*B,* 7.31 (modified), 7.35*A* & *B,* 7.41*B,* 7.59*B,* 7.61, 7.65*A,* 7.66, 7.69*B,* 7.72*A,* 7.78*A.*

Ger R. Albert Einstein College of Medicine, Bronx, NY. B7.12.

Ger R, Abrahams P, Olson T: *Essentials of Clinical Anatomy,* 3rd ed. New York: Parthenon, 1996. B7.12.

Hall-Craggs ECB: *Anatomy as the Basis of Clinical Medicine,* 3rd ed. Baltimore: Williams & Wilkins, 1995. 7.30*A,* 7.33 (modified).

Leung AKC, Wong AL, Robson WLLM: Ectopic thyroid gland simulating a thyroglossal duct cyst. *Can J Surg* 38:87, 1995. B7.29.

Moore KL, Persaud TVN: *The Developing Human: Clinically Oriented Embryology,* 6th ed. Philadelphia: Saunders, 1998. B7.14*B* (courtesy of Dr. Gerald S. Smyser, Altru Health System, Grand Forks, ND), B7.24, B7.26 (courtesy of Dr. John B Mullen, Hospital Boston, Harvard Medical School, Boston, MA).

Roche Lexikon Medizin, 3rd ed. Auflage, Munich, Germany: Urban & Schwarzenberg, 1998. B7.22, B7.31*B.*

Skin Cancer Foundation, New York, NY. B7.20.

Sadler TW. *Langman's Medical Embryology,* 7th ed. Baltimore: Williams & Wilkins, 1995. B7.28.

Smith Kline Corporation: *Essentials of Neurological Examination,* Philadelphia, PA, 1978. B7.18.

Visuals Unlimited, Amherst, NH. B7.14*A.*

Welch Allen, Inc., Skaneateles Falls, NY. B7.21, B7.30, B7.31*A.*

Chapter 8

Agur AMR: *Grant's Atlas of Anatomy,* 9th ed. Baltimore: Williams & Wilkins, 1991. 8.2, 8.47, 8.48, B8.7.

Agur AMR, Dalley AF: *Grant's Atlas of Anatomy,* 11th ed. Baltimore: Lippincott Williams & Wilkins, 2004. 8.5, 8.9, 8.10, 8.12*B,* 8.24, 8.27*C* & *D,* 8.29, 8.32, 8.35, 8.37 (bottom), 8.38*A,* 8.40*A* & *B,* 8.43*A* & *B,* 8.49, 8.52.

Agur AMR, Ming JL: *Grant's Atlas of Anatomy,* 10th ed. Baltimore: Williams & Wilkins, 1999. 8.2, 8.6, 8.7, 8.12*A,* 8.13, 8.14, 8.19*B,* 8.20*B,* 8.22, 8.23, 8.25*A,* 8.27*A* & *B,* 8.28, 8.30*A,* 8.38*B,* B8.9.

Moore KL, Persaud TVN: *The Developing Human: Clinically Oriented Embryology*, 6th ed. Philadelphia: Saunders, 1998. B8.14*B* (courtesy of Dr. DA Kernahan, The Children's Memorial Hospital, Chicago, IL).

Roche Lexikon Medizin, 4th ed. Munich: Urban & Schwarzenberg, 1998. B8.8.

Rohen JW, Yokochi C, Lutjen-Drecoll E, Romrell LJ: *Color Atlas of Anatomy: A Photographic Study of the Human Body*, 5th ed. Baltimore: Lippincott Williams & Wilkins, 2002. B8.10.

Rowland LP: *Merritt's Textbook of Neurology*, 9th ed. Baltimore: Williams & Wilkins, 1995. B8.1.

Stedman's Medical Dictionary, 27th ed. Baltimore: Lippincott Williams & Wilkins, 2000. B8.11.

Wicke L: *Atlas of Radiologic Anatomy*, 6th English ed. Ed and Trans: Taylor AN. Baltimore: Williams & Wilkins, 1998. [Wicke L: *Roentgen-Anatomie Normalbefunde*, 5th ed. Munich: Urban & Schwarzenberg, 1995.] 8.44, 8.45.

Willis MC: *Medical Terminology: The Language of Health Care.* Baltimore: Lippincott Williams & Wilkins, 1995. 8.52 (courtesy of Hoag Memorial Hospital Presbyterian, Newport Beach, CA), B8.3 (courtesy of Acuson Corp., Mt. View, CA).

Chapter 9

Agur AMR, Dalley AF: *Grant's Atlas of Anatomy,* 11th ed. Baltimore: Lippincott Williams & Wilkins, 2004. 9.1, 9.5, 9.6*A–C,* 9.7*A & B,* 9.9, 9.10, 9.13, 9.14 (modified), 9.15, B9.1.

Agur AMR, Ming JL: *Grant's Atlas of Anatomy,* 10th ed. Baltimore: Williams & Wilkins, 1999. Table 9.2 (brain orientation figures, modified).

List of Clinical Blue Boxes

2 Abdomen

3 Pelvis and Perineum

4 Back

5 Lower Limb

8 Neck

9 Summary of Cranial Nerves

Contents

Introduction to Clinically Oriented Anatomy

A Brief History of Anatomy

Anatomy—the study of the structure of the body—is one of the oldest basic medical sciences; it was first studied formally in Egypt (approximately 500 B.C.E. [B.C.]).

The earliest descriptions of anatomy were written on papyruses (paper reed) between 3000 and 2500 B.C.E. (Persaud, 1984). Much later, human anatomy was taught in Greece by *Hippocrates* (460–377 B.C.E.), who is regarded as the Father of Medicine and a founder of the science of anatomy. In addition to the *Hippocratic Oath*, Hippocrates wrote several books on anatomy. In one he stated, "The nature of the body is the beginning of medical science." *Aristotle* (384–322 B.C.E.) was the first person to use the term *anatome*, a Greek word meaning "cutting up or taking apart." The Latin word *dissecare* has a similar meaning.

Andreas Vesalius's (1514–1564 C.E [A.D.]) masterpiece *De Humani Corporis Fabrica*, published in 1543, marked a new era in the history of medicine. At that time, the study of anatomy became an objective discipline based on direct observations as well as scientific principles. Vesalius recognized anatomy "as the firm foundation of the whole art of medicine and its essential preliminary." *Hieronymus Fabricius* (1537–1619) was responsible for the construction in 1594 of the famous anatomical theater at Padua. He was one of the teachers of *William Harvey,* and it is believed that Fabricius's discovery of the valves in the veins led Harvey to the discovery of the circulation of blood. The publication in 1628 of Harvey's book *Exercitatio Anatomica de Motu Cordis et Sanguinis in Animalibus,* on the movements of the heart and the circulation of blood in animals, represents a milestone in the history of medicine (Persaud, 1997). By the 17th century, human dissections became an important feature in European medical schools, and anatomical museums were established in many cities.

During the 18th and 19th centuries, anatomists published impressive treatises and lavish atlases with illustrations that introduced new standards for depicting the human body. The shortage of cadavers for dissection and anatomical demonstrations led to illegal means of obtaining human bodies. Professional grave robbers supplied anatomy schools with corpses, in some cases by murdering their victims. Medical students and their teachers had also been involved in body snatching (Persaud, 1997). In Britain, the Anatomy Act was passed by Parliament in 1832. It made legal provisions for medical schools to receive unclaimed and donated bodies for anatomical studies. This paved the way for similar legislation in other countries.

Approaches to Studying Anatomy

Anatomy is the setting (structure) in which the events (functions) of life occur. Although historically and strictly speaking the primary concern of anatomy is structure, true understanding results when structure and function are considered together. Modern anatomy is functional anatomy. This book deals mainly with functional *human gross anatomy*—the examination of structures of the human that can be seen without a microscope. The three main approaches to studying anatomy are regional, systemic, and clinical (applied), reflecting the body's organization and the priorities and purposes for studying it.

Regional Anatomy

Regional anatomy (topographical anatomy) considers the organization of the human body as segments or major parts based on form and mass (Fig. I.1): a main body, consisting of the head, neck, and trunk (subdivided into thorax, abdomen, back, and pelvis/perineum), and paired upper limbs and lower limbs. All the major parts may be further subdivided into regions and zones. Regional anatomy is the method of studying the body's structure by focusing attention on a specific part (e.g., the head), region (the face), or subregion (the orbit); examining the arrangement and relationships of the various systemic structures (muscles, nerves, arteries, etc.) within it; and then usually continuing to study adjacent regions in an ordered sequence. It is the approach followed in this book, with each chapter addressing the anatomy of a major part of the body, and the approach usually taken in advanced anatomy courses that have a laboratory component involving dissection. When studying anatomy by this approach, it is important to make the effort routinely to put the regional anatomy into the context of that of adjacent regions and of the body as a whole.

Regional anatomy also recognizes the body's organization by layers: skin, subcutaneous tissue, and deep fascia covering the deeper structures of muscles, skeleton, and cavities, which contain *viscera* (internal organs). Many of these deeper structures are partially evident beneath the body's outer covering and may be studied and examined in living individuals via surface anatomy.

Surface anatomy is an essential part of the study of regional anatomy. It is specifically addressed in this book in "surface anatomy sections" (orange background) that provide knowledge of what lies under the skin and what structures are perceptible to touch (palpable) in the living body at rest and in action. We can learn much by observing the external form and surface of the body and observing or feeling the superficial aspects of structures beneath its surface. The aim of this method is to *visualize* (recall distinct mental images of) structures that confer contour to the surface or are palpable beneath it and, in clinical practice, to distinguish any unusual or abnormal findings. In other words, surface anatomy requires a thorough understanding of the anatomy of the structures beneath the surface. In people with stab wounds, for example, a physician must be able to visualize the deep structures that might be injured. Knowledge of surface anatomy can also decrease the need to memorize facts because the body is always available to observe and palpate.

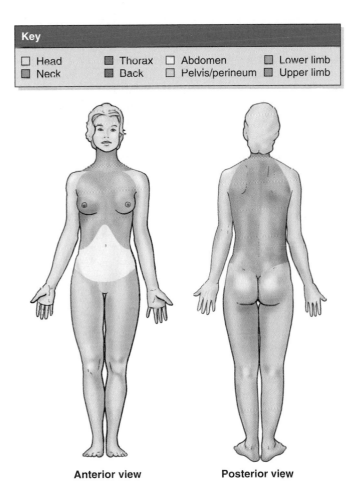

Key

☐ Head	■ Thorax	☐ Abdomen	■ Lower limb
■ Neck	■ Back	☐ Pelvis/perineum	■ Upper limb

Anterior view   Posterior view

Figure I.1. Major parts of the body as studied by regional anatomy. Anatomy is described relative to the anatomical position illustrated.

Physical examination is the clinical application of surface anatomy. *Palpation* is a clinical technique for examining living anatomy. *Palpation of arterial pulses,* for instance, is part of routine physical examinations. Students of many of the health sciences will learn to use instruments to facilitate examination of the body (such as an *ophthalmoscope* to observe features of the eyes) and to listen to functioning parts of the body (a *stethoscope* to listen to the heart and lungs). A *reflex hammer* may be used to examine the functional state of nerves and muscles. When reading the surface anatomy sections in this text, make an effort to associate living anatomy with the anatomy you learn from lectures, dissection, and/or demonstrations.

Regional study of deep structures and abnormalities in a living person is now also possible by means of radiological imaging. *Radiographic anatomy* provides useful information about normal structures in living individuals, as affected by muscle tone, body fluids and pressures, and gravity; *diagnostic radiology* reveals the effects of trauma, pathology, and aging on normal structures. In this book, the "medical imaging sections" (green background) at the end of each chapter provide an introduction to radiographic anatomy. However, the detailed and thorough learning of the three-dimensional anatomy of deep structures and their relationships is best accomplished by transecting or by removing the body's outer cover to observe the structures directly through the process of dissection. In clinical practice, surface anatomy, radiographic images, and your experience from studying anatomy will combine to provide you with knowledge of each patient's anatomy.

The computer is a useful adjunct in teaching regional anatomy (Cahill and Leonard, 1997) because it facilitates certain aspects of instruction and review. Computers aid learning by allowing interactivity and manipulation of two- and three-dimensional anatomical renderings; the sequential or side-by-side display of planar images, such as anatomical serial sections, computed tomography (CT), and magnetic resonance imaging (MRI); and layer separations of tissues in mock dissection. *Prosections,* carefully prepared dissections for the demonstration of anatomical structures, are also useful. However, learning is most efficient and retention is highest when didactic study is combined with the experience of actual dissection—that is, learning by doing (Amadio, 1996; Mutyala and Cahill, 1996). During dissection you observe, palpate, move, and sequentially reveal parts of the body. In 1770, Dr. *William Hunter,* a distinguished Scottish anatomist and obstetrician, stated: "Dissection alone teaches us where we may cut or inspect the living body with freedom and dispatch."

Systemic Anatomy

Systemic anatomy recognizes the organization of the body's organs into systems or collective apparatuses that work together to carry out complex functions; thus it is a sequential study of the functional systems of the body. The basic systems and the field of study or treatment of each (in parentheses) are

- The *integumentary system* (*dermatology*) consists of the skin (L. *integumentum,* a covering) and its appendages—hair, nails, and sweat glands, for example—and the subcutaneous tissue just beneath it. The skin, an extensive sensory organ, forms the body's outer, protective covering and container.

- The *skeletal system* (*osteology*) consists of bones and cartilage; it provides our basic shape and support for the body and is what the muscular system acts on to produce movement. It also protects vital organs such as the heart, lungs, and pelvic organs.

- The *articular system* (*arthrology*) consists of joints and their associated ligaments, connecting the bony parts of the skeletal system and providing the sites at which movements occur.

- The *muscular system* (*myology*) consists of muscles that act (contract) to move or position parts of the body (e.g., the bones that articulate at joints).

- The *nervous system* (*neurology*) consists of the *central nervous system* (brain and spinal cord) and the *peripheral nervous system* (nerves and ganglia, together with their motor and sensory endings). The nervous system controls and coordinates the functions of the organ systems, enabling the body's responses to and activities within its environment.

- The *circulatory system* (*angiology*) consists of the cardiovascular and lymphatic systems, which function in parallel to transport the body's fluids.

  - The *cardiovascular system* (*cardiology*) consists of the heart and blood vessels that propel and conduct blood through the body, delivering oxygen, nutrients, and hormones to cells and removing their waste products.

  - The *lymphatic system* is a network of lymphatic vessels that withdraws excess tissue fluid (lymph) from the body's interstitial (intercellular) fluid compartment, filters it through lymph nodes, and returns it to the bloodstream.

- The *digestive* or *alimentary system* (*gastroenterology*) consists of the organs and glands associated with ingestion, mastication (chewing), deglutition (swallowing), digestion, and absorption of food and the elimination of feces (solid waste) remaining after the nutrients have been absorbed.

- The *respiratory system* (*pulmonology*) consists of the air passages and lungs that supply oxygen to the blood for cellular respiration and eliminate carbon dioxide from it. The diaphragm and larynx control the flow of air through the system, which may also produce tone in the larynx that is further modified by the tongue, teeth, and lips into speech.

- The *urinary system* (*urology*) consists of the kidneys, ureters, urinary bladder, and urethra, which filter blood and subsequently produce, transport, store, and intermittently excrete urine (liquid waste).

- The *reproductive* or *genital system* (*gynecology* for females; *andrology* for males) consists of the gonads (ovaries and testes) that produce oocytes (eggs) and sperms, the ducts that transport them, and the genitalia that enable their union. After conception, the female reproductive tract nourishes and delivers the fetus.

- The *endocrine system* (*endocrinology*) consists of discrete ductless glands (such as the thyroid gland) as well as isolated and clustered cells of the gut and blood vessel walls and specialized nerve endings that secrete hormones. *Hormones* are organic molecules that are carried by the circulatory system to distant effector cells in all parts of the body. The influence of the endocrine system is thus as broadly distributed as that of the nervous system. These glands influence metabolism and other processes, such as the menstrual cycle.

The passive skeletal and articular systems and the active muscular system collectively constitute a *supersystem*, the *locomotor apparatus or system* (*orthopedics*), because they must work together to produce locomotion of the body. And although the structures directly responsible for locomotion are the muscles, bones, joints, and ligaments of the limbs, other systems are indirectly involved as well: the arteries and veins of the circulatory system supply oxygen and nutrients to and remove waste from these structures and the nerves of the nervous system stimulate them to act. In fact, none of the systems functions in isolation.

Systemic anatomy is the approach taken by most survey (introductory) courses not involving dissection and when the overall curriculum follows a systemic approach.

Clinical Anatomy

Clinical (applied) anatomy emphasizes aspects of bodily structure and function important in the practice of medicine, dentistry, and the allied health sciences. It incorporates the regional and systemic approaches to studying anatomy and stresses clinical application. *Endoscopic* and *imaging techniques* (e.g., examination of the interior of the stomach) also demonstrate living anatomy.

Clinical anatomy often involves inverting or reversing the thought process typically followed when studying regional or systemic anatomy. For example, instead of thinking, "The action of this muscle is to. . .," clinical anatomy asks, "How would the absence of this muscle's activity be manifest?" Instead of noting, "The . . . nerve provides innervation to this area of skin," clinical anatomy asks, "Numbness in this area indicates a lesion of which nerve?" Clinical anatomy is exciting to learn because of its role in solving clinical problems. The "clinical correlation (blue) boxes" (blue background) in this book describe practical applications of anatomy. "Case studies," such as those on the accompanying CD, are integral parts of the clinical approach to studying anatomy.

THE BOTTOM LINE: Anatomy is the study of the structure of the human body. Regional anatomy considers the body as organized into segments or parts; systemic anatomy sees the body as organized into organ systems. Surface anatomy provides information about structures that may be observed or palpated beneath the skin, and radiographic anatomy allows appreciation of structures in the living, as they are affected by muscle tone, body fluids and pressures, and gravity. Clinical anatomy emphasizes application of anatomical knowledge to the practice of medicine.

Anatomicomedical Terminology

An international vocabulary has been established for anatomy and medicine. Although you are familiar with common terms for parts and regions of the body, you must learn the correct nomenclature (e.g., axillary fossa instead of armpit and clavicle instead of collarbone) that enables precise communication among healthcare professionals worldwide as well as among scholars in basic and applied health sciences. You must also know the common and colloquial terms people are likely to use when they describe their complaints. Furthermore, you must be able to use terms people will understand when explaining their medical problems to them.

The terminology in this book conforms to the new *Terminologia Anatomica: International Anatomical Terminology* (Federative Committee on Anatomical Terminology, 1998)—the authorized international reference guide on anatomical language. *Terminologia Anatomica* (TA) lists anatomical terms both in Latin and as English equivalents (e.g., the common shoulder muscle is *musculus deltoideus* in Latin and *deltoid* in English). Most terms in this book are English equivalents. Unfortunately, the terminology commonly used in the clinical arena may differ from the official terminology. Because this discrepancy may be a source of confusion, this text clarifies commonly confused terms by placing the unofficial designations in parentheses when the terms are first used—for example, *pharyngotympanic tube* (auditory tube, eustachian tube) and *internal thoracic artery* (internal mammary artery). *Eponyms,* terms incorporating the names of people, are not used in the new terminology because they give no clue about the type or location of the structures involved. In addition, some eponyms are historically inaccurate—for example, Poupart was not the first anatomist to describe the inguinal ligament (Poupart ligament). Notwithstanding, commonly used eponyms appear in parentheses throughout the book when these terms are first used—such as *sternal angle* (angle of Louis)—since you will surely encounter them. Note that the eponymous term does not indicate that the angle is in the sternum.

Anatomical terminology introduces and makes up a large part of medical terminology. To be understood, you must express yourself clearly, using the proper terms in the correct way. Because most terms are derived from Latin and Greek, medical language may seem difficult at first; however, as you learn the origin of terms, the words make sense. For example, the term *decidua,* used to describe the lining of the pregnant uterus, is derived from Latin and means "a falling off." This term is appropriate because the endometrium "falls off" or is expelled after the baby is born, ending the pregnancy, just as the leaves of deciduous trees fall at the end of summer.

To describe the body clearly and to indicate the position of its parts and organs relative to each other, anatomists worldwide have agreed to use the same descriptive terms of position and direction. Because clinicians also use these terms, it is important to master the use of this vocabulary. Practice using proper terminology as you study and review so that your meaning will be clear when you describe parts of the body in patient histories or during discussions of patients with clinicians.

Anatomical Position

All anatomical descriptions are expressed in relation to one consistent anatomical position, ensuring that descriptions are not ambiguous (Figs. I.1 and I.2). The **anatomical position** refers to the body position as if the person were standing upright, regardless of the actual posture or position, with the:

- Head, gaze (eyes), and toes directed anteriorly (forward).

- Arms adjacent to the sides with the palms facing anteriorly.

- Lower limbs close together with the feet parallel and the toes directed anteriorly.

This anatomical position is adopted globally for anatomicomedical descriptions. By using this position and appropriate terminology, you can relate any part of the body precisely to any other part. Although gravity causes a downward shift of internal organs when the upright position is assumed, it is often necessary to describe the position of organs in the recumbent or supine position because this is the posture in which people are typically examined. Visualize the anatomical position in your mind's eye when describing patients (or cadavers), whether they are lying on their sides, supine (recumbent, lying down, face upward), or prone (face downward).

Anatomical Planes

Anatomical descriptions are based on four imaginary planes (median, sagittal, frontal, and transverse) that intersect the body in the anatomical position (Fig. I.2):

- The **median plane,** the vertical plane passing longitudinally through the body, divides the body into right and left halves. The plane intersects the midlines of the anterior and posterior surfaces of the body. *Midline* is often erroneously used as a synonym for the median plane.

- **Sagittal planes** are vertical planes passing through the body *parallel to the median plane.* It is helpful to give a point of reference by naming a structure intersected by the plane you are referring to, such as a sagittal plane through the midpoint of the clavicle. The term *midsagittal plane* is a superfluous term for the median plane (O'Rahilly, 1997). *Parasagittal,* commonly used by neuroanatomists and neurologists, is also unnecessary because any plane parallel and to either side of the median plane is sagittal by definition. However, a plane parallel and near to the median plane may be referred to as a *paramedian plane.*

- **Frontal (coronal) planes** are vertical planes passing through the body *at right angles to the median plane,* dividing the body into anterior (front) and posterior (back) parts. Again, a point of reference is necessary to indicate the position of the plane (e.g., a frontal plane through the heads of the mandible).

Figure I.2. Anatomical planes. The main planes of reference in the body are illustrated.

- **Transverse planes** are planes passing through the body *at right angles to the median and frontal planes,* dividing the body into superior (upper) and inferior (lower) parts. It is helpful to give a reference point to identify the level of the plane, such as a "transverse plane through the umbilicus" or through a specific vertebra. Radiologists refer to transverse planes as *transaxial,* which is commonly shortened to *axial planes.*

Commonly, sections of the body in frontal and transverse planes are symmetrical, passing through both the right and left members of paired structures, allowing some comparison. The number of sagittal, frontal, and transverse planes is unlimited. The main use of anatomical planes is to describe sections. Anatomists create sections of the body and its parts anatomically (Fig. I.3) and clinicians create them by planar imaging technologies, such as CT, to describe and display internal structures. Sections provide views of the body as if cut or sectioned along particular planes.

- **Longitudinal sections** run lengthwise or parallel to the long axis of the body or of any of its parts, and the term applies regardless of the position of the body.

- **Transverse sections,** or cross sections, are slices of the body or its parts that are cut at right angles to the longitudinal axis of the body or of any of its parts; because the long axis of the foot runs horizontally, a transverse section of the foot lies in the frontal plane (Fig. I.2*C*).

- **Oblique sections** are slices of the body or any of its parts that are not cut along one of the previously mentioned anatomical planes. In practice, many radiographic images and anatomical sections do not lie precisely in the sagittal, frontal, or transverse planes; often they are slightly oblique.

Terms of Relationship and Comparison

Various adjectives, arranged as pairs of opposites, describe the relationship of parts of the body in the anatomical position and compare the position of two structures relative to each other (Fig. I.4).

Superficial, intermediate, and **deep** describe the position of structures relative to the surface of the body or the relationship of one structure to another underlying or overlying structure.

Medial is used to indicate that (in the anatomical position) a structure, such as the 5th digit of the hand (little finger), is nearer to the median plane of the body than the other digits. Conversely, **lateral** stipulates that a structure, such as the 1st digit of the hand (thumb), is farther away from the median plane. Lateral and medial are not synonymous with the terms *external* (outer) and *internal* (inner). **External** and **internal** mean farther from and nearer to the center of an organ or cavity, respectively, regardless of direction.

Posterior (dorsal) denotes the back surface of the body or nearer to the back. **Anterior** (ventral) denotes the front

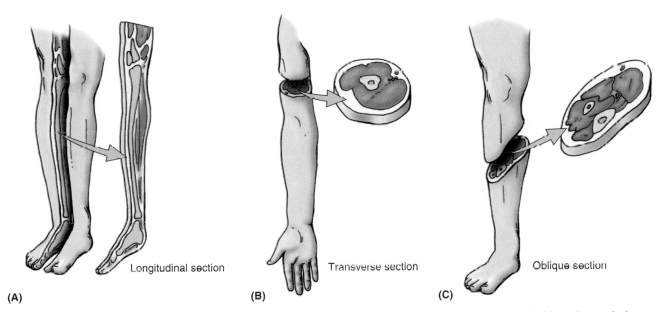

Figure I.3. Sections of the limbs. Sections may be obtained by anatomical sectioning or medical imaging techniques.

(A) Longitudinal section   (B) Transverse section   (C) Oblique section

surface of the body. **Rostral** is often used instead of anterior when describing parts of the brain; it means toward the rostrum (L. from beak); however, in humans it denotes nearer the anterior part of the head (e.g., the frontal lobe of the brain is rostral to the cerebellum).

Inferior refers to a structure that is situated nearer the sole of the foot. **Caudal** (L. *cauda,* tail) is a useful directional term that means toward the tail region, represented in humans by the coccyx, the small bone at the inferior (caudal) end of the vertebral column. The term *caudal* is used in embryology because the human embryo has a tail-like caudal eminence until the middle of the 8th week (Moore and Persaud, 2003). **Superior** refers to a structure that is nearer the **vertex,** the topmost point of the cranium. **Cranial** relates to the cranium (Mediev. L. skull) and is a useful directional term, meaning toward the head.

Combined terms describe intermediate positional arrangements: **inferomedial** means nearer to the feet and median plane—for example, the anterior parts of the ribs run inferomedially; **superolateral** means nearer to the head and farther from the median plane.

Proximal and **distal** are used when contrasting positions nearer to or farther from the attachment of a limb or the central aspect of a linear structure, respectively. **Dorsum** usually refers to the superior or **posterior** (back) surface of any part that protrudes anteriorly from the body, such as the dorsum of the tongue, nose, penis, or foot. It is also used to describe the back of the hand. It is easier to understand why these surfaces are considered posterior if one thinks of a quadripedal plantigrade animal that walks on its palms and soles, such as a bear. The **sole** indicates the inferior aspect or bottom of the foot, much of which is in contact with the ground when standing barefoot. The **palm** refers to the flat of the hand,

exclusive of the thumb and other fingers, and is the opposite of the dorsum of the hand.

Terms of Laterality

Paired structures having right and left members (e.g., the kidneys) are **bilateral,** whereas those occurring on one side only (e.g., the spleen) are **unilateral. Ipsilateral** refers to something occurring on the same side of the body as another structure; the right thumb and right great (big) toe are ipsilateral, for example. **Contralateral** means occurring on the opposite side of the body relative to another structure; the right hand is contralateral to the left hand.

Terms of Movement

Various terms describe movements of the limbs and other parts of the body (Fig. I.5). While most movements occur at joints where two or more bones or cartilages articulate with one another, several non-skeletal structures exhibit movement (e.g., tongue, lips, eyelids).

Flexion indicates bending or decreasing the angle between the bones or parts of the body. For most joints (e.g., elbow), flexion generally involves movement in an anterior direction; however, flexion at the knee joint involves posterior movement. **Dorsiflexion** describes flexion at the ankle joint, as occurs when walking uphill or lifting the toes off the ground. **Plantarflexion** turns the foot or toes toward the plantar surface (e.g., when standing on your toes).

Extension indicates straightening or increasing the angle between the bones or parts of the body. Extension usually occurs in a posterior direction, but extension of the knee joint occurs in an anterior direction. Extension of a limb or part

(cont'd on page 11)

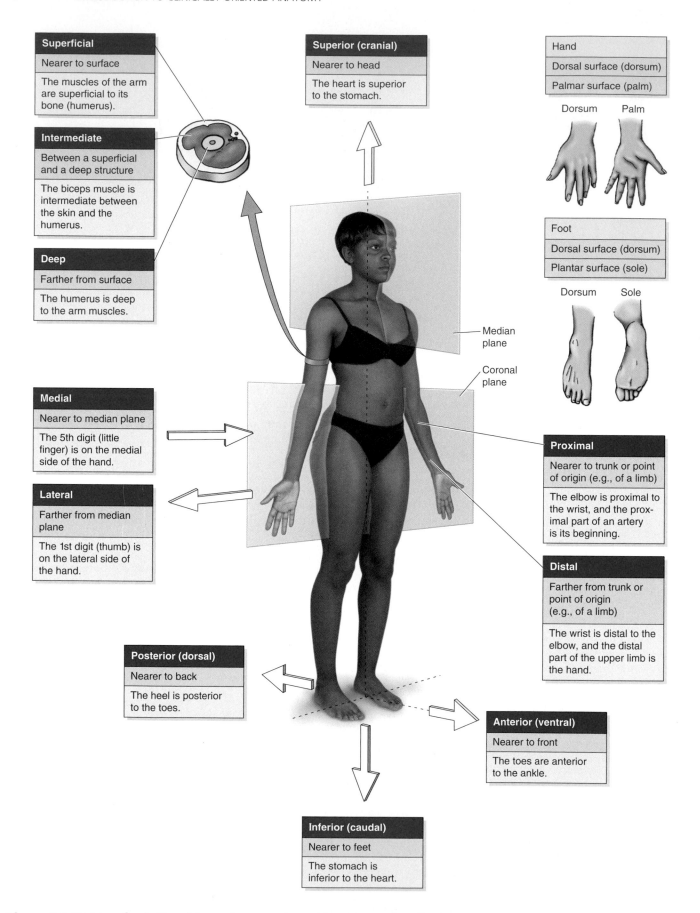

Superficial

Nearer to surface

The muscles of the arm are superficial to its bone (humerus).

Intermediate

Between a superficial and a deep structure

The biceps muscle is intermediate between the skin and the humerus.

Deep

Farther from surface

The humerus is deep to the arm muscles.

Superior (cranial)

Nearer to head

The heart is superior to the stomach.

Hand
Dorsal surface (dorsum)
Palmar surface (palm)

Dorsum   Palm

Foot
Dorsal surface (dorsum)
Plantar surface (sole)

Dorsum   Sole

Median plane

Coronal plane

Medial

Nearer to median plane

The 5th digit (little finger) is on the medial side of the hand.

Lateral

Farther from median plane

The 1st digit (thumb) is on the lateral side of the hand.

Proximal

Nearer to trunk or point of origin (e.g., of a limb)

The elbow is proximal to the wrist, and the proximal part of an artery is its beginning.

Distal

Farther from trunk or point of origin (e.g., of a limb)

The wrist is distal to the elbow, and the distal part of the upper limb is the hand.

Posterior (dorsal)

Nearer to back

The heel is posterior to the toes.

Anterior (ventral)

Nearer to front

The toes are anterior to the ankle.

Inferior (caudal)

Nearer to feet

The stomach is inferior to the heart.

Figure I.4. Terms of relationship and comparison. These terms describe the position of one structure relative to another.

Figure I.5. Terms of movement. These terms describe movements of the limbs and other parts of the body; the movements take place at joints, where two or more bones or cartilages articulate with one another.

Abduction and adduction of right limbs and rotation of left limbs at glenohumeral and hip joints, respectively

Circumduction (circular movement) of lower limb at hip joint

Dorsiflexion and plantarflexion of foot at ankle joint

Inversion and eversion of foot at subtalar and transverse tarsal joints

Lateral bending (lateral flexion) of trunk and rotation of upper trunk and neck

Elevation and depression of shoulders

Protrusion and retrusion of jaw at temporomandibular joints

Protraction and retraction of scapula on thoracic wall

Figure I.5. *(Continued)*

beyond the normal limit—**hyperextension** (overextension)—can cause injury, such as "whiplash" (i.e., hyperextension of the neck during a rear-end automobile collision). Note in Figure I.5 that when the foot is extended at the ankle joint, it is plantar*flexed* (e.g., when standing on your toes). Except for the thumb, from the anatomical position, flexion and extension are movements in the sagittal plane.

Abduction means moving away from the median plane in the frontal plane (e.g., when moving an upper limb away from the side of the body). In *abduction of the digits* (fingers or toes), the term means spreading them apart—moving the other fingers away from the neutrally positioned 3rd (middle) finger or moving the other toes away from the neutrally positioned 2nd toe. The 3rd finger and 2nd toe *medially* or *laterally abduct* away from the neutral position. Right and left lateral flexion (lateral bending) are special forms of abduction for only the neck and trunk. The face and upper trunk are directed anteriorly as the head and/or shoulders tilt to the right or left side, causing the midline of the body itself to become bent sideways. This is a compound movement occurring between many adjacent vertebrae.

Adduction means moving toward the median plane in a frontal plane (e.g., when moving an upper limb toward the side of the body). In *adduction of the digits,* the term means reapproximating the spread fingers or toes or moving the other digits toward the neutral position of the 3rd finger or 2nd toe. The medially or laterally abducted 3rd finger or 2nd toe adducts back to the neutral position. As you can see by noticing the way the thumbnail faces (laterally instead of posteriorly in the anatomical position), the thumb is rotated 90° relative to the other digits. Therefore, the thumb flexes and extends in the frontal plane, and abducts and adducts in the sagittal plane.

Circumduction is a circular movement that is a combination of flexion, extension, abduction, and adduction occurring in such a way that the distal end of the part moves in a circle. Circumduction can occur at any joint at which all the above-mentioned movements are possible (e.g., the hip joint).

Rotation involves turning or revolving a part of the body around its longitudinal axis, such as turning one's head to face sideways. *Medial rotation* (internal rotation) brings the anterior surface of a limb closer to the median plane, whereas *lateral rotation* (external rotation) takes the anterior surface away from the median plane.

Pronation is the rotational movement of the forearm and hand that swings the radius (the lateral long bone of the forearm) medially around its longitudinal axis so that the palm of the hand faces posteriorly and its dorsum faces anteriorly. When the elbow joint is flexed, pronation moves the hand so that the palm faces inferiorly (e.g., placing the palms flat on a table). When applied to the foot, pronation refers to a combination of eversion and abduction that results in lowering of the medial margin of the foot. (The feet of an individual with flat feet are pronated.)

Supination is the rotational movement of the forearm and hand that swings the radius laterally around its longitudinal axis so that the dorsum of the hand faces posteriorly and the palm faces anteriorly (i.e., moving them into the anatomical position). When the elbow joint is flexed, supination moves the hand so that the palm faces superiorly. (*Memory device:* You can hold soup in the palm of your hand when the flexed forearm is supinated but are prone [likely] to spill it if the forearm is then pronated!) When applied to the foot, supination generally implies movements resulting in raising the medial margin of the foot.

Opposition is the movement by which the pad of the 1st digit (thumb) is brought to another digit pad. This movement is used to pinch, button a shirt, and lift a teacup by the handle. **Reposition** describes the movement of the 1st digit from the position of opposition back to its anatomical position.

Protrusion is a movement anteriorly (forward) as in protruding the mandible (chin), lips, or tongue. **Retrusion** is a movement posteriorly (backward), as in retruding the mandible, lips, or tongue. The similar terms **protraction** and **retraction** are used most commonly for anterior and posterior movements of the shoulder.

Elevation raises or moves a part superiorly, as in elevating the shoulders when shrugging, the upper lid when opening the eye, or the tongue when pushing it up against the palate. **Depression** lowers or moves a part inferiorly, as in depressing the shoulders when standing at ease, the upper lid when closing the eye, or pulling the tongue away from the palate.

Eversion moves the sole of the foot away from the median plane (turning the sole laterally). When the foot is fully everted it is also dorsiflexed. **Inversion** moves the sole of the foot toward the median plane (facing the sole medially). When the foot is fully inverted it is also plantarflexed.

Structure of Terms

Anatomy is a descriptive science and necessarily requires names for the many structures and processes of the body. Students beginning their studies in anatomy often feel overwhelmed by the many new anatomicomedical terms. Fortunately, there are resources to help you learn these terms (Mehta et al., 1996; *Stedman's Medical Dictionary*, 2005; Willis, 1995). Many terms provide information about a structure's shape, size, location, or function or about the resemblance of one structure to another.

Some muscles have descriptive names to indicate their main characteristics—for example, the *deltoid muscle,* which covers the point of the shoulder, is triangular, like the symbol for *delta,* the fourth letter of the Greek alphabet. The suffix *-oid* means "like"; therefore, *deltoid* means like delta. *Biceps* means two-headed and *triceps* means three-headed. Some muscles are named according to their shape—the *piriformis muscle,* for example, is pear shaped (L. *pirum,* pear + L. *forma,* shape or form). Other muscles are named according to their location. The *temporal muscle* is in the temporal region (temple) of the cranium (skull). In some cases, actions are used to describe muscles—for example, the *levator scapulae* elevates the scapula (L. shoulder blade). Thus there are logical reasons for the names of muscles and other parts of the body, and if you learn their meanings and think about them as you read and dissect, you should have no difficulty remembering their names.

Abbreviations of Terms

Abbreviations of terms are used for brevity in medical histories and in this and other books, such as in tables of muscles, arteries, and nerves and even in speaking. Clinical abbreviations are used in discussions and descriptions of signs and symptoms. Learning to use these abbreviations also speeds note taking. Common anatomical and clinical abbreviations are provided in this text when the corresponding term is introduced—for example, temporomandibular joint (TMJ). They are also included in the lists of common medical abbreviations found in the appendices of comprehensive medical dictionaries (e.g., *Stedman's Medical Dictionary*).

THE BOTTOM LINE: Anatomical structural terms used in this book are derived from an international reference guide called *Terminologia Anatomica* (1998); however, colloquial terminology and eponymous terms are often used in the clinical setting. Anatomical directional terms are based on the body in the anatomical position. Four anatomical planes divide the body, and sections divide the planes into visually useful and descriptive parts. Other anatomic terms describe relationships of parts of the body, compare the positions of structures, and describe laterality and movement.

Anatomical Variations

Anatomy books describe (initially, at least) the structure of the body as it is usually observed in people—that is, the most common pattern. However, occasionally a particular structure demonstrates so much variation within the normal range that the most common pattern is found less than half the time! Beginning students are frequently frustrated because the bodies they are examining or dissecting do not conform to the atlas or text they are using (Bergman et al., 1988). Often students ignore the variations or inadvertently damage them by attempting to produce conformity. Therefore, you should *expect anatomical variations* when you dissect or inspect prosected specimens.

In a random group of people, individuals differ from each other in physical appearance. The bones of the skeleton vary not only in their basic shape but also in lesser details of surface structure. A wide variation is found in the size, shape, and form of the attachments of muscles. Similarly, considerable variation exists in the patterns of branching of veins, arteries, and nerves. Veins vary the most and nerves the least. Individual variation must be considered in physical examination, diagnosis, and treatment.

Most descriptions in this text assume a normal range of variation. However, the frequency of variation often differs among human groups, and variations collected in one population may not apply to members of another population. Some variations, such as those occurring in the origin and course of the cystic artery to the gallbladder, are clinically important (see Chapter 2), and any surgeon operating without knowledge of them is certain to have problems. In this book, clinically significant variations appear in the clinical correlation (blue) boxes.

Apart from racial and sexual differences, humans exhibit considerable genetic variation, such as polydactyly (extra digits). Approximately 3% of newborns show one or more significant congenital anomalies (Moore and Persaud, 2003). Other defects (e.g., atresia or blockage of the intestine) are not detected until symptoms occur. Discovering variations and congenital anomalies in cadavers is actually one of the many benefits of firsthand dissection, because it enables students to develop an awareness of the occurrence of variations and a sense of their frequency.

THE BOTTOM LINE: Anatomical variations are common and students should expect to encounter them during dissection. It is important to know how such variations may influence physical examination, diagnosis, and treatment.

Integumentary System

Because the skin is readily accessible and is one of the best indicators of general health (Swartz, 2001), careful observation of it is important in physical examinations. It is considered in the differential diagnosis of almost every disease. The skin provides

- *Protection* of the body from environmental effects, such as abrasions, fluid loss, harmful substances, ultraviolet radiation, and invading microorganisms.

- *Containment* for the body's structures (e.g., tissues and organs) and vital substances (especially extracellular fluids), preventing dehydration, which may be severe when extensive skin injuries (e.g., burns) are experienced.

- *Heat regulation* through the evaporation of sweat and/or the dilation or constriction of superficial blood vessels.

- *Sensation* (e.g., pain) by way of superficial nerves and their sensory endings.

- *Synthesis and storage* of vitamin D.

The skin, the body's largest organ, consists of the epidermis, a superficial cellular layer, and the dermis, a deep connective tissue layer (Fig. I.6).

The **epidermis** is a *keratinized epithelium*—that is, it has a tough, horny superficial layer that provides a protective outer surface overlying its regenerative and pigmented deep or *basal layer*. The epidermis has no blood vessels or lymphatics. The *avascular epidermis* is nourished by the underlying *vascular-*

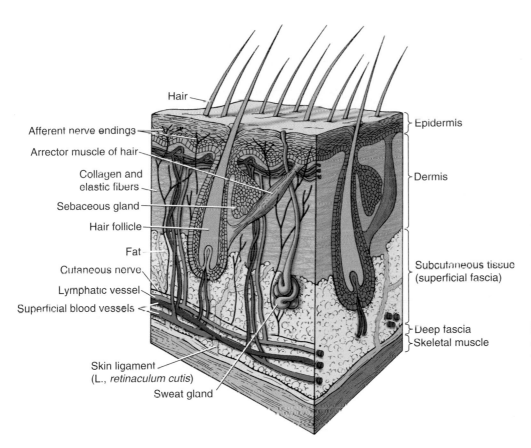

Hair

Afferent nerve endings

Arrector muscle of hair

Collagen and elastic fibers

Sebaceous gland

Hair follicle

Fat

Cutaneous nerve

Lymphatic vessel

Superficial blood vessels

Skin ligament (L., *retinaculum cutis*)

Sweat gland

Epidermis

Dermis

Subcutaneous tissue (superficial fascia)

Deep fascia
Skeletal muscle

Figure I.6. Skin and some of its specialized structures. The layered arrangement of the body's covering and the hairs and glands embedded within the skin and subcutaneous tissue are illustrated.

ized dermis, which is supplied by arteries that enter its deep surface to form a cutaneous plexus of anastomosing arteries. The skin is also supplied with afferent nerve endings that are sensitive to touch, irritation (pain), and temperature. Most nerve terminals are in the dermis, but a few penetrate into the epidermis.

The **dermis** is a dense layer of interlacing *collagen* and *elastic fibers.* These fibers provide skin tone and account for the strength and toughness of skin. The dermis of animals is removed and tanned to produce leather. *Karl Langer,* an Austrian anatomist, studied the skin of unembalmed cadavers and observed that, although the bundles of collagen fibers in the dermis run in all directions to produce a tough felt-like tissue, in any specific location most fibers run in the same direction. He noted that stab wounds in a cadaver's skin produced by an ice pick are slit-like rather than rounded because the pick splits the dermis in the predominate direction of the collagen fibers and allows the wound to gape.

The predominant pattern of collagen fibers determines the characteristic tension and wrinkle lines in the skin. The **tension lines** (also called cleavage lines or Langer lines) tend to spiral longitudinally in the limbs and run transversely in the neck and trunk (Fig. I.7). Tension lines at the elbows, knees, ankles, and wrists are parallel to the transverse creases that appear when the limbs are flexed; flex your wrist and you will see several of them. The elastic fibers of the dermis deteriorate with age and are not replaced; consequently, in older people the skin wrinkles and sags as it loses its elasticity.

The skin also contains many specialized structures (Fig. I.6). The deep layer of the dermis contains *hair follicles,* with associated smooth arrector muscles and sebaceous glands. Contraction of the **arrector muscles of hairs** (L. *musculi arrector pili*) erects the hairs, causing goose bumps. Hair follicles are generally slanted to one side, and several *sebaceous glands* lie on the side pointed to by the hair (as the hair appears to "enter" the skin—of course, it is emerging from rather than entering the skin). Thus contraction of the arrector muscles causes the hairs to stand up straighter, thereby compressing the sebaceous glands and helping them secrete their oily product onto the skin surface. The evaporation of the watery secretion (sweat) of the *sweat glands* from the skin provides a *thermoregulatory mechanism* for heat loss (cooling). Also involved in the loss or retention of body heat are the small arteries (arterioles) within the dermis. They dilate to fill superficial capillary beds to radiate heat (skin appears red) or constrict to minimize surface heat loss (skin, especially of lips and fingertips, appears blue). Other integumentary structures or derivatives include the hair, the nails (fingernails, toenails), the mammary glands, and the enamel of teeth.

Located between the overlying skin (dermis) and underlying deep fascia, the **subcutaneous tissue** (superficial fascia) is composed mostly of loose connective tissue and *stored fat,* and contains sweat glands, *superficial blood vessels, lymphatic vessels,* and *cutaneous nerves* (Fig. I.6). The neurovascular structures course in this layer, distributing only their terminal branches to the skin. The subcutaneous tissue provides for

Anterior view   Posterior view

Figure I.7. Tension (Langer) lines in the skin. The *dashed lines* indicate the predominant direction of the collagen fiber bundles in the dermis. Incisions or lacerations running parallel to these lines have less tendency to gape than those crossing them.

most of the body's fat storage, so its thickness varies greatly, depending on nutritional state. Nutritional state aside, the distribution of subcutaneous tissue varies considerably in different sites in the same individual. Compare, for example, the relative abundance of subcutaneous tissue evident by the thickness of the fold of skin that can be pinched at the waist or thighs with the anteromedial part of the leg (the shin, the anterior border of the tibia) or the back of the hand, the latter two being nearly devoid of it. Also consider the distribution of subcutaneous tissue and fat between the sexes: In

mature females, it tends to accumulate in the breasts and thighs and in males, in the lower abdominal wall. Subcutaneous tissue participates in thermoregulation, functioning as insulation, retaining heat in the body's core. It also provides padding that protects the skin from compression by bony prominences, such as in the buttocks.

Skin ligaments (L. *retinacula cutis*), numerous small fibrous bands, extend through the subcutaneous tissue and attach the deep surface of the dermis to the underlying deep fascia (Fig. I.6). The length and density of these ligaments determines the mobility of the skin over deep structures. Where skin ligaments are longer and sparse, the skin is more

(cont'd on page 16)

Skin Incisions and Scarring

The skin is always under tension. In general, lacerations or incisions that parallel the tension lines usually heal well with little scarring because there is minimal disruption of fibers. The uninterrupted fibers tend to retain the cut edges in place. However, a laceration or incision across the tension lines disrupts a greater number of collagen fibers. The disrupted lines of force cause the wound to gape, and it may heal with excessive (keloid) scarring. When other considerations, such as adequate exposure and access or avoidance of nerves, are not of greater importance, surgeons attempting to minimize scarring for cosmetic reasons may use surgical incisions that parallel the tension lines.

Stretch Marks in Skin

The collagen and elastic fibers in the dermis form a tough, flexible meshwork of tissue. Because the skin can distend considerably, a relatively small incision can be made during surgery compared with the much larger incision required to attempt the same procedure in an embalmed cadaver, which no longer exhibits elasticity. The skin can stretch and grow to accommodate gradual increases in size. However, marked and relatively fast size increases, such as the abdominal enlargement and weight gain accompanying pregnancy, can stretch the skin too far, damaging the collagen fibers in the dermis (Fig. BI.1). Bands of thin wrinkled skin, initially red but later becoming purple, and white stretch marks (L. *striae gravidarum*) appear on the abdomen, buttocks, thighs, and breasts during pregnancy. Stretch marks (L. *striae cutis distensae*) also form in obese individuals and result from loosening of the deep fascia and reduced cohesion between the collagen fibers as the skin stretches. Stretch marks generally fade after pregnancy and weight loss; they never disappear completely. ▶

Figure BI.1.

Skin Injuries and Their Classification

Lacerations

Accidental cuts and skin tears are superficial or deep. **Superficial lacerations** violate the epidermis and perhaps the superficial layer of the dermis; they bleed but do not interrupt the continuity of the dermis. **Deep lacerations** penetrate the deep layer of the dermis, extending into the subcutaneous tissue or beyond; they gape and require approximation of the cut edges of the dermis (by suturing, or stitches) to minimize scarring.

Burns

Burns, common injuries of skin, are caused by thermal trauma, ultraviolet or ionizing radiation, or chemical agents. Burns are classified, in increasing order of severity, based on the depth of skin injury (Fig. BI.2):

- *1st-degree (superficial) burn:* damage limited to epidermis; symptoms are *erythema* (hot red skin), pain, and *edema* (swelling); *desquamation* (peeling) of the superficial layer usually occurs several days later, but the layer is quickly replaced from the basal layer without significant scarring; example is sunburn.

- *2nd-degree (partial-thickness) burn:* epidermal and superficial dermis are damaged; blistering occurs; nerve endings are damaged, making this variety the most painful; except for their most superficial parts, the sweat glands and hair follicles are not damaged and can provide the source of replacement cells for the basal layer of the epidermis; healing will occur slowly (within 21 days or less), leaving scarring and some contracture, but it is usually complete.

2nd-degree (partial-thickness burn)

Figure BI.2.

- *3rd-degree (full-thickness) burn:* the entire thickness of the skin is damaged and perhaps underlying muscle; a minor degree of healing may occur at the edges, but the open, ulcerated portions require skin grafting; dead material (*eschar*) is removed and replaced with skin *harvested* (taken) from a non-burned location.

The extent of a burn (percent of total body surface affected) is generally more significant than the degree (severity in terms of depth) in estimating the effect on the well-being of the victim. ✚

mobile, such as on the back of the hand (Fig. I.8*A* & *C*). Where ligaments are short and abundant, the skin is firmly attached to the underlying deep fascia, such as in the palms and soles (Fig. I.8*B*). Skin ligaments are long but particularly well developed in the breasts, where they form weight-bearing *suspensory ligaments* (see Fig. 1.20).

Loose skin on dorsum of hand

(A)

Sparse subcutaneous tissue

Long, sparse skin ligaments

Skin incised to expose skin ligaments

(B)

Skin reflected to reveal short, stout, abundant skin ligaments traversing the relatively thin layer of subcutaneous tissue

(C)

Figure I.8. Skin ligaments of subcutaneous tissue. A. The thickness of subcutaneous tissue can be estimated as being approximately half that of a pinched fold of skin (i.e., a fold of skin includes a double thickness of subcutaneous tissue). The dorsum of the hand has relatively little subcutaneous tissue. **B.** Long, relatively sparse skin ligaments allow the mobility of the skin demonstrated in part **A. C.** The skin of the palm of the hand (like that of the soles of the feet) is firmly attached to the underlying deep fascia.

THE BOTTOM LINE: The integumentary system (the skin) consists of the epidermis, dermis, and specialized structures (hair follicles, sebaceous glands, and sweat glands). The skin plays important roles in protection, containment, heat regulation, and sensation; it also synthesizes and stores vitamin D. Tension (Langer) lines in the skin have implications in surgery and wound healing. Subcutaneous tissue, located beneath the dermis, contains most of the body's fat stores.

Fascias, Fascial Compartments, Bursae, and Potential Spaces

Fascias (L. *fasciae*) constitute the wrapping, packing, and insulating materials of the deep structures of the body. Underlying the *subcutaneous tissue* (also called *superficial fascia*) almost everywhere is the deep fascia (Fig. I.9). The **deep fascia** is a dense, organized connective tissue layer, devoid of fat, that covers most of the body parallel to (deep to) the skin and subcutaneous tissue. Extensions from its internal surface invest deeper structures, such as individual muscles and neurovascular bundles, as **investing fascia** (Gartner and Hiatt, 2001). Its thickness varies widely. In the face and ischioanal fossa, distinct layers of deep fascia are absent.

In the limbs, groups of muscles with similar functions sharing the same nerve supply are located in compartments, separated by thick sheets of deep fascia, called **intermuscular septa**, that extend centrally from the surrounding fascial sleeve to attach to the bones. These fascial compartments may contain or direct the spread of an infection or a tumor. In a few places, the deep fascia gives attachment (origin) to the underlying muscles (although it is not usually mentioned in lists or tables of origins and insertions); but in most places, the muscles are free to contract and glide deep to it. However, the deep fascia itself never passes freely over bone; where deep fascia contacts bone, it blends firmly with the *periosteum* (bone covering). The relatively unyielding deep fascia investing muscles, and especially that surrounding the fascial compartments in the limbs, limits the outward expansion of the bellies of contracting skeletal muscles. Blood is thus pushed out as the veins of the muscles and compartments are compressed. *Valves* within the veins allow the blood to flow only in one direction (toward the heart), preventing the backflow that might occur as the muscles relax. Thus deep fascia, contracting muscles, and venous valves work together as a *musculovenous pump* to return blood to the heart, especially in the lower limbs where blood must move against the pull of gravity (Fig. I.25).

Near certain joints (e.g., wrist and ankle), the deep fascia becomes markedly thickened, forming a **retinaculum** (plural = retinacula) to hold tendons in place where they cross the joint during flexion and extension, preventing them from taking a shortcut, or *bow stringing*, across the angle created (Fig. I.19).

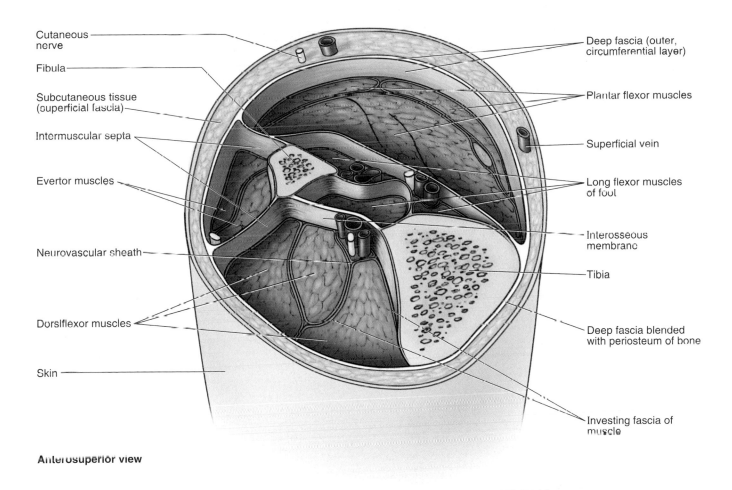

Cutaneous nerve

Fibula

Subcutaneous tissue (superficial fascia)

Intermuscular septa

Evertor muscles

Neurovascular sheath

Dorsiflexor muscles

Skin

Deep fascia (outer, circumferential layer)

Plantar flexor muscles

Superficial vein

Long flexor muscles of foot

Interosseous membrane

Tibia

Deep fascia blended with periosteum of bone

Investing fascia of muscle

Anterosuperior view

Figure I.9. Excavated section of the leg demonstrating the deep fascia and fascial formations. Deep to the skin and subcutaneous tissue, a circumferential layer of deep fascia covers the musculoskeletal structures. Thick intermuscular septa extend centrally from the outer layer, forming fascial compartments containing muscles of similar function. Individual muscles are covered by investing fascia.

Subscrous fascia, with varying amounts of fatty tissue, lies between the internal surfaces of the musculoskeletal walls and the serous membranes lining the body cavities. These are the *endothoracic, endoabdominal,* and *endopelvic fascias;* the latter two may be referred to collectively as *extraperitoneal fascia.*

Bursae (singular = bursa; Mediev. L., a purse) are closed sacs or envelopes of **serous membrane** (a delicate connective tissue membrane capable of secreting fluid to lubricate a smooth internal surface) that are collapsed or essentially "empty," except for a thin layer of lubricating fluid secreted by the membrane. Usually occurring in locations subject to friction, bursae enable one structure to move more freely over another. *Subcutaneous bursae* occur in the subcutaneous tissue between skin and bony prominences, such as at the elbow or knee; *subfascial bursae* lie beneath deep fascia; and *subtendinous bursae* facilitate the movement of tendons over bone. *Synovial tendon sheaths* are a specialized type of elongated bursae that wrap around tendons, usually enclosing them as they traverse osseofibrous tunnels that anchor the tendons in place (Fig. I.10A).

Bursae occasionally communicate with the synovial cavities of joints. Because they are formed only of delicate, transparent serous membrane and are collapsed, bursae are not easily noticed or dissected in the laboratory. It is possible to display bursae by injecting and distending them with colored fluid. In atlases and textbooks, they are typically illustrated as they would appear if injected with (usually blue) latex that has solidified so that it remains in place as a cast of the bursa when the surrounding tissues are removed.

As noted, bursae and synovial tendon sheaths are examples of empty, or potential, sacs or spaces, usually lined with or formed of a serous or synovial membrane, and are encountered in the study of anatomy. Unlike three-dimensional realized or actual spaces, these spaces are collapsed so that they have no depth; their walls are apposed with only a thin film of lubricating fluid between them. When the wall is interrupted at any point or when a fluid is secreted or formed within them in excess, they become realized spaces; however, this condition is abnormal or pathological.

Such collapsed bursal sacs surround many important organs (e.g., the heart, lungs, and abdominal viscera) and struc-

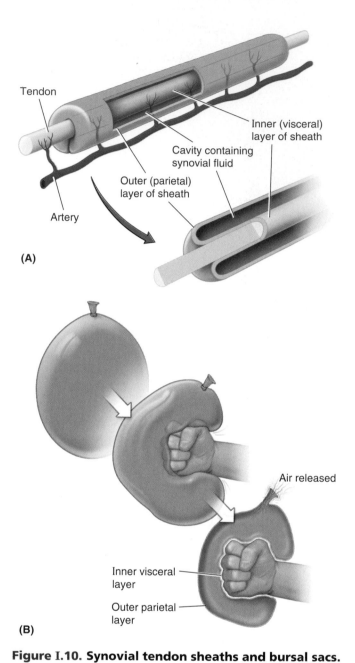

Tendon

Inner (visceral)
layer of sheath

Cavity containing
synovial fluid

Outer (parietal)
layer of sheath

Artery

(A)

Air released

Inner visceral
layer

Outer parietal
layer

(B)

Figure I.10. Synovial tendon sheaths and bursal sacs.
A. Synovial tendon sheaths are longitudinal bursae that surround tendons as they pass deep to retinacula or through fibrous digital sheaths. **B.** Bursal sacs enclose several structures, such as the heart, lungs, digestive tract, and tendons, much like this collapsed balloon encloses the fist. A thin film of lubricating fluid between the parietal and visceral layers confers mobility to the structure surrounded by the bursa within a confined compartment. The double folds of synovial membrane between the parietal and visceral layers surrounding the vessels (and other structures) passing to and from the intraperitoneal structure(s) are called mesenteries. In the case of a synovial tendon sheath, the mesentery is called a mesotendon.

tures (e.g., portions of tendons). This configuration is much like wrapping a large but empty balloon around a structure, such as a fist (Fig. I.10B). The object is surrounded by the two layers of the empty balloon, but is not inside the balloon; the balloon itself remains empty. For an even more exact com-

parison, the balloon should first be filled with water and then emptied, leaving the empty balloon wet inside. In exactly this way, the heart is surrounded by—but is not inside—the pericardial sac. Each lung is surrounded by—but is not inside—a pleural sac, and the abdominal viscera are surrounded by—but are not inside—the peritoneal sac. In such cases, the inner layer of the balloon or serous sac (the one adjacent to the fist, viscus, or viscera) is called the **visceral layer;** the outer layer of the balloon (or the one in contact with the body wall) is called the **parietal layer.** Such a surrounding double layer of membranes, moistened on their apposed surfaces, confers freedom of movement on the surrounded structure when it is contained within a confined space, such as the heart within the thorax and a tendon traversing an osseofibrous tunnel.

Fascial Planes

In living people, fascial planes (*interfascial* and *intrafascial*) exist that are potential spaces between adjacent fascias or fascia-lined structures or within loose areolar fascias, such as the *subserous fascias.* During operations, surgeons take advantage of these interfascial planes, separating structures to create actual spaces that allow movement and access to deeply placed structures. In some procedures, surgeons use extrapleural or extraperitoneal fascial planes, which allow them to operate outside the membranes lining the body cavities, minimizing the potential for contamination, the spread of infection, and consequent formation of adhesions within the cavities. Unfortunately, these planes are often fused and difficult to establish or appreciate in the embalmed cadaver. ✚

THE BOTTOM LINE: Deep fascia is an organized connective tissue layer that completely envelops the body beneath the subcutaneous tissue of the skin. Extensions of the deep fascia divide muscles into groups (intermuscular septa), invest individual muscles and neurovascular bundles (investing fascia), and lie between musculoskeletal walls and the serous membranes lining body cavities (subserous fascia). Retinacula are thickenings of deep fascia that hold tendons in place during joint movements. Bursae are closed sacs formed of serous membrane that occur in locations subject to friction; they enable one structure to move freely over another.

Skeletal System

The skeletal system may be divided into two functional parts (Fig. I.11):

- The **axial skeleton** consists of the bones of the head (*cranium* or *skull*), neck (*hyoid bone* and *cervical vertebrae*), and trunk (*ribs, sternum, vertebrae,* and *sacrum*).

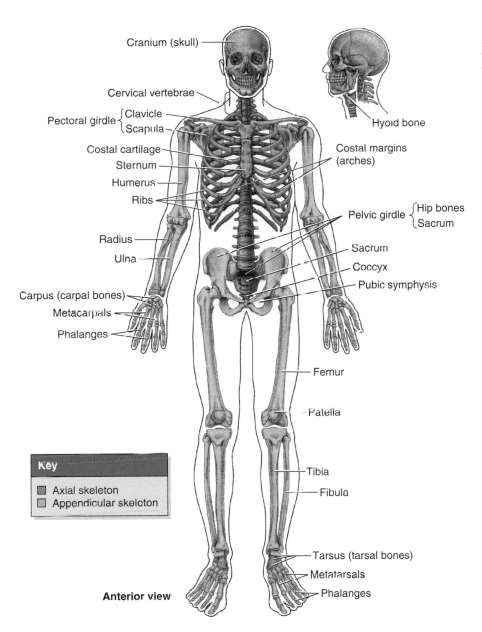

Cranium (skull)

Cervical vertebrae

Pectoral girdle { Clavicle
                  Scapula

Costal cartilage

Sternum

Humerus

Ribs

Radius

Ulna

Carpus (carpal bones)

Metacarpals

Phalanges

Hyoid bone

Costal margins (arches)

Pelvic girdle { Hip bones
                Sacrum

Sacrum

Coccyx

Pubic symphysis

Femur

Patella

Tibia

Fibula

Tarsus (tarsal bones)

Metatarsals

Phalanges

Key

▨ Axial skeleton
▨ Appendicular skeleton

Anterior view

Figure I.11. Skeletal system. The skeleton of the head, neck, and trunk forms the axial skeleton; the skeleton of the limbs forms the appendicular skeleton.

- The **appendicular skeleton** consists of the *bones of the limbs,* including those forming the pectoral (shoulder) and pelvic girdles.

Cartilage and Bones

The skeleton is composed of cartilages and bones. **Cartilage** is a resilient, semirigid form of connective tissue that forms parts of the skeleton where more flexibility is required—for example, where the costal cartilages attach the ribs to the sternum. Also, the articulating surfaces of bones participating in a synovial joint are capped with articular cartilages that provide smooth, low-friction, gliding surfaces for free movement (Fig. I.16). Blood vessels do not enter cartilage

(i.e., it is *avascular*); consequently, its cells obtain oxygen and nutrients by diffusion. The proportion of bone and cartilage in the skeleton changes as the body grows; the younger a person is, the more cartilage her or she has. The bones of a newborn are soft and flexible because they are mostly composed of cartilage.

Bone, a living tissue, is a highly specialized, hard form of connective tissue that makes up most of the skeleton. It is the chief supporting tissue of the body. Bones of the adult skeleton provide

- Support for the body and its vital cavities.

- Protection for vital structures.

Posterior view

Figure I.11. *(Continued)*

thin layer of compact bone around a central mass of spongy medullary bone, except where the latter is replaced by a *medullary (marrow) cavity.* Within the medullary cavity of adult bones, and between the **spicules** (trabeculae) of spongy bone, blood cells and blood platelets are formed (Ross et al., 2003). The architecture and proportion of compact and spongy bone vary according to function. Compact bone provides strength for weight bearing. In *long bones* designed for rigidity and attachment of muscles and ligaments, the amount of compact bone is greatest near the middle of the *shaft* where the bones are liable to buckle. In addition, long bones have elevations (e.g., *ridges, crests,* and *tubercles*) that serve as *buttresses* (supports) where large muscles attach. Living bones have some *elasticity* (flexibility) and great *rigidity* (hardness).

Classification of Bones

Bones are classified according to their shape.

- *Long bones* are tubular (e.g., the humerus in the arm).

- *Short bones* are cuboidal and are found only in the ankle (tarsus) and wrist (carpus).

- *Flat bones* usually serve protective functions (e.g., those forming the cranium protect the brain).

- *Irregular bones* (e.g., in the face) have various shapes other than long, short, or flat.

- The mechanical basis for movement (leverage).

- Storage for salts (e.g., calcium).

- A continuous supply of new blood cells (produced by the marrow contained within many bones).

A fibrous connective tissue covering surrounds each skeletal element like a sleeve, except where articular cartilage occurs; that surrounding bones is **periosteum** (Fig. I.15), whereas that around cartilage is **perichondrium.** The periosteum and perichondrium nourish the external aspects of the skeletal tissue. They are capable of laying down more cartilage or bone (particularly during fracture healing) and provide the interface for attachment of *tendons* and *ligaments.*

The two types of bone are **compact** bone and **spongy** (*trabecular* or *cancellous*) bone. They are distinguished by the relative amount of solid matter and by the number and size of the spaces they contain (Fig. I.12). All bones have a superficial

Figure I.12. Transverse sections of the humerus (upper arm bone). The shaft of a living bone is a tube of compact bone that surrounds a medullary cavity, which contains red or yellow bone marrow or a combination of both.

- *Sesamoid bones* (e.g., the patella or knee cap) develop in certain tendons and are found where tendons cross the ends of long bones in the limbs; they protect the tendons from excessive wear and often change the angle of the tendons as they pass to their attachments.

Accessory Bones

Accessory (supernumerary) bones develop when additional ossification centers appear and form extra bones. Many bones develop from several centers of ossification, and the separate parts normally fuse. Sometimes one of these centers fails to fuse with the main bone, giving the appearance of an extra bone; but careful study shows that the apparent extra bone is a missing part of the main bone. Circumscribed areas of bone are often seen along the sutures of the cranium where the flat bones abut, particularly those related to the parietal bone (see Chapter 7). These small, irregular, worm-like bones are **sutural bones** (wormian bones). It is important to know that accessory bones are common in the foot, to avoid mistaking them for bone fragments in radiographs and other medical images.

Heterotopic Bones

Bones sometimes form in soft tissues where they are not normally present (e.g., in scars). Horse riders often develop **heterotopic bones** in their thighs (*rider's bones*), probably because of chronic muscle strain resulting in small hemorrhagic (bloody) areas that undergo calcification and eventual ossification. ⊕

Bone Markings and Formations
Bone markings appear wherever tendons, ligaments, and fascias are attached or where arteries lie adjacent to or enter bones. Other formations occur in relation to the passage of a tendon (often to direct the tendon or improve its leverage) or to control the type of movement occurring at a joint. The various markings and features of bones are (Fig. I.13)

- *Capitulum:* small, round, articular head (e.g., the capitulum of the humerus).
- *Condyle:* rounded, knuckle-like articular area, usually occurring in pairs (e.g., the lateral femoral condyle).
- *Crest:* ridge of bone (e.g., the iliac crest).
- *Epicondyle:* eminence superior to a condyle (e.g., the lateral epicondyle of the humerus).
- *Facet:* smooth flat area, usually covered with cartilage, where a bone articulates with another bone (e.g., the superior costal facet on the body of a vertebra for articulation with a rib).

- *Foramen:* passage through a bone (e.g., the obturator foramen).
- *Fossa:* hollow or depressed area (e.g., the infraspinous fossa of the scapula).
- *Groove:* elongated depression or furrow (e.g., the radial groove of the humerus).
- *Head* (L. *caput*): large, round articular end (e.g., the head of the humerus).
- *Line:* linear elevation (e.g., the soleal line of the tibia).
- *Malleolus:* rounded process (e.g., the lateral malleolus of the fibula).
- *Notch:* indentation at the edge of a bone (e.g., the greater sciatic notch).
- *Protuberance:* projection of bone (e.g., the external occipital protuberance).
- *Spine:* thorn-like process (e.g., the spine of the scapula).
- *Spinous process:* projecting spine-like part (e.g., the spinous process of a vertebra).
- *Trochanter:* large blunt elevation (e.g., the greater trochanter of the femur).
- *Trochlea:* spool-like articular process or process that acts as a pulley (e.g., trochlea of the humerus).
- *Tubercle:* small raised eminence (e.g., the greater tubercle of the humerus).
- *Tuberosity:* large rounded elevation (e.g., the ischial tuberosity).

Trauma to Bone and Bone Changes

Bones are living organs that hurt when injured, bleed when fractured, remodel in relationship to stresses placed on them, and change with age. Like other organs, bones have blood vessels, lymphatic vessels, and nerves, and they may become diseased. Unused bones, such as in a paralyzed limb, *atrophy* (decrease in size). Bone may be absorbed, which occurs in the mandible when the teeth are extracted. Bones *hypertrophy* (enlarge) when they support increased weight for a long period.

Trauma to a bone (e.g., during an accident) may break it. For the fracture to heal properly, the broken ends must be brought together, approximating their normal position. This is called *reduction of a fracture*. During bone healing, the surrounding *fibroblasts* (connective tissue cells) proliferate and secrete collagen, which forms a *collar of callus* to hold the bones together ▶

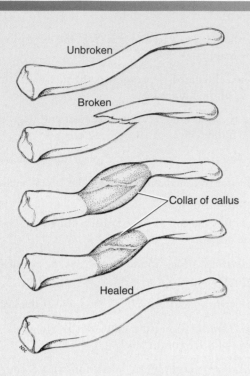

Figure BI.3.

(Fig. BI.3). Bone remodeling occurs in the fracture area, and the callus calcifies. Eventually, the callus is resorbed and replaced by bone. After several months, little evidence of the fracture remains, especially in young people. Fractures are more common in children than in adults because of the combination of their slender, growing bones and carefree activities. Fortunately, many of these breaks are *greenstick fractures* (incomplete breaks caused by bending the bones). Fractures in growing bones heal faster than those in adult bones.

Osteoporosis

During the aging process, the organic and inorganic components of bone both decrease, often resulting in *osteo-*

porosis, a reduction in the quantity of bone, or atrophy of skeletal tissue. (Fig. BI.4) Hence, the bones become brittle, lose their elasticity, and fracture easily.

Sternal Puncture

Examination of bone marrow provides valuable information for evaluating hematological diseases. Because it lies just beneath the skin (i.e., is subcutaneous) and is easily accessible, the sternum (breast bone) is a commonly used site for harvesting bone marrow. During a *sternal puncture*, a wide-bore (large-diameter) needle is inserted through the thin cortical bone of the sternum into the spongy bone, and a sample of *red bone marrow* (marrow that produces blood cells) is aspirated with a syringe for laboratory examination. *Bone marrow transplantation* is sometimes performed in the treatment of leukemia. ⊙

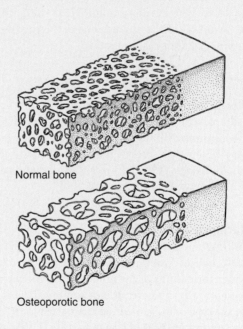

Normal bone

Osteoporotic bone

Figure BI.4.

THE BOTTOM LINE The skeletal system can be divided into the axial (bones of the head, neck, and trunk) and appendicular skeletons (bones of the limbs). The skeleton itself is composed of cartilage, a semirigid connective tissue, and bone, a hard form of connective tissue that provides support, protection, movement, storage (of certain electrolytes), and synthesis of blood cells. Periosteum, which surrounds bones, and perichondrium, which surrounds car-tilage, provide nourishment for these tissues and are the sites of new cartilage and bone formation. Two types of bone, spongy and compact, are distinguished by the amount of solid matter and the size and number of spaces they contain. Bones can be classified as long, short, flat, irregular, or sesamoid; standard terms for specific bone markings and features are used when describing the structure of individual bones.

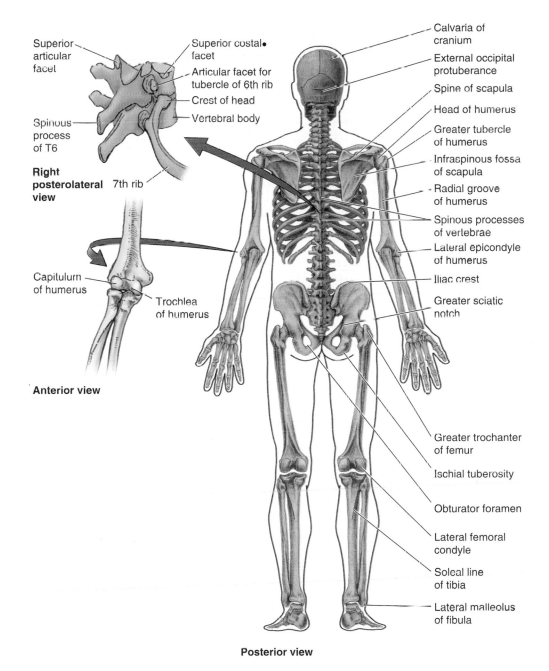

Right posterolateral view

Superior articular facet

Superior costal facet

Articular facet for tubercle of 6th rib

Crest of head

Vertebral body

Spinous process of T6

7th rib

Anterior view

Capitulum of humerus

Trochlea of humerus

Calvaria of cranium

External occipital protuberance

Spine of scapula

Head of humerus

Greater tubercle of humerus

Infraspinous fossa of scapula

Radial groove of humerus

Spinous processes of vertebrae

Lateral epicondyle of humerus

Iliac crest

Greater sciatic notch

Greater trochanter of femur

Ischial tuberosity

Obturator foramen

Lateral femoral condyle

Soleal line of tibia

Lateral malleolus of fibula

Posterior view

Figure I.13. Bone markings and formations. Markings appear on bones wherever tendons, ligaments, and fascia attach. Other formations relate to joints, the passage of tendons, and the provision of increased leverage.

Bone Development

Most bones take many years to grow and mature. The humerus (arm bone), for example, begins to ossify at the end of the embryonic period (8 weeks); however, ossification is not complete until age 20. All bones derive from *mesenchyme* (embryonic connective tissue) by two different processes: intramembranous ossification (directly from mesenchyme) and endochondral ossification (from cartilage derived from mesenchyme). The histology (microscopic structure) of a bone is the same either way (Cormack, 2001; Moore and Persaud, 2003).

- In *intramembranous ossification* (membranous bone formation), mesenchymal models of bones form during the embryonic period, and direct ossification of the mesenchyme begins in the fetal period.

- In *endochondral ossification* (cartilaginous bone formation), cartilage models of the bones form from mesenchyme during the fetal period, and bone subsequently replaces most of the cartilage.

A brief description of endochondral ossification helps explain

(A)

(B)

Figure I.14. Development and growth of a long bone.
A. The formation of primary and secondary ossification centers is shown. **B.** Growth in length occurs on both sides of the cartilaginous epiphysial plates (*blue arrows*). For growth to continue, the bone formed from the primary center in the diaphysis does not fuse with that formed from the secondary centers in the epiphyses until the bone reaches its adult size. When growth ceases, the epiphysial plate is replaced by a synostosis (bone-to-bone fusion), seen as an epiphysial line in radiographs.

how long bones grow (Fig. I.14). The mesenchymal cells condense and differentiate into *chondroblasts,* dividing cells in growing cartilage tissue, thereby forming a *cartilaginous bone model.* In the midregion of the model, the cartilage *calcifies* (becomes impregnated with calcium salts), and *periosteal capillaries* (capillaries from the fibrous sheath surrounding the model) grow into the calcified cartilage of the bone model and supply its interior. These blood vessels, together with as-

sociated *osteogenic (bone-forming) cells,* form a *periosteal bud* (Fig. I.14A). The capillaries initiate the **primary ossification center,** so named because the bone tissue it forms replaces most of the cartilage in the main body of the bone model. The shaft of a bone ossified from the primary ossification center is the **diaphysis,** which grows as the bone develops.

Most **secondary ossification centers** appear in other parts of the developing bone after birth; the parts of a bone ossified from these centers are **epiphyses.** The chondrocytes in the middle of the epiphysis hypertrophy, and the *bone matrix* (extracellular substance) between them calcifies. *Epiphysial arteries* grow into the developing cavities with associated osteogenic cells. The flared part of the diaphysis nearest the epiphysis is the **metaphysis.** For growth to continue, the bone formed from the primary center in the diaphysis does not fuse with that formed from the secondary centers in the epiphyses until the bone reaches its adult size. Thus, during growth of a long bone, *cartilaginous epiphysial plates* intervene between the diaphysis and epiphyses (Fig. I.14B). These growth plates are eventually replaced by bone at each of its two sides, diaphysial and epiphysial. When this occurs, bone growth ceases, and the diaphysis fuses with the epiphyses. The seam formed during this fusion process (*synostosis*) is particularly dense and is recognizable in radiographs as an *epiphysial line.* The epiphysial fusion of bones occurs progressively from puberty to maturity. *Ossification* of short bones is similar to that of the primary ossification center of long bones, and only one short bone, the calcaneus (heel bone), develops a secondary ossification center.

Bone Growth and the Assessment of Bone Age

Knowledge of the sites where ossification centers occur, the times of their appearance, the rates at which they grow, and the times of fusion of the sites (times when synostosis occurs) is important in clinical medicine, forensic science, and anthropology. A general index of growth during infancy, childhood, and adolescence is indicated by *bone age,* as determined from radiographs (negative images on X-ray films). The age of a young person can be determined by studying the ossification centers in bones (see "Medical Imaging of the Upper Limb" in Chapter 6 for examples). The main criteria are (1) the appearance of calcified material in the diaphysis and/or epiphyses and (2) the disappearance of the dark line representing the epiphysial plate (absence of this line indicates that epiphysial fusion has occurred; fusion occurs at specific times for each epiphysis). The fusion of epiphyses with the diaphysis occurs 1–2 ▶

years earlier in girls than in boys. Determining bone age can be helpful in predicting adult height in early- or late-maturing adolescents (Behrman et al., 2004). Assessment of bone age also helps establish the approximate age of human skeletal remains in medicolegal cases.

Effects of Disease and Diet on Bone Growth

Some diseases produce early epiphysial fusion (ossification time) compared with what is normal for the person's chronological age; other diseases result in delayed fusion. The growing skeleton is sensitive to relatively slight and transient illnesses and to periods of malnutrition. Proliferation of cartilage at the metaphysis slows down during starvation and illness, but the degeneration of cartilage cells in the columns continues, producing a dense line of provisional calcification. These lines later become bone with thickened trabeculae, or *lines of arrested growth.*

Displacement and Separation of Epiphyses

Without knowledge of bone growth and the appearance of bones in radiographic and other diagnostic images at various ages, a displaced epiphysial plate could be mistaken for a fracture, and separation of an epiphysis could be interpreted as a displaced piece of a fractured bone. Knowing the patient's age and the location of epiphyses can prevent these anatomical errors. The edges of the diaphysis and epiphysis are smoothly curved in the region of the epiphysial plate. Bone fractures always leave a sharp, often uneven edge of bone. An injury that causes a fracture in an adult usually causes the displacement of an epiphysis in a child. ✪

Vasculature and Innervation of Bones

Bones are richly supplied with blood vessels. Most apparent are the **nutrient arteries** (one or more per bone) that arise as independent branches of adjacent arteries outside the periosteum and pass obliquely through the compact bone of the shaft of a long bone via **nutrient foramina.** The nutrient artery divides in the medullary cavity into longitudinal branches that proceed toward each end, supplying the bone marrow, spongy bone, and deeper portions of the compact bone (Fig. I.15). However, many small branches from the periosteal arteries of the periosteum are responsible for nourishment of most of the compact bone. Consequently, a bone from which the periosteum has been removed dies. Blood reaches the *osteocytes* (bone cells) within the compact bone by means of microscopic canal systems (*haversian systems* or

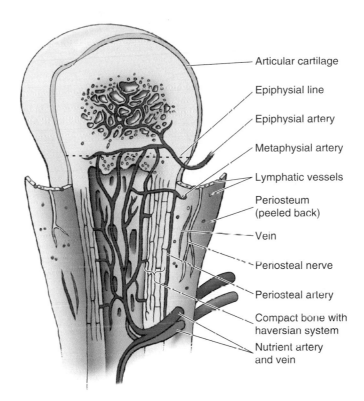

Figure I.15. Vasculature and innervation of a long bone. The large nutrient artery (or arteries) supplies the marrow, spongy bone, and deeper compact bone of the diaphysis and metaphyses. Small branches from the periosteal arteries supply most of the compact bone from the superficial aspect. The haversian canal systems enable blood to penetrate the compact bone to nourish the osteocytes (bone cells). Epiphysial and metaphysial arteries supply the ends of long bones. The periosteum is also rich in sensory (periosteal) nerves.

- Articular cartilage
- Epiphysial line
- Epiphysial artery
- Metaphysial artery
- Lymphatic vessels
- Periosteum (peeled back)
- Vein
- Periosteal nerve
- Periosteal artery
- Compact bone with haversian system
- Nutrient artery and vein

osteons) that house small blood vessels. The ends of the bones are supplied by metaphysial and epiphysial arteries that arise mainly from the arteries that supply the joints; in the limbs, these arteries are typically part of a *periarticular arterial plexus,* which surrounds the joint, ensuring blood flow distal to the joint regardless of the position assumed by the joint.

Veins accompany arteries through the nutrient foramina. Many large veins also leave through foramina near the articular ends of the bones. Bones containing red bone marrow have numerous large veins. *Lymphatic vessels* are abundant in the periosteum.

Nerves accompany blood vessels supplying bones. The periosteum is richly supplied with sensory nerves—**periosteal nerves**—that carry pain fibers. The periosteum is especially sensitive to tearing or tension, which explains the acute pain from bone fractures. Bone itself is relatively sparsely supplied with sensory endings. Within bones, **vasomotor nerves** cause constriction or dilation of blood vessels, regulating blood flow through the bone marrow.

Avascular Necrosis

Loss of the arterial supply to an epiphysis or other parts of a bone results in the death of bone tissue, or *avascular necrosis* (G. *nekrosis,* deadness). After every fracture, small areas of adjacent bone undergo necrosis. In some fractures, avascular necrosis of a large fragment of bone may occur. A number of clinical disorders of epiphyses in children result from avascular necrosis of unknown etiology (cause). These disorders are referred to as *osteochondroses* (Salter, 1998). ●

THE BOTTOM LINE: Bones grow through the processes of intramembraneous ossification, in which mesenchymal bone models are formed during the embryonic and prenatal periods, and endochondral ossification, in which cartilage models are formed during the fetal period, with bone subsequently replacing most of the cartilage after birth.

Joints

A **joint** (**articulation**) is a union or junction between two or more bones or rigid parts of the skeleton. Joints exhibit a variety of forms and functions. Some joints have no movement; others allow only slight movement, and some are freely movable, such as the glenohumeral (shoulder) joint.

Classification of Joints

Three classes of joints are described based on the manner or type of material by which the articulating bones are united.

1. The articulating bones of **synovial joints** are united by a joint (articular) capsule (composed of an outer fibrous layer or membrane lined by a serous synovial membrane) spanning and enclosing an articular cavity. The **articular cavity** of a synovial joint, like the knee, is a potential space that contains a small amount of lubricating synovial fluid, secreted by the synovial membrane. Inside the capsule, articular cartilage covers the articular surfaces (bearing surfaces) of the bones; all other internal surfaces are covered by synovial membrane. The bones in Figure I.16*A*, normally closely apposed, have been pulled apart for demonstration, and the joint capsule has been inflated. Consequently the normally potential joint cavity is exaggerated. The *periosteum* investing the participating bones external to the joint blends with the fibrous layer of the joint capsule.

2. The articulating bones of **fibrous joints** are united by fibrous tissue. The amount of movement occurring at a fibrous joint depends in most cases on the length of the fibers uniting the articulating bones. The sutures of the cranium are examples of fibrous joints (Fig. I.16*B*). These bones are close together, either interlocking along a wavy line or overlapping. A **syndesmosis type** of fibrous joint unites the bones with a sheet of fibrous tissue, either a ligament or a fibrous membrane. Consequently, this type of joint is partially movable. The interosseous membrane in the forearm is a sheet of fibrous tissue that joins the radius and ulna in a syndesmosis. A **gomphosis** (socket), or **dentoalveolar syndesmosis,** is a fibrous joint in which a peg-like process fits into a socket articulation between the root of the tooth and the alveolar process of the jaw. Mobility of this joint (a loose tooth) indicates a pathological state affecting the supporting tissues of the tooth. However, microscopic movements here give us information (via the sense of proprioception) about how hard we are biting or clenching our teeth and whether we have a particle stuck between our teeth.

3. The articulating structures of **cartilaginous joints** are united by hyaline cartilage or fibrocartilage. In **primary cartilaginous joints,** or synchondroses, the bones are united by hyaline cartilage, which permits slight bending during early life. Primary cartilaginous joints are usually temporary unions, such as those present during the development of a long bone (Figs. I.14 and I.16*C*), where the bony epiphysis and the shaft are joined by an epiphysial plate. Primary cartilaginous joints permit growth in the length of a bone. When full growth is achieved, the epiphysial plate converts to bone and the epiphyses fuse with the diaphysis. **Secondary cartilaginous joints,** or symphyses, are strong, slightly movable joints united by fibrocartilage. The fibrocartilaginous *intervertebral discs* (Fig. I.16*C*) between the vertebrae consist of binding connective tissue that joins the vertebrae together. Cumulatively, these joints provide strength and shock absorption as well as considerable flexibility to the vertebral column (spine).

Synovial joints, the most common type of joint, provide free movement between the bones they join; they are joints of locomotion, typical of nearly all limb joints. Synovial joints are usually reinforced by *accessory ligaments* that are either separate (*extrinsic*) or are a thickening of a portion of the joint capsule (*intrinsic*). Some synovial joints have other distinguishing features, such as fibrocartilaginous *articular discs* or menisci, which are present when the articulating surfaces of the bones are incongruous.

The six major types of synovial joints are classified according to the shape of the articulating surfaces and/or the type of movement they permit (Fig. I.17):

1. **Plane joints** permit gliding or sliding movements in the plane of the articular surfaces. The opposed surfaces of the bones are flat or almost flat, with movement limited by their tight joint capsules. Plane joints are numerous and are nearly always small. An example is the *acromioclavicular joint* between the acromion of the scapula and the clavicle.

2. **Hinge joints** permit flexion and extension only, movements that occur in one plane (sagittal) around a single axis that runs transversely; thus hinge joints are *uniaxial joints.*

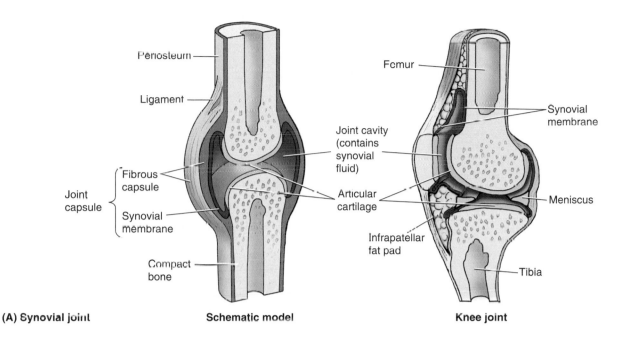

(A) Synovial joint   **Schematic model**   **Knee joint**

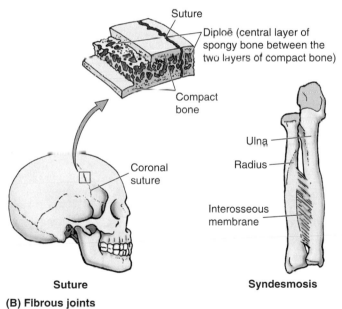

Suture   **Syndesmosis**

(B) Fibrous joints

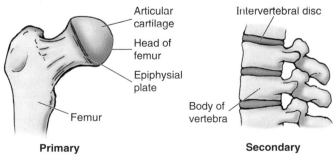

Primary   **Secondary**

(C) Cartilaginous joints

Figure I.16. Three classes of joints. Examples of each class are shown, as well as a model demonstrating the basic features of a synovial joint.

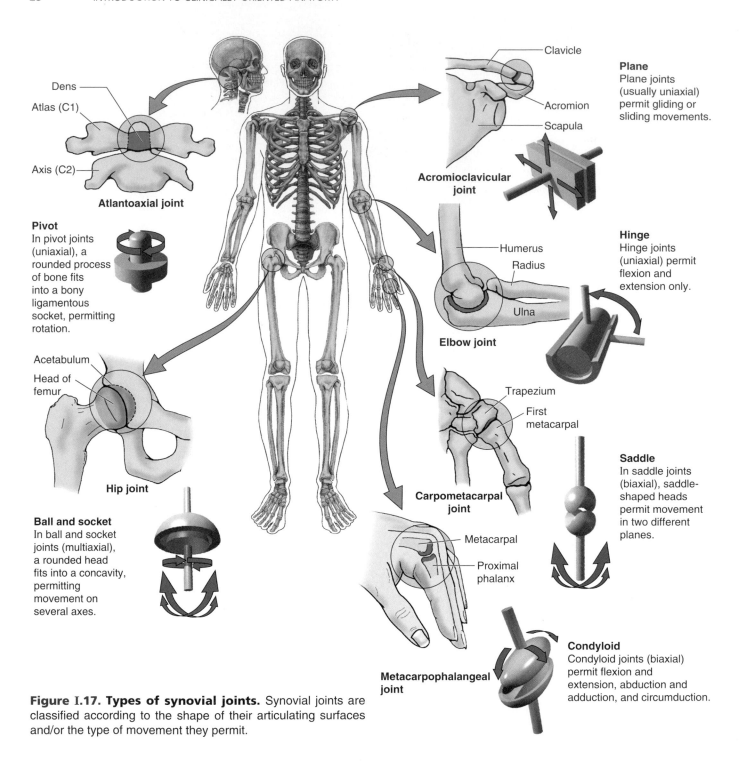

Figure I.17. Types of synovial joints. Synovial joints are classified according to the shape of their articulating surfaces and/or the type of movement they permit.

The joint capsule of these joints is thin and lax anteriorly and posteriorly where movement occurs; however, the bones are joined by strong, laterally placed collateral ligaments. An example is the *elbow joint.*

3. **Saddle joints** permit abduction and adduction as well as flexion and extension, movements occurring around two axes at right angles to each other; thus saddle joints are *biaxial joints* that allow movement in two planes, sagittal

and frontal. The performance of these movements in a circular sequence (circumduction) is also possible. The opposing articular surfaces are shaped like a saddle (i.e., they are reciprocally concave and convex). The *carpometacarpal joint* at the base of the 1st digit (thumb) is a saddle joint.

4. **Condyloid joints** permit flexion and extension as well as abduction and adduction; thus condyloid joints are also biaxial. However, movement in one plane (sagittal) is usually

greater (freer) than in the other. Circumduction, more restricted than that of saddle joints, is also possible. The *metacarpophalangeal joints* (knuckle joints) are examples.

5. **Ball and socket joints** allow movement in multiple axes and planes: flexion and extension, abduction and adduction, medial and lateral rotation, and circumduction; thus ball and socket joints are *multi-axial joints*. In these highly mobile joints, the spheroidal surface of one bone moves within the socket of another. An example is the *hip joint,* in which the spherical *head of the femur* rotates within the socket formed by the *acetabulum* of the hip bone.

6. **Pivot joints** permit rotation around a central axis; thus they are uniaxial. In these joints, a rounded process of bone rotates within a sleeve or ring. An example is the *central atlantoaxial joint,* in which the atlas (C1 vertebra) rotates around a finger-like process, the dens (odontoid process) of the axis (C2 vertebra) during rotation of the head.

Joint Vasculature and Innervation

Joints receive blood from *articular arteries* that arise from the vessels around the joint. The arteries often **anastomose** (communicate) to form networks (*periarticular arterial anasto-moses*) to ensure a blood supply to and across the joint in the various positions assumed by the joint. *Articular veins* are communicating veins that accompany arteries (L. *venae comitantes*) and, like the arteries, are located in the joint capsule, mostly in the synovial membrane.

Joints have a rich nerve supply; the nerve endings are in the joint capsule. In the distal parts of the limbs (hands and feet), the *articular nerves* are branches of the cutaneous nerves supplying the overlying skin. However, most articular nerves are branches of nerves that supply the muscles that cross and therefore move the joint. *Hilton's Law* states that the nerves supplying a joint also supply the muscles moving the joint or the skin covering their distal attachments.

Joints transmit a sensation called **proprioception,** which provides an awareness of movement and position of the parts of the body. The synovial membrane is relatively insensitive. Pain fibers are numerous in the fibrous layer and associated ligaments, causing considerable pain when the joint is injured. The sensory nerve endings respond to the twisting and stretching that occurs during sports activities such as basketball. People with arthritis will confirm that joints are well supplied with pain endings.

Joints of the Newborn Cranium

The bones of the *calvaria* (skullcap) of a newborn infant do not make full contact with each other (Fig. BI.5). At these sites, the sutures form wide areas of fibrous tissue called **fontanelles.** The *anterior fontanelle* is the most prominent; laypeople call it the baby's "soft spot." The fontanelles in a newborn are often felt as ridges because of the overlapping of the cranial bones by molding of the calvaria as it passes through the birth canal. Normally, the anterior fontanelle is flat. A bulging fontanelle may indicate increased intracranial pressure; however, the fontanelle normally bulges during crying. Pulsations of the fontanelle reflect the pulse. A depressed fontanelle may be observed when the baby is dehydrated (Swartz, 2001).

Degenerative Joint Disease

Synovial joints are well designed to withstand wear, but heavy use over several years can cause degenerative changes. Some destruction is inevitable during such activities as jogging, which wears away the articular cartilages and sometimes erodes the underlying articulating surfaces of the bones. The normal aging of articular cartilage begins early in adult life and progresses slowly thereafter, occurring on the ends of the articulating bones, particularly those of the hip, knee, vertebral column, and hands (Salter, 1998). These irreversible degenerative changes in joints result in the articular cartilage becoming less effective as a shock absorber and a lubricated surface. As a result, the articulation becomes increasingly vulnerable to the repeated friction that occurs during joint movements. In some people, these changes do not produce significant symptoms; in others, they cause considerable pain. ▶

Anterior fontanelle

Metopic suture

Internasal suture

Intermaxillary suture

Mandibular symphysis (intermandibular suture)

Figure BI.5.

Degenerative joint disease, **osteoarthritis,** is often accompanied by stiffness, discomfort, and pain. Osteoarthritis is common in older people and usually affects joints that support the weight of their bodies (e.g., the hips and knees). Most substances in the bloodstream, normal or pathological, easily enter the joint cavity. Similarly, traumatic infection of a joint may be followed by *arthritis,* inflammation of a joint, and *septicemia,* blood poisoning.

Arthroscopy

The cavity of a synovial joint can be examined by inserting a cannula and an arthroscope (a small telescope) into it. This surgical procedure—**arthroscopy**—enables an orthopedic surgeon to examine joints for abnormalities, such as torn articular discs. Some surgical procedures can also be performed during arthroscopy (e.g., by inserting instruments through small puncture incisions). Because the opening in the joint capsule for inserting the arthroscope is small, healing is more rapid after this procedure than after traditional joint surgery. ✪

THE BOTTOM LINE: A joint is a union between two or more bones or rigid parts of the skeleton. Three general types of joints are recognized: fibrous, cartilaginous, and synovial. Synovial joints are the most common type and can be classified into plane, hinge, saddle, condyloid, ball and socket, and pivot. Joints receive their blood supply from articular arteries that often form networks. Articular veins are usually located in the synovial membrane. Joints are richly innervated and transmit the sensation of proprioception, an awareness of movement and position of parts of the body.

Muscle Tissue and the Muscular System

The muscular system consists of all the muscles of the body. Although the muscles of the muscular system are all composed of one specific type of muscle tissue, other types of muscle tissue form important components of the organs of other systems, including the cardiovascular, digestive, genitourinary, and integumentary systems.

Types of Muscle (Muscle Tissue)

Muscle cells, often called *muscle fibers* because they are long and narrow when relaxed, are specialized contractile cells. They are organized into tissues that move body parts or temporarily alter the shape (reduce the circumference of all or part) of internal organs. Associated connective tissue conveys nerve fibers and capillaries to the muscle cells as it binds them

into bundles or fascicles. Three types of muscle are described based on distinct characteristics relating to:

- Whether it is normally willfully controlled (*voluntary* vs. *involuntary*).
- Whether it appears striped or unstriped when viewed under a microscope (*striated* vs. *smooth* or *unstriated*).
- Whether it is located in the body wall and limbs or makes up the hollow organs (*viscera*) of the body cavities or blood vessels (*somatic* vs. *visceral*).

As explained in "Nervous System" (later in this chapter), somatic muscle and visceral muscle are also distinct in regard to their innervation.

The three muscle types are (Table I.1) as follows:

- **Skeletal striated muscle** is voluntary somatic muscle that makes up the gross *skeletal muscles* that compose the muscular system, moving or stabilizing bones and other structures (e.g., the eyeballs).
- **Cardiac striated muscle** is involuntary visceral muscle that forms most of the walls of the heart and adjacent parts of the great vessels, such as the aorta, and pumps blood.
- **Smooth muscle** (unstriated or unstriped muscle) is involuntary visceral muscle that forms part of the walls of most vessels and hollow organs (viscera), moving substances through them by coordinated sequential contractions (pulsations or peristaltic contractions).

Skeletal Muscles

Form, Features, and the Naming of Muscles

All skeletal muscles, commonly referred to simply as "muscles," have fleshy, reddish, contractile portions (one or more heads or bellies) composed of skeletal striated muscle. Some muscles are fleshy throughout, but most also have white noncontractile portions (tendons), composed mainly of organized collagen bundles, that provide a means of attachment (Fig. I.18A). When referring to the length of a muscle, both the belly and the tendons are included. In other words, a muscle's length is the distance between its attachments. Most skeletal muscles are attached directly or indirectly to bones, cartilages, ligaments, or fascias or to some combination of these structures. Some muscles are attached to organs (the eyeball, for example), skin (such as facial muscles), and mucous membranes (intrinsic tongue muscles). Muscles are organs of locomotion (movement), but they also provide static support, give form to the body, and provide heat.

Figure I.19 identifies the skeletal muscles that lie most superficially. The deep muscles are identified when each region is studied.

The architecture and shape of muscles vary (Fig. I.18*B*). The tendons of some muscles form flat sheets, or **aponeuroses,** that anchor the muscle to the skeleton (usually a ridge or a series of spinous processes) and/or to deep fascia (such as

Table I.1. Types of Muscle

Muscle Type		Location	Appearance of Cells	Type of Activity	Stimulation
Skeletal striated muscle — Striation, Muscle fiber, Nucleus		Composes gross, named muscles (e.g., biceps of arm) attached to skeleton and fascia of limbs, body wall, and head/neck	Large, very long, unbranched, cylindrical fibers with transverse striations (stripes) arranged in parallel bundles; multiple, peripherally located nuclei	Strong, quick intermittent (phasic) contraction above a baseline tonus; acts primarily to produce movement or resist gravity	Voluntary (or reflexive) by somatic nervous system
Cardiac striated muscle — Nucleus, Intercalated disc, Striation, Muscle fiber		Muscle of heart (myocardium) and adjacent portions of great vessels (aorta, vena cava)	Branching and anastomosing shorter fibers with transverse striations (stripes) running parallel and connected end to end by complex junctions (intercalated discs), single, central nucleus	Strong, quick, continuous rhythmic contraction; acts to pump blood from heart	Involuntary; intrinsically (myogenically) stimulated and propagated; rate and strength of contraction modified by autonomic nervous system
Smooth (unstriated or unstriped) muscle — Smooth muscle fiber, Nucleus		Walls of hollow viscera and blood vessels, iris, and ciliary body of eye; attached to hair follicles of skin (arrector muscle of hair)	Single or agglomerated small, spindle-shaped fibers without striations; single, central nucleus	Weak, slow, rhythmic, or sustained tonic contraction; acts mainly to propel substances (peristalsis) and to restrict flow (vasoconstriction and sphincteric activity)	Involuntary by autonomic nervous system

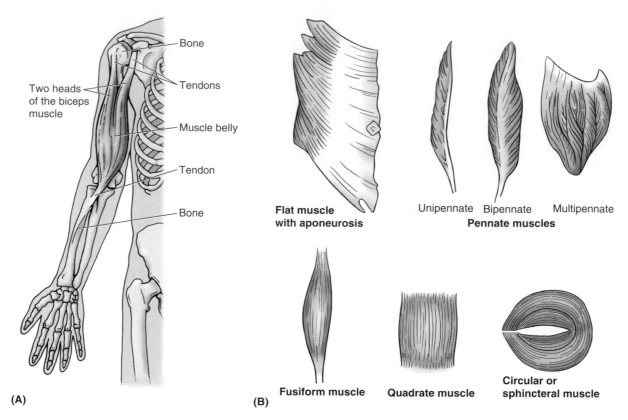

Figure I.18. Skeletal muscles. A. The belly is the fleshy contractile part of a muscle. This muscle has a belly with two heads; tendons provide attachment to bone at both ends. **B.** The architecture and shape of a skeletal muscle depend on the arrangement of its fibers.

the latissimus dorsi muscle), or to the aponeurosis of another muscle (such as the oblique muscles of the anterolateral abdominal wall) (Fig. I.19). Most muscles are named on the basis of their function or the bones to which they are attached. The abductor digiti minimi muscle, for example, abducts the little finger. The sternocleidomastoid muscle (G., *kleidos*, bolt or bar, clavicle) attaches inferiorly to the sternum and clavicle and superiorly to the mastoid process of the temporal bone of the cranium. Other muscles are named on the basis of their position (medial, lateral, anterior, posterior) or length (brevis, short; longus, long). Muscles may be described or classified according to their shape, for which a muscle may also be named (Figs. I.18 and I.19):

- **Flat muscles** have parallel fibers often with an aponeurosis—for example, external oblique.

- **Pennate muscles** are feather-like (L. *pennatus*, feather) in the arrangement of their fascicles, and may be unipennate, bipennate, or multi-pennate—for example, extensor digitorum longus (unipennate), bellies of the gastrocnemius (bipennate), and deltoid (multi-pennate).

- **Fusiform muscles** are spindle shaped with a round, thick belly (or bellies) and tapered ends—for example, biceps brachii.

- **Quadrate muscles** have four equal sides (L. *quadratus*, square)—for example, pronator quadratus.

- **Circular** or **sphincteral muscles** surround a body opening or orifice, constricting it when contracted—for example, orbicularis oris (closes the mouth).

- **Multi-headed** or **multi-bellied muscles** have more than one head of attachment or more than one contractile belly, respectively—for examples, biceps muscles (biceps brachii) have two heads of attachment, triceps muscles have three heads (triceps brachii), and the digastric and gastrocnemius muscles have two bellies (those of the former are tandem; those of the latter, parallel).

Contraction of Muscles

Skeletal muscles function by contracting; they pull and never push. However, certain phenomena—such as "popping of the ears" to equalize air pressure and the musculovenous pump (p. 43)—take advantage of the expansion of muscle bellies during contraction. When a muscle contracts and shortens, one of its attachments usually remains fixed while the other (more mobile) attachment is pulled toward it, often resulting in movement. Attachments of muscles are commonly described as the origin and insertion; the *origin* is usually the proximal end of the muscle, which remains fixed during muscular contraction, and the *insertion* is usually the distal end of the muscle, which is movable. However, this is not always the case. Some muscles can act in both directions under different circumstances. For example, when doing

Frontal belly of occipitofrontalis
Orbicularis oculi
Orbicularis oris
Zygomaticus major
Sternocleidomastoid
Infrahyoid ("strap") muscles
Trapezius
Deltoid
Pectoralis major
Biceps brachii
Serratus anterior
Rectus abdominis
External oblique
Brachioradialis
Flexor muscles of forearm
Flexor retinaculum
Iliacus and psoas major (iliopsoas)
Thenar muscles
Long flexor tendons
Hypothenar muscles
Fibrous tendinous sheaths of digits
Pectineus
Adductor longus
Sartorius
Rectus femoris
Vastus medialis
Vastus lateralis
Fibularis longus
Tibialis anterior
Extensor digitorum longus
Extensor hallucis longus
Extensor retinaculum (inferior)

Anterior

Figure I.19. Superficial skeletal muscles. Most of these muscles move the skeleton, but some muscles move other parts (e.g., the eyeballs and scalp). The sheath of the left rectus abdominis has been opened to reveal the muscle. The orbicularis oris encircles the mouth and plays important roles in controlling entrance and exit, chewing, speech, and facial expression.

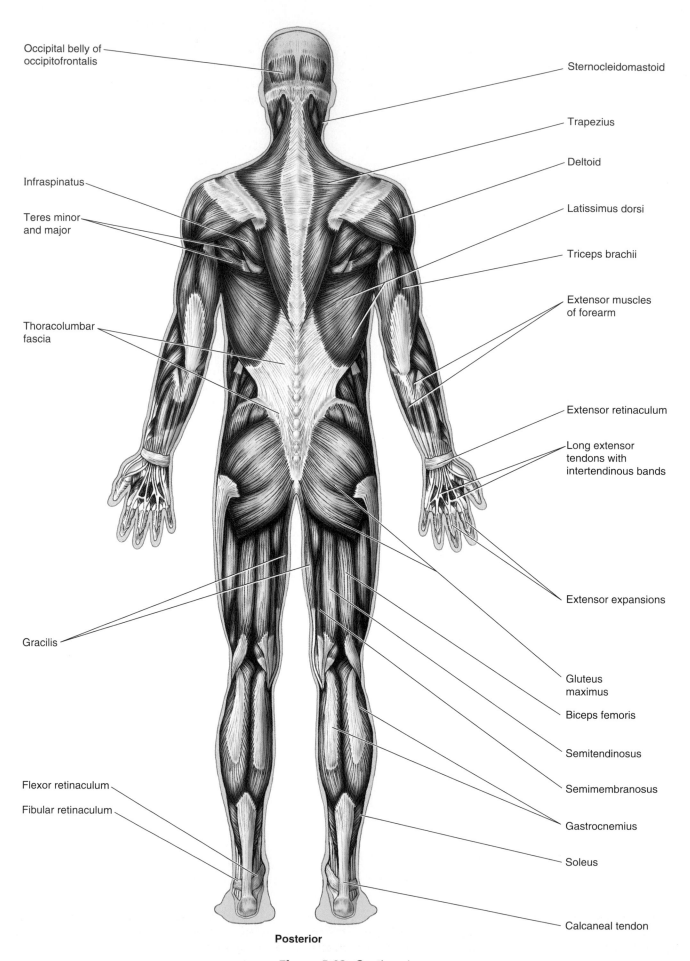

Occipital belly of occipitofrontalis

Sternocleidomastoid

Infraspinatus

Teres minor and major

Trapezius

Deltoid

Latissimus dorsi

Triceps brachii

Extensor muscles of forearm

Thoracolumbar fascia

Extensor retinaculum

Long extensor tendons with intertendinous bands

Gracilis

Extensor expansions

Gluteus maximus

Biceps femoris

Semitendinosus

Semimembranosus

Flexor retinaculum

Fibular retinaculum

Gastrocnemius

Soleus

Calcaneal tendon

Posterior

Figure I.19. *Continued*

push-ups, the distal end of the upper limb (the hand) is fixed (on the floor) and the proximal end of the limb and the trunk are being moved. Therefore, this book usually uses the terms *proximal* and *distal* or *medial* and *lateral* when describing most muscle attachments. Note that if the attachments of a muscle are known, the action of the muscle can usually be deduced (rather than memorized). When studying muscle attachments, act out the action; you are more likely to learn things you have experienced.

Reflexive Contraction. Although skeletal muscles are also referred to as voluntary muscles, certain aspects of their activity are automatic (reflexive) and therefore not voluntarily controlled. Examples are the respiratory movements of the diaphragm, controlled most of the time by reflexes stimulated by the levels of oxygen and carbon dioxide in the blood (although we can willfully control it within limits), and the *myotatic reflex*, which results in movement after a muscle stretch produced by tapping a tendon with a reflex hammer.

Tonic Contraction. Even when "relaxed" the muscles of a conscious individual are almost always slightly contracted. This slight contraction, called *muscle tone* (**tonus**), does not produce movement or active resistance (as *phasic contraction* does) but gives the muscle a certain firmness, assisting the stability of joints and the maintenance of posture, while keeping the muscle ready to respond to appropriate stimuli. Muscle tone is usually absent only when unconscious (as during deep sleep or under general anesthesia) or after a nerve lesion resulting in paralysis.

Phasic Contraction. There are two main types of **phasic (active) muscle contractions**: *isotonic contractions*, in which

the muscle changes length in relationship to the production of movement, and *isometric contractions*, in which muscle length remains the same—no movement occurs, but the force (muscle tension) is increased above tonic levels (Fig. I.20). The latter type of contraction is important in maintaining upright posture and when muscles act as fixators or shunt muscles.

There are two types of isotonic contractions. The type we most commonly think of is *concentric contraction*, in which movement occurs as a result of the muscle shortening—for example, when lifting a cup, pushing a door, or striking a blow. The ability to apply exceptional force by means of concentric contraction often is what distinguishes an athlete from an amateur. The other type is *eccentric contraction*, in which a contracting muscle lengthens—that is, it undergoes a controlled and gradual relaxation while continually exerting a (diminishing) force, like playing out a rope. While not as familiar, eccentric contractions are as important as concentric contractions for coordinated, functional movements such as walking, running, and setting objects (or one's self) down.

Often, when the main muscle of a particular movement (the *prime mover*) is undergoing a concentric contraction, its antagonist is undergoing a coordinated eccentric contraction. In walking, we contract concentrically to pull our center of gravity forward and then, as it passes ahead of the limb, we contract eccentrically to prevent a lurching during the transfer of weight to the other limb. Eccentric contractions require less metabolic energy at the same load but, with a maximal contraction, are capable of generating much higher tension levels than concentric contractions—as much as 50% higher (Marieb, 2004).

(A)

Deltoid holds arm in abduction

Isometric

Concentric

Deltoid shortens to raise arm in abduction

Eccentric

Deltoid lengthens to lower arm in adduction

(B)

Isometric

Concentric

Eccentric

Hamstrings hold thigh in flexion

Hamstrings shorten to raise thigh in extention

Hamstrings lengthen to lower thigh in flexion

Figure I.20. Isometric and isotonic contractions. Isometric contraction sustains the position of a joint without producing movement. Concentric and eccentric contractions are isotonic contractions in which the muscle changes length: concentric contractions by shortening, and eccentric contractions by actively controlled lengthening (relaxation).

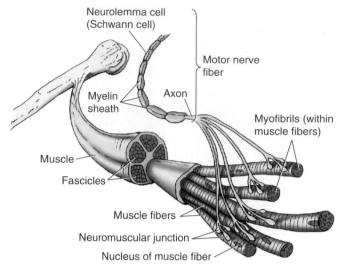

Figure I.21. Motor unit. A motor unit consists of a single motor neuron and the muscle fibers innervated by it.

Whereas the **structural unit** of a muscle is a skeletal striated muscle fiber, the **functional unit** of a muscle is a **motor unit**, consisting of a motor neuron and the muscle fibers it controls (Fig. I.21). When a *motor neuron* in the spinal cord is stimulated, it initiates an impulse that causes all the muscle fibers supplied by that motor unit to contract simultaneously. The number of muscle fibers in a motor unit varies from one to several hundred. The number of fibers varies according to the size and function of the muscle. Large motor units, in which one neuron supplies several hundred muscle fibers, are in the large trunk and thigh muscles. In the small eye and hand muscles, where precision movements are required, the motor units include only a few muscle fibers. Movement (phasic contraction) results from the activation of an increasing number of motor units, above the level required to maintain tonus.

Functions of Muscles

Muscles serve specific functions in moving and positioning the body.

- A **prime mover** or **agonist** is the main muscle responsible for producing a specific movement of the body. It contracts concentrically to produce the desired movement, doing most of the work (expending most of the energy) required. In most movements, there is a single prime mover, but some movements involve two prime movers working in equal measure.

- **Fixators** steady proximal parts of a limb through isometric contraction while movements are occurring in distal parts.

- A **synergist** complements the action of a prime mover. It may directly assist a prime mover, providing a weaker or less mechanically advantaged component of the same movement, or it may assist indirectly, by serving as a fixator of an intervening joint when a prime mover passes over more than one joint, for example. It is not unusual to have several synergists assisting a prime mover in a particular movement.

- An **antagonist** is a muscle that opposes the action of another muscle. A primary antagonist directly opposes the prime mover, but synergists may also be opposed by secondary antagonists. As the active movers concentrically contract to produce a movement, antagonists eccentrically contract, relaxing progressively in coordination to produce a smooth movement.

The same muscle may act as a prime mover, antagonist, synergist, or fixator under different conditions. Note also that the actual prime mover in a given position may be gravity. In such cases, a paradoxical situation may exist in which the prime mover usually described as being responsible for the movement is inactive (passive), while the controlled relaxation (eccentric contraction) of the antigravity antagonist(s) is the active (energy requiring) component in the movement. An example is lowering (adducting) the upper limbs from the abducted position (stretched out laterally at 90° to the trunk) when standing erect. The prime mover (adductor) is gravity; the muscles described as the prime movers for this movement (pectoralis major and latissimus dorsi) are inactive or passive; and the muscle being actively innervated (contracting eccentrically) is the deltoid (an abductor, typically described as the antagonist for this movement).

A muscle whose pull is exerted along a line that parallels the axis of the bones to which it is attached (e.g., the brachioradialis) is at a disadvantage for producing movement. Instead it acts to maintain contact between the articular surfaces of the joint it crosses (i.e., it resists dislocating forces); this type of muscle is a **shunt muscle**. The more oblique a muscle's line of pull is oriented to the bone it moves (i.e., the *less* parallel the line of pull is to the long axis of the bone, e.g., the biceps brachii during flexion of the elbow), the more capable it is of rapid and effective movement; this type of muscle is a **spurt muscle.**

Nerves and Arteries to Muscles

Variation in the nerve supply of muscles is rare; it is a nearly constant relationship. In the limb, muscles of similar actions are generally contained within a *common fascial compartment* and share innervation by the same nerves; therefore, you should learn the innervation of limb muscles in terms of the functional groups, making it necessary to memorize only the exceptions. Nerves supplying skeletal muscles (**motor nerves**) usually enter the fleshy portion of the muscle (vs. the tendon), almost always from the deep aspect (so it is protected by the muscle it supplies). The few exceptions will be pointed out in the text. When a nerve pierces a muscle, by passing through its fleshy portion or between two heads of attachment, it usually supplies that muscle. Exceptions are the cutaneous branches of posterior (dorsal) rami and the superficial muscles of the back.

The blood supply of muscles is not as constant as the nerve supply and is usually multiple. Arteries generally supply the structures they contact. Thus you should learn the course of the arteries and deduce that a muscle is supplied by all the arteries in its vicinity.

Muscle Dysfunction and Paralysis

From the clinical perspective, it is important not only to think in terms of the action normally produced by a given muscle but also to consider what loss of function would occur if the muscle failed to function (paralysis). How would the dysfunction of a given muscle or muscle group be manifest (i.e., what are the visible signs)?

Absence of Muscle Tone

Although a gentle force, muscle tone can have important effects; the tonus of muscles in the lips helps keep the teeth aligned, for instance. When this gentle but constant pressure is absent (owing to paralysis or a short lip that leaves the teeth exposed), teeth migrate, becoming everted ("buck teeth").

The absence of muscle tone in an unconscious patient (e.g., under a general anesthetic) may allow joints to be dislocated as he or she is being lifted or positioned. When a muscle is denervated (loses its nerve supply) it becomes *paralyzed* (flaccid, lacking both its tonus and its ability to contract phasically on demand or reflexively). In the absence of a muscle's normal tonus, that of opposing (*antagonist*) muscle(s) may cause a limb to assume an abnormal resting position. In addition, the denervated muscle will become fibrotic and lose its elasticity, also contributing to the abnormal position at rest.

Muscle Soreness and "Pulled" Muscles

Because eccentric contractions are capable of generating higher tension levels, eccentric contractions that are either excessive or associated with a novel task are often the cause of delayed-onset *muscle soreness.* Thus walking down many flights of stairs would actually result in more soreness, owing to the eccentric contractions, than walking up the same flights of stairs. The muscle stretching that occurs during the lengthening type of eccentric contraction appears to be more likely to produce microtears in the muscles and/or periosteal irritation than that associated with a shortening (concentric) contraction.

Skeletal muscles are limited in their ability to lengthen. Usually muscles cannot elongate beyond one third of their resting length without sustaining damage. This is reflected in their attachments to the skeleton, which usually do not permit excessive lengthening. An exception is the hamstring muscles of the posterior thigh. When the knee is extended, the hamstrings typically reach their maximum length before the hip is fully flexed (i.e., flexion at the hip is limited by the hamstring's ability to elongate). Undoubtedly this, as well as forces related to their eccentric contraction, explains why hamstrings muscles are "pulled" (sustain tears) more commonly than other muscles (Fig. BI.6).

Hamstrings tendon (torn and pulled from tuberosity)

Ischial tuberosity

Figure BI.6.

Growth and Regeneration of Skeletal Muscle

Skeletal striated muscle fibers cannot divide, but they can be replaced individually by new muscle fibers derived from *satellite cells of skeletal muscle.* Located inside the basement membranes of the muscle fibers, these satellite cells represent a potential source of *myoblasts,* precursors of muscle cells, which are capable of fusing with each other to form new skeletal muscle fibers if required (Cormack, 2001). The number of new fibers that can be produced is insufficient to compensate for major muscle degeneration or trauma. Instead of becoming regenerated effectively, the new skeletal muscle is composed of a disorganized mixture of muscle fibers and fibrous scar tissue. Skeletal muscles are able to grow larger in response to frequent strenuous exercise, such as body building. This growth results from *hypertrophy of existing fibers,* not from the addition of new muscle fibers. Hypertrophy lengthens and increases the *myofibrils* within the muscle fibers (Fig. I.21), thereby increasing the amount of work the muscle can perform.

Muscle Testing

Muscle testing helps an examiner diagnose nerve injuries. There are two common testing methods:

- The person performs movements that resist those of the examiner. For example, the person keeps the ▶

forearm flexed while the examiner attempts to extend it. This technique enables the examiner to gauge the power of the person's movements.

- The examiner performs movements that resist those of the person. When testing flexion of the forearm, the examiner asks the person to flex his or her forearm while the examiner resists the efforts. Usually muscles are tested in bilateral pairs for comparison.

Electromyography (EMG), the electrical stimulation of muscles, is another method for testing muscle action. The examiner places surface electrodes over a muscle, asks the person to perform certain movements, and then amplifies and records the differences in electrical action potentials of the muscles. A normal resting muscle shows only a baseline activity (tonus), which disappears only during deep sleep, paralysis, and when under anesthesia. Contracting muscles demonstrate variable peaks of phasic activity. EMG makes it possible to analyze the activity of an individual muscle during different movements. EMG may also be part of the treatment program for restoring the action of muscles. ✚

THE BOTTOM LINE: Muscles are categorized as skeletal striated, cardiac striated, or smooth. Skeletal muscles are further classified according to their shape as flat, pennate, fusiform, quadrate, circular or sphincteral, and multi-headed or multi-bellied. Skeletal muscle functions by contracting, enabling automatic (reflexive) movements, maintaining muscle tone (tonic contraction), and providing for phasic (active) contraction with (isotonic) or without (isometric) change in muscle length. Isotonic movements are either concentric (producing movement by shortening) or eccentric (allowing movement by controlled relaxation). Prime movers or agonists are the muscles primarily responsible for particular movements. Fixators "fix" a part of a limb while another part of the limb is moving. Synergists augment the action of prime movers. Antagonists oppose the actions of another muscle.

Cardiac Striated Muscle

Cardiac striated muscle forms the muscular wall of the heart, the **myocardium.** Some cardiac muscle is also present in the walls of the aorta, pulmonary vein, and superior vena cava (SVC). Cardiac striated muscle contractions are not under voluntary control. Heart rate is regulated intrinsically by a *pacemaker,* an impulse-conducting system composed of specialized cardiac muscle fibers; they in turn are influenced by the autonomic nervous system (ANS) (discussed later in this chapter). Cardiac striated muscle has a distinctly striped ap-

pearance under microscopy (Table I.1). Both types of striated muscle—skeletal and cardiac—are further characterized by the immediacy, rapidity, and strength of their contractions. *Note:* Even though the trait applies to both skeletal and cardiac striated muscle, in common use the terms *striated* and *striped* are used to designate voluntary skeletal striated muscle.

Cardiac muscle is distinct from skeletal muscle in both behavior and appearance. Unlike striated skeletal muscle fibers, cardiac muscle fibers:

- Contract spontaneously (without extrinsic stimuli) and rhythmically.

- Bifurcate (split or branch).

- Are traversed at intervals by intercalated discs (disks)—unique, specialized end-to-end junctions—where they are linked into a chain or mesh with other bifurcating cardiac muscle fibers.

To support its continuous level of high activity, the blood supply to cardiac muscle is twice as rich as that to skeletal muscle.

Smooth Muscle

Smooth muscle, named for the absence of striations in the appearance of the muscle fibers under microscopy, forms a large part of the middle coat or layer (*tunica media*) of the walls of blood vessels (above the capillary level) (Fig. I.23 and Table I.1). Consequently, it occurs in all vascularized tissue. It also makes up the muscular part of the walls of the digestive tract and ducts. Smooth muscle is found in skin, composing the arrector muscle of hair associated with hair follicles (Fig. I.6), and in the eyeball, where it controls lens thickness and pupil size.

Like cardiac striated muscle, smooth muscle is *involuntary muscle;* however, it is directly innervated by the ANS. Its contraction can also be initiated by hormonal stimulation or by local stimuli, such as stretching. Smooth muscle responds more slowly than striated muscle and with a delayed and more leisurely contraction. It can undergo partial contraction for long periods and has a much greater ability than striated muscle to elongate without suffering paralyzing injury. Both of these factors are important in regulating the size of sphincters and the caliber of the *lumina* (interior spaces) of tubular structures. In the walls of the digestive tract, uterine tubes, and ureters, smooth muscle cells are responsible for peristalsis, rhythmic contractions that propel the contents along these tubular structures.

Hypertrophy of the Myocardium and Myocardial Infarction

In *compensatory hypertrophy,* the myocardium responds to increased demands by increasing the size of its fibers. When cardiac striated muscle fibers are damaged by loss of their blood supply during a heart attack, the tissue ▶

becomes necrotic (dies) and the fibrous scar tissue that develops forms a *myocardial infarct* (MI), an area of *myocardial necrosis* (pathological death of cardiac tissue). Muscle cells that degenerate are not replaced, because cardiac muscle cells do not divide. Furthermore, there is no equivalent to the satellite cells of skeletal muscle that can produce new cardiac muscle fibers.

Hypertrophy and Hyperplasia of Smooth Muscle

Smooth muscle cells undergo compensatory hypertrophy in response to increased demands. Smooth muscle cells in the uterine wall during pregnancy increase not only in size but also in number (*hyperplasia*) because these cells retain the capacity for cell division. In addition, new smooth muscle cells can develop from incompletely differentiated cells (*pericytes*) that are located along small blood vessels (Cormack, 2001; Gartner and Hiatt, 2001). ○

THE BOTTOM LINE: Cardiac muscle is a striated muscle type found in the walls of the heart, or myocardium, as well as in some major blood vessels. Contraction of cardiac muscle is not under voluntary control but is instead activated by specialized cardiac muscle fibers forming the pacemaker, the activity of which is regulated by the autonomic nervous system. Smooth muscle does not have striations. It occurs in all vascular tissues and in the walls of the digestive tract and other organs. Smooth muscle is directly innervated by the autonomic nervous system and thus is not under voluntary control.

Cardiovascular System

The circulatory system transports fluids throughout the body; it consists of the cardiovascular and lymphatic systems. The heart and blood vessels make up the blood transportation network, the cardiovascular system (Fig. I.22). Through this system, the heart pumps blood through the body's vast system of blood vessels. The blood carries nutrients, oxygen, and waste products to and from the cells. There are three types of blood vessels: *arteries, veins,* and *capillaries.* Blood under high pressure leaves the heart and is distributed to the body by a branching system of thick-walled arteries. The final distributing vessels, *arterioles,* deliver oxygenated blood to capillaries. Capillaries form a *capillary bed,* where the interchange of oxygen, nutrients, waste products, and other substances with the extracellular fluid occurs. Blood from the capillary bed passes into thin-walled *venules,* which resemble wide capillaries.

Venules drain into small veins that open into larger veins. The largest veins, the superior and inferior venae cavae, return poorly oxygenated blood to the heart.

Most vessels of the circulatory system have three coats, or tunics (Fig. I.23):

- **Tunica intima,** an inner lining consisting of a single layer of extremely flattened epithelial cells, the *endothelium,* supported by delicate connective tissue. Capillaries consist only of this tunic, with blood capillaries also having a supporting basement membrane.

- **Tunica media,** a middle layer consisting primarily of smooth muscle.

- **Tunica adventitia,** an outer connective tissue layer or sheath.

The tunica media is the most variable. Arteries, veins, and lymphatic ducts are distinguished by the thickness of this layer relative to the size of the lumen, its organization, and, in the case of arteries, the presence of variable amounts of elastic fibers.

Arteries

Arteries carry blood from the heart and distribute it to the body. The blood passes through arteries of decreasing caliber. The different types of arteries are distinguished from each other on the basis of overall size, relative amounts of elastic tissue or muscle in the tunica media, the thickness of the wall relative to the lumen, and function. Artery size and type is a continuum—that is, there is a gradual change in morphological characteristics from one type to another. There are three types of arteries:

- Large elastic arteries (**conducting arteries**) have many elastic layers (sheets of elastic fibers) in their walls. These large arteries initially receive the cardiac output. Their elasticity enables them to expand when the heart contracts (when they receive the cardiac output), minimizing the pressure change, and return to normal size between cardiac contractions, pushing the blood into the medium arteries downstream. This maintains the blood pressure in the arterial system between cardiac contractions (at a time when ventricular pressure falls to zero). Overall, this minimizes the ebb in blood pressure as the heart contracts and relaxes. Examples of large elastic arteries are the aorta, the arteries that originate from the arch of the aorta (brachiocephalic, subclavian, and carotids arteries), and the pulmonary trunk and arteries.

- Medium muscular arteries (**distributing arteries**) have walls that consist chiefly of circularly disposed smooth muscle fibers. Their ability to decrease their diameter (vasoconstrict) regulates the flow of blood to different parts of the body as required by circumstance (e.g., activity, thermoregulation). Pulsatile contractions of their muscular walls (regardless of current diameter) temporarily

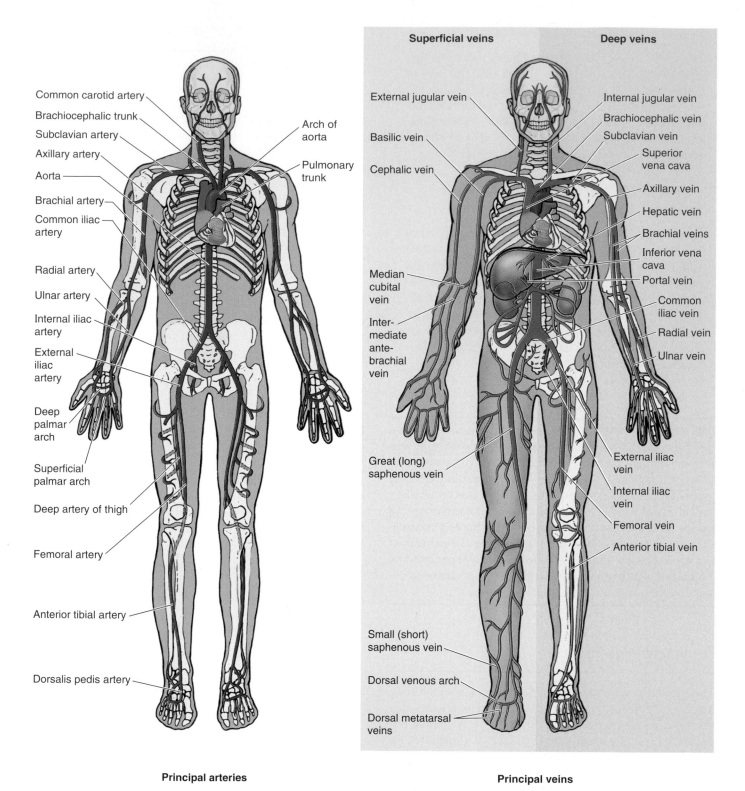

Principal arteries

Principal veins

Figure I.22. Cardiovascular system. Most arteries carry oxygenated blood away from the heart and most veins carry deoxygenated blood to the heart; however, the pulmonary arteries arising from the pulmonary trunk carry deoxygenated blood to the lungs, and the pulmonary veins carry oxygenated blood from the lungs to the heart. Although commonly depicted as a single vessel, as shown here, the deep veins of the limbs usually occur as a pair of accompanying veins (L. *venae comitantes*).

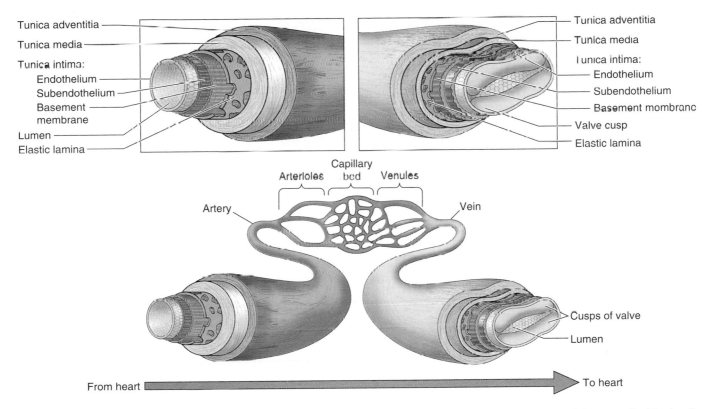

Figure I.23. Blood vessel structure. The walls of most blood vessels have three concentric layers of tissue, called tunics (L. *tunicae,* coats). With less muscle, veins are thinner walled than their companion arteries and have wide lumens (L. *luminae*) that usually appear flattened in tissue sections. Most medium veins that return blood to the heart against gravity (e.g., leg veins) have valves that break up the columns of blood and, if healthy, allow blood to flow only toward the heart.

and rhythmically constrict their lumina in progressive sequence, propelling and distributing blood to various parts of the body. Most of the named arteries, including those observed in the body wall and limbs during dissection such as the brachial or femoral arteries, are medium muscular arteries.

- **Small arteries and arterioles** have relatively narrow lumina and thick muscular walls. The degree of filling of the capillary beds and level of arterial pressure within the vascular system are regulated mainly by the degree of tonus (firmness) in the smooth muscle of the arteriolar walls. If the tonus is above normal, *hypertension* (high blood pressure) results. The small arteries are usually not named or specifically identified during dissection, and arterioles can be observed only under magnification.

Anastomoses (communications) between the multiple branches of an artery provide numerous potential detours for blood flow in case the usual pathway is obstructed by compression, the position of a joint, pathology, or surgical ligation. If a main channel is occluded, the smaller alternate channels can usually increase in size in a relatively short time, providing a *collateral circulation* that ensures the blood supply to structures distal to the blockage. However, collateral pathways require time to open adequately; they are usually insufficient to compensate for sudden occlusion or ligation. There are areas, however, where collateral circulation does not exist, or is inadequate to replace the main channel. Arteries that do not anastomose with adjacent arteries are anatomical or true terminal or end arteries. Occlusion of an end artery interrupts the blood supply to the structure or segment of an organ it supplies. True terminal arteries supply the retina, for example, where occlusion will result in blindness. While not true terminal arteries, *functional terminal arteries* (arteries with ineffectual anastomoses) supply segments of the brain, liver, kidneys, spleen, and intestines; they may also exist in the heart.

Arteriosclerosis: Ischemia and Infarction

The most common acquired disease of arteries—and a common finding in cadaver dissection—in developed countries is **arteriosclerosis** (hardening of the arteries), a group of diseases characterized by thickening and loss of elasticity of the arterial walls. A common form, *atherosclerosis,* is associated with the buildup of fat ▶

(mainly cholesterol) in the arterial walls. A calcium deposit forms an atheromatous plaque (*atheroma*)—well-demarcated, hardened yellow areas or swellings on the intimal surfaces of arteries (Fig. BI.7*A*). The consequent arterial narrowing and surface irregularity may result in *thrombosis* (local intravascular clotting), which may occlude the artery or be flushed into the bloodstream (forming a *thrombus*) and block smaller vessels distally (Fig. BI.7*B*). The consequences of atherosclerosis include *ischemia* (reduction of the blood supply to an organ or region) and *infarction* (local death, or necrosis, of an area of tissue or an organ resulting from the reduced blood supply). These consequences are particularly significant in regard to the heart (*ischemic heart disease* and *myocardial infarction* or heart attack), brain (*stroke*), and distal parts of limbs (*gangrene*). ☻

Figure BI.7.

Veins

Veins generally return deoxygenated (venous) blood from the capillary beds to the heart, which gives the veins a dark blue appearance. The large pulmonary veins are atypical in that they carry well-oxygenated blood (commonly called "arterial blood") from the lungs to the heart. Because of the lower blood pressure in the venous system, the walls (specifically, the tunica media) of veins are thinner than those of their companion arteries (Fig. I.23). Normally, veins do not pulsate and do not squirt or spurt blood when severed. There are three sizes of veins:

- **Venules** are the smallest veins. Venules drain capillary beds and join similar vessels to form small veins. Magnification is required to observe venules. Small veins are the tributaries of larger veins that unite to form *venous plexuses*, such as the posterior venous arch of the foot (Fig. I.22). Small veins are unnamed.

- **Medium veins** drain venous plexuses and accompany medium arteries. In the limbs, and in some other locations where the flow of blood is opposed by the pull of gravity, the medium veins have *flap valves* that permit blood to

flow toward the heart but not in the reverse direction. Examples of medium veins include the named superficial veins (cephalic and basilic veins of the upper limb and great and small saphenous veins of the lower limb) and the accompanying veins that are named according to the artery they accompany.

- **Large veins** are characterized by wide bundles of longitudinal smooth muscle and a well-developed tunica adventitia. An example is the superior vena cava.

Veins are more abundant than arteries. Although their walls are thinner, their diameters are usually larger than those of the corresponding artery. The thin walls allow veins to have a large capacity for expansion, and do so when blood return to the heart is impeded by compression or internal pressures (e.g., after taking a large breath and holding it; this is the *Valsalva maneuver*). Since the arteries and veins make up a circuit, it might be expected that half the blood volume would be in the arteries and half in the veins, but because of veins' larger diameter and ability to expand, typically only 20% of the blood occupies arteries, whereas 80% is in the veins.

Although often depicted as single vessels in illustrations for simplicity, veins tend to be double or multiple. Those that accompany deep arteries—**accompanying veins** (L. *venae comitantes*)—surround them in an irregular branching network (Fig. I.24). This arrangement serves as a *countercurrent heat exchanger,* the warm arterial blood warming the cooler venous blood as it returns to the heart from a cold extremity. The accompanying veins occupy a relatively unyielding fascial *vascular sheath* with the artery they accompany. As a result, they are stretched and flattened as the artery expands during contraction of the heart, which aids in driving venous blood toward the heart—an arteriovenous pump.

Systemic veins are more variable than arteries, and *venous anastomoses*—natural communications, direct or indirect, between two veins—occur more often between them. The outward expansion of the bellies of contracting skeletal mus-

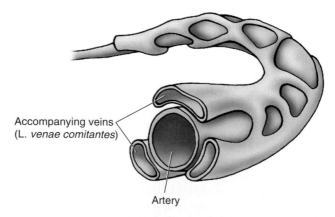

Accompanying veins
(L. *venae comitantes*)

Artery

Figure I.24. Accompanying veins (*venae comitantes*). Although most veins of the trunk occur as large single vessels, the veins in the limbs occur as two or more smaller vessels that accompany an artery in a common vascular sheath.

Blood pushed toward heart by compression

Deep fascia

Valve open

Vein compressed by contracting muscle

Valve closed

Contraction

Contraction

Retrograde flow obstructed by closed valve

Valve closed

Figure I.25. Musculovenous pump. Muscular contractions in the limbs function with the venous valves to move blood toward the heart. The outward expansion of the bellies of contracting muscles is limited by deep fascia and becomes a compressive force, propelling the blood against gravity. *Black arrows* indicate the direction of blood flow.

cles in the limbs, limited by the deep fascia, compresses the veins, "milking" the blood superiorly toward the heart; another (musculovenous) type of venous pump (Fig. I.25). The valves of the veins break up the columns of blood, thus relieving the more dependent parts of excessive pressure, allowing venous blood to flow only toward the heart. The venous congestion that hot and tired feet experience at the end of a busy day is relieved by resting the feet on a footstool that is higher than the trunk. This position of the feet also helps the veins return blood to the heart.

Varicose Veins

When the walls of veins lose their elasticity, they become weak. A weakened vein dilates under the pressure of supporting a column of blood against gravity. This results in *varicose veins*—abnormally swollen, twisted veins—most often seen in the legs (Fig. BI.8). Varicose veins have a caliber greater than normal, and their valve cusps do not meet or have been destroyed by inflammation. These veins have *incompetent valves;* thus the column of blood ascending toward the heart is unbroken, placing increased pressure on the weakened walls, further exacerbating the varicosity problem. Varicose veins also occur in the presence of degenerated deep fascia. Such incompetent fascia is incapable of containing the expansion of contracting muscles; thus the (musculofascial) musculovenous pump is ineffective. ✪

Figure BI.8.

Blood Capillaries

In order for the oxygen and nutrients carried by the arteries to benefit the cells that make up the tissues of the body, they must leave the transporting vessels and enter the *extravascular space* between the cells, the extracellular (intercellular) space in which the cells live. Capillaries are simple endothelial tubes connecting the arterial and venous sides of the circulation that allow the exchange of materials with the interstitial or *extracellular fluid* (ECF). Capillaries are generally arranged in capillary beds, networks that connect the arterioles and venules (Fig. I.23). The blood enters the capillary beds through arterioles that control the flow and is drained from them by venules. As the hydrostatic pressure in the arterioles forces blood into and through the capillary bed, it also forces fluid containing oxygen, nutrients, and other cellular materials out of the blood at the arterial end of the capillary bed (upstream) into the extracellular spaces, allowing exchange with cells of the surrounding tissue. Capillary walls are relatively impermeable, however, to plasma proteins. Downstream, at the venous end of the bed, most of this ECF—now containing waste products and carbon dioxide—is then reabsorbed into the blood as a result of the osmotic pressure from the higher concentrations of proteins within the capillary. (Although firmly established, this principle is referred to as the *Starling hypothesis*.)

In some regions, such as in the fingers, there are direct connections between the small arterioles and venules proximal to the capillary beds they supply and drain. The sites of such communications—arteriolovenular anastomoses (*AV shunts*)—permit blood to pass directly from the arterial to the venous side of the circulation without passing through capillaries. AV shunts are numerous in the skin, where they have an important role in conserving body heat.

In some situations, blood passes through two capillary beds before returning to the heart; a venous system linking two capillary beds constitutes a *portal venous system*. The venous system by which nutrient-rich blood passes from the capillary beds of the alimentary tract to the capillary beds or sinusoids of the liver—the *hepatic portal system*—is the major example (Chapter 2).

THE BOTTOM LINE: The cardiovascular system consists of the heart and blood vessels—the arteries, veins, and capillaries. Most of these vessels have three coats, or tunics—tunica intima, tunica media, and tunica adventitia. Arteries have both elastic and muscle fibers in their walls, which allow them to propel blood throughout the cardiovascular system. Veins have thinner walls than arteries and are distinguished by valves, which prevent backflow of blood. Capillaries are the smallest blood vessels and provide the linkage between the smallest arteries (arterioles) and veins (venules).

Lymphatic System

Although widely distributed throughout most of the body, most of the lymphatic (lymphoid) system is not apparent in the cadaver, yet it is essential to survival. Knowledge of the anatomy of the lymphatic system is important for clinicians. The *Starling hypothesis* (mentioned earlier) explains how most of the fluid and electrolytes entering the extracellular spaces from the blood capillaries is also reabsorbed by them. However, as much as 3 L each day fails to be reabsorbed by the blood capillaries. Furthermore, some plasma protein does leak into the extracellular spaces, and material originating from the tissue cells themselves that cannot pass through the walls of blood capillaries, such as cytoplasm from disintegrating cells, continually enters the space in which the cells live. If this material were to accumulate in the extracellular spaces, a reverse osmosis would occur, bringing even more fluid and resulting in *edema* (an excess of interstitial fluid, manifest as swelling). However, the amount of interstitial fluid remains fairly constant under normal conditions, and proteins and cellular debris normally do not accumulate in the extracellular spaces because of the lymphatic system.

The lymphatic system thus constitutes a sort of "overflow" system that provides for the drainage of surplus tissue fluid and leaked plasma proteins to the bloodstream, as well for the removal of debris from cellular decomposition and infection. The important components of the lymphatic system are (Fig. I.26):

- **Lymphatic plexuses,** networks of lymphatic capillaries that originate blindly in the extracellular (intercellular) spaces of most tissues. Because they are formed of a highly attenuated endothelium lacking a basement membrane, along with surplus tissue fluid, plasma proteins, bacteria, cellular debris, and even whole cells (especially lymphocytes) can readily enter them.

- **Lymphatic vessels** (lymphatics), a nearly bodywide network of thin-walled vessels with abundant lymphatic valves. In living individuals, the vessels bulge where each of the closely spaced valves occur, giving lymphatics a beaded appearance. Lymphatic capillaries and vessels occur almost everywhere blood capillaries are found, except, for example, teeth, bone, bone marrow, and the entire central nervous system (excess tissue fluid here drains into the cerebrospinal fluid).

- **Lymph** (L. *lympha,* clear water), the tissue fluid that enters lymph capillaries and is conveyed by lymphatic vessels. Usually clear, watery, and slightly yellow, lymph is similar in composition to blood plasma.

- **Lymph nodes,** small masses of lymphatic tissue located along the course of lymphatic vessels through which lymph is filtered on its way to the venous system.

- **Lymphocytes,** circulating cells of the immune system that react against foreign materials.

- **Lymphoid tissue,** sites that produce lymphocytes, such as that aggregated in the walls of the digestive tract (alimentary canal); in the spleen, thymus, and lymph nodes; and as myeloid tissue in red bone marrow.

Superficial lymphatic vessels, more numerous than veins in the subcutaneous tissue and anastomosing freely, converge

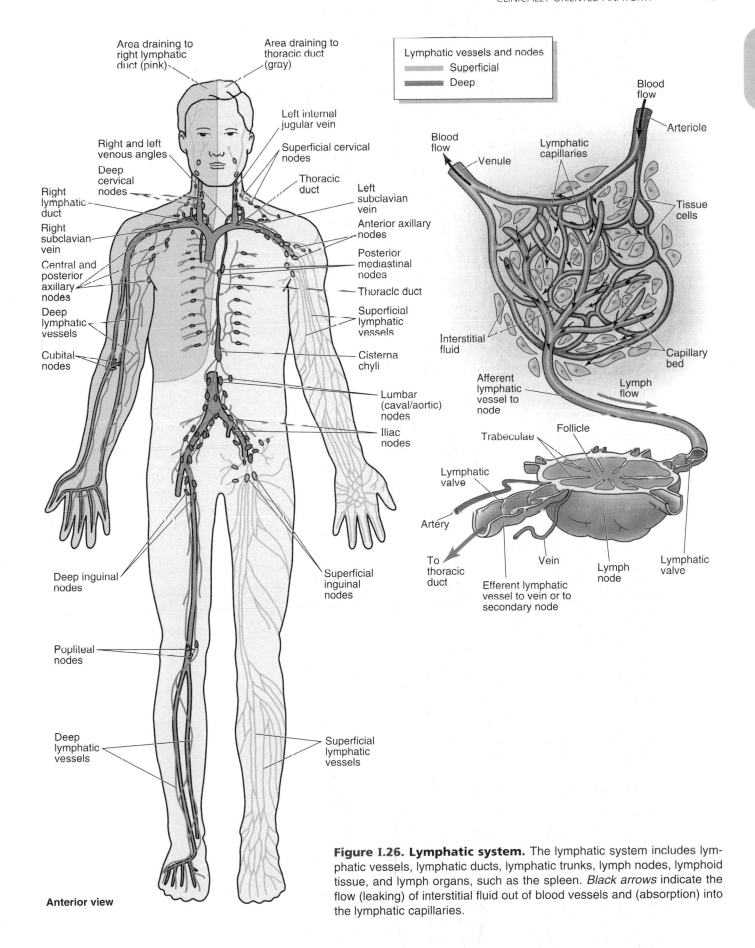

Area draining to right lymphatic duct (pink)

Area draining to thoracic duct (gray)

Right and left venous angles

Deep cervical nodes

Right lymphatic duct

Right subclavian vein

Central and posterior axillary nodes

Deep lymphatic vessels

Cubital nodes

Left internal jugular vein

Superficial cervical nodes

Thoracic duct

Left subclavian vein

Anterior axillary nodes

Posterior mediastinal nodes

Thoracic duct

Superficial lymphatic vessels

Cisterna chyli

Lumbar (caval/aortic) nodes

Iliac nodes

Deep inguinal nodes

Superficial inguinal nodes

Popliteal nodes

Deep lymphatic vessels

Superficial lymphatic vessels

Anterior view

Lymphatic vessels and nodes
- Superficial
- Deep

Blood flow

Arteriole

Blood flow

Venule

Lymphatic capillaries

Tissue cells

Interstitial fluid

Capillary bed

Afferent lymphatic vessel to node

Lymph flow

Trabeculae

Follicle

Lymphatic valve

Artery

To thoracic duct

Efferent lymphatic vessel to vein or to secondary node

Vein

Lymph node

Lymphatic valve

Figure I.26. Lymphatic system. The lymphatic system includes lymphatic vessels, lymphatic ducts, lymphatic trunks, lymph nodes, lymphoid tissue, and lymph organs, such as the spleen. *Black arrows* indicate the flow (leaking) of interstitial fluid out of blood vessels and (absorption) into the lymphatic capillaries.

toward and follow the venous drainage. These vessels eventually drain into deep lymphatic vessels that accompany the arteries and also receive the drainage of internal organs. It is likely that the deep lymphatic vessels are also compressed by the arteries they accompany, milking the lymph along these valved vessels in the same manner described earlier for accompanying veins. Both superficial and deep lymphatic vessels traverse lymph nodes (usually several sets) as they course proximally, becoming larger as they merge with vessels draining adjacent regions. The larger lymphatic vessels enter large collecting vessels, called lymphatic trunks, which unite to form either the right lymphatic duct or the thoracic duct (Fig. I.26):

- The **right lymphatic duct** drains lymph from the body's right upper quadrant (right side of the head, neck, and thorax plus the right upper limb). At the root of the neck, it enters the junction of the right internal jugular and right subclavian veins, called the right venous angle.

- The **thoracic duct** drains lymph from the remainder of the body. The lymphatic trunks draining the lower half of the body merge in the abdomen, sometimes forming a dilated collecting sac, the **chyle cistern** (L. *cisterna chyli*). From this sac (if present), or from the merger of the trunks, the thoracic duct ascends into and then through the thorax to enter the left venous angle (junction of left internal jugular and left subclavian veins).

Although this is the typical drainage pattern of most lymph, lymphatic vessels communicate with veins freely in many parts of the body. Consequently, ligation of a lymphatic trunk or even the thoracic duct itself may have only a transient effect as a new pattern of drainage is established through more peripheral lymphaticovenous—and later interlymphatic—anastomoses.

Additional functions of the lymphatic system include:

- *Absorption and transport of dietary fat.* Special lymphatic capillaries, called *lacteals* (L. *lacteus,* milk), receive all lipid and lipid-soluble vitamins absorbed by the intestine. Visceral lymphatics then convey the milky fluid, *chyle* (G. *chylos,* juice), to the thoracic duct and into the venous system.

- *Formation of a defense mechanism for the body.* When foreign protein drains from an infected area, antibodies specific to the protein are produced by immunologically competent cells and/or lymphocytes and dispatched to the infected area.

The Spread of Cancer

Cancer invades the body by *contiguity* (growing into adjacent tissue) or by *metastasis* (the dissemination of tumor cells to sites distant from the original or primary tumor). Metastasis occurs by one of three ways:

- *Direct seeding* of the serous membranes of body cavities.

- *Lymphogenous spread* (via lymphatic vessels).

- *Hematogenous spread* (via blood vessels).

It is surprising that often even a thin fascial sheet or serous membrane deflects tumor invasion. However, once a malignancy penetrates into a potential space, the direct seeding of cavities—that is, of its serous membranes—is likely. Lymphogenous spread is the most common route for the initial dissemination of *carcinomas* (epithelial tumors), the most common type of cancer. Cells loosened from the primary tumor enter and travel via lymphatics. The lymph-borne cells are filtered through and trapped by the lymph nodes, which thus become secondary (metastatic) cancer sites. The pattern of lymph node involvement follows the natural routes of lymph drainage. Thus when removing a potentially metastatic tumor, surgeons *stage* the metastasis (determine the degree to which cancer has spread) by removing and examining lymph nodes that receive drainage from the organ or region in the order the lymph normally passes through them. Therefore, it is important for the physician to know the lymphatic drainage backward and forward—that is, to know what nodes are likely to be affected when a tumor is identified in a certain site or organ (and the order in which they receive lymph) and to be able to determine likely sites of tumors (sources of metastasis) when an enlarged node is detected. *Cancerous nodes* become enlarged as the tumor(s) within them grows; however, unlike swollen infected nodes, they are not usually painful when compressed.

Hematogenous spread is the most common route for the metastasis of the less common (but more malignant) *sarcomas* (connective tissue cancers). Because veins are more abundant and have thinner walls that offer less resistance, metastasis occurs more often by venous than arterial routes. Since the blood-borne cells follow venous flow, the liver and lungs are the most common sites of secondary sarcomas. Typically, the treatment or removal of a primary tumor is not difficult, but the treatment or removal of all the affected lymph nodes or other secondary (metastatic) tumors may be impossible (Cotran et al., 1999)

Lymphangitis, Lymphadenitis, and Lymphedema

Lymphangitis and *lymphadenitis* are the secondary inflammation of lymphatic vessels and lymph nodes, respectively. These conditions may occur when the lymphatic system is involved in chemical or bacterial transport after severe injury or infection. The lymphatic vessels, not normally evident, may become apparent as red streaks in the skin, ▶

and the nodes become painfully enlarged. This is potentially dangerous because the uncontained infection may lead to *septicemia* (blood poisoning). *Lymphedema* (or edema), the localized accumulation of interstitial fluid, occurs when lymph does not drain from an area of the body. For instance, if cancerous lymph nodes are surgically removed from the axilla (armpit), lymphedema of the limb may occur. Solid cell growths may permeate lymphatic vessels and form minute *cellular emboli* (plugs), which may break free and pass to regional lymph nodes. In this way, further lymphogenous spread to other tissues and organs may occur. ☉

THE BOTTOM LINE: The lymphatic system drains surplus fluid from the extracellular spaces to the bloodstream. It also functions as the body's defense system. Important components of the lymphatic system are networks of lymphatic capillaries, the lymphatic plexuses; lymphatic vessels; lymph; lymph nodes; lymphocytes; and lymphoid tissue. The lymphatic system provides a (relatively) predictable route for the spread of certain types of cancerous cells throughout the body. Inflammation of the lymphatic vessels and lymph nodes is an important harbinger of injury or inflammation.

Nervous System

The nervous system enables the body to react to continuous changes in its internal and external environments. It also controls and integrates the various activities of the body, such as circulation and respiration. For descriptive purposes, the nervous system is divided:

- Structurally into the *central nervous system* (CNS) and *peripheral nervous system* (PNS).

- Functionally into the *somatic nervous system* (SNS) and *autonomic nervous system* (ANS).

Nervous tissue consists of two main cell types: neurons (*nerve cells*) and neuroglia (*glial cells*), which support the neurons.

- **Neurons** are the structural and functional units of the nervous system specialized for rapid communication (Fig. I.27). A neuron is composed of a cell body with processes (extensions) called **dendrites** and an **axon**, which carry impulses to and away from the cell body, respectively. *Myelin,* layers of lipid, and protein substances form a *myelin sheath* around some axons, greatly increasing the velocity of impulse conduction. Neurons communicate with each other at **synapses,** points of contact between neurons. The communication occurs by means of *neurotransmitters,* chemical agents released or secreted by one neuron, which may excite or inhibit another neuron, continuing or terminating the relay of impulses or the response to them.

- **Neuroglia** (glial cells or glia), approximately five times as abundant as neurons, are non-neuronal, non-excitable cells that form a major component (scaffolding) of nervous tissue, supporting, insulating, and nourishing the neurons. In the CNS, neuroglia include *oligodendroglia, astrocytes, ependymal cells,* and *microglia* (small glial cells). In the PNS, neuroglia include *satellite cells* around the neurons in the spinal (posterior root) and autonomic ganglia and *neurolemma* (*Schwann*) cells.

Central Nervous System

The central nervous system consists of the brain and spinal cord (Fig. I.28). The principal roles of the CNS are to integrate and coordinate incoming and outgoing neural signals and to carry out higher mental functions, such as thinking and learning.

A collection of nerve cell bodies in the CNS is called a **nucleus.** A bundle of nerve fibers (axons) connecting neighboring or distant nuclei of the CNS is a **tract.** The brain and spinal cord are composed of gray matter and white matter. The nerve cell bodies lie within and constitute the **gray matter;** the interconnecting fiber tract systems form the **white matter** (Fig. I.29). In transverse sections of the spinal cord, the gray matter appears roughly as an H-shaped area embedded in a matrix of white matter. The struts (supports) of the H are *horns;* hence there are right and left posterior (dorsal) and anterior (ventral) gray horns.

Three membranous layers—pia mater, arachnoid mater, and dura mater—collectively constitute the meninges. The meninges and the cerebrospinal fluid (CSF) surround and protect the CNS. The brain and spinal cord are intimately covered on their outer surface by the innermost meningeal layer, a delicate, transparent covering, the **pia mater.** The CSF is located between the pia mater and the **arachnoid mater.** External to the pia mater and arachnoid mater is the thick, tough dura mater. The **dura mater** of the brain is intimately related to the internal aspect of the bone of the surrounding *neurocranium* (braincase); that of the spinal cord is separated from the surrounding bone of the vertebral column by a fat-filled *epidural space.*

Damage to the CNS

When the brain or spinal cord is damaged, the injured axons do not recover in most circumstances. Their proximal stumps begin to regenerate, sending sprouts into the area of the lesion; however, this growth is blocked by *astrocyte proliferation* at the injury site, and the axonal sprouts are soon retracted. As a result, permanent disability follows destruction of a tract in the CNS. For discussions of axonal degeneration and regeneration in the CNS, see Hutchins et al. (2002). ☉

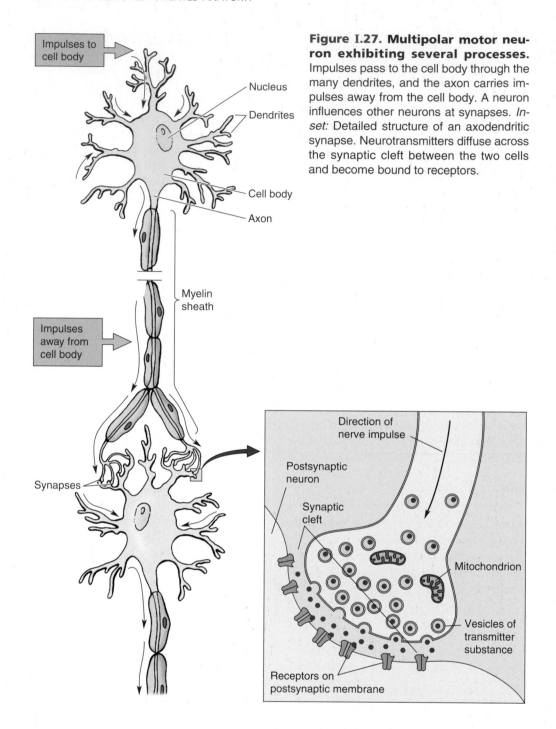

Figure I.27. Multipolar motor neuron exhibiting several processes. Impulses pass to the cell body through the many dendrites, and the axon carries impulses away from the cell body. A neuron influences other neurons at synapses. *Inset:* Detailed structure of an axodendritic synapse. Neurotransmitters diffuse across the synaptic cleft between the two cells and become bound to receptors.

Peripheral Nervous System

The peripheral nervous system consists of nerve fibers and cell bodies outside the CNS that conduct impulses to or away from the CNS (Fig. I.28). The PNS is organized into nerves that connect the CNS with peripheral structures. It is important to distinguish between *nerve fibers* and *nerves,* which are sometimes depicted diagrammatically as being one and the same.

A **peripheral nerve fiber** consists of an axon, its neurolemma (G. *neuron,* nerve + G. *lemma,* husk), and

surrounding endoneurial connective tissue (Figs. I.30). The neurolemma (also spelled neurilemma) consists of the neurolemma (Schwann) cells that immediately surround the axon, separating it from other axons. In the PNS, the neurolemma may take two forms, creating two classes of nerve fibers:

1. The neurolemma of myelinated nerve fibers consists of neurolemma cells specific to an individual axon, organized into a continuous series of enwrapping cells that form myelin.

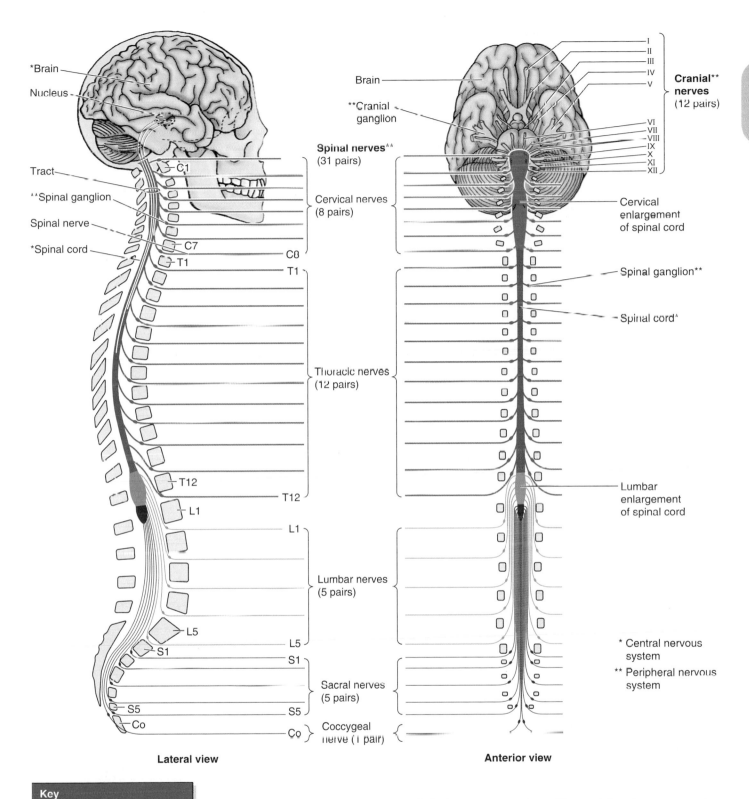

Lateral view

Anterior view

Brain

Cranial** nerves (12 pairs)

I
II
III
IV
V
VI
VII
VIII
IX
X
XI
XII

*Brain

Nucleus

Tract

**Spinal ganglion

Spinal nerve

*Spinal cord

**Cranial ganglion

Spinal nerves** (31 pairs)

Cervical nerves (8 pairs)

Cervical enlargement of spinal cord

Spinal ganglion**

Spinal cord*

Lumbar enlargement of spinal cord

C1

C7

T1

C8

T1

T12

L1

L5

S1

S5

Co

T1

T12

L1

L5

S1

S5

Co

Thoracic nerves (12 pairs)

Lumbar nerves (5 pairs)

Sacral nerves (5 pairs)

Coccygeal nerve (1 pair)

* Central nervous system

** Peripheral nervous system

Key

- Cervical nerves and ganglia
- Thoracic nerves and ganglia
- Lumbar nerves and ganglia
- Sacral and coccygeal nerves and ganglia
- Cranial nerves and ganglia

Figure I.28. Basic organization of the nervous system. The peripheral nervous system consists of nerve fibers and ganglia. Peripheral nerves are either cranial nerves or spinal nerves. Except in the cervical region, each spinal nerve bears the same letter–numeral designation as the vertebra forming the superior boundary of its exit from the vertebral column. In the cervical region, each spinal nerve bears the same letter–numeral designation as the vertebra forming its inferior boundary. Spinal nerve C8 exits between vertebrae C7 and T1. The cervical and lumbar enlargements of the spinal cord occur in relationship to the innervation of the limbs.

Anterolateral view

Figure I.29. Spinal cord and spinal meninges. The dura mater and arachnoid mater are incised and reflected to show the posterior and anterior roots and the denticulate ligament (a bilateral, longitudinal, toothed thickening of the pia that anchors the cord in the center of the vertebral canal). The spinal cord is sectioned to show its horns of gray matter. These membranes or coverings extend along the nerve roots to the point where the posterior and anterior roots join, forming the dural root sleeves that enclose the sensory (posterior root) ganglia.

2. The neurolemma of unmyelinated nerve fibers is composed of cells that do not make up such an apparent series; multiple axons are separately embedded within the cytoplasm of each cell. These neurolemma cells do not produce myelin. Most fibers in cutaneous nerves are unmyelinated.

A peripheral nerve consists of (1) a bundle of peripheral nerve fibers (or a "bundle of bundled fibers," or *fascicles,* in the case of a larger nerve), (2) the connective tissue coverings that surround and bind the nerve fibers and fascicles together, and (3) the blood vessels (vasa nervorum) that nourish the nerve

fibers and their coverings (Fig. I.31). Peripheral nerves are fairly strong and resilient because the nerve fibers are supported and protected by three connective tissue coverings:

1. **Endoneurium,** delicate connective tissue immediately surrounding the neurolemma cells and axons.

2. **Perineurium,** a layer of dense connective tissue that encloses a fascicle of peripheral nerve fibers, providing an effective barrier against penetration of the nerve fibers by foreign substances.

3. **Epineurium,** a thick connective tissue sheath that surrounds and encloses a bundle of fascicles, forming the outermost covering of the nerve; it includes fatty tissue, blood vessels, and lymphatics.

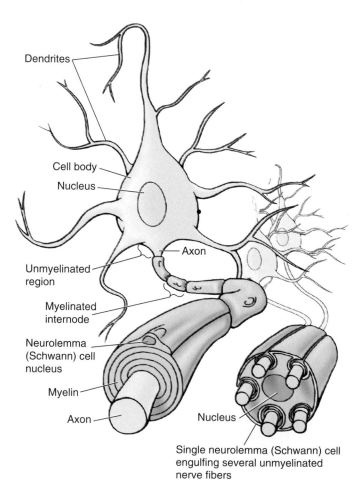

Figure I.30. Myelinated and unmyelinated peripheral nerve fibers. Myelinated nerve fibers have a sheath composed of a continuous series of neurolemma (Schwann) cells that surround the axon and form a series of myelin segments. Multiple unmyelinated nerve fibers are individually engulfed within a single neurolemma cell that does not produce myelin.

A peripheral nerve is organized much like a telephone cable: the axons are like individual wires insulated by the neurolemma and endoneurium; the insulated wires are bundled by the perineurium, and the bundles are surrounded by the epineurium forming the cable's outer wrapping.

A collection of nerve cell bodies outside the CNS is a **ganglion**. There are both motor (autonomic) and sensory ganglia.

Types of Peripheral Nerves

The PNS is anatomically and operationally continuous with the CNS (Fig. I.28). Its *afferent* (sensory) *fibers* convey neural impulses to the CNS from the sense organs (e.g., the eyes) and from sensory receptors in various parts of the body (e.g., in the skin). Its *efferent* ("motor") *fibers* convey neural impulses from the CNS to *effector organs* (muscles and glands).

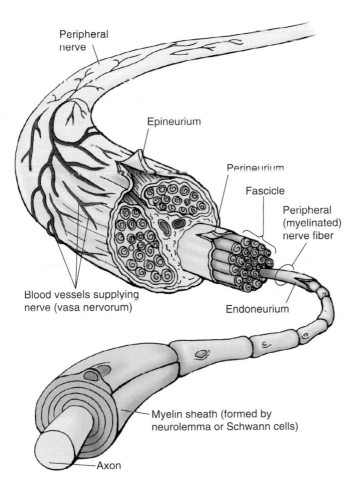

Peripheral nerve

Epineurium

Perineurium

Fascicle

Peripheral (myelinated) nerve fiber

Blood vessels supplying nerve (vasa nervorum)

Endoneurium

Myelin sheath (formed by neurolemma or Schwann cells)

Axon

Figure I.31. Arrangement and ensheathment of peripheral, myelinated nerve fibers. All but the smallest peripheral nerves are arranged in bundles called fascicles. The peripheral nerve consists of the bundles of nerve fibers, the layers of connective tissue binding them together, and the blood vessels (vasa nervorum) that serve them.

Peripheral nerves are either cranial nerves or spinal nerves.

- **Cranial nerves** exit the cranial cavity through foramina (openings) in the cranium (G. *kranion*, skull) and are identified by a descriptive name (e.g., trochlear) or a Roman numeral (e.g., CN IV). Only 11 of the 12 pairs of cranial nerves arise from the brain; the other pair (CN XI) arises from the superior part of the spinal cord.

- **Spinal nerves** exit the vertebral column (spine) through intervertebral foramina. All 31 pairs arise from the spinal cord and are identified by a letter and number (e.g., T4) designating the order of their origin from the 31 consecutive *spinal cord segments* (*C,* cervical; *T,* thoracic; *L,* lumbar; *S,* sacral; *Co,* coccygeal).

Spinal Nerves. Spinal nerves initially arise from the spinal cord as rootlets (commonly omitted from diagrams for the sake of simplicity), which converge to form two nerve roots (Fig. I.32):

1. An **anterior (ventral) root,** consisting of motor (efferent) fibers passing from nerve cell bodies in the anterior horn of spinal cord gray matter to effector organs located peripherally.

2. A **posterior (dorsal) root,** consisting of sensory (afferent) fibers from cell bodies in the spinal sensory or posterior (dorsal) root ganglion (commonly abbreviated DRG) that extend peripherally to sensory endings and centrally to the posterior horn of spinal cord gray matter.

The posterior and anterior nerve roots unite, within or just proximal to the intervertebral foramen, to form a *mixed spinal nerve,* which immediately divides into two primary rami (L. branches): a posterior (dorsal) ramus and an anterior (ventral) ramus. As branches of the mixed spinal nerve, the posterior and anterior rami carry both motor and sensory fibers, as do all their subsequent branches. The terms *motor nerve* and *sensory nerve* are almost always relative terms, referring to the *majority* of fiber types conveyed by that nerve. Nerves supplying muscles of the trunk or limbs (motor nerves) also contain about 40% sensory fibers, which convey pain and proprioceptive information. Conversely, cutaneous (sensory) nerves contain motor fibers, which serve sweat glands and the smooth muscle of blood vessels and hair follicles.

The unilateral area of skin innervated by the fibers of a single spinal nerve is called a **dermatome**; the unilateral muscle mass receiving innervation from the fibers conveyed by a single spinal nerve is a **myotome** (Fig. I.33*A*). From clinical studies of lesions of the posterior roots or spinal nerves, dermatome maps have been devised to indicate the typical pattern of innervation of the skin by specific spinal nerves (Fig. I.33*B*). However, a lesion of a single posterior root or spinal nerve would rarely result in numbness over the area demarcated for that nerve in these maps because the fibers conveyed by adjacent spinal nerves overlap almost completely as they

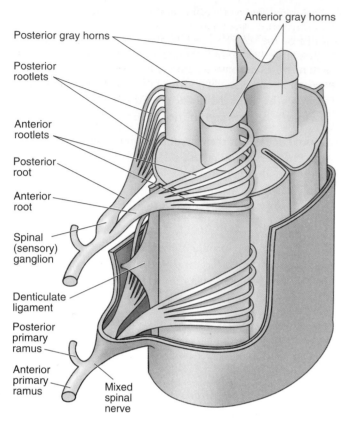

Posterior gray horns

Anterior gray horns

Posterior rootlets

Anterior rootlets

Posterior root

Anterior root

Spinal (sensory) ganglion

Denticulate ligament

Posterior primary ramus

Anterior primary ramus

Mixed spinal nerve

Figure I.32. Spinal cord gray matter, spinal roots, and spinal nerves. The meninges are incised and reflected to show the H-shaped gray matter in the spinal cord and the posterior and anterior rootlets and roots of two spinal nerves. The posterior and anterior rootlets enter and leave the posterior and anterior gray horns, respectively. The posterior and anterior nerve roots unite distal to the spinal ganglion to form a mixed spinal nerve, which immediately divides into posterior and anterior rami.

are distributed to the skin, providing a type of double coverage. The lines indicating dermatomes on dermatome maps would thus be better represented by smudges or gradations of color. Generally, at least two adjacent spinal nerves (or posterior roots) must be interrupted to produce a discernible area of numbness.

The posterior rami remain separate from each other, supplying nerve fibers to the synovial joints of the vertebral column, deep muscles of the back, and the overlying skin in a segmental pattern. The anterior rami supply nerve fibers to the much larger remaining area, consisting of the anterior and lateral regions of the trunk and the upper and lower limbs.

The anterior rami distributed exclusively to the trunk remain separate from each other, also innervating muscles and skin in a segmental pattern (Figs. I.33C and I.34). However, primarily in relationship to the innervation of the limbs, the

majority of anterior rami merge with all or portions of one or more adjacent anterior rami, forming *nerve plexuses* (networks) in which their fibers intermingle and from which a new set of **multisegmental peripheral nerves** emerges (Figs. I.34 and I.35A & B). The anterior rami of segmental nerves participating in plexus formation contribute fibers to multiple peripheral nerves arising from the plexus (Fig. I.35A); therefore, peripheral nerves arising from the plexus contain fibers from multiple spinal nerves (Fig. I.35B).

Although the spinal nerves lose their identity as they split and merge in the plexus, the fibers arising from a specific spinal cord segment and conveyed from it by a single spinal nerve are ultimately distributed to one segmental dermatome, although they may reach it by means of a multisegmental peripheral nerve arising from the plexus that also conveys fibers to all or parts of other adjacent dermatomes (Fig. I.35C).

It thus becomes important to distinguish between the distribution of the fibers carried by spinal nerves (spinal nerve innervation or segmental distribution—i.e., dermatomes and myotomes labeled with a letter and a number, such as T4) and of the fibers carried by branches of a plexus (peripheral nerve innervation or distribution, labeled with the names of peripheral nerves, such as the median nerve) (Fig. I.33B & C). Mapping segmental innervation (dermatomes, determined by clinical experience) and mapping the distribution of peripheral nerves (determined by dissecting the branches of a named nerve distally) produce entirely different maps, except for most of the trunk where, in the absence of plexus formation, segmental and peripheral distributions are the same. (Overlapping also occurs in the cutaneous distribution of peripheral nerves derived from plexuses.)

Cranial Nerves. Some cranial nerves convey only sensory fibers, some only motor fibers (initially, at least), and some carry a mixture of both types of fibers. Communication occurs between cranial nerves, and between cranial nerves and upper cervical (spinal) nerves; thus a nerve that initially conveys only motor fibers may receive sensory fibers distally in its course, and vice versa. Except for the first two (those involved in the senses of smell and sight), cranial nerves that convey sensory fibers into the brain bear sensory ganglia (similar to spinal sensory or posterior root ganglia), where the cell bodies of those fibers are located. Although, by definition, the term *dermatome* applies only to spinal nerves, similar areas of skin supplied by single cranial nerves can be identified and mapped. Unlike dermatomes, however, there is little overlap in the innervation of zones of skin supplied by cranial nerves.

Somatic and Visceral Fibers

The types of fibers conveyed by cranial or spinal peripheral nerves are as follows (Fig. I.36):

- Somatic fibers

  - *General sensory fibers* (*general somatic afferent* [*GSA*] *fibers*) transmit sensations from the body to the CNS;

(cont'd on page 56)

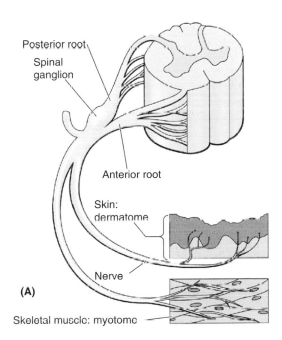

(A)

Figure I.33. Dermatomes, myotomes, and cutaneous distribution of multi-segmental peripheral nerves. A. A single dermatome (the unilateral area of skin) and myotome (portion of skeletal muscle of one side) innervated by a single spinal nerve are shown. **B.** Dermatome maps of the body are based on an accumulation of clinical findings following spinal nerve injuries; this map is based on the studies of Keegan and Garrett (1948). Spinal nerve C1 lacks a significant afferent component and does not supply the skin; therefore, no C1 dermatome is depicted. **C.** Maps of the cutaneous distribution of peripheral nerves are based on dissection and supported by clinical findings.

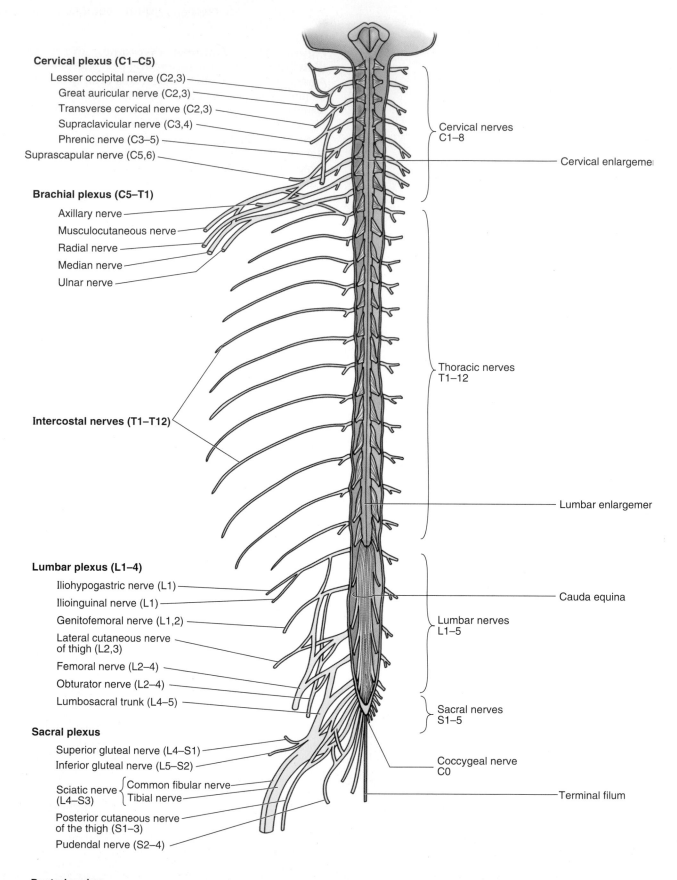

Cervical plexus (C1–C5)
- Lesser occipital nerve (C2,3)
- Great auricular nerve (C2,3)
- Transverse cervical nerve (C2,3)
- Supraclavicular nerve (C3,4)
- Phrenic nerve (C3–5)
- Suprascapular nerve (C5,6)

Brachial plexus (C5–T1)
- Axillary nerve
- Musculocutaneous nerve
- Radial nerve
- Median nerve
- Ulnar nerve

Intercostal nerves (T1–T12)

Lumbar plexus (L1–4)
- Iliohypogastric nerve (L1)
- Ilioinguinal nerve (L1)
- Genitofemoral nerve (L1,2)
- Lateral cutaneous nerve of thigh (L2,3)
- Femoral nerve (L2–4)
- Obturator nerve (L2–4)
- Lumbosacral trunk (L4–5)

Sacral plexus
- Superior gluteal nerve (L4–S1)
- Inferior gluteal nerve (L5–S2)
- Sciatic nerve (L4–S3) { Common fibular nerve / Tibial nerve
- Posterior cutaneous nerve of the thigh (S1–3)
- Pudendal nerve (S2–4)

Cervical nerves C1–8

Cervical enlargeme[nt]

Thoracic nerves T1–12

Lumbar enlargeme[nt]

Cauda equina

Lumbar nerves L1–5

Sacral nerves S1–5

Coccygeal nerve C0

Terminal filum

Posterior view

Figure I.34. Anterior rami and their participation in plexus formation. Although the posterior rami (not shown) remain separate from each other and follow a distinctly segmental pattern of distribution, most anterior rami (20 of 31 pairs) participate in the formation of plexuses, which are primarily involved in the innervation of the limbs. The anterior rami distributed only to the trunk do, however, remain separate and follow a segmental distribution similar to that of the posterior rami.

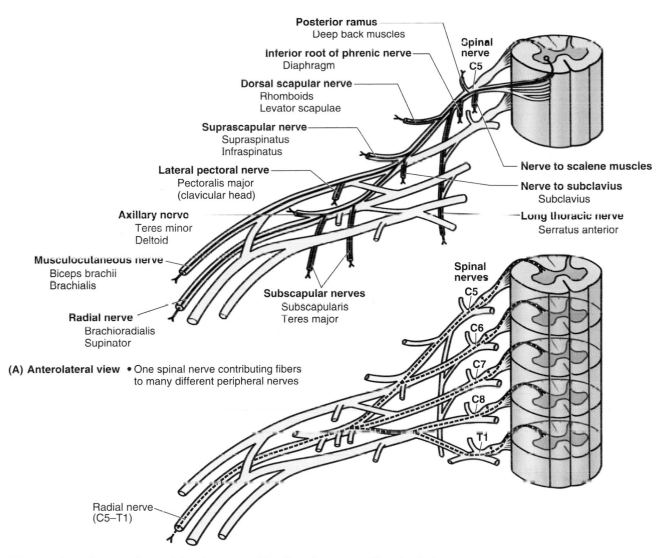

Posterior ramus
Deep back muscles

Inferior root of phrenic nerve
Diaphragm

Dorsal scapular nerve
Rhomboids
Levator scapulae

Suprascapular nerve
Supraspinatus
Infraspinatus

Lateral pectoral nerve
Pectoralis major
(clavicular head)

Axillary nerve
Teres minor
Deltoid

Musculocutaneous nerve
Biceps brachii
Brachialis

Radial nerve
Brachioradialis
Supinator

Subscapular nerves
Subscapularis
Teres major

Spinal nerve
C5

Nerve to scalene muscles

Nerve to subclavius
Subclavius

Long thoracic nerve
Serratus anterior

Spinal nerves
C5
C6
C7
C8
T1

(A) Anterolateral view • One spinal nerve contributing fibers to many different peripheral nerves

Radial nerve
(C5–T1)

(B) Anterolateral view • One peripheral nerve receiving fibers from many different spinal nerves

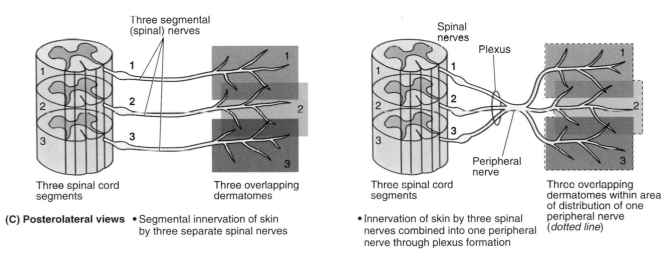

Three segmental (spinal) nerves

1
2
3

Three spinal cord segments

Three overlapping dermatomes

(C) Posterolateral views • Segmental innervation of skin by three separate spinal nerves

Spinal nerves

Plexus

1
2
3

Peripheral nerve

Three spinal cord segments

Three overlapping dermatomes within area of distribution of one peripheral nerve (*dotted line*)

• Innervation of skin by three spinal nerves combined into one peripheral nerve through plexus formation

Figure I.35. Plexus formation. Adjacent anterior rami merge to form plexuses in which their fibers are exchanged and redistributed, forming a new set of multisegmental peripheral (named) nerves. **A.** The fibers of a single spinal nerve entering the plexus are distributed to multiple branches of the plexus. **B.** The peripheral nerves derived from the plexus contain fibers from multiple spinal nerves. **C.** Although segmental nerves merge and lose their identity in the plexus formation that results in multisegmental peripheral nerves, the segmental (dermatomal) pattern of nerve fiber distribution remains.

they may be *exteroceptive sensations* from the skin (pain, temperature, touch, and pressure) or pain and *proprioceptive sensations* from muscles, tendons, and joints. Proprioceptive sensations are usually subconscious, providing information regarding joint position and the tension of tendon and muscles that is combined with

input from the vestibular apparatus of the internal ear, resulting in awareness of the orientation of the body and limbs in space, independent of visual input.

- *Somatic motor fibers* (*general somatic efferent* [GSE] *fibers*) transmit impulses to skeletal (voluntary) muscles.

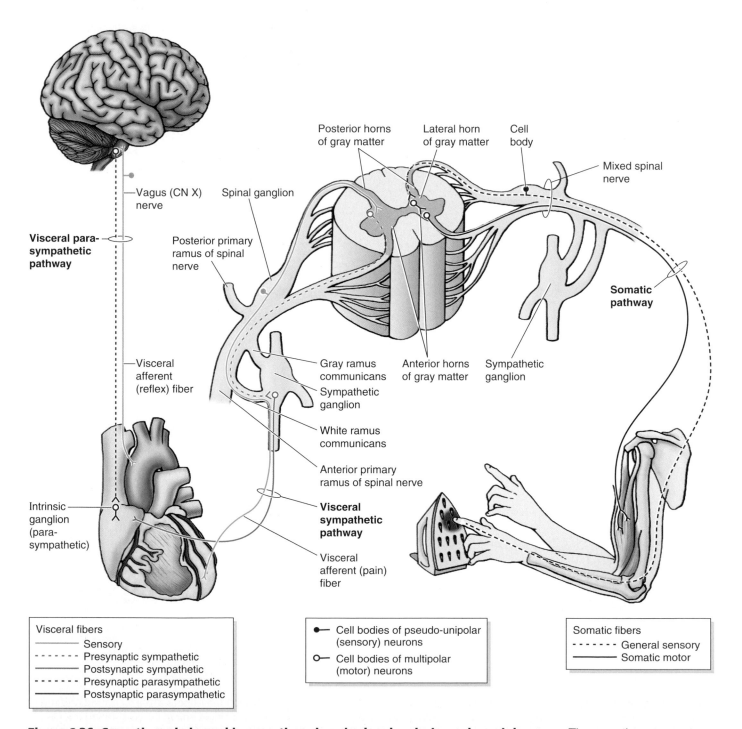

Figure I.36. Somatic and visceral innervation via spinal, splanchnic, and cranial nerves. The somatic motor system permits voluntary and reflexive movement caused by contraction of skeletal muscles, such as occurs when one touches a hot iron.

- Visceral fibers

  - *Visceral sensory fibers* (*general visceral afferent* [GVA] *fibers*) transmit pain or subconscious visceral *reflex sensations* (information concerning distension, blood gas, and blood pressure levels, for example) from hollow organs and blood vessels to the CNS.

  - *Visceral motor fibers* (*general visceral efferent* [GVE] *fibers*) transmit impulses to smooth (involuntary) muscle and glandular tissues. Two varieties of fibers, *presynaptic* and *postsynaptic,* work together to conduct impulses from the CNS to smooth muscle or glands (explained later in this chapter).

Both types of sensory fibers—visceral sensory and general sensory—are processes of pseudo-unipolar neurons with cell bodies located outside of the CNS in spinal or cranial sensory ganglia (Figs. I.36 and I.37). The motor fibers of peripheral nerves are axons of multi-polar neurons. The cell bodies of somatic motor and presynaptic visceral motor neurons are located in the gray matter of the spinal cord. Cell bodies of postsynaptic motor neurons are located outside the CNS in autonomic ganglia.

In addition to the fiber types listed above, some cranial nerves also convey special sensory fibers for the special senses (smell, sight, hearing, balance, and taste). (On the basis of the embryologic/phylogenetic derivation of certain muscles of the head and neck, some motor fibers conveyed by cranial nerves to striated muscle have traditionally been classified as "special visceral"; however, the designation is confusing and not applied clinically, and its practicality is questionable. That term will not be used here. When it is appropriate to do so, these fibers will be designated as *branchial motor,* referring to muscle tissue derived from the pharyngeal arches in the embryo.)

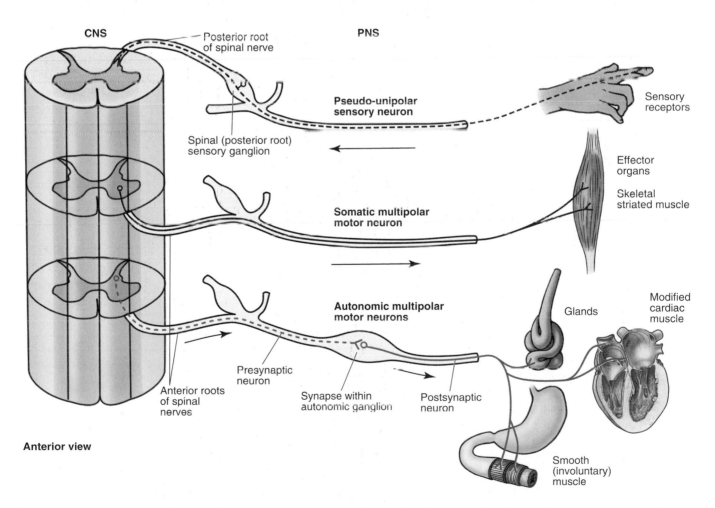

Figure I.37. Neurons of the PNS. Note the types of neurons involved in the somatic and visceral nervous systems, the general location of their cell bodies in relation to the CNS, and their receptors or effector organs.

Rhizotomy

The posterior and anterior roots are the only sites where the motor and sensory fibers of a spinal nerve are segregated. Therefore, only at these locations can the surgeon selectively section either functional element for the relief of intractable pain or spastic paralysis (*rhizotomy*).

Peripheral Nerve Degeneration and Ischemia of Nerves

Neurons do not proliferate in the adult nervous system, except those related to the sense of smell in the olfactory epithelium. Therefore, neurons destroyed through disease or trauma are not replaced (Hutchins et al., 2002). When peripheral nerves are stretched, crushed, or severed, their axons degenerate mainly distal to the lesion because they depend on their cell bodies for survival. If the axons are damaged but the cell bodies are intact, regeneration and return of function may occur in certain circumstances. The chance of survival is best when a peripheral nerve is compressed. Pressure on a nerve commonly causes **paresthesia**, the pins-and-needles sensation that occurs when you sit too long with your legs crossed, for example.

A *crushing nerve injury* damages or kills the axons distal to the injury site; however, the neuronal cell bodies usually survive, and the nerve's connective tissue coverings remain intact. No surgical repair is needed for this type of nerve injury because the intact connective tissue coverings guide the growing axons to their destinations. Regeneration is less likely to occur in a severed peripheral nerve. Sprouting occurs at the proximal ends of the axons, but the growing axons may not reach their distal targets. A *cutting nerve injury* requires surgical intervention because regeneration of the axon requires apposition of the cut ends by sutures through the epineurium. The individual nerve bundles are realigned as accurately as possible. *Anterograde* (*wallerian*) *degeneration* is the degeneration of axons detached from their cell bodies (Hutchins et al., 2002). The degenerative process involves the axon and its myelin sheath, even though this sheath is not part of the injured neuron.

Compromising a nerve's blood supply for a long period by *compression of the vasa nervorum* (Fig. I.31) can also cause nerve degeneration. Prolonged *ischemia* (inadequate blood supply) of a nerve may result in damage no less severe than that produced by crushing or even cutting the nerve. The Saturday night syndrome, named after an intoxicated individual who "passes out" with a limb dangling across the arm of a chair or the edge of a bed, is an example of a more serious, often permanent, paresthesia. This condition can also result from the sustained use of a tourniquet during a surgical procedure. If the ischemia is not too prolonged, temporary numbness or paresthesia results. *Transient paresthesias* are familiar to anyone who has had an injection of anesthetic for dental repairs. ⊕

THE BOTTOM LINE: The nervous system can be functionally divided into the central nervous system, which consists of the brain and spinal cord, and the peripheral nervous system, which consists of the nerve fibers and their cell bodies that reside outside the central nervous system. Neurons are the functional units of the nervous system. They are composed of a cell body, dendrites, and axons. The neuronal axons (nerve fibers) transmit impulses to other neurons or to a target organ or muscle or, in the case of sensory nerves, transmit impulses to the CNS from peripheral sensory organs. Neuroglia are the non-neuronal, supporting cells of the nervous system. Within the CNS, a collection of nerve cell bodies is called a nucleus; within the PNS, it is called a ganglion. In the CNS, a bundle of nerve fibers that connect the nuclei is called a tract; in the PNS, a bundle of nerve fibers, the connective tissue holding it together, and the blood vessels serving it (vasa nervorum) constitute a nerve. Nerves exiting the cranium are cranial nerves; those exiting the vertebral column (formerly, the spine), are spinal nerves. Although some cranial nerves convey a single type of fiber, most nerves convey a variety of visceral or somatic and sensory or motor fibers.

Somatic Nervous System

The somatic nervous system, composed of somatic parts of the CNS and PNS, provides sensory and motor innervation to all parts of the body (G. *soma*), except the viscera in the body cavities, smooth muscle, and glands (Figs. I.36 and I.37). The *somatic sensory system* transmits sensations of touch, pain, temperature, and position from sensory receptors. Most of these sensations reach conscious levels (i.e., we are aware of them). The *somatic motor system* innervates only skeletal muscle, stimulating voluntary and reflexive movement by causing the muscle to contract, as occurs in response to touching a hot iron.

Autonomic Nervous System

The autonomic nervous system, classically described as the *visceral nervous system* or *visceral motor system* (Figs. I.33 and I.37), consists of motor fibers that stimulate smooth (involuntary) muscle, modified cardiac muscle (the intrinsic stimulating and conducting tissue of heart), and glandular (secretory) cells. However, the visceral efferent fibers of the ANS are accompanied by visceral afferent fibers. As the afferent component of autonomic reflexes and in conducting visceral pain impulses, these fibers also play a role in the regulation of visceral function. Thus some authors consider the visceral afferent fibers to be part of the ANS. In any case, these fibers should be considered along with this system.

The efferent nerve fibers and ganglia of the ANS are organized into two systems or divisions: the *sympathetic* (thoracolumbar) division and the *parasympathetic* (craniosacral) division. Unlike sensory and somatic motor innervation, in which the passage of impulses between the CNS and the sensory ending or effector involves a single neuron, in both divisions of the ANS, conduction of impulses from the CNS to the effector organ involves a series of two *multi-polar neurons* (Fig. I.37). The cell body of the first *presynaptic (preganglionic) neuron* is located in the gray matter of the CNS. Its fiber (axon) synapses only on the cell body of a *postsynaptic (postganglionic) neuron*, the second neuron in the series. The cell bodies of these second neurons are located outside the CNS in autonomic ganglia, with fibers terminating on the effector organ (smooth muscle, modified cardiac muscle, or glands).

The anatomical distinction between the two divisions of the ANS is based primarily on (1) the location of the presynaptic cell bodies and (2) which nerves conduct the presynaptic fibers from the CNS. A functional distinction of pharmacological importance for medical practice is that the postsynaptic neurons of the two divisions generally liberate different neurotransmitter substances: *norepinephrine* by the sympathetic division (except in the case of sweat glands) and *acetylcholine* by the parasympathetic division.

Sympathetic (Thoracolumbar) Division of the ANS

The cell bodies of the presynaptic neurons of the sympathetic division of the ANS are found in only one location: the *intermediolateral cell columns* (IMLs) or nuclei of the spinal cord (Fig. I.38). The paired (right and left) IMLs are a part of the gray matter of the thoracic (T1–12) and the upper lumbar (T1–L2 or 3) segments of the spinal cord (hence the alternate name for the division). In transverse sections of this part of the spinal cord, the IMLs appear as small lateral horns of the H-shaped gray matter, looking somewhat like an extension of the cross-bar of the H between the posterior and the anterior horns. The IMLs are organized *somatotopically* (i.e., arranged like the body, the cell bodies involved with innervation of the head located superiorly, and those involved with innervation of the pelvic viscera and lower limbs located inferiorly). Thus it is possible to deduce the location of the presynaptic

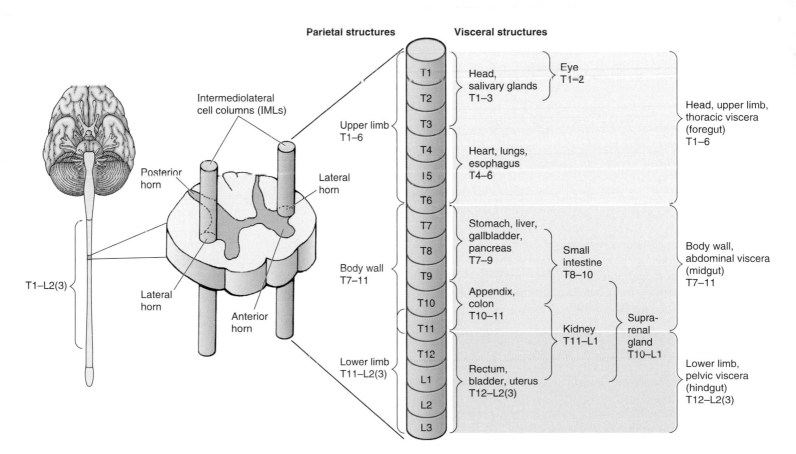

Figure I.38. Intermediolateral cell columns. Each IML or nucleus constitutes the lateral horn of gray matter of spinal cord segments T1–L2 or 3 and consists of the cell bodies of the presynaptic neurons of the sympathetic nervous system, which are somatotopically arranged.

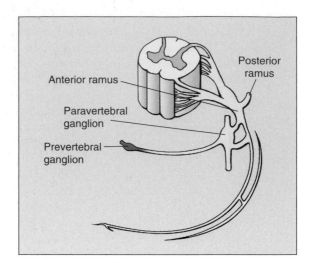

Figure I.39. Ganglia of the sympathetic nervous system. Paravertebral ganglia are linked to form right and left sympathetic trunks on each side of the vertebral column. Paravertebral ganglia are associated with all spinal nerves, although at the cervical levels, eight spinal nerves share three ganglia—superior, middle, and inferior. Prevertebral (preaortic) ganglia occur in the plexuses that surround the origins of the main branches of the abdominal aorta, such as the celiac artery, and are specifically involved in the innervation of abdominopelvic viscera.

sympathetic cell bodies involved in innervation of a specific part of the body.

The cell bodies of postsynaptic neurons of the sympathetic nervous system occur in two locations, the paravertebral and prevertebral ganglia (Fig. I.39):

- **Paravertebral ganglia** are linked to form right and left *sympathetic trunks* (*chains*) on each side of the vertebral column and extend essentially the length of this column. The *superior paravertebral ganglion* (the superior cervical ganglion of each sympathetic trunk) lies at the base of the cranium. The *ganglion impar* forms inferiorly where the two trunks unite at the level of the coccyx.

- **Prevertebral ganglia** are in the plexuses that surround the origins of the main branches of the abdominal aorta (for

which they are named), such as the two large celiac ganglia that surround the origin of the *celiac trunk* (a major artery arising from the aorta).

Because they are motor fibers, the axons of presynaptic neurons leave the spinal cord through anterior roots and enter the anterior rami of spinal nerves T1–L2 or 3 (Fig. I.40). Almost immediately after entering, all the presynaptic sympathetic fibers leave the anterior rami of these spinal nerves and pass to the sympathetic trunks through *white rami communicantes.* Within the sympathetic trunks, presynaptic fibers follow one of four possible courses:

- Ascend in the sympathetic trunk to synapse with a postsynaptic neuron of a higher paravertebral ganglion.

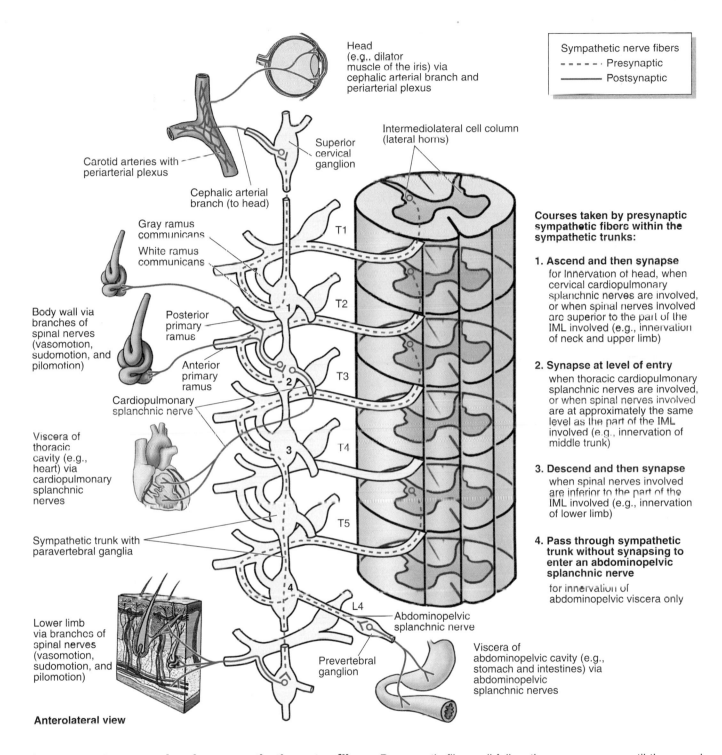

Head
(e.g., dilator
muscle of the iris) via
cephalic arterial branch and
periarterial plexus

Intermediolateral cell column
(lateral horns)

Carotid arteries with
periarterial plexus

Superior
cervical
ganglion

Cephalic arterial
branch (to head)

Gray ramus
communicans

White ramus
communicans

Body wall via
branches of
spinal nerves
(vasomotion,
sudomotion, and
pilomotion)

Posterior
primary
ramus

Anterior
primary
ramus

Cardiopulmonary
splanchnic nerve

Viscera of
thoracic
cavity (e.g.,
heart) via
cardiopulmonary
splanchnic
nerves

Sympathetic trunk with
paravertebral ganglia

Lower limb
via branches of
spinal nerves
(vasomotion,
sudomotion, and
pilomotion)

Prevertebral
ganglion

Abdominopelvic
splanchnic nerve

Viscera of
abdominopelvic cavity (e.g.,
stomach and intestines) via
abdominopelvic
splanchnic nerves

T1
T2
T3
T4
T5
L4

Anterolateral view

Sympathetic nerve fibers
- - - - - Presynaptic
——— Postsynaptic

**Courses taken by presynaptic
sympathetic fibers within the
sympathetic trunks:**

1. Ascend and then synapse
for innervation of head, when
cervical cardiopulmonary
splanchnic nerves are involved,
or when spinal nerves involved
are superior to the part of the
IML involved (e.g., innervation
of neck and upper limb)

2. Synapse at level of entry
when thoracic cardiopulmonary
splanchnic nerves are involved,
or when spinal nerves involved
are at approximately the same
level as the part of the IML
involved (e.g., innervation of
middle trunk)

3. Descend and then synapse
when spinal nerves involved
are inferior to the part of the
IML involved (e.g., innervation
of lower limb)

**4. Pass through sympathetic
trunk without synapsing to
enter an abdominopelvic
splanchnic nerve**
for innervation of
abdominopelvic viscera only

Figure I.40. Courses taken by sympathetic motor fibers. Presynaptic fibers all follow the same course until they reach the sympathetic trunks. In the sympathetic trunks, they follow one of four possible courses. Fibers involved in providing sympathetic innervation to the body wall and limbs or viscera above the level of the diaphragm follow paths 1–3. They synapse in the paravertebral ganglia of the sympathetic trunks. Fibers involved in innervating abdominopelvic viscera follow path 4 to prevertebral ganglion via abdominopelvic splanchnic nerves.

- Descend in the sympathetic trunk to synapse with a post-synaptic neuron of a lower paravertebral ganglion.

- Enter and synapse immediately with a postsynaptic neuron of the paravertebral ganglion at that level.

- Pass through the sympathetic trunk without synapsing, continuing through an abdominopelvic splanchnic nerve (a branch of the trunk involved in innervating abdominopelvic viscera) to reach the prevertebral ganglia.

Presynaptic sympathetic fibers that provide autonomic innervation within the head, neck, body wall, limbs, and thoracic cavity follow one of the first three courses, synapsing within the paravertebral ganglia. Presynaptic sympathetic fibers innervating viscera within the abdominopelvic cavity follow the fourth course.

Postsynaptic sympathetic fibers greatly outnumber the presynaptic fibers; each presynaptic sympathetic fiber synapses with 30 or more postsynaptic fibers. Those postsynaptic sympathetic fibers, destined for distribution within the neck, body wall, and limbs, pass from the paravertebral ganglia of the sympathetic trunks to adjacent anterior rami of spinal nerves through gray rami communicantes (Fig. I.41). By this means, they enter all branches of all 31 pairs of spinal nerves, including the posterior rami, to stimulate contraction of the blood vessels (*vasomotion*) and arrector muscles associated with hairs (*pilomotion*, resulting in "goose bumps"), and to cause sweating (*sudomotion*). Postsynaptic sympathetic fibers that perform these functions in the head (plus innervation of the dilator muscle of the iris) all have their cell bodies in the *superior cervical ganglion* at the superior end of the sympathetic trunk. They pass from the ganglion by means of a cephalic arterial branch to form periarterial plexuses of nerves, which follow the branches of the carotid arteries, or they may pass directly to nearby cranial nerves, to reach their destination in the head (Maklad et al., 2001).

Splanchnic nerves convey visceral efferent (autonomic) and afferent fibers to and from the viscera of the body cavities. Postsynaptic sympathetic fibers destined for the viscera of the thoracic cavity (e.g., the heart, lungs, and esophagus) pass through *cardiopulmonary splanchnic nerves* to enter the cardiac, pulmonary, and esophageal plexuses (Fig. I.40). The presynaptic sympathetic fibers involved in the innervation of viscera of the abdominopelvic cavity (e.g., the stomach and intestines) pass to the prevertebral ganglia through abdominopelvic splanchnic nerves (making up the greater, lesser, least, and lumbar splanchnic nerves) (Figs. I.40–I.42). All presynaptic sympathetic fibers of the *abdominopelvic splanchnic nerves,* except those involved in innervating the suprarenal (adrenal) glands, synapse here. The postsynaptic fibers from the prevertebral ganglia form periarterial plexuses, which follow branches of the abdominal aorta to reach their destination.

Some presynaptic sympathetic fibers pass through the prevertebral (celiac) ganglia without synapsing, continuing to terminate directly on cells of the medulla of the suprarenal

gland (Fig. I.42). The suprarenal medullary cells function as a special type of postsynaptic neuron that, instead of releasing their neurotransmitter substance onto the cells of a specific effector organ, release it into the bloodstream to circulate throughout the body, producing a widespread sympathetic response. Thus the sympathetic innervation of this gland is exceptional.

As described earlier, postsynaptic sympathetic fibers are components of virtually all branches of all spinal nerves. By this means and via periarterial plexuses, they extend to and innervate all the body's blood vessels (the sympathetic system's primary function) as well as sweat glands, arrector muscles of hairs, and visceral structures. Thus the sympathetic nervous system reaches virtually all parts of the body, with the rare exception of such avascular tissues as cartilage and nails. Because the two sets of sympathetic ganglia are centrally placed in the body and are close to the midline (hence relatively close to the spinal cord), in this division the presynaptic fibers are relatively short, whereas the postsynaptic fibers are relatively long, having to extend to all parts of the body.

Parasympathetic (Craniosacral) Division of the ANS
Presynaptic parasympathetic neuron cell bodies are located in two sites within the CNS, their fibers exiting by two routes. This arrangement accounts for the alternate name of the parasympathetic (craniosacral) division of the ANS (Fig. I.43):

- In the gray matter of the brainstem, the fibers exit the CNS within cranial nerves (CN) III, VII, IX, and X; these fibers constitute the *cranial parasympathetic outflow.*

- In the gray matter of the sacral segments of the spinal cord (S2–4), the fibers exit the CNS through the anterior roots of sacral spinal nerves S2–4 and the pelvic splanchnic nerves that arise from their anterior rami; these fibers constitute the *sacral parasympathetic outflow.*

Not surprisingly, the cranial outflow provides parasympathetic innervation of the head, and the sacral outflow provides the parasympathetic innervation of the pelvic viscera. However, in terms of the innervation of thoracic and abdominal viscera, the cranial outflow through the vagus nerve (CN X) is dominant. It provides innervation to all the thoracic viscera and most of the gastrointestinal (GI) tract from the esophagus through most of the large intestine (to its left colic flexure). The sacral outflow to the GI tract supplies only the descending and sigmoid colon and rectum.

Regardless of the extensive influence of its cranial outflow, the parasympathetic system is much more restricted than the sympathetic system in its distribution. The parasympathetic system distributes only to the head, visceral cavities of the trunk, and erectile tissues of the external genitalia. With the exception of the latter, it does not reach the body wall or limbs; and except for the initial parts of the anterior rami of spinal nerves S2–4, its fibers are not components of spinal nerves or their branches.

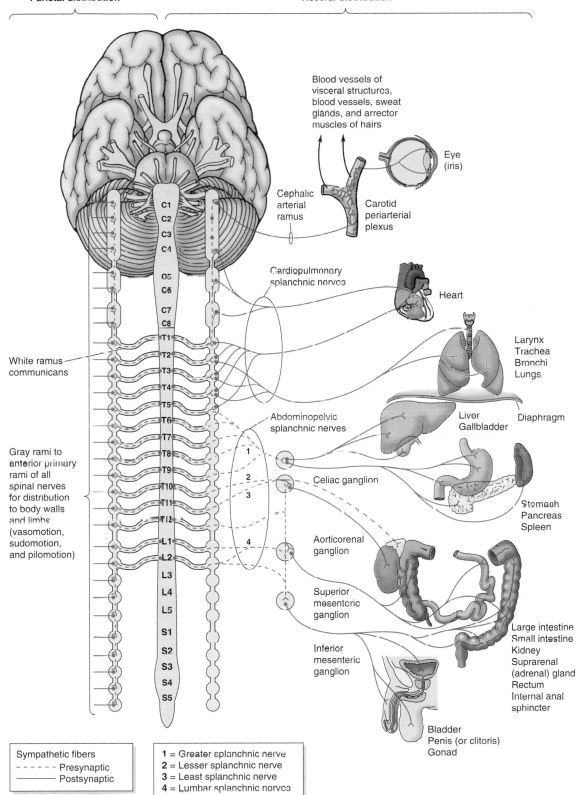

Parietal distribution

Visceral distribution

Blood vessels of visceral structures, blood vessels, sweat glands, and arrector muscles of hairs

Eye (iris)

Cephalic arterial ramus

Carotid periarterial plexus

C1
C2
C3
C4
C5
C6
C7
C8

Cardiopulmonary splanchnic nerves

Heart

White ramus communicans

T1
T2
T3
T4
T5
T6
T7
T8
T9
T10
T11
T12

Larynx
Trachea
Bronchi
Lungs

Abdominopelvic splanchnic nerves

Liver
Gallbladder

Diaphragm

Gray rami to anterior primary rami of all spinal nerves for distribution to body walls and limbs (vasomotion, sudomotion, and pilomotion)

1
2
3

Celiac ganglion

Stomach
Pancreas
Spleen

L1
L2
L3
L4
L5

4

Aorticorenal ganglion

Superior mesenteric ganglion

S1
S2
S3
S4
S5

Inferior mesenteric ganglion

Large intestine
Small intestine
Kidney
Suprarenal (adrenal) gland
Rectum
Internal anal sphincter

Bladder
Penis (or clitoris)
Gonad

Sympathetic fibers
- - - - - Presynaptic
———— Postsynaptic

1 = Greater splanchnic nerve
2 = Lesser splanchnic nerve
3 = Least splanchnic nerve
4 = Lumbar splanchnic nerves

Figure I.41. The sympathetic (thoracolumbar) division of the ANS. Postsynaptic sympathetic fibers exit from the sympathetic trunks by different means, depending on their destination: Those destined for parietal distribution within the neck, body wall, and limbs pass from the sympathetic trunks to adjacent anterior rami of all spinal nerves through gray rami communicantes; those destined for the head pass from cervical ganglia by means of cephalic arterial rami to form a carotid periarterial plexus; and those destined for viscera of the thoracic cavity (e.g., the heart) pass through cardiopulmonary splanchnic nerves. Presynaptic sympathetic fibers involved in the innervation of viscera of the abdominopelvic cavity (e.g., the stomach) pass through the sympathetic trunks to the prevertebral ganglia by means of abdominopelvic splanchnic nerves. Postsynaptic fibers from the prevertebral ganglia form periarterial plexuses, which follow branches of the abdominal aorta to reach their destination.

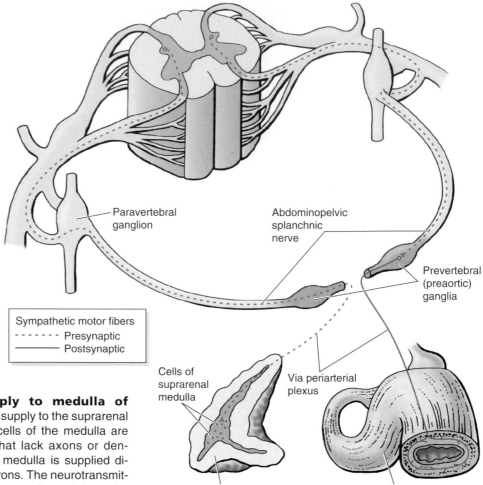

Figure I.42. Sympathetic supply to medulla of suprarenal gland. The sympathetic supply to the suprarenal gland is exceptional. The secretory cells of the medulla are postsynaptic sympathetic neurons that lack axons or dendrites. Consequently, the suprarenal medulla is supplied directly by presynaptic sympathetic neurons. The neurotransmitters produced by medullary cells are released into the bloodstream to produce a widespread sympathetic response.

Four discrete pairs of parasympathetic ganglia occur in the head (see Chapters 7 and 9). Elsewhere, presynaptic parasympathetic fibers synapse with postsynaptic cell bodies, which occur singly in or on the wall of the target organ (*intrinsic or enteric ganglia*). Consequently, in this division, most presynaptic fibers are very long, extending from the CNS to the effector organ, whereas the postsynaptic fibers are very short, running from a ganglion located near or embedded in the effector organ.

Functions of the Divisions of the ANS

Although both sympathetic and parasympathetic systems innervate involuntary (and often affect the same) structures, they have different, usually contrasting yet coordinated, effects (Figs. I.41 and I.43). In general, the sympathetic system is a **catabolic** (energy-expending) system that enables the body to deal with stresses, such as when preparing the body for the fight-or-flight response. The parasympathetic system is primarily a **homeostatic** or **anabolic** (energy-conserving) system, promoting the quiet and orderly processes of the body, such as those that allow the body to feed and assimilate.

Table I.2 summarizes the specific functions of the ANS and its divisions.

The primary function of the sympathetic system is to regulate blood vessels. This is accomplished by several means having different effects. Blood vessels throughout the body are tonically innervated by sympathetic nerves, maintaining a resting state of moderate vasoconstriction. In most vascular beds, an increase in sympathetic signals causes increased vasoconstriction, and a decrease in the rate of sympathetic signals allows vasodilation. However, in certain regions of the body, sympathetic signals are vasodilatory (i.e., sympathetic transmitter substances inhibit active vasoconstriction, allowing the blood vessels to be passively dilated by the blood pressure). In the coronary vessels, the vessels of skeletal muscles, and the external genitals, sympathetic stimulation results in vasodilation (Wilson-Pauwels et al., 1997).

Visceral Sensation

Visceral afferent fibers have important relationships to the ANS, both anatomically and functionally. We are usually unaware of the sensory input of these fibers, which provides

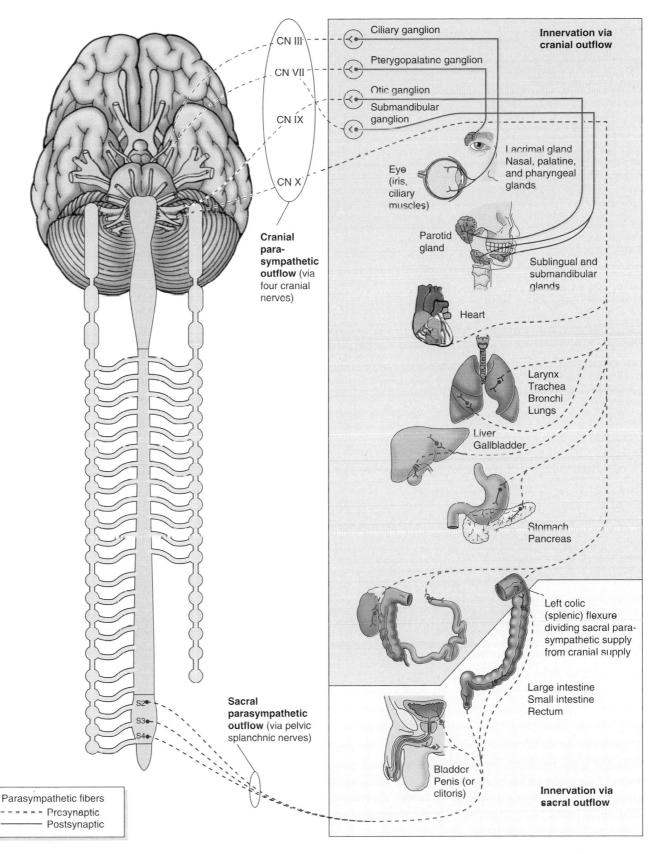

Figure I.43. Parasympathetic (craniosacral) division of the ANS. Presynaptic parasympathetic nerve cell bodies are located in opposite ends of the CNS and their fibers exit by two different routes: (1) in the gray matter of the brainstem, with fibers exiting the CNS within cranial nerves II, VII, IX, and X (these fibers constitute the cranial parasympathetic outflow), and (2) in the gray matter of the sacral (S2–4) segments of the spinal cord, with fibers exiting the CNS via the anterior roots of spinal nerves S2–4 and the pelvic splanchnic nerves that arise from their anterior rami (these fibers constitute the sacral parasympathetic outflow). The cranial outflow provides parasympathetic innervation of the head, neck, and most of the trunk; the sacral outflow provides the parasympathetic innervation of the pelvic viscera.

Table I.2. Functions of the Autonomic Nervous System (ANS)

Organ, Tract, or System		Effect of Sympathetic Stimulation[a]	Effect of Parasympathetic Stimulation[b]
Eyeballs	Pupil	Dilates pupil (admits more light for increased acuity at a distance)	Constricts pupil (protects pupil from excessively bright light)
	Ciliary body		Contracts ciliary muscle, allowing lens to thicken for near vision (accommodation)
Skin	Arrector muscle of hair	Causes hairs to stand on end (gooseflesh or goose bumps)	No effect (does not reach)[c]
	Peripheral blood vessels	Vasoconstricts (blanching of skin, lips, and turning fingertips blue)	No effect (does not reach)[c]
	Sweat glands	Promotes sweating[d]	No effect (does not reach)[c]
Other glands	Lacrimal glands	Slightly decreases secretion[e]	Promotes secretion
	Salivary glands	Secretion decreases, becomes thicker, more viscous[e]	Promotes abundant, watery secretion
Heart		Increases rate and strength of contraction; inhibits effect of parasympathetic system on coronary vessels, allowing them to dilate[e]	Decreases the rate and strength of contraction (conserving energy); constricts coronary vessels in relation to reduced demand
Lungs		Inhibits effect of parasympathetic system, resulting in bronchodilation and reduced secretion, allowing for maximum air exchange	Constricts bronchi (conserving energy) and promotes bronchial secretion
Digestive tract		Inhibits peristalsis and constricts blood vessels to digestive tract so that blood is available to skeletal muscle; contracts internal anal sphincter to aid fecal continence	Stimulates peristalsis and secretion of digestive juices; contracts rectum; inhibits internal anal sphincter to cause defecation
Liver and gallbladder		Promotes breakdown of glycogen to glucose (for increased energy)	Promotes building/conservation of glycogen; increases secretion of bile
Urinary tract		Vasoconstriction of renal vessels slows urine formation; internal sphincter of bladder contracted to maintain urinary continence	Inhibits contraction of internal sphincter of bladder; contracts detrusor muscle of bladder wall causing urination
Genital system		Causes ejaculation and vasoconstriction resulting in remission of erection	Produces engorgement (erection) of erectile tissues of external genitals
Suprarenal medulla		Release of adrenaline into blood	No effect (does not innervate)

[a] In general, the effects of sympathetic stimulation are catabolic, preparing body for the fight-or-flight response.
[b] In general, the effects of parasympathetic stimulation are anabolic, promoting normal function and conserving energy.
[c] The parasympathetic system is restricted in its distribution to the head, neck, and body cavities (except for erectile tissues of genitalia); otherwise, parasympathetic fibers are never found in the body wall and limbs. Sympathetic fibers, by comparison, are distributed to all vascularized portions of the body.
[d] With the exception of the sweat glands, glandular secretion is parasympathetically stimulated.
[e] With the exception of the coronary arteries, vasoconstriction is sympathetically stimulated; the effects of sympathetic stimulation on glands (other than sweat glands) are the indirect effects of vasoconstriction.

information about the condition of the body's internal environment. This information is integrated in the CNS, often triggering visceral or somatic reflexes or both. Visceral reflexes regulate blood pressure and chemistry by altering such functions as heart and respiratory rates and vascular resistance.

Visceral sensation that reaches a conscious level is generally perceived as pain that is either poorly localized or felt as cramps or that may convey a feeling of hunger, fullness, or nausea. Surgeons operating on patients who are under local anesthesia may handle, cut, clamp, or even burn (cauterize) visceral organs without evoking conscious sensation. However, adequate stimulation, such as the following, may elicit true pain:

- Sudden distension.

- Spasms or strong contractions.

- Chemical irritants.

- Mechanical stimulation, especially when the organ is active.

- Pathological conditions (especially ischemia) that lower the normal thresholds of stimulation.

Normal activity usually produces no sensation but may do so when the blood supply is inadequate (ischemia). Most visceral reflex (unconscious) sensation and some pain travel in visceral afferent fibers that accompany the parasympathetic fibers retrograde. Most visceral pain impulses (from the heart and most organs of the peritoneal cavity) travel centrally along visceral afferent fibers accompanying sympathetic fibers.

THE BOTTOM LINE: The autonomic nervous system is a subdivision of the motor nervous system that controls functions of the body not under conscious control. Two neurons, a presynaptic and a postsynaptic fiber, connect the CNS with an end organ, consisting of smooth muscle, gland, or modified cardiac muscle. Based on the location of the cell body of the presynaptic fibers, the ANS can be subdivided into two divisions: the sympathetic and parasympathetic. Presynaptic cell bodies of the sympathetic division are found only in the intermediolateral cell columns of gray matter in the thoracolumbar spinal cord, which are organized somatotopically. The presynaptic sympathetic nerve fibers terminate in sympathetic ganglia formed of the cell bodies of postsynaptic sympathetic neurons. Sympathetic ganglia occur in the sympathetic trunks (paravertebral ganglia) or around the roots of the major branches of the abdominal aorta (prevertebral ganglia). Cell bodies of the presynaptic neurons of the parasympathetic division are located in the gray matter of the brainstem and sacral segments of the spinal cord. Cell bodies of postsynaptic parasympathetic neurons of the trunk are located in or on the structure being innervated, whereas those in the head are organized into discrete ganglia. The sympathetic and parasympathetic divisions usually have opposite but coordinated effects. The sympathetic system facilitates emergency (flight-or-fight) responses. The parasympathetic system—distributed only to the viscera of the head, neck, and cavities of the trunk and the erectile tissues of the genitalia—is primarily concerned with body conservation, often reversing the effects of sympathetic stimulation. Some nerves distributing autonomic fibers ANS to the body cavities also convey visceral sensory fibers carrying impulses for pain or reflexes.

Medical Imaging Techniques

Radiological anatomy is the study of the structure and function of the body using medical imaging techniques. It has become an important part of anatomy and is the anatomical basis of radiology, the branch of medical science dealing with the use of radiant energy in the diagnosis and treatment of disease. Being able to identify normal structures on radiographs (X-rays) makes it easier to recognize the changes caused by disease and injury. Familiarity with medical imaging techniques commonly used in clinical settings enables one to recognize congenital anomalies, tumors, and fractures. The most commonly used medical imaging techniques are

- Conventional radiography (ordinary X-ray images).

- Computerized tomography (CT).

- Ultrasonography (US).

- Magnetic resonance imaging (MRI).

- Nuclear medicine imaging.

Although the techniques differ, each is based on the receipt of attenuated beams of energy that have been passed through, reflected off of, or generated by the body's tissues. Learn to interpret medical images. Along with surface anatomy, they are the only views of a person's anatomy that are commonly available after completion of the gross anatomy course. Medical imaging techniques permit the observation of anatomical structures in living people and the study of their movements in normal and abnormal activities (e.g., the heart and stomach).

Conventional Radiography

Wilhelm Roentgen, a German physicist and Nobel laureate, discovered X-rays in 1895. His discovery enabled observation of the living structure of the human skeletal system, readily visualized on radiographs (roentgenograms). A conventional radiograph, in which special techniques such as contrast media have not been used, is referred to clinically as a *plain film* (Fig. I.44). In a radiological examination, a highly penetrating beam of X-rays transilluminates the patient, showing tissues of differing densities of mass within the body as images of differing intensities (areas of relative light and dark) on the film or monitor (Fig. I.45). A tissue or organ that is relatively dense in mass (e.g., compact bone) absorbs or reflects more X-rays than does a less dense tissue (e.g., spongy bone). Consequently, a dense tissue or organ produces a somewhat transparent area on the X-ray film because fewer X-rays reach the film or detector. Therefore, relatively fewer grains of silver are developed at this area when the film is processed. A dense substance is *radiopaque,* whereas a substance of less density is *radiolucent.*

Many of the same principles that apply to making a shadow apply to conventional radiography. When making a shadow of your hand on a wall, the closer your hand is to the wall, the sharper the shadow produced. The farther your hand is from the wall (and therefore the closer to ▶

Trachea

1st rib

Superior vena cava

Rib

Right atrium

Right dome of diaphragm

Clavicle

Coracoid process of scapula

Arch of aorta

Pulmonary artery

Left auricle

Left ventricle

Apex of heart

Figure I.44. Radiograph of thorax (chest). AP view of a PA projection radiograph demonstrates the arch of the aorta, parts of the heart, and domes of the diaphragm. Note that the dome of the diaphragm is higher on the right side. (Courtesy of Dr. E. L. Lansdown, Professor of Medical Imaging, University of Toronto, Toronto, ON, Canada.)

light source), the more the shadow is magnified. Radiographs are made with the part of the patient's body being studied close to the X-ray film or detector to maximize the clarity of the image and minimize magnification artifacts. In basic radiological nomenclature, *posteroanterior* (*PA*) *projection* refers to a radiograph in which the X-rays traversed the patient from posterior (P) to anterior (A); the X-ray tube was posterior to the patient and the X-ray film was anterior (Fig. I.46*A*). A radiograph using *anteroposterior* (*AP*) *projection* radiography is the opposite. Both PA and AP projection radiographs are viewed as if you and the patient were facing each other (the patient's right side is opposite your left); this is referred to as an *anteroposterior* (*AP*) *view.* (Thus the standard chest X-ray, taken to examine the heart and lungs, is an AP view of a PA projection.) For lateral radiographs, radiopaque letters (R or L) are used to indicate the side placed closest to the film or detector, and the image is viewed from the same direction that the beam was projected (Fig. I.46*B*).

The introduction of contrast media (radiopaque fluids such as iodine compounds or barium) allows the study of various luminal or vascular organs and potential or actual spaces—such as the digestive tract, blood vessels, kidneys, synovial cavities, and the subarachnoid space—that are not visible in plain films (Fig. I.47). Most radiological examinations are performed in at least two projections at right angles to each other. Because each radiograph presents a two-dimensional representation of a three-dimensional structure, structures sequentially penetrated by the X-ray beam overlap each other. Thus more than one view is usually necessary to detect and localize an abnormality accurately.

Computerized Tomography

In computerized tomography, the scans show radiographic images of the body that resemble transverse anatomical sections (Fig. I.48). In this technique, a beam of X-rays passes through the body as the X-ray tube and detector ▶

Figure I.45. Principles of X-ray image formation. Portions of the beam of X-rays traversing the body become attenuated to varying degrees based on tissue thickness and density. The beam is diminished by structures that absorb or reflect it, causing less reaction on the film or by the detector, compared with areas that allow the beam to pass relatively uninterrupted.

Figure I.46. Orientation of patient's thorax during radiography. A. When taking a PA projection, the X-rays from the X-ray tube pass through the thorax from the back to reach the X-ray film or detector anterior to the person. **B.** When taking a lateral projection, the X-rays pass through the thorax from the side to reach the X-ray film adjacent to the person's other side.

rotate around the axis of the body. Multiple overlapping radial energy absorptions are measured, recorded, and compared by a computer to determine the radiodensity of each volume element (*voxel*) of the chosen body plane. The radiodensity of (amount of radiation absorbed by) each voxel is determined by factors that include the amount of air, water, fat, or bone in that element. The computer maps the voxels into a planar image (slice) that is displayed on a monitor or printout. CT images relate well to conventional radiographs, in that areas of great absorption (e.g., bone) are relatively transparent (white) and those with little absorption are black (Fig. I.48). CT scans are always displayed as if the viewer were standing at a supine patient's feet.

Ultrasonography

Ultrasonography or sonography is a technique that visualizes superficial or deep structures in the body by recording pulses of ultrasonic waves reflecting off the tissues (Fig. I.49). Ultrasonography has the advantage of a lower cost than CT and MRI, and the machine is portable. The technique can be performed virtually anywhere, including the clinic examination room, bedside, or on the operating table. A transducer in contact with the skin generates high-frequency soundwaves that pass through the body and reflect off tissue interfaces between tissues of differing characteristics, such as soft tissue and bone. Echoes from the body reflect into the transducer and convert to electrical energy. The electrical signals are recorded and displayed on a monitor as a cross-sectional image, which can be viewed in real time and recorded as a single image or on videotape.

A major advantage of ultrasonography is its ability to produce real-time images, demonstrating motion of structures and flow within blood vessels. In *Doppler ultrasonography*, the shifts in frequency between emitted ultrasonic waves and their echoes are used to measure the velocities of moving objects. This technique is based on the principle of the *Doppler effect*. Blood flow through vessels is displayed in color, superimposed on the two-dimensional cross-sectional image.

Scanning of the pelvic viscera from the surface of the abdomen requires a fully distended bladder. The urine serves as an "acoustical window," transmitting soundwaves to and from the posteriorly placed pelvic viscera with minimal attenuation. The distended bladder also displaces gas-filled intestinal loops out of the pelvis. *Transvaginal sonography* permits the positioning of the transducer closer to the organ of interest (e.g., the ovary) and avoids fat and gas, which absorb or reflect soundwaves. Bone reflects nearly all ultrasound waves, whereas air conducts them poorly. Consequently, the CNS and lungs of adults cannot be examined by ultrasonography. ▶

Gallbladder

Duodenal cap

Pylorus of stomach

Pyloric antrum of
stomach

Jejunum

Fundus of stomach

Peristaltic wave

Rugae

Greater curvature

Figure I.47. Radiograph of stomach, small intestine, and gallbladder. Observe the gastric folds, or rugae (longitudinal folds of the mucous membrane). Also note the peristaltic wave that is moving the gastric contents toward the duodenum, which is closely related to the gallbladder. (Courtesy of Dr. J. Heslin, Toronto, ON, Canada.)

The appeal of ultrasonography in obstetrics is that it is a non-invasive procedure that does not use radiation; it can yield useful information about the pregnancy, such as determining whether it is intrauterine or extrauterine (ectopic) and whether the embryo is living. It has also become a standard method of evaluating the growth and development of the embryo and fetus.

Magnetic Resonance Imaging

Magnetic resonance imaging provides images of the body similar to those of CT scans, but MRI is better for tissue differentiation. MRI studies closely resemble anatomical sections, especially in the brain (Fig. I.50). The person is placed in a scanner with a strong magnetic field, and the body is pulsed with radiowaves. Signals subsequently emitted from the patient's tissues are stored in a computer and reconstructed into various images of the body. The appearance of tissues on the generated images can be varied by controlling how radiofrequency pulses are sent and received.

Free protons in the tissues that become aligned by the surrounding magnetic field are excited (flipped) with a radiowave pulse. As the protons flip back, minute but measurable energy signals are emitted. Tissues that are high in proton density, such as fat and water, emit more signals than tissues that are low in proton density. The tissue signal is based primarily on three properties of protons in a particular region of the body. These are referred to as T1 relaxation, T2 relaxation, and proton density. Although liquids have a high density of free protons, the excited free protons in moving fluids such as blood tend to move out of the field before they flip and give off their signal and are replaced by unexcited protons. Consequently, moving fluids appear black.

Computers associated with MRI scanners have the capacity to reconstruct tissues in any plane from the data acquired: transverse, median, sagittal, frontal, and even arbitrary oblique planes. The data may also be used to generate three-dimensional reconstructions. MRI scanners produce good images of soft tissues without the use of ionizing radiation. Motion made by the patient during long ▶

X-ray tube

Head of pancreas

Stomach

Descending
part of
duodenum

Body of
pancreas

Left colic
flexure

Portal
vein

Splenic artery

Celiac trunk

Liver

Inferior
vena cava

Abdominal
aorta

Spleen

Detectors

Diaphragm
(right crus)

Tail of
pancreas

Right kidney

Diaphragm
(left crus)

Left suprarenal
gland

Left kidney

CT image of the upper abdomen

Figure I.48. Technique for producing an abdominal CT scan. The X-ray tube rotates around the person in the CT scanner and sends a fan-shaped beam of X-rays through the upper abdomen from a variety of angles. X-ray detectors on the opposite side of the body measure the amount of radiation that passes through a horizontal section. A computer reconstructs the images from several scans, and an abdominal CT scan is produced. The scan is oriented so it appears the way an examiner would view it when standing at the foot of the bed and looking toward a supine person's head.

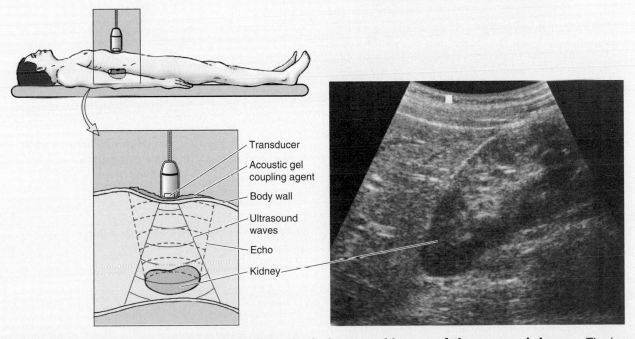

Transducer

Acoustic gel
coupling agent

Body wall

Ultrasound
waves

Echo

Kidney

Figure I.49. Technique for producing an abdominal ultrasound image of the upper abdomen. The image results from the echo of ultrasound waves from abdominal structures of different densities. The ultrasound image of the right kidney is displayed on a monitor.

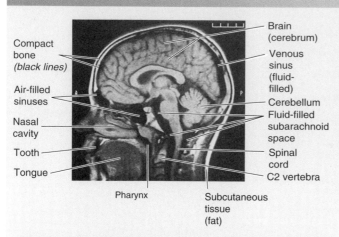

Compact bone *(black lines)*
Air-filled sinuses
Nasal cavity
Tooth
Tongue
Pharynx

Brain (cerebrum)
Venous sinus (fluid-filled)
Cerebellum
Fluid-filled subarachnoid space
Spinal cord
C2 vertebra
Subcutaneous tissue (fat)

Figure I.50. Median MRI of the head. Many details of the CNS and structures in the nasal and oral cavities and upper neck are seen in this study. The black low signal areas superior to the anterior and posterior aspects of the nasal cavity are the air-filled frontal and sphenoidal sinuses.

scanning sessions created problems for early-generation scanners, but fast scanners now in use can be gated or paced to visualize moving structures, such as the heart and blood flow, in real time.

Nuclear Medicine Imaging

Nuclear medicine imaging techniques provide information about the distribution or concentration of trace amounts of radioactive substances introduced into the body. Nuclear medicine scans show images of specific organs after intravenous (I.V.) injection of a small dose of radioactive material. The radionuclide is tagged to a compound that is selectively taken up by an organ, such as technetium-99m methylene diphosphonate (^{99m}Tc-MDP) for bone scanning (Fig. I.51).

Positron emission tomography (PET) scanning uses cyclotron-produced isotopes of extremely short half-life that emit positrons. PET scanning is used to evaluate the physiological function of organs, such as the brain, on a

dynamic basis. Areas of increased brain activity will show selective uptake of the injected isotope. Images can be viewed as the whole organ or in cross sections, which are referred to as single-photon emission computerized tomography (SPECT) scans. ✪

Figure I.51. Bone scans of the head and neck, thorax, and pelvis. These nuclear medicine images can be viewed as a whole or in cross section.

THE BOTTOM LINE: Medical imaging techniques enable the visualization of normal anatomy in the living. This allows us to view structures with their normal tonus, fluid volumes, internal pressures, etc., which are not present in the cadaver. The primary goal of medical imaging is, of course, to detect pathology. However, a sound knowledge of radiological anatomy is required to distinguish pathologies and abnormalities from normal anatomy.

References and Suggested Readings

Amadio PC: Reaffirming the importance of dissection. *Clin Anat* 9:136, 1996.

Behrman RE, Kliegman RM, Jenson HB (eds): *Nelson Textbook of Pediatrics,* 17th ed. Philadelphia, Saunders, 2004.

Bergman RA, Thompson SA, Afifi AK, Saadeh FA: *Compendium of Human Anatomic Variation: Text, Atlas, and World Literature.* Baltimore, Urban & Schwarzenberg, 1988.

This useful source has been updated and is available from the Virtual Hospital's Web site *Illustrated Encyclopedia of Human Anatomic Variation* at www.vh.org/Providers/Textbooks/ AnatomicVariants/AnatomyHP.html (accessed May 2004).

Cahill DR, Leonard RJ: The role of computers and dissection in teaching anatomy: A comment. *Clin Anat* 10:140, 1997.

Cormack DH: *Essential Histology,* 2nd ed. Baltimore, Lippincott Williams & Wilkins, 2001.

Cotran RS, Kumar V, Collins T: *Robbin's Pathologic Basis of Disease,* 6th ed. Philadelphia, Saunders, 1999.

Federative Committee on Anatomical Terminology: *Terminologia Anatomica: International Anatomical Nomenclature.* Stuttgart, Thieme, 1998.

Gartner LP, Hiatt JL: *Color Textbook of Histology,* 2nd ed. Philadelphia, Saunders, 2001.

Haines DE (ed): *Fundamental Neuroscience,* 2nd ed. New York, Churchill Livingstone, 2002.

Hutchins JB, Naftel JP, Ard MD: The cell biology of neurons and glia. *In* Haines DE (ed): *Fundamental Neuroscience,* 2nd ed. New York, Churchill Livingstone, 2002.

Keegan JJ, Garrett FD: The segmental distribution of the cutaneous nerves in the limbs of man. *Anat Rec* 102:409, 1948.

Maklad A, Quinn T, Fritsch B: Intracranial distribution of the sympathetic system in mice: DiI tracing and immunocytochemical labeling. *Anat Rec* 263:99, 2001.

Marieb, E: *Human Anatomy and Physiology,* 6th ed. Menlo Park, CA, Benjamin/Cummings, 2004.

Mehta LA, Natrajan M, Korhari ML: Understanding anatomical terms. *Clin Anat* 9:330, 1996.

Moore KL, Persaud TVN: *The Developing Human: Clinically Oriented Embryology,* 7th ed. Philadelphia, Saunders, 2003.

Mutyala S, Cahill DR: Catching up. *Clin Anat* 9:53, 1996.

O'Rahilly R: Making planes plain. *Clin Anat* 10:129, 1997.

Persaud TVN: *Early History of Human Anatomy from Antiquity to the Beginning of the Modern Era.* Springfield, IL, Thomas, 1984.

Persaud TVN: *A History of Anatomy. The Post-Vesalian Era.* Springfield, IL, Thomas, 1997.

Ross MH, Kaye G, Pawlina W: *Histology. A Text and Atlas,* 4th ed. Baltimore, Lippincott Williams & Wilkins, 2003.

Salter RB: *Textbook of Disorders and Injuries of the Musculoskeletal System,* 3rd ed. Baltimore, Lippincott Williams & Wilkins, 1998.

Stedman's Medical Dictionary, 28th ed. Baltimore, Lippincott Williams & Wilkins, 2005.

Swartz MH: *Textbook of Physical Diagnosis, History and Examination,* 4th ed. Philadelphia, Saunders, 2001.

Willis MC: *Medical Terminology: The Language of Health Care.* Baltimore, Lippincott Williams & Wilkins, 1995.

Wilson-Pauwels L, Stewart PA, Akesson E: *Autonomic Nerves: Basic Science, Clinical Aspects, Case Studies.* Hamilton, ON, Decker, 1997.

1 Thorax

he **thorax** is the superior part of the trunk between the neck and abdomen. Commonly the term *chest* is used as a synonym for *thorax,* but our concept of the chest (upper part of the torso) is much more extensive than the thoracic wall and cavity contained within it. The **chest** is generally conceived as being broadest superiorly owing to the presence of the *pectoral,* or *shoulder, girdle* (clavicles and scapulae), with much of its girth accounted for by the associated pectoral and scapular (upper limb) musculature. Our concept of the well-formed chest is one that narrows inferiorly to the waist and, in adult females, gains further dimension from the breasts.

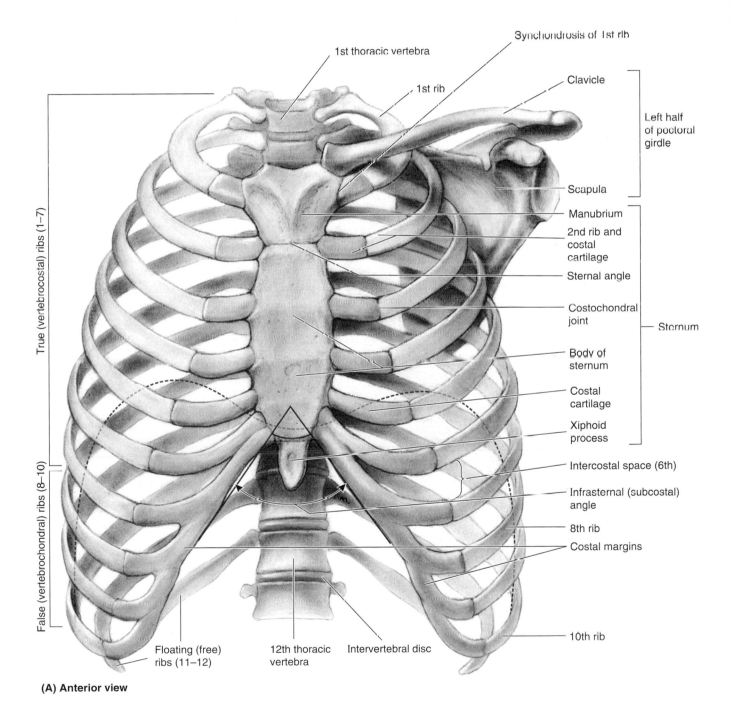

(A) Anterior view

Figure 1.1. Thoracic skeleton. A and B. The osteocartilaginous thoracic cage includes the sternum, 12 pairs of ribs and costal cartilages, and 12 thoracic vertebrae and intervertebral discs. The clavicles and scapulae form the pectoral (shoulder) girdle. The dotted line indicates the position of the diaphragm, which separates the thoracic and abdominal cavities. The thoracic cavity is much smaller than the surrounding thoracic cage.

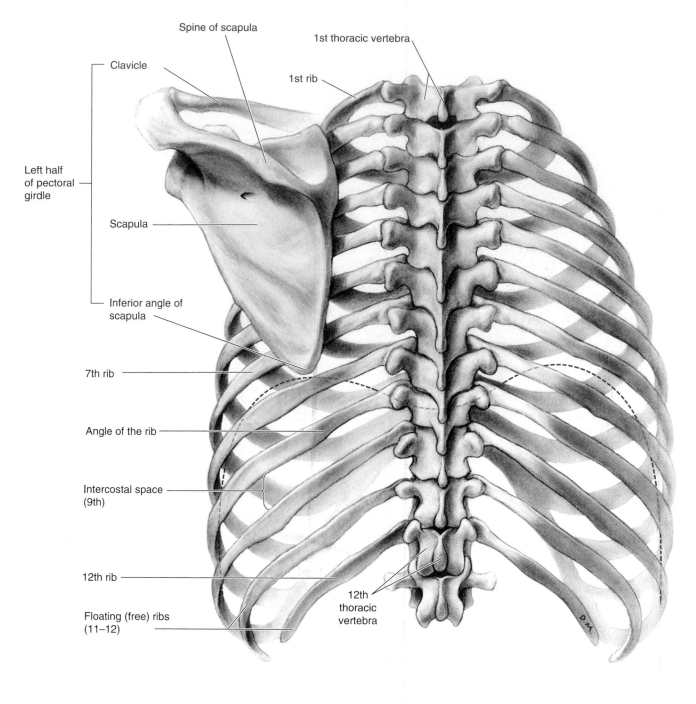

Spine of scapula

1st thoracic vertebra

Clavicle

1st rib

Left half
of pectoral
girdle

Scapula

Inferior angle of
scapula

7th rib

Angle of the rib

Intercostal space
(9th)

12th rib

12th
thoracic
vertebra

Floating (free) ribs
(11–12)

(B) Posterior view

Figure 1.1. *(Continued)*

The **thoracic cavity** and the wall specific to it are actually the opposite of this. They have the shape of a truncated cone, being narrowest superiorly, with the circumference increasing inferiorly, and reaching its maximum at the junction with the abdominal portion of the trunk. The wall of the thoracic cavity is relatively thin, essentially as thick as its skeleton. The thoracic skeleton takes the form of a domed birdcage, the **thoracic cage** (rib cage), with the horizontal bars formed by ribs and costal cartilages supported by the vertical sternum (breastbone) and thoracic vertebrae (Fig. 1.1). Furthermore, the floor of the thoracic cavity (the diaphragm) is deeply invaginated inferiorly (i.e., is pushed upward) by viscera of the abdominal cavity. Consequently, nearly the lower half of the thoracic wall surrounds and protects abdominal rather than thoracic viscera. Thus the true thorax and especially the thoracic cavity are much smaller than one might expect based on external appearances of the chest.

The thorax includes the primary organs of the respiratory and cardiovascular systems. The thoracic cavity is divided into three major spaces: The central compartment, or *mediastinum,* houses the conducting structures that make up the thoracic viscera, except for the lungs. The *lungs* occupy the lateral compartments or *pulmonary cavities* that lie on each side of the mediastinum. Thus the majority of the thoracic cavity is occupied by the lungs, which provide for the exchange of oxygen and carbon dioxide between air and blood, whereas most of the remainder of the thoracic cavity is occupied with structures involved in conducting the air and blood to and from the lungs. Nutrients (food) traverse the thoracic cavity via the esophagus, passing from the intake organ (mouth) to the site of digestion and absorption (abdomen).

Although in terms of function and development the mammary glands are most related to the reproductive system, the breasts are located on the thoracic wall and thus are included in this chapter.

Chest Pain

Although chest pain can result from pulmonary disease, it is probably the most important symptom of cardiac disease (Swartz, 2002). However, chest pain may also occur in intestinal, gallbladder, and musculoskeletal disorders. When evaluating a patient with chest pain, the examination is largely concerned with discriminating between serious conditions and the many minor causes of pain. People who have had a *heart attack* usually describe the associated pain as a "crushing" substernal pain (deep to the sternum) that does not disappear with rest. ⊕

THE BOTTOM LINE: The thorax, consisting of the thoracic cavity, its contents, and the wall that surrounds it, is the part of the trunk between neck and abdomen. The shape and size of the thoracic cavity and the wall specific to it are much different from (especially smaller than) that of the chest (upper torso), because the latter includes some upper limb bones and muscles and, in adult females, the breasts.

Thoracic Wall

The true **thoracic wall** includes the thoracic cage and the muscles that extend between its elements as well as the skin, subcutaneous tissue, muscles, and fascia covering its anterolateral aspect; the same structures covering its posterior aspect are considered to belong to the back. The mammary glands of the breasts lie within the subcutaneous tissue of

the thoracic wall. Although the shoulders are clearly part of the upper limb, the anterolateral thoracoappendicular muscles (see Chapter 6) that overlie the thoracic cage and form the bed of the breast (pectoralis major and serratus anterior—distinctly upper limb muscles based on function and innervation) are encountered in the thoracic wall and may be considered part of it (but will be mentioned only briefly here). Similar thoracoappendicular muscles placed posteriorly (trapezius and latissimus dorsi) have commonly been considered to be superficial muscles of the back, although in terms of function they are clearly upper limb muscles (and are also covered in Chapter 6).

The domed shape of the thoracic cage provides remarkable rigidity, given the light weight of its components, enabling it to:

* Protect vital thoracic and abdominal internal organs (most air or fluid filled) from external forces
* Resist the negative (sub-atmospheric) internal pressures generated by the elastic recoil of the lungs and inspiratory movements.
* Provide attachment for and support the weight of the upper limbs.
* Provide the anchoring attachment (origin) of many of the muscles that move and maintain the position of the upper limbs relative to the trunk as well as provide the attachments for muscles of the abdomen, neck, back, and respiration.

Although the shape of the thoracic cage provides rigidity, its joints and the thinness and flexibility of the ribs allow remarkable flexibility, permitting it to absorb many external blows and compressions without fracture and to change its shape repetitively and sufficiently as required for respiration. Because the most important structures within the thorax (heart, great vessels, lungs, and trachea) as well as its floor and walls are constantly in motion, the thorax is one of the most dynamic regions of the body. With each breath, the muscles of the thoracic wall—working in concert with the diaphragm and muscles of the abdominal wall—vary the volume of the thoracic cavity, first by expanding the capacity of the cavity, thereby causing the lungs to expand and draw air in and then (mostly owing to lung elasticity and muscle relaxation) decreasing the volume of the cavity, compressing the lungs, and causing them to expel air.

Skeleton of the Thoracic Wall

The **thoracic skeleton** forms the osteocartilaginous *thoracic cage* (Fig. 1.1), which protects the thoracic viscera and some abdominal organs. The thoracic skeleton includes 12 pairs of ribs and associated costal cartilages, 12 thoracic vertebrae and the intervertebral (IV) discs interposed between them, and the sternum. The ribs and costal cartilages form the largest part of the thoracic cage.

Ribs, Costal Cartilages, and Intercostal Spaces

Ribs (L. *costae*) are curved, flat bones that form most of the thoracic cage (Figs. 1.1 and 1.2). They are remarkably light in weight yet highly resilient. Each rib has a spongy interior containing *bone marrow* (hematopoietic tissue), which forms blood cells. There are three types of rib:

- **True (vertebrocostal) ribs** (1st–7th ribs): They attach directly to the sternum through their own costal cartilages.

- **False (vertebrochondral) ribs** (8th, 9th, and usually 10th ribs): Their cartilages are connected to the cartilage of the rib above them; thus their connection with the sternum is indirect.

- **Floating (vertebral, free) ribs** (11th, 12th, and sometimes 10th ribs): The rudimentary cartilages of these ribs do not connect even indirectly with the sternum; instead they end in the posterior abdominal musculature.

Typical ribs (3rd–9th) have the following components:

- **Head:** wedge-shaped and has two facets, separated by the **crest of the head** (Figs. 1.2 and 1.3); one facet for articulation with the numerically corresponding vertebra and one facet for the vertebra superior to it.

- **Neck:** connects the head with the body at the level of the tubercle.

- **Tubercle:** at the junction of the neck and body and has a smooth *articular part,* for articulating with the corresponding transverse process of the vertebra, and a rough *non-articular part,* for attachment of the costotransverse ligament.

- **Body** (shaft): thin, flat, and curved, most markedly at the **costal angle** where the rib turns anterolaterally (also the point of the lateral limit of attachment of the erector spinae muscles to the ribs; see Chapter 4); the concave internal surface of the body has a **costal groove** paralleling the inferior border of the rib, which provides some protection for the intercostal nerve and vessels.

Atypical ribs (1st, 2nd, and 10th–12th) are dissimilar (Fig. 1.3):

- The *1st rib* is the broadest (i.e., its body is widest and nearly horizontal), shortest, and most sharply curved of the seven true ribs. It has a single facet on its head for articulation with the T1 vertebra only and two transversely directed grooves crossing its superior surface for the subclavian vessels; the grooves are separated by a **scalene tubercle** and ridge, to which the anterior scalene muscle is attached.

- The *2nd rib* is more typical; its body is thinner, less curved, and substantially longer than the 1st rib, and its head has two facets for articulation with the bodies of the T1 and T2 vertebrae; its main atypical feature is a rough area on its upper surface, the **tuberosity for serratus anterior,** from which part of that muscle originates.

- The *10th–12th ribs,* like the 1st rib, have only one facet on their heads and articulate with a single vertebra.

- The *11th and 12th ribs* are short and have no neck or tubercle.

Costal cartilages prolong the ribs anteriorly and contribute to the elasticity of the thoracic wall, providing a flexible attachment for their anterior or distal ends (tips). The cartilages increase in length through the first 7 and then gradually decrease. The first 7 cartilages (and sometimes the 8th; Fig. 1.16) attach directly and independently to the sternum; the 8th, 9th, and 10th articulate with the costal cartilages just superior to them, forming a continuous, articulated, cartilaginous *costal margin* (Fig. 1.1A). The 11th and 12th cartilages form caps on the anterior ends of these ribs and do not reach or attach to any other bone or cartilage. The costal

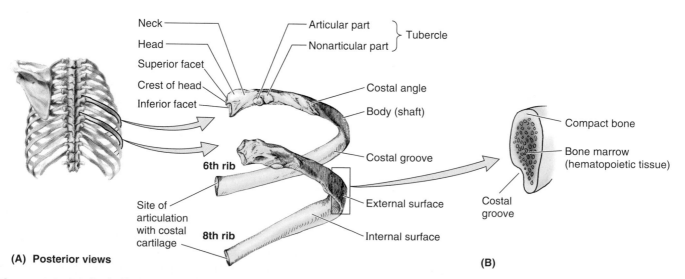

(A) Posterior views

(B)

Figure 1.2. Typical ribs. A. The 3rd–9th ribs have common characteristics. Each rib has a head, neck, tubercle, and body (shaft). **B.** Cross section of a rib at midbody.

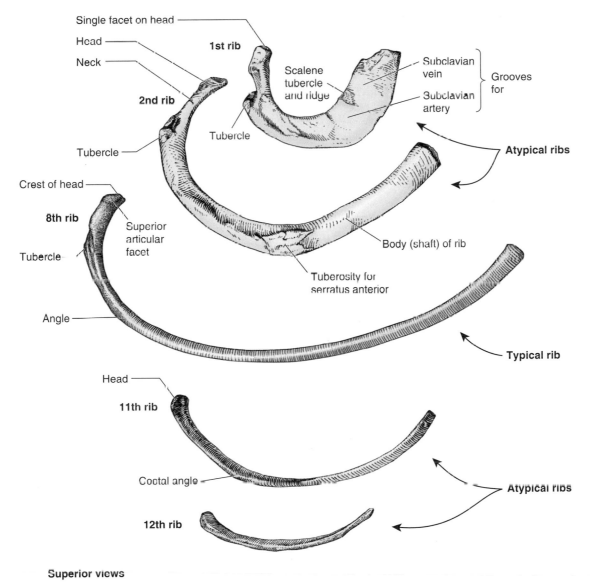

Single facet on head

Head

Neck

1st rib

2nd rib

Scalene
tubercle
and ridge

Tubercle

Subclavian
vein

Subclavian
artery

Grooves
for

Atypical ribs

Tubercle

Crest of head

8th rib

Superior
articular
facet

Tubercle

Body (shaft) of rib

Angle

Tuberosity for
serratus anterior

Typical rib

Head

11th rib

Costal angle

Atypical ribs

12th rib

Superior views

Figure 1.3. Atypical ribs. The atypical 1st, 2nd, 11th, and 12th ribs differ from typical ribs (e.g., the 8th rib, shown in center). The 1st rib is short and flattened and the tubercle merges with the angle. The body of the 2nd rib bears a tuberosity for attachment of the serratus anterior. The 11th and 12th ribs lack a neck and tubercle, and the 12th rib is shorter than most ribs.

cartilages of ribs 1–10 clearly anchor the anterior end (tips) of the rib to the sternum, limiting its overall movement as the posterior end rotates around the transverse axis of the rib (Fig. 1.5).

   Intercostal spaces separate the ribs and their costal cartilages from one another (Fig. 1.1*A*). The spaces are named according to the rib forming the superior border of the space— for example, the 4th intercostal space lies between rib 4 and rib 5. There are 11 intercostal spaces and 11 intercostal nerves. Intercostal spaces are occupied by intercostal muscles and membranes, and two sets (main and collateral) of intercostal blood vessels and nerves, identified by the same number assigned to the space. The space below the 12th rib does not lie between ribs and thus is referred to as the **subcostal**

space, and the anterior ramus of spinal nerve T12 is the subcostal nerve. The intercostal spaces are widest anterolaterally, and they widen with inspiration. They can be further widened by extension and/or lateral flexion of the thoracic vertebral column to the contralateral side.

Rib Fractures

The short, broad 1st rib, posteroinferior to the clavicle, is rarely fractured because of its protected position (it cannot be palpated). When it is broken, however, injury to the brachial plexus of nerves and subclavian ▶

vessels may occur. The middle ribs are most commonly fractured. *Rib fractures* usually result from blows or from crushing injuries. The weakest part of a rib is just anterior to its angle; however, direct violence may fracture a rib anywhere, and its broken end may injure internal organs such as a lung and/or the spleen. *Lower rib fractures* may tear the diaphragm and result in a *diaphragmatic hernia* (see Chapter 2). Rib fractures are painful because the broken parts move during respiration, coughing, laughing, and sneezing.

Flail Chest

Multiple rib fractures may allow a sizable segment of the anterior and/or lateral thoracic wall to move freely. The loose segment of the wall moves paradoxically (inward on inspiration and outward on expiration). *Flail chest* (stove-in chest) is an extremely painful injury and impairs ventilation, thereby affecting oxygenation of the blood. During treatment, the loose segment is often fixed by hooks and/or wires so that it cannot move.

Thoracotomy, Intercostal Space Incisions, Rib Excision, and Bone Grafting

The surgical creation of an opening through the thoracic wall to enter a pleural cavity is a *thoracotomy* (Fig. B1.1). ▶

Figure B1.1

An *anterior thoracotomy* may involve making H-shaped cuts through the perichondrium of one or more costal cartilages and then shelling out segments of costal cartilage to gain entrance to the thoracic cavity (Fig 1.16). The posterolateral aspects of the 5th–7th intercostal spaces are important sites for *posterior thoracotomy* incisions. In general, a lateral approach is most satisfactory for entry into the thoracic cage. With the patient lying on the contralateral side, the upper limb is fully abducted, placing the forearm behind the patient's head. This elevates and laterally rotates the inferior angle of scapula, allowing access as high as the 4th intercostal space. Surgeons use an H-shaped incision to incise the superficial aspect of the periosteum that ensheaths the rib, strip the periosteum from the rib, and then remove a wide segment of the rib to gain better access, as might be required to enter the thoracic cavity and remove a lung (*pneumonectomy*), for example. In the rib's absence, entry into the thoracic cavity can be made through the deep aspect of the periosteal sheath, sparing the adjacent intercostal muscles. After the operation, the missing pieces of ribs regenerate from the intact periosteum, although imperfectly. Sometimes surgeons use a piece of rib so removed for autogenous bone grafting in procedures such as reconstruction of the mandible (lower jaw) after tumor excision.

Supernumerary Ribs

People usually have 12 ribs on each side, but the number is increased by the presence of cervical and/or lumbar ribs, or decreased by failure of the 12th pair to form (see Chapter 4 for details). Cervical ribs are relatively common (0.5–2%), but lumbar ribs are less common. Cervical ribs may interfere with neurovascular structures exiting the superior thoracic aperture (See "Thoracic Outlet Syndromes," in Chapter 6.) *Supernumerary* (extra) *ribs* also have clinical significance in that they may confuse the identification of vertebral levels in radiographs and other diagnostic images.

Protective Function and Aging of Costal Cartilages

Costal cartilages provide resilience to the thoracic cage, preventing many blows from fracturing the sternum and/or ribs. Because of the remarkable elasticity of the ribs and costal cartilages in children, chest compression may produce injury within the thorax even in the absence of a rib fracture. In elderly people, the costal cartilages lose some of their elasticity and become brittle; they may undergo calcification, making them radiopaque (e.g., in radiographs). ○

Thoracic Vertebrae

Thoracic vertebrae are typical vertebrae in that they are independent, have bodies, vertebral arches, and seven processes for muscular and articular connections (Figs. 1.4 and 1.5). Characteristic features of thoracic vertebrae include

- Bilateral costal facets (demifacets) on their bodies, usually occurring in inferior and superior pairs, for articulation with the heads of ribs.

- Costal facets on their transverse processes for articulation with the tubercles of ribs, except for the inferior two or three thoracic vertebrae.

- Long, inferiorly slanting spinous processes.

Superior and *inferior costal facets,* most of which actually occur in the form of **demifacets**, make up only a portion of a compound articular surface. They occur as bilaterally paired, planar surfaces on the superior and inferior posterolateral margins of typical (T2–T9) thoracic vertebrae. Functionally, the facets are arranged in pairs on adjacent vertebrae, flanking an interposed IV disc: an inferior (demi)facet of the superior vertebra and a superior (demi)facet of the inferior vertebra. Typically, two demifacets paired in this manner and the posterolateral margin of the IV disc between them form a single socket to receive the head of the rib that is assigned the same number as the inferior vertebra. Atypical

thoracic vertebrae bear whole costal facets in place of demifacets:

- The superior costal facets of vertebra T1 are not demifacets because there are no demifacets on the C7 vertebra above, and rib 1 articulates only with vertebra T1. T1 has a typical inferior costal (demi)facet.

- T10 has only one bilateral pair of (whole) costal facets, located partly on its body and partly on its pedicle.

- T11 and T12 also have only a single pair of (whole) costal facets, located on their pedicles.

The *spinous processes* projecting from the vertebral arches of typical thoracic vertebrae are long and slope inferiorly, usually overlapping the vertebra below (Fig. 1.4D). They cover the intervals between the **laminae** of adjacent vertebrae, thereby preventing sharp objects such as a knife from entering the *vertebral canal* and injuring the spinal cord. The **superior articular facets** of the **superior articular processes** face mainly posteriorly and slightly laterally, whereas the **inferior articular facets** of the **inferior articular processes** face mainly anteriorly and slightly medially. The bilateral joint planes between the respective articular facets of the adjacent vertebrae describe an arc, centering on an axis of rotation within the vertebral body (Fig. 1.4A–C). Thus small rotatory movements are permitted between adjacent vertebra, but they are limited by the attached rib cage.

Figure 1.4. Thoracic vertebrae. A. T1 has a vertebral foramen and body similar to a cervical vertebra. **B.** T5–T9 vertebrae have typical characteristics of thoracic vertebrae. **C.** T12 has bony processes and a body size similar to a lumbar vertebra. The planes of the articular facets of thoracic vertebrae define an arc (*red arrows*) that centers on an axis traversing the vertebral bodies vertically. **D.** Superior and inferior costal facets (demifacets) on the vertebral body, costal facets on the transverse processes, and long sloping spinous processes are characteristic of thoracic vertebrae.

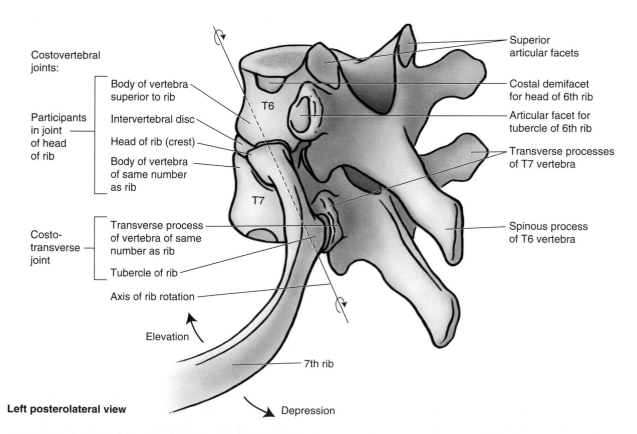

Figure 1.5. Costovertebral articulations of a typical rib. The costovertebral joints include the joint of head of rib, in which the head articulates with two adjacent vertebral bodies and the intervertebral disc between them, and the costotransverse joint, in which the tubercle of the rib articulates with the transverse process of a vertebra. The rib moves (elevates and depresses) around an axis that traverses the head and neck of the rib (*arrows*).

The Sternum

The sternum (G. *sternon*, chest) is the flat, elongated bone that forms the middle of the anterior part of the thoracic cage (Fig. 1.6). The sternum consists of three parts: manubrium, body, and xiphoid process.

The **manubrium** (L. handle, as in the handle of a sword, the sternal body forming the blade) is a roughly trapezoidal bone. The manubrium is the widest and thickest of the three parts of the sternum. The easily palpated concave center of the superior border of the manubrium is the **jugular notch** (**suprasternal notch**). The notch is deepened in an articulated skeleton (and in life) by the medial (sternal) ends of the clavicles, which are much larger than the relatively small **clavicular notches** in the manubrium that receive them, forming the sternoclavicular (SC) joints. Inferolateral to the clavicular notch, the costal cartilage of the 1st rib is tightly attached to the lateral border of the manubrium—the *synchondrosis of the first rib* (Fig. 1.1*A*). The manubrium and body of the sternum lie in slightly different planes superior and inferior to their junction, the **manubriosternal joint** (Fig. 1.6*A* & *B*); hence, their junction forms a projecting **sternal angle** (of Louis).

The **body** of the sternum, which is longer, narrower, and thinner than the manubrium, is located at the level of the T5–T9 vertebrae (Fig. 1.6*A–C*). Its width varies because of the scalloping of its lateral borders by the **costal notches**. In young people, four *sternebrae* (primordial segments of the sternum) are obvious. The sternebrae articulate with each other at primary cartilaginous joints (*sternal synchondroses*). These joints begin to fuse from the inferior end between puberty (sexual maturity) and age 25. The nearly flat anterior surface of the body of the sternum is marked in adults by three variable **transverse ridges** (Fig. 1.6*A*), which represent the lines of fusion (*synostosis*) of its four originally separate sternebrae.

The **xiphoid process**, the smallest and most variable part of the sternum, is thin and elongated. It lies at the level of T10 vertebra. Although often pointed, the process may be blunt, bifid, curved, or deflected to one side or anteriorly. It is cartilaginous in young people but more or less ossified in adults older than age 40. In elderly people, the xiphoid process may fuse with the sternal body.

The xiphoid process is an important landmark in the median plane because

- Its junction with the sternal body at the **xiphisternal joint** indicates the inferior limit of the central part of the thoracic cavity projected onto the anterior body wall; this joint is also the site of the **infrasternal angle** (subcostal angle) of the inferior thoracic aperture (Fig. 1.1).

- It is a midline marker for the superior limit of the liver, the central tendon of the diaphragm, and the inferior border of the heart.

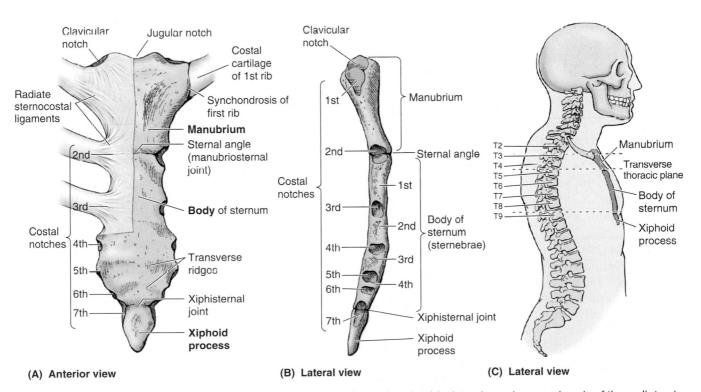

(A) Anterior view   **(B) Lateral view**   **(C) Lateral view**

Figure 1.6. Sternum. A. The felt-like covering of the sternum—formed as the thin, broad membranous bands of the radiate sternocostal ligaments pass from the costal cartilages to the anterior and posterior surfaces of the sternum—is shown on the upper right side. **B.** Observe the thickness of the superior third of the manubrium between the clavicular notches. **C.** The relationship of the sternum to the vertebral column is shown.

Ossified Xiphoid Processes

Many people in their early 40s suddenly become aware of their partly *ossified xiphoid process* and consult their physician about the hard lump in the "pit of their stomach" (*epigastric fossa*). Never having been aware of their xiphoid process before, they fear they have developed a tumor, such as "stomach cancer."

Sternal Fractures

Despite the subcutaneous location of the sternum, *sternal fractures* are not common. Crush injuries can occur after traumatic compression of the thoracic wall in automobile accidents when the driver's chest is forced into the steering column, for example. The installation and use of air bags in vehicles has reduced the number of sternal fractures. A fracture of the sternal body is usually a *comminuted fracture* (the sternum is broken into several pieces). Displacement of the bone fragments is uncommon because the sternum is invested by *deep fascia* (fibrous continuities of radiate sternocostal ligaments; Fig. 1.6*A*) and the sternal attachment of the pectoralis major muscles. The most common site of sternal fracture is at the sternal angle, after the manubriosternal joint has fused in elderly people, resulting in *dislocation of the* (re-established) *manubriosternal joint.*

In sternal injuries, the concern is not primarily for the fracture itself but for the likelihood of heart injury (myocardial contusion, cardiac rupture, tamponade) or pulmonary injury. The mortality (death rate) associated with sternal fractures is reported as 25–45%, largely owing to these underlying injuries. All patients with sternal contusion should be evaluated for underlying visceral injury (Rosen, 1998).

Median Sternotomy

To gain access to the thoracic cavity for surgical operations in the mediastinum—for example, for *coronary artery bypass grafting*—the sternum is divided (split) in the median plane and retracted. The flexibility of ribs and costal cartilages enables spreading of the halves of the sternum. *Sternal splitting* also gives good exposure for removal of tumors in the superior lobes of the lungs. After surgery, the halves of the sternum are joined (e.g., with wire sutures).

Sternal Biopsy

The sternal body is often used for *bone marrow needle biopsy* because of its breadth and subcutaneous position. The needle pierces the thin cortical bone and enters the vascular trabecular (cancellous) bone. Sternal biopsy is commonly used to obtain specimens of marrow for transplantation and for detection of metastatic cancer and *blood dyscrasias* (abnormalities).

Sternal Anomalies

The cartilaginous halves of the sternum of the fetus (sternal plates) may not fuse because of defective ossification. *Complete sternal cleft* is uncommon. Sternal clefts involving the manubrium and superior half of the body are V- or U-shaped and can be repaired during infancy by direct apposition and fixation of the cartilaginous sternal halves.

Sometimes there is a perforation (*sternal foramen*) in the sternal body because of incomplete fusion of the fetal sternal plates. It is not clinically significant; however, one should be aware of its possible presence so that it will not be misinterpreted on a medical image of the thorax as a bullet wound. Although the xiphoid process is commonly perforated in elderly persons because of age-related changes, this perforation is not clinically significant. Similarly, a protruding xiphoid process in infants is not unusual; when it occurs, it usually does not require correction. ✺

THE BOTTOM LINE: The functions of the thoracic wall are to protect the contents of the thoracic cavity; to provide the mechanics for breathing; and to provide for attachment of neck, back, upper limb and abdominal musculature. Its domed shape endows the thoracic cage with the necessary strength, and its light, relatively flexible osteocartilaginous elements and joints enable the flexibility necessary especially for respiration. Posteriorly, the thoracic cage consists of a column of 12 thoracic vertebrae and interposed IV discs. Laterally and anteriorly, it consists of 12 ribs, most continuous with a costal cartilage anteriorly that articulates directly or indirectly with the sternum. The ribs, the intercostal spaces between them, and vertical lines extrapolated from visible or palpable structures provide a grid for precisely locating related structures or pathologies.

Thoracic Apertures

While the thoracic cage provides a complete wall peripherally, it is open superiorly and inferiorly. The much smaller superior opening is a passageway that allows communication with the neck and upper limb. The larger inferior opening provides the ring-like origin of the diaphragm, which completely occludes the opening, and the excursions of which primarily control the volume/internal pressure of the thoracic cavity, providing the basis for tidal respiration.

Superior Thoracic Aperture

The **superior thoracic aperture**, the anatomical *thoracic inlet,* is bounded as follows (Fig. 1.7):

- Posteriorly, by vertebra T1 (protruding or convex posterior boundary/landmark).

- Laterally, by the 1st pair of ribs and their costal cartilages.

- Anteriorly, by the superior border of the manubrium (anterior landmark).

Structures that pass between the thoracic cavity and the neck through the oblique, kidney-shaped superior thoracic aperture include the trachea, esophagus, nerves, and vessels that supply and drain the head, neck, and upper limbs. The adult superior thoracic aperture measures approximately 6.5 cm anteroposteriorly and 11 cm transversely. To visualize the size of this opening, note that it is slightly larger than necessary to allow the passage of a 2×4 piece of lumber. Because of the obliquity of the 1st pair of ribs, the aperture slopes anteroinferiorly.

Inferior Thoracic Aperture

The **inferior thoracic aperture**, the anatomical *thoracic outlet,* is bounded as follows:

- Posteriorly, by the 12th thoracic vertebra (posterior landmark).

- Posterolaterally, by the 11th and 12th pairs of ribs.

- Anterolaterally, by the joined costal cartilages of ribs 7–10, forming the costal margins.

- Anteriorly, by the xiphisternal joint (anterior landmark).

The inferior thoracic aperture is much more spacious than the superior thoracic aperture and is irregular in outline. It is also oblique because the posterior thoracic wall is much longer than the anterior wall. In closing the inferior thoracic aperture, the diaphragm separates the thoracic and abdominal cavities almost completely. Structures passing from or to the thorax from the abdomen pass through openings that traverse the diaphragm (e.g., esophagus and inferior vena cava), or pass posterior to it (e.g., aorta).

Just as the size of the thoracic cavity (or its contents) is often overestimated, its inferior extent (corresponding to the boundary between thoracic and abdominal cavities) is often incorrectly estimated because of the discrepancy between the inferior thoracic aperture and the location of the diaphragm (the floor of the thoracic cavity) in living persons. Although the diaphragm takes origin from the structures that make up the inferior thoracic aperture, the domes of the diaphragm rise to the level of the 4th intercostal space, and abdominal visceral, including the large liver, spleen, and stomach, lie superior to the plane of the inferior thoracic aperture, within the thoracic wall (Fig. 1.1*A* & *B*).

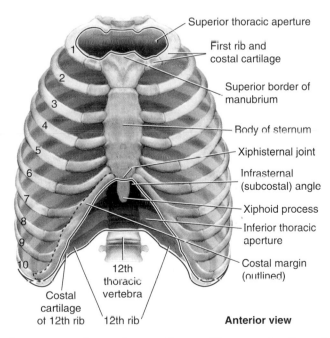

Figure at bottom labels:
Superior thoracic aperture
First rib and costal cartilage
Superior border of manubrium
Body of sternum
Xiphisternal joint
Infrasternal (subcostal) angle
Xiphoid process
Inferior thoracic aperture
Costal margin (outlined)
12th thoracic vertebra
Costal cartilage of 12th rib
12th rib
Anterior view

Figure 1.7. Thoracic apertures. The superior thoracic aperture is the "doorway" between the thoracic cavity and the neck and upper limb. The inferior thoracic aperture (thoracic outlet) provides attachment for the diaphragm, which protrudes upward so that upper abdominal viscera receive protection from the thoracic cage. The continuous cartilaginous bar formed by the articulated cartilages of the 7th–10th (false) ribs makes up the costal margin.

Thoracic Outlet Syndrome

Anatomists refer to the superior thoracic aperture as the *thoracic inlet* because non-circulating substances (air and food) may enter the thorax only through this aperture. When clinicians refer to the superior thoracic aperture as the *thoracic outlet,* they are emphasizing the arteries and T1 spinal nerves that emerge from the thorax through this aperture to enter the lower neck and upper limbs. Hence, various types of *thoracic outlet syndrome* (TOS) exist in which emerging structures are affected by obstructions of the superior thoracic aperture (Rowland, 2000). Although TOS implies a thoracic location, the obstruction actually occurs outside the aperture in the root of the neck (see Chapter 8), and the manifestations of the syndromes involve the upper limb (see Chapter 6). ✪

THE BOTTOM LINE: Although the thoracic wall is complete peripherally, the thoracic cage is open superiorly and inferiorly. The superior thoracic aperture is a relatively small passageway for the transmittal of structures to and from the neck and upper limbs, and the inferior thoracic aperture provides a rim to which the diaphragm is attached.

Joints of the Thoracic Wall

Although movements of the joints of the thoracic wall are frequent—for example, in association with normal respiration—the range of movement at the individual joints is relatively small; nonetheless, any disturbance that reduces the mobility of these joints interferes with respiration. During deep breathing, the excursions of the thoracic cage (anteriorly, superiorly, or laterally) are considerable. Extending the vertebral column farther increases the anteroposterior (AP) diameter of the thorax. Joints of the thoracic wall (Table 1.1) occur between the

- Vertebrae (intervertebral joints).

- Ribs and vertebrae (costovertebral joints: joints of heads of ribs and costotransverse joints).

- Ribs and costal cartilages (costochondral joints).

- Costal cartilages (interchondral joints).

- Sternum and costal cartilages (sternocostal joints).

- Sternum and clavicle (sternoclavicular joints).

- Parts of the sternum (manubriosternal and xiphisternal joints) in young people—the manubriosternal (and sometimes the xiphisternal) joint usually fuses in the elderly.

The *intervertebral joints* between the bodies of adjacent vertebrae are joined together by longitudinal ligaments and *intervertebral discs*. These joints are discussed with the back in Chapter 4; the sternoclavicular joints are discussed in Chapter 6. The manubriosternal and xiphisternal joints were discussed earlier in this chapter, with the sternum.

Costovertebral Joints

A typical rib articulates with the vertebral column at two joints: the joints of heads of ribs and the costotransverse joints (Fig. 1.8).

Joints of Heads of Ribs The head of each typical rib articulates with demifacets or costal facets of two adjacent thoracic vertebrae (Fig. 1.4) and the IV disc between them. The head articulates with the superior part of the corresponding (same-numbered) vertebra, the inferior part of the vertebra superior to it, and the adjacent IV disc uniting the two vertebrae. For example, the head of the 6th rib articulates with the superior part of the body of the T6 vertebra, the inferior part of T5, and the IV disc between these vertebrae (Fig. 1.8). The crest of the head of the rib attaches to the IV disc by an *intra-articular ligament* within the joint, dividing the enclosed space into two synovial cavities. Exceptions to this general arrangement of articulation occur with the heads of the 1st, sometimes the 10th, and usually the 11th and 12th ribs; they articulate only with their own vertebral bodies (bodies of the same number as the rib). In these cases no intra-articular ligaments exist, and the joint cavities are not divided.

A *joint capsule* surrounds each joint and connects the head of the rib with the circumference of the joint cavity.

The fibrous layer of the capsule is strongest anteriorly, where it forms a **radiate sternocostal ligament** that fans out from the anterior margin of the head of the rib to the sides of the bodies of two vertebrae and the IV disc between them. The heads of the ribs connect so closely to the vertebral bodies that only slight gliding movements occur at the (demi)facets (pivoting around the intra-articular ligament) of the joints of the heads of ribs; however, even slight movement here may produce a relatively large excursion of the distal (sternal or anterior) end of a rib.

Costotransverse Joints The tubercle of a typical rib articulates with the transverse costal facet on the anterior surface of the end of the transverse process of its own vertebra (vertebra of the same number). These small synovial joints are surrounded by thin joint capsules that attach to the edges of the articular facets. A **costotransverse ligament** passing from the neck of the rib to the transverse process and a **lateral costotransverse ligament** passing from the tubercle of the rib to the tip of the transverse process strengthen the anterior and posterior aspects of the joint, respectively. A **superior costotransverse ligament** is a broad band that joins the crest of the neck of the rib to the transverse process superior to it. The aperture between this ligament and the vertebra permits passage of the spinal nerve and the posterior branch of the intercostal artery. The superior costotransverse ligament may be divided into a strong *anterior costotransverse ligament* and a weak *posterior costotransverse ligament*. The strong costotransverse ligaments binding these joints limit their movements to slight gliding. However, the articular surfaces on the tubercles of the superior 6 ribs are convex and fit into concavities on the transverse processes (Fig. 1.8C). As a result, rotation occurs around a mostly transverse axis that traverses the intra-articular ligament and the head and neck of the rib (Fig. 1.8A & B). This results in elevation and depression movements of the distal (sternal) ends of the ribs (and the sternum to which they attach) in the sagittal plane (*pump-handle movement*) (Fig. 1.9A & C). Flat articular surfaces of tubercles and transverse processes of the 7th–10th ribs allow gliding here (Fig. 1.8C), resulting in elevation and depression of the lateral-most portions of these ribs in the transverse plane (*bucket-handle movement*) (Fig. 1.9B & C).

The floating 11th and 12th ribs do not articulate with transverse processes and have even freer movements as a result.

Costochondral Joints

The costochondral articulations are *hyaline cartilaginous joints*. Each rib has a cup-shaped depression in its sternal end into which the costal cartilage fits (Table 1.1). The rib and its cartilage are firmly bound together by the continuity of the periosteum of the rib with the perichondrium of the cartilage. No movement normally occurs at these joints.

Interchondral Joints

The interchondral joints—articulations between the adjacent borders of the 6th and 7th, 7th and 8th, and 8th and 9th costal cartilages—are *plane synovial joints* (Table 1.1). Each of

Table 1.1. Joints of Thoracic Wall

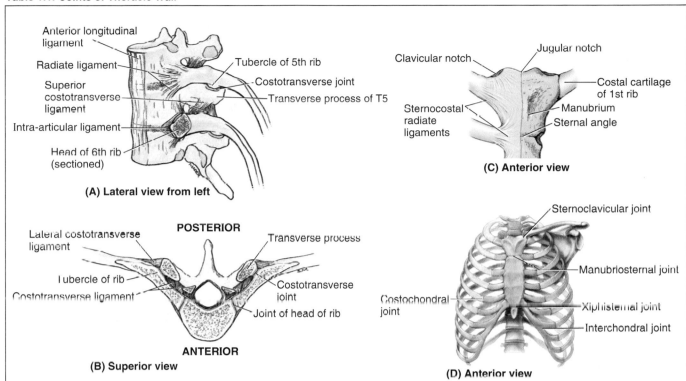

(A) Lateral view from left

(B) Superior view

(C) Anterior view

(D) Anterior view

Joint	Type	Articulation	Ligaments	Comments
Intervertebral	Symphysis (secondary cartilaginous)	Adjacent vertebral bodies bound together by IV disc	Anterior and posterior longitudinal	
Costovertebral Joints of head of rib	Synovial plane joint	Head of each rib with superior demifacet or costal facet of corresponding vertebral body and inferior demifacet or costal facet of vertebral body superior to it	Radiate and intra-articular ligaments of head of rib	Heads of 1st, 11th, and 12th ribs (sometimes 10th) articulate only with corresponding vertebral body
Costotransverse		Articulation of tubercle of rib with transverse process of corresponding vertebra	Lateral and superior costotransverse	11th and 12th ribs do not articulate with transverse process of corresponding vertebrae
Costochondral	Primary cartilaginous joint	Articulation of lateral end of costal cartilage with sternal end of rib	Cartilage and bone bound together by periosteum	No movement normally occurs at this joint
Interchondral	Synovial plane joint	Articulation between costal cartilages of 6th and 7th, 7th and 8th, and 8th and 9th ribs	Interchondral ligaments	Articulation between costal cartilages of 9th and 10th ribs is fibrous
Sternocostal	1st: primary cartilaginous joint (synchondrosis)	Articulation of 1st costal cartilages with manubrium of sternum		
	2nd–7th: synovial plane joint	Articulation of the 2nd–7th pairs of costal cartilages with sternum	Anterior and posterior radiate sternocostal	
Sternoclavicular	Saddle type of synovial joint	Sternal end of clavicle with manubrium of sternum and 1st costal cartilage	Anterior and posterior sternoclavicular ligaments; costoclavicular ligament	This joint is divided into two compartments by an articular disc
Manubriosternal	Secondary cartilaginous joint (symphysis)	Articulation between manubrium and body of sternum		This joint often fuses and becomes a synostosis in older individuals
Xiphisternal	Primary cartilaginous joint (synchondrosis)	Articulation between xiphoid process and body of sternum		

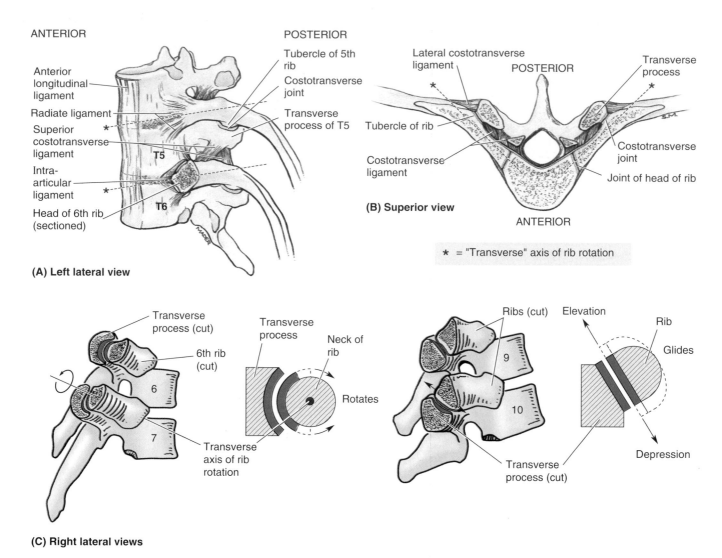

Figure 1.8 Costovertebral joints. A and B. The ligaments of the costovertebral articulations with transverse axes of rib rotation (*asterisks, dotted lines*). **C.** Conformation of articular surfaces, revealed in sagittal sections of the costotransverse joints, demonstrates how the 1st–7th ribs rotate about an axis that runs longitudinally through the neck of the rib to change thoracic volume for respiration (*left*), whereas the 8th–10th ribs glide (*right*).

these joints usually has a synovial cavity that is enclosed by a joint capsule. The joints are strengthened by interchondral ligaments. The articulation between the 9th and the 10th costal cartilages is a fibrous joint.

Sternocostal Joints

The 1st–7th ribs articulate through their costal cartilages with the lateral borders of the sternum; in mature adults, the articulations are (Fig. 1.1; Table 1.1):

- The 1st pair of cartilages with the manubrium only.

- The 2nd pair of cartilages with the manubrium and body of the sternum (i.e., with components of manubriosternal joint).

- The 3rd–6th pairs of cartilages with the body of the sternum.

- The 7th pair of cartilages with the body of the sternum and the xiphoid process (i.e., with the components of the xiphisternal joint).

The 1st pair of costal cartilages articulates with the manubrium by means of a thin dense layer of tightly adherent fibrocartilage interposed between cartilage and the manubrium, the **synchondrosis of the 1st rib** (Williams et al., 1995). The 2nd–7th pairs of costal cartilages articulate with the sternum at synovial joints with fibrocartilaginous articular surfaces on both the chondral and sternal aspects, allowing movement during respiration. The weak joint capsules of these joints are reinforced (thickened) anteriorly and posteriorly to form **radiate sternocostal ligaments**. These continue as thin, broad membranous bands passing from the costal cartilages to the anterior and posterior surfaces of the sternum, forming a felt-like covering for this bone (Fig. 1.6*A*; Table 1.1).

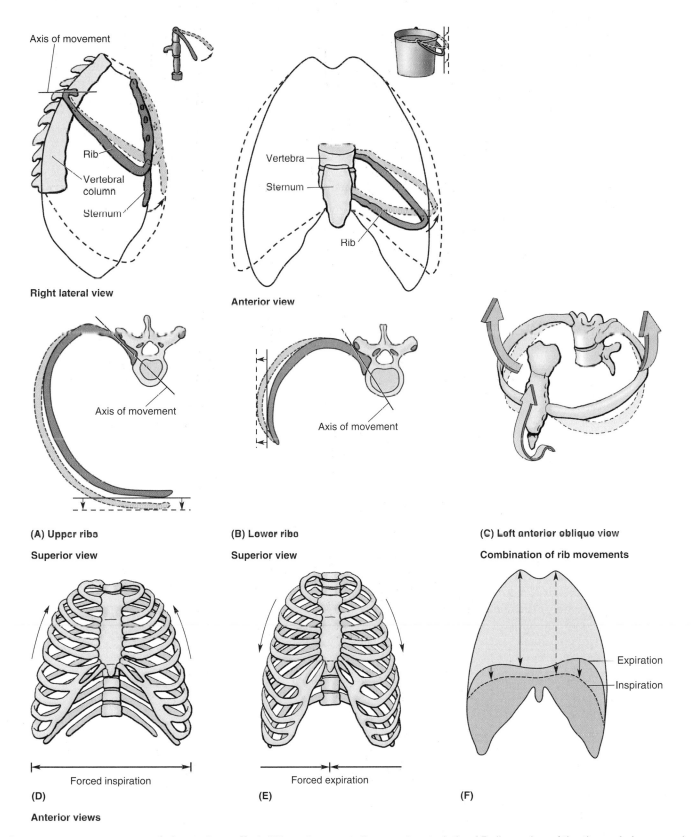

Axis of movement

Rib

Vertebral column

Sternum

Right lateral view

Vertebra

Sternum

Rib

Anterior view

Axis of movement

(A) Upper ribs

Superior view

Axis of movement

(B) Lower ribs

Superior view

(C) Left anterior oblique view

Combination of rib movements

Forced inspiration

(D)

Forced expiration

(E)

Expiration

Inspiration

(F)

Anterior views

Figure 1.9. Movements of thoracic wall. A. When the upper ribs are elevated, the AP dimension of the thorax is increased (pump-handle movement), with a greater excursion (increase) occurring inferiorly, at the end of the pump handle. **B.** The middle parts of the lower ribs move laterally when they are elevated, increasing the transverse dimension (bucket-handle movement). **C.** The combination of rib movements (*arrows*) that occur during forced inspiration increase the AP and transverse dimensions of the thoracic cage. **D.** The thorax widens during forced inspiration as the ribs are elevated (*arrows*). **E.** The thorax narrows during expiration as the ribs are depressed (*arrows*). **F.** The primary movement of inspiration (resting or forced) is contraction of the diaphragm, which increases the vertical dimension of the thoracic cavity (*arrows*). When the diaphragm relaxes, decompression of the abdominal viscera pushes the diaphragm upward, reducing the vertical dimension for expiration.

Dislocation of Ribs

A *rib dislocation* (*slipping rib syndrome*) is the displacement of a costal cartilage from the sternum—*dislocation of a sternocostal joint* or the displacement of the interchondral joints. Rib dislocations are common in body-contact sports; complications may result from pressure on or damage to nearby nerves, vessels, and muscles. *Displacement of interchondral joints* usually occurs unilaterally and involves ribs 8, 9, and 10. Trauma sufficient to displace these joints often injures underlying structures such as the diaphragm and/or liver, causing severe pain, particularly during deep inspiratory movements. The injury produces a lump-like deformity at the displacement site.

Separation of Ribs

Rib separation refers to *dislocation of a costochondral junction* between the rib and its costal cartilage. In separations of the 3rd–10th ribs, tearing of the perichondrium and periosteum usually occurs. As a result, the rib may move superiorly, overriding the rib above and causing pain. ✚

Movements of the Thoracic Wall

Movements of the thoracic wall and diaphragm during inspiration produce increases in the intrathoracic volume and diameters of the thorax (Fig. 1.9D & F). Consequent pressure changes result in air being alternately drawn into the lungs (inspiration) through the nose, mouth, larynx, and trachea and expelled from the lungs (expiration) through the same passages. During passive expiration, the diaphragm, intercostal muscles, and other muscles relax, decreasing intrathoracic volume and increasing the *intrathoracic pressure* (Fig. 1.9E & C). Concurrently, *intra-abdominal pressure* decreases and abdominal viscera are decompressed. This allows the stretched elastic tissue of the lungs to recoil, expelling most of the air.

The *vertical dimension* (height) of the central part of the thoracic cavity increases during inspiration as contraction of the diaphragm causes it to descend, compressing the abdominal viscera (Fig. 1.9F). During expiration, the vertical dimension returns to the neutral position as the elastic recoil of the lungs produces sub-atmospheric pressure in the pleural cavities, between the lungs and the thoracic wall. As a result of this and the absence of resistance to the previously compressed viscera, the domes of the diaphragm ascend, diminishing the vertical dimension. The *AP dimension* of the thorax increases considerably when the intercostal muscles contract: Movement of the ribs (primarily 2nd–6th) at the costovertebral joints around an axis passing through the necks of the ribs causes the anterior ends of the ribs to rise—the pump-handle movement (Fig. 1.9A & C). Because the ribs slope in-

feriorly, their elevation also results in anterior–posterior movement of the sternum, especially its inferior end, with slight movement occurring at the manubriosternal joint in young people, in whom it has not yet synostosed.

The *transverse dimension* of the thorax also increases slightly when the intercostal muscles contract, raising the middle (lateral-most parts) of the ribs (especially the lower ones)—the bucket-handle movement (Fig. 1.9B & C). The combination of all these movements moves the thoracic cage anteriorly, superiorly, and laterally (Fig. 1.9C & F).

Paralysis of the Diaphragm

Paralysis of half of the diaphragm (one dome or hemidiaphragm) because of injury to its motor supply from the *phrenic nerve* does not affect the other half because each dome has a separate nerve supply. One can detect paralysis of the diaphragm radiographically by noting its paradoxical movement. Instead of descending as it normally would during inspiration owing to diaphragmatic contraction (Fig. B1.2A), the paralyzed dome ascends as it is pushed superiorly by the abdominal viscera that are being compressed by the active contralateral dome (Fig. B1.2B). Instead of ascending during expiration, the paralyzed dome descends in response to the positive pressure in the lungs. ✚

■ Inspiration   ■ Resting (normal expiration)

Resting
Normal inspiration
Paralyzed inspiration

(A) Normal inspiration   **(B) Paralysis of right hemidiaphragm**

Figure B1.2

THE BOTTOM LINE: The movements of most ribs occur around a generally transverse axis that passes through the head, neck, and tubercle. This axis, plus the slope and curvature of the ribs, results in bucket-handle-type movements that alter the transverse diameter of the thorax and pump-handle-type movements that alter its AP diameter. Most important, however, is contraction and relaxation of the superiorly convex diaphragm that alters its vertical dimensions. Increasing dimensions result in inhalation, and decreasing dimensions produce exhalation.

Surface Anatomy of the Thoracic Wall Skeleton

The **clavicles** (collar bones) lie subcutaneously, forming bony ridges at the junction of the thorax and neck (Fig. SA1.1). They can be palpated easily throughout their length, especially where their medial ends articulate with the manubrium of the sternum. *The clavicles demarcate the superior divide between zones of lymphatic drainage:* above the clavicles, lymph flows ultimately to inferior jugular lymph nodes; below them, parietal lymph (that from the body wall and upper limb) flows to the axillary lymph nodes.

The **sternum** lies subcutaneously in the anterior median line and is palpable throughout its length. Between the prominences of the medial ends of the clavicles at the sternoclavicular joints, the **jugular notch** in the manubrium can be palpated between the prominent medial ends of the clavicles. The notch lies at the level of the inferior border of the body of T2 vertebra and the space between the 1st and 2nd thoracic spinous processes.

The **manubrium**, approximately 4 cm long, lies at the level of the bodies of T3 and T4 vertebrae (Fig. SA1.2). The **sternal angle** is palpable and often visible in young people because of the slight movement that occurs at the manubriosternal joint during forced respiration. The sternal angle lies at the level of the T4–T5 IV disc and the space between the 3rd and 4th thoracic spinous processes. The sternal angle marks the level of the 2nd pair of costal cartilages. The left side of the manubrium is anterior to the arch

of the aorta, and its right side directly overlies the merging of the brachiocephalic veins to form the **superior vena cava** (SVC). Because it is common clinical practice to insert catheters into the SVC for feeding extremely ill patients and other purposes (Ger et al., 1996), it is essential to know the surface anatomy of this large vein. The SVC passes inferiorly deep to the manubrium and manubriosternal junction but projects as much as a fingerbreadth to the right of the margin of the bony structures. The SVC enters the right atrium of the heart opposite the right 3rd costal cartilage.

The **body of the sternum**, approximately 10 cm long, lies anterior to the right border of the heart and vertebrae T5–T9. The **intermammary cleft** (midline depression or cleavage between the mature female breasts) overlies the sternal body. The **xiphoid process** lies in a slight depression, the **epigastric fossa**, where the converging costal margins form the **infrasternal angle**. This angle is used in cardiopulmonary resuscitation (CPR) for locating the proper hand position on the inferior part of the sternal body. You can feel the **xiphisternal joint**, often seen as a ridge, at the level of the inferior border of T9 vertebra.

The **costal margins**, formed by the joined costal cartilages of the 7th–10th costal cartilages, are easily palpable because they extend inferolaterally from the xiphisternal joint. The costal margins form the sides of the infrasternal angle.

The **ribs** and **intercostal spaces** provide a basis for locating or describing the position of structures or sites of trauma or pathology on or deep to the thoracic wall, much like lines of latitude are used in navigation. For example, ▶

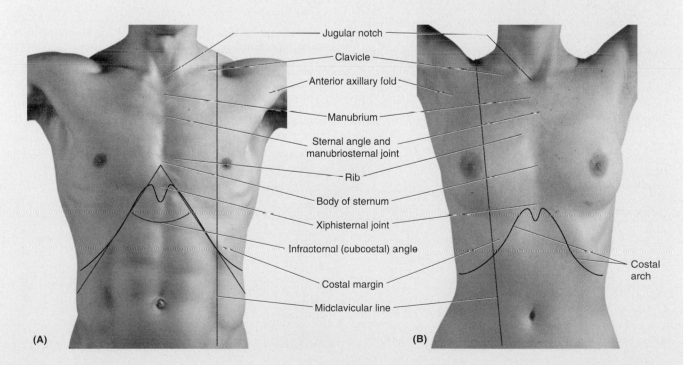

Jugular notch
Clavicle
Anterior axillary fold
Manubrium
Sternal angle and manubriosternal joint
Rib
Body of sternum
Xiphisternal joint
Infrasternal (subcostal) angle
Costal margin
Midclavicular line
Costal arch

(A)   (B)

Figure SA1.1

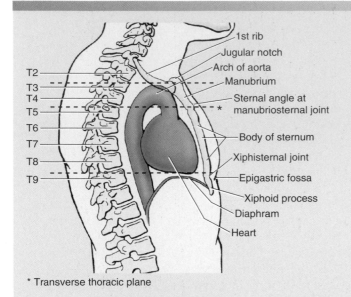

* Transverse thoracic plane

Figure SA1.2

"the beat of the mitral valve of the heart may be heard by placing the stethoscope in the intercostal space between the 5th and 6th ribs inferior to the left nipple." Because the 1st rib is not palpable, rib counting in physical examinations starts with the 2nd rib adjacent to the subcutaneous and easily palpated sternal angle.

To count the ribs and intercostal spaces anteriorly, slide the fingers laterally from the sternal angle onto the 2nd costal cartilage and begin counting the ribs and spaces by moving the digits from here. The 1st intercostal space is that superior to the 2nd costal cartilage—that is, intercostal spaces are numbered according to the rib forming their superior boundary. Generally, it is more reliable to count intercostal spaces, since the fingertip tends to rest in (slip into) the gaps between ribs. One finger should remain in place while another is used to locate the next space. Using all the fingers, it is possible to locate four spaces at a time. The spaces are widest anterolaterally (approximately

in the midclavicular line). If the fingers are removed from the thoracic wall while counting spaces, the finger may easily be returned to the same space, mistaking it for the one below. Posteriorly, the medial end of the spine of the scapula overlies the 4th rib.

While the ribs and/or intercostal spaces provide the "latitude" for navigation and localization on the thoracic wall, several imaginary lines facilitate anatomical and clinical descriptions by providing "longitude." The following lines are extrapolated over the thoracic wall based on visible or palpable superficial features:

- The **anterior median (midsternal) line** (AML) indicates the intersection of the median plane with the anterior thoracic wall (Fig. SA1.3A).

- The **midclavicular line** (MCL) passes through the midpoint of the clavicle, parallel to the AML.

- The **anterior axillary line** (AAL) runs vertically along the anterior axillary fold that is formed by the inferolateral border of the pectoralis major as it spans from the thoracic cage to the humerus in the arm (Fig. SA1.3B).

- The **midaxillary line** (MAL) runs from the apex (deepest part) of the axillary fossa, parallel to the AAL.

- The **posterior axillary line** (PAL), also parallel to the AAL, is drawn vertically along the posterior axillary fold formed by the latissimus dorsi and teres major muscles as they span from the back to the humerus.

- The **posterior median (midvertebral) line** (PML) is a vertical line along the tips of the spinous processes of the vertebrae (Fig. SA1.3C).

- The **scapular line** (SL) is parallel to the posterior median line and intersects the inferior angles of the scapula.

Additional lines (not illustrated) are extrapolated along the borders of palpable bony formations such as the sternum and vertebral column, such as the **parasternal** and **paravertebral lines** (G. *para,* alongside of, adjacent to). ☉

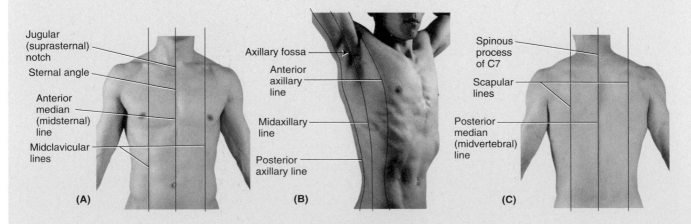

Figure SA1.3

Muscles of the Thoracic Wall

Several upper limb (*thoracoappendicular*) muscles attach to the thoracic cage—including the pectoralis major, pectoralis minor, subclavius, and serratus anterior muscles anteriorly and latissimus dorsi muscles posteriorly—as do the anterolateral abdominal muscles and some back and neck muscles (Fig. 1.10). The thoracoappendicular muscles usually act on the upper limbs (see Chapter 6). But several, including the **pectoralis major** and **pectoralis minor** and the inferior part of the **serratus anterior** may also function as accessory muscles of respiration, helping elevate the ribs to expand the thoracic cavity when inspiration is deep and forceful (e.g., after a 100-m dash). The **scalene muscles** of the neck, which descend to the 1st and 2nd ribs, also serve as accessory respiratory muscles by fixing these ribs and enabling the muscles connecting the ribs below to be more effective in elevating the lower ribs during forced inspiration.

The serratus posterior, levatores costarum, intercostal, subcostal, and transverse thoracic are muscles of the thoracic wall (Table 1.2).

The *serratus posterior muscles,* extending from the vertebrae to the ribs, have traditionally been described as inspiratory muscles, but this function is not supported by electromyography or other evidence. The **serratus posterior superior** lies at the junction of the neck and back. It arises from the inferior part of the nuchal ligament (L. *ligamentum nuchae*) in the neck and the spinous processes of the C6 or C7 through T2 or T3 vertebrae. This muscle runs inferolaterally and attaches by a series of digitations to the superior borders of the 2nd–5th ribs, immediately lateral to their angles. On the basis of its attachments and disposition, the serratus posterior superior was said to elevate the superior four ribs, thus increasing the AP diameter of the thorax and raising the sternum.

The **serratus posterior inferior** lies at the junction of the thoracic and lumbar regions (see Chapter 4). It arises from the spinous processes of the last two thoracic spinous processes, the first two lumbar spinous processes, and the thoracolumbar fascia. It runs superolaterally and attaches to the inferior borders of the inferior three or four ribs, also just lateral to their angles. On the basis of its attachments and disposition, the serratus posterior inferior was said to depress the inferior ribs, preventing them from being pulled superiorly by the diaphragm. However, recent studies (Vilensky et al., 2001) suggest that these muscles, which span the superior and inferior thoracic apertures as well as the transitions from the relatively inflexible thoracic vertebral column to the much more flexible cervical and lumbar segments of the column, may not be primarily motor in function. Rather, they may have a proprioceptive function. These muscles, particularly the superior one, have been implicated as a source of chronic pain in myofascial pain syndromes.

Anterior view

Figure 1.10. Thoracoappendicular and anterolateral abdominal muscles overlying thoracic wall. The pectoralis major has been removed on the left side to expose the pectoralis minor, subclavius, and external intercostal muscles. When the upper limb muscles are removed, the domed shape of the thoracic cage is revealed.

Table 1.2. Muscles of Thoracic Wall

Muscle	Superior Attachment	Inferior Attachment	Innervation	Main Action[a]
Serratus posterior superior	Nuchal ligament, spinous processes of C7 to T3 vertebrae	Superior borders of 2nd to 4th ribs	2nd to 5th intercostal nerves	Elevate ribs[b]
Serratus posterior inferior	Spinous processes of T11 to L2 vertebrae	Inferior borders of 8th to 12th ribs near their angles	Anterior rami of T9 to T12 thoracic spinal nerves	Depress ribs[b]
Levator costarum	Transverse processes of T7–11	Subjacent ribs between tubercle and angle	Posterior primary rami of C8–T11 nerves	Elevate ribs
External intercostal	Inferior border of ribs	Superior border of ribs below	Intercostal nerve	Elevate ribs during forced inspiration[a]
Internal intercostal				Interosseous part: depresses ribs ⎤ During active Interchondral part: elevates ribs ⎦ (forced) respiration[a]
Innermost intercostal				
Subcostal	Internal surface of lower ribs near their angles	Superior borders of 2nd or 3rd ribs below		Probably act in same manner as internal intercostal muscles
Transverse thoracic	Posterior surface of lower sternum	Internal surface of costal cartilages 2–6		Weakly depress ribs[b]

[a]All intercostal muscles keep intercostal spaces rigid, thereby preventing them from bulging out during expiration and from being drawn in during inspiration. The role of individual intercostal muscles and accessory muscles of respiration in moving the ribs is difficult to interpret despite many electromyographic studies
[b]Action traditionally assigned based on attachments; appear to be largely proprioceptive in function.

The **levatores costarum muscles** are attached to the transverse processes of the C7 and T1–T11 vertebrae (Fig. 1.14) and pass inferolaterally to attach to the ribs, close to their tubercles. As their name indicates, these 12 fan-shaped muscles elevate the ribs; but their role, if any, in normal inspiration is uncertain. They may play a role in vertebral movement and/or proprioception.

The *intercostal muscles* occupy the intercostal spaces (Figs. 1.10–1.12; Table 1.2). The superficial layer is formed by the external intercostals, the inner layer by the internal intercostals. The deepest fibers of the latter, lying internal to the intercostal vessels are somewhat artificially designated as a separate muscle, the *innermost intercostals*.

- The **external intercostal muscles** (11 pairs) occupy the intercostal spaces from the tubercles of the ribs posteriorly to the costochondral junctions anteriorly (Figs. 1.10, 1.11, and 1.13). Anteriorly, the muscle fibers are replaced by the **external intercostal membranes** (Fig. 1.13*A*). These muscles run inferoanteriorly from the rib above to the rib below. Each muscle attaches superiorly to the inferior border

of the rib above and inferiorly to the superior border of the rib below (Fig. 1.13*C*). These muscles are continuous inferiorly with the *external oblique muscles* in the anterolateral abdominal wall. The external intercostals are most active during inspiration; they maintain or increase the tonus of the intercostal space. They elevate the ribs during forced inspiration.

- The **internal intercostal muscles** (11 pairs) run deep to and at right angles to the external intercostals (Figs. 1.12 and 1.13*C*). Their fibers run inferoposteriorly from the floors of the costal grooves to the superior borders of the ribs inferior to them. The internal intercostals attach to the bodies of the ribs and their costal cartilages as far anteriorly as the sternum and as far posteriorly as the angles of the ribs. Between the ribs posteriorly, medial to the angles, the internal intercostals are replaced by the **internal intercostal membranes** (Fig. 1.13*A*). The inferior internal intercostals are continuous with the *internal oblique muscles* in the anterolateral abdominal wall. The internal intercostals—weaker than the external intercostal muscles—are most

Scaleni — Posterior / Medius / Anterior

Subclavian vein

Sternothyroid / Sternohyoid

1st intercostal nerve

2nd intercostal nerve

Internal thoracic vein and artery

External intercostal muscle

Internal intercostal muscle deep to external intercostal membrane

Transverse thoracic muscle

Brachial plexus / Axillary artery / Axillary vein

Parasternal lymph node

Serratus anterior muscle

Anterior aspect of anterior thoracic wall

Anterior view

Figure 1.11. Dissection of anterior aspect of anterior thoracic wall. The external intercostal muscles are replaced by membranes between costal cartilages. The H-shaped cuts through the perichondrium of the 3rd and 4th costal cartilages are used to shell out pieces of cartilage, as was done with the 4th costal cartilage, illustrating how one type of thoracotomy is performed. It is not uncommon for the 8th rib to attach to the sternum, as in this specimen. The internal thoracic vessels and the parasternal lymph nodes (*green*) lie inside the thoracic cage lateral to the sternum.

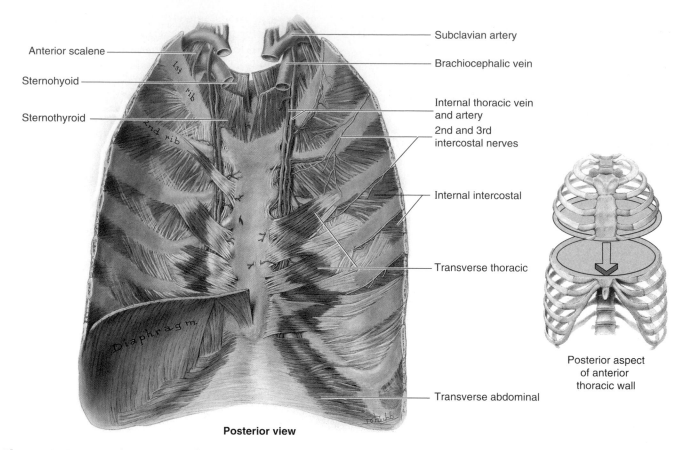

Anterior scalene
Sternohyoid
Sternothyroid

Subclavian artery
Brachiocephalic vein
Internal thoracic vein and artery
2nd and 3rd intercostal nerves
Internal intercostal
Transverse thoracic
Posterior aspect of anterior thoracic wall
Transverse abdominal

Posterior view

Figure 1.12. Posterior aspect of anterior thoracic wall. The internal thoracic arteries arise from the subclavian arteries and have paired accompanying veins (L. *venae comitantes*) inferiorly. Superior to the 2nd costal cartilage, there is only a single internal thoracic vein on each side, which drains into the brachiocephalic vein. The continuity of the transverse thoracic with the transverse abdominal becomes apparent when the diaphragm is removed, as has been done here on the right side.

active during expiration; they maintain or increase the tonus of the intercostal space. Their interosseous (vs. interchondral) portions may depress ribs during forced respiration (Fig. 1.13*C*). The interchondral portion of the internal intercostals appears to act with the external intercostals during active inspiration (discussed later in this chapter).

- The **innermost intercostal muscles** are similar to the internal intercostals and are essentially their deeper parts. The innermost intercostals are separated from the internal intercostals by the intercostal nerves and vessels (Fig. 1.13). These muscles pass between the internal surfaces of adjacent ribs and occupy the lateralmost parts of the intercostal spaces. It is likely (but undetermined) that their actions are the same as those of the internal intercostal muscles.

The **subcostal muscles** are variable in size and shape, usually being well developed only in the lower thoracic wall. These thin muscular slips extend from the internal surface of the angle of one rib to the internal surface of the second or third rib inferior to it. Crossing one or two intercostal spaces, the subcostals run in the same direction as the internal intercostals

and blend with them (Fig. 1.13*B*). Thus it is assumed that the subcostals act with the internal intercostals, and that they may depress ribs.

The **transverse thoracic** (L. *transversus thoracis*) **muscles,** consist of four or five slips that attach posteriorly to the xiphoid process, the inferior part of the body of the sternum, and the adjacent costal cartilages (Figs. 1.11 and 1.12). They pass superolaterally and attach to the 2nd–6th costal cartilages. The transverse thoracic muscles are continuous inferiorly with the *transverse abdominal muscles* in the anterolateral body wall. These muscles appear to have a weak expiratory function, drawing downward on the costal cartilages to which they attach. They may provide proprioceptive information.

Although the external and internal intercostals are active during inspiration and expiration, respectively, most activity is isometric; the role of these muscles in producing movement of the ribs appears to be related mainly to forced respiration. The diaphragm is the primary muscle of inspiration. Expiration is passive unless one is exhaling against resistance (e.g., inflating a balloon) or trying to expel air more rapidly than usual (e.g., coughing, sneezing, blowing one's nose, or shouting), the elastic recoil of the lungs and decompression of

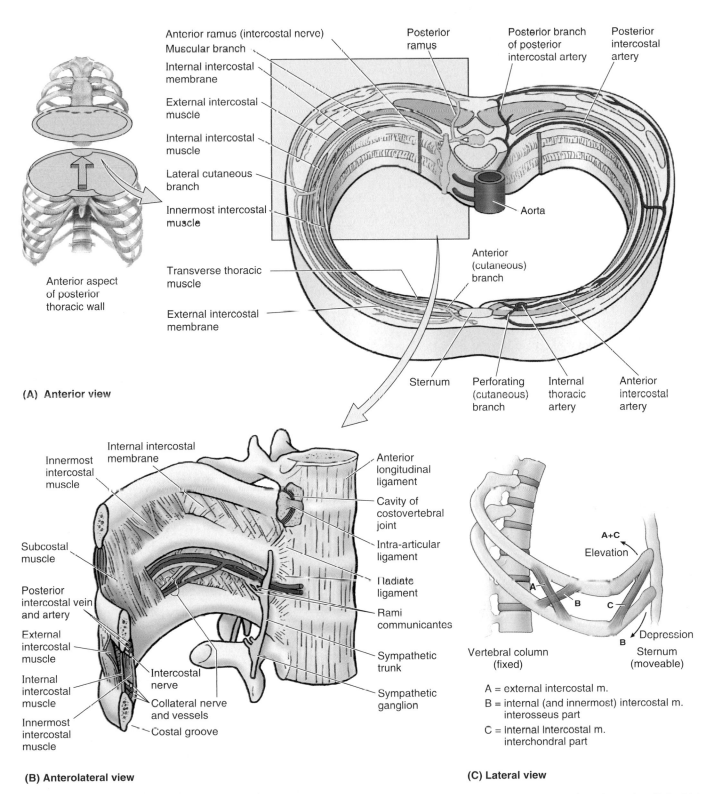

(A) Anterior view

(B) Anterolateral view

(C) Lateral view

A = external intercostal m.
B = internal (and innermost) intercostal m.
        interosseus part
C = Internal Intercostal m.
        interchondral part

Figure 1.13. Contents of an intercostal space. A. This transverse section shows nerves (*right side*) and arteries (*left side*) in relation to the intercostal muscles. **B.** The posterior part of an intercostal space is shown. The joint capsule (radiate ligament) of one costovertebral joint has been removed. Innermost intercostal muscles bridge one intercostal space; subcostal muscles bridge two. The mnemonic for the order of the neurovascular structures in the intercostal space from superior to inferior is VAN—vein, artery, and nerve. Communicating branches (L. *rami communicantes*) extend between the intercostal nerves and the sympathetic trunk. **C.** A simple model of the action of the intercostal muscles is shown. Contraction of the muscle fibers that most closely parallel the slope of the ribs at a given point (fibers *A* and *C*) will elevate the ribs and sternum; contraction of muscle fibers that are approximately perpendicular to the slope of the ribs (fibers *B*) will depress the ribs.

abdominal viscera expel previously inhaled air. The primary role of the intercostal muscles in respiration is to support (increase the tonus or rigidity of) the intercostal space, resisting paradoxical movement especially during inspiration when internal thoracic pressures are lowest (most negative). This is most apparent following a high spinal cord injury, when there is an initial flaccid paralysis of the entire trunk but the diaphragm remains active. In these circumstances, the vital capacity is markedly compromised by the paradoxical incursion of the thoracic wall during inspiration. Several weeks later, the paralysis becomes spastic; the thoracic wall stiffens and vital capacity rises (Williams et al., 1995).

The mechanical action of the intercostal muscles in rib movement, especially during forced respiration, can be appreciated by means of a simple model (Fig. 1.13C). A pair of curved levers, representing the ribs bordering an intercostal space, are hinged posteriorly to a fixed, vertical (vertebral) column; their anterior ends (costal cartilages) are hinged to a moveable, vertical column (the sternum). The ribs (and intervening intercostal space) descend as they run anteriorly, reaching their low point approximately at the costochondral junction, and then ascend to the sternum. The concentric contraction of the muscle fibers that most closely approximate the slope of the ribs at their attachments (fibers A and C in Fig. 1.13C) rotate the ribs superiorly at their posterior axes, elevating the ribs and sternum. The concentric contraction of muscle fibers that are approximately perpendicular to the slope of the ribs at their attachment (fibers B in the figure) rotate the ribs inferiorly at their posterior axes, depressing the ribs and sternum. Fibers A represent the external intercostal muscles, and fibers B represent the interosseous portion of the internal intercostal muscles. Fibers A run nearly perpendicular to fibers B. Thus the external intercostal muscles elevate and the interosseous internal intercostal muscles depress the ribs. Note that even though the fibers of the interchondral portion of the internal interosseous muscles (fibers C) run parallel to the fibers of the interosseous portion (fibers B), they approximate the slope of the ribs (instead of being perpendicular to the slope). Therefore, the interchondral portion of the internal intercostal muscles (fibers C) act with the external intercostal muscles (fibers A) to elevate the ribs (Slaby et al., 1994).

The **diaphragm** is a shared wall (actually floor/ceiling) separating the thorax and abdomen. Although it has functions related to both compartments of the trunk, its most important (vital) function is serving as the primary muscle of inspiration. The detailed description of the thoracic diaphragm appears in Chapter 2 because the attachments of its crura occur at abdominal levels (i.e., to lumbar vertebrae) and all of its attachments are best observed from its inferior (abdominal) aspect; they are essentially inaccessible from the thoracic side if the abdominal viscera are still in place. Consequently, the diaphragm is usually most fully studied when, during dissections, the abdominal viscera and kidneys have been removed. However, you may wish to read about the diaphragm at this time.

Dyspnea: Difficult Breathing

When people with respiratory problems (e.g., *asthma*) or with *heart failure* struggle to breathe, they use their accessory respiratory muscles to assist the expansion of their thoracic cavity. They lean on their knees or on the arms of a chair to fix their pectoral girdle so these muscles are able to act on their rib attachments and expand the thorax. ☉

THE BOTTOM LINE: The thorax is overlapped by the thoracoappendicular muscles of the upper limb. These muscles account for many of the anatomical features of its surface, along with the breasts. Most of these muscles can effect deep respiration when the pectoral girdle is fixed. The muscles that are truly thoracic, however, provide few if any surface features. The serratus posterior muscles are thin with small bellies that may be proprioceptive organs. The costal muscles can move the ribs and do so during forced respiration, but most of the time they function to support (provide tonus for) the intercostal spaces, resisting negative and positive intrathoracic pressures. The diaphragm is the primary muscle of respiration.

Fascia of the Thoracic Wall

Each part of the deep fascia is named for the muscle it invests or the structure(s) to which it is attached. Consequently, a large portion of the deep fascia overlying the anterior thoracic wall, forming a major part of the **bed of the breast** (area or structures immediately deep to the breast, i.e., on which the breast lies), is called **pectoral or pectoralis fascia** for its association with the pectoralis major muscles (Fig. 1.15). Deep to the pectoralis major and its fascia is another layer of deep fascia suspended from the clavicle and investing the pectoralis minor muscle, the **clavipectoral fascia.** (The pectoral and clavipectoral fascias are explained and illustrated in Chapter 6 in relation to the axillary fossa or armpit.) The thoracic cage is lined internally with **endothoracic fascia.** This thin fibroareolar layer attaches the adjacent portion of the lining of the lung cavities (the costal parietal pleura) to the thoracic wall. It becomes more fibrous over the apices of the lungs as the *suprapleural membrane* (see clinical correlation [blue] box "Extrapleural Intrathoracic Surgical Access."

Extrapleural Intrathoracic Surgical Access

Fixation makes it difficult to appreciate in the embalmed cadaver, but in surgery the relatively loose nature of the thin endothoracic fascia provides a natural ▶

cleavage plane, allowing the surgeon to separate the costal parietal pleura lining the lung cavity from the thoracic wall. This allows intrathoracic access to extrapleural structures (e.g., lymph nodes) and instrument placement without opening and perhaps contaminating the potential space (pleural cavity) that surrounds the lungs. ✪

THE BOTTOM LINE: Deep fascia overlies and invests the muscles of the thoracic wall, as it does elsewhere. Where the fleshy portions of the intercostal muscles are absent, their fascia is continued as intercostal membranes, so that the wall is complete. The endothoracic fascia is a thin, fibroareolar layer between the internal aspect of the thoracic cage and the lining of the pulmonary cavities, which can be opened surgically to gain access to intrathoracic structures.

Nerves of the Thoracic Wall

The 12 pairs of thoracic spinal nerves supply the thoracic wall. As soon as they leave the IV foramina in which they are formed, the mixed thoracic spinal nerves divide into anterior and posterior primary rami (Fig. 1.13A). The anterior rami of nerves T1–T11 form the intercostal nerves that run along the extent of the intercostal spaces. The anterior ramus of nerve T12, coursing inferior to the 12th rib, is the *subcostal nerve* (see Chapter 2). The posterior rami of thoracic spinal nerves pass posteriorly, immediately lateral to the articular processes of the vertebrae (Fig. 1.14), to supply the joints, muscles, and skin of the back in the thoracic region (see Chapter 4).

Typical Intercostal Nerves

The 3rd–6th intercostal nerves enter the medial-most parts of the posterior intercostal spaces, running initially within the endothoracic fascia between the parietal pleura (serous lining of the pulmonary cavity) and the internal intercostal membrane nearly in the middle of the intercostal spaces (Figs. 1.13

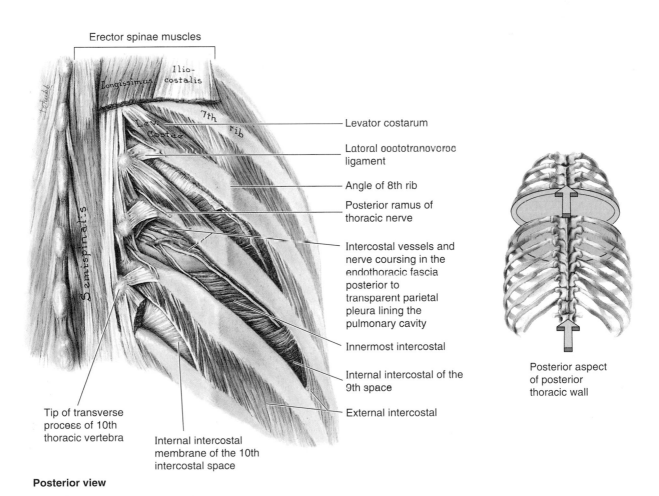

Erector spinae muscles

Ilio-costalis

Longissimus

7th rib

Lev. Costae

Semispinalis

Levator costarum

Lateral costotransverse ligament

Angle of 8th rib

Posterior ramus of thoracic nerve

Intercostal vessels and nerve coursing in the endothoracic fascia posterior to transparent parietal pleura lining the pulmonary cavity

Innermost intercostal

Internal intercostal of the 9th space

External intercostal

Tip of transverse process of 10th thoracic vertebra

Internal intercostal membrane of the 10th intercostal space

Posterior aspect of posterior thoracic wall

Posterior view

Figure 1.14. Dissection of posterior aspect of thoracic wall. The iliocostalis and longissimus muscles (two of the three components of the erector spinae muscles of the back) have been removed to expose the levatores costarum muscles. In the 8th and 10th intercostal spaces, varying parts of the external intercostal muscle have been removed to expose the underlying internal intercostal membrane, which is continuous with the internal intercostal muscle. In the 9th intercostal space, the levator costae has been removed to expose the intercostal vessels and nerve.

and 1.14). Near the angles of the ribs, the nerves pass between the internal intercostal and the innermost intercostal muscles. At this point, the intercostal nerves pass to and then continue to course within the *costal grooves*, running inferior to the intercostal arteries (which, in turn, run inferior to the intercostal veins) (Fig. 1.13*B*). The neurovascular bundles are thus sheltered by the inferior margins of the overlying ribs. Collateral branches of these nerves arise near the angles of the ribs and run along the superior border of the rib below. The nerves continue anteriorly between the internal and the innermost intercostal muscles, giving branches to these and other muscles and giving rise to lateral cutaneous branches in approximately the MAL. Anteriorly, the nerves appear on the internal surface of the internal intercostal muscle. Near the sternum, the intercostal nerves turn anteriorly, passing between the costal cartilages to become anterior cutaneous branches.

Through its posterior ramus and the lateral and anterior cutaneous branches of its anterior ramus, each spinal nerve supplies a strip-like *dermatome* extending from the posterior median line to the anterior median line (Fig. 1.16). The group of muscles supplied by the posterior ramus and anterior ramus (intercostal nerve) of each pair of thoracic spinal nerves constitutes a *myotome*. Constituting the myotome supplied by the *muscular branches of a typical intercostal nerve* is the intercostal, subcostal, transverse thoracic, levatores costarum, and

serratus posterior muscles associated with the intercostal space that includes the nerve. The branches of a typical intercostal nerve are:

- **Rami communicantes**, or communicating branches, that connect each intercostal nerve to the ipsilateral sympathetic trunk (Fig. 1.13*A* & *B*). Presynaptic fibers leave the initial portions of the anterior ramus of each thoracic (and upper lumbar) spinal nerve by means of a white communicating ramus and pass to the *sympathetic trunk*. Postsynaptic fibers distributed to the body wall and limbs pass from the ganglia of the sympathetic trunk via gray rami to join the anterior ramus of the nearest spinal nerve, including all intercostal nerves. Sympathetic nerve fibers are distributed through all branches of all spinal nerves (anterior and posterior rami) to reach the blood vessels, sweat glands, and smooth muscle of the body wall and limbs.

- **Collateral branches** that arise near the angles of the ribs and descend to course along the superior margin of the lower rib, helping supply intercostal muscles and parietal pleura (Fig. 1.13*B*).

- **Lateral cutaneous branches** that arise near the MAL and pierce the internal and external intercostal muscles approximately halfway around the thorax (Figs. 1.13*A* & *B*, 1.15, and 1.16). The lateral cutaneous branches divide in

Supraclavicular nerves (C3 and C4)

Deltoid

Deltopectoral triangle
Cephalic vein

Skin

Subcutaneous tissue

Anterior branches of lateral cutaneous nerves (derived from intercostal nerves)

Pectoral fascia covering pectoralis major

Anterior cutaneous nerves

Platysma

Pectoralis

Major

6th Cart.

Intercostobrachial nerve (T2)

Anterior and posterior branches of lateral cutaneous nerves (derived from intercostal nerves)

Serratus anterior

External oblique and nerve supply

Anterior view (slightly oblique)

Figure 1.15. Superficial dissection of male pectoral region. The platysma is cut short on the right side and is reflected on the left side, together with the underlying supraclavicular nerves. Observe the filmy, deep fascia covering the right pectoralis major. The fascia has been removed on the left side. The cutaneous branches of the intercostal nerves that supply the breast are shown.

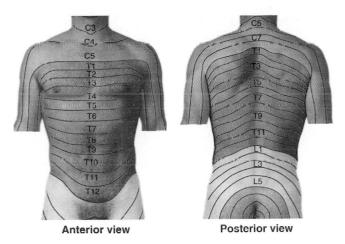

Anterior view   **Posterior view**

Figure 1.16. Segmental innervation (dermatomes) of thoracic wall. Spinal nerve C5 supplies skin at the level of the clavicles and immediately below. Anteriorly, the dermatome immediately inferior to the C5 dermatome is that of spinal nerve T1. Dermatomes C6–C7 are located mostly in the upper limbs and are represented on the posterior, but not the anterior, body wall. Since the anterior rami of spinal nerves T2–T12 are not involved in plexus formation, there is no difference between the dermatomes and the zones of peripheral nerve distribution here. Dermatome T4 includes the nipple; dermatome T10 includes the umbilicus.

turn into anterior and posterior branches that supply the skin of the lateral thoracic and abdominal walls.

- **Anterior cutaneous branches** that supply the skin on the anterior aspect of the thorax and abdomen. After penetrating the muscles and membranes of the intercostal space in the parasternal line, the anterior cutaneous branches divide into medial and lateral branches.

- **Muscular branches** that supply the intercostal, subcostal, transverse thoracic, levatores costarum, and serratus posterior muscles (Fig. 1.13*A*).

Atypical Intercostal Nerves

Although the anterior ramus of most thoracic spinal nerves is simply the intercostal nerve for that level, the anterior ramus of the 1st thoracic (T1) spinal nerve first divides into a large superior and a small inferior part. The superior part joins the **brachial plexus**, the nerve plexus supplying the upper limb (see Chapter 6), and the inferior part becomes the 1st intercostal nerve. Other atypical features of specific intercostal nerves include the following:

- The *1st and 2nd intercostal nerves* course on the internal surface of the 1st and 2nd ribs, instead of along the inferior margin in costal grooves (Fig. 1.12).

- The *1st intercostal nerve* has no anterior cutaneous branch and often no lateral cutaneous branch. When there is a lateral cutaneous branch, it supplies the skin of the axilla and may communicate with either the intercostobrachial nerve or the medial cutaneous nerve of the arm.

- The *2nd* (and sometimes 3rd) *intercostal nerve* gives rise to a large lateral cutaneous branch, the *intercostobrachial nerve;* it emerges from the 2nd intercostal space at the MAL, penetrates the serratus anterior, and enters the axilla and arm. The intercostobrachial nerve usually supplies the floor—skin and subcutaneous tissue—of the axilla and then communicates with the *medial brachial cutaneous nerve* to supply the medial and posterior surfaces of the arm. The lateral cutaneous branch of the 3rd intercostal nerve frequently gives rise to a second intercostobrachial nerve.

- The *7th–11th intercostal nerves,* after giving rise to lateral cutaneous branches, cross the costal margin posteriorly and continue on to supply abdominal skin and muscles. No longer being between ribs (intercostal), they now become the **thoracoabdominal nerves** of the anterior abdominal wall (see Chapter 2). Their anterior cutaneous branches pierce the rectus sheath, becoming cutaneous close to the median plane.

Herpes Zoster Infection of the Spinal Ganglia

A *herpes zoster infection* causes a classic, dermatomally distributed skin lesion—*shingles*—an agonizingly painful condition (Fig. B1.3). Herpes zoster is primarily a viral disease of spinal ganglia, usually a reactivation of the varicella zoster virus (VZV), or chickenpox virus. After invading a ganglion, the virus produces a sharp burning pain in the dermatome supplied by the involved nerve (Fig. 1.16). The affected skin area becomes red, and vesicular eruptions appear. The pain may precede or follow the skin eruptions. Although primarily a *sensory neuropathy* (pathological change in the nerve) weakness from motor involvement occurs in ▶

Figure B1.3

0.5–5.0% of people, commonly in elderly cancer patients (Rowland, 2000). Muscular weakness usually occurs in the same myotomal distribution, as do the dermatomal pain and vesicular eruptions.

Intercostal Nerve Block

Local anesthesia of an intercostal space is produced by injecting a local anesthetic agent around the intercostal nerves between the paravertebral line and the area of required anesthesia. This procedure, *an intercostal nerve block,* involves infiltration of the anesthetic around the intercostal nerve trunk and its collateral branches (Fig. B1.4). The word *block* indicates that the nerve endings in the skin and the transmission of impulses through the sensory nerves carrying information about pain are interrupted (blocked) before the impulses reach the spinal cord and brain. Because any particular area of skin usually receives innervation from two adjacent nerves, considerable overlapping of contiguous dermatomes oc-

curs. Therefore, complete loss of sensation usually does not occur unless two or more intercostal nerves are anesthetized. ✚

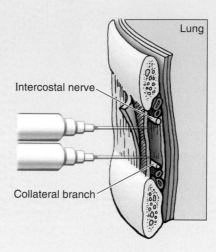

Figure B1.4

Vasculature of the Thoracic Wall

In general, the pattern of vascular distribution in the thoracic wall reflects the structure of the thoracic cage—that is, it runs in the intercostal spaces, parallel to the ribs.

Arteries of the Thoracic Wall

The arterial supply to the thoracic wall (Fig. 1.17; Table 1.3) derives from the:

- *Thoracic aorta,* through the posterior intercostal and subcostal arteries.
- *Subclavian artery,* through the internal thoracic and supreme intercostal arteries.

- *Axillary artery,* through the superior and lateral thoracic arteries.

The intercostal arteries course through the thoracic wall between the ribs. With the exception of the 10th and 11th intercostal spaces, each intercostal space is supplied by three arteries: a large posterior intercostal artery (and its collateral branch) and a small pair of anterior intercostal arteries.

The **posterior intercostal arteries:**

- Of the 1st and 2nd intercostal spaces arise from the **supreme (superior) intercostal artery,** a branch of the costocervical trunk of the subclavian artery.
- Of the 3rd–11th intercostal spaces (and the subcostal arteries of the subcostal space) arise posteriorly from the tho-

Table 1.3. Arterial Supply of Thoracic Wall

Artery	Origin	Course	Distribution
Posterior intercostals	Superior intercostal artery (intercostal spaces 1 and 2) and thoracic aorta (remaining intercostal spaces)	Pass between internal and innermost intercostal muscles	Intercostal muscles, overlying skin, and parietal pleura
Anterior intercostals	Internal thoracic (intercostal spaces 1–6) and musculophrenic arteries (intercostal spaces 7–9)		
Internal thoracic	Subclavian artery	Passes inferiorly and lateral to sternum between costal cartilages and transverse thoracic muscle to divide into superior epigastric and musculophrenic arteries	By way of anterior intercostal arteries to intercostal spaces 1–6
Subcostal	Thoracic aorta	Courses along inferior border of 12th rib	Muscles of anterolateral abdominal wall

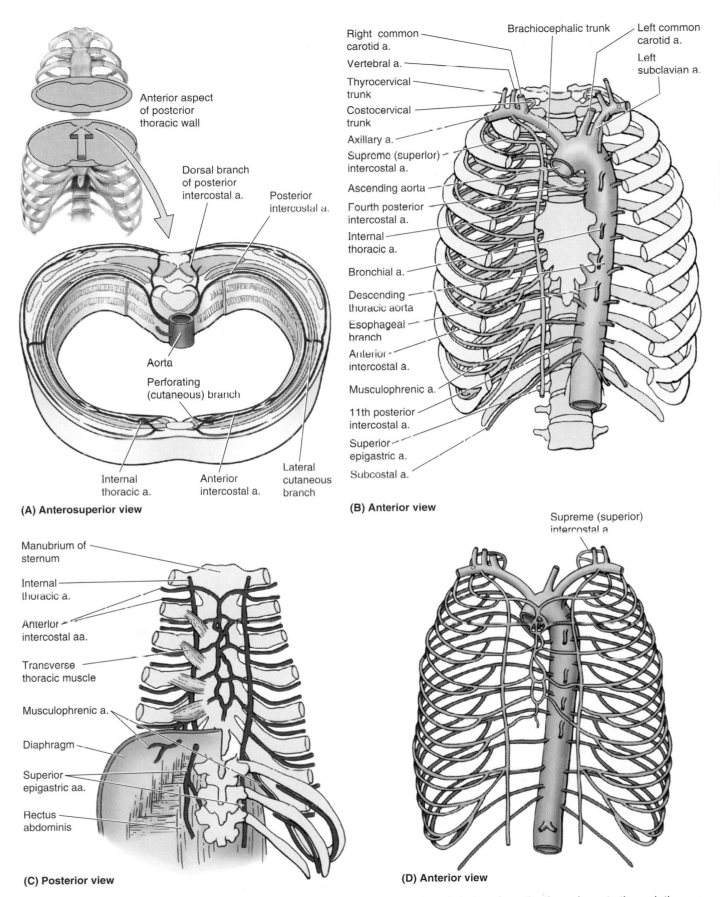

(A) Anterosuperior view

Anterior aspect of posterior thoracic wall

Dorsal branch of posterior intercostal a.

Posterior intercostal a.

Aorta

Perforating (cutaneous) branch

Internal thoracic a.

Anterior intercostal a.

Lateral cutaneous branch

(B) Anterior view

Right common carotid a.

Brachiocephalic trunk

Left common carotid a.

Left subclavian a.

Vertebral a.

Thyrocervical trunk

Costocervical trunk

Axillary a.

Supreme (superior) intercostal a.

Ascending aorta

Fourth posterior intercostal a.

Internal thoracic a.

Bronchial a.

Descending thoracic aorta

Esophageal branch

Anterior intercostal a.

Musculophrenic a.

11th posterior intercostal a.

Superior epigastric a.

Subcostal a.

(C) Posterior view

Manubrium of sternum

Internal thoracic a.

Anterior intercostal aa.

Transverse thoracic muscle

Musculophrenic a.

Diaphragm

Superior epigastric aa.

Rectus abdominis

(D) Anterior view

Supreme (superior) intercostal a

Figure 1.17. Arteries of thoracic wall. The arterial supply to the thoracic wall derives from the thoracic aorta through the posterior intercostal and subcostal arteries (**A**, **B**, and **D**), from the axillary artery (**B**), and from the subclavian artery through the internal thoracic (**C**) and supreme (superior) intercostal arteries (**B**). Connections (anastomoses) between the arteries permit collateral circulation pathways to develop (**D**) racic aorta (Fig. 1.17). Because the aorta is slightly to the left of the vertebral column, the right 3rd–11th intercostal arteries have a longer course than those on the left side. The right arteries cross the vertebrae and pass posterior to the esophagus, thoracic duct, azygos vein (Fig. 1.27), and the right lung and pleura.

- All give off a posterior branch that accompanies the posterior ramus of the spinal nerve to supply the spinal cord, vertebral column, back muscles, and skin.

- Give rise to a small collateral branch that crosses the intercostal space and runs along the superior border of the rib.

- Accompany the intercostal nerves through the intercostal spaces. Close to the angle of the rib, the arteries enter the costal grooves, where they lie between the intercostal vein and nerve. At first the arteries run in the endothoracic fascia between the parietal pleura and the internal intercostal membrane (Fig. 1.14); then they run between the innermost intercostal and internal intercostal muscles.

- Have terminal and collateral branches that anastomose anteriorly with anterior intercostal arteries (Fig. 1.17A).

The **internal thoracic arteries** (historically, the internal mammary arteries):

- Arise in the root of the neck from the inferior surfaces of the first parts of the *subclavian arteries.*

- Descend into the thorax posterior to the clavicle and 1st costal cartilage (Figs. 1.11, 1.12, and 1.17).

- Are crossed near their origins by the ipsilateral phrenic nerve.

- Descend on the internal surface of the thorax slightly lateral to the sternum and posterior to the upper six costal cartilages and intervening internal intercostal muscles. After descending past the 2nd costal cartilage, the internal thoracic artery runs anterior to the transverse thoracic muscle (Figs. 1.13A and 1.17C). Between slips of the transverse thoracic muscle, the artery contacts parietal pleura posteriorly.

- Terminate in the 6th intercostal space by dividing into the **superior epigastric** and the **musculophrenic arteries.**

- Directly give rise to the anterior intercostal arteries supplying the superior six intercostal spaces.

Ipsilateral pairs of **anterior intercostal arteries:**

- Supply the anterior parts of the upper 9 intercostal spaces.

- Pass laterally in the intercostal space, one near the inferior margin of the superior rib and the other near the superior margin of the inferior rib.

- Of the first 2 intercostal spaces lie initially in the endothoracic fascia between the parietal pleura and the internal intercostal muscles.

- Supplying the 3rd–6th intercostal spaces are separated from the pleura by slips of the transverse thoracic muscle.

- Of the 7th–9th intercostal spaces derive from the *musculophrenic arteries,* also branches of the internal thoracic arteries.

- Supply the intercostal muscles and send branches through them to supply the pectoral muscles, breasts, and skin.

- Are absent from the inferior two intercostal spaces; these spaces are supplied only by the posterior intercostal arteries and their collateral branches.

Veins of the Thoracic Wall

The *intercostal veins* accompany the intercostal arteries and nerves and lie most superior in the costal grooves (Figs. 1.13 and 1.18). There are 11 **posterior intercostal veins** and one **subcostal vein** on each side. The posterior intercostal veins anastomose with the **anterior intercostal veins** (tributaries of internal thoracic veins). As they approach the vertebral column, the posterior intercostal veins receive a posterior branch, which accompanies the posterior ramus of the spinal nerve of that level, and an intervertebral vein draining the vertebral venous plexuses. Most posterior intercostal veins (4–11) end in the *azygos/hemiazygos venous system,* which conveys venous blood to the SVC (see "Vessels and Lymph Nodes of the Posterior Mediastinum" in this chapter). The posterior intercostal veins of the 1st intercostal space usually

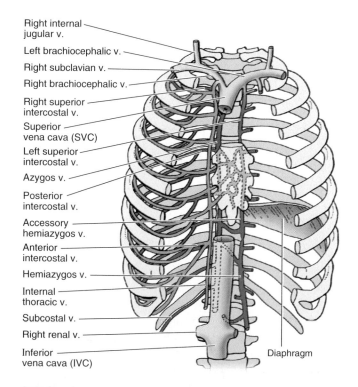

Anterior view

Figure 1.18. Veins of thoracic wall. Although depicted here as continuous channels, the anterior and posterior intercostal veins are separate vessels, normally draining in opposite directions, the tributaries of which communicate (anastomose) in approximately the anterior axillary line. Because these veins lack valves, however, flow can be reversed.

enter directly into the corresponding and nearby brachio-cephalic veins. The posterior intercostal veins of the 2nd and 3rd (and occasionally 4th) intercostal spaces unite to form a trunk, the *superior intercostal vein* (Fig. 1.60*A* & *B*). The **right superior intercostal vein** is typically the final tributary of the azygos vein, before it enters the SVC. The **left superior intercostal vein**, however, usually empties into the *left brachiocephalic vein*. This requires the vein to pass anteriorly along the left side of the superior mediastinum, specifically across the arch of the aorta or the root of the great vessels arising from it and between the vagus and phrenic nerves (Fig. 1.60*B*). It usually receives the left bronchial veins and may receive the left pericardiacophrenic vein as well. Typically, it communicates inferiorly with the accessory hemiazygos vein. The **internal thoracic veins** are the companion veins (L. *venae comitantes*) of the internal thoracic arteries.

THE BOTTOM LINE: The pattern of distribution of neurovascular structures to the thoracic wall reflects the construction of the thoracic cage. These structures course in the intercostal spaces, parallel to the ribs, and serve the intercostal muscles as well as the integument and parietal pleura on their superficial and deep aspects. Because plexus formation does not occur in relationship to the thoracic wall, the pattern of peripheral and segmental (dermatomal) innervation is identical in this region. The intercostal nerves run a posterior to anterior course along the length of each intercostal space, and the anterior and posterior intercostal arteries and veins converge toward and anastomose in approximately the anterior axillary line. The posterior vessels arise from the thoracic aorta and drain to the azygos venous system, and the anterior vessels arise from the internal thoracic artery, branches, and tributaries and drain to the internal thoracic vein, branches, and tributaries.

Breasts

Both men and women have **breasts** (L. *mammae*); normally they are well developed only in women (Fig. 1.19). The **mammary glands** in the breasts are accessory to reproduction in women but are rudimentary and functionless in men, consisting of only a few small ducts or epithelial cords. Usually, the fat present in the male breast is not different from that of subcutaneous tissue elsewhere, and the glandular system does not normally develop. The breasts are the most prominent superficial structures in the anterior thoracic wall, especially in women. The mammary glands are in the subcutaneous tissue overlying the pectoralis major and minor muscles. The amount of fat surrounding the glandular tissue determines the size of non-lactating breasts. At the greatest prominence of the breast is the *nipple,* surrounded by a circular pigmented area of skin, the **areola** (L. small area).

Female Breasts

The roughly circular body of the female breast rests on a bed that extends transversely from the lateral border of the ster-

num to the midaxillary line and vertically from the 2nd through 6th ribs. Two thirds of the bed of the breast are formed by the **pectoral fascia** overlying the pectoralis major; the other third, by the fascia covering the serratus anterior (Figs. 1.19 and 1.20). Between the breast and the pectoral fascia is a loose connective tissue plane or potential space—the **retromammary space** (bursa). This plane, containing a small amount of fat, allows the breast some degree of movement on the pectoral fascia. A small part of the mammary gland may extend along the inferolateral edge of the pectoralis major toward the axillary fossa (armpit), forming an **axillary process** or **tail** (of Spence). Some women discover this (especially when it may enlarge during a menstrual cycle) and become concerned that it may be a lump (tumor) or enlarged lymph nodes. The mammary gland is firmly attached to the dermis of the overlying skin, especially by substantial skin ligaments (L. *retinacula cutis*), the **suspensory ligaments** (of Cooper). These condensations of fibrous connective tissue, particularly well developed in the superior part of the gland, help support the **mammary gland lobules.**

During puberty (ages 8–15 years), the breasts normally enlarge, owing in part to glandular development but primarily from increased fat deposition. The areolae and nipples also enlarge. Breast size and shape are determined by genetic, ethnic, and dietary factors. The **lactiferous ducts** give rise to buds that form 15–20 **lobules** of glandular tissue, which constitute the *parenchyma of the mammary gland.* Each lobule is drained by a lactiferous duct, which usually opens independently on the nipple. The ducts converge toward the nipple like the spokes of a bicycle wheel. Deep to the areola, each duct has a dilated

Anterior view

Figure 1.19. Superficial dissection of female pectoral region. The pectoral fascia has been removed, except where it lies deep to the breast. The bed of the breast extends from the 2nd through the 6th ribs. The axillary tail of the breast extends toward or into the axillary fossa. The non-lactating breast consists primarily of fat.

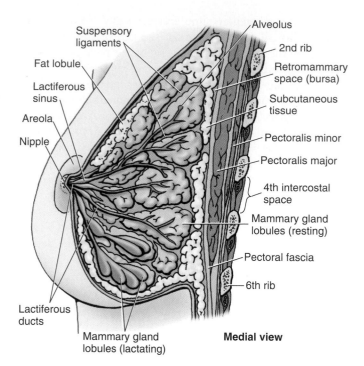

Figure labels (clockwise from top):
Suspensory ligaments — Alveolus — 2nd rib — Retromammary space (bursa) — Subcutaneous tissue — Pectoralis minor — Pectoralis major — 4th intercostal space — Mammary gland lobules (resting) — Pectoral fascia — 6th rib — **Medial view** — Mammary gland lobules (lactating) — Lactiferous ducts — Nipple — Areola — Lactiferous sinus — Fat lobule

Figure 1.20. Sagittal section of female breast and anterior thoracic wall. The breast consists of glandular tissue and fibrous and adipose tissue between the lobes and lobules of glandular tissue, together with blood vessels, lymphatic vessels, and nerves. The superior two thirds of the figure demonstrates the suspensory ligaments and alveoli of the breast with resting mammary gland lobules; the inferior part shows lactating mammary gland lobules.

portion, the **lactiferous sinus,** in which a small droplet of milk accumulates or remains in the nursing mother. As the infant begins to suckle, compression of the areola (and the lactiferous sinus beneath it) expresses the accumulated droplets and encourages the infant to continue nursing as the hormonally mediated *let-down reflex* ensues and the mother's milk is secreted into—not sucked from the gland by—the baby's mouth.

The areolae contain numerous **sebaceous glands,** which enlarge during pregnancy and secrete an oily substance that provides a protective lubricant for the areola and nipple, which are particularly subject to chaffing and irritation as mother and baby begin the nursing experience. The **nipples** are conical or cylindrical prominences in the centers of the areolae. The nipples have no fat, hair, or sweat glands. The tips of the nipples are fissured with the lactiferous ducts opening into them. The nipples are composed mostly of circularly arranged smooth muscle fibers that compress the lactiferous ducts during lactation and erect the nipples in response to stimulation, as when a baby begins to suckle.

The mammary glands are modified sweat glands; therefore, they have no special capsule or sheath. The rounded contour and most of the volume of the breasts are produced by subcutaneous fat, except during pregnancy when the mammary glands enlarge and new glandular tissue forms. The milk-

secreting **alveoli** (L. small hollow spaces) are arranged in grapelike clusters. In most women, the breasts enlarge slightly during the menstrual period from increased release of the gonadotropic hormones—follicle-stimulating hormone (FSH) and luteinizing hormone (LH)—on the glandular tissue.

Changes in the Breasts

Changes, such as branching of the lactiferous ducts, occur in the breast tissues during menstrual periods and pregnancy (Ferguson et al., 1992). Although mammary glands are prepared for secretion by midpregnancy, they do not produce milk until shortly after the baby is born. *Colostrum,* a creamy white to yellowish premilk fluid, may secrete from the nipples during the last trimester of pregnancy and during initial episodes of nursing. Colostrum is believed to be especially rich in protein, immune agents, and a growth factor affecting the infant's intestines. In multiparous women, the breasts often become large and pendulous. The breasts in elderly women are usually small because of the decrease in fat and the atrophy of glandular tissue.

Breast Quadrants

For the anatomical location and description of tumors and cysts, the surface of the breast is divided into four quadrants (Fig. B1.5). For example, a physician's record might state: "A hard irregular mass was felt in the superior medial quadrant of the breast at the 2 o'clock position, approximately 2.5 cm from the margin of the areola." ✪

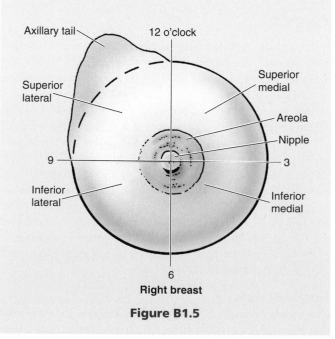

Figure labels: Axillary tail — 12 o'clock — Superior lateral — Superior medial — Areola — Nipple — 9 — 3 — Inferior lateral — Inferior medial — 6 — **Right breast**

Figure B1.5

Vasculature of the Breast

The *arterial supply of the breast* (Fig. 1.21*A* & *B*) derives from the:

- Medial mammary branches of perforating branches and *anterior intercostal branches of the internal thoracic artery,* originating from the subclavian artery.

- **Lateral thoracic** and **thoracoacromial arteries,** branches of the axillary artery.

- *Posterior intercostal arteries,* branches of the thoracic aorta in the 2nd, 3rd, and 4th intercostal spaces.

The *venous drainage of the breast* is mainly to the **axillary vein,** but there is some drainage to the internal thoracic vein (Fig. 1.21*C*).

The *lymphatic drainage of the breast* is important because of its role in the metastasis of cancer cells. Lymph passes from the nipple, areola, and lobules of the gland to the **subareolar lymphatic plexus** (Fig. 1.22*A* & *B*). From this plexus:

- Most lymph (> 75%), especially from the lateral breast quadrants, drains to the *axillary lymph nodes,* initially to the *anterior* or *pectoral nodes* for the most part. However,

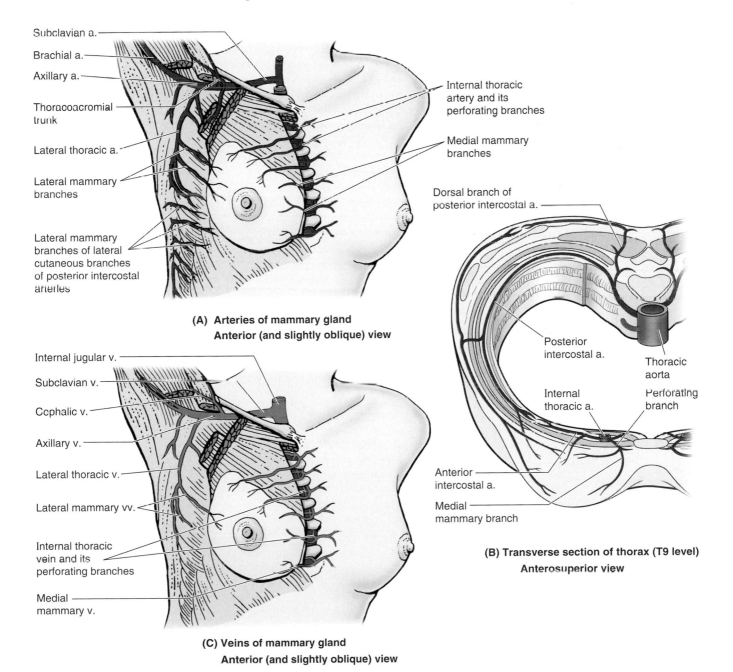

(A) **Arteries of mammary gland**
Anterior (and slightly oblique) view

(B) **Transverse section of thorax (T9 level)**
Anterosuperior view

(C) **Veins of mammary gland**
Anterior (and slightly oblique) view

Figure 1.21. Vasculature of breast. A. The mammary gland is supplied from its medial aspect mainly by perforating branches of the internal thoracic artery and by several branches of the axillary artery (principally the lateral thoracic artery) superiorly and laterally. **B.** The breast is supplied deeply by branches arising from the intercostal arteries. **C** Venous drainage is to the axillary (mainly) and internal thoracic veins.

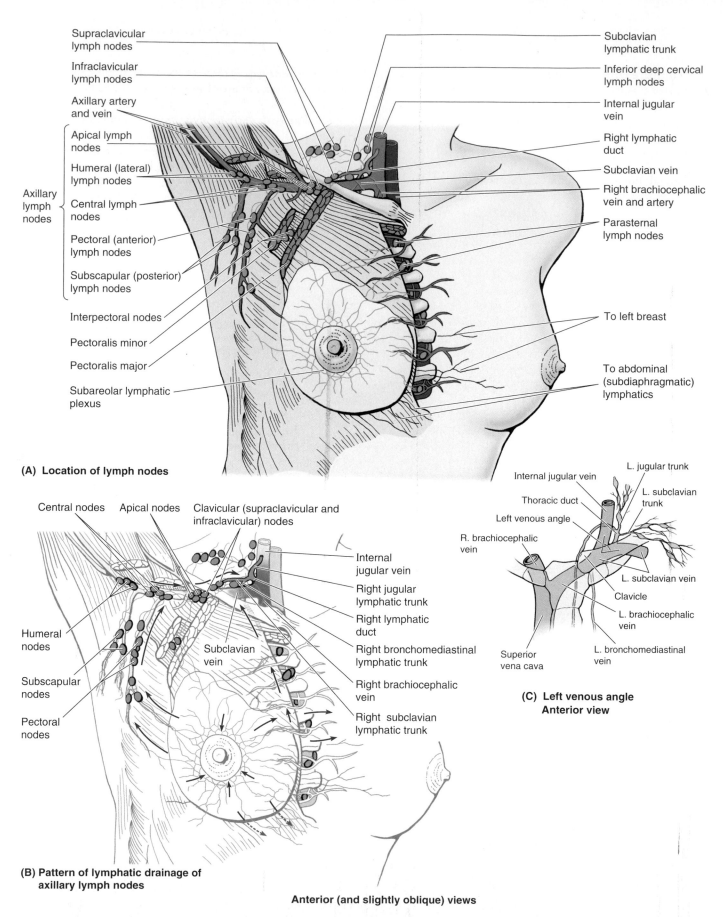

(A) Location of lymph nodes

Supraclavicular lymph nodes

Infraclavicular lymph nodes

Axillary artery and vein

Axillary lymph nodes

Apical lymph nodes

Humeral (lateral) lymph nodes

Central lymph nodes

Pectoral (anterior) lymph nodes

Subscapular (posterior) lymph nodes

Interpectoral nodes

Pectoralis minor

Pectoralis major

Subareolar lymphatic plexus

Subclavian lymphatic trunk

Inferior deep cervical lymph nodes

Internal jugular vein

Right lymphatic duct

Subclavian vein

Right brachiocephalic vein and artery

Parasternal lymph nodes

To left breast

To abdominal (subdiaphragmatic) lymphatics

(B) Pattern of lymphatic drainage of axillary lymph nodes

Central nodes

Apical nodes

Clavicular (supraclavicular and infraclavicular) nodes

Humeral nodes

Subscapular nodes

Pectoral nodes

Subclavian vein

Internal jugular vein

Right jugular lymphatic trunk

Right lymphatic duct

Right bronchomediastinal lymphatic trunk

Right brachiocephalic vein

Right subclavian lymphatic trunk

Anterior (and slightly oblique) views

(C) Left venous angle Anterior view

Internal jugular vein

Thoracic duct

Left venous angle

R. brachiocephalic vein

Superior vena cava

L. jugular trunk

L. subclavian trunk

L. subclavian vein

Clavicle

L. brachiocephalic vein

L. bronchomediastinal vein

Figure 1.22. Lymphatic drainage of breast. A. The lymph nodes in the region are shown. **B.** The *red arrows* indicate lymph flow from the right breast. Most lymph, especially that from the superior lateral quadrant and center of the breast, drains to the axillary lymph nodes, which, in turn, are drained by the subclavian lymphatic trunk and then into the venous system via the right lymphatic duct. **C.** Most lymph from the left breast returns to the venous system via the thoracic duct, which enters the left venous angle.

some lymph may drain directly to other axillary nodes or even to interpectoral, deltopectoral, supraclavicular, or inferior deep cervical nodes. (The axillary lymph nodes are covered in detail in Chapter 6.)

- Most of the remaining lymph, particularly from the medial breast quadrants, drains to the *parasternal lymph nodes* or to the opposite breast, whereas lymph from the inferior quadrants may pass deeply to abdominal lymph nodes (subdiaphragmatic *inferior phrenic lymph nodes*).

Lymph from the skin of the breast, except the nipple and areola, drains into the ipsilateral axillary, inferior deep cervical, and infraclavicular lymph nodes and also into the parasternal lymph nodes of both sides.

Lymph from the axillary nodes drains into *clavicular* (*infraclavicular* and *supraclavicular*) *lymph nodes* and from them into the **subclavian lymphatic trunk**, which also drains lymph from the upper limb. Lymph from the parasternal nodes enters the **bronchomediastinal lymphatic trunk**, which also drains lymph from the thoracic viscera. The termination of these lymphatic trunks varies; traditionally, these trunks are described as merging with each other and with the **jugular lymphatic trunk**, draining the head and neck to form a short *right lymphatic duct* on the right side or entering the termination at the *thoracic duct* on the left side. However, in many (perhaps most) cases, the trunks open independently into the *junction of the internal jugular and subclavian vein*, the **venous angle**, to form the brachiocephalic veins (Fig. 1.22C). In some cases, they open into both of these veins.

Nerves of the Breast

The *nerves of the breast* derive from anterior and lateral cutaneous branches of the **4th–6th intercostal nerves** (Fig. 1.13). The anterior primary rami of T1–T11 are called *intercostal nerves* because they run within the intercostal spaces. Rami communicantes connect each anterior ramus to a sympathetic trunk. The branches of the intercostal nerves pass through the deep fascia covering the pectoralis major to reach the skin, including the breast in the subcutaneous tissue overlying this muscle. The branches of the intercostal nerves thus convey sensory fibers to the skin of the breast and sympathetic fibers to the blood vessels in the breasts and smooth muscle in the overlying skin and nipple.

Carcinoma of the Breast

Understanding the lymphatic drainage of the breasts is of practical importance in predicting the metastasis of *carcinoma of the breast* (breast cancer). Carcinomas of the breast are malignant tumors, usually adenocarcinomas arising from the epithelial cells of the lactiferous ducts in the mammary gland lobules (Fig. B1.6A). Metastatic cancer cells that enter a lymphatic vessel usually pass through two or three groups of lymph nodes before entering the venous system.

Interference with the lymphatic drainage by cancer may cause *lymphedema* (edema, excess fluid in the subcutaneous tissue), which in turn may result in deviation of the nipple and a thickened, leather-like appearance of the skin. Prominent or "puffy" skin between dimpled pores give it an orange-peel appearance (*peau d'orange sign*). Larger dimples (fingertip size or bigger) result from cancerous invasion of the glandular tissue and fibrosis (fibrous degeneration), which causes shortening or places traction on the suspensory ligaments. *Subareolar breast cancer* may cause inversion of the nipple by a similar mechanism involving the lactiferous ducts.

Breast cancer typically spreads by means of lymphatic vessels (*lymphogenic metastasis*), which carry cancer cells from the breast to the lymph nodes, chiefly those in the axilla. The cells lodge in the nodes, producing nests of tumor cells (*metastases*). Abundant communications among lymphatic pathways and among axillary, cervical, and parasternal nodes may also cause metastases from the breast to develop in the supraclavicular lymph nodes, the opposite breast, or the abdomen. Because most of lymphatic drainage of the breast is to the axillary lymph nodes, they are the most common site of metastasis from a breast cancer. Enlargement of these palpable nodes suggests the possibility of breast cancer and may be key to early detection. However, the absence of enlarged axillary lymph nodes is no guarantee that metastasis from a breast cancer has not occurred because the malignant cells may have passed to other nodes, such as the infraclavicular and supraclavicular lymph nodes.

The posterior intercostal veins drain into the *azygos/hemiazygos system of veins* alongside the bodies of the vertebrae (Fig. 1.31B) and communicate with the internal vertebral venous plexus surrounding the spinal cord. Cancer cells can also spread from the breast by these venous routes to the vertebrae and from there to the cranium and brain. Cancer also spreads by contiguity (invasion of adjacent tissue). When breast cancer cells invade the retromammary space (Fig. 1.20), attach to or invade the deep pectoral fascia overlying the pectoralis major, or metastasize to the interpectoral nodes, the breast elevates when the muscle contracts. This movement is a clinical sign of advanced cancer of the breast. To observe this upward movement, the physician has the patient place her hands on her hips and press while pulling her elbows forward to tense her pectoral muscles.

Mammography

Radiographic examination of the breasts, or *mammography,* is one of the techniques used to detect breast masses (Fig. B1.6B). A carcinoma appears as a large, jagged density in the *mammogram* (*upper two arrows* in Fig. B1.6C). ▶

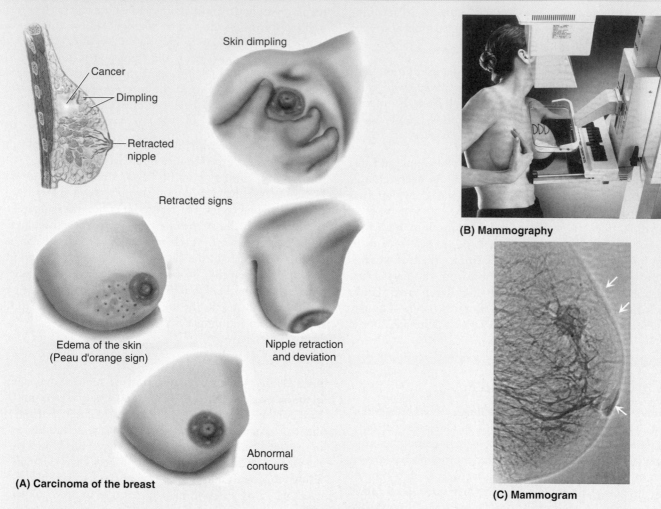

(A) Carcinoma of the breast

Skin dimpling

Cancer

Dimpling

Retracted nipple

Retracted signs

Edema of the skin (Peau d'orange sign)

Nipple retraction and deviation

Abnormal contours

(B) Mammography

(C) Mammogram

Figure B1.6

The skin is thickened over the tumor. The *lower arrow* points to the depressed nipple. Surgeons use mammography as a guide when removing breast tumors, cysts, and abscesses.

Surgical Incisions of the Breast

Incisions are placed in the inferior breast quadrants when possible because these quadrants are less vascular than the superior ones. The transition between the thoracic wall and breast is most abrupt inferiorly, producing a line, crease, or deep skin fold—the *inferior cutaneous crease*. Incisions made along this crease will be least evident and may actually be hidden by overlap of the breast. Incisions that must be made near the areola or on the breast itself are usually directed radially to either side of the nipple (Langer tension lines run transversely here; see the Introduction) or circumferentially.

Mastectomy (breast excision) is not as common as it once was as a treatment for breast cancer. In *simple mastectomy*, the breast is removed down to the retromammary

space. *Radical mastectomy*, a more extensive surgical procedure, involves removal of the breast, pectoral muscles, fat, fascia, and as many lymph nodes as possible in the axilla and pectoral region. In current practice, often only the tumor and surrounding tissues are removed—a *lumpectomy* or *quadrantectomy* (known as *breast-conserving surgery*, a wide local excision)—followed by radiation therapy (Goroll, 2000).

Polymastia, Polythelia, and Amastia

Polymastia (supernumerary breasts) or **polythelia** (accessory nipples) may occur superior or inferior to the normal pair, occasionally developing in the axillary fossa or anterior abdominal wall (Figs. B1.7 and SA1.5). Supernumerary breasts usually consist of only a rudimentary nipple and areola, which may be mistaken for a mole (nevus) until they change pigmentation with the normal nipples during pregnancy. However, glandular tissue may also be present and further develop with lactation. Extra breasts may appear ▶

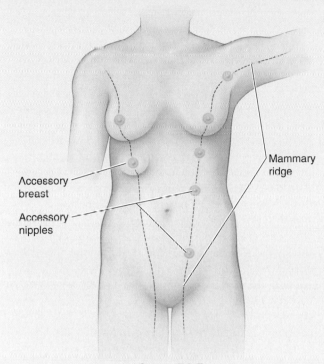

Accessory breast

Accessory nipples

Mammary ridge

Figure B1.7

anywhere along a line extending from the axilla to the groin—the location of the *embryonic mammary ridge* (the milk line) from which the breasts develop (Moore and Persaud, 2003), and along which breasts develop in animals with multiple breasts. In either sex, there may be no breast development (*amastia*), or there may be a nipple and/or areola, but no glandular tissue.

Breast Cancer in Men

Approximately 1.5% of breast cancers occur in men. As in women, the cancer usually metastasizes to lymph nodes but also to bone, pleura, lung, liver, and skin. Carcinoma of the breast affects approximately 1000 men per year in the United States (Swartz, 2002). A visible and/or palpable subareolar mass or secretion from a nipple may indicate a *malignant tumor*. Breast cancer in males tends to infiltrate the pectoral fascia, pectoralis major, and apical lymph nodes in the axilla. Although breast cancer is uncommon in men, the consequences are serious because they are frequently not detected until extensive metastases have occurred—for example, in bone.

Gynecomastia

Slight temporary enlargement of the breasts is a normal occurrence (frequency = 70%) in males at puberty (age 10–12 years). Breast hypertrophy in males after puberty (**gynecomastia**) is relatively rare (< 1%) and may be age related or drug related (e.g., after treatment with diethylstilbestrol for prostate cancer). Gynecomastia may also result from an imbalance between estrogenic and androgenic hormones or from a change in the metabolism of sex hormones by the liver. Thus a finding of gynecomastia should be regarded as a symptom, and an evaluation must be initiated to rule out important potential causes, such as suprarenal and testicular cancers or cirrhosis (Goroll, 2000). Approximately 40% of postpubertal males with Klinefelter syndrome (XXY trisomy) have gynecomastia (Moore et al., 2000). ☉

THE BOTTOM LINE: The mammary glands are in the subcutaneous tissue of the breast, overlying the pectoralis major and serratus anterior muscles and associated deep fascia (the bed of the breast). Lobules of glandular tissue converge toward the nipple, each having its own lactiferous duct, which opens there. The superior lateral quadrant of the breast has the most glandular tissue, largely owing to an extension toward or into the axilla (axillary process) and, therefore, is the site of most tumors. The breast is served by the internal thoracic and lateral thoracic vessels, and the 2nd–6th intercostal vessels and nerves. Most lymph from the breast drains to the axillary lymph nodes; this is significant in breast cancer. Because the mammary glands and the axillary lymph nodes are superficial, the ability to palpate primary and metastatic tumors during routine breast examination enables early detection and treatment.

Surface Anatomy of the Thoracic Wall Musculature and Breasts

The **breasts** are the most prominent surface features of the anterior thoracic wall, especially in women. Except when there is an overabundance of subcutaneous tissue, the breasts in men are mostly an accentuation of the contour of the **pectoralis major muscles,** highlighted by the presence of the nipple in the 4th intercostal space, lateral to the MCL. In the moderately athletic individual, the contour of the pectoralis major muscles is apparent, separated in the midline by the **intermammary cleft** overlying the **sternum**, with the lateral border forming the **anterior axillary fold** (Fig. SA1.4). Inferolaterally, forming about a third of the bed of the breast, finger-like slips, or **digitations of the serratus anterior**, have a ▶

- Axilla
- Lateral border of pectoralis major
- Lateral border of latissimus dorsi
- Digitations of serratus anterior
- External abdominal oblique
- Ribs

Figure SA1.4

serrated (sawtooth) appearance as they attach to the ribs and interdigitate with the **external oblique**. The **inferior ribs** and **costal margins** are often apparent, especially when the abdominal muscles are contracted to pull the belly in. The intercostal musculature per se is not normally evident; however, in (rare) cases in which there is an absence or atrophy of the intercostal musculature, the intercostal spaces become apparent during inspiration, when they are concave, and expiration, when they protrude.

Variation in the size, shape, and symmetry of female finger-like slips, or **digitations of the serratus anterior,** have a serrated (sawtooth) appearance as they attach to the ribs and intergitate with the **external oblique**. The **inferior ribs** and **costal margins** are often apparent, especially when the abdominal muscles are contracted to "pull the belly in." The intercostal musculature per se is not evident

normally; however, in (rare) cases where there is an absence or atrophy of the intercostal musculature, the intercostal spaces become apparent during inspiration, when they are concave, and expiration, when they protrude.

Variation in the size, shape, and symmetry of female breasts—even between the two breasts of one person—is the rule, not the exception. Their flattened superior surfaces show no sharp demarcation from the anterior surface of the thoracic wall, but laterally and inferiorly, their borders are well defined (Fig. SA1.5). The median depression separating the breasts is the *intermammary cleft.* A venous pattern over the breasts is often visible, especially during pregnancy. The **nipple** is surrounded by the slightly raised and circular pigmented **areola,** the color of which depends on the woman's complexion. The areola usually darkens during pregnancy and retains the darkened pigmentation thereafter. The areola is normally dotted with the papular openings of the **areolar glands** (sebaceous glands in the skin forming the areola). On occasion, one or both nipples are inverted; this minor congenital anomaly may make breast feeding difficult.

In men and young *nulliparous women*—those who have never borne a viable child—with moderate breast size, the nipple lies anterior to the 4th intercostal space, approximately 10 cm from the AML. However, the position of nipples varies considerably with breast size in women, especially *multiparous women*—those who have given birth to viable children at least twice. Consequently, because of variations in size and shape, the nipples are not a reliable guide to the 4th intercostal spaces in adult females. **○**

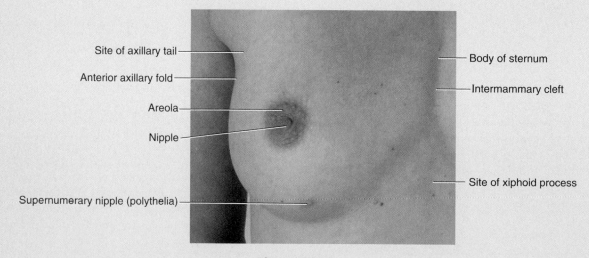

- Site of axillary tail
- Anterior axillary fold
- Areola
- Nipple
- Supernumerary nipple (polythelia)
- Body of sternum
- Intermammary cleft
- Site of xiphoid process

Figure SA1.5

Viscera of the Thoracic Cavity

When sectioned transversely, it is apparent that the *thoracic cavity* is kidney shaped: a transversely ovoid space deeply indented posteriorly by the thoracic vertebral column and the posteromedial parts of the ribs (heads and necks), which ar-

ticulate with it (Fig. 1.23*A*). The thoracic cavity is divided into three compartments (Figs. 1.23*A* & *C*):

- Right and left *pulmonary cavities,* bilateral compartments, which contain the lungs and *pleurae* (lining membranes) and occupy the majority of the thoracic cavity.

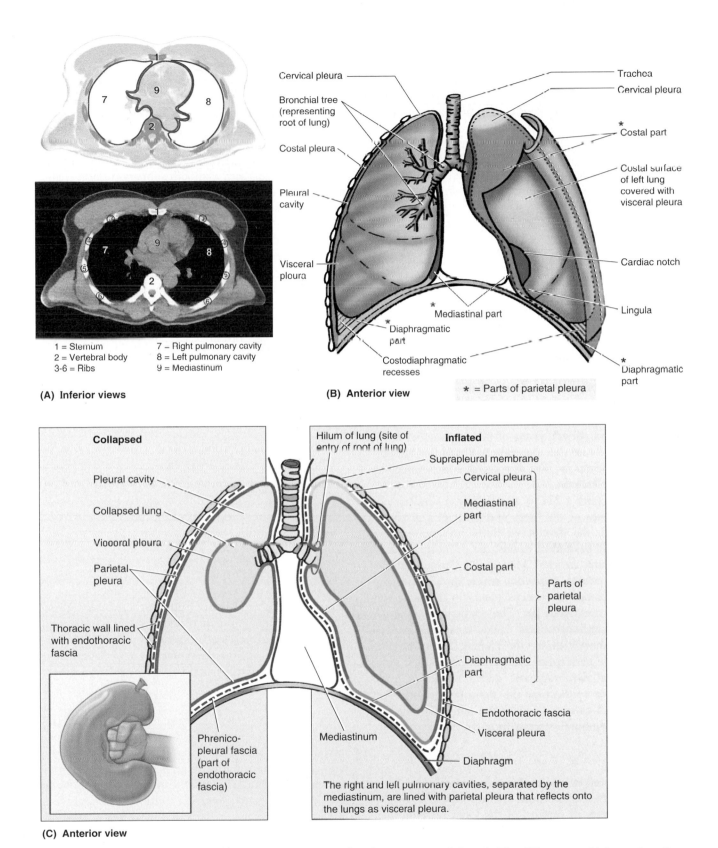

(A) Inferior views

1 = Sternum
2 = Vertebral body
3-6 = Ribs
7 – Right pulmonary cavity
8 = Left pulmonary cavity
9 = Mediastinum

(B) Anterior view

Cervical pleura
Bronchial tree (representing root of lung)
Costal pleura
Pleural cavity
Visceral pleura
Trachea
Cervical pleura
* Costal part
Costal surface of left lung covered with visceral pleura
Cardiac notch
Lingula
* Mediastinal part
* Diaphragmatic part
Costodiaphragmatic recesses
* Diaphragmatic part
* = Parts of parietal pleura

(C) Anterior view

Collapsed
Pleural cavity
Collapsed lung
Visceral pleura
Parietal pleura
Thoracic wall lined with endothoracic fascia
Phrenico-pleural fascia (part of endothoracic fascia)

Hilum of lung (site of entry of root of lung)
Inflated
Suprapleural membrane
Cervical pleura
Mediastinal part
Costal part
Parts of parietal pleura
Diaphragmatic part
Endothoracic fascia
Visceral pleura
Diaphragm
Mediastinum

The right and left pulmonary cavities, separated by the mediastinum, are lined with parietal pleura that reflects onto the lungs as visceral pleura.

Figure 1.23. Divisions of thoracic cavity and lining of pulmonary cavities. A. The CT scan and interpretive diagram of a transverse cross-sectional view of the thoracic cavity demonstrates the kidney-like shape and division into three compartments. (From Dean and Herbener, 2000.) The dimensional (**B**) and coronal cross-sectional (**C**) views demonstrate the linings of the pleural cavities and lungs (pleurae). The parts of the parietal pleura are named after the portion of the wall of the pulmonary cavity that they cover. Each lung is invested by the inner layer of a closed sac that has been invaginated by the lung. The cervical pleura, extending above the ribs, is reinforced by an overlying fibrous portion of the endothoracic fascia, the suprapleural membrane. Another portion of the endothoracic fascia, the phrenicopleural fascia, attaches the diaphragmatic part of the parietal pleura to the diaphragm. **Inset:** A fist invaginating an underinflated balloon demonstrates the relationship of the lung (represented by the fist) to walls of the pleural sac (parietal and visceral layers of pleura).

- A *central mediastinum,* a compartment intervening between and completely separating the two pulmonary cavities, which contains essentially all other thoracic structures—the heart, thoracic parts of the great vessels, thoracic part of the trachea, esophagus, thymus, and other structures (e.g., lymph nodes). It extends vertically from the superior thoracic aperture to the diaphragm and anteroposteriorly from the thoracic vertebral bodies to the sternum.

Pleurae and Lungs

The **pulmonary cavities** are lined by pleural membranes (**pleurae**) that also reflect onto and cover the external surface of the lungs contained within the cavities (Fig. 1.23*B* & *C*). To visualize the relationship of the pleurae and lungs, push your fist into an underinflated balloon (Fig. 1.23*C*). The inner part of the balloon wall (adjacent to your fist), which represents the lung, is comparable to the *visceral pleura;* the remaining outer wall of the balloon represents the *parietal pleura.* The cavity between the layers of the balloon is analogous to the pleural cavity. At your wrist (root of the lung), the inner and outer walls of the balloon are continuous, as are the visceral and parietal layers of pleura, together forming a pleural sac. Note that the lung is outside of but surrounded by the pleural sac, just as your fist is surrounded by but outside of the balloon.

The inset in Figure 1.23*C* is also helpful in understanding the development of the lungs and pleurae. During the embryonic period, the developing lungs invaginate (grow into) the **pericardioperitoneal canals,** the primordia (beginnings) of the pleural cavities (Moore and Persaud, 2003). The invaginated *coelomic epithelium* covers the primordia of the lungs and becomes the visceral pleura in the same way that the balloon covers your fist. The epithelium lining the walls of the pericardioperitoneal canals forms the parietal pleura. During embryogenesis, the pleural cavities become separated from the pericardial and peritoneal cavities; however, a congenital diaphragmatic defect results in a *diaphragmatic hernia* connecting the peritoneal cavity with one of the pleural cavities (usually the left one), and the herniation of abdominal viscera into the thorax (Moore et al., 2000).

Pleurae
Each lung is invested by and enclosed in a serous pleural sac that consists of two continuous membranes: the *visceral pleura,* which invests all surfaces of the lungs forming their shiny outer surface, and the *parietal pleura,* which lines the pulmonary cavities (Fig. 1.23*B* & *C*). The **pleural cavity**—the potential space between the layers of pleura—contains a capillary layer of **serous pleural fluid,** which lubricates the pleural surfaces and allows the layers of pleura to slide smoothly over each other during respiration. Its surface tension also provides the cohesion that keeps the lung surface in contact with the thoracic wall; consequently, the lung expands and fills with air when the thorax expands while still

allowing sliding to occur, much like a layer of water between two glass plates.

The **visceral pleura** (pulmonary pleura) closely covers the lung and is adherent to all its surfaces, including the surfaces within the horizontal and oblique fissures; it cannot be dissected from their surfaces (Fig. 1.24*A*). The visceral pleura provides the lung with a smooth slippery surface, enabling it to move freely on the parietal pleura. The visceral pleura is continuous with the parietal pleura at the **hilum of the lung,** where structures making up the *root of the lung* (e.g., the bronchus and pulmonary vessels) enter and leave the lung.

The **parietal pleura** lines the pulmonary cavities, thereby adhering to the thoracic wall, the mediastinum, and the diaphragm. It is more substantial than the visceral pleura, and in surgery and in cadaver dissections, it may be separated from the surfaces it covers. The parietal pleura consists of four parts:

- The **costal part** covers the internal surfaces of the thoracic wall.

- The **mediastinal part** covers the lateral aspects of the mediastinum—the mass of tissues and organs separating the pulmonary cavities and their pleural sacs.

- The **diaphragmatic part** covers the superior or thoracic surface of the diaphragm on each side of the mediastinum.

- The **cervical pleura** extends through the superior thoracic aperture into the root of the neck, forming a cup-shaped pleural dome over the apex of the lung (the part extending above the 1st rib).

The *costal part of the parietal pleura* (costovertebral or costal pleura) is separated from the internal surface of the thoracic wall (sternum, ribs and costal cartilages, intercostal muscles and membranes, and sides of thoracic vertebrae) by *endothoracic fascia.* This thin, extrapleural layer of loose connective tissue forms a natural cleavage plane for the surgical separation of the costal pleura from the thoracic wall (see clinical correlation [blue] box "Extrapleural Intrathoracic Surgical Access," in this chapter).

The *mediastinal part of the parietal pleura* (mediastinal pleura) covers the lateral aspects of the mediastinum, the partition between the pulmonary cavities. It continues superiorly into the root of the neck as cervical pleura. It is continuous with costal pleura anteriorly and posteriorly and with the diaphragmatic pleura inferiorly. Superior to the root of the lung, the mediastinal pleura is a continuous sheet passing anteroposteriorly between the sternum and the vertebral column. At the *hilum of the lung,* the mediastinal pleura reflects laterally onto the structures making up the root of the lung and becomes continuous with the visceral pleura.

Inferior to the root of the lung, this continuity between parietal and visceral pleura is an "empty" double layer of pleura, the **pulmonary ligament,** extending between the lung and the mediastinum, immediately anterior to the esophagus (Fig. 1.26). When the root of the lung is severed and the lung is removed, this double layer of pleura appears to hang from the root, similar to the manner in which the large sleeve of a Chinese robe hangs from the forearm. To visualize the root of the lung, the pleural sleeve surrounding it, and the pulmonary ligament hanging from it, put on an extra-large lab coat and abduct your upper limb. Your forearm is comparable to the root of the lung,

and the coat sleeve represents the pleural sleeve surrounding the root. The pulmonary ligament is comparable to the slack of the sleeve as it hangs from your forearm; and your wrist, hand, and abducted fingers represent the branching structures of the root—the bronchi and pulmonary vessels.

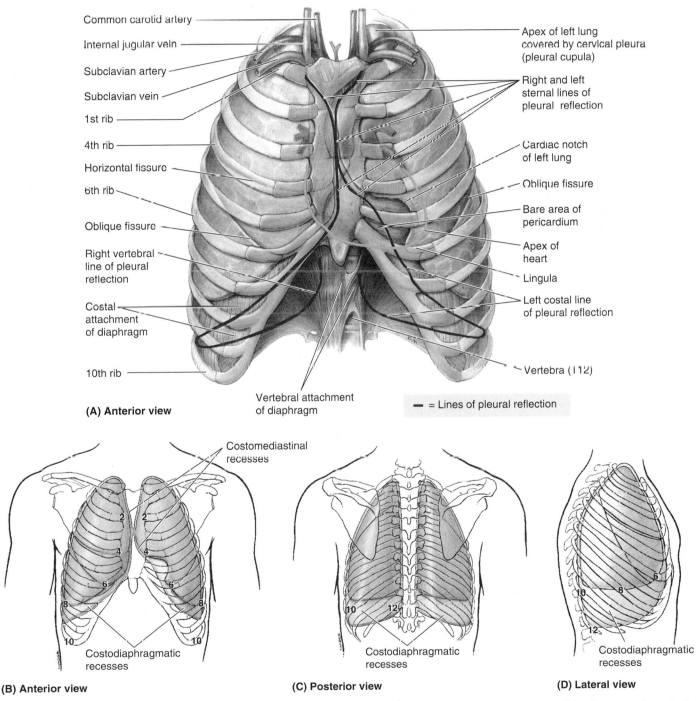

Common carotid artery

Internal jugular vein

Subclavian artery

Subclavian vein

1st rib

4th rib

Horizontal fissure

6th rib

Oblique fissure

Right vertebral line of pleural reflection

Costal attachment of diaphragm

10th rib

Vertebral attachment of diaphragm

(A) Anterior view

Apex of left lung covered by cervical pleura (pleural cupula)

Right and left sternal lines of pleural reflection

Cardiac notch of left lung

Oblique fissure

Bare area of pericardium

Apex of heart

Lingula

Left costal line of pleural reflection

Vertebra (T12)

▬ = Lines of pleural reflection

Costomediastinal recesses

Costodiaphragmatic recesses

(B) Anterior view

Costodiaphragmatic recesses

(C) Posterior view

Costodiaphragmatic recesses

(D) Lateral view

Figure 1.24. Relationship of thoracic contents and linings of thoracic cage. A. The apices of the lungs and cervical pleura extend into the neck. The left sternal reflection of parietal pleura deviates away from the median plane toward the left side in the region of the lung's cardiac notch, leaving a bare area, where the pericardial sac is accessible for needle puncture without traversing the lung or pleural cavity. **B–D.** The shapes of the parietal pleura and lungs during quiet respiration are demonstrated. The costodiaphragmatic recesses, not occupied by lung, are where pleural exudate accumulates when the body is erect. Observe that the outline of the horizontal fissure in the right lung clearly parallels the 4th rib. (Ribs are identified by number.)

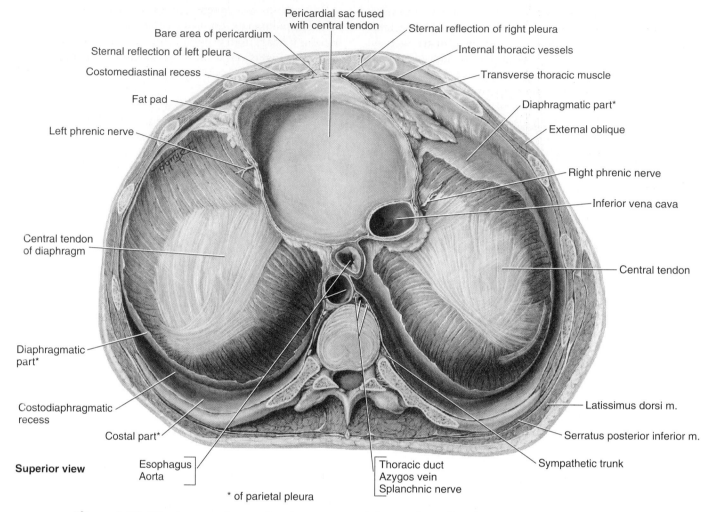

Pericardial sac fused
with central tendon

Bare area of pericardium

Sternal reflection of left pleura

Costomediastinal recess

Fat pad

Left phrenic nerve

Central tendon
of diaphragm

Diaphragmatic
part*

Costodiaphragmatic
recess

Costal part*

Superior view

Esophagus
Aorta

Sternal reflection of right pleura

Internal thoracic vessels

Transverse thoracic muscle

Diaphragmatic part*

External oblique

Right phrenic nerve

Inferior vena cava

Central tendon

Latissimus dorsi m.

Serratus posterior inferior m.

Sympathetic trunk

Thoracic duct
Azygos vein
Splanchnic nerve

* of parietal pleura

Figure 1.25. Diaphragm, base of pulmonary cavities and mediastinum, and costodiaphragmatic recesses. Most of the diaphragmatic pleura has been removed. At this level, the mediastinum consists of the pericardial sac (middle mediastinum) and the posterior mediastinum, mainly containing the esophagus and aorta. The deep groove surrounding the convexity of the diaphragm is the costodiaphragmatic recess, lined with parietal pleura. The pericardium and costomediastinal recesses and, between them, an area of pericardium only (the bare area) lie between the heart and the thoracic wall at this level.

The *diaphragmatic part of the parietal pleura* (diaphragmatic pleura) covers the superior surface of the diaphragm, except along its costal attachments (origins) and where the diaphragm is fused to the *pericardium,* the fibroserous membrane surrounding the heart (Fig. 1.23B & C). A thin, more elastic layer of endothoracic fascia, the **phrenicopleural fascia,** connects the diaphragmatic pleura with the muscular fibers of the diaphragm (Fig. 1.23C).

The *cervical pleura* (pleural cupula, dome of pleura) is the dome-shaped cap of the pleural sac and is the superior continuation of the costal and mediastinal parts of the parietal pleura. The cervical pleura covers the apex of the lung that extends superiorly through the superior thoracic aperture into the root of the neck (Fig. 1.24A). The summit of the cervical pleura is 2–3 cm superior to the level of the medial third of the clavicle at the level of the neck of the 1st

rib. The cervical pleura is reinforced by a fibrous extension of the endothoracic fascia—the **suprapleural membrane** (Sibson fascia), which attaches to the internal border of the 1st rib and the transverse process of C7 vertebra (Fig. 1.23C).

The relatively abrupt lines along which the parietal pleura changes direction as it passes (reflects) from one wall of the pleural cavity to another are the *lines of pleural reflection* (Figs. 1.24 and 1.25):

- The **sternal line** of pleural reflection is sharp or abrupt and occurs where the costal pleura becomes continuous with the mediastinal pleura anteriorly.

- The **costal line** of pleural reflection is also sharp and occurs where the costal pleura becomes continuous with diaphragmatic pleura inferiorly.

- The **vertebral line** of pleural reflection is a much rounder, gradual reflection and occurs where the costal pleura becomes continuous with the mediastinal pleura posteriorly.

The right and left sternal reflections of pleura are indicated by lines that pass inferomedially from the sternoclavicular joints to the AML at the level of the sternal angle. Between the levels of costal cartilages 2–4, the pleural sacs come in contact and may even slightly overlap each other.

The *sternal line of pleural reflection on the right side* passes inferiorly in the median plane to the posterior aspect of the xiphoid process (level of the 6th costal cartilage), where it turns laterally (Fig. 1.24). The *sternal line of reflection on the left side* passes inferiorly in the median plane only to the level of the 4th costal cartilage. Here it passes to the left margin of the sternum and then continues inferiorly to the 6th costal cartilage, creating a notch, which is shallower than the cardiac notch of the lung and allows a part of the pericardium (heart sac) to be in direct contact with the anterior thoracic wall. This is important for *pericardiocentesis* (see clinical correlation [blue] box, "Pericardiocentesis," in this chapter).

The costal line of pleural reflection passes obliquely across the 8th rib in the MCL, the 10th rib in the MAL, and the 12th rib at its neck or inferior to it. The vertebral line of pleural reflection parallels the vertebral column, running in the paravertebral plane from vertebral level T1 through T12.

The lungs do not occupy the pulmonary cavities completely during expiration; thus the peripheral diaphragmatic pleura is in contact with the lowermost parts of the costal pleura. The potential pleural spaces here are the **costodiaphragmatic recesses,** pleura-lined "gutters," which surround the upward convexity of the diaphragm inside the thoracic wall (Figs. 1.23C and 1.25). Similar but smaller pleural recesses are located posterior to the sternum where the costal pleura is in contact with the mediastinal pleura. The potential pleural spaces here are the **costomediastinal recesses;** the left recess is potentially larger (less occupied) because of the *cardiac notch* in the left lung. The inferior borders of the lungs move farther into the pleural recesses during deep inspiration and retreat from them during expiration.

Injuries to the Cervical Pleura and Apex of Lung

Because of the inferior slope of the 1st pair of ribs and the superior thoracic aperture they form, the cervical pleura and apex of the lung project through this opening into the neck, posterior to the inferior attachments of the sternocleidomastoid muscles. Consequently, the lungs and pleural sacs may be injured in wounds to the base of the neck resulting in a **pneumothorax,** the presence of air (G. *pneuma*) in the pleural cavity. The cervical pleura reaches a relatively higher level in infants and young children because of the shortness of their necks. Consequently, the cervical pleura is especially vulnerable to injury during the first few years after birth.

Injury to Other Parts of the Pleurae

The pleurae descend inferior to the costal margin in three regions, where an abdominal incision might inadvertently enter a pleural sac: the right part of the infrasternal angle and right and left costovertebral angles. The small areas of pleura exposed in the costovertebral angles inferomedial to the 12th ribs are posterior to the superior poles of the kidneys. The pleura is in danger here (i.e., a pneumothorax may occur) from an incision in the posterior abdominal wall when surgical procedures expose a kidney, for example.

Pulmonary Collapse

The lungs (more specifically, the air sacs that collectively make up the lung) are comparable to an inflated balloon when they are distended. If the distension is not maintained, their inherent elasticity will cause them to collapse (*secondary atelectasis* is the collapse of a previously inflated lung; *primary atelectasis* refers to the failure of a lung to inflate at birth). An inflated balloon remains distended only as long as its outlet is closed. Normal lungs in situ remain distended even when their outlet (the airway) is open because their outer surfaces (visceral pleura) adhere to the inner surface of the thoracic walls (parietal pleura) as a result of the surface tension consequent to the pleural fluid between them. The elastic recoil of the lungs causes the pressure in the pleural cavities to be sub-atmospheric. The pressure is usually about −2 mm Hg; during inspiration, it drops to about −8 mm Hg.

If a penetrating wound (hole) opens through the thorax or in the lungs, air will be sucked into the pleural cavity because of the negative pressure (Fig. B1.8). The surface tension adhering visceral to parietal pleura (lung to thoracic wall) will be broken, and the lung will collapse, expelling most of its air because of its inherent elasticity (elastic recoil). When a lung collapses, the pleural cavity (normally a potential space) becomes a real space. The pleural sacs do not normally communicate; thus one lung may be collapsed after surgery, for example, without ▶

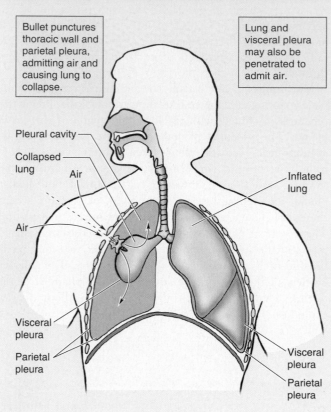

Bullet punctures thoracic wall and parietal pleura, admitting air and causing lung to collapse.

Lung and visceral pleura may also be penetrated to admit air.

Pleural cavity

Collapsed lung

Air

Air

Inflated lung

Visceral pleura

Parietal pleura

Visceral pleura

Parietal pleura

Figure B1.8

the other lung collapsing. Laceration or rupture of the surface of a lung (and its visceral pleura) or penetration of the thoracic wall (and its parietal pleura) results in hemorrhage and the entrance of air into the pleural cavity. The amount of blood and air that accumulates determines the extent of pulmonary collapse.

When the lung collapses, it occupies less volume within the pulmonary cavity and the pulmonary cavity does not increase in size (in fact, it may decrease in size) during inspiration. This reduction in size will be evident radiographically on the affected side by elevation of the diaphragm above usual levels, intercostal space narrowing (ribs closer together), and displacement of the mediastinum (*mediastinal shift;* most evident via the air-filled trachea within it) toward the affected side. In addition, the collapsed lung will probably appear more dense (whiter) surrounded by more radiolucent (blacker) air.

In *open-chest surgery,* respiration and lung inflation must be maintained by intubating the trachea with a cuffed tube and using a positive-pressure pump, varying the pressure to alternately inflate and deflate the lungs.

Pneumothorax, Hydrothorax, and Hemothorax

Entry of air into the pleural cavity (*pneumothorax*), resulting from a penetrating wound of the parietal pleura from a bullet, for example, or from rupture of a pulmonary lesion into the pleural cavity (*bronchopulmonary fistula*), results in collapse of the lung (Fig. B1.8). Fractured ribs may also tear the visceral pleura and lung, thus producing pneumothorax. The accumulation of a significant amount of fluid in the pleural cavity (**hydrothorax**) may result from **pleural effusion** (escape of fluid into the pleural cavity). With a chest wound, blood may also enter the pleural cavity (**hemothorax**) (Fig. B1.9). Hemothorax results more commonly from injury to a major intercostal or internal thoracic vessel than from laceration of a lung. If both air and fluid (*hemopneumothorax,* if the fluid is blood) accumulate in the pleural cavity, an *air–fluid level* or interface (sharp line, horizontal regardless of the patient's position, indicating the upper surface of the fluid) will be seen on a radiograph.

Thoracentesis

Sometimes it is necessary to insert a hypodermic needle through an intercostal space into the pleural cavity (**thoracentesis**) to obtain a sample of fluid or to remove blood or pus (Fig. B1.10). To avoid damage to the intercostal nerve and vessels, the needle is inserted superior to the rib, high enough to avoid the collateral branches. The needle passes through the intercostal muscles and costal parietal pleura into the pleural cavity. When the patient is in the upright position, intrapleural fluid accumulates in the costodiaphragmatic recess. Inserting the needle into the 9th intercostal space in the midaxillary line during expiration will avoid the inferior border of the lung. The needle ▶

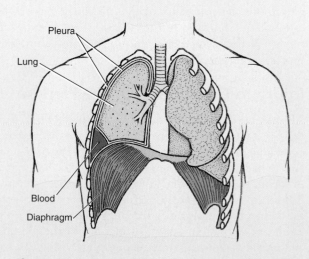

Pleura

Lung

Blood

Diaphragm

Figure B1.9. Hemothorax in right lung cavity.

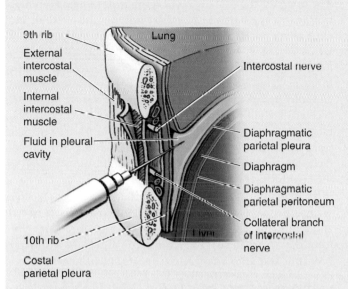

9th rib
External intercostal muscle
Internal intercostal muscle
Fluid in pleural cavity
10th rib
Costal parietal pleura
Lung
Intercostal nerve
Diaphragmatic parietal pleura
Diaphragm
Diaphragmatic parietal peritoneum
Collateral branch of intercostal nerve
Liver

Figure B1.10. Technique for thoracentesis (in MAL)

should be angled upward, to avoid penetrating the deep side of the recess (a thin layer of diaphragmatic parietal pleura and diaphragm overlying the liver).

Insertion of a Chest Tube

Major amounts of air, blood, serous fluid, pus or any combination of these substances in the pleural cavity are typically removed by placement of a chest tube. A short incision is made in the 5th or 6th intercostal space in the midaxillary line (which is approximately at nipple level). The tube may be directed superiorly (toward to the cervical pleura or pleural cupula) for air removal or inferiorly (toward the costodiaphragmatic recess) for fluid drainage. The extracorporeal end of the tube (i.e., the end that is outside of the body) is connected to an underwater drainage system, often with controlled suction, to prevent air from being sucked back into the pleural cavity. Removal of air allows reinflation of a collapsed lung. Failure to remove fluid may cause the lung to develop a resistant fibrous covering that inhibits expansion unless it is peeled (*lung decortication*).

Thoracoscopy

Thoracoscopy is a diagnostic and sometimes therapeutic procedure in which the pleural cavity is examined with a thoracoscope (Fig. B1.11). Small incisions are made into the pleural cavity via an intercostal space. In addition to observation, biopsies can be taken and some thoracic conditions can be treated (e.g., disrupting adhesions or removing plaques).

Pleuritis (Pleurisy)

During inspiration and expiration, the sliding of normally smooth, moist pleurae makes no detectable sound during **auscultation of the lungs** (listening to breath sounds); however, inflammation of the pleura, **pleuritis** or **pleurisy**, makes the lung surfaces rough. The resulting friction (*pleural rub*) is detectable with a stethoscope. It sounds ▶

Monitor showing excision of pleura (pleurectomy)
Forceps
Thoracoscope
(A)

Lung covered with visceral pleura
Intercostal vessels external to costal part of parietal pleura
(B) Thoracoscopic view

Figure B1.11

like a clump of hair being rolled between the fingers. The inflamed surfaces of pleura may also cause the parietal and visceral layers of pleura to adhere (*pleural adhesion*). Acute pleuritis is marked by sharp, stabbing pain, especially on exertion, such as climbing stairs, when the rate and depth of respiration may be increased even slightly.

Pleurectomy and Pleurodesis

Obliteration of a pleural cavity by disease such as *pleuritis* (inflammation of pleura) or during surgery (**pleurectomy,** or excision of a part of the pleura, for example (Fig. B1.11) does not cause appreciable functional consequences; however, it may produce pain during exertion. In other procedures, adherence of the parietal and visceral layers of pleura is induced by covering the apposing layers of pleura with an irritating powder or sclerosing agent (**pleurodesis**). Pleurectomy and pleurodesis are performed to prevent recurring *spontaneous secondary atelectasis* (spontaneous lung collapse) caused by chronic pneumothorax or malignant effusion resulting from lung disease (Ahya et al., 2001). ○

THE BOTTOM LINE: The thoracic cavity is divided into three compartments: two bilateral pulmonary cavities that are entirely separated by the central mediastinum. The pulmonary cavities are completely lined by membranous parietal pleura that reflects onto the lungs at their roots, becoming the visceral pleura that intimately invests the lungs' outer surface. The pleural cavity between the two layers of the pleural sac is empty, except for a lubricating film of pleural fluid. The pleural fluid also maintains the surface tension that keeps the surface of the lung applied to the internal surface of the thoracic wall, preventing collapse of the open respiratory system, and causing the lungs to expand when the thorax expands for inhalation. Most of the parietal pleura is named for the structures it covers: costal, mediastinal, and diaphragmatic. The cervical pleura extends as a peak or dome above the anterior aspect of the 1st rib and clavicle into the root of the neck. Parietal pleura is sensitive, being innervated by the phrenic and intercostal nerves. Because the lungs do not completely fill the pulmonary cavities, and because of the protrusion of the diaphragm and underlying abdominal viscera into the inferior thoracic aperture, a peripheral gutter—the costodiaphragmatic recess—is formed. Extrapulmonary fluids (exudates) accumulate in this space when the trunk is erect. Awareness of the extent of the lungs and pleural cavities is important for physical examination and detection of disease.

Lungs

The **lungs** are the vital organs of respiration. Their main function is to oxygenate the blood by bringing inspired air into close relation with the venous blood in the pulmonary capillaries. Although cadaveric lungs may be shrunken, firm or hard to the touch, and discolored in appearance, healthy lungs in living people are normally light, soft, and spongy, and fully occupy the pulmonary cavities. They are also elastic and recoil to approximately one third their size when the thoracic cavity is opened (Fig. 1.23*C*). The lungs are separated from each other by the mediastinum, to which they are attached by the **roots of the lungs**—that is, the bronchi (and associated bronchial vessels), pulmonary arteries, superior and inferior pulmonary veins, the pulmonary plexuses of nerves (sympathetic, parasympathetic, and visceral afferent fibers), and lymphatic vessels (Fig. 1.26). If the root is sectioned before the (medial to) branching of the main (primary) bronchus and pulmonary artery, its general arrangement is

- Pulmonary artery, superiormost on left (the superior lobar or "eparterial" bronchus may be superiormost on the right).

- Superior and inferior pulmonary veins, anteriormost and inferiormost, respectively.

- Bronchus, against and approximately in the middle of the posterior boundary, with the bronchial vessels immediately surrounding (usually on posterior aspect at this point).

Medial to the hilum, the root is enclosed within the area of continuity between the parietal and the visceral layers of pleura—the **pleural sleeve,** or **mesopneumonium** (mesentery of the lung). The *hilum of the lung* is a wedge-shaped area of the medial surface of each lung, the point at which the structures forming the root enter and leave the lung. The hilum (doorway) can be likened to the area of earth where a plant's roots enter the ground.

The **horizontal** and **oblique fissures** divide the lungs into **lobes** (Figs. 1.26 and 1.27). The right lung has three lobes, the left lung has two. The right lung is larger and heavier than the left, but it is shorter and wider because the right dome of the diaphragm is higher and the heart and pericardium bulge more to the left. The anterior border of the right lung is relatively straight, whereas this border of the left lung has a deep **cardiac notch,** an indentation consequent to the deviation of the apex of the heart to the left side. This notch primarily indents the anteroinferior aspect of the superior lobe of the left lung. This indentation often creates a thin, tongue-like process of the superior lobe, the **lingula** (L. dim. of *lingua,* tongue), which extends below the cardiac notch and slides in and out of the costomediastinal recess during inspiration and expiration (Figs. 1.23*B*, 1.24*A,* and 1.26*C*). Each lung has (Figs. 1.26 and 1.27)

- *An apex,* the blunt superior end of the lung ascending above the level of the 1st rib into the root of the neck that is covered by cervical pleura.

(*cont'd on page 123*)

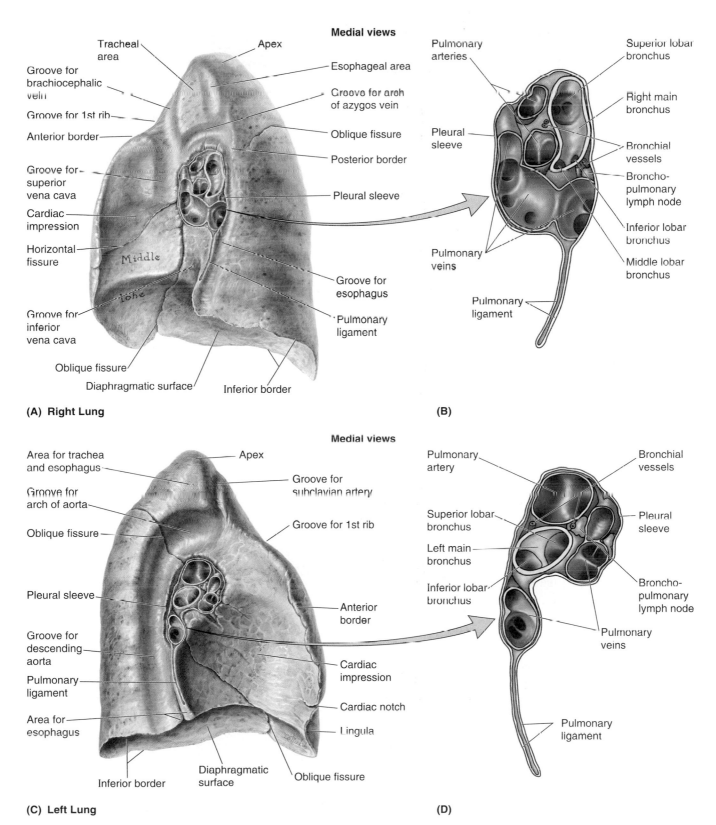

Medial views

(A) Right Lung

- Tracheal area
- Groove for brachiocephalic vein
- Groove for 1st rib
- Anterior border
- Groove for superior vena cava
- Cardiac impression
- Horizontal fissure
- Middle lobe
- Groove for inferior vena cava
- Oblique fissure
- Diaphragmatic surface
- Apex
- Esophageal area
- Groove for arch of azygos vein
- Oblique fissure
- Posterior border
- Pleural sleeve
- Groove for esophagus
- Pulmonary ligament
- Inferior border

(B)

- Pulmonary arteries
- Pleural sleeve
- Pulmonary veins
- Pulmonary ligament
- Superior lobar bronchus
- Right main bronchus
- Bronchial vessels
- Broncho-pulmonary lymph node
- Inferior lobar bronchus
- Middle lobar bronchus

Medial views

(C) Left Lung

- Area for trachea and esophagus
- Groove for arch of aorta
- Oblique fissure
- Pleural sleeve
- Groove for descending aorta
- Pulmonary ligament
- Area for esophagus
- Inferior border
- Diaphragmatic surface
- Apex
- Groove for subclavian artery
- Groove for 1st rib
- Anterior border
- Cardiac impression
- Cardiac notch
- Lingula
- Oblique fissure

(D)

- Pulmonary artery
- Superior lobar bronchus
- Left main bronchus
- Inferior lobar bronchus
- Bronchial vessels
- Pleural sleeve
- Broncho-pulmonary lymph node
- Pulmonary veins
- Pulmonary ligament

Figure 1.26. Mediastinal surfaces and hila of lungs. The hilum of each lung is centered in the mediastinal surface. At the hilum (**B and D**), the root of each lung is surrounded by a pleural sleeve that descends inferior to the root as the pulmonary ligament. The pulmonary veins are the most anterior and inferior in the root, with the bronchi central and posteriorly placed. Impressions are formed in embalmed lungs by contact with adjacent structures. Superior to the root of the right lung (**A**), a groove is formed as the arch of the azygos vein courses anteriorly to enter the SVC; whereas in the left lung (**C**), a similar but larger groove is formed superior to the root as the aorta arches posteriorly and descends as the thoracic aorta.

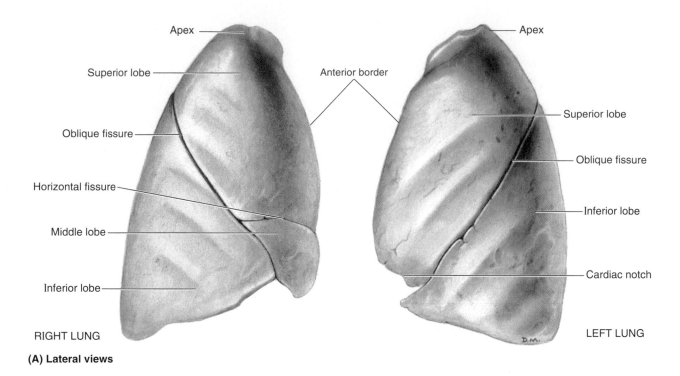

Apex

Superior lobe

Anterior border

Apex

Superior lobe

Oblique fissure

Oblique fissure

Horizontal fissure

Inferior lobe

Middle lobe

Inferior lobe

Cardiac notch

RIGHT LUNG

LEFT LUNG

(A) Lateral views

Right vagus nerve

Trachea

Left vagus nerve

Superior lobe of right lung

Phrenic nerve

Origin of left recurrent
laryngeal nerve

Costal surface of lung

Superior lobe of left lung

Root of lung

Horizontal fissure

Parietal layer of
serous pericardium

Middle lobe
of right lung

Fibrous pericardium

Oblique fissure

Oblique fissure

Inferior lobe
of right lung

Mediastinal surface of lung

Inferior lobe of left lung

Costal part of
parietal pleura

Costodiaphragmatic recess

Diaphragm

(B) Anterior view

Figure 1.27. Costal surfaces of lungs. A. The lungs are shown in isolation. **B.** The heart and lungs are shown in situ. Although clearly defined here, the oblique and horizontal fissures may be incomplete or absent in some specimens. In part **B,** the left lung is retracted from the heart (fibrous pericardium) revealing the phrenic nerve as it passes anterior to the root of the lung, while the vagus nerve (CN X) passes posterior to the root.

- Three *surfaces* (costal, mediastinal, and diaphragmatic).

- Three *borders* (anterior, inferior, and posterior).

The lungs of an embalmed cadaver, usually firm to the touch, have impressions that are formed by the structures adjacent to them, such as the ribs (Fig. 1.27A & B). These markings provide clues to the relationships of the lungs; however, they are not visible during surgery or in fresh cadaveric or postmortem specimens.

The *costal surface of the lung* is large, smooth, and convex. It is related to the costal pleura, which separates it from the ribs, costal cartilages, and the innermost intercostal muscles. The posterior part of the costal surface is related to the bodies of the thoracic vertebrae and is sometimes referred to as the *vertebral part of the costal surface.*

The *mediastinal surface of the lung* is concave because it is related to the middle mediastinum, which contains the pericardium and heart (Fig. 1.26). The mediastinal surface includes the hilum and thus receives the root of the lung, around which the pleura forms the pleural sleeve. The *pulmonary ligament* hangs inferiorly from the pleural sleeve around the lung root. If embalmed, there is a *groove for the esophagus* and a *cardiac impression for the heart* on the medi-

astinal surface of the right lung. Because two thirds of the heart lies to the left of the midline, the cardiac impression on the mediastinal surface of the left lung is much larger. This surface of the left lung also features a prominent, continuous groove for the *arch of the aorta* and the *descending* (thoracic) *aorta* as well as a smaller groove for the esophagus.

The *diaphragmatic surface of the lung,* which is also concave, forms the *base of the lung,* which rests on the dome of the diaphragm. The concavity is deeper in the right lung because of the higher position of the right diaphragmatic dome, which overlies the large liver. Laterally and posteriorly, the diaphragmatic surface is bounded by a thin, sharp margin (inferior border) that projects into the *costodiaphragmatic recess* of the pleura (Figs. 1.26 and 1.27B).

The *anterior border of the lung* is where the costal and mediastinal surfaces meet anteriorly and overlap the heart; the cardiac notch indents this border of the left lung. The *inferior border of the lung* circumscribes the diaphragmatic surface of the lung and separates this surface from the costal and mediastinal surfaces. The *posterior border of the lung* is where the costal and mediastinal surfaces meet posteriorly; it is broad and rounded and lies in the cavity at the side of the thoracic region of the vertebral column.

Variations in the Lobes of the Lung

Occasionally, an extra fissure divides a lung or a fissure is absent. For example, the left lung sometimes has three lobes and the right lung only two. The most common "accessory" lobe is the *azygos lobe,* which appears in the right lung in approximately 1% of people. In these cases, the azygos vein arches over the apex of the right lung and not over the right hilum, isolating the medial part of the apex as an azygos lobe.

Appearance of the Lungs and Inhalation of Carbon Particles and Irritants

The lungs are light pink in healthy children and people who are non-smokers and live in a clean environment (e.g., Pacific islanders). The lungs are commonly dark and mottled in most adults who live in either urban or agricultural areas, especially those who smoke, because of the accumulation of carbon and dust particles in the air and irritants in tobacco that are inhaled. *Smoker's cough* results from the inhalation of these irritants. However, the lungs are capable of accumulating a considerable amount of carbon without being adversely affected. Lymph from the lungs carries special "dust cells" (*phagocytes*) that remove carbon from the gas-exchanging surfaces and deposit it in the "in-

active" connective tissue, which supports the lung or in lymph nodes receiving lymph from the lungs.

Auscultation of the Lungs and Percussion of the Thorax

Auscultation of the lungs (listening to their sounds with a stethoscope) and **percussion of the thorax** (tapping the thorax over the lungs with the fingers to detect sounds in the lungs) (Fig. B1.12A) are important techniques of physical examination. Auscultation assesses airflow through the tracheobronchial tree into the lobes of the lung. Percussion helps establish whether the underlying tissues are air filled (resonant sound), fluid filled (dull sound), or solid (flat sound). An awareness of normal anatomy, particularly the projection of the lungs and the portions that are overlapped by bone with associated muscles (e.g., the scapula) enable the examiner to know where flat and resonant sounds should be expected (Fig. B1.12B). Auscultation and percussion should always include the root of the neck where the apices of the lungs are located. When clinicians refer to "auscultating the base of the lung," they are not usually referring to its diaphragmatic surface or anatomical base. They are usually referring to the inferoposterior part of the inferior lobe. To auscultate this area, the clinician applies a stethoscope to the posterior thoracic wall at the level of the 10th thoracic vertebra. ▶

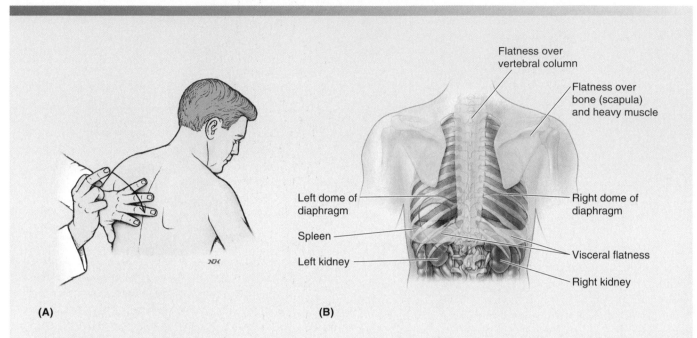

Figure B1.12. Percussion of the lungs. A. Bimanual percussion is shown. **B.** Areas of flatness (yellow) and resonance are shown.

Lung Cancer and Mediastinal Nerves

Lung cancer involving a phrenic nerve may result in paralysis of the hemidiaphragm. Because of the intimate relationship of the *recurrent laryngeal nerve* to the apex of the lung (Fig. 1.27*B*), this nerve may be involved in *apical lung cancers.* This involvement usually results in hoarseness owing to paralysis of a vocal fold (cord) because the recurrent laryngeal nerve supplies all but one of the laryngeal muscles (see Chapter 8). ☉

THE BOTTOM LINE: The lungs are the vital organs of respiration in which venous blood exchanges oxygen and carbon dioxide with a tidal airflow. Air and blood are delivered to each lung via its root, consisting of a pulmonary artery and vein and a main bronchus and their branches/tributaries that enter the lung at its hilum. Both lungs are pyramidal, having an apex, a base, three surfaces, and three borders. The right lung has three lobes that are separated by horizontal and oblique fissures; the left lung has two lobes, separated by an oblique fissure, and features a marked cardiac notch in its anterior border owing to the asymmetrical placement of the heart.

Trachea and Bronchi

Beginning at the *larynx,* the walls of the airway are supported by horseshoe- or C-shaped rings of hyaline cartilage. The sublaryngeal airway constitutes the **tracheobronchial tree.** The *trachea,* located within the superior mediastinum, constitutes the trunk of the tree. (The trachea will be described in greater detail with the *superior mediastinum,* later in this chapter.) It bifurcates at the level of the transverse thoracic plane (or sternal angle) into *main (primary) bronchi,* one to each lung, passing inferolaterally to enter the lungs at the hila (singular = hilum) (Fig. 1.28*B*).

• The **right main bronchus** is wider, shorter, and runs more vertically than the left main bronchus as it passes directly to the hilum of the lung.

• The **left main bronchus** passes inferolaterally, inferior to the arch of the aorta and anterior to the esophagus and thoracic aorta, to reach the hilum of the lung.

Within the lungs, the bronchi branch in a constant fashion to form the roots of the tracheobronchial tree, as components of the root of each lung (consisting of branches of the pulmonary artery and veins as well as the bronchi). Each main bronchus divides into **lobar bronchi** (secondary bronchi), two on the left and three on the right, each of which supplies a lobe of the lung. Each lobar bronchus divides into several **segmental bronchi** (tertiary bronchi) that supply the bronchopulmonary segments (Figs. 1.28 and 1.29).

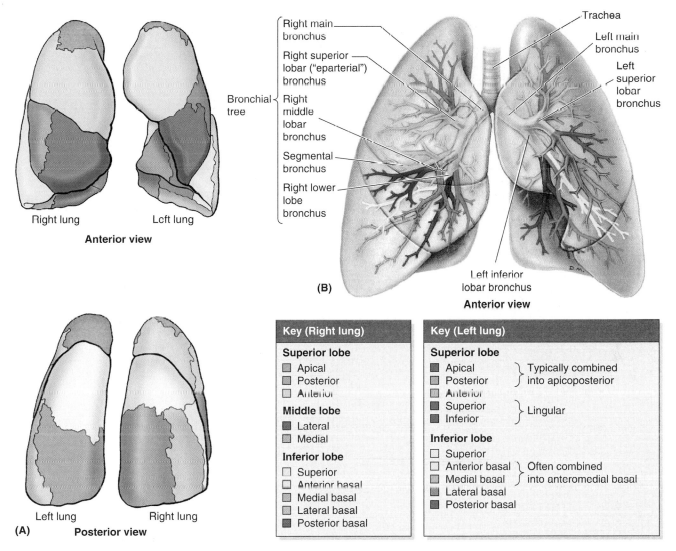

Bronchial tree

(B)
Anterior view

Key (Right lung)

Superior lobe
- ☐ Apical
- ☐ Posterior
- ☐ Anterior

Middle lobe
- ☐ Lateral
- ☐ Medial

Inferior lobe
- ☐ Superior
- ☐ Anterior basal
- ☐ Medial basal
- ☐ Lateral basal
- ☐ Posterior basal

Key (Left lung)

Superior lobe
- ☐ Apical   ⎫ Typically combined
- ☐ Posterior   ⎬ into apicoposterior
- ☐ Anterior
- ☐ Superior   ⎫ Lingular
- ☐ Inferior   ⎭

Inferior lobe
- ☐ Superior
- ☐ Anterior basal   ⎫ Often combined
- ☐ Medial basal   ⎬ into anteromedial basal
- ☐ Lateral basal
- ☐ Posterior basal

Figure 1.28. Tracheobronchial tree and bronchopulmonary segments. A, C, and D. The bronchopulmonary segments are demonstrated after injection of a different color latex into each segmental bronchus. **B.** The right main bronchus is more vertical and shorter than the left main bronchus. Although not apparent here, the right main bronchus gives off the right superior lobar (lobe) bronchus before entering the hilum of the lung. The lobar bronchi divide into segmental bronchi (colored), each of which serves a bronchopulmonary segment of the same name (and color).

The **bronchopulmonary segments** are

- Pyramidal-shaped segments of the lung, with their apices facing the lung root and their bases at the pleural surface.
- The largest subdivisions of a lobe.
- Separated from adjacent segments by connective tissue septa.
- Supplied independently by a segmental bronchus and a tertiary branch of the pulmonary artery.
- Named according to the segmental bronchi supplying them.
- Drained by intersegmental parts of the pulmonary veins that lie in the connective tissue between and drain adjacent segments.

- Surgically resectable.
- Usually 18–20 in number (10 in the right lung; 8–10 in the left lung, depending on the combining of segments).

Beyond the direct branches of the lobar bronchi—that is, beyond the segmental bronchi (Fig. 1.28B)—are from 20 to 25 generations of branches that eventually end in **terminal bronchioles** (Fig. 1.29). Each terminal bronchiole gives rise to several generations of **respiratory bronchioles,** and each respiratory bronchiole provides 2–11 **alveolar ducts,** each of which gives rise to 5–6 **alveolar sacs** lined by alveoli. The **pulmonary alveolus** is the basic structural unit of gas exchange in the lung. New alveoli continue to develop until about age 8 years, by which time there are approximately 300 million alveoli.

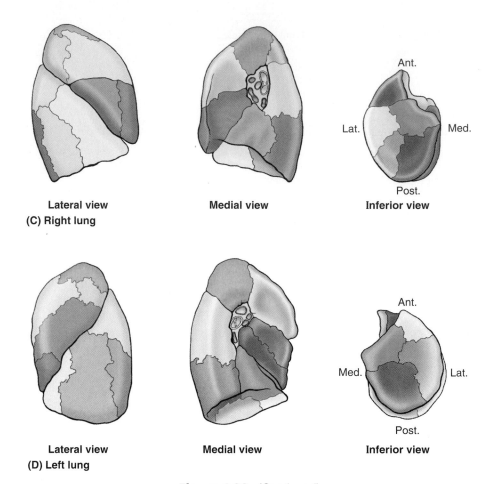

Lateral view
(C) Right lung

Medial view

Ant.

Lat.   Med.

Post.
Inferior view

Lateral view
(D) Left lung

Medial view

Ant.

Med.   Lat.

Post.
Inferior view

Figure 1.28. *(Continued)*

Aspiration of Foreign Bodies

Because the right bronchus is wider and shorter and runs more vertically than the left bronchus, foreign material (e.g., a foreign body or food) is more likely to enter and lodge in it or one of its branches. A potential hazard encountered by dentists is an aspirated foreign body, such as a piece of tooth or filling material, that is likely to enter the right main bronchus. To create a sterile environment and avoid aspiration of foreign objects, dentists may insert a thin rubber dam into the oral cavity during procedures.

Bronchoscopy

As a *bronchoscope* proceeds down the trachea to enter a main bronchus, a keel-like ridge, the **carina** (L. keel of a boat) is observed between the orifices of the main bronchi (Fig. B1.13). A cartilaginous projection of the last tracheal ring, the carina normally lies in a sagittal plane and has a fairly definite edge. If the tracheobronchial lymph nodes in the angle between the main bronchi are enlarged because cancer cells have metastasized from a *bronchogenic carcinoma,* for example, the carina is distorted, widened posteriorly, and immobile. Hence, morphological changes in the carina are important diagnostic signs to bronchoscopists in assisting with the differential diagnosis of respiratory disease.

The mucous membrane covering the carina is one of the most sensitive areas of the tracheobronchial tree and is associated with the *cough reflex.* For example, when children aspirate a peanut, they choke and cough. Once the peanut passes the carina, coughing usually stops. If the choking victim is inverted to make use of gravity to expel the foreign body (postural drainage of the lungs), lung ▶

(cont'd on page 128)

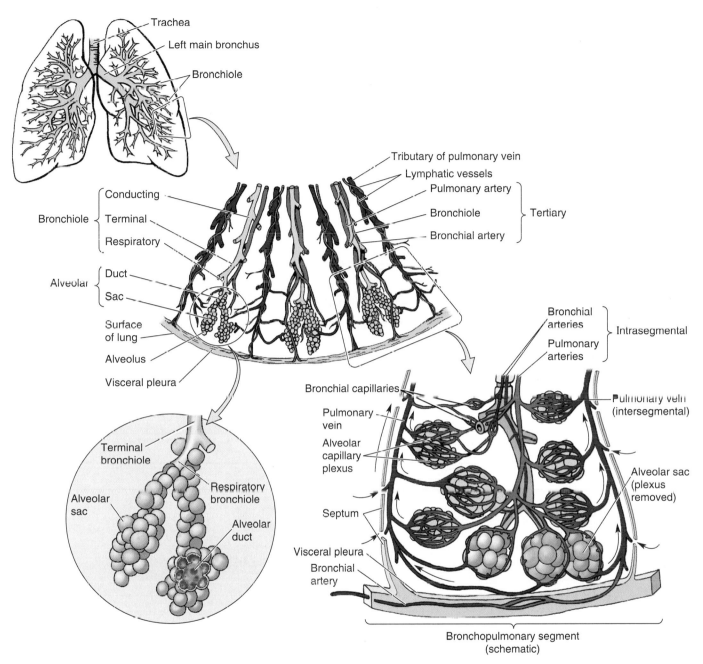

Figure 1.29. Internal structure and organization of lungs. Within the lungs, the bronchi and pulmonary arteries are paired and branch in unison. Segmental (tertiary) branches supply the bronchopulmonary segments, the smallest resectable units of the lungs. Each intrasegmental pulmonary artery, carrying poorly oxygenated blood, ends in a capillary plexus in the walls of the alveolar sacs and alveoli, where oxygen and carbon dioxide are exchanged. The pulmonary veins arise from the pulmonary capillaries and drain toward and then course within the septa between adjacent segments, carrying well-oxygenated blood to the heart. Bronchial arteries are distributed along and supply the bronchial tree. Their distalmost branches supply capillary beds drained by the pulmonary veins, such as those of the visceral pleura (even though this small amount of blood is poorly oxygenated).

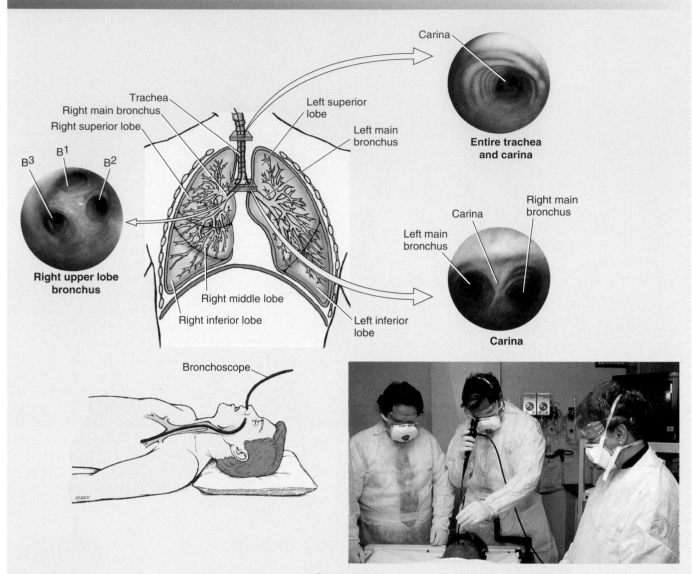

Figure B1.13

secretions passing the carina also cause coughing, which assists the expellation.

Lung Resections

Knowledge of the anatomy of the bronchopulmonary segments is essential for precise interpretation of radiographs and other medical images of the lungs. Knowledge of these segments is also essential for surgical resection of diseased segments. Bronchial and pulmonary disorders such as tumors or abscesses (collections of pus) often localize in a bronchopulmonary segment, which may be surgically resected. During treatment of *lung cancer*, the surgeon may remove a whole lung (**pneumonectomy**), a lobe (**lobectomy**), or a bronchopulmonary segment (**segmentectomy**).

Segmental Atelectasis

Blockage of a segmental bronchus, as by an aspirated object, will prevent air from reaching the bronchopulmonary segment it supplies. The air within the blocked segment will gradually be absorbed into the blood, and the segment will collapse. A segmental collapse does not require compensating space (air) in the pleural cavity to be realized because adjacent segments will expand to compensate for the reduced volume of the collapsed segment. ✪

Vasculature of the Lungs and Pleurae

Each lung has a large pulmonary artery supplying blood to it and two pulmonary veins draining blood from it (Fig. 1.30). The **right** and **left pulmonary arteries** arise from the *pulmonary trunk* at the level of the *sternal angle* and carry poorly oxygenated ("venous") blood to the lungs for oxygenation. (They are usually colored blue, like veins, in anatomical illustrations.) Each pulmonary artery becomes part of the root of the corresponding lung and gives off its first branch to the superior lobe before entering the hilum. Within the lung, each artery descends posterolateral to the main bronchus and divides into **lobar** and **segmental arteries**. Consequently, an arterial branch goes to each lobe and bronchopulmonary segment of the lung, usually on the anterior aspect of the corresponding bronchus. The arteries and bronchi are paired in the lung, branching simultaneously and running parallel courses.

The **pulmonary veins**, two on each side, carry well-oxygenated ("arterial") blood from the lungs to the left atrium of the heart. (They are commonly colored red or purple, like arteries, in anatomical illustrations.) Beginning in the pulmonary capillaries, the veins unite into larger and larger vessels. The pulmonary veins run independently of the arteries and bronchi, coursing between and receiving blood from adjacent segments as they run toward the hilum. The veins from the visceral pleura drain into the pulmonary veins, and the veins from the parietal pleura join systemic veins in adjacent parts of the thoracic wall.

The **bronchial arteries** supply blood for nutrition of the structures making up the root of the lungs, the supporting tissues of the lungs, and the visceral pleura (Fig. 1.31A). The two *left bronchial arteries* usually arise directly from the thoracic aorta. The single *right bronchial artery* may arise directly from the aorta. Most commonly it arises indirectly, either by way of the proximal part of one of the upper posterior intercostal arteries (usually the right 3rd posterior intercostal artery) or from a common trunk with the left superior bronchial artery.

The small bronchial arteries provide branches to the upper esophagus and then typically pass along the posterior aspects of the main bronchi, supplying them and their branches as far distally as the respiratory bronchioles. (However, see the variation shown in Figs. 1.53 and 1.59, drawn from a cadaver dissection.) The distalmost branches of the bronchial arteries anastomose with branches of the pulmonary arteries in the walls of the bronchioles and in the visceral pleura. The parietal pleura is supplied by the arteries that supply the thoracic wall (see "Arteries of the Thoracic Wall," in this chapter).

The **bronchial veins** (Fig. 1.31B) drain only part of the blood supplied to the lungs by the bronchial arteries, primar-

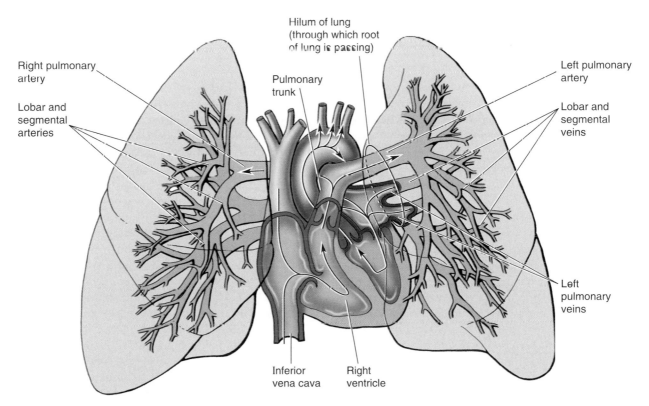

Figure 1.30. Pulmonary circulation. Although the intrapulmonary relationships are accurately demonstrated, the separation of the vessels of the root of the lung has been exaggerated in the hilar region to show them as they enter and leave the lung. Note that the right pulmonary artery passes under the arch of the aorta to reach the right lung and that the left pulmonary artery lies completely to the left of the arch.

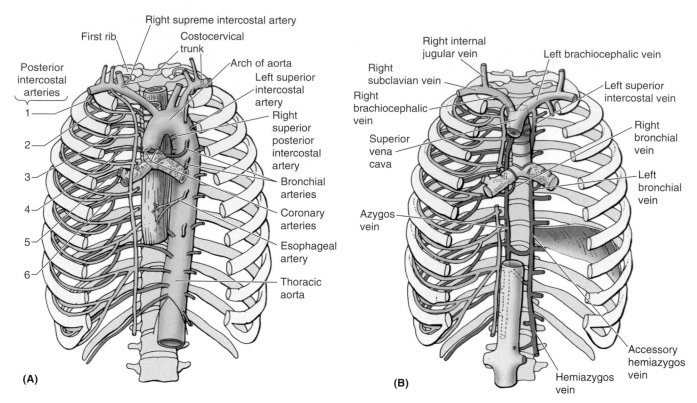

Figure 1.31. Bronchial arteries and veins. A. The bronchial arteries supply the supporting tissues of the lungs and visceral pleura. Left bronchial arteries arise from the superior thoracic aorta, but the origin of the right bronchial artery is variable; in order of frequency, it may arise (1) from a right posterior intercostal artery (usually the 3rd), (2) from a common trunk shared with the left superior bronchial artery, or (3) directly from the aorta. **B.** The bronchial veins drain the more proximal capillary beds supplied by the bronchial arteries; the rest is drained by the pulmonary veins. The right bronchial vein drains into the azygos vein and the left bronchial vein drains into the accessory hemiazygos vein or the left superior intercostal vein.

ily that distributed to or near the more proximal part of the roots of the lungs. The remainder of the blood is drained by the pulmonary veins, specifically that returning from the visceral pleura, the more peripheral regions of the lung, and the distal components of the root of the lung. The *right bronchial vein* drains into the *azygos vein* and the *left bronchial vein* drains into the *accessory hemiazygos vein* or the *left superior intercostal vein.* Bronchial veins also receive some blood from esophageal veins.

The *pulmonary lymphatic plexuses* communicate freely (Fig. 1.32). The **superficial** (subpleural) **lymphatic plexus** lies deep to the visceral pleura and drains the lung parenchyma (tissue) and visceral pleura. Lymphatic vessels from this superficial plexus drain into the **bronchopulmonary lymph nodes** (hilar lymph nodes) in the hilum of the lung.

The **deep lymphatic plexus** is located in the submucosa of the bronchi and in the peribronchial connective tissue. It is largely concerned with draining the structures that form the root of the lung. Lymphatic vessels from this deep plexus drain initially into the **pulmonary lymph nodes,** located along the lobar bronchi. Lymphatic vessels from these nodes continue to follow the bronchi and pulmonary vessels to the hilum of the lung, where they also drain into the bron-

chopulmonary (hilar) lymph nodes. From them, lymph from both the superficial and deep lymphatic plexuses drains to the **superior** and **inferior tracheobronchial lymph nodes,** superior and inferior to the bifurcation of the trachea and main bronchi, respectively. The right lung drains primarily through the respective sets of nodes on the right side, and the superior lobe of the left lung drains primarily through respective nodes of the left side. Many, but not all, of the lymphatics from the lower lobe of the left lung, however, drain to the right superior tracheobronchial nodes; the lymph then continues to follow the right-side pathway.

Lymph from the tracheobronchial lymph nodes passes to the *right* and *left bronchomediastinal lymph trunks.* These trunks usually terminate on each side at the *venous angles* (junctions of the subclavian and internal jugular veins); however, the right bronchomediastinal trunk may first merge with other lymphatic trunks, converging here to form the short **right lymphatic duct.** The left bronchomediastinal trunk may terminate in the **thoracic duct.** Lymph from the parietal pleura drains into the lymph nodes of the thoracic wall (intercostal, parasternal, mediastinal, and phrenic). A few lymphatic vessels from the cervical parietal pleura drain into the axillary lymph nodes.

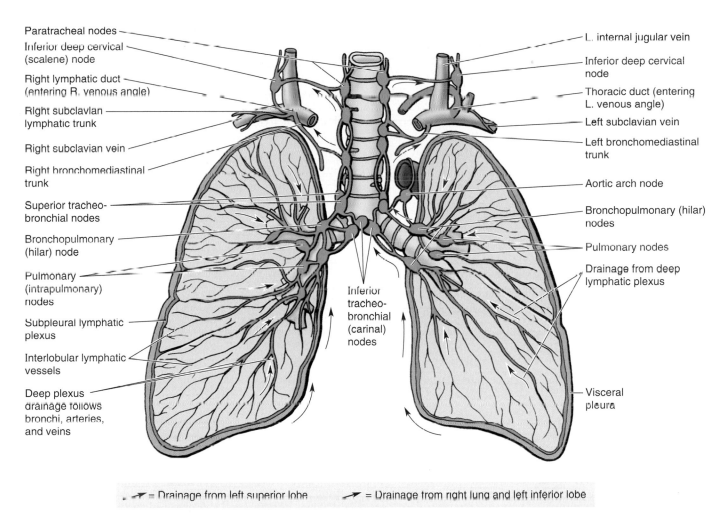

Paratracheal nodes
Inferior deep cervical (scalene) node
Right lymphatic duct (entering R. venous angle)
Right subclavian lymphatic trunk
Right subclavian vein
Right bronchomediastinal trunk
Superior tracheo-bronchial nodes
Bronchopulmonary (hilar) node
Pulmonary (intrapulmonary) nodes
Subpleural lymphatic plexus
Interlobular lymphatic vessels
Deep plexus drainage follows bronchi, arteries, and veins

L. internal jugular vein
Inferior deep cervical node
Thoracic duct (entering L. venous angle)
Left subclavian vein
Left bronchomediastinal trunk
Aortic arch node
Bronchopulmonary (hilar) nodes
Pulmonary nodes
Drainage from deep lymphatic plexus
Visceral pleura

Inferior tracheo-bronchial (carinal) nodes

✈ = Drainage from left superior lobe   ➤ = Drainage from right lung and left inferior lobe

Figure 1.32. Lymphatic drainage of lungs. The lymphatic vessels originate in superficial subpleural and deep lymphatic plexuses. All lymph from the lung leaves along the root of the lung and drains to the inferior or superior tracheobronchial lymph nodes. The inferior lobe of *both* lungs drain to the centrally placed inferior tracheobronchial (carinal) nodes, which primarily drain to the right side. The other lobes of each lung drain primarily to the ipsilateral superior tracheobronchial lymph nodes. From here the lymph traverses a variable number of paratracheal nodes and enters the bronchomediastinal trunks.

Pulmonary Embolism

Obstruction of a pulmonary artery by a blood clot (*embolus*) is a common cause of morbidity (sickness) and mortality (death). An embolus in a pulmonary artery forms when a blood clot, fat globule, or air bubble travels in the blood to the lungs from a leg vein, for example, after a compound fracture. The embolus passes through the right side of the heart to a lung through a pulmonary artery. It may block a pulmonary artery—**pulmonary embolism** (PE)—or one of its branches. The pulmonary arteries carry all of the blood that has been returned to the right heart via the vena caval system. Consequently, the immediate result of PE is partial or complete obstruction of blood flow to the lung. The blockage results in a lung or a sector of lung that is ventilated with air but not perfused with blood.

When a large embolus occludes a pulmonary artery, the patient suffers *acute respiratory distress* because of a major decrease in the oxygenation of blood, owing to blockage of blood flow through the lung. Conversely, the right side of the heart may become acutely dilated because the volume of blood arriving from the systemic circuit cannot be pushed through the pulmonary circuit (*acute cor pulmonale*). In either case, death may occur in a few minutes. A medium-size embolus may block an artery supplying a bronchopulmonary segment, producing a *pulmonary infarct*, an area of necrotic (dead) lung tissue.

In physically active people, a collateral circulation—an indirect, accessory blood supply—often exists and develops further when there is a PE so that infarction is not as likely to occur, or at least not be as devastating. Anastomoses with branches of the bronchial arteries abound in ▶

the region of the terminal bronchioles. In ill people with impaired circulation in the lung, such as *chronic congestion,* PE commonly results in lung infarction. When an area of visceral pleura is also deprived of blood, it becomes inflamed (*pleuritis*) and irritates or becomes fused to the sensitive parietal pleura, resulting in pain. Pain from the parietal pleura is referred to the cutaneous distribution of the intercostal nerves to the thoracic wall, or, in the case of inferior nerves, to the anterior abdominal wall.

Lymphatic Drainage after Pleural Adhesion

If the parietal and visceral layers of pleura adhere (*pleural adhesion*), the lymphatic vessels in the lung and visceral pleura may drain into the axillary lymph nodes. The presence of carbon particles in these nodes is presumptive evidence of pleural adhesion.

Bronchogenic Carcinoma

The term *bronchogenic carcinoma* once was a specific designation for cancer arising in the bronchus—usually squamous- (oat) or small-cell carcinoma (cancer)—but now the term refers to any lung cancer. **Lung cancer** is mainly caused by cigarette smoking; most cancers arise in the mucosa of the large bronchi and produce a persistent, productive cough or *hemoptysis* (spitting of blood). Malignant (cancer) cells can be detected in the sputum (saliva-borne matter).

The primary tumor, observed radiologically as an enlarging lung mass, metastasizes early to the bronchopulmonary (hilar) lymph nodes and subsequently to other thoracic lymph nodes. Common sites of *hematogenous metastases* (spreading through the blood) of cancer cells from a bronchogenic carcinoma are the brain, bones, lungs, and suprarenal (adrenal) glands. The tumor cells probably enter the systemic circulation by invading the wall of a sinusoid or venule in a lung and are transported through the pulmonary veins, left heart, and aorta to these structures. Often the lymph nodes superior to the clavicle—the *supraclavicular lymph nodes*—are enlarged when bronchogenic carcinoma develops owing to metastases of cancer cells from the tumor. Consequently, the supraclavicular lymph nodes are called *sentinel lymph nodes* because their enlargement alerts the physician to the possibility of malignant disease in the thoracic and/or abdominal organs. ⊙

Nerves of the Lungs and Pleurae

The *nerves of the lungs and visceral pleura* are derived from the pulmonary plexuses anterior and (mainly) posterior to the roots of the lungs (Fig. 1.33). These nerve networks contain parasympathetic fibers from the **vagus nerves** (CN X) and sympathetic fibers from the *sympathetic trunks*. The **parasympathetic ganglion cells** (cell bodies of postsynaptic parasympathetic neurons) are in the *pulmonary plexuses* and along the branches of the bronchial tree. The **sympathetic ganglion cells** (cell bodies of postsynaptic sympathetic neurons) are in the *paravertebral sympathetic ganglia of the sympathetic trunks.* The parasympathetic fibers from the vagus nerves are motor to the smooth muscle of the bronchial tree (*bronchoconstrictor*), inhibitory to the pulmonary vessels (*vasodilator*), and secretory to the glands of the bronchial tree (*secretomotor*). Reflexive visceral afferent fibers of CN X are distributed to the:

- Bronchial mucosa, probably in association with tactile sensation for cough reflexes.

- Bronchial muscles, possibly involved in stretch reception.

- Interalveolar connective tissue, in association with Hering-Breuer reflexes (a mechanism that tends to limit respiratory excursions).

- Pulmonary arteries, serving pressor receptors (receptors sensitive to blood pressure).

- Pulmonary veins, serving chemoreceptors (receptors sensitive to blood gas levels).

Visceral afferent fibers mediating *nociceptive impulses* (impulses generated in response to painful or injurious stimuli) from the visceral pleura and bronchi accompany the sympathetic fibers, whereas those from the trachea accompany the parasympathetic fibers of the vagus. The sympathetic fibers are inhibitory to the bronchial muscle (*bronchodilator*), motor to the pulmonary vessels (*vasoconstrictor*), and inhibitory to the alveolar glands of the bronchial tree—type II secretory epithelial cells of the alveoli (Fig. 1.29).

The *nerves of the parietal pleura* derive from the intercostal and phrenic nerves. The *costal pleura* and the peripheral part of the *diaphragmatic pleura* are supplied by the **intercostal nerves.** They mediate the sensations of touch and pain. The central part of the diaphragmatic pleura and the *mediastinal pleura* are supplied by the **phrenic nerves** (Figs. 1.25 and 1.27*B*).

Pleural Pain

The visceral pleura is insensitive to pain because it receives no nerves of general sensation. The parietal pleura (particularly the costal part) is extremely sensitive to pain. The parietal pleura is richly supplied by branches of the intercostal and phrenic nerves. Irritation of the parietal pleura may produce local pain or referred ▶

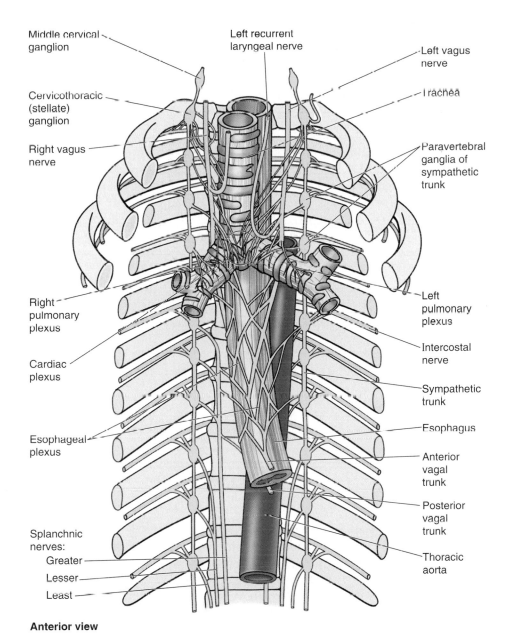

Middle cervical ganglion

Cervicothoracic (stellate) ganglion

Right vagus nerve

Left recurrent laryngeal nerve

Left vagus nerve

Trachea

Paravertebral ganglia of sympathetic trunk

Right pulmonary plexus

Cardiac plexus

Esophageal plexus

Splanchnic nerves:
   Greater
   Lesser
   Least

Left pulmonary plexus

Intercostal nerve

Sympathetic trunk

Esophagus

Anterior vagal trunk

Posterior vagal trunk

Thoracic aorta

Anterior view

Figure 1.33. Nerves of lungs and visceral pleura. The right and left pulmonary plexuses, anterior and posterior to the roots of the lungs, receive sympathetic contributions from the right and left sympathetic trunks and parasympathetic contributions from the right and left vagus nerves (CN X). After contributing to the posterior pulmonary plexus, the vagi continue inferiorly and become part of the esophageal plexus, often losing their identity and then reforming as anterior and posterior vagal trunks. Branches of the pulmonary plexuses accompany pulmonary arteries and especially bronchi to and within the lungs.

pain projected to dermatomes supplied by the same spinal (posterior root) ganglia and segments of the spinal cord. Irritation of the costal and peripheral parts of the diaphragmatic pleura results in local pain and referred pain to the dermatomes of the thoracic and abdominal walls. Irritation of the mediastinal and central diaphragmatic areas of parietal pleura results in referred pain to the root of the neck and over the shoulder (C3–C5 dermatomes). ✪

Surface Anatomy of the Pleurae and Lungs

The cervical pleurae and apices of the lungs pass through the superior thoracic aperture into the **supraclavicular fossae,** which are located posterior and superior to the clavicles and lateral to the tendons of the sternocleidomastoid muscles (Fig. SA1.6). The anterior borders of the lungs lie adjacent to the anterior line ▶

of reflection of the parietal pleura between the 2nd and 4th costal cartilages. Here the margin of the left pleural reflection moves laterally and then inferiorly at the cardiac notch to reach the 6th costal cartilage. The anterior border of the left lung is more deeply indented by its cardiac notch. On the right side, the pleural reflection continues inferiorly from the 4th to the 6th costal cartilage, paralleled closely by the anterior border of the right lung. Both pleural reflections and anterior lung borders pass laterally at the 6th costal cartilages. The pleural reflections reach the MCL at the level of the 8th costal cartilage, the 10th rib at the MAL, and the 12th rib at the SL; however, the inferior margins of the lungs reach the MCL at the level of

the 6th rib, the MAL at the 8th rib, and the scapular line at the 10th rib, proceeding toward the spinous process of T10 vertebra. They then proceed toward the spinous process of T12 vertebra. Thus the parietal pleura generally extends approximately two ribs inferior to the lung.

The *oblique fissure* of the lungs extends from the level of the spinous process of T2 vertebra posteriorly to the 6th costal cartilage anteriorly, which coincides approximately with the medial border of the scapula when the upper limb is elevated above the head (causing the inferior angle to rotate laterally). The *horizontal fissure* of the right lung extends from the oblique fissure along the 4th rib and costal cartilage anteriorly. ⊙

Figure SA1.6

THE BOTTOM LINE: The tracheobronchial tree is distinguished grossly by cartilage in its walls. The bifurcation of the trachea (at the level of the sternal angle) is asymmetrical: the right main bronchus is more vertical and of greater caliber than the left. The bronchi and pulmonary arteries course and branch together: the main bronchi/arteries each serve a lung, second-order lobar branches supply the two to three lobes, and third-order segmental branches supply the 8–10 bronchopulmonary segments of each lung. The bronchopulmonary segment is the smallest resectable division of the lung. The pulmonary veins run independent intersegmental courses, draining adjacent bronchopulmonary segments. The structures of the root of the lung and supporting tissues (and part of the esophagus) are supplied by bronchial arteries. The lymphatic drainage of the lungs follows a mostly predictable course, with most of the right lung and the superior lobe of the left lung following ipsilateral pathways to the right lymphatic trunk and thoracic duct. However, much of the drainage from the left inferior lobe passes to the right. Nerve fibers of the pulmonary plexuses are autonomic (bronchioconstrictive, vasoinhibitory, and secretomotor) and reflexive visceral afferent.

Mediastinum

The **mediastinum** (Mod. L. middle septum), occupied by the mass of tissue between the two pulmonary cavities, is the central compartment of the thoracic cavity (Fig. 1.34). It is covered on each side by *mediastinal pleura* and contains all the thoracic viscera and structures except the lungs. The mediastinum extends from the superior thoracic aperture to the di-

aphragm inferiorly and from the sternum and costal cartilages anteriorly to the bodies of the thoracic vertebrae posteriorly. Unlike the rigid structure observed in the embalmed cadaver, the mediastinum in living people is a highly mobile region, because it consists primarily of hollow (liquid- or air-filled) visceral structures united only by loose connective tissue, often infiltrated with fat. The major structures in the mediastinum are also surrounded by blood and lymphatic vessels, lymph nodes, nerves, and fat.

The looseness of the connective tissue and the elasticity of the lungs and parietal pleura on each side of the mediastinum enable it to accommodate movement as well as volume and pressure changes in the thoracic cavity–such as those resulting from movements of the diaphragm, thoracic wall, and tracheobronchial tree during respiration, contraction (beating) of the heart and pulsations of the great arteries, and passage of ingested substances through the esophagus. Connective tissue here becomes more fibrous and rigid with age; hence the mediastinal structures become less mobile.

The mediastinum is artificially divided into superior and inferior parts for purposes of description. The *superior mediastinum* extends inferiorly from the superior thoracic aperture to the horizontal plane that includes the sternal angle anteriorly and passes approximately through the junction (IV disc) of the T4 and T5 vertebrae posteriorly, often referred to as the **transverse thoracic plane** (Fig. 1.34). The **inferior mediastinum**—between this plane and the diaphragm—is further subdivided by the pericardium into anterior, middle, and posterior parts. The pericardium and its contents (the heart and roots of its great vessels) constitute the **middle mediastinum**. Some structures, such as the esophagus, pass vertically through the mediastinum and therefore lie in more than one mediastinal compartment.

Figure 1.34. Subdivisions and levels of mediastinum. The subdivisions of the mediastinum are demonstrated as if the person were in the supine position. The level of the viscera relative to the subdivisions as defined by thoracic cage landmarks depends on the individual's position because the soft tissue of the mediastinum sags with the pull of gravity

Levels of the Viscera Relative to the Mediastinal Divisions

The division between the superior and the inferior mediastinum (the *transverse thoracic plane*) is defined in terms of bony body wall structures and are mostly independent of gravitational effects. The level of the viscera relative to the subdivisions of the mediastinum depends on the position of the person (i.e., gravity). When a person is supine or when a cadaver is being dissected, the viscera are positioned higher (more superior) relative to the subdivisions of the mediastinum than when the person is upright (Figs. 1.34 and B1.14*A*). In other words, gravity pulls the viscera downward when we are vertical. Anatomical descriptions traditionally describe the level of the viscera as if the person were in the *supine position*—that is, lying in bed or on the operating or dissection table. In this position, the abdominal viscera spread horizontally, pushing the mediastinal structures superiorly. However, when the individual is standing or sitting erect, the levels of the viscera are as shown in Figure B1.14*B*. This occurs because the soft structures in the mediastinum (especially the pericardium and its contents), the heart and great vessels, and the abdominal viscera supporting them sag inferiorly under the influence of gravity.

In the supine position, the:

- Arch of the aorta lies superior to the transverse thoracic plane.

- Bifurcation of the trachea is transected by the transverse thoracic plane.

- Central tendon of the diaphragm (or the diaphragmatic surface or inferior extent of the heart) lies at the level of the xiphisternal junction and vertebra T9.

When standing or sitting upright, the:

- Arch of the aorta is transected by the transverse thoracic plane.

- Tracheal bifurcation lies inferior to the transverse thoracic plane.

- Central tendon of the diaphragm may fall to the level of the middle of the xiphoid process and the T9–T10 IV disc.

This vertical movement of mediastinal structures must be considered during physical and radiological examinations in the erect and supine positions. In addition, when lying on one's side, the mediastinum sags toward the lower side under the pull of gravity.

Mediastinoscopy and Mediastinal Biopsies

Using an endoscope (**mediastinoscope**), surgeons can see much of the mediastinum and conduct minor surgical procedures. They insert the endoscope through a ▶

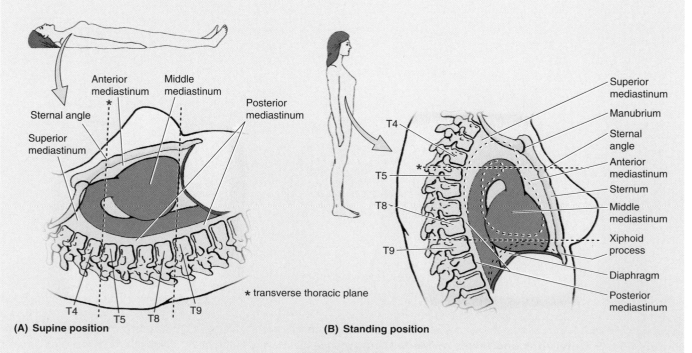

(A) Supine position

Anterior mediastinum
Middle mediastinum
Posterior mediastinum
Sternal angle
Superior mediastinum
T4
T5
T8
T9

* transverse thoracic plane

(B) Standing position

Superior mediastinum
Manubrium
Sternal angle
Anterior mediastinum
Sternum
Middle mediastinum
Xiphoid process
Diaphragm
Posterior mediastinum
T4
T5
T8
T9

Figure B1.14

small incision at the root of the neck, just superior to the jugular notch of the manubrium, into the potential space anterior to the trachea. During **mediastinoscopy,** surgeons can view or biopsy mediastinal lymph nodes to determine if cancer cells have metastasized to them from a bronchogenic carcinoma, for example. The mediastinum can also be explored and biopsies taken through an *anterior thoracotomy* (removing part of a costal cartilage; see clinical correlation [blue] box "Thoracotomy, Intercostal Space Incisions, Rib Excision, and Bone Grafting," in this chapter).

Widening of the Mediastinum

Radiologists and emergency physicians sometimes observe widening of the mediastinum when viewing chest radiographs (Sauerland, 1999). Any structure in the mediastinum may contribute to pathological widening. It is often observed after trauma resulting from a head-on collision, for example, which produces hemorrhage into the mediastinum from lacerated great vessels such as the aorta or SVC. Frequently, *malignant lymphoma* (cancer of lymphatic tissue) produces massive enlargement of mediastinal lymph nodes and widening of the mediastinum. Enlargement (hypertrophy) of the heart (occurring with congestive heart failure) is a common cause of widening of the inferior mediastinum. ○

THE BOTTOM LINE: The mediastinum is the central compartment of the thoracic cavity and contains all thoracic viscera except the lungs. Occupying structures are hollow (fluid or air filled), and although contained between bony formations anteriorly and posteriorly, lie between "pneumatic packing," inflated to constantly changing volumes on each side. Thus the mediastinum is a pliable, dynamic structure that is moved by structures contained within it (the heart) and surrounding it (the diaphragm and other movements of respiration) as well as the effect of gravity and body position. The superior mediastinum (above the transverse thoracic plane) is occupied by the trachea and upper parts of the great vessels; the middle part (most) of the inferior mediastinum is occupied by the heart; and most of the posterior mediastinum is occupied by structures vertically traversing all or much of the thorax.

Pericardium

The middle mediastinum includes the pericardium, heart, and roots of its great vessels (Fig. 1.34)—ascending aorta, pulmonary trunk, and SVC—passing to and from the heart. The **pericardium** is a fibroserous membrane that covers the heart and the beginning of its great vessels (Figs. 1.27*B* and 1.35). The pericardium is a closed sac composed of two layers. The tough external layer, the *fibrous pericardium,* is continuous with (blends with) the central tendon of the diaphragm (Fig. 1.25). The internal surface of the fibrous pericardium is lined with a glistening serous membrane, the **parietal layer of serous pericardium.** This layer is reflected onto the heart at the great

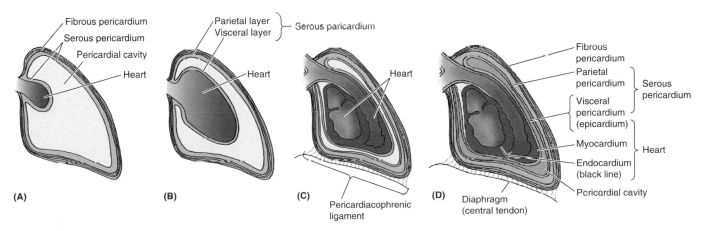

Diagrammatic right lateral views

Figure 1.35. Pericardium and heart. A. The heart occupies the middle mediastinum and is enclosed by the pericardium, composed of two parts. The tough, outer fibrous pericardium stabilizes the heart and helps prevent it from overdilating. Within the fibrous pericardium is a "collapsed" sac, the serous pericardium. The embryonic heart invaginates the wall of the serous sac (**B**) and soon practically obliterates the pericardial cavity (**C**), leaving only a potential space between the layers of serous pericardium. **C** and **D.** The continuity of the fibrous pericardium with the central tendon of the diaphragm constitutes the pericardiacophrenic ligament.

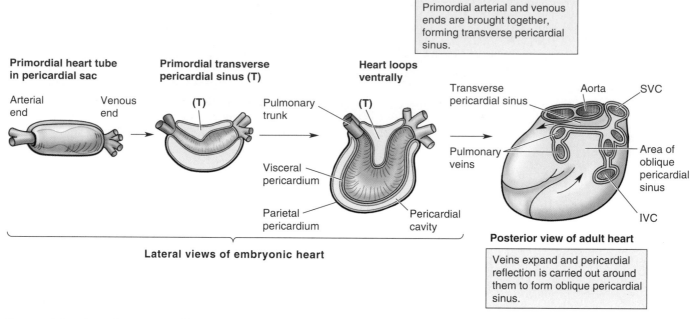

Primordial heart tube in pericardial sac

Arterial end   Venous end

Primordial transverse pericardial sinus (T)

(T)

Heart loops ventrally

(T)

Pulmonary trunk

Visceral pericardium

Parietal pericardium

Pericardial cavity

Primordial arterial and venous ends are brought together, forming transverse pericardial sinus.

Transverse pericardial sinus   Aorta   SVC

Pulmonary veins

Area of oblique pericardial sinus

IVC

Posterior view of adult heart

Veins expand and pericardial reflection is carried out around them to form oblique pericardial sinus.

Lateral views of embryonic heart

Figure 1.36. Development of heart and pericardium. The longitudinal, embryonic heart tube invaginates the double-layered pericardial sac (somewhat like placing a wiener in a hot-dog bun). The primordial heart tube then "loops" ventrally, bringing the primordial arterial and venous ends of the heart together and creating the primordial transverse pericardial sinus (*T*) between them. With growth of the embryo, the veins expand and spread apart, inferiorly and laterally. The pericardium reflected around them forms the boundaries of the oblique pericardial sinus. *IVC,* inferior vena cava; *SVC,* superior vena cava.

vessels—aorta, pulmonary trunk and veins, and superior and inferior venae cavae—as the **visceral layer of serous pericardium.** The *serous pericardium* is composed mainly of mesothelium, a single layer of flattened cells forming an epithelium that lines both the internal surface of the fibrous pericardium and the external surface of the heart.

The **fibrous pericardium** is

- Continuous superiorly with the *tunica adventitia* of the great vessels entering and leaving the heart and with the pretracheal layer of deep cervical fascia.

- Attached anteriorly to the posterior surface of the sternum by the *sternopericardial ligaments,* which are highly variable in their development.

- Bound posteriorly by loose connective tissue to structures in the posterior mediastinum.

- Continuous inferiorly with the central tendon of the diaphragm (Fig. 1.35*C* & *D*).

The inferior wall (floor) of the fibrous pericardial sac is firmly attached and confluent (partially blended) centrally with the central tendon of the diaphragm. The site of continuity has been referred to as the **pericardiacophrenic ligament;** however, the fibrous pericardium and central tendon are not two separate structures that fused together secondarily, nor are they separable by dissection. As a result of the at-tachments just described, the heart is relatively well tethered in place inside this fibrous sac. The pericardium is influenced by movements of the heart and great vessels, the sternum, and diaphragm.

The fibrous pericardium protects the heart against sudden overfilling because it is so unyielding and closely related to the great vessels that pierce it superiorly. The ascending aorta carries the pericardium superiorly beyond the heart to the level of the sternal angle.

The **pericardial cavity** is the potential space between opposing layers of the parietal and visceral layers of serous pericardium. It normally contains a thin film of fluid that enables the heart to move and beat in a frictionless environment.

The *visceral layer of serous pericardium* makes up the *epicardium,* the outermost of three layers of the heart wall. It extends onto the beginning of the great vessels, becoming continuous with the parietal layer of serous pericardium, (1) where the aorta and pulmonary trunk leave the heart and (2) where the SVC, IVC, and pulmonary veins enter the heart. The *transverse pericardial sinus* lies between these two groups of vessels and the reflections of serous pericardium around them, and the reflection of the serous pericardium around the second group of vessels defines the *oblique pericardial sinus.* The pericardial sinuses form during development of the heart as a consequence of the folding of the primordial heart tube. As the heart tube folds, its venous end moves postero-superiorly (Fig. 1.36) so that the venous end of the tube lies adjacent to the arterial end, separated only by the **transverse pericardial sinus,** a transversely running passage in the pericardial sac between the origins of the afferent and the efferent great vessels (Fig. 1.37). Thus the transverse sinus is posterior to the intrapericardial parts of the pulmonary trunk and ascending aorta and anterior to the SVC and superior to the atria of the heart.

As the veins of the heart develop and expand, a pericardial reflection surrounding them forms the **oblique pericardial sinus,** a wide pocket-like recess in the pericardial cavity posterior to the base (posterior aspect) of the heart, formed by the left atrium (Fig. 1.42C & D). The oblique sinus is bounded laterally by the pericardial reflections surrounding the pulmonary veins and IVC and posteriorly by the pericardium overlying the anterior aspect of the esophagus. The oblique sinus can be entered inferiorly and will admit several fingers; however, they cannot pass around any of these structures because the sinus is a blind sac (cul-de-sac).

The *arterial supply of the pericardium* (Fig. 1.38) is mainly from a slender branch of the internal thoracic artery, the peri-

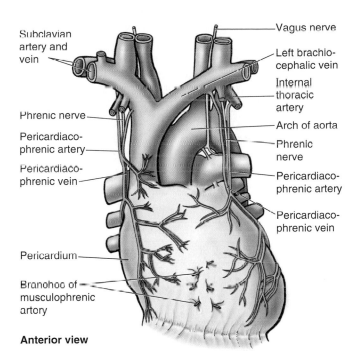

Anterior view

Figure 1.38. Arterial supply and venous drainage of pericardium. The arteries of the pericardium derive primarily from the internal thoracic arteries with minor contributions from its musculophrenic branch and the thoracic aorta. The veins are tributaries of the brachiocephalic veins.

cardiacophrenic artery, that often accompanies or at least parallels the phrenic nerve to the diaphragm. Smaller contributions of blood come from the:

- *Musculophrenic artery,* a terminal branch of the internal thoracic artery.

- *Bronchial, esophageal,* and *superior phrenic arteries,* branches of the thoracic aorta.

- *Coronary arteries* (visceral layer of serous pericardium only), the first branches of the aorta.

The *venous drainage of the pericardium* is from the:

- *Pericardiacophrenic veins,* tributaries of the brachiocephalic (or internal thoracic) veins.

- Variable tributaries of the *azygos venous system* (discussed later in this chapter).

The *nerve supply of the pericardium* is from the:

- *Phrenic nerves* (C3–C5), primary source of sensory fibers; pain sensations conveyed by these nerves are commonly referred to the skin (C3–C5 dermatomes) of the ipsilateral supraclavicular region (top of the shoulder of the same side).

- *Vagus nerves,* function uncertain.

- *Sympathetic trunks,* vasomotor.

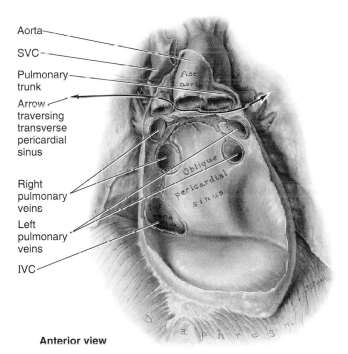

Anterior view

Figure 1.37. Interior of pericardial sac. To remove the heart from the sac, the eight vessels piercing the sac were severed. The oblique pericardial sinus is circumscribed by five veins. The superior vena cava (*SVC*), pulmonary trunk, and especially the aorta have intrapericardial portions. The peak of the pericardial sac occurs at the junction of the ascending aorta and the arch of the aorta. The transverse pericardial sinus is bounded anteriorly by the serous pericardium covering the posterior aspect of the pulmonary trunk and ascending aorta, posteriorly by that covering the SVC, and inferiorly by the visceral pericardium covering the atria of the heart. *IVC,* inferior vena cava.

The innervation of the pericardium by the phrenic nerves (they are somatic—not visceral—nerves, despite their location) and the course of these somatic nerves between the heart and the lungs make little sense unless the development of the fibrous pericardium is considered. It is split or separated from the developing body wall by the developing pleural cavities, which extend to accommodate the rapidly growing lungs. The lungs develop within the pericardioperitoneal canals that run on both sides of the foregut, connecting the thoracic and abdominal cavities on each side of the septum transversum. The canals (primordial pleural cavities) are too small to ac-

commodate the rapid growth of the lungs, and they begin to invade the mesenchyme of the body wall posteriorly, laterally, and anteriorly, splitting it into two layers: an outer layer that becomes the definitive thoracic wall (ribs and intercostal muscles) and an inner or deep layer (the pleuropericardial membranes) that contains the phrenic nerves and form the fibrous pericardium (Moore and Persaud, 2003). Thus the pericardial sac can be a source of pain just as the rib cage or parietal pleura can be, although that pain tends to be referred to dermatomes of the body wall—areas from which we more commonly receive sensation.

Surgical Significance of the Transverse Pericardial Sinus

The *transverse pericardial sinus* is especially important to cardiac surgeons. After the pericardial sac is opened anteriorly, a finger can be passed through the transverse pericardial sinus posterior to the aorta and pulmonary trunk (Fig. B1.15). By passing a surgical clamp or placing a ligature around these vessels, inserting the tubes of a coronary bypass machine, and then tightening the ligature, surgeons can stop or divert the circulation of blood in these large arteries while performing cardiac surgery, such as *coronary artery bypass grafting.*

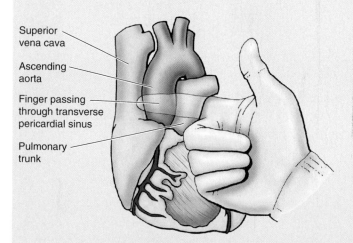

Superior
vena cava

Ascending
aorta

Finger passing
through transverse
pericardial sinus

Pulmonary
trunk

Figure B1.15

Exposure of the IVC and SVC

After passing through the diaphragm, the entire thoracic part of the IVC (approximately 2 cm) is enclosed by the pericardium. Consequently, the pericardial sac must be opened to expose the superior part of the IVC. The same is true for the terminal part of the SVC, which is partly inside and partly outside the pericardial sac.

Pericarditis, Pericardial Rub, and Pericardial Effusion

The pericardium may be involved in several disease processes. Inflammation of the pericardium (**pericarditis**) usually causes chest pain. It may also make the serous pericardium rough. Usually the smooth opposing layers of serous pericardium make no detectable sound during auscultation, but in pericarditis friction of the roughened surfaces sounds like the rustle of silk when listening with a stethoscope over the left sternal border and upper ribs (**pericardial friction rub**). A chronically inflamed and thickened pericardium may actually calcify, seriously hampering cardiac efficiency (Sauerland, 1999). Some inflammatory diseases produce **pericardial effusion** (passage of fluid from pericardial capillaries into the pericardial cavity, or an accumulation of pus). As a result, the heart becomes compressed (unable to expand and fill fully) and ineffective. Non-inflammatory pericardial effusions often occur with **congestive heart failure**, inadequacy owing to a heart that fails to pump out blood at the same rate that it receives it (i.e., that fails to maintain blood circulation).

Cardiac Tamponade

The *fibrous pericardium* is a tough, inelastic, closed sac that contains the heart, normally the only occupant other than a thin lubricating layer of pericardial fluid. If extensive pericardial effusion exists, the compromised volume of the sac does not allow full expansion of the heart, limiting the amount of blood the heart can receive, which in turn reduces cardiac output. This phenomenon, **cardiac tamponade** (heart compression), is a potentially lethal condition because heart volume is increasingly compromised by the fluid outside the heart but inside the pericardial cavity.

Blood in the pericardial cavity, *hemopericardium*, likewise produces cardiac tamponade. Hemopericardium may result from perforation of a weakened area of heart muscle owing to a previous **myocardial infarction** (MI) or heart attack, from bleeding into the pericardial ▶

cavity after cardiac operations, or from stab wounds. This situation is especially lethal because of the high pressure involved and the rapidity with which the fluid accumulates. The heart is increasingly compressed and circulation fails. The veins of the face and neck become engorged because of the backup of blood, beginning where the SVC enters the pericardium.

In patients with pneumothorax—air or gas in the pleural cavity—the air may dissect along connective tissue planes and enter the pericardial sac, producing a **pneumopericardium,** which can be demonstrated radiographically (Sauerland, 1999).

Pericardiocentesis

Drainage of fluid from the pericardial cavity, **pericardiocentesis,** is usually necessary to relieve cardiac tamponade. To remove the excess fluid, a wide-bore needle may be inserted through the left 5th or 6th intercostal space near the sternum. This approach to the pericardial sac is possible because the cardiac notch in the left lung and the shallower notch in the left pleural sac leaves part of the pericardial sac exposed—the bare area" of the pericardium (Figs. 1.24*A* and 1.25). The pericardial sac may also be reached by entering the infrasternal angle and passing the needle superoposteriorly (Fig. B1.16). At this site, the needle avoids the lung and pleurae and enters the pericardial cavity; however, care must be taken not to puncture the internal thoracic artery or its terminal branches. In acute cardiac tamponade from hemopericardium, an emergency thoracotomy may be performed (the thorax is rapidly opened) so that the pericardial sac may be incised to immediately relieve the tamponade and establish *stasis of the hemorrhage* (stop the escape of blood) from the heart (see clinical correlation [blue] box "Thoracotomy, Intercostal Space Incisions, Rib Excision, and Bone Grafting," in this chapter). ⊙

Figure B1.16

THE BOTTOM LINE The pericardium is a fibroserous sac, invaginated by the heart and roots of the great vessels, that encloses the serous cavity surrounding the heart. The fibrous pericardium is inelastic, attached anteriorly and inferiorly to the sternum and diaphragm, and blends with the adventitia of the great vessels as they enter or leave the sac. Thus it holds the heart in its middle mediastinal position and limits expansion (filling) of the heart. If fluid or a tumor occupies the pericardial space, the capacity of the heart is compromised. The serous pericardium lines the fibrous pericardium and the exterior of the heart. This glistening lubricated surface allows the heart (attached only by its afferent and efferent vessels and related reflections of serous membrane) the free movement required for its "wringing-out" contraction motions. The parietal layer of the serous pericardium is sensitive. Pain impulses conducted from it by the somatic phrenic nerves result in referred pain sensations.

Heart and Great Vessels

The **heart,** slightly larger than a clenched fist, is a double, self-adjusting, suction and pressure pump, the parts of which work in unison to propel blood to all parts of the body. The right side of the heart (*right heart*) receives poorly oxygenated (venous) blood from the body through the SVC and IVC and pumps it through the pulmonary trunk to the lungs for oxygenation (Fig. 1.39*A*). The left side of the heart (*left heart*) receives well-oxygenated (arterial) blood from the lungs through the pulmonary veins and pumps it into the aorta for distribution to the body.

The heart has four chambers: **right** and **left atria** and **right** and **left ventricles.** The atria are receiving chambers that pump blood into the ventricles (the discharging chambers). The synchronous pumping actions of the heart's two atrioventricular (AV) pumps (right and left chambers) constitute the **cardiac cycle** (Fig. 1.39*B–F*). The cycle begins with a period of ventricular elongation and filling (**diastole**) and ends with a period of ventricular shortening and emptying (**systole**). Two heart sounds are heard with a stethoscope: a *lub* sound as the blood is transferred (sucked) from the atria into the ventricles and a *dub* sound as the ventricles expel blood from the heart. The heart sounds are produced by the snapping shut of the oneway valves that normally keep blood from flowing backward during contractions of the heart.

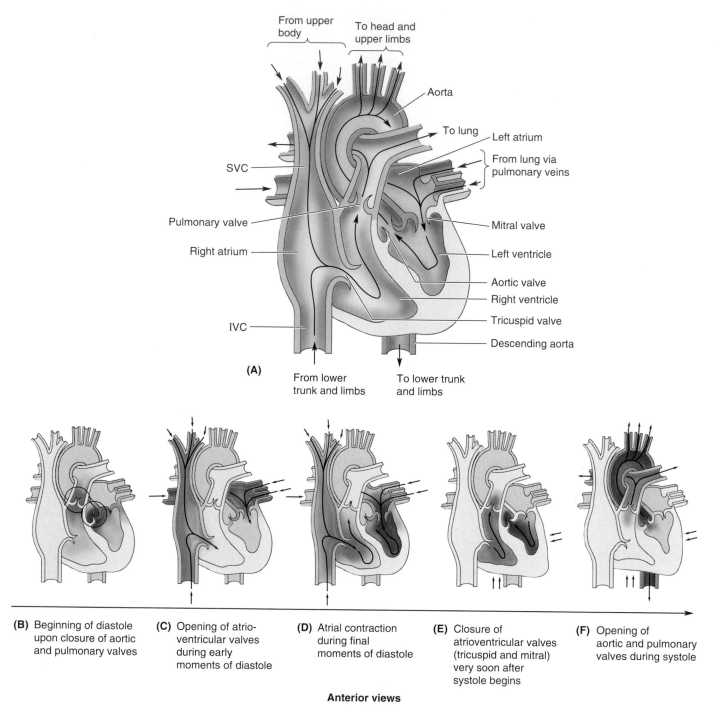

From upper body

To head and upper limbs

Aorta

To lung
Left atrium

From lung via pulmonary veins

SVC

Pulmonary valve

Mitral valve

Right atrium

Left ventricle

Aortic valve

Right ventricle

Tricuspid valve

IVC

Descending aorta

(A)

From lower trunk and limbs

To lower trunk and limbs

(B) Beginning of diastole upon closure of aortic and pulmonary valves

(C) Opening of atrio-ventricular valves during early moments of diastole

(D) Atrial contraction during final moments of diastole

(E) Closure of atrioventricular valves (tricuspid and mitral) very soon after systole begins

(F) Opening of aortic and pulmonary valves during systole

Anterior views

Figure 1.39. Cardiac cycle. The cardiac cycle describes the complete movement of the heart or heartbeat and includes the period from the beginning of one heartbeat to the beginning of the next one. The cycle consists of diastole (ventricular relaxation and filling) and systole (ventricular contraction and emptying). The right heart (blue side) is the pump for the pulmonary circuit; the left heart (red side) is the pump for the systemic circuit.

The wall of each heart chamber consists of three layers (Fig. 1.35):

- **Endocardium,** a thin internal layer (endothelium and subendothelial connective tissue) or lining membrane of the heart that also covers its valves.

- **Myocardium,** a thick, helical middle layer composed of cardiac muscle.

- **Epicardium,** a thin external layer (mesothelium) formed by the visceral layer of serous pericardium.

The walls of the heart consist mostly of thick myocardium, especially in the ventricles.

When the ventricles contract, they produce a wringing motion because of the double helical orientation of the cardiac muscle fibers (Torrent-Guasp et al., 2001) (Fig. 1.40*A*).

Figure 1.40 Arrangement of the myocardium and the fibrous skeleton of heart. A. The helical (double spiral) arrangement of the myocardium. (Modified from Torrent-Guasp et al., 2001). *1,* When the superficial myocardium is incised along the anterior interventricular groove (*dashed red line*) and peeled back starting at its origin from the fibrous ring of the pulmonary artery (*PA*), the thick double spirals of the ventricular myocardial band are revealed (*2*). It can be seen that a band of nearly horizontal fibers forms an outer basal spiral (*dark brown*) that comprises the outer wall of the right ventricle (right segment; *rs*) and external layer of the outer wall of the left ventricle (left segment; *ls*). *3.* After the left ventricle has been rotated to bring the interventricular septum anteriorly, it can be seen that the myocardium then abruptly turns more vertically, descending to the apex (descending segment; *ds*) and then ascends (ascending segment; *as*) to insert onto the fibrous ring of the aorta (*Ao*). The ds and as form the deeper apical spiral (*light brown*), which comprises the internal layer of the outer wall of the left ventricle, while the criss-crossing as and ds fibers make up the interventricular septum. Thus the septum, like the outer wall of the left ventricle, is also double layered. *4* and *5.* The ventricular myocardial band is progressively unwrapped. *6.* It is completely uncoiled and its segments are identified. The sequential contraction of the myocardial band enables the ventricles to function as parallel, sucking and propelling pumps; on contraction, the ventricles do not merely collapse inward but rather wring themselves out. *apm,* anterior papillary muscles; *pg1* and *pg2,* posterior interventricular groove; *ppm,* posterior papillary muscles. **B.** The isolated fibrous skeleton is composed of four fibrous rings (or two rings and two "coronets"), each encircling a valve; two trigones; and the membranous portions of the interatrial, interventricular, and atrioventricular septa.

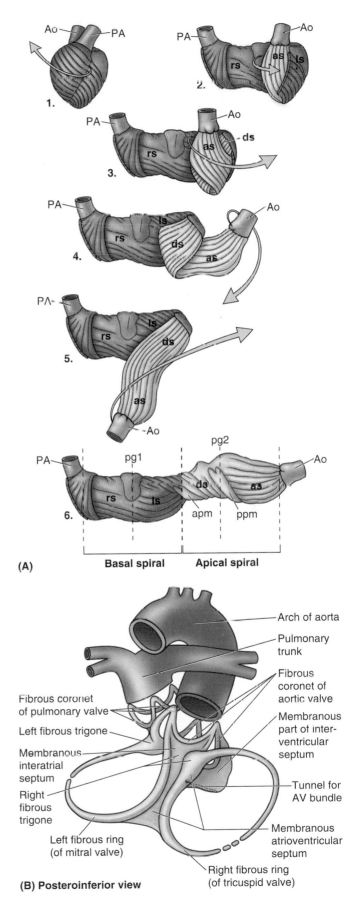

(A)

(B) Posteroinferior view

This motion initially ejects the blood from the ventricles as the outer (basal) spiral contracts, first narrowing and then shortening the heart, reducing the volume of the ventricular chambers. Continued sequential contraction of the inner (apical) spiral elongates the heart, followed by widening as the myocardium briefly relaxes, increasing the volume of the chambers to draw blood from the atria. The muscle fibers are anchored to the **fibrous skeleton of the heart** (Fig. 1.40*B*). This is a complex framework of dense collagen forming four **fibrous rings** (L. *anuli fibrosi*) that surround the orifices of the valves, a right and left **fibrous trigone** (formed by connections between rings), and the membranous parts of the interatrial and interventricular septa. The fibrous skeleton of the heart:

- Keeps the orifices of the AV and semilunar valves patent and prevents them from being overly distended by an increased volume of blood pumping through them.

- Provides attachments for the leaflets and cusps of the valves.

- Provides attachment for the myocardium, which, when uncoiled, forms a continuous **ventricular myocardial band** that originates primarily from the fibrous ring of the pulmonary valve and inserts primarily into the fibrous ring of the aortic valve (Torrent-Guasp et al., 2001) (Fig. 1.40*A*).

- Forms an electrical "insulator," by separating the myenterically conducted impulses of the atria and ventricles so that they contract independently and by surrounding and providing passage for the initial part of the AV bundle of the conducting system of the heart (discussed later in this chapter).

The heart and roots of the great vessels within the pericardial sac are related anteriorly to the sternum, costal cartilages, and anterior ends of the 3rd–5th ribs on the left side (Fig. 1.41). The heart and pericardial sac are situated obliquely, approximately two thirds to the left and one third to the right of the median plane (Figs. 1.41 and 1.42*A*). If you turn your face to the left about 45° without rotating your shoulders, the rotation of your head approximates that of the heart relative to the trunk. Externally, the atria are demarcated from the ventricles by the **coronary** or **atrioventricular groove** (L. *sulcus*), and the right and left ventricles are demarcated from each other by **anterior** and **posterior interventricular (IV) grooves** (Figs. 1.42*B* & *D*). The heart appears trapezoidal from an anterior or posterior view (Fig. 1.42*A*), but in three dimensions it is shaped like a tipped-over pyramid with an apex (directed anteriorly and to the left), a base (opposite the apex, facing mostly posteriorly), and four sides.

The **apex of the heart** (Fig. 1.42*B*):

- Is formed by the inferolateral part of the left ventricle.

- Lies posterior to the left 5th intercostal space in adults, usually approximately 9 cm (a hand's breadth) from the median plane.

- Remains motionless throughout the cardiac cycle.

- Is where the sounds of mitral valve closure are maximal (**apex beat**); the apex underlies the site where the heartbeat may be auscultated on the thoracic wall.

The **base of the heart** (Fig. 1.42*C* & *D*):

- Is the heart's posterior aspect (opposite the apex).

- Is formed mainly by the left atrium, with a lesser contribution by the right atrium.

- Faces posteriorly toward the bodies of vertebrae T6–T9 and is separated from them by the pericardium, oblique pericardial sinus, esophagus, and aorta.

- Extends superiorly to the bifurcation of the pulmonary trunk and inferiorly to the coronary groove.

- Receives the pulmonary veins on the right and left sides of its left atrial portion and the superior and inferior venae cavae at the superior and inferior ends of its right atrial portion.

The four *surfaces of the heart* (Fig. 1.44*A*–*D*) are the:

- **Anterior (sternocostal) surface,** formed mainly by the right ventricle.

- **Diaphragmatic (inferior) surface,** formed mainly by the left ventricle and partly by the right ventricle; it is related mainly to the central tendon of the diaphragm.

- **Right pulmonary surface,** formed mainly by the right atrium.

- **Left pulmonary surface,** formed mainly by the left ventricle; it forms the cardiac impression of the left lung.

The heart appears trapezoidal in both anterior (Fig. 1.42*A* & *B*) and posterior views (Fig. 1.42*C* & *D*). Its four *borders* are the:

- **Right border** (slightly convex), formed by the right atrium and extending between the SVC and the IVC.

- **Inferior border** (oblique, nearly vertical), formed mainly by the right ventricle and slightly by the left ventricle.

- **Left border** (nearly horizontal), formed mainly by the left ventricle and slightly by the left auricle.

- **Superior border,** formed by the right and left atria and auricles in an anterior view; the ascending aorta and pulmonary trunk emerge from this border and the SVC enters its right side. Posterior to the aorta and pulmonary trunk and anterior to the SVC, this border forms the inferior boundary of the transverse pericardial sinus.

The **pulmonary trunk,** approximately 5 cm long and 3 cm wide, is the arterial continuation of the right ventricle and divides into right and left pulmonary arteries. The pulmonary trunk and arteries conduct poorly oxygenated blood to the lungs for oxygenation (Fig. 1.39*A*).

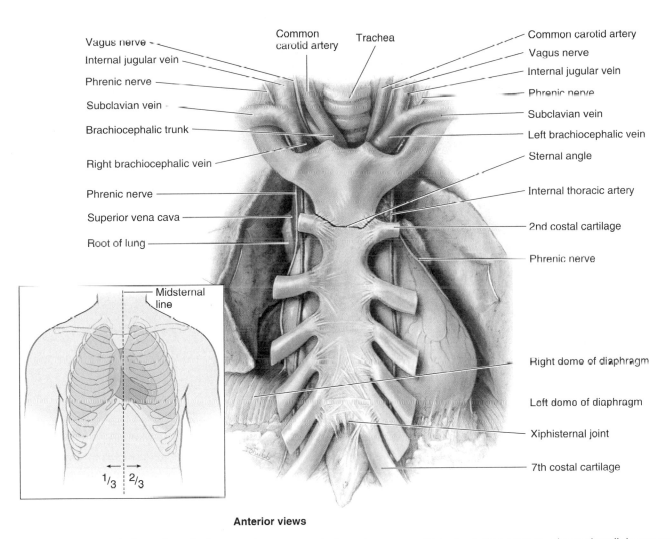

Vagus nerve
Internal jugular vein
Phrenic nerve
Subclavian vein
Brachiocephalic trunk
Right brachiocephalic vein
Phrenic nerve
Superior vena cava
Root of lung

Common carotid artery
Trachea

Common carotid artery
Vagus nerve
Internal jugular vein
Phrenic nerve
Subclavian vein
Left brachiocephalic vein
Sternal angle
Internal thoracic artery
2nd costal cartilage
Phrenic nerve

Right dome of diaphragm
Left dome of diaphragm
Xiphisternal joint
7th costal cartilage

Midsternal line

1/3   2/3

Anterior views

Figure 1.41. Pericardial sac in relation to sternum and phrenic nerves. This dissection exposes the pericardial sac posterior to the body of the sternum from just superior to the sternal angle to the level of the xiphisternal joint. The pericardial sac lies approximately one third to the right of the midsternal line and two thirds to the left.

Positional Abnormalities of the Heart

Abnormal folding of the embryonic heart may cause the position of the heart to be completely reversed so that the apex is directed to the right instead of the left—**dextrocardia** (Moore and Persaud, 2003). This congenital anomaly is the most common positional abnormality of the heart, but it is still relatively uncommon. Dextrocardia is associated with mirror image positioning of the great vessels and the arch of the aorta. This anomaly may be part of a general transposition of the thoracic and abdominal viscera (*situs inversus*), or the transposition may affect only the heart (*isolated dextrocardia*). In dextrocardia with situs inversus, the incidence of accompanying cardiac defects is low, and the heart usually functions normally. In isolated dextrocardia, how-

ever, the congenital anomaly is complicated by severe cardiac anomalies, such as *transposition of the great arteries*. For a discussion of the prognosis and treatment of dextrocardia, see Behrman et al. (2000).

Percussion of the Heart

Percussion defines the density and size of the heart. The classical percussion technique is to create vibration by tapping the chest with a finger while listening and feeling for differences in soundwave conduction. Percussion is performed at the 3rd, 4th, and 5th intercostal spaces from the left anterior axillary line to the right anterior axillary line (Fig. B1.17) Normally, the percussion note changes from resonance to dullness (because of the presence of ▶

(cont'd on page 147)

Figure 1.42. Shape, orientation, surfaces, and borders of heart. A and B. The sternocostal surface of the heart and the relationship of the great vessels are shown. The ventricles dominate this surface (two thirds right ventricle, one third left ventricle). The entire right auricle and much of the right atrium are visible, but only a small part of the left auricle is seen. **C and D.** The pulmonary (left) and diaphragmatic (inferior) surfaces and the base of the heart are shown as well as the relationship of the great vessels.

the heart) approximately 6 cm lateral to the left border of the sternum. ⊕

Figure B1.17. Areas of flatness and resonance.

(Labels in figure: Resonance; Flatness over bones and heavy muscles; Cardiac dullness; Liver dullness; Stomach tympany)

Right Atrium

The right atrium forms the right border of the heart and receives venous blood from the SVC, IVC, and coronary sinus (Fig. 1.42*B* & *D*). The ear-like **right auricle** is a conical muscular pouch that projects from this chamber like an add-on room, increasing the capacity of the atrium as it overlaps the ascending aorta.

The interior of the right atrium (Fig. 1.43*A* & *B*) has a:

- Smooth, thin-walled, posterior part (the **sinus venarum**) on which the venae cavae (SVC and IVC) and coronary sinus open, bringing poorly oxygenated blood into the heart.

- Rough, muscular anterior wall composed of pectinate muscles (L. *musculi pectinati*).

- Right AV orifice through which the right atrium discharges the poorly oxygenated blood it has received into the right ventricle.

The smooth and rough parts of the atrial wall are separated externally by a shallow vertical groove, the **sulcus terminalis** or terminal groove (Fig. 1.42*C*), and internally by a vertical ridge, the **crista terminalis** or terminal crest (Fig. 1.43*A*). The SVC opens into the superior part of the right atrium at the level of the right 3rd costal cartilage. The IVC opens into the inferior part of the right atrium almost in line with the SVC at approximately the level of the 5th costal cartilage. The **opening of the coronary sinus,** a short venous trunk receiving most of the cardiac veins, is between the right AV orifice and the IVC orifice. The **interatrial septum** separating the atria has an oval, thumbprint-size depression, the **oval fossa** (L. *fossa ovalis*), which is a remnant of the **oval foramen** (L. *foramen ovale*) and its valve in the fetus.

Embryology of the Right Atrium

Understanding the development of the right atrium makes its adult anatomy easier to learn and remember (Moore and Persaud, 2003). The primordial atrium is represented in the adult by the right auricle. The definitive atrium is enlarged by incorporation of most of the embryonic **venous sinus** (L. *sinus venosus*). The coronary sinus is also a derivative of this venous sinus. The part of the venous sinus incorporated into the primordial atrium becomes the smooth-walled sinus venarum of the adult right atrium (Fig. 1.45*A*) into which all the veins drain, including the coronary sinus. The line of fusion of the primordial atrium (the adult auricle) and the sinus venarum (the derivative of the venous sinus) is indicated internally by the *crista terminalis* and externally by the *sulcus terminalis.* The sinuatrial (SA) node (discussed later in this chapter) is located just in front of the opening of the SVC at the superior end of the crista terminalis—that is, in the border between the primordial atrium and the sinus venosus; hence its name.

Before birth, the valve of the IVC directs most of the oxygenated blood returning from the placenta in the umbilical vein and IVC toward the oval foramen in the interatrial septum, through which it passes into the left atrium. The oval foramen has a flap-like valve that permits a right to left shunt of blood but prevents a left to right shunt. At birth, when the baby takes its first breath, the lungs expand with air and pressure in the right heart falls below that in the left heart. Consequently, the oval foramen closes for its first and last time, and its valve usually fuses with the interatrial septum. The closed oval foramen is represented in the postnatal interatrial septum by the depressed oval fossa. The **border of the oval fossa** (L. *limbus fossae ovalis*) surrounds the fossa. The floor of the fossa is formed by the valve of the oval foramen. The rudimentary **IVC valve,** a semilunar crescent of tissue, has no function after birth; it varies considerably in size and is occasionally absent. ⊕

Right Ventricle

The right ventricle forms the largest part of the anterior surface of the heart, a small part of the diaphragmatic surface, and almost the entire inferior border of the heart (Fig. 1.42*B*). Superiorly it tapers into an arterial cone, the **conus arteriosus** (infundibulum), which leads into the pulmonary trunk (Fig. 1.44). The interior of the right ventricle has irregular muscular elevations (**trabeculae carneae**). A thick muscular ridge, the **supraventricular crest,** separates the ridged muscular wall of the inflow part of the chamber from the smooth wall of the *conus arteriosus,* or outflow part. The inflow part of the ventricle receives blood from the right atrium through the

Superior vena cava (SVC)

Pectinate muscles

Border of oval fossa

Interatrial septum

Oval fossa

Crista terminalis

Sinus venarum

Opening of coronary sinus

Right ventricle

(A)

Valve of coronary sinus

Inferior vena cava (IVC) and valve

Right atrioventricular orifice

Right anterolateral views

SVC

Oval fossa

IVC

Opening of coronary sinus

(B)

Figure 1.43. Right atrium of heart. A. The smooth-walled part of the atrium, the sinus venarum, is derived from absorption of the venous sinus of the embryonic heart. All of the venous structures entering the right atrium (superior and inferior vena cavae and coronary sinus) open into the sinus venarum. The rough-walled part of the atrium is derived from the primordial atrium. The shallow oval fossa is the site of fusion of the embryonic valve of the oval foramen with the interatrial septum. **B.** The inflow from the superior vena cava (*SVC*) is directed toward the right atrioventricular orifice, whereas blood from the inferior vena cava (*IVC*) is directed toward the oval fossa, as it was before birth.

right AV (tricuspid) orifice (Fig. 1.45*A*), located posterior to the body of the sternum at the level of the 4th and 5th intercostal spaces. The right AV orifice is surrounded by one of the fibrous rings of the *fibrous skeleton of the heart* (discussed earlier in this chapter). The fibrous ring keeps the caliber of the orifice constant (large enough to admit the tips of three fingers), resisting the dilation that might otherwise result from blood being forced through it at varying pressures.

The **tricuspid valve** (Fig. 1.45) guards the right AV orifice. The bases of the valve cusps are attached to the fibrous ring around the orifice. Because the fibrous ring maintains the caliber of the orifice, the attached valve cusps contact each other in the same way with each heartbeat. **Tendinous cords** (L. *chordae tendineae*) attach to the free edges and ventricular surfaces of the anterior, posterior, and septal cusps, much like the cords attaching to a parachute (Fig. 1.44). The tendinous cords arise from the apices of *papillary muscles,* which are conical muscular projections with bases attached to the ventricular wall. The papillary muscles begin to contract before contraction of the right ventricle, tightening the tendinous cords and drawing the cusps together. Because the cords are attached to adjacent sides of two cusps, they prevent separation

of the cusps and their inversion when tension is applied to the tendinous cords and maintained throughout ventricular contraction (*systole*)—that is, the cusps of the tricuspid valve are prevented from prolapsing (being driven into the right atrium) as ventricular pressure rises. Thus regurgitation of blood (backward flow of blood) from the right ventricle back into the right atrium is blocked by the valve cusps.

Three papillary muscles in the right ventricle correspond to the cusps of the tricuspid valve:

- The **anterior papillary muscle,** the largest and most prominent of the three, arises from the anterior wall of the right ventricle; its tendinous cords attach to the anterior and posterior cusps of the tricuspid valve.

- The **posterior papillary muscle,** smaller than the anterior muscle, may consist of several parts; it arises from the inferior wall of the right ventricle, and its tendinous cords attach to the posterior and septal cusps of the tricuspid valve.

- The **septal papillary muscle** arises from the interventricular septum, and its tendinous cords attach to the anterior and septal cusps of the tricuspid valve.

Pulmonary trunk

Aorta

Superior vena cava

Right atrium

Anterior cusp

Septal cusp

Tendinous cords (L. *chordae tendineae*)

Posterior cusp of tricuspid valve

(A) Anterior view

The three cusps of the valve of the pulmonary trunk

Conus arteriosus (infundibulum)

Supraventricular crest

Septal papillary muscles

Trabeculae carneae

Opened chamber is right ventricle

Interventricular septum (left leader = membranous part)

Septomarginal trabecula (moderator band)

Pulmonary trunk

Pulmonary valve

Conus arteriosus (outflow part of right ventricle)

Supraventricular crest

Anterior cusp of tricuspid valve

Inflow part of right ventricle

SVC

Right atrium

IVC

(B) Anterior view

Figure 1.44. Interior of right ventricle of heart. A. The entrance to the ventricle, the right atrioventricular orifice, is situated inferiorly and posteriorly. The smooth funnel-shaped outflow tract of the chamber, the conus arteriosus, lies superiorly and leads to the pulmonary orifice, the exit to the pulmonary trunk, where the ventricular aspect of the cusps of the tricuspid valve are shown. Tendinous cords extend from the papillary muscles to the cusps of the tricuspid valve. **B.** The inflow of blood enters the chamber from its posterior and inferior aspect, flowing anteriorly and to the left (toward the apex); the outflow of blood to the pulmonary trunk leaves superiorly and posteriorly.

The **interventricular septum (IVS)**, composed of muscular and membranous parts, is a strong, obliquely placed partition between the right and left ventricles (Figs. 1.42*A* and 1.44), forming part of the walls of each. Because of the much higher blood pressure in the left ventricle, the *muscular part of the IVS*, which forms the majority of the septum, has the thickness of the remainder of the wall of the left ventricle (two to three times as thick as the wall of the right ventricle) and bulges into the cavity of the right ventricle. Superiorly and posteriorly, a thin membrane, part of the fibrous skeleton of the heart (Fig. 1.40), forms the much smaller *membranous part of the IVS*. On the right side, the septal cusp of the tricuspid valve is attached to the middle of this membranous part of the fibrous skeleton (Fig. 1.44). This means that inferior to the cusp the membrane is an interventricular septum, but superior to the cusp it is an atrioventricular septum, separating the right atrium from the left ventricle.

The **septomarginal trabecula (moderator band)** is a curved muscular bundle that traverses the right ventricular chamber from the inferior part of the IVS to the base of the anterior papillary muscle. This trabecula is important because it carries part of the **right branch of the AV bundle,** a part of the conducting system of the heart to the anterior papillary muscle (see "Conducting System of the Heart," in this chapter). This "shortcut" across the chamber seems to facilitate conduction time, allowing coordinated contraction of the anterior papillary muscle.

The right atrium contracts when the right ventricle is empty and relaxed; thus blood is forced through this orifice into the right ventricle, pushing the cusps of the tricuspid valve aside like curtains. The inflow of blood into the right ventricle (*inflow tract*) enters posteriorly; and when the ventricle contracts, the outflow of blood into the pulmonary trunk (*outflow tract*) leaves superiorly and to the left (Fig.

Figure 1.45. Valves of heart and great vessels. A. The coronary valves are shown in situ. *AV,* atrioventricular. **B.** At the beginning of diastole (ventricular relaxation and filling), the aortic and pulmonary valves are closed; shortly thereafter, the tricuspid and mitral valves open (also shown in Fig. 1.39). **C.** Shortly after systole (ventricular contraction and emptying) begins, the tricuspid and mitral valves close and the aortic and pulmonary valves open.

1.44*B*). Consequently, the blood takes a U-shaped path through the right ventricle, changing direction about 140°. This change in direction is accommodated by the *supraventricular crest,* which deflects the incoming flow into the main cavity of the ventricle, and the outgoing flow into the conus arteriosus toward the pulmonary orifice. The inflow (AV) orifice and outflow (pulmonary) orifice are approximately 2 cm apart.

The **pulmonary valve** (Figs. 1.44 and 1.45) at the apex of the conus arteriosus is at the level of the left 3rd costal cartilage. The *semilunar valves* (pulmonary and aortic) are discussed later in this chapter, after discussion of the heart chambers.

Septal Defects

Atrial Septal Defects

A congenital anomaly of the interatrial septum, usually incomplete closure of the oval foramen, is an **atrial septal defect** (ASD). A probe-size patency is present in the superior part of the oval fossa in 15–25% of adults (Moore and Persaud, 2003). These small openings, by themselves, cause no hemodynamic abnormalities and are, therefore, of no clinical ▶

significance and should not be considered forms of ASDs. *Clinically significant ASDs* vary widely in size and location and may occur as part of more complex congenital heart disease. Large ASDs allow oxygenated blood from the lungs to be shunted from the left atrium through the ASD into the right atrium, causing enlargement of the right atrium and ventricle and dilation of the pulmonary trunk (Fig B1.18*A*). This left to right shunt of blood overloads the pulmonary vascular system, resulting in *hypertrophy of the right atrium and ventricle* and pulmonary arteries.

Ventricular Septal Defects

The membranous part of the IVS develops separately from the muscular part and has a complex embryological origin (Moore and Persaud, 2003). Consequently, this part is the common site of **ventricular septal defects** (VSDs), although defects also occur in the muscular part (Fig. B1.18*B*). VSDs rank first on all lists of cardiac defects. Isolated VSDs account for approximately 25% of all forms of congenital heart disease. The size of the defect varies from 1 to 25 mm. A VSD causes a left to right shunt of blood through the defect. A large shunt increases pulmonary blood flow, which causes severe pulmonary disease (*hypertension,* or increased blood pressure) and may cause *cardiac failure.* The much less common VSD in the muscular part of the septum frequently closes spontaneously during childhood (Creasy and Resnik, 1999). ✪

(A)

(B)

Figure B1.18. Septal defects. A. An atrial septal defect is shown. **B.** A ventricular septal defect is shown.

Left Atrium

The left atrium forms most of the base of the heart (Fig. 1.42*C* & *D*). The valveless pairs of right and left pulmonary veins enter the smooth-walled atrium (Fig. 1.46). In the embryo, there is only one common pulmonary vein, just as there is a single pulmonary trunk. The wall of this vein and four of its tributaries were incorporated into the wall of the left atrium, in the same way that the sinus venosus was incorporated into the right atrium. The part of the wall derived from the embryonic pulmonary vein is smooth walled. The tubular, muscular **left auricle,** its wall trabeculated with *pectinate muscles,* forms the superior part of the left border of the heart and overlaps the root of the *pulmonary trunk* (Fig. 1.42*A* & *B*). It represents the remains of the left part of the primordial atrium (Moore and Persaud, 2003). A *semilunar depression* in the interatrial septum indicates the floor of the oval fossa (Fig. 1.46*A*); the surrounding ridge is the valve of the oval fossa (L. *valvulae foramen ovale*).

The interior of the left atrium has

- A larger smooth-walled part and a smaller muscular auricle containing pectinate muscles.

- Four pulmonary veins (two superior and two inferior) entering its smooth posterior wall (Fig. 1.46*A–C*).

- A slightly thicker wall than that of the right atrium.

- An interatrial septum that slopes posteriorly and to the right.

- A left AV orifice through which the left atrium discharges the oxygenated blood it receives from the pulmonary veins into the left ventricle (Fig. 1.46*B*).

Stroke or Cerebrovascular Accident

Thrombi (clots) form on the walls of the left atrium in certain types of heart disease. If these thrombi detach or pieces break off of them, they pass into the systemic circulation and occlude peripheral arteries. Occlusion of an artery supplying the brain results in a **stroke** or **cerebrovascular accident** (CVA), which may affect vision, cognition, or the motor function of parts of the body previously controlled by the now-damaged (ischemic) area of the brain. ✪

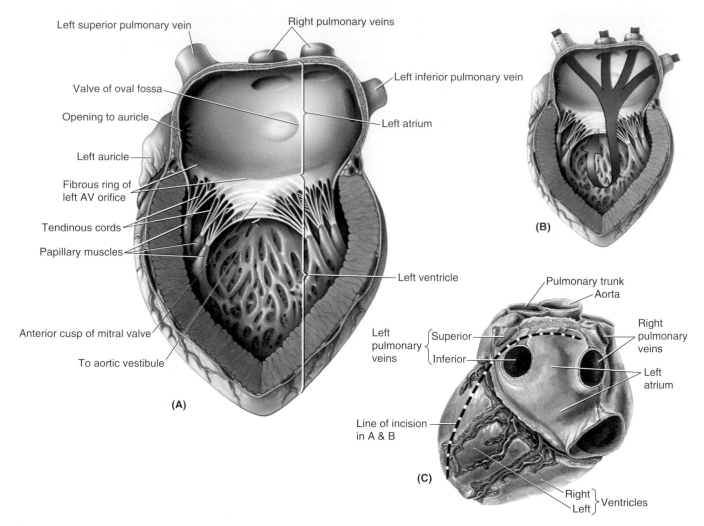

Figure 1.46. Interior of left atrium and ventricle of heart. A. The features of the internal aspects of the left atrium and the inflow tract of the left ventricle are shown. *AV,* atrioventricular. **B.** The pattern of blood flow through the left side of the heart is demonstrated. **C.** The heart in parts A and B was incised vertically along its left border and then transversely across the superior part of its base, passing between the superior and the inferior left pulmonary veins.

Left Ventricle

The left ventricle forms the apex of the heart, nearly all its left (pulmonary) surface and border, and most of the diaphragmatic surface (Figs. 1.42 and 1.47). Because arterial pressure is much higher in the systemic than in the pulmonary circulation, the left ventricle performs more work than the right ventricle.

The interior of the left ventricle has (Fig. 1.47)

• Walls that are two to three times as thick as that of the right ventricle.

• Walls that are mostly covered with a mesh of *trabeculae carneae* that are finer and more numerous than those of the right ventricle.

• A conical cavity that is longer than that of the right ventricle.

• Anterior and posterior *papillary muscles* that are larger than those in the right ventricle.

• A smooth-walled, non-muscular, superoanterior, outflow part, the **aortic vestibule,** leading to the aortic orifice and *aortic valve.*

• A double-leaflet *mitral valve* that guards the left AV orifice (Figs. 1.45 and 1.47A).

• An **aortic orifice** that lies in its right posterosuperior part and is surrounded by a fibrous ring to which the right, posterior, and left cusps of the aortic valve are attached; the ascending aorta begins at the aortic orifice.

The **mitral valve** has two cusps, anterior and posterior. The adjective *mitral* derives from the valve's resemblance to a bishop's miter (headdress). The mitral valve is located posterior to the sternum at the level of the 4th costal cartilage. Each of its cusps receives tendinous cords from more than one papillary muscle. These muscles and their cords support the mitral valve, allowing the cusps to resist the pressure developed during contractions (pumping) of the left ventricle.

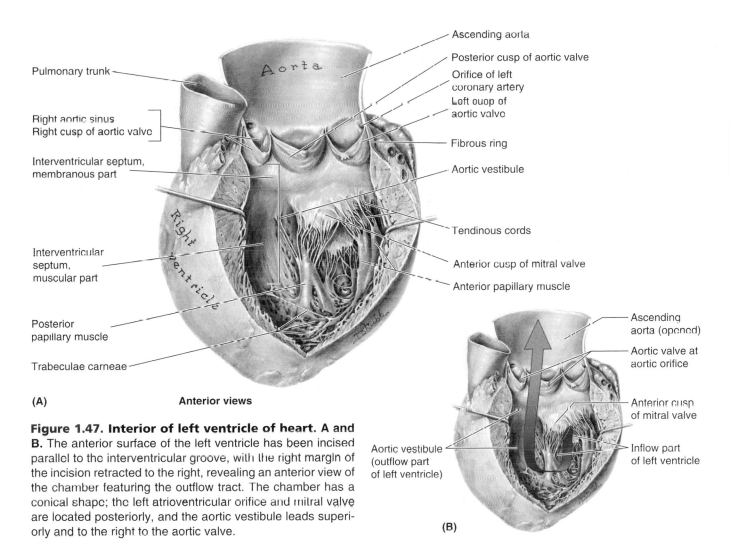

Pulmonary trunk

Right aortic sinus
Right cusp of aortic valve

Interventricular septum,
membranous part

Interventricular
septum,
muscular part

Posterior
papillary muscle

Trabeculae carneae

Ascending aorta
Posterior cusp of aortic valve
Orifice of left
coronary artery
Left cusp of
aortic valve
Fibrous ring
Aortic vestibule
Tendinous cords
Anterior cusp of mitral valve
Anterior papillary muscle

Ascending
aorta (opened)
Aortic valve at
aortic orifice
Anterior cusp
of mitral valve
Inflow part
of left ventricle

Aortic vestibule
(outflow part
of left ventricle)

(A)   **Anterior views**

(B)

**Figure 1.47. Interior of left ventricle of heart. A and
B.** The anterior surface of the left ventricle has been incised
parallel to the interventricular groove, with the right margin of
the incision retracted to the right, revealing an anterior view of
the chamber featuring the outflow tract. The chamber has a
conical shape; the left atrioventricular orifice and mitral valve
are located posteriorly, and the aortic vestibule leads superiorly and to the right to the aortic valve.

The tendinous cords become taut just before and during
systole, preventing the cusps from being forced into the
left atrium. As it traverses the left ventricle, the bloodstream undergoes two right angle turns, which together
result in a 180° change in direction. This reversal of
flow takes place around the anterior cusp of the mitral valve
(Fig. 1.47*B*).

The semilunar **aortic valve,** between the left ventricle and
the ascending aorta, is obliquely placed (Fig. 1.45). It is located posterior to the left side of the sternum at the level of
the 3rd intercostal space.

Semilunar Valves

Each of three **semilunar cusps of the pulmonary valve** (*anterior, right,* and *left*), like the **semilunar cusps of the aortic
valve** (*posterior, right,* and *left*), is concave when viewed superiorly (Figs 1.45*B* and 1.47*A*). Semilunar cusps do not have
tendinous cords to support them. They are smaller in area
than the cusps of the AV valves, and the force exerted on them
is less than half that exerted on the cusps of the tricuspid and
mitral valves. The cusps project into the artery but are pressed
toward (and not against) its walls as blood leaves the ventricle

(Fig. 1.48). After relaxation of the ventricle (*diastole*), the elastic recoil of the wall of the pulmonary trunk or aorta forces
the blood back toward the heart. However, the cusps open up
like pockets as they catch the reversed blood flow, coming together to completely close the orifice, supporting each other
and preventing any significant amount of blood from returning to the ventricle.

The edge of each cusp is thickened in the region of contact, forming the **lunule;** the apex of the angulated free edge
is thickened further as the **nodule.** Immediately superior to
each semilunar cusp, the walls of the origins of the pulmonary
trunk and aorta are slightly dilated, forming a sinus. The *pulmonary* and *aortic sinuses* are the spaces at the origin of the
pulmonary trunk and ascending aorta between the dilated
wall of the vessel and each cusp of the semilunar valves (Figs.
1.45*B* and 1.47*A*). The blood in the sinuses and the dilation
of the wall prevent the cusps from sticking to the wall of the
vessel, which might prevent closure.

The mouth of the right coronary artery is in the **right aortic sinus,** the mouth of the left coronary artery is in the **left
aortic sinus,** and no artery arises from the **posterior aortic
(non-coronary) sinus.**

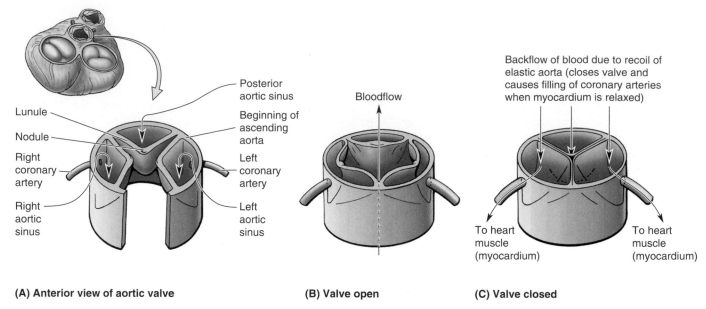

(A) Anterior view of aortic valve   **(B) Valve open**   **(C) Valve closed**

Figure 1.48. Aortic valve, aortic sinuses, and coronary arteries. A. Like the pulmonary valve, the aortic valve has three semilunar cusps: right, posterior, and left. Each cusp has a fibrous nodule at the midpoint of its free edge and a thin connective tissue area, the lunule, to each side of the nodule. **B.** Blood ejected from the left ventricle forces the cusps apart. **C.** When the valve closes, the nodules and lunules meet in the center. The coronary arteries arise from the right and left aortic sinuses (spaces superior to the cusps).

Basis for Naming the Cusps of the Aortic and Pulmonary Valves

The following account explains the embryological basis for naming the pulmonary and aortic valves. The **truncus arteriosus,** the common arterial trunk from both ventricles of the embryonic heart, has four cusps (Fig. B1.19*A*). The truncus arteriosus divides into two vessels, each with its own three-cusp valve (pulmonary and aortic) (Fig. B1.19*B*). The heart undergoes partial rotation so that its apex becomes directed to the left, resulting in the arrangement of cusps as shown in Figure B1.19*C*. Consequently, the cusps are named according to their embryological origin, not their postnatal anatomical position. Thus the pulmonary valve has right, left, and anterior cusps, and the aortic valve has right, left, and posterior cusps. Similarly, the aortic sinuses are named right, left, and posterior.

This terminology also agrees with the coronary arteries. Note that the right coronary artery arises from the right aortic sinus, superior to the right cusp of the aortic valve, and that the left coronary has a similar relation to the left cusp and sinus. The posterior cusp and sinus do not give rise to a coronary artery; thus they are also referred to as a "non-coronary" cusp and sinus.

Valvular Heart Disease

Disorders involving the valves of the heart disturb the pumping efficiency of the heart. Valvular heart disease produces either stenosis (narrowing) or insufficiency. ▶

Figure B1.19

Stenosis is the failure of a valve to open fully, slowing blood flow from a chamber. **Insufficiency** or **regurgitation**, on the other hand, is failure of the valve to close completely, usually owing to nodule formation on (or scarring and contraction of) the cusps so that the edges do not meet or align. This allows a variable amount of blood (depending on the severity) to flow back into the chamber it was just ejected from. Both stenosis and insufficiency result in an increased workload for the heart. Restriction of high pressure blood flow (stenosis) or passage of blood through a narrow opening into a larger vessel or chamber (stenosis and regurgitation) produce turbulence. Turbulence sets up *eddies* (small whirlpools) that produce vibrations that are audible as **murmurs**. Superficial vibratory sensations (**thrills**) may be felt on the skin over an area of turbulence.

The clinical significance of a valvular dysfunction ranges from slight and physiologically insignificant to severe and rapidly fatal. Factors such as degree, duration and etiology (cause) affect secondary changes in the heart, blood vessels, and other organs, both proximal and distal to the valve lesion. Valvular disorders may be congenital or acquired. Insufficiency may result from pathology of the valve itself or its supporting structures (anulus, tendinous cords, dilation of chamber wall, etc.). It may occur *acutely* (suddenly—for example, from a rupture of the cords) or *chronically* (over a relatively long time—for example, scarring and retraction). Valvular stenosis, on the other hand, is almost always the result of a valve abnormality and is essentially always a chronic process (Cotran et al., 1999).

Because valvular diseases are mechanical problems, damaged or defective cardiac valves are often replaced surgically in a procedure called **valvuloplasty**. Most commonly, artificial **valve prostheses** made of synthetic materials are used in these valve-replacement procedures, but xenografted valves (valves transplanted from other species, such as pigs) are also used.

Mitral Valve Insufficiency (Mitral Valve Prolapse)

A **prolapsed mitral valve** is an insufficient or incompetent valve with one or both leaflets enlarged, redundant or "floppy," and extending back into the left atrium during systole. As a result, blood regurgitates into the left atrium when the left ventricle contracts, producing a characteristic murmur. This is an extremely common condition, occurring in up to 1 in every 20 people, most often in young females. Usually, it is an incidental finding on physical examination; but it is of clinical importance in a small fraction of those affected, with the patient suffering chest pain and fatigue.

Pulmonary Valve Stenosis

With **pulmonary valve stenosis**, the valve cusps are fused, forming a dome with a narrow central opening. In **infundibular pulmonary stenosis**, the conus arteriosus is underdeveloped. Both types of pulmonary stenoses produce a restriction of right ventricular outflow and may occur together. The degree of hypertrophy of the right ventricle is variable.

Pulmonary Valve Incompetence

If the free margins (*lunules*) of the cusps of a semilunar valve thicken and become inflexible or are damaged by disease, the valve will not close completely. An **incompetent pulmonary valve** results in a backrush of blood under high pressure into the right ventricle during diastole. Pulmonic regurgitation may be heard through a stethoscope as a *heart murmur*, an abnormal sound from the heart, produced in this case by damage to the cusps of the pulmonary valve.

Aortic Valve Stenosis

Aortic valve stenosis is the most frequent valve abnormality. In the 20th century, rheumatic fever was a common cause but now accounts for < 10% of cases of aortic stenosis. The great majority of aortic stenoses is a result of degenerative calcification and comes to clinical attention in the 6th decade of life or later. Aortic stenosis causes extra work for the heart, resulting in *left ventricular hypertrophy*.

Aortic Valve Insufficiency

Insufficiency of the aortic valve results in aortic regurgitation (backrush of blood into the left ventricle), producing a heart murmur and a **collapsing pulse** (forcible impulse that rapidly diminishes). ✪

THE BOTTOM LINE: The heart is a dual suction and pressure pump that propels blood through the infinite double loop formed by the pulmonary and systemic circuits. The right heart serves the former and the left heart the latter. The heart is shaped like a tipped-over pyramid, with the apex directed anteroinferiorly and to the left and the base opposite the apex (posterior). Each side of the heart includes a receiving chamber (atrium) and a suction, compression, expulsion chamber (ventricle). The bilateral chambers (and thus the high-pressure systemic and lower-pressure pulmonary circuits) are separated by an oblique cardiac septum that is largely muscular but partly membranous. AV valves are placed between unilateral chambers to facilitate two-stage (accumulate and then eject) pumping. Oneway semilunar valves (pulmonic and aortic) placed at the exit on each side prevent backflow (except that which fills the coronary arteries) and maintains the diastolic pressure of the arteries. The chambers have a glistening endothelial lining, the endocardium; a muscular wall or myocardium, the thickness of which is proportional to the internal pressures occurring within the specific chamber; and a glistening outer covering (the visceral layer of serous pericardium, or epicardium). The myocardium of the atria and ventricles (and the myogenic propagation of contracting stimuli through it) is attached to and separated by the connective tissue of the fibrous skeleton of the heart. The fibrous skeleton consists of four fibrous rings, two trigones, and the membranous parts of the cardiac septa. Only specialized muscle conducting contractile impulses from the atria to the ventricles penetrates the skeleton at defined sites. The fibrous skeleton provides attachment for the myocardium and cusps of the valves, and maintains the integrity of the orifices.

Vasculature and Innervation of the Heart

The blood vessels of the heart comprise the coronary arteries and cardiac veins, which carry blood to and from most of the myocardium (Figs. 1.49 and 1.50). The endocardium and some subendocardial tissue located immediately external to the endocardium receive oxygen and nutrients by diffusion or microvasculature directly from the chambers of the heart. The blood vessels of the heart, normally embedded in fat, course across the surface of the heart just deep to the epicardium. Occasionally, parts of the vessels become embedded within the myocardium. The blood vessels of the heart are affected by both sympathetic and parasympathetic innervation.

Arterial Supply of the Heart The **coronary arteries**, the first branches of the aorta, supply the myocardium and epicardium. The right and left coronary arteries arise from the corresponding aortic sinuses at the proximal part of the ascending aorta, just superior to the aortic valve, and pass around opposite sides of the pulmonary trunk (Figs. 1.49 and 1.50; Table 1.4). The coronary arteries supply both the atria and the ventricles; however, the atrial branches are usually small and not readily apparent in the cadaveric heart. The ventricular distribution of each coronary artery is not sharply demarcated.

The **right coronary artery** (RCA) arises from the right aortic sinus of the ascending aorta and passes to the right side of the pulmonary trunk, running in the coronary groove (Figs. 1.48 and 1.49A). Near its origin, the RCA usually gives off an ascending **sinuatrial nodal branch**, which supplies the *SA node* (Fig. 1.49A). The RCA then descends in the coronary groove and gives off the **right marginal branch**, which supplies the right border of the heart as it runs toward (but does not reach) the apex of the heart. After giving off this branch, the RCA turns to the left and continues in the coronary groove to the posterior aspect of the heart. At the **crux** (L. cross) **of the heart**—the junction of the septa and walls of the four heart chambers—the RCA gives rise to the **atrioventricular nodal branch**, which supplies the *AV node* (Fig. 1.49A–C). The SA and AV nodes are part of the *conducting system of the heart* (discussed later in this chapter).

Dominance of the coronary arterial system is defined by which artery gives rise to the posterior interventricular (IV)

branch (posterior descending artery). Dominance of the right coronary artery is typical (approximately 67%) (Fig. 1.49A); the right coronary artery gives rise to the large **posterior interventricular branch**, which descends in the posterior IV groove toward the apex of the heart. This branch supplies adjacent areas of both ventricles and sends perforating **interventricular septal branches** into the IV septum (Fig. 1.49C). The terminal (left ventricular) branch of the RCA then continues for a short distance in the coronary groove. Thus, in the most common pattern of distribution, the RCA supplies the diaphragmatic surface of the heart.

Typically, the RCA supplies

- The right atrium.

- Most of right ventricle.

- Part of the left ventricle (the diaphragmatic surface).

- Part (usually the posterior third) of the IV septum.

- The SA node (in approximately 60% of people).

- The AV node (in approximately 80% of people).

The **left coronary artery** (LCA) arises from the *left aortic sinus* of the ascending aorta (Fig. 1.48), passes between the left auricle and the left side of the pulmonary trunk, and runs in the coronary groove (Fig. 1.49A & B). In approximately 40% of people, the **SA nodal branch** arises from the circumflex branch of the LCA and ascends on the posterior surface of the left atrium to the SA node. As it enters the coronary groove, at the superior end of the anterior IV groove (Fig. 1.42B), the LCA divides into two branches, the **anterior IV branch** (left anterior descending [LAD] branch) and the **circumflex branch** (Fig. 1.49A & C). The anterior IV branch passes along the IV groove to the apex of the heart. Here it turns around the inferior border of the heart and commonly anastomoses with the posterior IV branch of the right coronary artery (Fig. 1.49B). The anterior IV branch supplies adjacent parts of both ventricles and, via IV septal branches, the anterior two thirds of the IVS (Fig. 1.49C). In many people, the anterior IV branch gives rise to a **lateral (diagonal) branch,** which descends on the anterior surface of the heart (Fig. 1.49A).

The smaller *circumflex branch of the LCA* follows the coronary groove around the left border of the heart to the posterior surface of the heart. The **left marginal artery,** a branch of the circumflex branch, follows the left margin of the heart and supplies the left ventricle. Most commonly, the circumflex branch of the LCA terminates in the coronary groove on the posterior aspect of the heart before reaching the crux (Fig. 1.49B), but in approximately one third of hearts it continues to supply a branch that runs in or adjacent to the posterior IV groove.

Typically, the LCA supplies

- The left atrium.

- Most of the left ventricle.

(cont'd on page 159)

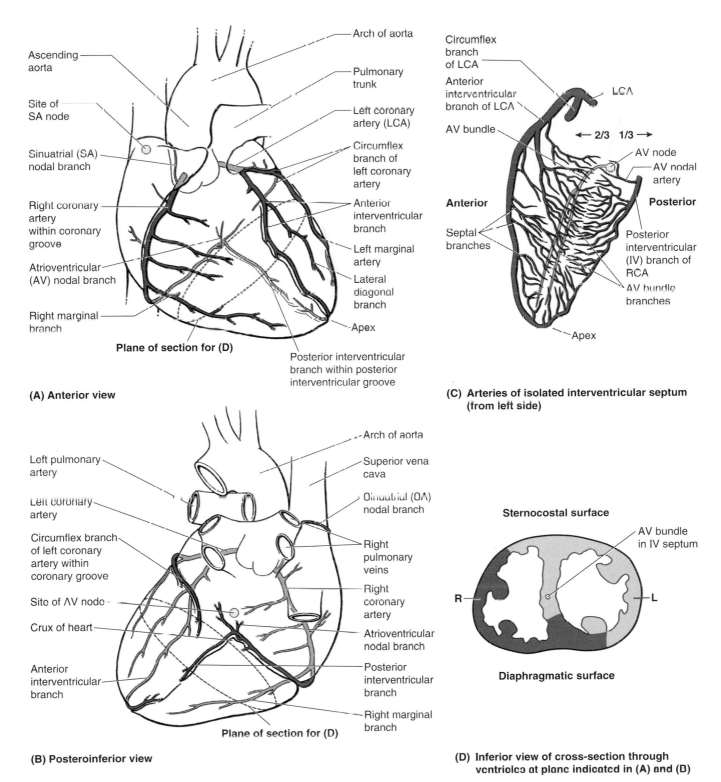

(A) Anterior view

Ascending aorta

Site of SA node

Sinuatrial (SA) nodal branch

Right coronary artery within coronary groove

Atrioventricular (AV) nodal branch

Right marginal branch

Plane of section for (D)

Arch of aorta

Pulmonary trunk

Left coronary artery (LCA)

Circumflex branch of left coronary artery

Anterior interventricular branch

Left marginal artery

Lateral diagonal branch

Apex

Posterior interventricular branch within posterior interventricular groove

(C) Arteries of isolated interventricular septum (from left side)

Circumflex branch of LCA

Anterior interventricular branch of LCA

AV bundle

LCA

← 2/3   1/3 →

AV node

AV nodal artery

Anterior   **Posterior**

Septal branches

Posterior interventricular (IV) branch of RCA

AV bundle branches

Apex

(B) Posteroinferior view

Left pulmonary artery

Left coronary artery

Circumflex branch of left coronary artery within coronary groove

Site of AV node

Crux of heart

Anterior interventricular branch

Plane of section for (D)

Arch of aorta

Superior vena cava

Sinuatrial (SA) nodal branch

Right pulmonary veins

Right coronary artery

Atrioventricular nodal branch

Posterior interventricular branch

Right marginal branch

(D) Inferior view of cross-section through ventricles at plane indicated in (A) and (B)

Sternocostal surface

AV bundle in IV septum

R   L

Diaphragmatic surface

Figure 1.49. Coronary arteries. A and B. In the most common pattern of distribution, the right coronary artery anastomoses with the circumflex branch of the left coronary artery (*LCA*) (anastomoses are not shown) after the RCA has given rise to the posterior interventricular (*IV*) artery. The RCA gives rise to branches supplying both the sinuatrial (*SA*) and the atrioventricular (*AV*) nodes; that to the AV node is the first of many septal branches of the posterior IV artery. The anterior IV artery (left anterior descending branch) hooks around the apex of the heart to anastomose with the posterior IV artery. **C.** Arteries of the interventricular septum are shown. The septal branches of the anterior interventricular branch of the LCA supply the anterior two thirds of the IVS, whereas the septal branches of the posterior interventricular artery (usually a branch of the RCA) supply the posterior third. Because the AV bundle and bundle branches are centrally placed in and on the IVS, the LCA typically provides most blood to this conducting tissue. **D.** A cross-section of the right and left ventricles demonstrates the most common pattern of distribution of blood from the RCA (*red*) and LCA (*pink*) to the ventricular walls and IVS.

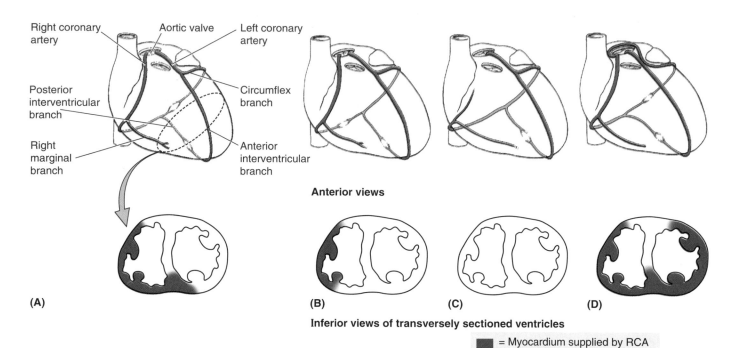

Anterior views

Inferior views of transversely sectioned ventricles

■ = Myocardium supplied by RCA

Figure 1.50. Variations in distribution of coronary arteries. A. In the most common pattern (67%), the right coronary artery is dominant, giving rise to the posterior interventricular branch. **B and C.** The left coronary artery gives rise to the posterior interventricular branch in approximately 15% of individuals. **D.** Many other variations occur.

Table 1.4. Arterial Supply to Heart

Artery/Branch	Origin	Course	Distribution	Anastomoses
Right coronary	Right aortic sinus	Follows coronary (AV) groove between atria and ventricles	Right atrium, SA and AV nodes, and posterior part of IVS	Circumflex and anterior IV branches of left coronary artery
SA nodal	Right coronary artery near its origin (in 60%)	Ascends to SA node	Pulmonary trunk and SA node	
Right marginal	Right coronary artery	Passes to inferior margin of heart and apex	Right ventricle and apex of heart	IV branches
Posterior interventricular	Right coronary artery (in 67%)	Runs in posterior IV groove to apex of heart	Right and left ventricles and posterior third of IVS	Anterior IV branch of left coronary artery (at apex)
AV nodal	Right coronary artery near origin of posterior IV artery	Passes to AV node	AV node	
Left coronary	Left aortic sinus	Runs in AV groove and gives off anterior IV and circumflex branches	Most of left atrium and ventricle, IVS, and AV bundles; may supply AV node	Right coronary artery
SA nodal	Circumflex branch (in 40%)	Ascends on posterior surface of left atrium to SA node	Left atrium and SA node	
Anterior interventricular	Left coronary artery	Passes along anterior IV groove to apex of heart	Right and left ventricles and anterior two thirds of IVS	Posterior IV branch of right coronary artery (at apex)
Circumflex	Left coronary artery	Passes to left in AV groove and runs to posterior surface of heart	Left atrium and left ventricle	Right coronary artery
Left marginal	Circumflex branch	Follows left border of heart	Left ventricle	IV branches
Posterior interventricular	Left coronary artery (in 33%)	Runs in posterior IV groove to apex of heart	Right and left ventricles and posterior third of IVS	Anterior IV branch of left coronary artery (at apex)

AV, atrioventricular; *IV,* interventricular; *IVS,* interventricular septum; *SA,* sinuatrial.

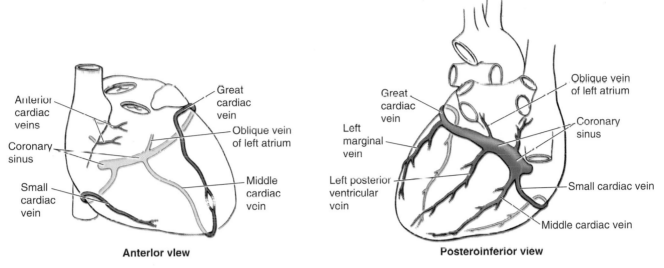

Figure 1.51. Cardiac veins. The great, middle, and small cardiac veins; the oblique vein of the left atrium; and the left posterior ventricular vein are the main vessels draining into the coronary sinus. The coronary sinus, in turn, empties into the right atrium. The anterior cardiac veins drain directly into the auricle of the right atrium.

Coronary Artery Disease or Coronary Heart Disease

Coronary artery disease (CAD) is one of the leading causes of death. CAD has many causes, all of which result in a reduced blood supply to the vital myocardial tissue.

Myocardial Infarction

With sudden occlusion of a major artery by an embolus (G. *embolos,* plug), the region of myocardium supplied by the occluded vessel becomes **infarcted**(rendered virtually bloodless) and undergoes **necrosis** (pathological tissue death).

The three most common sites of coronary artery occlusion and the percentage of occlusions involving each artery are (Fig. B1.20*A* & *B*) the:

- Anterior IV (LAD) branch of the LCA (40–50%).
- RCA (30–40%).
- Circumflex branch of the LCA (15–20%).

An area of myocardium that has undergone necrosis constitutes a **myocardial infarction** (MI). The most common cause of *ischemic heart disease* is coronary artery insufficiency resulting from atherosclerosis. ▶

- Part of the right ventricle.
- Most of the IVS (usually its anterior two thirds), including the AV bundle of the conducting system of the heart, through its perforating IV septal branches.
- The SA node (in approximately 40% of people).

Variations of the Coronary Arteries Variations in the branching patterns and distribution of the coronary arteries are common. In the most common *right dominant pattern,* present in approximately 67% of people, the RCA and LCA share about equally in the blood supply of the heart (Fig. 1.50*A*). In approximately 15% of hearts, the LCA is dominant in that the posterior IV branch is a branch of the circumflex artery (Fig. 1.50*B*). There is codominance in approximately 18% of people, in which branches of both the right and left coronary arteries reach the crux and give rise to branches that course in or near the posterior IV groove. A few

people have only a single coronary artery (Fig. 1.50*C*). In other people, the circumflex branch arises from the right aortic sinus (Fig. 1.50*D*). Approximately 4% of people have an accessory coronary artery.

Coronary Collateral Circulation The branches of the coronary arteries are generally considered to be **end arteries**, arteries that supply regions of the myocardium lacking sufficient anastomoses from other large branches to maintain viability of the tissue should occlusion occur. However, anastomoses do exist between branches of the coronary arteries, subepicardial or myocardial, and between these arteries and extracardiac vessels such as thoracic vessels (Williams et al., 1995). Anastomoses exist between the terminations of the right and the left coronary arteries in the coronary groove and between the IV branches around the apex in approximately 10% of apparently normal hearts. The potential for the development of this collateral circulation probably exists in most if not all hearts.

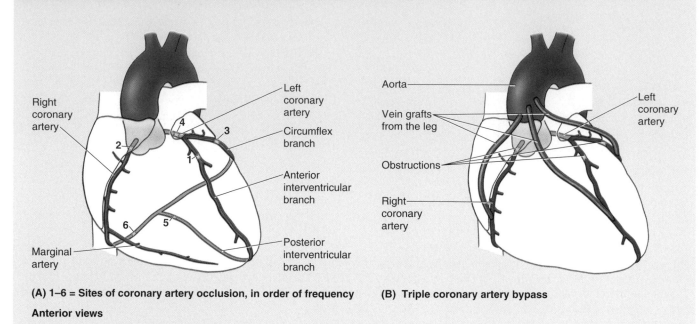

(A) 1–6 = Sites of coronary artery occlusion, in order of frequency

Anterior views

(B) Triple coronary artery bypass

Figure B1.20

Coronary Atherosclerosis

The **atherosclerotic process**, which results in lipid accumulations on the internal walls of the coronary arteries, begins during early adulthood and slowly results in stenosis of the lumina of the coronary arteries. As **coronary atherosclerosis** progresses, the collateral channels connecting one coronary artery with the other expand, which may initially permit adequate perfusion of the heart during relative inactivity. Despite this compensatory mechanism, the myocardium may not receive enough oxygen when the heart needs to perform increased amounts of work. Strenuous exercise, for example, increases the heart's activity and its need for oxygen. The insufficiency of blood supply to the heart (**myocardial ischemia**) may result in MI.

Slowly Progressive Coronary Artery Disease

In slow occlusion of a coronary artery, the collateral circulation has time to increase so that adequate perfusion of the myocardium can occur when a potentially ischemic event occurs. Consequently, MI may not result. On sudden blockage of a large coronary branch, some infarction is probably inevitable, but the extent of the area damaged depends on the degree of development of collateral anastomotic channels. If large branches of both coronary arteries are partially obstructed, an extracardiac collateral circulation may be used to supply blood to the heart. These collaterals connect the coronary arteries with the vasa vasorum in the tunica adventitia of the aorta and pulmonary arteries and with branches of the internal thoracic, bronchial,

and phrenic arteries. Clinical studies show that anastomoses cannot provide collateral routes quickly enough to prevent the effects of sudden coronary artery occlusion. The functional value of these anastomoses thus appears to be more effective in slowly progressive CAD.

Angina Pectoris

Pain that originates in the heart is called **angina** or **angina pectoris** (L. *angina,* strangling pain + L. *pectoris,* of the chest). Individuals with angina commonly describe the transient (15 sec to 15 min) but moderately severe constricting pain as tightness in the thorax, deep to the sternum. The pain is the result of ischemia of the myocardium that falls short of inducing the cellular necrosis that defines infarction. Most often, angina results from narrowed and hardened coronary arteries. The reduced blood flow results in less oxygen being delivered to cardiac muscle cells (myocytes). As a result of the limited anaerobic metabolism of the myocytes, lactic acid accumulates and the pH is reduced in affected areas of the heart. Pain receptors in muscle are stimulated by lactic acid. Strenuous exercise (especially after a heavy meal), sudden exposure to cold, and stress all require increased activity on the part of the heart, but the occluded vessels cannot provide it. When food enters the stomach, blood flow to it and other parts of the digestive tract is increased. As a result, some blood is diverted from other organs, including the heart.

Anginal pain is relieved by a period of rest (1–2 min are often adequate). Sublingual nitroglycerin ▶

(medication placed or sprayed under the tongue for absorption through the oral mucosa) may be administered because it dilates the coronary (and other) arteries. This increases blood flow to the heart, while decreasing the workload and the heart's need for oxygen because the heart is pumping against less resistance. Furthermore, the dilated vessels accommodate more of the blood volume, and so less blood arrives in the heart that needs to be pumped out again. Thus the angina is usually relieved. Such angina provides a warning that the coronary arteries are compromised and that there is a need for a change of lifestyle, a healthcare intervention, or both.

The pain resulting from MI is usually more severe than with angina pectoris, and the pain resulting from MI does not disappear after 1–2 min of rest. MI may also follow excessive exertion by a person with stenotic (narrowed) coronary arteries. The straining heart muscle demands more oxygen than the stenotic arteries can provide; as a result, the ischemic area of myocardium undergoes infarction and a **heart attack** occurs. Occlusion of any but the smallest branches of a coronary artery usually results in death of the cardiac muscle fibers it supplies. The damaged muscle is replaced by fibrous tissue and a scar forms.

Coronary Bypass Graft

Some patients with obstruction of the coronary circulation and severe angina undergo a **coronary bypass graft** operation. A segment of an artery or a vein is connected to the ascending aorta or to the proximal part of a coronary artery and then to the coronary artery distal to the stenosis (Fig. B1.20B). The *great saphenous vein* is commonly harvested for coronary bypass surgery because (1) it has a diameter equal to or greater than that of the coronary arteries, (2) can be easily dissected from the lower limb, (3) and offers relatively lengthy portions with a minimum occurrence of valves or branching. Reversal of the implanted segment of vein can negate the effect of a valve if a valved segment must be used. Use of the *radial artery* in bypass surgery has become increasingly more common. A coronary bypass graft shunts blood from the aorta to a stenotic coronary artery to increase the flow distal to the obstruction. Simply stated, it provides a detour around the stenotic area (arterial stenosis) or blockage (arterial atresia). Revascularization of the myocardium may also be achieved by surgically anastomosing an internal thoracic artery with a coronary artery.

Coronary Angioplasty

In selected patients, surgeons use **percutaneous transluminal coronary angioplasty** in which they pass a catheter with a small inflatable balloon attached to its tip into the obstructed coronary artery (Fig. B1.21). When the catheter reaches the obstruction, the balloon is inflated, flattening the atherosclerotic plaque against the vessel's wall, and the vessel is stretched to increase the size of the lumen, thus improving blood flow. In other cases, *thrombokinase* is injected through the catheter; this enzyme dissolves the blood clot. Intraluminal instruments with rotating blades and lasers have also been employed. After dilation of the vessel, an *intravascular* stent may be introduced to maintain the dilation. Intravascular stents are composed of rigid or semi-rigid tubular meshes, collapsed during introduction. Once in place, they expand or are expanded with a balloon catheter, to maintain luminal patency. Complications of angioplastic procedures include reoccurrence and formation of clots in the coronary artery. ○

Balloon catheter headed toward coronary artery

Deflated balloon catheter approaches blockage

Inflated balloon crushes blockage

Circulation re-established

Figure B1.21. Percutaneous transluminal angioplasty.

Venous Drainage of the Heart The heart is drained mainly by veins that empty into the coronary sinus and partly by small veins that empty into the right atrium (Fig. 1.51). The **coronary sinus,** the main vein of the heart, is a wide venous channel that runs from left to right in the posterior part of the coronary groove. The coronary sinus receives the great cardiac vein at its left end and the middle cardiac vein and small cardiac veins at its right end. The left posterior ventricular vein and left marginal vein also open into the coronary sinus.

The **great cardiac vein** is the main tributary of the coronary sinus. Its first part (**anterior interventricular vein**) begins near the apex of the heart and ascends with the anterior IV branch of the LCA. At the coronary groove it turns left, and its second part runs around the left side of the heart with the circumflex branch of the LCA to reach the coronary sinus. (An unusual situation is occurring here: Blood is flowing in the same direction within a paired artery and vein!) The great cardiac vein drains the areas of the heart supplied by the LCA. The **middle cardiac vein** (**posterior IV vein**) accompanies the posterior interventricular branch (usually arising from the RCA), and a **small cardiac vein** accompanies the right marginal branch of the RCA. Thus these two veins drain most of the areas commonly supplied by the RCA. The **oblique vein of the left atrium** (of Marshall) is a small vessel, relatively unimportant postnatally, that descends over the posterior wall of the left atrium and merges with the great cardiac vein to form the coronary sinus (defining the beginning of the sinus). The oblique vein is the remnant of the embryonic left SVC, which usually atrophies during the fetal period, but occasionally persists in adults, replacing or augmenting the right SVC (Moore and Persaud, 2003).

Some cardiac veins do not drain via the coronary sinus. Several small **anterior cardiac veins** begin over the anterior surface of the right ventricle, cross over the coronary groove, and usually end directly in the right atrium; sometimes they enter the small cardiac vein. The **smallest cardiac veins** (L. *venae cordis minimae*) are minute vessels that begin in the capillary beds of the myocardium and open directly into the chambers of the heart, chiefly the atria. Although called veins, they are valveless communications with the capillary beds of the myocardium and may carry blood from the heart chambers to the myocardium.

Collateral Circulation via the Smallest Cardiac Veins

Reversal of flow in the anterior and *smallest cardiac veins* may bring **luminal blood** (blood from the heart chambers) to the capillary beds of the myocardium in some regions, providing some additional collateral circulation. However, unless these collaterals have dilated in response to pre-existing ischemic heart disease, they are unlikely to be able to supply sufficient blood to the heart during an acute event and thus prevent MI. ○

Lymphatic Drainage of the Heart Lymphatic vessels in the myocardium and subendocardial connective tissue pass to the **subepicardial lymphatic plexus.** Vessels from this plexus pass to the coronary groove and follow the coronary arteries. A single lymphatic vessel, formed by the union of various vessels from the heart, ascends between the pulmonary trunk and left atrium and ends in the inferior **tracheobronchial lymph nodes,** usually on the right side.

THE BOTTOM LINE: The circulatory system of the myocardium is unique in that the coronary arteries fill during ventricular diastole as a result of aortic recoil. They are typically (but not necessarily) functional end arteries. The right coronary artery (RCA) and circumflex branch of the left coronary artery (LCA) supply the walls of the atria via small branches. The RCA typically supplies the SA and AV nodes, the myocardium of the external wall of the right ventricle (except its anterior surface), the diaphragmatic surface of the left ventricle, and the posterior third of the IVS. The LCA typically supplies the anterior two thirds of the IVS (including the AV bundle of conductive tissue), the anterior wall of the right ventricle, and the external wall of the left ventricle (except the diaphragmatic surface). The capillary beds of the myocardium drain primarily into the right atrium via veins emptying into the coronary sinus. However, the vein also may enter directly into the chambers via the smallest cardiac veins. Both pathways lack valves.

Conducting System of the Heart In the ordinary sequence of events in the cardiac cycle, the atrium and ventricle work together as one pump on each side of the heart. The **conducting system of the heart** (Fig. 1.52), which coordinates the *cardiac cycle* (discussed earlier in this chapter), consists of cardiac muscle cells and highly specialized conducting fibers for initiating impulses and conducting them rapidly through the heart. Nodal tissue initiates the heartbeat and coordinates contractions of the four heart chambers.

The **sinuatrial (SA) node** is located anterolaterally just deep to the epicardium at the junction of the SVC and right atrium, near the superior end of the *sulcus terminalis* (Figs. 1.49*A* and 1.52*A*). The SA node—a small collection of nodal tissue, specialized cardiac muscle fibers, and associated fibroelastic connective tissue—is the *pacemaker of the heart*. The SA node initiates and regulates the impulses for contraction, giving off an impulse approximately 70 times per minute in most people. The contraction signal from the SA node spreads myogenically (through the musculature) of both atria. The SA node is supplied by the **sinuatrial nodal artery,** which usually arises as an atrial branch of the RCA (in 60% of people), but it may arise from the LCA (in 40%). The SA node is stimulated by the sympathetic division of the autonomic nervous system to accelerate the heart rate and is inhibited by the parasympathetic division to return to or toward its basal rate.

Anterosuperior views

Figure 1.52. Conducting system of heart. A. Impulses (*arrows*) initiated at the sinuatrial node, located at the superior end of the sulcus (internally, crista) terminalis, are propagated through the atrial musculature to the atrioventricular node. **B.** Impulses (*arrows*) received by the atrioventricular node, in the inferior part of the interatrial septum, are conducted through the AV bundle and its branches to the myocardium. The AV bundle begins at the AV node and divides into right and left bundles at the junction of the membranous and muscular parts of the IVS.

The **atrioventricular (AV) node** is a smaller collection of nodal tissue than the SA node. The AV node is located in the posteroinferior region of the interatrial septum near the opening of the coronary sinus (Figs. 1.49A–C and 1.52B). The signal generated by the SA node passes through the walls of the right atrium, propagated by the cardiac muscle (**myogenic conduction**), which transmits the signal rapidly from the SA node to the AV node. The AV node then distributes the signal to the ventricles through the **AV bundle** (Fig. 1.52B). Sympathetic stimulation speeds up conduction, and parasympathetic stimulation slows it down. The AV bundle, the only bridge between the atrial and ventricular myocardium, passes from the AV node through the insulating *fibrous skeleton of the heart* and along the membranous part of the IVS.

At the junction of the membranous and muscular parts of the septum, the AV bundle divides into **right** and **left bundles.** These branches proceed on each side of the muscular IVS deep to the endocardium and then ramify into **subendocardial branches** (Purkinje fibers), which extend into the walls of the respective ventricles. The subendocardial branches of the right bundle stimulate the muscle of the IVS, the anterior papillary muscle through the septomarginal trabecula (moderator band), and the wall of the right ventricle. The left bundle divides near its origin into approximately six smaller tracts, which give rise to subendocardial branches that stimulate the IVS, the anterior and posterior papillary muscles, and the wall of the left ventricle.

The AV node is supplied by the **AV nodal artery,** the largest and usually the first IV septal branch of posterior IV artery, a branch of the RCA in 80% of people (Fig. 1.49A–C). Thus the arterial supply to both the SA and AV nodes is usually derived from the RCA. However, the AV bundle traverses the center of the IVS, the anterior two thirds of which is supplied by the IVS branches of the anterior IV branch of the LCA (Fig. 1.49C & D).

Impulse generation and conduction can be summarized as follows:

- The SA node initiates an impulse that is rapidly conducted to cardiac muscle fibers in the atria, causing them to contract (Fig. 1.52A).

- The impulse spreads by myogenic conduction, which rapidly transmits the impulse from the SA node to the AV node.

- The signal is distributed from the AV node through the AV bundle and its branches (the right and left bundles), which pass on each side of the IVS to supply subendocardial branches to the papillary muscles and the walls of the ventricles (Fig. 1.52B).

Innervation of the Heart The heart is supplied by autonomic nerve fibers from the **cardiac plexus** (Figs. 1.53 and 1.58B & C), which is often quite artificially divided into superficial and deep portions. This nerve network is most commonly described as lying on the anterior surface of the bi-

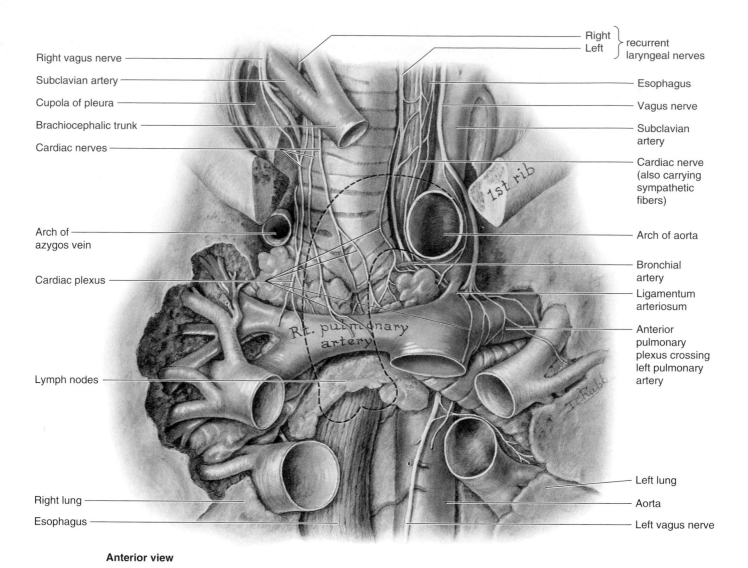

Right vagus nerve

Subclavian artery

Cupola of pleura

Brachiocephalic trunk

Cardiac nerves

Arch of azygos vein

Cardiac plexus

Lymph nodes

Right lung

Esophagus

Right · Left } recurrent laryngeal nerves

Esophagus

Vagus nerve

Subclavian artery

Cardiac nerve (also carrying sympathetic fibers)

Arch of aorta

Bronchial artery

Ligamentum arteriosum

Anterior pulmonary plexus crossing left pulmonary artery

Left lung

Aorta

Left vagus nerve

Rt. pulmonary artery

1st rib

Anterior view

Figure 1.53. Cardiac nerves and plexus. This dissection of the superior and posterior mediastina demonstrates cardiac branches of the vagus nerve (CN X) and sympathetic trunks running down the sides of the trachea to form the cardiac plexus. Although shown lying anterior to the tracheal bifurcation here, the primary relationship of the cardiac plexus is to the ascending aorta (*broken lines*) and pulmonary trunk, the former having been removed to expose the plexus.

furcation of the *trachea* (a respiratory structure), since it is most commonly observed in dissection after removal of the ascending aorta and the bifurcation of the pulmonary trunk. However, its primary relationship is to the posterior aspect of the latter two (cardiovascular) structures, especially the ascending aorta. The cardiac plexus is formed of both sympathetic and parasympathetic fibers en route to the heart. Fibers are distributed along and to the coronary vessels and to components of the conducting system, particularly the SA node.

The *sympathetic supply* is from presynaptic fibers, with cell bodies in the intermediolateral cell columns (IMLs) of the superior five or six thoracic segments of the spinal cord, and postsynaptic sympathetic fibers, with cell bodies in the cervical and superior thoracic paravertebral ganglia of the sympathetic trunks. The postsynaptic fibers traverse *cardiopul-*

monary splanchnic nerves and the cardiac plexus to end in the SA and AV nodes and in relation to the terminations of parasympathetic fibers on the coronary arteries. *Sympathetic stimulation* causes increased heart rate; impulse conduction; force of contraction; and, at the same time, increased blood flow through the coronary vessels to support the increased activity. Adrenergic stimulation of the SA node and conducting tissue increases the rate of depolarization of the pacemaker cells while increasing atrioventricular conduction. Direct adrenergic stimulation from the sympathetic nerve fibers, as well as indirect suprarenal (adrenal) hormone stimulation, increases atrial and ventricular contractility. Most adrenergic receptors on coronary blood vessels are β_2-receptors which, when activated, cause relaxation (or perhaps inhibition) of vascular smooth muscle and, therefore, dilation of the arteries (Wilson-Pauwels et al., 1997). This supplies more oxygen and nutrients to the myocardium during periods of increased activity.

The *parasympathetic supply* is from presynaptic fibers of the vagus nerves. Postsynaptic parasympathetic cell bodies (intrinsic ganglia) are located in the atrial wall and interatrial septum near the SA and AV nodes and along the coronary arteries. *Parasympathetic stimulation* slows the heart rate, reduces the force of the contraction, and constricts the coronary arteries, saving energy between periods of increased demand. Postsynaptic parasympathetic fibers release acetylcholine, which binds with *muscarinic receptors* to slow the rates of depolarization of the pacemaker cells and atrioventricular conduction and decrease atrial contractility.

Electrocardiography

The passage of impulses over the heart from the SA node can be amplified and recorded as an **electrocardiogram** (ECG or EKG) (Fig. B1.22). Functional testing of the heart includes *exercise tolerance tests* (treadmill stress tests), primarily to check the consequences of possible coronary artery disease. Exercise tolerance tests are of considerable importance in detecting the cause of heartbeat irregularities. Heart rate, ECG, and blood pressure readings are monitored as the patient does increasingly demanding exercise on a treadmill. The results show the maximum effort a patient's heart can safely tolerate.

Coronary Occlusion and the Conducting System of the Heart

Damage to the conducting system of the heart, often resulting from ischemia caused by coronary artery disease, produces disturbances of cardiac muscle contraction. Since the anterior IV branch (LAD) gives rise to the septal branches supplying the AV bundle in most people, and branches of the RCA supply both the SA and AV nodes (Figs. B1.23 and 1.49C), parts of the conducting system of the heart are likely to be affected by their occlusion, and a **heart block** may occur. In this case (if the patient survives the initial stages), the ventricles will begin to contract independently at their own rate: 25–30 times per minute (much slower than the slowest normal rate (40–45 times per minute). The atria continue to contract at the normal rate if the SA node has been spared, but the impulse generated by the SA node no longer reaches the ventricles.

Damage to one of the bundle branches results in a *bundle branch block,* in which excitation passes along the unaffected branch and causes a normally timed systole of that ventricle only. The impulse then spreads to the ▶

(A) Electrocardiography (ECG)

(B) Events of the cardiac cycle (P, Q, R, S, and T)

Figure B1.22

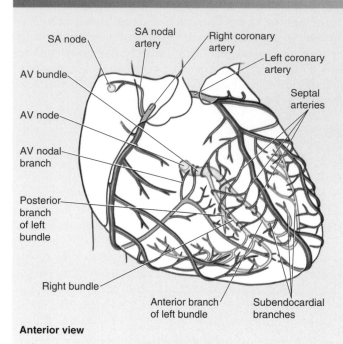

SA node
SA nodal artery
Right coronary artery
Left coronary artery
AV bundle
Septal arteries
AV node
AV nodal branch
Posterior branch of left bundle
Right bundle
Anterior branch of left bundle
Subendocardial branches

Anterior view

Figure B1.23

other ventricle via *myogenic* (muscle propagated) conduction, producing a late asynchronous contraction. In these cases, a *cardiac pacemaker* (artificial heart regulator) may have to be implanted to increase the ventricular rate of contraction to 70–80 per minute (see clinical correlation [blue] box "Artificial Cardiac Pacemaker").

With a ventricular septal defect, the AV bundle usually lies in the margin of the VSD. Obviously, this vital part of the conducting system must be preserved during surgical repair of the defect. Destruction of the AV bundle would cut the only physiological link between the atrial and ventricular musculature, also producing a heart block as described above.

Artificial Cardiac Pacemaker

In some people with a heart block, an **artificial cardiac pacemaker** (approximately the size of a pocket watch) is inserted subcutaneously. The pacemaker consists of a pulse generator or battery pack, a wire (lead), and an electrode. Pacemakers produce electrical impulses that initiate ventricular contractions at a predetermined rate. An electrode with a catheter connected to it is inserted into a vein and its progression through the venous pathway is followed with a **fluoroscope**, a device for examining deep structures in real time (as motion occurs) by means of radiographs. The terminal of the electrode is passed through the SVC to the right atrium and through the tricuspid valve into the right ventricle. Here the electrode is firmly fixed to the trabeculae carneae in the ventricular wall and placed in contact with the endocardium.

Restarting the Heart

In most cases of cardiac arrest, first-aid workers perform **cardiopulmonary resuscitation** to restore cardiac output and pulmonary ventilation. By applying firm pressure to the thorax over the inferior part of the sternal body (external or closed chest cardiac massage), the sternum moves posteriorly 4–5 cm. The increased intrathoracic pressure forces blood out of the heart into the great arteries. When the external pressure is released and the intrathoracic pressure falls, the heart again fills with blood. If the heart stops beating (**cardiac arrest**) during heart surgery, the surgeon attempts to restart it using internal or open chest (direct) heart massage.

Fibrillation of the Heart

Fibrillation is multiple, rapid, circuitous contractions or twitchings of muscular fibers, including cardiac muscle. In **atrial fibrillation,** the normal regular rhythmical contractions of the atria are replaced by rapid irregular and uncoordinated twitchings of different parts of the atrial walls. The ventricles respond at irregular intervals to the dysrhythmic impulses received from the atria, but usually circulation remains satisfactory. In **ventricular fibrillation,** the normal ventricular contractions are replaced by rapid, irregular twitching movements that do not pump (i.e., they do not maintain the systemic circulation, including the coronary circulation). The damaged conducting system of the heart does not function normally. As a result, an irregular pattern of uncoordinated contractions occurs in the ventricles, except in those areas that are infarcted. Ventricular fibrillation is the most disorganized of all *dysrhythmias,* and in its presence no effective cardiac output occurs. The condition is fatal if allowed to persist.

Defibrillation of the Heart

An electric shock may be given to the heart through the thoracic wall via large electrodes (paddles). This shock causes cessation of all cardiac movements and a few seconds later the heart may begin to beat more normally. As coordinated contractions and hence pumping of the heart is re-established, some degree of systemic (including coronary) circulation results.

Cardiac Referred Pain

The heart is insensitive to touch, cutting, cold, and heat; however, ischemia and the accumulation of metabolic products stimulate pain endings in the myocardium. The afferent pain fibers run centrally in the middle and inferior cervical branches and especially in the thoracic ▶

Figure B1.24

cardiac branches of the sympathetic trunk. The axons of these primary sensory neurons enter spinal cord segments T1 through T4 or T5, especially on the left side.

Cardiac referred pain is a phenomenon whereby noxious stimuli originating in the heart are perceived by a person as pain arising from a superficial part of the body—the skin on the left upper limb, for example. **Visceral referred pain** is transmitted by visceral afferent fibers accompanying sympathetic fibers and is typically referred to somatic structures or areas such as a limb having afferent fibers with cell bodies in the same spinal ganglion, and central processes that enter the spinal cord through the same posterior roots (Hardy and Naftel, 2001).

Anginal pain is commonly felt as radiating from the substernal and left pectoral regions to the left shoulder and the medial aspect of the left upper limb (Fig. B1.24A). This part of the limb is supplied by the medial cutaneous nerve of the arm. Often the lateral cutaneous branches of the 2nd and 3rd intercostal nerves (the intercostobrachial nerves) join or overlap in their distribution with the medial cutaneous nerve of the arm. Consequently, cardiac pain is referred to the upper limb because the spinal cord segments of these cutaneous nerves (T1–T3) are also common to the visceral afferent terminations for the coronary arteries. Synaptic contacts may also be made with commissural (connector) neurons, which conduct impulses to neurons on the right side of comparable areas of the spinal cord. This occurrence explains why pain of cardiac origin, although usually referred to the left side, may be referred to the right side, both sides, or the back (Fig. B.21B & C). ⊕

Surface Anatomy of the Heart and Great Vessels

The heart and great vessels are approximately in the middle of the thorax, surrounded laterally and posteriorly by the lungs and anteriorly by the sternum and the central part of the thoracic cage (Fig. SA 1.7A & B). The borders of the heart are variable and depend on the position of the diaphragm and the build and physical condition of the person. The outline of the heart can be traced on the anterior surface of the thorax by using the following guidelines (Fig. SA1.7C):

* The *superior border* corresponds to a line connecting the inferior border of the 2nd left costal cartilage to the superior border of the 3rd right costal cartilage.

* The *right border* corresponds to a line drawn from the 3rd right costal cartilage to the 6th right costal cartilage; this border is slightly convex to the right.

* The *inferior border* corresponds to a line drawn from the inferior end of the right border to a point in the 5th intercostal space close to the left MCL; the left end of this line corresponds to the location of the apex of the heart and the apex beat.

* The *left border* corresponds to a line connecting the left ends of the lines representing the superior and inferior borders.

* The valves are located posterior to the sternum; however, the sounds produced by them are projected to the areas shown in Figure SA1.7B—pulmonary (*P*), aortic (*A*), mitral (*M*), and tricuspid (*T*)—where the stethoscope may be placed to avoid intervening bone. ▶

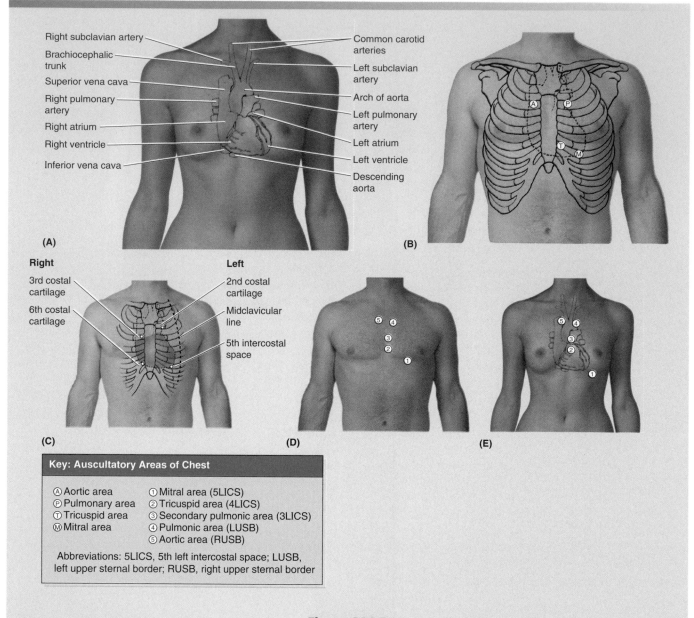

Right subclavian artery
Brachiocephalic trunk
Superior vena cava
Right pulmonary artery
Right atrium
Right ventricle
Inferior vena cava

Common carotid arteries
Left subclavian artery
Arch of aorta
Left pulmonary artery
Left atrium
Left ventricle
Descending aorta

(A)

(B)

Right
3rd costal cartilage
6th costal cartilage

Left
2nd costal cartilage
Midclavicular line
5th intercostal space

(C)

(D)

(E)

Key: Auscultatory Areas of Chest

Ⓐ Aortic area
Ⓟ Pulmonary area
Ⓣ Tricuspid area
Ⓜ Mitral area

① Mitral area (5LICS)
② Tricuspid area (4LICS)
③ Secondary pulmonic area (3LICS)
④ Pulmonic area (LUSB)
⑤ Aortic area (RUSB)

Abbreviations: 5LICS, 5th left intercostal space; LUSB, left upper sternal border; RUSB, right upper sternal border

Figure SA1.7

The **apex beat** is the impulse that results from the apex of the heart being forced against the anterior thoracic wall when the left ventricle contracts. The location of the apex beat (mitral area, M) varies in position and may be located in the 4th or 5th intercostal spaces, 6–10 cm from the AML.

Auscultatory Areas

Clinicians' interest in the surface anatomy of the heart and cardiac valves results from their need to listen to valve sounds. The five areas (two areas are for the pulmonary valve) are as wide apart as possible so that the sounds produced at any given valve may be clearly distinguished from those produced at other valves (Fig. SA1.7D & E). Blood tends to carry the sound in the direction of its flow; consequently, each area is situated superficial to the chamber or vessel into which the blood has passed and in a direct line with the valve orifice. ✪

THE BOTTOM LINE: The conducting system of the heart consists of specialized intrinsic nodes that rhythmically generate stimuli and of bundles of modified cardiac muscle that conduct the impulses, resulting in the coordinated contraction of the atria and ventricles. The rate of gener-ation and speed of conductivity are increased by the sympathetic division, and inhibited by the parasympathetic division, of the ANS to meet demands or conserve energy. The impulse-generating sinuatrial node and the relaying atrioventricular node are typically supplied by nodal branches of the RCA, whereas the atrioventricular bundle and its branches are primarily supplied by septal branches of the LCA. Occlusion of either artery with subsequent infarction of nodal or conductive tissue may require placement of an artificial cardiac pacemaker. The effect of the ANS on the coronary arteries is paradoxical, with sympathetic stimulation producing vasodilation and parasympathetic stimulation producing vasoconstriction.

Superior Mediastinum

The **superior mediastinum** is superior to the transverse thoracic plane, passing through the sternal angle and the junction (IV disc) of vertebrae T4 and T5 (Fig. 1.54). From anterior to posterior, the contents of the superior mediastinum are (Figs. 1.55A & B and 1.56) the:

- Thymus.

- Great vessels, with the veins (brachiocephalic veins and SVC) anterior to the arteries (arch of the aorta and the roots of its major branches—the brachiocephalic trunk, left common carotid artery, and left subclavian artery) and related nerves (vagus and phrenic nerves and the cardiac plexus of nerves).

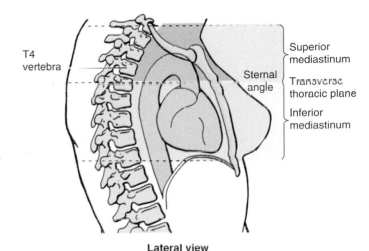

Lateral view

Figure 1.54 Boundaries of superior mediastinum. The superior mediastinum extends interiorly from the superior thoracic aperture to the transverse thoracic plane, which passes through the sternal angle anteriorly and the intervertebral disc of vertebrae T4 and T5 posteriorly.

- Inferior continuation of the cervical viscera (trachea anteriorly and esophagus posteriorly) and related nerves (left recurrent laryngeal nerve).

- Thoracic duct and lymphatic trunks.

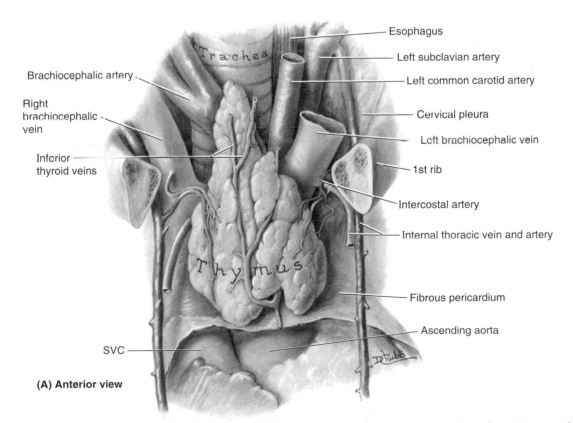

(A) Anterior view

Figure 1.55. Dissections of superior mediastinum. A. In this superficial dissection, the sternum and ribs have been excised and the pleurae removed. It is unusual to see such a distinct thymus in an adult; usually it is impressive during puberty but subsequently regresses and becomes largely replaced by fat and fibrous tissue. *SVC*, superior vena cava.

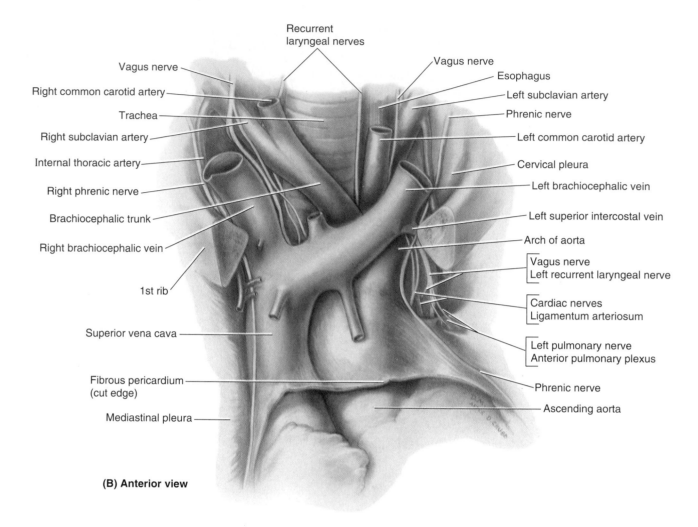

Recurrent
laryngeal nerves

Vagus nerve
Esophagus
Left subclavian artery
Phrenic nerve
Left common carotid artery
Cervical pleura
Left brachiocephalic vein
Left superior intercostal vein
Arch of aorta
Vagus nerve
Left recurrent laryngeal nerve
Cardiac nerves
Ligamentum arteriosum
Left pulmonary nerve
Anterior pulmonary plexus
Phrenic nerve
Ascending aorta

Vagus nerve
Right common carotid artery
Trachea
Right subclavian artery
Internal thoracic artery
Right phrenic nerve
Brachiocephalic trunk
Right brachiocephalic vein
1st rib
Superior vena cava
Fibrous pericardium
(cut edge)
Mediastinal pleura

(B) Anterior view

Figure 1.55. *(Continued)* **B.** In this deep dissection of the root of the neck and superior mediastinum, the thymus has been removed. The right vagus nerve (CN X) crosses anterior to the right subclavian artery and gives off the right recurrent laryngeal nerve, which passes medially to reach the trachea and esophagus. The left recurrent laryngeal nerve passes inferior and then posterior to the arch of the aorta and ascends between the trachea and esophagus to the larynx.

To summarize systemically, the major structures in the superior mediastinum, from anterior to posterior, are the thymus, veins, arteries, airway, alimentary tract, and lymphatic trunks.

Thymus

The **thymus**, a primary lymphoid organ, is located in the inferior part of the neck and the anterior part of the superior mediastinum (Figs. 1.55*A* and 1.56). It lies posterior to the manubrium and extends into the anterior mediastinum, anterior to the fibrous pericardium. After puberty, the thymus undergoes gradual involution and is largely replaced by fat. The rich *arterial supply of the thymus* is derived mainly from the anterior intercostal and **anterior mediastinal branches of the internal thoracic arteries**. The *veins of the thymus* end in the left brachiocephalic, internal thoracic, and inferior thyroid veins. The *lymphatic vessels of the thymus* end in the parasternal, brachiocephalic, and tracheobronchial lymph nodes.

Age Changes in the Thymus

The flat, flask-shaped lobes of the thymus are a prominent feature of the superior mediastinum during infancy and childhood. In some infants, the thymus may compress the trachea. The thymus plays an important role in the development and maintenance of the immune system. As puberty is reached, the thymus begins to diminish in relative size. By adulthood, it is usually replaced by adipose tissue and is often scarcely recognizable; however, it continues to produce T-lymphocytes. ✪

Great Vessels

The *brachiocephalic veins* are formed posterior to the sternoclavicular (SC) joints by the union of the internal jugular and subclavian veins. At the level of the inferior border of the

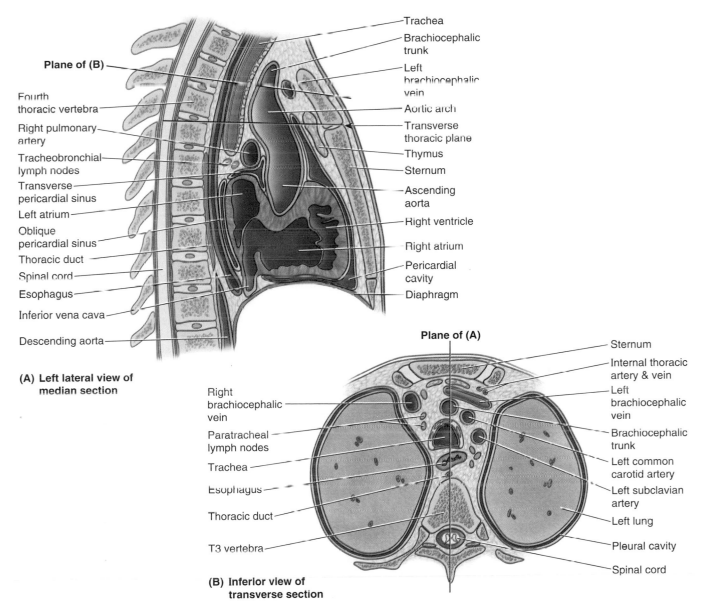

(A) Left lateral view of median section

(B) Inferior view of transverse section

Figure 1.56. Relationships of structures of superior mediastinum. A. A median section of the thorax is shown. **B.** A transverse section of the superior mediastinum at the level of the sternoclavicular joints is shown. The order of systemic structures in the superior mediastinum, from anterior to posterior, is demonstrated in both views: thymus, veins, arteries, airway (trachea), alimentary tract (esophagus), lymphatic ducts, vertebral bodies/IV discs, and spinal cord.

1st right costal cartilage, the brachiocephalic veins unite to form the SVC (Figs. 1.55B and 1.56B). The **left brachiocephalic vein** is more than twice as long as the right vein because it passes from the left to the right side, passing over the anterior aspects of the roots of the three major branches of the arch of the aorta (Fig. 1.55B). It shunts blood from the head, neck, and left upper limb to the right atrium.

The **superior vena cava** returns blood from all structures superior to the diaphragm, except the lungs and heart. It passes inferiorly and ends at the level of the 3rd costal cartilage, where it enters the right atrium of the heart. The SVC lies in the right side of the superior mediastinum, anterolateral to the trachea and posterolateral to the ascending aorta.

The *right phrenic nerve* lies between the SVC and the mediastinal pleura. The terminal half of the SVC is in the middle mediastinum, where it lies beside the ascending aorta and forms the posterior boundary of the transverse pericardial sinus (Fig. 1.37).

The **ascending aorta,** approximately 2.5 cm in diameter, begins at the aortic orifice (Table 1.5). Its only branches are the coronary arteries, arising from the aortic sinuses (discussed under "Semilunar Valves," earlier in this chapter). The ascending aorta is intrapericardial (Fig. 1.55B); for this reason and because it lies inferior to the transverse thoracic plane, it is considered a content of the middle mediastinum (part of the inferior mediastinum).

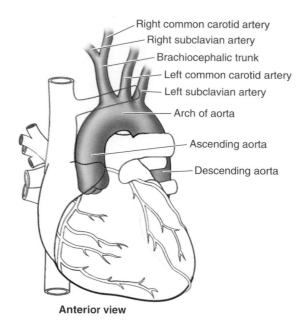

Right common carotid artery
Right subclavian artery
Brachiocephalic trunk
Left common carotid artery
Left subclavian artery
Arch of aorta
Ascending aorta
Descending aorta

Anterior view

Figure 1.57. Common pattern of branches of arch of aorta. The pattern shown is present in approximately 65% of people. The largest branch (brachiocephalic trunk) arises from the beginning of the arch and divides into two branches (right subclavian artery and right common carotid artery). The next artery (left common carotid artery) arises from the superior part of the arch. The third branch (left subclavian artery) arises from the arch approximately 1 cm distal to the left common carotid.

The **arch of the aorta** (aortic arch), the curved continuation of the ascending aorta (Figs. 1.56*A* and 1.57; Table 1.5), begins posterior to the 2nd right sternocostal (SC) joint at the level of the sternal angle and arches superiorly, posteriorly and to the left, and then inferiorly. The arch of the aorta ascends anterior to the right pulmonary artery and the bifurcation of the trachea, reaching its apex at the left side of the trachea and esophagus as it passes over the root of the left lung. The arch descends posterior to the root of the lung on the left side of the body of the T4 vertebra. The arch of the aorta ends by becoming the **thoracic aorta** posterior to the 2nd left sternocostal joint. The arch of the azygos vein occupies a corresponding position on the right side of the trachea over the root of the right lung, although its contents are flowing in the opposite direction (Fig. 1.53). The **ligamentum arteriosum,** the remnant of fetal ductus arteriosus, passes from the root of the left pulmonary artery to the inferior surface of the arch of the aorta. The usual branches of the arch of the aorta are the *brachiocephalic trunk, left common carotid artery,* and *left subclavian artery* (Figs. 1.57 and 1.58*A*).

The **brachiocephalic trunk,** the first and largest branch of the arch of the aorta, arises posterior to the manubrium, where it is anterior to the trachea and posterior to the left brachiocephalic vein (Figs. 1.55*B*, 1.56*A* & *B*, and 1.58*A*). It ascends superolaterally to reach the right side of the trachea and the right SC joint, where it divides into the right common carotid and right subclavian arteries.

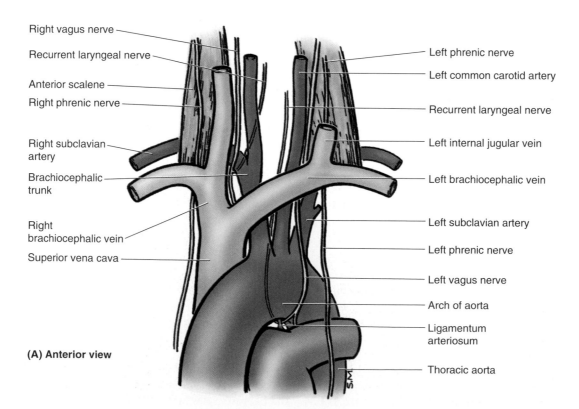

Right vagus nerve
Recurrent laryngeal nerve
Anterior scalene
Right phrenic nerve
Right subclavian artery
Brachiocephalic trunk
Right brachiocephalic vein
Superior vena cava

Left phrenic nerve
Left common carotid artery
Recurrent laryngeal nerve
Left internal jugular vein
Left brachiocephalic vein
Left subclavian artery
Left phrenic nerve
Left vagus nerve
Arch of aorta
Ligamentum arteriosum
Thoracic aorta

(A) Anterior view

Figure 1.58 Great vessels and nerves. A. The relationships of the great vessels and nerves in the inferior neck and superior mediastinum are shown. The ligamentum arteriosum is the remnant of the fetal shunt that bypasses the prefunctional lungs (ductus arteriosus).

(1) (2) (3) (4)

(B) Anterior views

Right vagus nerve

Right recurrent laryngeal nerve

Right pulmonary plexus

Left vagus nerve

Left recurrent laryngeal nerve

Cardiac plexus

Left pulmonary plexus

Esophageal nerve plexus

(C) Anterior view

Figure 1.58. *(Continued)* **B.** The relationships at the bifurcation of the trachea from superficial to deep are shown. *1* (most anterior). The left brachiocephalic vein passes across the roots of the three major branches of the arch of the aorta. *2.* The ascending aorta and arch pass anterior and superior, respectively, to the right pulmonary artery. *3.* The bifurcation of the pulmonary trunk and right pulmonary artery lie directly anterior to the bifurcation of the trachea. *4.* The cardiac plexus remains on the anterior aspect of the tracheal bifurcation after removal of the pulmonary trunk and arteries and the ascending aorta and arch of the aorta, to which the plexus is primarily related. **C.** The nerves in the superior and posterior mediastina are seen after the viscera that lie anterior to the trachea and esophagus have been removed.

The **left common carotid artery**, the second branch of the arch of the aorta, arises posterior to the manubrium, slightly posterior and to the left of the brachiocephalic trunk. It ascends anterior to the left subclavian artery and is at first anterior to the trachea and then to its left. It enters the neck by passing posterior to the left SC joint.

The **left subclavian artery**, the third branch of the arch, arises from the posterior part of the arch of the aorta, just posterior to the left common carotid artery. It ascends lateral to the trachea and left common carotid artery through the superior mediastinum; it has no branches in the mediastinum. As it leaves the thorax and enters the root of the neck, it passes posterior to the left SC joint.

Aneurysm of the Ascending Aorta

The distal part of the ascending aorta receives a strong thrust of blood when the left ventricle contracts. Because its wall is not reinforced by fibrous pericardium (the fibrous pericardium blends with the aortic adventitia at the beginning of the arch; Fig. 1.55*B*), an **aneurysm** (localized dilation) may develop. The aneurysm will be evident on a chest film (radiograph of the thorax) as an enlarged ascending aorta silhouette. Individuals with an aneurysm usually complain of chest pain that radiates to the back.

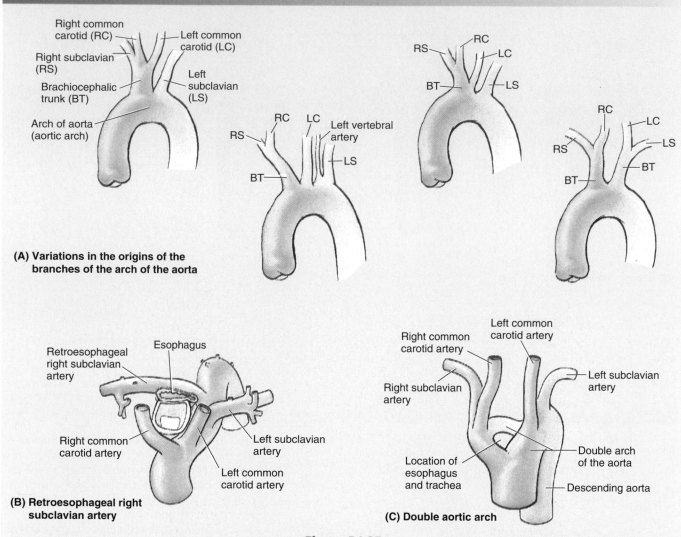

(A) Variations in the origins of the branches of the arch of the aorta

(B) Retroesophageal right subclavian artery

(C) Double aortic arch

Figure B1.25

Variations in the Great Arteries

Branches of the Arch of the Aorta

The usual pattern of branches of the arch of the aorta is present in approximately 65% of people (Fig. 1.57). Variations in the origin of the branches of the arch of the aorta are fairly common (Fig. B1.25A). In approximately 27% of people, the left common carotid originates from the brachiocephalic trunk. A brachiocephalic trunk fails to form in approximately 2.5% of people; in these cases each of the four arteries (right and left common carotid and subclavian arteries) originate independently from the arch of the aorta. The left vertebral artery originates from the arch of the aorta in approximately 5% of people. Both right and left brachiocephalic trunks originate from the arch in approximately 1.2% of people. For a description of other variations in the origins of the branches of the arch of the aorta, see Bergman et al. (1988).

A **retroesophageal right subclavian artery** sometimes arises as the last (most-left-sided) branch of the arch of the aorta (Fig. B1.25B). The artery crosses posterior to the esophagus to reach the right upper limb and may compress the esophagus, causing difficulty in swallowing (dysphagia). An accessory artery to the thyroid gland, the **thyroid ima artery** (L. *arteria thyroidea ima*), may arise from the arch of the aorta or the brachiocephalic artery.

Anomalies of the Arch of the Aorta

The most superior part of the arch of the aorta is usually approximately 2.5 cm inferior to the superior border of the manubrium, but it may be more superior or inferior. Sometimes the arch of the aorta curves over the root of the right lung and passes inferiorly on the right side, forming a **right arch of the aorta**. In some cases, the abnormal arch, after passing over the root of the right lung, passes posterior to the esophagus to reach ▶

its usual position on the left side. Less frequently, a **double arch of the aorta** forms a vascular ring around the esophagus and trachea (Fig. B1.25C). A trachea that is compressed enough to affect breathing may require surgical division of the vascular ring. An *aneurysm of the arch of the aorta* may also exert pressure on the trachea and esophagus, causing difficulty in breathing and swallowing (see clinical correlation [blue] box "Aneurysm of Ascending Aorta.)"

Coarctation of the Aorta

In **coarctation of the aorta,** the arch of the aorta or descending aorta has an abnormal narrowing (stenosis) that diminishes the caliber of the aortic lumen, producing an obstruction to blood flow to the inferior part of the body (Fig. B1.26). The most common site for a coarctation is near the site of the ductus or ligamentum arteriosum. When the coarctation is inferior to this site (*postductal coarctation*), a good collateral circulation usually develops between the proximal and distal parts of the aorta through the intercostal and internal thoracic arteries. This type of coarctation is compatible with many years of life because the collateral circulation carries blood to the thoracic aorta inferior to the stenosis. The collateral vessels may become so large that they cause notable pulsation in the intercostal spaces and erode the adjacent surfaces of the ribs, which is visible in radiographs of the thorax. ○

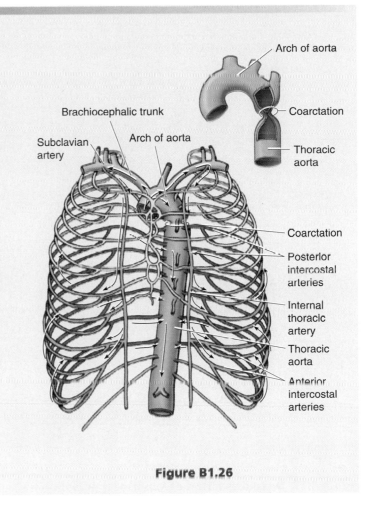

Figure B1.26

Nerves in the Superior Mediastinum

The *vagus nerves* exit the cranium and descend through the neck posterolateral to the common carotid arteries (Fig. 1.58A; Table 1.6). Each nerve enters the superior mediastinum posterior to the respective SC joint and brachiocephalic vein. The **right vagus nerve** enters the thorax anterior to the right subclavian artery, where it gives rise to the **right recurrent laryngeal nerve** (Fig. 1.58A–C). This nerve hooks around the right subclavian artery and ascends between the trachea and esophagus to supply the larynx. The right vagus nerve runs posteroinferiorly through the superior mediastinum on the right side of the trachea. It then passes posterior to the right brachiocephalic vein, SVC, and root of the right lung. Here it divides into many branches, which contribute to the **right pulmonary plexus** (Fig. 1.58C). Usually, the right vagus nerve leaves this plexus as a single nerve and passes to the esophagus, where it again breaks up and contributes fibers to the **esophageal nerve plexus.** The right vagus nerve also gives rise to nerves that contribute to the *cardiac plexus.*

The **left vagus nerve** descends in the neck posterior to the left common carotid artery (Fig. 1.58A). It enters the mediastinum between the left common carotid artery and left subclavian artery. When it reaches the left side of the arch of the aorta, the nerve diverges posteriorly from the left phrenic nerve. It is separated laterally from the phrenic nerve by the left superior intercostal vein. As the left vagus nerve curves medially at the inferior border of the arch of the aorta, it gives off the **left recurrent laryngeal nerve.** This nerve passes inferior to the arch of the aorta, immediately lateral to the ligamentum arteriosum, and ascends to the larynx in the groove between the trachea and the esophagus (Figs. 1.53, 1.55B, 1.58A–C, and 1.59). The left vagus nerve passes posterior to the root of the left lung, where it breaks up into many branches that contribute to the **left pulmonary plexus.** The nerve leaves this plexus as a single trunk and passes to the esophagus, where it joins fibers from the right vagus in the *esophageal nerve plexus* (Fig. 1.58B & C).

The *phrenic nerves* (Fig. 1.58A) supply the diaphragm with motor and sensory fibers, the latter accounting for approximately one third of the nerve's fibers. The phrenic nerves also supply sensory fibers to the pericardium and mediastinal pleura. Each nerve enters the superior mediastinum between the subclavian artery and the origin of the brachiocephalic vein (Table 1.6). The fact that the phrenic nerves pass anterior to the roots of the lungs provides an important means of distinguishing them from the vagus nerves, which pass posterior to the roots. The **right phrenic nerve** passes along the right side of the

Vertebral column

Longus colli

Cervical pleura

Arch of
azygos vein

Esophagus

Anterior view

Vagus nerve

Esophagus

Left recurrent laryngeal nerve

Thoracic duct

Trachea

1st rib

Arch of aorta

Bronchial arteries

Root of lung
(entering lung at hilum)

Intrapulmonary bronchi

Thoracic aorta

Right bronchus

Left bronchus

Figure 1.59. Deep dissection of superior mediastinum. Four structures run parallel as they traverse the superior thoracic aperture: trachea, esophagus, left recurrent laryngeal nerve, and thoracic duct. The right main bronchus is more vertical, shorter, and wider than the left main bronchus. The course of the right bronchial artery shown here is aberrant; usually it passes posterior to the bronchus.

right brachiocephalic vein, SVC, and pericardium over the right atrium. It also passes anterior to the root of the right lung and descends on the right side of the IVC to the diaphragm, which it pierces near the caval opening (Fig. 1.60*A*). The **left phrenic nerve** descends between the left subclavian and left common carotid arteries. It crosses the left surface of the arch of the aorta anterior to the left vagus nerve and passes over the left superior intercostal vein. It then descends anterior to the root of the left lung and runs along the fibrous pericardium, superficial to the left atrium and ventricle of the heart, where it pierces the diaphragm to the left of the pericardium (Fig. 1.60*B*). Most branching of the phrenic nerves for distribution to the diaphragm occurs on the diaphragm's inferior (abdominal) surface.

Trachea

The **trachea** descends anterior to the esophagus and enters the superior mediastinum, inclining a little to the right of the median plane (Figs. 1.55*A* & *B* and 1.58*B* & *C*, and 1.59). The posterior surface of the trachea is flat where it is applied to the esophagus (Fig. 1.56*B*). The trachea ends at the level of

Injury to the Recurrent Laryngeal Nerves

The recurrent laryngeal nerves supply all intrinsic muscles of the larynx, except one. Consequently, any investigative (diagnostic) procedure (e.g., *mediastinotomy*) or disease process in the superior mediastinum may injure these nerves and affect the voice. Because the left recurrent laryngeal nerve winds around the arch of the aorta and ascends between the trachea and esophagus, it may be involved in a bronchogenic or esophageal carcinoma, enlargement of mediastinal lymph nodes, or an *aneurysm of the arch of the aorta*. In the latter condition, the nerve may be stretched by the dilated arch. ⊙

the sternal angle by dividing into the right and left main bronchi (Figs. 1.56*A* and 1.59). The trachea terminates superior to the level of the heart and is not a component of the posterior mediastinum.

Table 1.5. Aorta and Its Branches in Thorax

Artery	Origin	Course	Branches
Ascending aorta	Aortic orifice of left ventricle	Ascends approximately 5 cm to sternal angle where it becomes arch of aorta	Right and left coronary arteries
Arch of aorta	Continuation of ascending aorta	Arches posteriorly on left side of trachea and esophagus and superior to left main bronchus	Brachiocephalic, left common carotid, left subclavian
Thoracic aorta	Continuation of arch of aorta	Descends in posterior mediastinum to left of vertebral column; gradually shifts to right to lie in median plane at aortic hiatus	Posterior intercostal arteries, subcostal, some phrenic arteries and visceral branches (e.g., esophageal)
Posterior intercostal	Posterior aspect of thoracic aorta	Pass laterally and then anteriorly parallel to ribs	Lateral and anterior cutaneous branches
Bronchial (1–2 branches)	Anterior aspect of aorta or posterior intercostal artery	Run with the tracheobronchial tree	Bronchial and peribronchial tissue, visceral pleura
Esophageal (4–5 branches)	Anterior aspect of thoracic aorta	Run anteriorly to esophagus	To esophagus
Superior phrenic (vary in number)	Anterior aspects of thoracic aorta	Arise at aortic hiatus and pass to superior aspect of diaphragm	To diaphragm

Esophagus

The **esophagus** is a fibromuscular tube that extends from the pharynx to the stomach (Figs. 1.56A & B, 1.58B & C, 1.59, 1.60A, and 1.61). It enters the superior mediastinum between the trachea and the vertebral column, where it lies anterior to the bodies of the T1–T4 vertebrae. It is usually flattened anteroposteriorly. Initially, it inclines to the left but is pushed back to the median plane by the arch of the aorta. It is then compressed anteriorly by the root of the left lung. In the superior mediastinum, the *thoracic duct* usually lies on the left side of the esophagus, deep (medial) to the arch of the aorta (Figs. 1.59 and 1.60B). Inferior to the arch, the esophagus again inclines to the left as it approaches and passes through the **esophageal hiatus** in the diaphragm (Fig. 1.61).

THE BOTTOM LINE: The superior mediastinum extends between the superior thoracic aperture and the transverse thoracic plane. The only organ that belongs exclusively to this region is the adult thymus. The remainder of the structures traverse this space, passing through the superior thoracic aperture to the root of the neck, or passing between the neck and abdomen. Within the superior mediastinum, structures occur in systemic layers, proceeding from anterior to posterior: (1) lymphoid system (thymus), (2) blood vascular system (veins first, then arteries), (3) respiratory system (trachea), (4) alimentary system (esophagus), and (5) lymph vascular system (thoracic duct, bronchomediastinal trunks, posterior mediastinal lymph nodes). The nervous system does not have its own layer in the superior mediastinum, but it is integrated with layer 2 (phrenic and vagus nerves) and lies between layers 3 and 4 (recurrent laryngeal nerves). The pattern of the branches of the arch of the aorta is atypical in approximately 35% of people.

Posterior Mediastinum

The **posterior mediastinum** (the posterior part of the inferior mediastinum) is located inferior to the transverse thoracic plane, anterior to the T5–T12 vertebrae, posterior to the pericardium and diaphragm, and between the parietal pleura of the two lungs (Figs. 1.56A and 1.58C). The posterior mediastinum contains the thoracic aorta, thoracic duct and lymphatic trunks, posterior mediastinal lymph nodes, azygos and hemiazygos veins, and esophagus and esophageal nerve plexus. Some authors also include the thoracic sympathetic trunks and thoracic splanchnic nerves; however, these structures lie lateral to the vertebral bodies and are not within the posterior mediastinal compartment or space per se.

Thoracic Aorta

The thoracic aorta is the continuation of the arch of the aorta (Figs. 1.58C, 1.59, 1.60B, 1.61, and 1.62; Table 1.5). It begins on the left side of the inferior border of the body of the T4 vertebra and descends in the posterior mediastinum on the left sides of the T5–T12 vertebrae. As it descends, it approaches the median plane and displaces the esophagus to the right. The **thoracic aortic plexus** (Fig. 1.60B), an autonomic nerve network, surrounds it. The thoracic aorta lies posterior to the root of the left lung (Figs. 1.59 and 1.60B), pericardium, and esophagus. The thoracic aorta terminates (with a name change to *abdominal aorta*) anterior to the inferior border of the T12 vertebra and enters the abdomen through the **aortic hiatus** in the diaphragm (Fig. 1.61). The thoracic duct and azygos vein ascend on its right side and accompany it through this hiatus.

In a pattern that will be more evident in the abdomen, the *branches of the descending aorta* arise and course within three "vascular planes" (Fig. 1.62A):

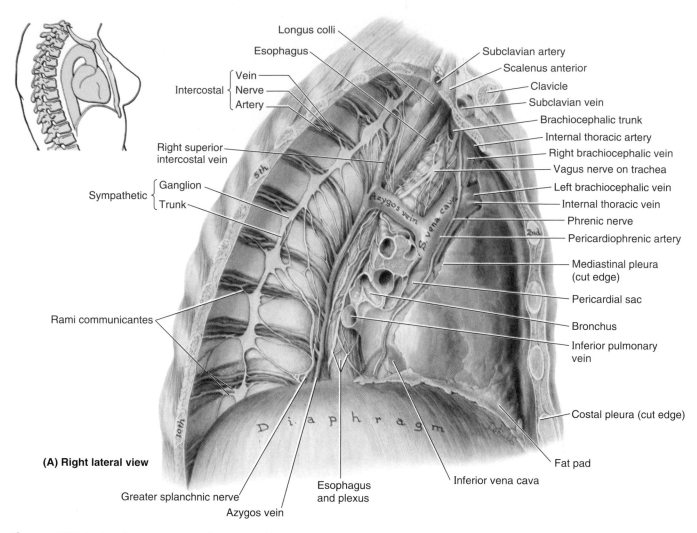

Longus colli

Esophagus

Intercostal { Vein — Nerve — Artery —

Right superior intercostal vein

Sympathetic { Ganglion — Trunk —

Rami communicantes

(A) Right lateral view

Greater splanchnic nerve

Azygos vein

Esophagus and plexus

Subclavian artery

Scalenus anterior

Clavicle

Subclavian vein

Brachiocephalic trunk

Internal thoracic artery

Right brachiocephalic vein

Vagus nerve on trachea

Left brachiocephalic vein

Internal thoracic vein

Phrenic nerve

Pericardiophrenic artery

Mediastinal pleura (cut edge)

Pericardial sac

Bronchus

Inferior pulmonary vein

Costal pleura (cut edge)

Fat pad

Inferior vena cava

Figure 1.60 Lateral exposures of the mediastinum. A. In this right side view, most of the costal and mediastinal pleura has been removed to expose the underlying structures. This side of the mediastinum, the "blue side," is dominated by venous structures: the azygos vein and arch, SVC, right atrium, and IVC.

- An anterior, midline plane of unpaired visceral branches to the gut and its derivatives.

- Lateral planes of paired visceral branches serving viscera other than the gut and its derivatives.

- Posterolateral planes of paired, segmental, parietal branches to the body wall.

In the thorax, the unpaired visceral branches of the anterior vascular plane are the **esophageal arteries**—usually two, but as many as five (Fig. 1.62B and Table 1.5). The paired visceral branches of the lateral plane are represented in the thorax by the *bronchial arteries* (Fig. 1.59). Although the right and left bronchial arteries may arise directly from the aorta, most commonly only the paired left bronchial

arteries do so, the right arising indirectly as branches of a right posterior intercostal artery (usually the 3rd). The paired, parietal branches of the thoracic aorta that arise posterolaterally are the nine posterior intercostal arteries that supply all but the upper two intercostal spaces and the subcostal arteries (Fig. 1.62B). The latter vessels arise from the thoracic aorta but course below the diaphragm. They are in series with the posterior intercostal arteries.

Exceptions to this pattern include the:

- **Superior phrenic arteries,** paired parietal branches that pass anterolaterally to the superior surface of the diaphragm (which is actually facing posteriorly at this level owing to the convexity of the diaphragm), where they

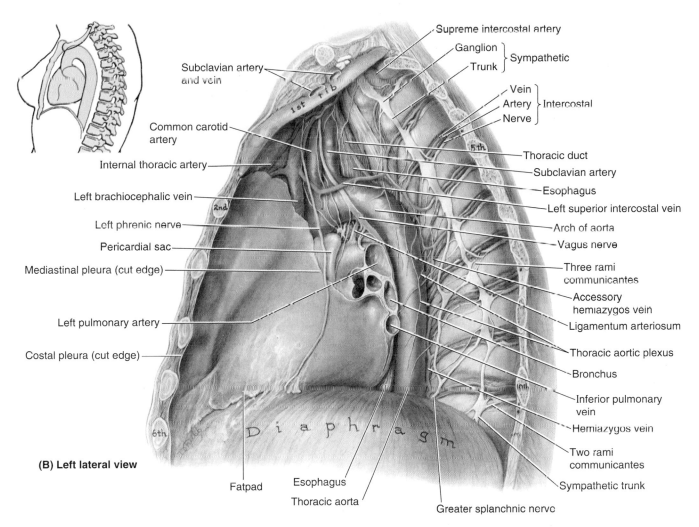

Figure 1.60. *(Continued)* **B.** The left side of the mediastinum, the "red side," is dominated by arterial structures: the arch of aorta and thoracic aorta, left common carotid and subclavian arteries, and left ventricle (plus the pulmonary trunk and left pulmonary artery). At the thoracic and superior lumbar levels, the sympathetic trunk is attached to intercostal nerves by paired (white and gray) rami communicantes. The left superior intercostal vein, draining the upper two to three intercostal spaces, passes anteriorly to enter the left brachiocephalic vein.

anastomose with the musculophrenic and pericardia-cophrenic branches of the internal thoracic artery.

- **Pericardial branches,** unpaired branches that arise anteriorly but, instead of passing to the gut, send twigs to the pericardium. The same is true for the small **mediastinal arteries** that supply the lymph nodes and other tissues of the posterior mediastinum.

Esophagus

The esophagus descends into the posterior mediastinum from the superior mediastinum, passing posterior and to the right of the arch of the aorta (Figs. 1.58C, 1.59, and 1.61) and posterior to the pericardium and left atrium. The esophagus

constitutes the primary posterior relationship of the base of the heart. It then deviates to the left and passes through the esophageal hiatus in the diaphragm at the level of the T10 vertebra, anterior to the aorta. The esophagus may have three impressions, or "constrictions," in its thoracic part. These may be observed as narrowings of the lumen in oblique chest radiographs that are taken as barium is swallowed. The esophagus is compressed by three structures: (1) the arch of the aorta, (2) the left main bronchus, and (3) the diaphragm. The first two occur in close proximity; the former is most evident in a posteroanterior (PA) radiograph after a barium swallow, and the latter is more evident in lateral views. No constrictions are visible in the empty esophagus; however, as it expands during filling, the structures noted above compress its walls.

Blockage of the Esophagus

The impressions produced in the esophagus by adjacent structures are of clinical interest because of the slower passage of substances at these sites. The impressions indicate where swallowed foreign objects are most likely to lodge and where a stricture may develop after the accidental drinking of a caustic liquid such as lye. ⊙

Thoracic Duct and Lymphatic Trunks

In the posterior mediastinum, the thoracic duct lies on the anterior aspect of the bodies of the inferior 7 thoracic vertebrae (Fig. 1.63). It is the largest lymphatic channel in the body. The thoracic duct conveys most lymph of the body to the venous system, that from the lower limbs; pelvic cavity; abdominal cavity; left upper limb; and left side of the thorax, head, and neck—that is, all but the right superior quadrant (see Introduction). The thoracic duct originates from the **chyle cistern** (L. *cisterna chyli*) in the abdomen and ascends through the aortic hiatus in the diaphragm (Fig. 1.61). The thoracic duct is usually thin walled and dull white; often it is beaded because of its numerous valves. It ascends in the

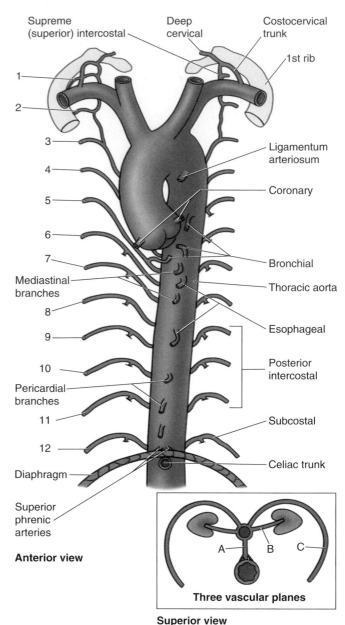

Anterior view

Superior view

Figure 1.62 Branches of thoracic aorta. In a pattern that will be more obvious and strictly adhered to in the abdomen, branches of the thoracic aorta tend to arise within three vascular planes (*inset*). Esophageal and pericardial branches represent unpaired visceral branches (*A* in inset) arising anteriorly; the bronchial arteries represent paired lateral visceral branches (*B* in inset); posterior intercostal and subcostal arteries (*1–12*) represent paired, segmental parietal branches that mostly arise posterolaterally (*C* in inset). The paired superior phrenic arteries arising from the inferior part of the thoracic aorta that supply the diaphragm are exceptions to the pattern.

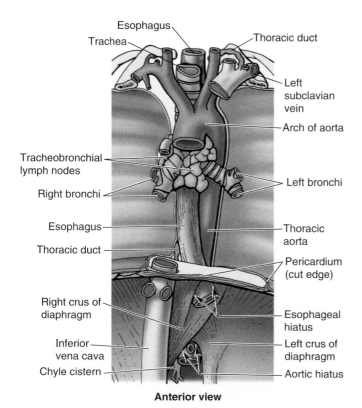

Anterior view

Figure 1.61 Anterior view of esophagus, trachea, bronchi, and aorta. The arch of aorta curves posteriorly on the left side of the trachea and esophagus. Enlargement of the inferior tracheobronchial (carinal) nodes may widen the angle between the main primary bronchi. In this specimen, the thoracic duct enters the left subclavian vein.

posterior mediastinum among the thoracic aorta on its left, the azygos vein on its right, the esophagus anteriorly, and the vertebral bodies posteriorly. At the level of the T4, T5, or T6 vertebra, the thoracic duct crosses to the left, posterior to the

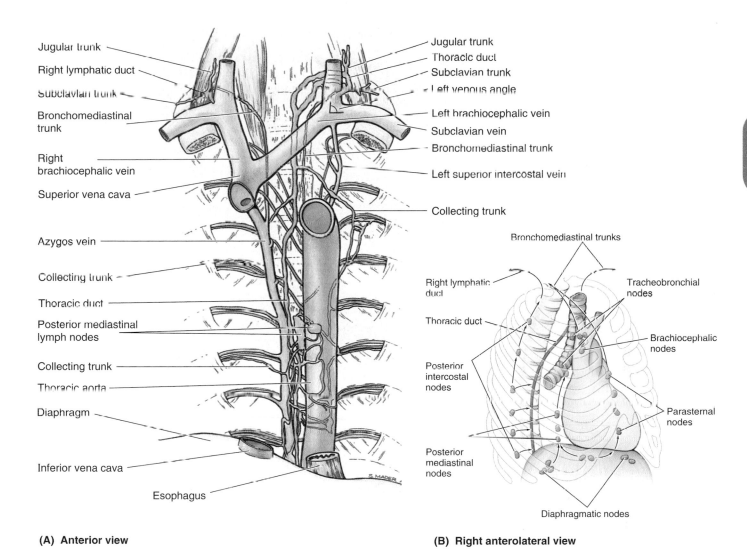

(A) Anterior view

(B) Right anterolateral view

Figure 1.63. Thoracic duct and bronchomediastinal trunks. A. The thoracic aorta has been pulled slightly to the left and the azygos vein slightly to the right to expose the thoracic duct, which ascends on the vertebral column between the azygos vein and the thoracic aorta. At approximately the transverse thoracic plane (sternal angle, T4–T5 IV disc level), the thoracic duct passes to the left and continues its ascent to the neck where it arches laterally to open near, or at, the angle of union of the internal jugular and subclavian veins (left venous angle). The thoracic duct receives branches from the intercostal spaces of both sides through several collecting trunks and branches from posterior mediastinal structures. Near its termination, the thoracic duct receives the jugular, subclavian, and bronchomediastinal trunks. The right lymphatic duct is formed by the union of the right jugular, subclavian, and bronchomediastinal trunks. **B.** Lymph nodes and pathways providing lymphatic drainage of the thoracic cavity are shown.

esophagus, and ascends into the superior mediastinum. The thoracic duct receives branches from the middle and superior intercostal spaces of both sides through several collecting trunks. It also receives branches from posterior mediastinal structures. Near its termination, it often receives the *jugular, subclavian,* and *bronchomediastinal lymphatic trunks* (although any or all these vessels may terminate independently). The thoracic duct usually empties into the venous system near the union of the left internal jugular and subclavian veins—the left *venous angle* or origin of the left brachiocephalic vein (Figs. 1.62 and 1.63*A*)—but it may open into the left subclavian vein as shown in Figure 1.61.

Laceration of the Thoracic Duct

Because the thoracic duct is thin walled and may be colorless, it may be difficult to identify. Consequently, it is vulnerable to inadvertent injury during investigative and/or surgical procedures in the posterior mediastinum. Laceration of the thoracic duct during an accident or lung surgery results in lymph escaping into the thoracic cavity at rates ranging from 75 to 200 mL per hour. Lymph or chyle from the lacteals of the ▶

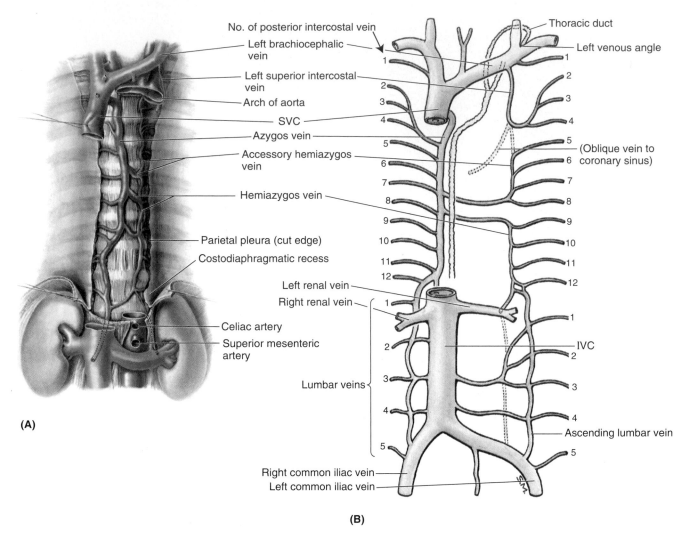

No. of posterior intercostal vein
Left brachiocephalic vein
Left superior intercostal vein
Arch of aorta
SVC
Azygos vein
Accessory hemiazygos vein
Hemiazygos vein
Parietal pleura (cut edge)
Costodiaphragmatic recess
Left renal vein
Right renal vein
Celiac artery
Superior mesenteric artery
Lumbar veins

(A)

Thoracic duct
Left venous angle
(Oblique vein to coronary sinus)
IVC
Ascending lumbar vein
Right common iliac vein
Left common iliac vein

(B)

Figure 1.64. Azygos system of veins. The azygos vein forms a direct connection between the inferior vena cava (*IVC*) and the superior vena cava (*SVC*). The azygos and hemiazygos veins are also continuous inferiorly (below diaphragm) with the ascending lumbar veins.

intestine (see Chapter 2) may also enter the pleural cavity, producing *chylothorax.* This fluid may be removed by a needle tap or by thoracentesis; in some cases it may be necessary to ligate the thoracic duct. The lymph then returns to the venous system by other lymphatic channels that join the thoracic duct superior to the ligature.

Variations of the Thoracic Duct

Variations of the thoracic duct are common because the superior part of the duct represents the original left member of a pair of vessels in the embryo (Moore and Persaud, 2003). Sometimes two thoracic ducts are present for a short distance. ⊙

Vessels and Lymph Nodes of the Posterior Mediastinum

The thoracic aorta and its branches were discussed earlier in this chapter. **Posterior mediastinal lymph nodes** (Fig. 1.63A & B) lie posterior to the pericardium, where they are related to the esophagus and thoracic aorta. There are several nodes posterior to the inferior part of the esophagus and more (up to eight) anterior and lateral to it. The posterior mediastinal lymph nodes receive lymph from the esophagus, the posterior aspect of the pericardium and diaphragm, and the middle posterior intercostal spaces. They drain to the right or left venous angles via the right lymphatic duct or the thoracic duct.

The **azygos system of veins,** on each side of the vertebral column, drains the back and thoracoabdominal walls (Figs. 1.63A and 1.64A & B) as well as the mediastinal viscera. The azygos system exhibits much variation in its origin, course, tributaries, and anastomoses. The *azygos vein* (G., *azygos,* unpaired) and its

Table 1.6. Nerves of Thorax

Nerve	Origin	Course	Distribution
Vagus (CN X)	8–10 rootlets from medulla of brainstem	Enters superior mediastinum posterior to sternoclavicular joint and brachiocephalic vein; gives rise to recurrent laryngeal nerve; continues into abdomen	Pulmonary plexus, esophageal, plexus, and cardiac plexus
Phrenic	Anterior rami of C3–C5 nerves	Passes through superior thoracic aperture and runs between mediastinal pleura and pericardium	Central portion of diaphragm
Intercostals (1–11)	Anterior rami of T1–T11 nerves	Run in intercostal spaces between internal and innermost layers of intercostal muscles	Muscles in and skin over intercostal space; lower nerves supply muscles and skin of anterolateral abdominal wall
Subcostal	Anterior ramus of T12 nerve	Follows inferior border of 12th rib and passes into abdominal wall	Abdominal wall and skin of gluteal region
Recurrent laryngeal	Vagus nerve	Loops around subclavian on right; on left runs around arch of aorta and ascends in tracheoesophageal groove	Intrinsic muscles of larynx (except cricothyroid); sensory inferior to level of vocal folds
Cardiac plexus	Cervical and cardiac branches of vagus nerve and sympathetic trunk	From arch of aorta and posterior surface of heart, fibers extend along coronary arteries and to sinuatrial node	Impulses pass to sinuatrial node; parasympathetic fibers slow rate, reduce force of heartbeat, and constrict coronary arteries; sympathetic fibers have the opposite effect
Pulmonary plexus	Vagus nerve and sympathetic trunk	Forms on root of lung and extends along bronchial subdivisions	Parasympathetic fibers constrict bronchioles; sympathetic fibers dilate them; afferents convey reflexes
Esophageal plexus	Vagus nerve, sympathetic ganglia, greater splanchnic nerve	Distal to tracheal bifurcation; vagus and sympathetic nerves form a plexus around esophagus	Vagal and sympathetic fibers to smooth muscle and glands of inferior two thirds of esophagus

Figure 1.65. Autonomic nerves of superior and posterior mediastina. The cervicothoracic (stellate) ganglion is formed by the fusion of the inferior cervical ganglion and the first thoracic ganglion. The second ganglion is often larger than the adjacent ganglia.

Alternate Venous Routes to the Heart

The azygos, hemiazygos, and accessory hemiazygos veins offer alternate means of venous drainage from the thoracic, abdominal, and back regions when *obstruction of the IVC* occurs. In some people, an accessory azygos vein parallels the azygos vein on the right side. Other people have no hemiazygos system of veins. A clinically important variation, although uncommon, is when the azygos system receives all the blood from the IVC except that from the liver. In these people, the azygos system drains nearly all the blood inferior to the diaphragm, except from the digestive tract. If *obstruction of the SVC* occurs superior to the entrance of the azygos vein, blood can drain inferiorly into the veins of the abdominal wall and return to the right atrium through the azygos venous system and the IVC. ⊕

main tributary, the *hemiazygos vein,* usually arise from "roots" arising from the posterior aspect of the IVC and/or renal vein, respectively, which merge with the ascending *lumbar veins.*

The **azygos vein** forms a collateral pathway between the SVC and IVC and drains blood from the posterior walls of the thorax and abdomen. It ascends in the posterior mediastinum, passing close to the right sides of the bodies of the inferior 8 thoracic vertebrae. It arches over the superior aspect of the root of the right lung to join the SVC, similar to the way the arch of the aorta passes over the root of the left lung. In addition to the *posterior intercostal veins,* the azygos vein communicates with the vertebral venous plexuses that drain the back, vertebrae, and structures in the vertebral canal (see Chapter 4). The azygos vein also receives the mediastinal, esophageal, and bronchial veins.

The **hemiazygos vein** arises on the left side by the junction of the left subcostal and ascending lumbar veins. It ascends on the left side of the vertebral column, posterior to the thoracic aorta as far as the T9 vertebra. Here it crosses to the right, posterior to the aorta, thoracic duct, and esophagus, and joins the azygos vein. The hemiazygos vein receives the inferior three posterior intercostal veins, the inferior esophageal veins, and several small mediastinal veins.

The **accessory hemiazygos vein** begins at the medial end of the 4th or 5th intercostal space and descends on the left side of the vertebral column from T5 through T8. It receives tributaries from veins in the 4th–8th intercostal spaces and sometimes from the left bronchial veins. It crosses over the T7 or T8 vertebra, posterior to the thoracic aorta and thoracic duct, where it joins the azygos vein. Sometimes the accessory hemiazygos vein joins the hemiazygos vein and opens with it into the azygos vein. The accessory hemiazygos is frequently connected to the left superior intercostal vein, as shown in Figure 1.64. The left superior intercostal vein, which drains the 1st–3rd intercostal spaces, may communicate with the accessory hemiazygos vein; however, it drains primarily into the left brachiocephalic vein.

Nerves of the Posterior Mediastinum

The sympathetic trunks and their associated ganglia form a major portion of the autonomic nervous system (Fig. 1.65, Table 1.6). The **thoracic sympathetic trunks** are in continuity with the cervical and lumbar sympathetic trunks. The thoracic trunks lie against the heads of the ribs in the superior part of the thorax, the costovertebral joints in the midthoracic level, and the sides of the vertebral bodies in the inferior part of the thorax. The **lower thoracic splanchnic nerves**—also known as greater, lesser, and least splanchnic nerves—are part of the *abdominopelvic splanchnic nerves* because they supply viscera inferior to the diaphragm. They consist of presynaptic fibers from the 5th through the 12th sympathetic ganglia, which pass through the diaphragm and synapse in prevertebral ganglia in the abdomen. They supply sympathetic innervation for most of the abdominal viscera. These splanchnic nerves are discussed further in Chapter 2.

Anterior Mediastinum

The **anterior mediastinum,** the smallest subdivision of the mediastinum (Fig. 1.34), lies between the body of the sternum and the transverse thoracic muscles anteriorly and the pericardium posteriorly. It is continuous with the superior mediastinum at the sternal angle and is limited inferiorly by the diaphragm. The anterior mediastinum consists of loose connective tissue (**sternopericardial ligaments**), fat, lymphatic vessels, a few lymph nodes, and branches of the internal thoracic vessels. In infants and children, the anterior mediastinum contains the inferior part of the thymus. In unusual cases, this lymphoid organ may extend to the level of the 4th costal cartilages.

THE BOTTOM LINE The posterior mediastinum is the narrow passageway posterior to the heart and diaphragm and between the lungs for conduction structures passing from thorax to abdomen or vice versa. Contents include the esophagus and esophageal nerve plexus, thoracic aorta, thoracic duct and lymphatic trunks, posterior mediastinal lymph nodes, and azygos and hemiazygos veins. Branches of the thoracic aorta occur primarily within three vascular planes. The azygos/hemiazygos venous system constitutes the venous counterpart to the thoracic aorta and its posterior mediastinal branches. The thoracic portion of the sympathetic trunks and thoracic splanchnic nerves may or may not be considered components of the posterior mediastinum.

Medical Imaging of the Thorax

The main imaging methods for examination of the thorax are radiography, echocardiography, CT, and MRI.

Radiography

The most common radiographic study of the thorax is the **posteroanterior (PA) projection** (Fig. 1.66A), producing a **PA radiograph** (Fig. 1.66B). The radiologist or technician places the anterior aspect of the patient's thorax against the X-ray detector or film cassette and rotates the shoulders anteriorly to move the scapulae away from

the superior parts of the lungs (Fig. 1.66A). The person takes a deep breath and holds it. The deep inspiration causes the diaphragmatic domes to descend, filling the lungs with air (increasing their radiolucency), and moving the costodiaphragmatic parts of the lungs into the costodiaphragmatic recesses.

A PA radiograph, which is viewed as if you were facing the patient (an **anteroposterior [AP] view**), is a composite of the images cast by the soft tissues and bones of the thoracic wall. Soft tissues, including those of the breasts, cast shadows of varying density, depending on their composition and thickness. Paralleling the superior margins of the clavicles are shadows cast by the skin and subcutaneous tis-

(A)

(B) PA radiograph of thorax (viewed in AP position)

(D) Lateral radiograph of thorax (chest)

(F)

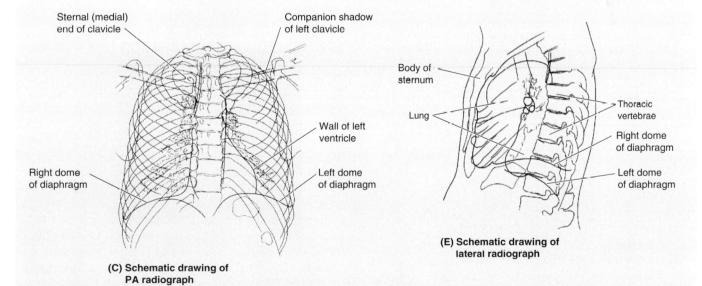
(C) Schematic drawing of PA radiograph

(E) Schematic drawing of lateral radiograph

Figure 1.66 Radiographs of thorax. A. The orientation of the person's thorax relative to the film cassette or detector and the X-ray beam (*arrow*) for a PA projection is demonstrated. **B.** An example of a PA radiograph (PA projection/AP view) of the thorax is shown. **C.** The main structures visible in the PA radiograph are outlined. Note that the right dome is usually higher than the left dome. **D.** An example of a lateral radiograph of the thorax is shown. **E.** The principal structures visible in the lateral radiograph are outlined. **F.** The orientation of the person's thorax relative to the film cassette or detector and the X-ray beam (*arrow*) for a lateral radiograph is demonstrated.

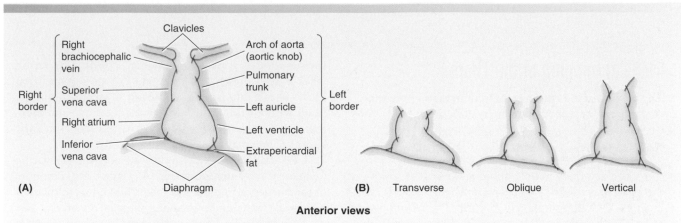

(A)

Right border

Clavicles

Right brachiocephalic vein

Superior vena cava

Right atrium

Inferior vena cava

Arch of aorta (aortic knob)

Pulmonary trunk

Left auricle

Left ventricle

Extrapericardial fat

Diaphragm

Left border

(B) Transverse Oblique Vertical

Anterior views

Figure 1.67 Cardiovascular shadows (mediastinal silhouettes). A. The composition of the margins of the cardio-vascular shadow is identified. **B.** The common types of cardiovascular shadow are shown.

Left coronary artery

Circumflex artery

Anterior interventricular artery

(A) Left lateral view

Sinuatrial nodal artery

Right coronary artery

Posterior interventricular branch

(B) Left anterior oblique view

Figure 1.68. Coronary arteriograms. Radiopaque dye has been injected into the LCA (**A**) and the RCA (**B**) via a catheter passed through the aorta (visible here as it traverses the arch of the aorta and descends to the heart via the as-cending aorta) from the femoral artery (just inferior to the midpoint of inguinal ligament). The orientation drawings show the course of the coronary arteries as demonstrated by the arteriograms. In part **B**, observe the sinuatrial nodal artery arising from the right coronary artery. (Courtesy of Dr. I. Morrow, Department of Radiology, Health Sciences Centre, University of Manitoba, Winnipeg, Manitoba, Canada.)

Right subclavian artery

Right common carotid artery

Left common carotid artery

Left subclavian artery

Brachiocephalic trunk (artery)

Aortic arch

Ascending aorta

Thoracic aorta

Left anterior oblique view

Figure 1.69. Aortic angiogram. The arch of aorta and the typical arrangement of its branches are visible. Note the major branches of the subclavian arteries arising within the superior thoracic aperture. (Courtesy of Dr. E. L. Lansdown, Professor of Medical Imaging, University of Toronto, Toronto, Ontario, Canada.)

sues covering these bones. The clavicles, ribs, and inferior cervical and superior thoracic vertebrae are visible. In PA radiographs, most ribs stand out clearly against the background of the relatively lucent lungs (Fig. 1.66B & C). The inferior ribs tend to be obscured by the diaphragm and the superior contents of the abdomen (e.g., liver), depending on the phase of respiration when the radiograph was taken. Usually only lateral margins of the manubrium are visible in these projections. The lower thoracic vertebrae are more or less obscured by the sternum and mediastinum. Uncommonly, cervical ribs, missing ribs, forked ribs, and fused ribs are visible. Occasionally, the costal cartilages are calcified in older people (especially the inferior cartilages).

In PA projections, the right and left domes of the diaphragm are separated by the central tendon, which is obscured by the heart. The right dome of the diaphragm, formed by the underlying liver, is usually approximately half an intercostal space higher than the left dome. The lungs, because of their low density, are relatively lucent compared with surrounding structures. The lungs exhibit a radiodensity similar to that of air and, therefore, produce paired radiolucent areas. In PA projections, the lungs are obscured

inferior to the domes of the diaphragm and anterior and posterior to the mediastinum. The pulmonary arteries are visible in the hilum of each lung. Intrapulmonary vessels are slightly larger in caliber in the inferior lobes. Transverse sections of the air-filled bronchi have lucent centers and thin walls.

The areas obscured in PA projections are usually visible in lateral radiographs. In **lateral projections**, the middle and inferior thoracic vertebrae are visible, although they are partially obscured by the ribs (Fig. 1.66D & F). The three parts of the sternum are also visible. **Lateral radiographs** allow better viewing of a lesion or anomaly confined to one side of the thorax. In a lateral projection, both domes of the diaphragm are often visible as they arch superiorly from the sternum. A lateral radiograph is made using a lateral projection, with the side of the thorax against the film cassette or X-ray detector and the upper limbs elevated over the head (Fig. 1.66E).

The heart casts most of the central radiopaque shadow in PA projections (Fig. 1.66B), but the separate

(cont'd on page 190)

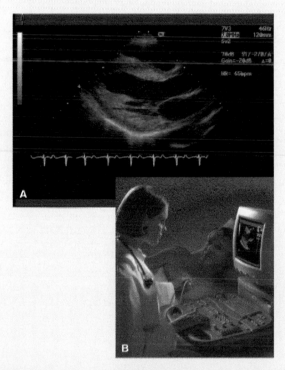

Figure 1.70. Echocardiography. A. A normal two-dimensional view echocardiogram is shown. The transducer is placed in a left intercostal space in the parasternal line, overlying the heart, and oriented so that it produces a longitudinal cross-sectional image of the heart. Note the thick ventricular wall and IVS. **B.** The technique is demonstrated.

Apex of right lung

Right dome of diaphragm

Liver

Gallbladder

Left lung

Spleen

Stomach

(B)
(C)
(D)
(E)

(A) Anterior view

Figure 1.71. Serial transverse CT scans of thorax. A. The level of each scan is indicated (broken lines). **B.** At the level of the sternoclavicular joints, the left brachiocephalic vein (*2*) crosses the midline anterior to the three branches of the arch of the aorta (*3, 4,* and *5*) to join the right brachiocephalic vein (*1*), forming the SVC (*22*) at a more inferior level. **C.** The arch of the aorta (*20*) is obliquely placed (more sagittal than transverse), with the ascending end anteriorly in the midline, and the descending end posteriorly and to the left of the vertebral bodies (*17*). The SVC (*22*) on the right side receives the arch of the azygos vein (*23*) from its posterior aspect. **D.** The pulmonary trunk (*27*) forms the stem of an inverted Y, with the arms formed by the right (*28*) and left (*29*) pulmonary arteries. The right pulmonary artery (*28*) passes beneath the arch of the aorta [between ascending (*24*) and descending (*25*) aortae]. **E.** A scan at the level of the maximum diameter of the heart demonstrates all four chambers (*32–35*) and the diagonal slant of the IVS (between *33* and *35*).

Key to Structures in Transverse CT Scans of Thorax		
1 = Right brachiocephalic vein	14 = Right lung	26 = Conus arteriosus
2 = Left brachiocephalic vein	15 = Left lung	27 = Pulmonary trunk
3 = Brachiocephalic artery	16 = T4 vertebral body	28 = Right pulmonary artery
4 = Left common carotid artery	17 = T5 vertebral body	29 = Left pulmonary artery
5 = Left subclavian artery	18 = T6 vertebral body	30 = Hemiazygos vein
6 = Esophagus	19 = T8 vertebral body	31 = Internal thoracic vessels
7 = Trachea	20 = Arch of aorta	32 = Right atrium
8 = Right main bronchus	21 = Anterior mediastinum	33 = Right ventricle
9 = Left main bronchus	(region of thymic remnant)	34 = Left atrium
10 = Costal cartilage	22 = Superior vena cava	35 = Left ventricle
11 = Sternum	23 = Arch of azygos vein	36 = Inferior right pulmonary
12 = Clavicle	24 = Ascending aorta	vein
13 = Axillary vein	25 = Descending aorta	37 = Inferior left pulmonary vein

Figure 1.71. *(Continued)*

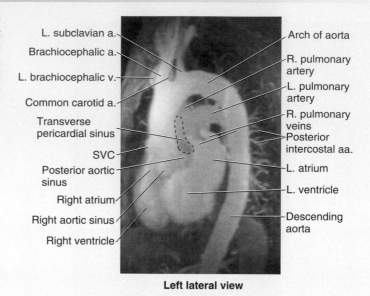

Figure 1.72 Magnetic resonance reconstructed angiogram of heart and great vessels. The study is a lateral view (from left and slightly anterior). This non-invasive, non-ionizing image is reconstructed from data generated and accumulated by spiral MRI. All chambers of the heart and great vessels are clearly visible. *SVC,* superior vena cava.

Labels: L. subclavian a.; Brachiocephalic a.; L. brachiocephalic v.; Common carotid a.; Transverse pericardial sinus; SVC; Posterior aortic sinus; Right atrium; Right aortic sinus; Right ventricle; Arch of aorta; R. pulmonary artery; L. pulmonary artery; R. pulmonary veins; Posterior intercostal aa.; L. atrium; L. ventricle; Descending aorta

Left lateral view

chambers of the heart are not distinguishable. Knowledge of the structures forming the **cardiovascular shadow** or silhouette is important because changes in the shadow may indicate anomalies or functional disease (Fig. 1.67*A*). In PA radiographs (AP views), the borders of the cardiovascular shadow are as follows:

- *Right border,* right brachiocephalic vein, SVC, right atrium, and IVC.
- *Left border,* terminal part of the arch of aorta (aortic knob), pulmonary trunk, left auricle, and left ventricle.

The left inferior part of the cardiovascular shadow presents the region of the apex. The typical anatomical apex, if present, is often inferior to the shadow of the diaphragm. Three main types of cardiovascular shadows occur, depending primarily on body type or habitus (Fig. 1.67*B*):

- *Transverse type,* observed in obese persons, pregnant women, and infants.
- *Oblique type,* characteristic of most people.
- *Vertical type,* present in people with narrow chests.

Fluoroscopy

The movements of different organs (e.g., heart, lungs, and diaphragm) may be studied by means of fluoroscopy. In this system, the X-rays impinge on the input screen of an image-intensifier tube, which is coupled to a television monitor. This image-intensifier television system gives superior resolution along with reduced radiation exposure.

Bronchography

Bronchography, a radiographic examination of the tracheobronchial tree after introduction of an oily radiopaque material (by means of aerosol or drip), is rarely performed now. It has been superseded by high-resolution CT and bronchoscopy.

Cardiac Catheterization

In cardiac catheterization, a radiopaque catheter is inserted into a peripheral vein (e.g., the femoral vein) and passed under fluoroscopic control into the right atrium, right ventricle, pulmonary trunk, and pulmonary arteries, respectively. Using this technique, intracardiac pressures can be recorded and blood samples may be removed. If a radiopaque contrast medium is injected, it can be followed through the heart and great vessels using serially exposed X-ray films. Alternatively, **cineradiography** can be performed to observe the flow of dye in real time. Both techniques permit study of the circulation through the functioning heart and are helpful in the study of congenital cardiac defects.

Coronary Angiography

Using **coronary angiography,** the coronary arteries can be visualized with **coronary arteriograms** (Fig. 1.68). A long, narrow catheter is passed into the ascending aorta via the femoral or brachial artery in the inguinal or elbow region, respectively. Under fluoroscopic control, the tip of the catheter is placed just inside the opening of a coronary artery. A small injection of radiopaque contrast material is made, and cineradiographs are taken to show the lumen of the artery and its branches as well as any stenotic areas that may be present. In a similar manner, an **aortic angiogram** can be made by injecting radiopaque contrast material into the aorta and into openings of the arteries arising from the arch of the aorta (Fig. 1.69).

Echocardiography

Echocardiography (ultrasonic cardiography) is a method of graphically recording the position and motion of the heart by the echo obtained from beams of ultrasonic waves directed through the thoracic wall (Fig. 1.70). Echocardiography delineates valvular stenosis and regurgitation, especially on the left side of the heart. This technique may detect as little as 20 mL of fluid in the pericardial cavity, such as that resulting from pericardial effusion. **Doppler echocardiography** is a technique that records the flow of blood through the heart and great vessels by Doppler ultrasonography.

CT and MRI

CT and MRI are commonly used to examine the thorax (Figs. 1.71 and 1.72). CT is sometimes combined with mammography for detection of breast cancer. Before CT scans are taken, an iodide contrast material is given intravenously. Because breast cancer cells have an unusual affinity for iodide, they become recognizable. MRI is usually better for detecting and delineating soft tissue lesions. Transverse (axial) CT and MR scans are always oriented to show how a horizontal section of a patient's body lying on an examination table would appear to the physician who is at the patient's feet. Therefore, the top of the image is anterior, and the left lateral edge of the image represents the right lateral surface of the patient's body. Data from CT and MR scans can be graphically reconstructed by the computer as transverse, sagittal, oblique, or coronal sections of the body. ●

References and Suggested Readings

Ahya SN, Flood K, Paranjothi S: *Washington Manual of Medical Therapeutics,* 30th ed. Baltimore, Lippincott Williams & Wilkins, 2001.

Behrman RE, Kliegman RM, Jenson HB (eds): *Nelson Textbook of Pediatrics,* 16th ed. Philadelphia, Saunders, 2000.

Bergman RA, Thompson SA, Afifi AK, Saadeh FA: *Compendium of Human Anatomic Variation: Text, Atlas, and World Literature.* Baltimore, Urban & Schwarzenberg, 1988.

This useful source has been updated and is available from the Virtual Hospital's Web site Illustrated Encyclopedia of Human Anatomic Variation at www.vh.org/Providers/Textbooks/ AnatomicVariants/AnatomyHP.html (accessed May 2004).

Cotran RS, Kumar V, Collins T: *Robbins Pathological Basis of Disease,* 6th ed. Philadelphia, Saunders, 1999.

Creasy RK, Resnik R: *Maternal-Fetal Medicine,* 4th ed. Philadelphia, Saunders, 1999.

Dean DX, Herbener TE: *Cross-Sectional Human Anatomy,* Lippincott Williams & Wilkins, 2000.

Ferguson JE, Schor AM, Howell A, Ferguson MW: Changes in the extracellular matrix of the normal breast during the menstrual cycle. *Cell Tissue Res* 268:167–177, 1992.

Ger R, Abrahams P, Olson T: *Essentials of Clinical Anatomy,* 3rd ed. New York, Parthenon, 1996.

Goroll AH: *Primary Care Medicine: Office Evaluation and Management of the Adult Patient,* 4th ed. Philadelphia: Lippincott Williams & Wilkins, 2000.

Hardy SGP, Nattel JP: Viscerosensory pathways. *In* Haines DE (ed): *Fundamental Neuroscience,* 2nd ed. New York, Churchill Livingstone, 2001.

Moore KL, Persaud TVN: *The Developing Human. Clinically Oriented Embryology,* 7th ed. Philadelphia, Saunders, 2003.

Moore, KL, Persaud TVN, Shiota K: *Color Atlas of Clinical Embryology,* 2nd ed. Philadelphia, Saunders, 2000.

Rosen P: *Emergency Medicine: Concepts and Clinical Practice,* 4th ed. St. Louis, Mosby, 1998.

Rowland LP (ed): *Merritt's Neurology,* 10th ed. Baltimore, Lippincott Williams & Wilkins, 2000.

Sauerland EK: *Grant's Dissector,* 12th ed. Baltimore, Lippincott Williams & Wilkins, 1999.

Slaby FJ, McCune SK, Summers RW: *Gross Anatomy in the Practice of Medicine.* Philadelphia: Lea & Febiger, 1994.

Swartz MH: *Textbook of Physical Diagnosis, History and Examination,* 4th ed. Philadelphia, Saunders, 2002.

Torrent-Guasp F, Buckberg GD, Clemente C, Cox JL, Coghlan HC, Gharib M: The structure and function of the helical heart and its buttress wrapping. I. The normal macroscopic structure of the heart. *Semin Thoracic Cardiovasc Surg* 13:301–319, 2001.

Vilensky JA, Baltes M, Weikel L, Fortin JD, Fourie LJ: Serratus posterior muscles: Anatomy, clinical relevance, and function. *Clin Anat* 14:237–241, 2001.

Williams PL, Bannister LH, Berry MM, Collins P, Dyson M, Dussek JE, Ferguson MWJ (eds): *Gray's Anatomy. The Anatomical Basis of Medicine and Surgery,* 38th ed. New York, Churchill Livingstone, 1995.

Wilson-Pauwels L, Stewart PA, Akesson EJ: *Autonomic Nerves—Basic Science, Clinical Aspects, Case Studies.* Hamilton, ON, Canada, Decker, 1997.

2 Abdomen

The **abdomen** is the part of the trunk between the thorax and the pelvis (Fig. 2.1).

It is a flexible, dynamic container, housing most of the organs of the digestive system and part of the urogenital system. Containment of the abdominal organs and their contents is provided by musculoaponeurotic walls anterolaterally, the diaphragm superiorly, and the muscles of the pelvis inferiorly, which are suspended between and supported by two bony rings (the inferior margin of the thoracic skeleton superiorly and pelvic girdle inferiorly) linked by a semirigid lumbar vertebral column in the posterior abdominal wall. The abdomen is thus able to enclose and protect its contents while allowing the flexibility between the more rigid thorax and pelvis required by respiration, posture, and locomotion. Through voluntary or reflexive contraction, its muscular roof, anterolateral walls, and floor can raise internal (intra-abdominal) pressure to aid expulsion from the abdominopelvic cavity or from the adjacent thoracic cavity, expulsion of air from the thoracic cavity (lungs and bronchi) or of fluid (e.g., urine or vomitus), flatus, feces, or fetuses from the abdominopelvic cavity.

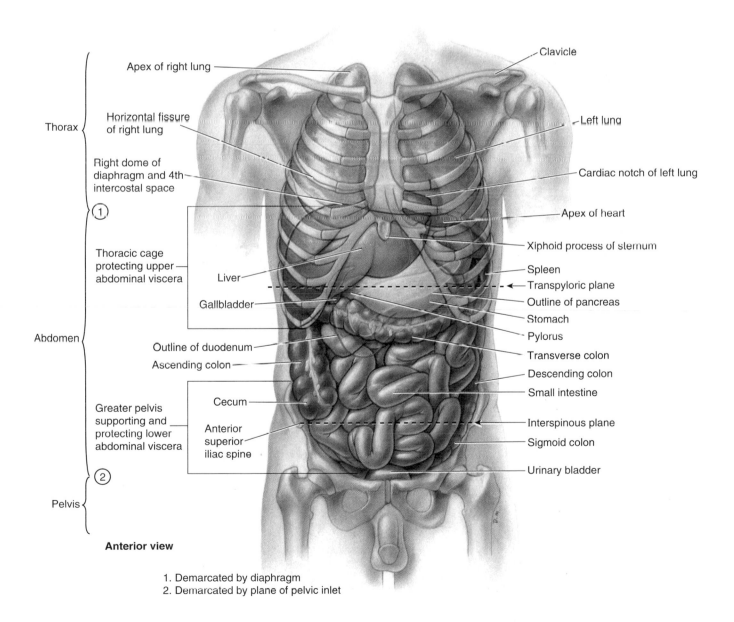

Anterior view

1. Demarcated by diaphragm
2. Demarcated by plane of pelvic inlet

Figure 2.1. Overview of viscera of thorax and abdomen in situ.

Overview: Walls, Cavities, Regions, and Planes

The dynamic musculoaponeurotic **abdominal walls** not only contract to increase intra-abdominal pressure but also distend considerably, accommodating expansions caused by ingestion, pregnancy, fat deposition, or pathology. The *anterolateral abdominal walls* and several organs lying against the *posterior wall* are covered on their internal aspects with a serous membrane or *peritoneum* (serosa) that also *reflects* (turns sharply and continues) onto the contained **abdominal viscera** (L. soft parts, internal organs), such as the stomach, intestine, liver, and spleen. Thus a bursal sac or lined potential space (the *peritoneal cavity*) is formed between the walls and the viscera that normally contains only enough extracellular (parietal) fluid to lubricate the membrane covering most of the surfaces of the structures forming or occupying the abdominal cavity. Visceral movement associated with digestion occurs freely, and the double-layered reflections of peritoneum passing between the walls and the viscera provide passage for the blood vessels, lymphatics, and nerves. Variable amounts of fat may also occur between the walls and viscera and the peritoneum lining them.

The **abdominal cavity** forms the superior and major part of the **abdominopelvic cavity** (Fig. 2.2), the continuous cavity that extends between the *thoracic diaphragm* and the *pelvic diaphragm.* The abdominal cavity has no floor of its own because it is continuous with the *pelvic cavity.* The plane of the *pelvic inlet* (superior pelvic aperture) arbitrarily, but not physically, separates the abdominal and the pelvic cavities. The abdominal cavity extends superiorly into the osseocartilaginous *thoracic cage* to the 4th intercostal space (Fig. 2.1). Consequently, the more superiorly placed abdominal organs (spleen, liver, part of the kidneys, and stomach) are protected by the thoracic cage. The greater pelvis (expanded part of the pelvis superior to the pelvic inlet) supports and partly protects the lower abdominal viscera (part of the ileum, cecum, and sigmoid colon).

In summary, the abdominal cavity is

- The major part of the abdominopelvic cavity.

- Located between the diaphragm and the pelvic inlet.

- Separated from the thoracic cavity by the thoracic diaphragm.

- Continuous inferiorly with the pelvic cavity.

- Under cover of the thoracic cage superiorly.

- Supported and partially protected inferiorly by the greater pelvis.

- Enclosed anterolaterally by multi-layered, musculoaponeurotic, abdominal walls.

- The location of most digestive organs, parts of the urogenital system (kidneys and most of the ureters), and the spleen.

Clinicians refer to nine regions of the abdominal cavity to describe the location of abdominal organs, pains, or pathologies (Table 2.1*A* & *B*). The nine regions are delineated by four planes: two sagittal (vertical) and two transverse (horizontal) planes. The two sagittal planes are usually the **midclavicular planes** that pass from the midpoint of the clavicles (approximately 9 cm from the midline) to the **midinguinal points,** midpoints of the lines joining the *anterior superior iliac spine* (ASIS) and the superior edge of the *pubic symphysis* (L. *symphysis pubis*) on each side. Sometimes planes intersecting the **semilunar lines,** the surface markings (shallow grooves) of the lateral borders of the rectus abdominis muscles, are used as the vertical delineations. However, this is practical only in lean people who have distinct surface definition of the underlying muscles.

There is also some variation in the transverse planes that are used to define abdominal regions. Most commonly, the transverse planes are the **subcostal plane,** passing through the inferior border of the 10th costal cartilage on each side, and

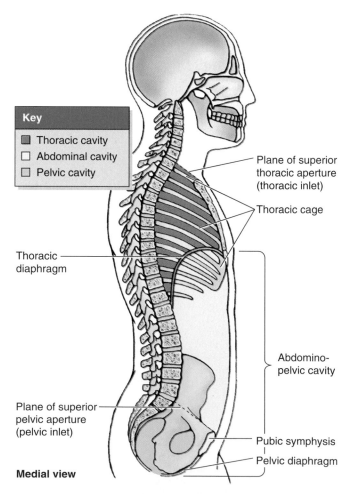

Key
- ☐ Thoracic cavity
- ☐ Abdominal cavity
- ☐ Pelvic cavity

Plane of superior thoracic aperture (thoracic inlet)

Thoracic cage

Thoracic diaphragm

Abdomino-pelvic cavity

Plane of superior pelvic aperture (pelvic inlet)

Pubic symphysis

Pelvic diaphragm

Medial view

Figure 2.2. Abdominopelvic cavity. The body has been sectioned in the median plane to show the abdominal and pelvic cavities as subdivisions of the continuous abdominopelvic cavity.

Table 2.1. Abdominal Regions (A), Reference Planes (B), and Quadrants (C)

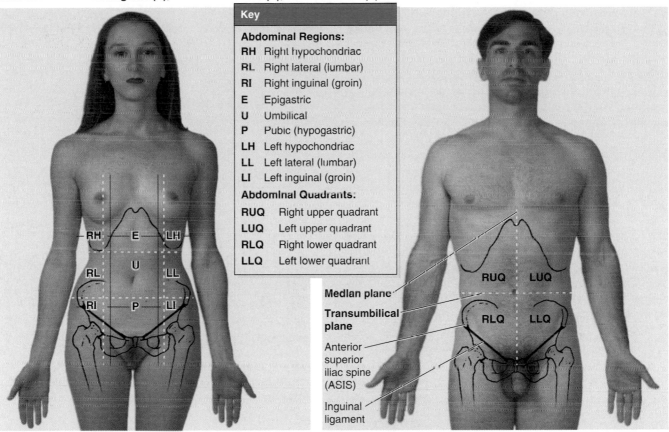

Key

Abdominal Regions:

RH	Right hypochondriac
RL	Right lateral (lumbar)
RI	Right inguinal (groin)
E	Epigastric
U	Umbilical
P	Pubic (hypogastric)
LH	Left hypochondriac
LL	Left lateral (lumbar)
LI	Left inguinal (groin)

Abdominal Quadrants:

RUQ	Right upper quadrant
LUQ	Left upper quadrant
RLQ	Right lower quadrant
LLQ	Left lower quadrant

(A) Abdominal regions

(C) Abdominal quadrants

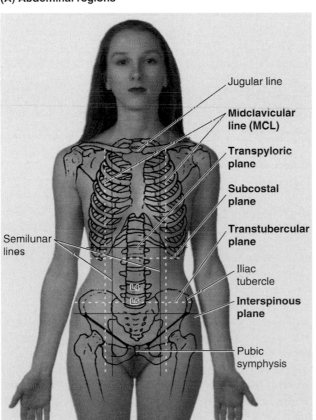

(B) Abdominal reference planes

Right upper quadrant (RUQ)	**Left upper quadrant (LUQ)**
Liver: right lobe	Liver: left lobe
Gallbladder	Spleen
Stomach: pylorus	Stomach
Duodenum: parts 1–3	Jejunum and proximal ileum
Pancreas: head	Pancreas: body and tail
Right suprarenal gland	Left kidney
Right kidney	Left suprarenal gland
Right colic (hepatic) flexure	Left colic (splenic) flexure
Ascending colon: superior part	Transverse colon: left half
Transverse colon: right half	Descending colon: superior part

Right lower quadrant (RLQ)	**Left lower quadrant (LLQ)**
Cecum	Sigmoid colon
Vermiform appendix	Descending colon: inferior part
Most of ileum	Left ovary
Ascending colon: inferior part	Left uterine tube
Right ovary	Left ureter: abdominal part
Right uterine tube	Left spermatic cord:
Right ureter: abdominal part	abdominal part
Right spermatic cord:	Uterus (if enlarged)
abdominal part	Urinary bladder (if very full)
Uterus (if enlarged)	
Urinary bladder (if very full)	

the **transtubercular plane,** passing through the iliac tubercles (approximately 5 cm posterior to the ASIS on each side) and the body of the L5 vertebra. Both of these planes have the advantage of intersecting palpable structures. However, other clinicians use the transpyloric and interspinous planes to establish the nine regions. The **transpyloric plane,** extrapolated midway between the superior borders of the manubrium of the sternum and the pubic symphysis (typically the L1 vertebral level), commonly transects the *pylorus* (the distal, more tubular part of the stomach) when the patient is recumbent (supine or prone) (Fig. 2.1). Because the viscera sag with the pull of gravity, the pylorus usually lies at a lower level when the individual is standing erect. The transpyloric plane is a useful landmark because it also transects many other important structures: the fundus of the gallbladder, neck of the pancreas, origins of the superior mesenteric artery (SMA) and portal vein, root of the transverse mesocolon, duodenojejunal junction, and hila of the kidneys. The **interspinous plane** passes through the easily palpated ASIS of each side (Table 2.1*B*).

For more general clinical descriptions, four quadrants of the abdominal cavity (right and left upper and lower quadrants) are defined by two readily defined planes: (1) the transverse **transumbilical plane,** passing through the umbilicus (and the intervertebral [IV] disc between the L3 and L4 vertebrae), dividing it into upper and lower halves, and (2) the vertical **median plane,** passing longitudinally through the body, dividing it into right and left halves (Table 2.1*C*).

It is important to know what organs are located in each abdominal region or quadrant so that one knows where to auscultate, percuss, and palpate them (Table 2.1). Knowledge of the location of the organs is also essential for recording findings during a physical examination.

Anterolateral Abdominal Wall

Although the abdominal wall is continuous, it is subdivided into the *anterior wall, right and left lateral walls (flanks),* and *posterior wall* for descriptive purposes (Fig. 2.3). The wall is *musculoaponeurotic,* except for the posterior wall, which includes the lumbar vertebral column. Because the boundary between the anterior and the lateral walls is indefinite, the term **anterolateral abdominal wall** is often used; some structures, such as the muscles and cutaneous nerves, are in both the anterior and the lateral walls. The anterolateral abdominal wall extends from the thoracic cage to the pelvis.

During a physical examination, the anterolateral wall is inspected, palpated, percussed, and auscultated. Surgeons usually incise this wall during abdominal surgery. The anterolateral abdominal wall is bounded superiorly by the cartilages of the 7th–10th ribs and the xiphoid process of the sternum and inferiorly by the inguinal ligament and the superior margins of the anterolateral aspects of the pelvic girdle (iliac crests, pubic crests, and pubic symphysis) (Fig. 2.4*A*).

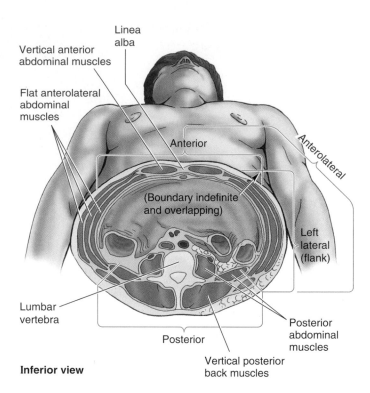

Figure 2.3. Subdivisions of abdominal wall. This transverse section of the abdomen demonstrates various aspects of the wall and its components.

The wall consists of skin and subcutaneous tissue (superficial fascia) composed mainly of fat, muscles and their aponeuroses and deep fascia, extraperitoneal fat, and parietal peritoneum (Fig. 2.4*B*). The skin attaches loosely to the subcutaneous tissue, except at the umbilicus, where it adheres firmly. Most of the anterolateral wall includes three musculotendinous layers; the fibers of each layer run in different directions. This three-ply structure is similar to that of the intercostal spaces in the thorax (see Chapter 1).

Fascia of the Anterolateral Abdominal Wall

The subcutaneous tissue over most of the wall includes a variable amount of fat. It is a major site of fat storage. Males are especially susceptible to subcutaneous accumulation in the lower anterior abdominal wall and may have disproportional amounts of fat here while having more normal amounts elsewhere. In morbid obesity, the fat is many inches thick, often forming one or more sagging folds (L. *panniculi;* singular = *panniculus,* apron). Inferior to the umbilicus, the deepest part of the subcutaneous tissue is reinforced by many elastic and collagen fibers, so the subcutaneous tissue here has two layers: a **superficial fatty layer** (Camper fascia) and a **deep membranous layer** (Scarpa fascia). The membranous layer continues inferiorly into the perineal region as the superficial perineal fascia (Colles fascia), but not into the thighs. In many individuals, the membranous layer is sufficiently complete that

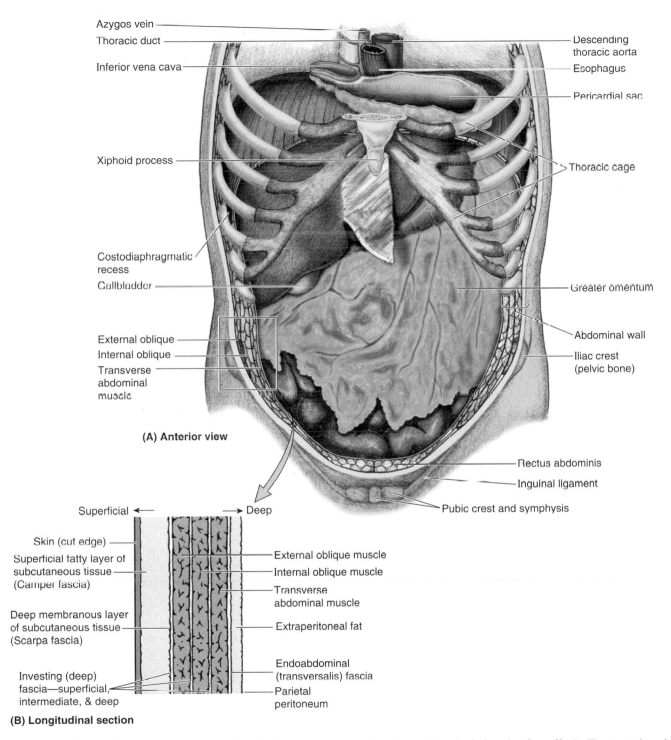

Azygos vein

Thoracic duct

Inferior vena cava

Xiphoid process

Costodiaphragmatic recess

Gallbladder

External oblique

Internal oblique

Transverse abdominal muscle

(A) Anterior view

Descending thoracic aorta

Esophagus

Pericardial sac

Thoracic cage

Greater omentum

Abdominal wall

Iliac crest (pelvic bone)

Rectus abdominis

Inguinal ligament

Pubic crest and symphysis

Superficial ← → Deep

Skin (cut edge)

Superficial fatty layer of subcutaneous tissue (Camper fascia)

Deep membranous layer of subcutaneous tissue (Scarpa fascia)

Investing (deep) fascia—superficial, intermediate, & deep

External oblique muscle

Internal oblique muscle

Transverse abdominal muscle

Extraperitoneal fat

Endoabdominal (transversalis) fascia

Parietal peritoneum

(B) Longitudinal section

Figure 2.4. Abdominal contents, undisturbed, and layers of anterolateral abdominal wall. A. The anterior abdominal wall and soft tissues of the anterior thoracic wall have been removed. Most of the intestine is covered by the apron-like greater omentum, a peritoneal fold hanging from the stomach. **B.** Layers of the anterolateral abdominal wall, including the trilaminar flat muscles, are shown.

fluids escaping from a ruptured vessel or urethra (blood and/or urine) may accumulate deep to it (see the clinical correlation [blue] box "Rupture of the Urethra and Extravasation of Urine," in Chapter 3).

Superficial, intermediate, and deep layers of **investing fascia** cover the external aspects of the three muscle layers of the an-

terolateral abdominal wall and their **aponeuroses** (flat expanded tendons) and cannot be easily separated from them. The investing fascias here are extremely thin, being represented mostly by the epimysium superficial to or between muscles. The internal aspect of the abdominal wall is lined with a membranous sheet of varying thickness called the **endoabdominal** fascia. Although continuous, different parts of this fascia are named according to the muscle or aponeurosis it is lining. The portion lining the deep surface of the transverse abdominal muscle and its aponeurosis, the **transversalis fascia**, is relatively firm. The lining of the abdominal cavity, the *parietal peritoneum*, is internal to the transversalis fascia and is separated from it by a variable amount of **extraperitoneal fat**.

Clinical Significance of Fascia and Fascial Spaces of Abdominal Wall

Liposuction is a surgical method for removing unwanted subcutaneous fat using a percutaneously placed suction tube and high vacuum pressure. The tubes are inserted subdermally through small skin incisions.

When closing lower abdominal skin incisions, surgeons include the membranous layer of subcutaneous tissue when suturing because of its strength. Between this layer and the deep fascia covering the rectus abdominis and external oblique muscles is a potential space where fluid may accumulate (e.g., urine from a ruptured urethra). Although there are no barriers (other than gravity) to prevent fluid from spreading superiorly from this space, it cannot spread inferiorly into the thigh because the membranous layer fuses with the deep fascia of the thigh (*fascia lata*) along a line approximately 2.5 cm inferior and parallel to the inguinal ligament.

The potential or fat-filled space between the endoabdominal fascia is of special importance in surgery. It provides a plane that can be opened, enabling the surgeon to approach structures on or in the anterior aspect of the posterior abdominal wall, such as the kidneys or bodies of lumbar vertebrae, without entering the membranous peritoneal sac containing the abdominal viscera. Thus the risk of contamination is minimized. An anterolateral part of this potential space between the transversalis fascia and the parietal peritoneum (the *space of Bogros*) is used for placing prostheses, for example, when repairing inguinal hernias (Skandalakis et al., 1996) (Fig. 2.12*A* & *B*). ☉

THE BOTTOM LINE: The fascia of the anterolateral abdominal wall consists of subcutaneous (superficial), investing (deep), and intra-abdominal (endoabdominal) portions. The subcutaneous layer is modified in the lower abdomen to include a superficial fatty layer and a deep membranous layer. The superficial fatty layer is specialized, particularly in males, for lipid storage, whereas the deep membranous layer is sufficiently complete to compartmentalize extravasated fluids (blood or urine) and allow place-

ment of sutures during surgery. The investing layer is typical of deep fascias ensheathing voluntary muscles, and here reflects the trilaminar arrangement of the flat abdominal muscles and their aponeuroses. The endoabdominal fascia is of particular importance in surgery, enabling the establishment of an extraperitoneal space that allows anterior access to retroperitoneal structures (e.g., kidneys, ureters and bodies of lumbar vertebra) without entering the peritoneal cavity.

Muscles of the Anterolateral Abdominal Wall

There are five (bilaterally paired) muscles in the anterolateral abdominal wall (Fig. 2.3): three flat muscles and two vertical muscles. Their attachments, nerve supply, and main actions are listed in Table 2.2. The three flat muscles are the *external oblique, internal oblique,* and *transverse abdominal* (Fig. 2.4). The muscle fibers of these concentric layers crisscross each other, with the fibers of the outer two layers running diagonally and perpendicular to each other for the main part, and the fibers of the deep layer running transversely (Fig. 2.5*A*). All three flat muscles are continued anteriorly and medially as strong, sheet-like aponeuroses. Between the midclavicular line (MCL) and the midline, the aponeuroses form the tough, aponeurotic, tendinous *rectus sheath* enclosing the rectus abdominis muscle (Fig. 2.5*B*). The aponeuroses then interweave with their fellows of the opposite side, forming a midline raphe (G. *rhaphe,* suture, seam), the *linea alba* (L. white line), which extends from the xiphoid process to the pubic symphysis. The decussation and interweaving of the fibers here is not only between right and left sides but also between superficial and intermediate and intermediate and deep layers.

The two vertical muscles of the anterolateral abdominal wall, contained within the rectus sheath, are the *rectus abdominis* and *pyramidalis.*

External Oblique Muscle

The **external oblique muscle** is the largest and most superficial of the three flat anterolateral abdominal muscles (Fig. 2.6). The attachments, nerve supply, and main actions of the external oblique are presented in Table 2.2. In contrast to the two deeper layers, the external oblique does not originate posteriorly from the thoracolumbar fascia; its posteriormost fibers (the thickest part of the muscle) have a free edge where they span between its costal origin and the iliac crest (Table 2.2*D*). The fleshy part of the muscle contributes primarily to the lateral part of the abdominal wall. Its aponeurosis contributes to the anterior part of the wall.

Although the posteriormost fibers from rib 12 are nearly vertical as they run to the iliac crest, more anterior fibers fan out, taking an increasingly medial direction, so that most of the fleshy fibers run inferomedially—in the same direction as the fingers do when the hands are in one's side pockets—with the most anterior and superior fibers approaching a horizontal course. The muscle fibers become aponeurotic

Table 2.2. Muscles of the Anterolateral Abdominal Wall

Muscle	Origin	Insertion	Innervation	Main Action[a]
Rectus abdominis (A)	Pubic symphysis and pubic crest	Xiphoid process and 5th–7th costal cartilages	Thoracoabdominal nerves (anterior rami of inferior 6 thoracic nerves)	Flexes trunk (lumbar vertebrae) and compresses abdominal viscera;[b] stabilizes and controls tilt of pelvis (antilordosis)
Transverse abdominal (B)	Internal surfaces of 7th–12th costal cartilages, thoracolumbar fascia, iliac crest, and lateral third of inguinal ligament	Linea alba with aponeurosis of internal oblique, pubic crest, and pecten pubis via conjoint tendon	Thoracoabdominal nerves (anterior rami of inferior 6 thoracic nerves) and first lumbar nerves	Compresses and supports abdominal viscera[b]
Internal oblique (C)	Thoracolumbar fascia, anterior two-thirds of iliac crest, and lateral half of inguinal ligament	Inferior borders of 10th–12th ribs, linea alba, and pecten pubis via conjoint tendon		Compress and support abdominal viscera,[b] flex and rotate trunk
External oblique (D)	External surfaces of 5th–12th ribs	Linea and alba, pubic tubercle, and anterior half of iliac crest	Thoracoabdominal nerves (inferior 5 [T7–T11] thoracic nerves) and subcostal nerve	

[a] Approximately 80% of people have an insignificant muscle, *the pyramidalis*, which is located in the rectus sheath anterior to the most inferior part of the rectus abdominis. It extends from the pubic crest of the hip bone to the linea alba. This small muscle draws down on the linea alba.
[b] In so doing, these muscles act as antagonists of the diaphragm to produce expiration.

approximately at the MCL medially and at the **spinoumbilical line** (line running from the umbilicus to the ASIS) inferiorly, forming a sheet of tendinous fibers that decussate at the linea alba, most becoming continuous with tendinous fibers of the contralateral internal oblique (Fig. 2.5*A*). Thus the contralateral external and internal oblique muscles together form a "digastric muscle," a two-bellied muscle sharing a common central tendon that works as a unit. For example, the right external oblique and left internal oblique work together when flexing and rotating to bring the right shoulder toward the left hip (torsional movement of trunk).

Inferiorly, the external oblique aponeurosis attaches to the **pubic crest** medial to the **pubic tubercle**. The inferior margin of the external oblique aponeurosis is thickened as an under

(cont'd on page 202)

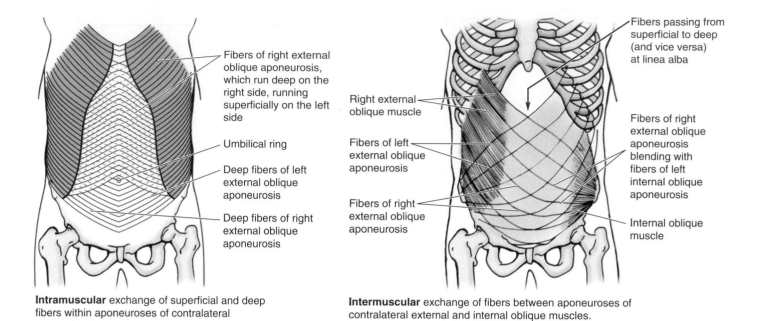

Fibers of right external oblique aponeurosis, which run deep on the right side, running superficially on the left side

Umbilical ring

Deep fibers of left external oblique aponeurosis

Deep fibers of right external oblique aponeurosis

Fibers passing from superficial to deep (and vice versa) at linea alba

Right external oblique muscle

Fibers of left external oblique aponeurosis

Fibers of right external oblique aponeurosis

Fibers of right external oblique aponeurosis blending with fibers of left internal oblique aponeurosis

Internal oblique muscle

Intramuscular exchange of superficial and deep fibers within aponeuroses of contralateral external oblique muscles.

Intermuscular exchange of fibers between aponeuroses of contralateral external and internal oblique muscles.

(A) Anterior views

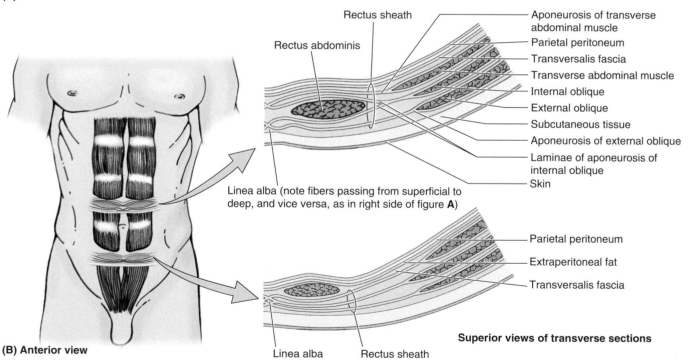

Rectus sheath

Rectus abdominis

Aponeurosis of transverse abdominal muscle
Parietal peritoneum
Transversalis fascia
Transverse abdominal muscle
Internal oblique
External oblique
Subcutaneous tissue
Aponeurosis of external oblique
Laminae of aponeurosis of internal oblique
Skin

Linea alba (note fibers passing from superficial to deep, and vice versa, as in right side of figure **A**)

Parietal peritoneum

Extraperitoneal fat

Transversalis fascia

Superior views of transverse sections

(B) Anterior view

Linea alba   Rectus sheath

Figure 2.5. Structure of anterolateral abdominal wall. A. Intramuscular and intermuscular fiber exchanges within the bilaminar aponeuroses of the external and the internal oblique muscles are shown. **B.** Transverse sections of the wall superior and inferior to the umbilicus show the makeup of the rectus sheath.

(A) Anterior view

Serratus anterior

5th costal cartilage

Anterior layer of rectus sheath

Anterior layer of rectus sheath

Linea alba

External oblique muscle

Rectus abdominis muscle

External oblique muscle

Lateral abdominal cutaneous branches

Anterior abdominal cutaneous branches

Tendinous intersection

Anterior superior iliac spine

External oblique aponeurosis

Superficial circumflex iliac artery and vein

Superficial epigastric artery and vein

External pudendal artery and vein

Great saphenous vein

Deep membranous layer of subcutaneous tissue

Intercrural fibers

Superficial inguinal ring

Ilioinguinal nerve
Spermatic cord

(B) Anterior view

Internal oblique muscle

External oblique muscle

Anterior superior iliac spine

External oblique aponeurosis

Musculoaponeurotic arcade of transverse abdominal muscle

Incurved lower margin (gutter) of aponeurosis forming inguinal ligament (floor of inguinal canal)

Femoral { Nerve Artery Vein

Anterior superior iliac spine

Transverse abdominal muscle

Deep inguinal ring (transversalis fascia)

Spermatic cord

Pubic crest

Inguinal ligament (passing anterior to pecten pubis)

Pubic tubercle

Testis

Figure 2.6. Anterolateral abdominal wall. A. In this superficial dissection, the anterior layer of the rectus sheath is reflected on the left side. Observe the anterior cutaneous nerves (T7–T12) piercing the rectus abdominis and the anterior layer of the rectus sheath. **B.** The three flat abdominal muscles and the formation of the inguinal ligament are demonstrated.

curving fibrous band with a free posterior edge that spans between the ASIS and the pubic tubercle as the *inguinal ligament* (Poupart ligament) (Figs. 2.6B and 2.7). Palpate your inguinal ligament by pressing deeply into the center of the crease between the thigh and trunk and moving the fingertips up and down. Inferiorly the inguinal ligament is continuous with the deep fascia of the thigh. The inguinal ligament is therefore not a freestanding structure, although—as a useful landmark—it is frequently depicted as such. It serves as a *retinaculum* (a retaining band) for the structures passing deep to it to enter the thigh (iliopsoas muscle and femoral vessels and nerve). The lateral portion of the inguinal ligament provides the origin for the inferior parts of the two deeper anterolateral abdominal muscles. The modifications and attachments of the inguinal ligament and of the inferomedial portions of the aponeuroses of the anterolateral abdominal wall muscles are complex and most significant in relation to the inguinal canal; they are discussed in detail with the inguinal region (later in this chapter).

Internal Oblique Muscle

The intermediate of the three flat abdominal muscles, the **internal oblique muscle** is a thin muscular sheet that fans out anteromedially (Figs. 2.7 and 2.8A; Table 2.2B). Except for its lowermost fibers, which arise from the lateral half of the inguinal ligament, its fleshy fibers run perpendicular to those of the external oblique, running superomedially (like your fingers when the hand is placed over your chest). Its fibers also become aponeurotic in roughly the same (midclavicular) line as the external oblique and participate in the formation of the rectus sheath. The attachments, nerve supply, and main actions of the internal oblique are listed in Table 2.2.

Figure 2.7. Inferior abdominal wall and inguinal region of a male. The aponeurosis of the external oblique is partly cut away and the spermatic cord has been cut and removed from the inguinal canal. The reflected (reflex) inguinal ligament is formed by aponeurotic fibers of the external oblique. The iliohypogastric and ilioinguinal nerves (branches of the first lumbar nerve) pass between the external and the internal oblique muscles. The ilioinguinal nerve traverses the inguinal canal and is vulnerable during repair of an inguinal hernia.

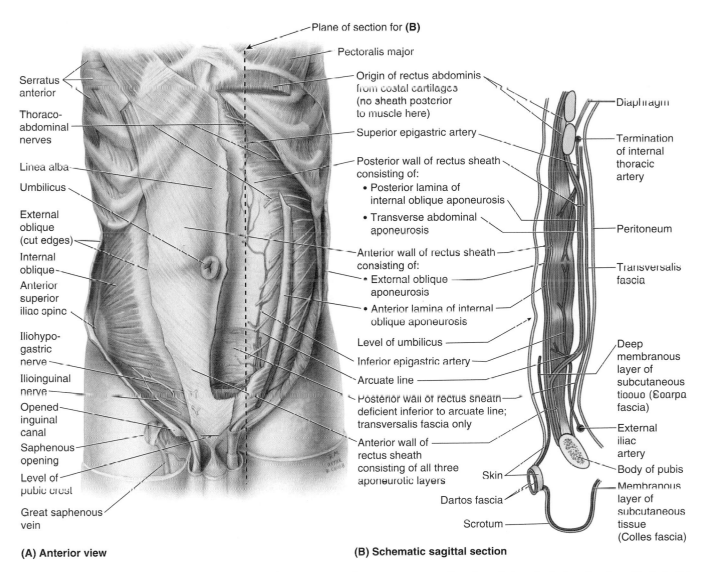

(A) Anterior view

(B) Schematic sagittal section

Figure 2.8. Formation of rectus sheath and neurovascular structures of anterolateral abdominal wall. A. In this deep dissection, the fleshy portion of the external oblique is excised on the right side, but its aponeurosis and the anterior wall of the rectus sheath are intact. The anterior wall of the sheath and the rectus abdominis are removed on the left side so that the posterior wall of the sheath is seen. Lateral to the left rectus sheath, the fleshy part of the internal oblique has been cut longitudinally; the edges of the cut are retracted to reveal the thoracoabdominal nerves coursing in the neurovascular plane between the internal oblique and the transverse abdominal. **B.** A sagittal section through the rectus sheath of the anterior abdominal wall is shown. The anastomosis between the superior and the inferior epigastric arteries indirectly unites the arteries of the upper limb (subclavian artery) and lower limb (external iliac artery).

Transverse Abdominal Muscle

The fibers of the **transverse abdominal muscle** (L. *musculus transversus abdominis*), the innermost of the three flat abdominal muscles (Fig. 2.6*B*, Table 2.2*B*), run more or less transversally, except for the inferior ones, which run parallel to those of the internal oblique. This transverse, circumferential orientation is ideal for compressing the abdominal contents, increasing intra-abdominal pressure. The fibers of the transverse abdominal muscle also end in an aponeurosis, which contributes to the formation of the rectus sheath (Fig. 2.8). The attachments, nerve supply, and main actions of the transverse abdominal muscle are listed in Table 2.2.

Between the internal oblique and the transverse abdominal muscles is a **neurovascular plane,** which corresponds with a similar plane in the intercostal spaces. In both regions, the plane lies between the middle and the deepest layers of muscle (Fig. 2.8*A*). The neurovascular plane of the anterolateral abdominal wall contains the nerves and arteries supplying the anterolateral abdominal wall. In the anterior part of the abdominal wall, the nerves and vessels leave the neurovascular plane and lie mostly in the subcutaneous tissue.

Rectus Abdominis Muscle

A long, broad, strap-like muscle, the **rectus abdominis** (L. *rectus,* straight) is the principal vertical muscle of the anterior abdominal wall (Figs. 2.6*A* and 2.8*B;* Table 2.2*A*). The attachments, nerve supply, and main actions of the rectus abdominis are listed in Table 2.2. The paired rectus muscles, separated by the linea alba, lie close together inferiorly. The rectus abdominis is three times as wide superiorly as inferiorly; it is broad and thin superiorly and narrow and thick inferiorly. Most of the rectus abdominis is enclosed in the rectus sheath. The rectus muscle is anchored transversely by attachment to the anterior layer of the rectus sheath at three or more **tendinous intersections.** When tensed in muscular people, the stretches of muscle between the tendinous intersections bulge outward. The intersections, indicated by grooves in the skin between the muscular bulges, usually occur at the level of the xiphoid process, umbilicus, and halfway between these structures.

Pyramidalis

The **pyramidalis** is a small triangular muscle that is absent in approximately 20% of people. It lies anterior to the inferior part of the rectus abdominis and attaches to the anterior surface of the pubis and the anterior pubic ligament. It ends in the linea alba, which is especially thickened for a variable distance superior to the pubic symphysis. The pyramidalis tenses the linea alba; when present, surgeons use the attachment of the pyramidalis to the linea alba as a landmark for an accurate median abdominal incision (Skandalakis et al., 1995).

Rectus Sheath, Linea Alba, and Umbilicus

The **rectus sheath** is the strong, incomplete fibrous compartment of the rectus abdominis and pyramidalis muscles (Figs. 2.5–2.8). Also found in the rectus sheath are the superior and inferior epigastric arteries and veins, lymphatic vessels, and distal portions of the thoracoabdominal nerves (abdominal portions of the anterior rami of spinal nerves T7–T12). The sheath is formed by the decussation and interweaving of the aponeuroses of the flat abdominal muscles. The external oblique aponeurosis contributes to the anterior wall of the sheath throughout its length. The superior two thirds of the internal oblique aponeurosis splits into two layers, or laminae, at the lateral border of the rectus abdominis; one lamina passing anterior to the muscle and the other passing posterior to it. The anterior lamina joins the aponeurosis of the external oblique to form the anterior layer of the rectus sheath. The posterior lamina joins the aponeurosis of the transverse abdominal muscle to form the posterior layer of the rectus sheath.

Beginning at approximately one third of the distance from the umbilicus to the pubic crest, the aponeuroses of the three flat muscles pass anterior to the rectus abdominis to form the anterior layer of the rectus sheath, leaving only the relatively thin transversalis fascia to cover the rectus abdominis posteriorly. A crescentic line, called the **arcuate line,** demarcates the transition between the aponeurotic posterior wall of the sheath covering the superior three quarters of the rectus and the transversalis fascia covering the inferior quarter. Throughout the length of the sheath, the fibers of the anterior and posterior layers of the sheath interlace in the anterior median line to form the complex linea alba.

The posterior layer of the rectus sheath is also deficient superior to the costal margin because the transverse abdominal muscle passes internal to the costal cartilages and the internal oblique attaches to the costal margin. Hence, superior to the costal margin, the rectus abdominis lies directly on the thoracic wall.

The **linea alba,** running vertically the entire length of the anterior abdominal wall and separating the bilateral rectus sheaths, narrows inferior to the umbilicus to the width of the pubic symphysis and widens superiorly to the width of the xiphoid process. The linea alba transmits small vessels and nerves to the skin. In thin muscular people, a groove is visible in the skin overlying the linea alba. At its middle, underlying the umbilicus, the linea alba contains the **umbilical ring,** a defect in the linea alba through which the fetal umbilical vessels passed to and from the umbilical cord and placenta. All layers of the anterolateral abdominal wall fuse at the umbilicus. As fat accumulates in the subcutaneous tissue postnatally, the skin becomes raised around the umbilical ring and the umbilicus becomes depressed. This occurs 7–14 days after birth, when the atrophic umbilical cord "falls off."

Functions and Actions of the Anterolateral Abdominal Muscles

The muscles of the anterolateral abdominal wall:

- Form a strong expandable support for the anterolateral abdominal wall.

- Protect the abdominal viscera from injury.

- Compress the abdominal contents to maintain or increase the intra-abdominal pressure and, in so doing, oppose the diaphragm (increased intra-abdominal pressure facilitates expulsion).

- Move the trunk and help maintain posture.

The anterolateral abdominal muscles protect and support the abdominal viscera. The oblique and transverse muscles, acting together bilaterally, form a muscular girdle that exerts firm pressure on the abdominal viscera. The rectus abdominis participates little, if at all, in this action. Compressing the abdominal viscera and increasing intra-abdominal pressure elevates the relaxed diaphragm to expel air during respiration and more forcibly for coughing, sneezing, nose blowing, voluntary eructation (burping), and yelling or screaming. When the diaphragm contracts during inspiration, the anterolateral abdominal wall expands as its muscles relax to make room for the organs, such as the liver, that are pushed inferiorly. The combined actions of the anterolateral muscles also produce the force required for defecation (evacuation of fecal material from the rectum), micturition (urination), vomiting, and parturition (childbirth). Increased intra-abdominal (and intrathoracic) pressure is also involved in heavy lifting, the resulting force sometimes producing a hernia.

The anterolateral abdominal muscles are also involved in movements of the trunk at the lumbar vertebrae and in controlling the tilt of the pelvis when standing for maintenance of posture (resisting lumbar lordosis). Consequently, strengthening the anterolateral abdominal wall musculature improves standing and sitting posture. The rectus abdominis is a powerful flexor of the thoracic region and especially of the lumbar region of the vertebral column, pulling the anterior costal margin and pubic crest toward each other. The oblique abdominal muscles also assist in movements of the trunk, especially lateral flexion and rotation of the lumbar and lower thoracic vertebral column. The transverse abdominal muscle probably has no appreciable effect on the vertebral column (Williams et al., 1995).

Protuberance of the Abdomen

A prominent abdomen is normal in infants and young children because their gastrointestinal (GI) tracts contain considerable amounts of air. In addition, their anterolateral abdominal cavities are enlarging and their abdominal muscles are gaining strength. An infant's and young child's relatively large liver also accounts for some bulging. Abdominal muscles protect and support the viscera most effectively when they are well toned; thus the well-conditioned adult of normal weight has a flat or scaphoid (lit. boat shaped; i.e., hollowed or concave) abdomen when in the supine position. The six common causes of abdominal protrusion begin with the letter *F*: food, fluid, fat, feces, flatus, and fetus. Eversion of the umbilicus may be a sign of increased intra-abdominal pressure, usually resulting from ascites (abnormal accumulation of serous fluid in the peritoneal cavity) or a large mass (e.g., a tumor, a fetus, or an enlarged organ such as the liver).

Excess fat accumulation owing to overnourishment most commonly involves the subcutaneous fatty layer; however, there may also be excessive depositions of extraperitoneal fat in some types of obesity.

Tumors and organomegaly (organ enlargement such as splenomegaly, or enlargement of the spleen) also produce abdominal enlargement. When the anterior abdominal muscles are underdeveloped or become atrophic, as a result of old age or insufficient exercise. They provide insufficient tonus to resist the increased weight of a protuberant abdomen on the anterior pelvis. The pelvis tilts anteriorly at the hip joints when standing (the pubis descends and the sacrum ascends) producing excessive *lordo-sis* of the lumbar region of the vertebral column (see Chapter 4 for details).

Abdominal Hernias

The anterolateral abdominal wall may be the site of *hernias*. Most hernias occur in the inguinal, umbilical, and epigastric regions (see clinical correlation [blue] box "Inguinal Hernias," in this chapter) *Umbilical hernias* are common in newborns because the anterior abdominal wall is relatively weak in the umbilical ring, especially in low-birth-weight infants. Umbilical hernias are usually small and result from increased intra-abdominal pressure in the presence of weakness and incomplete closure of the anterior abdominal wall after ligation of the umbilical cord at birth. Herniation occurs through the umbilical ring. *Acquired umbilical hernias* occur most commonly in women and obese people. Extraperitoneal fat and/or peritoneum protrude into the hernial sac. The lines along which the fibers of the abdominal aponeuroses interlace are also potential sites of herniation (Fig. 2.5B). Occasionally, gaps exist where these fiber exchanges occur—for example, in the midline or in the transition from aponeurosis to rectus sheath. These gaps may be congenital, the result of the stresses of obesity and aging, or the consequence of surgical or traumatic wounds. An *epigastric hernia*, a hernia in the epigastric region through the linea alba, occurs in the midline between the xiphoid process and the umbilicus. *Spigelian hernias* are those occurring along the semilunar lines. These types of hernia tend to occur in people > 40 years and are usually associated with obesity. The hernial sac, composed of peritoneum, is covered with only skin and fatty subcutaneous tissue. ⊕

THE BOTTOM LINE: The anterolateral abdominal muscles consist of concentric, flat muscles located anterolaterally and vertical muscles placed anteriorly adjacent to the midline. A trilaminar arrangement of the flat muscles, like that in the thorax, also occurs here; however, other than their innervation by multiple but separate segmental nerves, the metamerism (segmentation) characteristic of the thoracic intercostal musculature is not apparent in the abdomen. The fleshy portions of the flat muscles become aponeurotic anteriorly. The fibers of the aponeuroses interlace in the midline, forming the linea alba, and continue into the aponeuroses of the contralateral muscles. The aponeurotic fibers of the external obliques are also continuous across the midline with those of the contralateral internal oblique muscles. Thus three layers of flat, bilateral digastric muscles encircle the trunk, forming oblique and transverse girdles that enclose the abdominal cavity. In the upper two thirds of the abdominal wall, the aponeurotic layers separate on each side of the linea alba to form longitudinal pockets, or sheaths, that contain the rectus muscles. This brings them into a functional relationship with the flat muscles in which the vertical muscles brace the girdles anteriorly. In the lower third of the anterior abdominal wall, the aponeuroses of all three layers of flat muscles pass anterior to the rectus muscles (recti). As flexors of the trunk, the recti are the antagonistic partners of the deep (extensor) muscles of the back. Balance in the development and tonus of these partners affects posture (and thus weakness of the abdominal muscles may result in excessive lumbar lordosis). The special arrangements of the anterolateral abdominal muscles enable them to provide flexible containing walls for the abdominal contents, to increase intra-abdominal pressure or decrease abdominal volume for expulsion, and to produce anterior and lateral flexion and torsional (rotatory) movements of the trunk.

Nerves of the Anterolateral Abdominal Wall

The map of dermatomes of the anterolateral abdominal wall is almost identical to the map of peripheral nerve distribution (Table 2.3). This is because the anterior rami of spinal nerves T7–T12, which supply most of the abdominal wall, do not participate in plexus formation. The exception occurs at the L1 level, where the L1 anterior ramus bifurcates into two named peripheral nerves. Each dermatome begins posteriorly overlying the intervertebral foramen by which the spinal nerve exits the vertebral column and follows the slope of the ribs around the trunk. Dermatome T10 includes the umbilicus, whereas dermatome L1 includes the inguinal fold.

The skin and muscles of the anterolateral abdominal wall are supplied mainly by the following nerves (Fig. 2.8*A*; Table 2.3):

- **Thoracoabdominal nerves:** the distal, abdominal parts of the anterior rami of the inferior six thoracic spinal nerves (T7–T11); these are the former inferior intercostal nerves distal to the costal margin.

- **Lateral (thoracic) cutaneous branches:** of the thoracic spinal nerves T7–T9 or T10.

- **Subcostal nerve:** the large anterior ramus of spinal nerve T12.

- **Iliohypogastric** and **ilioinguinal nerves:** terminal branches of the anterior ramus of spinal nerve L1.

The thoracoabdominal nerves pass inferoanteriorly from the intercostal spaces and run in the neurovascular plane between the internal oblique and the transverse abdominal muscles to supply the abdominal skin and muscles. The lateral cutaneous branches emerge from the musculature of the anterolateral wall to enter the subcutaneous tissue along the anterior axillary line (as anterior and posterior divisions), whereas the anterior abdominal cutaneous branches pierce the rectus sheath to enter the subcutaneous tissue a short distance from the me-

dian plane. Of the *anterior abdominal cutaneous branches of thoracoabdominal nerve(s):*

- *T7–T9* supply the skin superior to the umbilicus.

- *T10* innervates the skin around the umbilicus.

- *T11,* plus the cutaneous branches of the subcostal (T12), iliohypogastric, and ilioinguinal (L1), supply the skin inferior to the umbilicus.

During their course through the wall, the thoracoabdominal, subcostal, and iliohypogastric nerves communicate with each other.

Palpation of the Anterolateral Abdominal Wall

Warm hands are especially important when palpating the abdominal wall because cold hands make the anterolateral abdominal muscles tense, producing involuntary spasms of the muscles, known as **guarding**. Intense guarding, board-like reflexive muscular rigidity that cannot be willfully suppressed, occurs during palpation when an organ (such as the appendix) is inflamed and in itself constitutes a clinically significant sign of *acute abdomen*. The involuntary muscular spasms attempt to protect the viscera from pressure, which is painful when an abdominal infection is present. The common nerve supply of the skin and muscles of the wall explains why these spasms occur. Palpation of abdominal viscera is performed with the patient in the supine position with thighs and knees semiflexed to enable adequate relaxation of the anterolateral abdominal wall. Otherwise, the deep fascia of the thighs pulls on the membranous layer of abdominal subcutaneous tissue, tensing the abdominal wall. Some people tend to place their hands behind their heads when lying supine, which also tightens the muscles and makes the examination difficult. Placing the upper limbs at the sides and putting a pillow under the person's knees tends to relax the anterolateral abdominal muscles.

Superficial Abdominal Reflexes

Physicians and surgeons examine the reflexes of the abdominal wall to determine if there is abdominal disease, such as appendicitis. The abdominal wall is the only protection most of the abdominal organs have. Consequently, it will react if an organ is diseased or injured. With the person supine and the muscles relaxed, the superficial abdominal reflex is elicited by quickly stroking horizontally, lateral to medial, toward the umbilicus. Usually, contraction of the abdominal muscles is felt; this reflex may not be observed in obese people. ▶

Table 2.3. Nerves of the Anterolateral Abdominal Wall

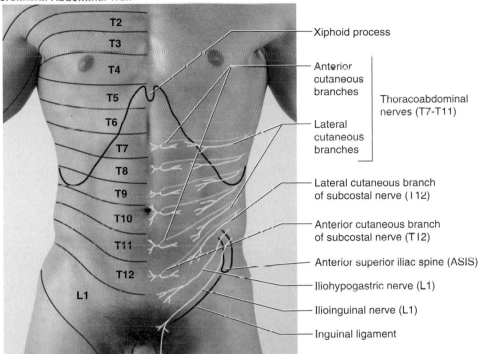

Anterior view

Nerves	Origin	Course	Distribution
Thoracoabdominal (T7–T11)	Continuation of lower (7th–11th) intercostal nerves distal to costal margin	Run between second and third layers of abdominal muscles; branches enter subcutaneous tissue as lateral cutaneous branches of T10–T11 (in anterior axillary line) and anterior cutaneous branches of T7–T11 (parasternal line)	Muscles of anterolateral abdominal wall and overlying skin
7th–9th lateral cutaneous branches	7th–9th intercostal nerves (anterior rami of spinal nerves T7–T9)	Anterior divisions continue across costal margin in subcutaneous tissue	Skin of right and left hypochondriac regions
Subcostal (anterior ramus of T12)	Spinal nerve T12	Runs along inferior border of 12th rib; then onto subumbilical abdominal wall between second and third layers of abdominal muscles	Muscles of anterolateral abdominal wall (including most inferior slip of external oblique) and overlying skin, superior to iliac crest and inferior to umbilicus
Iliohypogastric (L1)	As superior terminal branch of anterior ramus of spinal nerve L1	Pierces transverse abdominal muscle to course between second and third layers of abdominal muscles; branches pierce external oblique aponeuroses of most inferior abdominal wall	Skin overlying iliac crest, upper inguinal, and hypogastric regions; internal oblique and transverse abdominal muscles
Ilioinguinal (L1)	As inferior terminal branch of anterior ramus of spinal nerve L1	Passes between second and third layers of abdominal muscles; then traverses inguinal canal	Skin of lower inguinal region, mons pubis, anterior scrotum or labium majus, and adjacent medial thigh; inferiormost internal oblique and transverse abdominal

Similarly, any injury to the abdominal skin results in a rapid reflex contraction of the abdominal muscles.

Injury to Nerves of the Anterolateral Abdominal Wall

The inferior thoracic spinal nerves (T7–T12) and the iliohypogastric and ilioinguinal nerves (L1) approach the abdominal musculature separately to provide the multi-segmental innervation of the abdominal muscles (versus the limbs, in which multi-segmental peripheral nerves provide innervation). Thus they are distributed across the anterolateral abdominal wall, where they run oblique but mostly horizontal courses and are susceptible to injury in surgical incisions or from trauma at any level of the abdominal wall. Injury to them during surgery or from an abdominal injury may result in weakening of the muscles. In the inguinal region, such a weakness may predispose an individual to development of an inguinal hernia (see clinical correlation [blue] box "Inguinal Hernias," in this chapter).

Abdominal Surgical Incisions

Surgeons use various incisions to gain access to the abdominal cavity. When possible, the incisions follow the cleavage lines (Langer lines) in the skin (see Introduction for discussion of these lines). The incision that allows adequate exposure and, secondarily, the best possible cosmetic effect, is chosen. The location of the incision also depends on the type of operation, the location of the organ(s) the surgeon wants to reach, bony or cartilaginous boundaries, avoidance of (especially motor) nerves, maintenance of blood supply, and minimizing injury to muscles and fascia of the wall while aiming for favorable healing. Thus before making an incision, the surgeon considers the direction of the muscle fibers and the location of the aponeuroses and nerves. Consequently, a variety of incisions are routinely used, each having specific advantages and limitations.

Instead of transecting muscles, causing irreversible necrosis (death) of muscle fibers, the surgeon splits them in the direction of (and between) their fibers. The rectus abdominis is an exception; it can be transected because its muscle fibers run short distances between tendinous intersections and its segmental innervation enters at the lateral part of the rectus sheath. Therefore, the nerves can be easily located and preserved. The surgeon chooses the part of the anterolateral abdominal wall that gives the freest access to the targeted organ with the least disturbance to the nerve supply to the muscles. Muscles and viscera are retracted toward, not away from, their neurovascular supply. Cutting a motor nerve paralyzes the muscle fibers supplied by it, thereby weakening the anterolateral abdominal wall. However, because of overlapping areas of innervation between

nerves, one or two small branches of nerves may usually be cut without a noticeable loss of motor supply to the muscles or loss of sensation to the skin. Little if any communication occurs between nerves from the lateral border of the rectus abdominis to the anterior midline.

Longitudinal Incisions

Longitudinal incisions are used centrally in the abdomen, because muscle and vasculature are primarily longitudinally oriented here and the nerves, which have been approaching circumferentially or transversely, diminish in size and significance near the midline. Longitudinal incisions, such as median and paramedian incisions (Fig. B2.1), are preferred for exploratory operations because they offer good exposure of and access to the viscera and can be extended as necessary with minimal complication.

Median or *midline incisions* can be made rapidly without cutting muscle, major blood vessels, or nerves. They cut ▶

McBurney point

Key

- ■ Median or midline incision
- ■ Left paramedian incision
- ■ Gridiron (muscle-splitting) incision (traditional McBurney incision and horizontal incision)
- □ Suprapubic (Pfannenstiel) incision
- ▨ Transverse (abdominal) incision
- ■ Subcostal incision

Figure B2.1.

through the fibrous tissue of the linea alba, superior and/or inferior to the umbilicus. Because the linea alba transmits only small vessels and nerves to the skin, a midline incision is relatively bloodless and avoids major nerves; however, incisions in some people may reveal abundant and well-vascularized fat, particularly in the falciform ligament of the liver (discussed later in this chapter). Conversely, because of its relatively poor blood supply, the linea alba may undergo necrosis and subsequent degeneration after incision if its edges are not aligned properly during closure. Median incisions can be made along any part or the length of the linea alba from the xiphoid process to pubic symphysis. Lower median incisions (below the umbilicus) are frequently used for reaching female pelvic viscera.

Paramedian incisions (lateral, left or right, to the median plane) are made in the sagittal plane and may extend from the costal margin to the pubic hairline. After the incision passes through the anterior layer of the rectus sheath, the muscle is freed and retracted laterally to prevent tension and injury to the vessels and nerves. The posterior layer of the rectus sheath and the peritoneum are then incised to enter the peritoneal cavity.

Oblique and Transverse Incisions

Oblique and *transverse incisions* are used most commonly on one side of the midline and especially in the more peripheral abdomen where their direction is related to muscle fiber orientation, nearby hard tissue (costal margin or iliac or pubic crest), or minimizing potential nerve damage.

Gridiron (muscle-splitting) incisions are often used for an appendectomy. The oblique *McBurney incision* is made at the *McBurney point*, approximately 2.5 cm superomedial to the ASIS on the *spinoumbilical line*. This incision is currently less popular than an almost transverse incision in the line of a skin crease. In either case, the external oblique aponeurosis is incised inferomedially in the direction of its fibers and retracted. The musculoaponeurotic fibers of the internal oblique and transverse abdominal are then split in the line of their fibers and retracted. The iliohypogastric nerve, running deep to the internal oblique, is identified and preserved. Carefully made, the entire exposure cuts no musculoaponeurotic fibers; therefore, when the incision is closed, the muscle fibers move together and the abdominal wall is as strong after the operation as it was before. When kept relatively small and done carefully, the gridiron incision provides good access and avoids cutting, tearing, and stretching of nerves.

Suprapubic (Pfannenstiel) incisions ("bikini" incisions) are made at the pubic hairline. These incisions—horizontal with a slight convexity—are used for most gynecological and obstetrical operations (e.g., for cesarean section and removal of a tubal pregnancy). The linea alba and the anterior layers of the rectus sheaths are transected and resected superiorly, and the rectus muscles are retracted laterally or

divided through their tendinous parts allowing reattachment without muscle fiber injury. The iliohypogastric and ilioinguinal nerves are identified and preserved.

Transverse incisions through the anterior layer of the rectus sheath and rectus abdominis provide good access and cause the least possible damage to the nerve supply of the rectus abdominis. This muscle may be divided transversely without serious damage because a new transverse band forms that, when the muscle segments are rejoined, is similar to a tendinous intersection. Transverse incisions are not made through the tendinous intersections because cutaneous nerves and branches of the superior epigastric vessels pierce these fibrous regions of the muscle. Transverse incisions are most useful above the level of the umbilicus. They can be increased laterally as needed to increase exposure but are not good for exploratory procedures because superior and inferior extension is difficult.

Subcostal incisions provide access to the gallbladder and biliary ducts on the right side and the spleen on the left. The incision is made parallel but at least 2.5 cm inferior to the costal margin to avoid the 7th and 8th thoracic spinal nerves (Table 2.3).

High-Risk Incisions

High-risk incisions include pararectus and inguinal incisions. *Pararectus incisions* along the lateral border of the rectus sheath are undesirable because they are likely to cut the nerve supply to the rectus abdominis. Blood supply from the inferior epigastric artery also may be compromised. *Inguinal incisions* for repairing hernias may injure the ilioinguinal nerve directly or it may be inadvertently included in the suture during closure of the incision. In such cases, people may feel pain in the L1 dermatome region, which includes the scrotum (or the labium majus).

Incisional Hernia

An *incisional hernia* is a protrusion of *omentum* (a fold of peritoneum) or an organ through a surgical incision. Surgeons who make incisions based on a thorough knowledge of anterolateral abdominal wall anatomy will only occasionally have to deal with this problem. However, if the muscular and aponeurotic layers of the abdomen do not heal properly, an incisional hernia can result. Factors predisposing a patient to incisional hernia include advanced age or debility of the patient, obesity, and postoperative wound infection.

Minimally Invasive (Endoscopic) Surgery

Many abdominopelvic surgical procedures are now performed using an *endoscope*, in which tiny perforations of the abdominal wall allow the entry of remotely operated instruments, replacing the larger conventional incisions. Thus the potential for nerve injury, incisional hernia, or contamination through the open wound and the time required for healing are minimized. ⊕

THE BOTTOM LINE: The anterolateral abdominal muscles receive multi-segmental innervation via the anterior rami of lower thoracic (T7–T12) and the L1 spinal nerves. The rami pass separately to the muscles (i.e., without uniting into multi-segmental peripheral nerves as occurs in the limbs) as five thoracoabdominal nerves (T7–T11), a subcostal nerve (T12), and iliohypogastric and ilioinguinal nerves (L1) that course in a plane between the second and third layers. Lateral cutaneous branches supply the overlying abdominal skin lateral to the MCL; anterior cutaneous branches supply skin medial to the MCL. Except for L1, the maps of the abdominal dermatomes and of the peripheral nerves are thus identical. Landmark dermatomes are dermatome T10, which includes the umbilicus, and dermatome L1, which includes the inguinal fold.

Vessels of the Anterolateral Abdominal Wall

The skin and subcutaneous tissue of the abdominal wall is served by an intricate subcutaneous venous plexus, draining superiorly to the internal thoracic vein medially and the lateral thoracic vein laterally and inferiorly to the superficial and inferior epigastric veins, tributaries of the femoral and external iliac veins, respectively (Fig. 2.9). Cutaneous veins surrounding the umbilicus anastomose with **parumbilical veins,** small tributaries of the *portal vein* that parallel the **obliterated umbilical vein** (round ligament of the liver). A relatively direct lateral superficial anastomotic channel, the **thoracoepigastric vein,** may exist or develop (as a result of altered venous flow) between the *superficial epigastric vein* (a femoral vein tributary) and the *lateral thoracic vein* (an axillary vein tributary). The deeper veins of the anterolateral abdominal wall accompany the arteries, bearing the same name. A deeper, medial venous anastomosis may exist or develop between the *inferior epigastric vein* (an external iliac vein tributary) and the *superior epigastric/internal thoracic veins* (subclavian vein tributaries). The superficial and deep anastomoses may afford collateral circulation during blockage of either vena cava.

The primary blood vessels (arteries and veins) of the anterolateral abdominal wall are the

- *Superior epigastric vessels* and branches of the *musculophrenic vessels* from the internal thoracic vessels.

- *Inferior epigastric* and *deep circumflex iliac vessels* from the external iliac vessels.

- *Superficial circumflex iliac* and *superficial epigastric vessels* from the femoral artery and greater saphenous vein, respectively.

- *Posterior intercostal vessels* of the 11th intercostal space and the anterior branches of *subcostal vessels*

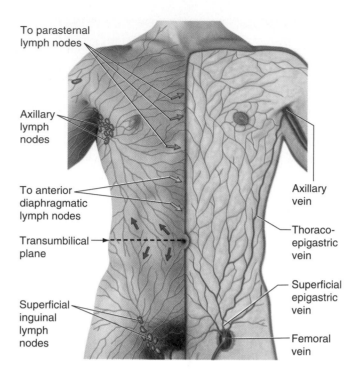

Anterior view

Figure 2.9. Lymphatics and superficial veins of anterolateral abdominal wall. Most superficial lymphatic vessels superior to the umbilicus drain to the axillary lymph nodes; a few drain medially and deeply to the parasternal and anterior diaphragmatic lymph nodes. Superficial lymphatic vessels inferior to the umbilicus drain to the superficial inguinal lymph nodes. The pattern of superficial venous drainage is more vertical than transverse (circumferential). The thoracoepigastric vein, formed of anastomosing tributaries of the lateral thoracic (axillary) and superficial epigastric (femoral) veins, is capable of providing collateral circulation between the superior and the inferior vena caval systems.

The arterial supply to the anterolateral abdominal wall is summarized in Table 2.4. The distribution of the deep abdominal blood vessels reflects the arrangement of the muscles: The vessels of the anterolateral abdominal wall have an oblique, circumferential pattern (similar to the intercostal vessels above), whereas the vessels of the central anterior abdominal wall are oriented more vertically.

The **superior epigastric artery** is the direct continuation of the *internal thoracic artery.* It enters the rectus sheath superiorly through its posterior layer and supplies the superior part of the rectus abdominis and anastomoses with the inferior epigastric artery approximately in the umbilical region (Fig. 2.8, Table 2.4)

The **inferior epigastric artery** arises from the *external iliac artery* just superior to the inguinal ligament. It runs superiorly in the transversalis fascia to enter the rectus sheath below the arcuate line. It enters the lower rectus abdominis and anastomoses with the superior epigastric artery.

Table 2.4. Arteries of the Anterolateral Abdominal Wall

Musculophrenic a.
Superior epigastric a.
10th posterior intercostal a.
External oblique m.
11th posterior intercostal a.
Internal oblique m.
Subcostal a.
Transverse abdominal m.
Inferior epigastric a.
Deep circumflex iliac a.
Superficial epigastric a.
Superficial circumflex iliac a.
External iliac a.
Femoral a.
Transversalis fascia

Artery	Origin	Course	Distribution
Musculophrenic	Internal thoracic artery	Descends along costal margin	Superficial and deep abdominal wall of hypochondriac region; anterolateral diaphragm
Superior epigastric		Descends in rectus sheath deep to rectus abdominis	Rectus abdominis muscle; superficial and deep abdominal wall of epigastric and upper umbilical regions
10th and 11th posterior intercostal arteries	Aorta	Arteries continue beyond ribs to descend in abdominal wall between internal oblique and transverse abdominal muscles	Superficial and deep abdominal wall of lateral (lumbar or flank) region
Subcostal artery			
Inferior epigastric	External iliac artery	Runs superiorly and enters rectus sheath; runs deep to rectus abdominis	Rectus abdominis muscle; deep abdominal wall of pubic and inferior umbilical regions
Deep circumflex iliac		Runs on deep aspect of anterior abdominal wall, parallel to inguinal ligament	Iliacus muscle and deep abdominal wall of inguinal region; iliac fossa
Superficial circumflex iliac	Femoral artery	Runs in subcutaneous tissue along inguinal ligament	Superficial abdominal wall of inguinal region and adjacent anterior thigh
Superficial epigastric		Runs in subcutaneous tissue toward umbilicus	Superficial abdominal wall of pubic and inferior umbilical region

Lymphatic drainage of the anterolateral abdominal wall follows the following patterns (Fig. 2.9):

- *Superficial lymphatic vessels* accompany the subcutaneous veins; those superior to the transumbilical plane drain mainly to the **axillary lymph nodes**; however, a few drain to the **parasternal lymph nodes.** Superficial lymphatic vessels inferior to the transumbilical plane drain to the **superficial inguinal lymph nodes.**

- *Deep lymphatic vessels* accompany the deep veins of the abdominal wall and drain to the *external iliac, common iliac,* and *right* and *left lumbar (caval* and *aortic)* **lymph nodes.**

For an overview of superficial and deep lymphatic drainage, see the Introduction.

Reversal of Venous Flow and Collateral Pathways of Superficial Abdominal Veins

When flow in the superior or inferior vena cava is obstructed, anastomoses between the tributaries of these systemic veins, such as the thoracoepigastric vein, may provide collateral pathways by which the obstruction may be bypassed, allowing blood to return to the heart (Fig. B2.2). Small cutaneous (systemic) veins surrounding the umbilicus also anastomose with the paraumbilical veins (tributaries of the portal vein), which run with the obliterated umbilical vein (round ligament of the liver). During either caval or portal obstruction, these anastomosing veins may also become distended, causing the *caput medusae* appearance (referring to the head of Medusa, who had writhing snakes for hair). ☉

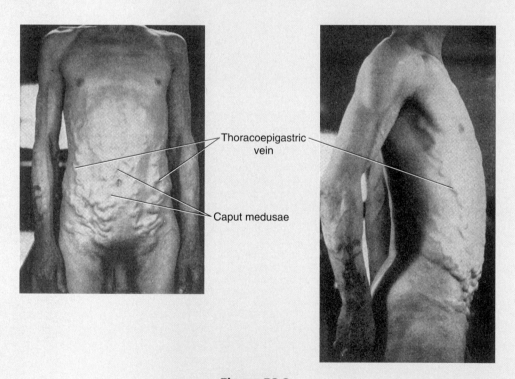

Thoracoepigastric vein

Caput medusae

Figure B2.2.

THE BOTTOM LINE: The skin and subcutaneous tissue of the abdominal wall drain superiorly (ultimately to the superior vena caval system) via the internal thoracic vein medially and the lateral thoracic vein laterally, and inferiorly (ultimately to the inferior vena caval system) via the superficial and inferior epigastric veins. Cutaneous veins surrounding the umbilicus anastomose with small tributaries of the portal vein. The distribution of the deeper abdominal blood vessels reflects the arrangement of the muscles: an oblique, circumferential pattern (similar to the intercostal vessels above) over the anterolateral abdominal wall and a vertical pattern anteriorly. The circumferential vessels of the anterolateral wall are continuations of the 11th posterior intercostal vessels, subcostal vessels, and deep circumflex iliac vessels. An anastomosis between the superior and the inferior epigastric vessels within the rectus sheath includes the vertical vessels. A superficial anastomotic channel, the thoracoepigastric vein, and the deeper medial pathway between the inferior and the superior epigastric veins afford collateral circulation during blockage of either vena cava.

Superficial abdominal lymphatic vessels superior to the transumbilical plane drain primarily to the axillary lymph nodes; those inferior to the plane drain to the superficial inguinal lymph nodes. Deep lymphatic vessels accompany deep veins of the abdominal wall to the iliac and right and left lumbar (caval and aortic) lymph nodes.

Internal Surface of the Anterolateral Abdominal Wall

The internal (posterior) surface of the anterolateral abdominal wall is covered with transversalis fascia, a variable amount of extraperitoneal fat, and parietal peritoneum (Fig. 2.10). The infraumbilical part of this surface exhibits several peritoneal folds, some of which contain remnants of vessels that carried blood to and from the fetus (Moore and Persaud, 2003). Five *umbilical peritoneal folds*—two on each side and one in the median plane—pass toward the umbilicus:

- The **median umbilical fold** extends from the apex of the urinary bladder to the umbilicus and covers the **median umbilical ligament,** the remnant of the *urachus,* which joined the apex of the fetal bladder to the umbilicus.

- Two **medial umbilical folds,** lateral to the median umbilical fold, cover the **medial umbilical ligaments,** formed by *occluded parts of the umbilical arteries.*

- Two **lateral umbilical folds,** lateral to the medial umbilical folds, cover the *inferior epigastric vessels* and therefore bleed if cut.

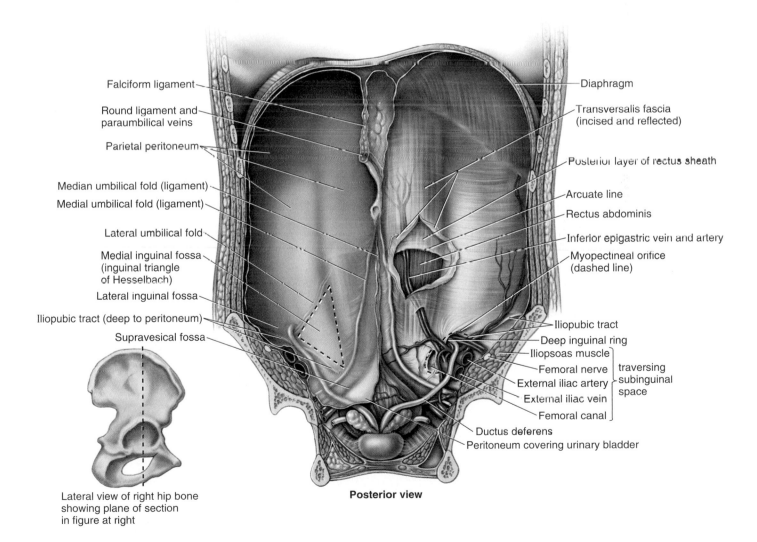

Lateral view of right hip bone showing plane of section in figure at right

Posterior view

Figure 2.10. Posterior aspect of anterolateral abdominal wall of a male. The peritoneal ligaments, folds, and fossae are the main features of this aspect.

The depressions lateral to the umbilical folds are the *peritoneal fossae,* each of which is a potential site for a hernia. The location of a hernia in one of these fossae determines how the hernia is classified. The shallow fossae between the umbilical folds are the:

- **Supravesical fossae** between the median and the medial umbilical folds, formed as the peritoneum reflects from the anterior abdominal wall onto the bladder. The level of the supravesical fossae rises and falls with filling and emptying of the bladder.

- **Medial inguinal fossae** between the medial and the lateral umbilical folds, areas also commonly called **inguinal triangles (Hesselbach triangles)**, which are potential sites for the less common direct inguinal hernias.

- **Lateral inguinal fossae,** lateral to the lateral umbilical folds, include the *deep inguinal rings* and are potential sites for the most common type of hernia in the lower abdominal wall, the *indirect inguinal hernia* (see clinical correlation [blue] box "Inguinal Hernias," in this chapter).

The supraumbilical part of the internal surface of the anterior abdominal wall has a sagittally oriented peritoneal reflection, the **falciform ligament,** that extends between the superior anterior abdominal wall and the liver. It encloses the **round ligament of the liver** (L. *ligamentum teres hepatis*) and paraumbilical veins in its inferior free edge. The round ligament is a fibrous remnant of the umbilical vein, which extended from the umbilicus to the liver prenatally (Moore and Persaud, 2003).

External Supravesical Hernia

An *external supravesical hernia* leaves the peritoneal cavity through the supravesical fossa. The site of this hernia is medial to that of a direct inguinal hernia (see clinical correlation [blue] box "Inguinal Hernias," in this chapter). The iliohypogastric nerve is in danger of injury during the repair of this rare type of hernia.

Postnatal Patency of the Umbilical Vein

Before the birth of a fetus, the umbilical vein carries well-oxygenated, nutrient-rich blood from the placenta to the fetus. Although reference is often made to the "occluded" umbilical vein forming the round ligament of the liver, this vein is patent for some time after birth and is used for *umbilical vein catheterization* for exchange transfusion during early infancy—for example, in infants with *erythroblastosis fetalis* or *hemolytic disease* of the newborn (Behrman et al., 2000). ○

THE BOTTOM LINE: The primary features of the internal surface of the anterolateral abdominal wall are peritoneal folds overlying structures radiating from the umbilical ring and the peritoneal fossae formed in relation to the folds. Of the umbilical peritoneal folds, the central three (median and medial umbilical folds) cover remnants of embryological structures, whereas the lateral umbilical folds cover the inferior epigastric vessels, making them the most significant of the folds postnatally. The peritoneal fossae formed in relation to them include the transitional supravesical fossae, the height of which changes with bladder filling, and the medial and lateral inguinal fossa, overlying potential weak areas in the anterior abdominal wall where direct and indirect inguinal hernias, respectively, may occur. The supraumbilical falciform ligament encloses the remnant of the embryological umbilical vein and the accompanying paraumbilical veins (tributaries of the portal vein) in its free edge.

Inguinal Region

The **inguinal region** (groin), extending between the ASIS and pubic tubercle, is an important area anatomically and clinically; anatomically because it is a region where structures exit and enter the abdominal cavity and clinically because the pathways of exit and entrance are potential sites of herniation. In fact, the majority of abdominal hernias occur in this region, with inguinal hernias in particular accounting for 75% of all abdominal hernias. These hernias occur in both sexes, but most inguinal hernias (approximately 86%) occur in males because of the passage of the spermatic cord through the *inguinal canal.*

Although the testis is located in the perineum postnatally, the male gonad originally forms in the abdomen. Its migration out of the abdomen into the perineum through the inguinal canal accounts for many of the structural features of the region. Traditionally, the testis and scrotum are dissected and studied in relation to the anterior abdominal wall, and the inguinal region in particular, in spite of their postnatal perineal location.

For these reasons, male anatomy receives greater emphasis in this section.

The Inguinal Ligament and Iliopubic Tract

Thickened fibrous bands, or *retinacula,* occur in relationship to many joints that have a wide range of movement to retain structures against the skeleton during the various positions of the joint (see the Introduction). The *inguinal ligament* and *iliopubic tract,* extending from the ASIS to the *pubic tubercle,* constitute a bilaminar anterior (flexor) retinaculum of the hip joint (Figs. 2.10 and 2.11). The retinaculum spans the **subinguinal space,** through which pass flexors of the hip and the neurovascular structures serving much of the lower limb. Consequently, the subinguinal space will be treated in greatest detail in Chapter 5. These fibrous bands are the thickened inferolateral-most portions of the external and internal layers of

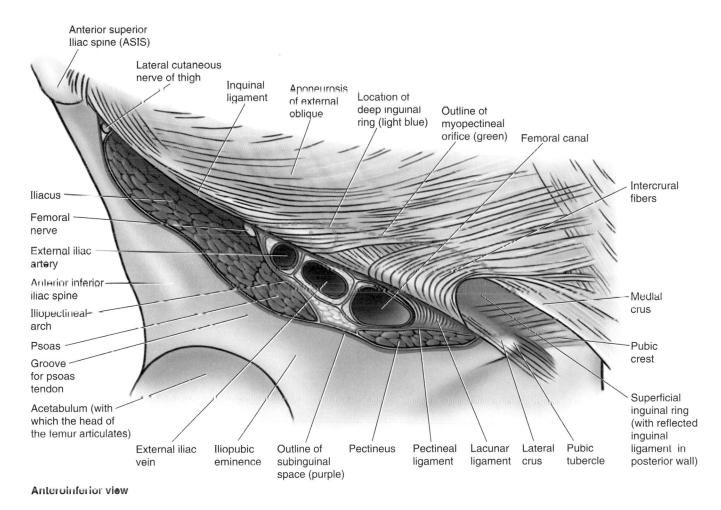

Anteroinferior view

Figure 2.11. Formations of inguinal region. The inguinal ligament is the thickened, underturned, inferior margin of the aponeurosis of the external oblique, forming a retinaculum that bridges the subinguinal space. A slit-like gap between the medial and the lateral crura of the external oblique aponeurosis, bridged by intercrural fibers, forms the superficial inguinal ring.

the anterolateral abdominal wall (integumentary and extraperitoneal structures excepted) and are major landmarks of the region.

The **inguinal ligament** is a dense band constituting the inferiormost part of the external oblique aponeurosis. Although most of the fibers of the ligament's medial end insert into the pubic tubercle, some follow other courses (Fig. 2.11):

- Some of the deeper fibers pass posteriorly to attach to the *superior pubic ramus* lateral to the tubercle, forming the arching **lacunar ligament** (of Gimbernat), which forms the medial boundary of the subinguinal space. The most lateral of these fibers continue to run along the *pecten pubis* as the **pectineal ligament** (of Cooper).

- Some of the more superior fibers fan upward, bypassing the *pubic tubercle* and crossing the linea alba to blend with the lower fibers of the contralateral external oblique aponeurosis. These fibers form the **reflected inguinal ligament** (Figs. 2.7, 2.11, and 2.12A).

The **iliopubic tract** is the thickened inferior margin of the transversalis fascia, which appears as a fibrous band running parallel and posterior (deep) to the inguinal ligament (Figs. 2.10 and 2.12B). The iliopubic tract, seen in the place of the inguinal ligament when the inguinal region is viewed from its internal (posterior) aspect (e.g., during laparoscopy), reinforces the posterior wall and floor of the inguinal canal as it bridges the structures traversing the subinguinal space.

The inguinal ligament and iliopubic tract span an area of innate weakness in the body wall in the region of the groin called the **myopectineal orifice** (Fruchaud, 1956). This weak area, occurring in relation to structures traversing the body wall, is the site of groin hernias (direct and indirect inguinal and femoral hernias).

Inguinal Canal

The **inguinal canal** is formed in relation to the descent of the testis during fetal development. The inguinal canal in

(A) Anterior view

* Musculoaponeurotic arcades of
internal oblique & transverse abdominal

Peritoneum
Transversalis fascia
Transverse abdominal muscle
Internal oblique muscle
External oblique muscle
Testicular artery and veins
External oblique aponeurosis
Ductus deferens
Ilioinguinal nerve
Inferior epigastric vessels
Space of Bogros
Deep inguinal ring
Plane of section for (B)
Intercrural fibers

Internal
spermatic fascia
*
Inguinal
ligament
Origin of
cremasteric muscle
Inguinal falx
(conjoint tendon)
Femoral vessels
Superficial inguinal ring
External spermatic fascia
Reflected inguinal ligament
Cremasteric muscle and fascia
Internal spermatic
fascia
Spermatic cord
External spermatic fascia
Testis

(B) Schematic sagittal section

Aponeuroses of:
external
internal } oblique
Skin
Fatty layer
Spermatic cord
Membranous
layer of sub-
cutaneous
tissue
Anterior wall
of inguinal canal
(intercrural
fibers)
Transverse
abdominal
Transversalis fascia
Space of Bogros
Peritoneum
Inguinal falx (conjoint
tendon) forming
posterior wall of canal
Iliopubic tract
Inguinal ligament
forming "gutter" (floor
of inguinal canal)
Superior ramus
of pubis
Fascia lata
of thigh

(C) Anterior view

Musculoaponeurotic arcades of
Internal oblique   Superficial inguinal ring
Transverse abdominal
Relaxed   Contracted

Figure 2.12. Inguinal canal and spermatic cord. *A.* The layers of the abdominal wall and the coverings of the spermatic cord and testis derived from them, as a result of the passage of the testis and spermatic cord through the canal during development, are shown. The inguinal falx, the common tendon of the transverse and internal oblique muscles, forms the posterior wall of the medial part of the inguinal canal. It is frequently muscular rather than aponeurotic (as shown here) and it may be poorly developed. *B.* This sagittal section of the anterior abdominal wall and inguinal canal is at the plane shown in part *A.* *C.* The inguinal canal consists of a series of three musculoaponeurotic arcades traversed by the spermatic cord or round ligament of the uterus (*arrow*). The muscular contraction that increases intra-abdominal pressure also causes the roof of the canal to descend, narrowing the canal as it is simultaneously collapsed anteroposteriorly by the increased internal pressure.

adults is an oblique passage approximately 4 cm long directed inferomedially through the inferior part of the anterolateral abdominal wall. It lies parallel and superior to the medial half of the inguinal ligament (Figs. 2.11 and 2.12). The main occupant of the inguinal canal is the spermatic cord in males and the round ligament of the uterus in females. These are functionally and developmentally distinct structures that occur in the same location. The inguinal canal also contains blood and lymphatic vessels and the ilioinguinal nerve in both sexes. The inguinal canal has an opening at each end:

- The **deep (internal) inguinal ring** (internal entrance to the inguinal canal), located superior to the middle of the inguinal ligament and lateral to the inferior epigastric artery, is the beginning of an evagination in the transversalis fascia, forming an opening like the entrance to a cave (Figs. 2.6B, 2.10, and 2.12). Through this opening, the extraperitoneal ductus deferens (vas deferens) and testicular vessels in males (or round ligament of the uterus in females) pass to enter the inguinal canal. The transversalis fascia itself continues into the canal, forming the innermost covering (internal fascia) of the structures traversing the canal.

- The **superficial (external) inguinal ring** is the exit by which the spermatic cord in males, or the round ligament in females, emerges from the inguinal canal (Figs. 2.6A, 2.11, and 2.12). The superficial ring is a split that occurs in the diagonal, otherwise parallel fibers of the external oblique aponeurosis just superolateral to the pubic tubercle. The parts of the aponeurosis that lie lateral and medial to, and form the margins of, the superficial ring are *crura* (L. leg-like parts). The **lateral crus** attaches to the pubic tubercle and the **medial crus** to the pubic crest. Fibers of the superficial layer of investing (deep) fascia overlying the external oblique muscle and aponeurosis, running perpendicular to the fibers of the aponeurosis, pass from one crus to the other across the superolateral part of the ring; these **intercrural fibers** help prevent the crura from spreading apart (i.e., they keep the "split" in the aponeurosis from expanding).

Although normally collapsed anteroposteriorly against the structures it conveys, between its two openings (rings) the inguinal canal has two walls (anterior and posterior), as well as a roof and floor (Figs. 2.11 and 2.12A & B). The structures forming these boundaries are listed in Table 2.5.

Two musculoaponeurotic arches bound the canal. The inferior parts of the internal oblique and transverse abdominal, arising as muscular fibers from the inguinal ligament, arch over the inguinal canal forming its roof (Fig. 2.12A). The fibers become aponeurotic as they descend to attach to the superior margin (crest and pecten) of the pubic bone (Fig. 2.6B), forming the posterior wall of the medial half of the canal, including that part posterior to the superficial inguinal ring (Fig. 2.7). Frequently, the most inferior, medial tendinous fibers of the internal oblique merge with aponeurotic fibers of the transverse abdominal muscle here to form the **inguinal falx (conjoint tendon)**. The extent of their fusion and the width of their insertions here are quite variable, however; and the two aponeuroses may insert separately with no falx being formed.

As the inguinal ligament and the iliopubic tract span the myopectineal orifice, they demarcate the inferior boundaries of the inguinal canal and its openings as well as the inguinal triangle, separating these formations from the structures of the femoral sheath (the femoral vessels and femoral canal) that traverse the medial part of the subinguinal space. The iliopubic tract is a useful landmark during laparoscopic hernia repair (Skandalakis et al., 1996). Most groin hernias in males pass superior to the iliopubic tract (inguinal hernias), whereas most pass inferior to it in females (femoral hernias). Because of its relative weakness, the myopectineal orifice is the formation overlaid with mesh placed in the extraperitoneal "space of Bogros" in many laparoscopic hernia repairs employing prosthetic materials.

Development of the Inguinal Canal. The testes develop in the extraperitoneal connective tissue in the superior lumbar region of the posterior abdominal wall (Fig. 2.13A). The **male gubernaculum** is a fibrous cord connecting the **primordial testis** to the anterolateral abdominal wall at the site of the future deep ring of the inguinal canal (Moore and Persaud, 2003). A peritoneal diverticulum, the **processus vaginalis**,

Table 2.5. Boundaries of the Inguinal Canal

Boundary	Deep Ring/Lateral Third	Middle Third	Lateral Third/Superficial Ring
Posterior wall	Transversalis fascia	Transversalis fascia	Inguinal falx (conjoint tendon) plus reflected inguinal ligament
Anterior wall	Internal oblique plus lateral crus of aponeurosis of external oblique	Aponeurosis of external oblique (lateral crus and intercrural fibers)	Aponeurosis of external oblique (intercrural fibers), with fascia of external oblique continuing onto cord as external spermatic fascia
Roof	Transversalis fascia	Musculoaponeurotic arches of internal oblique and transverse abdominal	Medial crus of aponeurosis of external oblique
Floor	Iliopubic tract	Inguinal ligament	Lacunar ligament

Figure 2.13. Formation of the inguinal canals and descent of testes. A. In a 7-week embryo, the testis has not yet descended from the posterior abdominal wall. **B.** A fetus at 28 weeks (seventh month) shows the processus vaginalis and the testis passing through the inguinal canal. The processus vaginalis carries fascial layers of the abdominal wall before it. Observe that the testis passes posterior to the processus vaginalis, not through it. **C.** In a newborn infant, obliteration of the stalk of the processus vaginalis has occurred. The remains of the processus vaginalis have formed the tunica vaginalis of the testis, and the remnant of the gubernaculum has formed the scrotal ligament or disappeared.

Sagittal section to right of midline

(A) Seventh week

(B) Seventh month

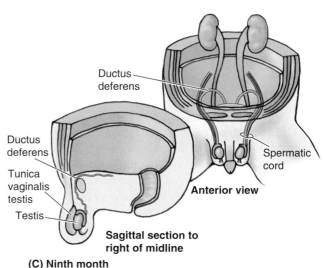

(C) Ninth month

traverses the developing inguinal canal, carrying muscular and fascial layers of the anterolateral abdominal wall before it as it enters the **primordial scrotum.** By the 12th week of development, the testis is in the pelvis, and by 28 weeks (7th month) it lies close to the developing deep inguinal ring (Fig. 2.13*B*). The testis begins to pass through the inguinal canal during the 28th week and takes approximately 3 days to traverse it. Approximately 4 weeks later, the testis enters the scrotum (Fig. 2.13*C*). As the testis, its duct (the *ductus deferens*), and its vessels and nerves descend, they are ensheathed by musculofascial extensions of the anterolateral abdominal wall, which account for the presence of their derivatives in the adult scrotum: the internal and external spermatic fasciae and cremaster muscle (Fig. 2.12). The stalk of the processus vaginalis normally degenerates; however, its distal saccular part

forms the **tunica vaginalis testis,** the serous sheath of the testis and epididymis.

The **ovaries** also develop in the superior lumbar region of the posterior abdominal wall and migrate to the lateral wall of the pelvis (Fig. 2.14). The processus vaginalis of the peritoneum traverses the transversalis fascia at the site of the deep inguinal ring, forming the inguinal canal as in the male, and protrudes into the developing labium majus.

The **female gubernaculum,** a fibrous cord connecting the ovary and primordial uterus to the developing labium majus, is represented postnatally by the **ovarian ligament,** between the ovary and the uterus, and the **round ligament of the uterus** (L. *ligamentum teres uteri*), between the uterus and the labium majus. Because of the attachment of the ovarian ligaments to the uterus, the ovaries do not descend to the inguinal region; however, the round ligament passes through the inguinal canal and attaches to the subcutaneous tissue of the labium majus (Fig. 2.14*B* & *C*).

Except for its most inferior part, which becomes a serous sac engulfing the testis, the *tunica vaginalis,* the processus vaginalis usually obliterates by the 6th month of fetal development. (For a review of the embryology of the female genital tract, see Moore and Persaud, 2003.) The inguinal canals in females are narrower than those in males, and the canals in

infants of both sexes are shorter and much less oblique than in adults. The superficial inguinal rings in infants lie almost directly anterior to the deep inguinal rings.

The Inguinal Canal and Increased Intra-Abdominal Pressure. The deep and superficial inguinal rings in the adult do not overlap because of the oblique path of the inguinal canal. Consequently, increases in intra-abdominal pressure act on the inguinal canal, forcing the posterior wall of the canal against the anterior wall and strengthening this

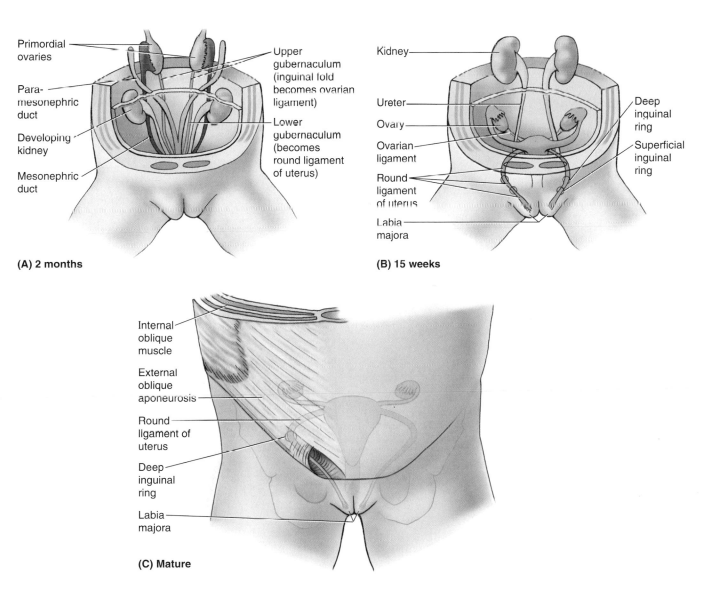

(A) 2 months

(B) 15 weeks

(C) Mature

Anterior views

Figure 2.14. Formation of inguinal canals in females. A. The undifferentiated gonads (primordial ovaries) at 2 months are located on the dorsal abdominal wall. **B.** The ovaries at 15 weeks have descended into the greater pelvis. The gubernaculum has become the ovarian ligament and round ligament of the uterus. The processus vaginalis (not shown) passes through the abdominal wall forming the inguinal canal on each side as in the male fetus. The round ligament passes through the canal and attaches to the subcutaneous tissue of the labium majus. **C.** In the mature female, the processus vaginalis has degenerated but the round ligament and ilioinguinal nerve (not shown) pass through the inguinal canal.

wall, thereby decreasing the likelihood of herniation until the pressures overcome the resistant effect of this mechanism. Simultaneously, contraction of the external oblique approximates the anterior wall of the canal to the posterior wall. It also increases tension on the medial and lateral crura, resisting enlargement (dilation) of the superficial inguinal ring. Contraction of the musculature that forms the lateral part of the arcades of the internal oblique and transverse abdominal muscles makes the roof of the canal descend, constricting the canal (Fig. 2.12C).

Maldescent of Testis

The testes are undescended in approximately 3% of full-term and 30% of premature infants (Moore and Persaud, 2003). About 95% of maldescended testes occur unilaterally. If a testis has not descended or is not retractable (capable of being drawn down), the condition is *cryptorchidism* (G. *orchis*, testis + L. from G. *kryptos*, hidden). The undescended testis usually lies somewhere along the normal path of its prenatal descent, commonly in the inguinal canal. The importance of cryptorchidism is a greatly increased risk for developing malignancy in the undescended testis, particularly problematic because it is not palpable and is not usually detected until cancer has progressed.

Cancer of the Uterus and Labium Majus

Lymphogenous metastasis of cancer most commonly occurs along lymphatic pathways that parallel the venous drainage of the organ that is the site of the primary tumor. This is also true of the uterus, the veins and lymph vessels of which mostly drain via deep routes. However, some lymphatic vessels follow the course of the round ligament through the inguinal canal. Thus, while occurring less often, metastatic uterine cancer cells (especially from tumors adjacent to the proximal attachment of the round ligament) can spread from the uterus to the labium majus (the developmental homologue of the scrotum and site of distal attachment of the round ligament) and from there to the superficial inguinal nodes, which receive lymph from the skin of the perineum (including the labia). ✪

THE BOTTOM LINE: The inguinal region extends from the ASIS to the pubic tubercle, its superficial inguinal fold demarcating the abdomen from the lower limb. It lies within the L1 dermatome. Most of the structures and formations of the region relate to a double (bilaminar) retinaculum formed by the inguinal ligament and iliopubic

tract as they extend between the two bony points. These two bands are thickenings of the inferior margins of the external (external oblique aponeurosis) and internal (transversalis fascia) layers of the abdominal wall, respectively (the integumentary and peritoneal coverings excluded).

To allow the testis to descend prenatally to a subcutaneous location that will be cooler postnatally (a requirement for the development of sperms), the inguinal canal traverses the abdominal wall superior and parallel to the medial half of the inguinal ligament. In females, only the inferior portion of the gubernaculum traverses the canal, becoming the round ligament of the uterus. The canal itself consists of a deep ring internally, a superficial ring externally, and two musculoaponeurotic arches in between. The oblique passageway through the offset rings and arches collapses when intra-abdominal pressure increases. Collapse of the canal, combined with the prenatal occlusion of the peritoneal evagination (processus vaginalis) and the contraction of the arches, normally resists the tendency for abdominal contents to herniate (protrude through) the canal. However, failure of the processus vaginalis to occlude, or defective anatomy, or degeneration of tissues may result in the development of inguinal hernias.

Spermatic Cord

The **spermatic cord** contains structures running to and from the testis and suspends the testis in the scrotum (Fig. 2.12 and Table 2.6). The spermatic cord begins at the deep inguinal ring lateral to the inferior epigastric vessels, passes through the inguinal canal, exits at the superficial inguinal ring, and ends in the scrotum at the posterior border of the testis. Fascial coverings derived from the anterolateral abdominal wall during prenatal development surround the spermatic cord.

The coverings of the spermatic cord include the following:

- **Internal spermatic fascia:** derived from the transversalis fascia.

- **Cremasteric fascia:** derived from the fascia of both the superficial and the deep surfaces of the internal oblique muscle.

- **External spermatic fascia:** derived from the external oblique aponeurosis and its investing fascia.

The cremasteric fascia contains loops of the **cremaster muscle**, which is formed by the lowermost fascicles of the internal oblique muscle arising from the inguinal ligament (Figs. 2.7 and 2.12A). The cremaster muscle reflexively draws the testis superiorly in the scrotum, particularly in response to cold. In a warm environment, such as a hot bath, the cremaster relaxes and the testis descends deeply in the scrotum. Both responses occur in an attempt to regulate the temperature of the testis for **spermatogenesis** (formation of sperms), which requires a constant temperature approximately one degree cooler than

Table 2.6. Corresponding Layers of the Anterior Abdominal Wall, Scrotum, and Spermatic Cord

Layers of Anterior Abdominal Wall
- Skin
- Subcutaneous tissue or superficial fascia
- External oblique muscle
- Internal oblique muscle
- Fascia of both superficial and deep surfaces of the internal oblique muscle
- Transverse abdominal muscle
- Transversalis fascia
- Extraperitoneal fat
- Peritoneum

Medial umbilical fold

Inferior epigastric vessels

Testicular artery and vein and ductus deferens

Obliterated umbilical artery

Urinary bladder

Conjoint tendon

Membranous layer (Scarpa) } Subcutaneous tissue (dartos fascia)

Fatty layer (Camper)

Deep inguinal ring formed by transversalis fascia

Cremasteric vessels

Intercrural fibers

Superficial inguinal ring

Scrotum and Coverings of Testis
- Skin
- Subcutaneous tissue (dartos fascia) and dartos muscle
- External spermatic fascia
- Cremaster muscle
- Cremasteric fascia
- Internal spermatic fascia
- Tunica vaginalis | Parietal layer
- | Visceral layer (covering testis and epididymis

Coverings of Spermatic Cord
- Scrotum (and scrotal septum)
- External spermatic fascia
- Cremaster muscle
- Cremasteric fascia
- Internal spermatic fascia
- Vestige of processus vaginalis

Pampiniform plexus of veins

Testicular artery

Ductus deferens

core temperature, or during sexual activity as a protective response. The cremaster typically acts coincidentally with the **dartos muscle,** smooth muscle of the fat-free subcutaneous tissue of the scrotum (the *dartos fascia*), which inserts into the skin, assisting testicular elevation as it produces contraction of the skin of the scrotum in response to the same stimuli. The cremaster is innervated by the **genital branch of the genitofemoral nerve** (L1, L2), a derivative of the lumbar plexus (Fig 2.15). The cremaster is striated muscle receiving somatic innervation, whereas the dartos is smooth muscle receiving autonomic innervation. Although less well developed and usually indistinct, the round ligament of the female receives similar contributions from the layers of the abdominal wall as it traverses the canal.

The constituents of the spermatic cord are the following (Figs. 2.15 and 2.16; Table 2.6):

- **Ductus deferens** or deferent duct: a muscular tube approximately 45 cm long that conveys sperms from the epididymis to the ejaculatory duct.

- **Testicular artery:** arising from the aorta and supplying the testis and epididymis.

- **Artery of the ductus deferens:** arising from the inferior vesical artery.

- *Cremasteric artery:* arising from the inferior epigastric artery.

- *Pampiniform venous plexus:* a network formed by up to 12 veins that converge superiorly as right or left testicular veins.

- Sympathetic *nerve fibers* on arteries and sympathetic and parasympathetic nerve fibers: on the ductus deferens.

- *Genital branch of the genitofemoral nerve:* supplying the cremaster muscle.

- *Lymphatic vessels:* draining the testis and closely associated structures and passing to the lumbar lymph nodes.

- **Vestige of the processus vaginalis:** may be seen as a fibrous thread in the anterior part of the spermatic cord extending between the abdominal peritoneum and the tunica vaginalis; it may not be detectable.

Because it is a not a homolog of the spermatic cord, the round ligament does not contain comparable structures. It includes only vestiges of the lower part of the ovarian gubernaculum and the processus vaginalis.

Anterior view

Lymphatic drainage
———————▶ From testis
• • • • • • • •▶ From scrotum

Figure 2.15. Arterial supply and lymphatic drainage of testis and scrotum; innervation of scrotum. The course of the testicular artery, arising from the abdominal aorta near the renal artery, results from the descent of the fetal testis from the posterior abdominal wall into the scrotum. Lymph draining from the testis and scrotum follow different courses. The anterior aspect of the scrotum is innervated by branches of the lumbar plexus that pass anteriorly to reach it, whereas the posterior aspect of the scrotum is innervated from branches of the sacral plexus that pass posteriorly.

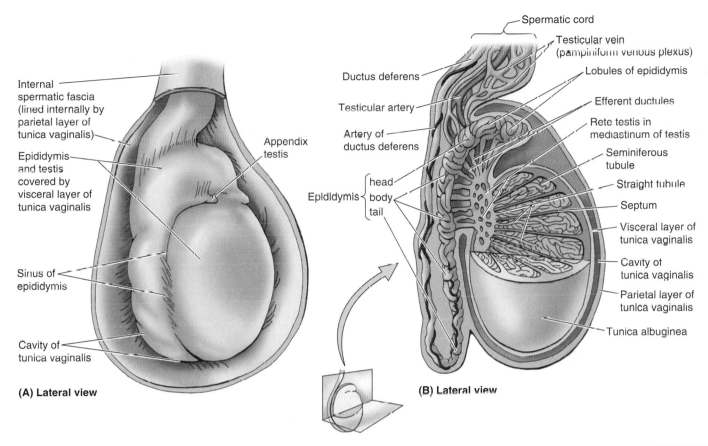

Figure 2.16. Structures of testis and epididymis. A. The distal part of the spermatic cord, the epididymis, and most of the testis are covered by the two layers of the tunica vaginalis: the visceral layer, which directly covers these structures, and the outer parietal layer, which lines the internal spermatic fascia (cut open). The two layers are separated by the collapsed cavity (opened in part **A** and highly exaggerated in part **B**) of the tunica vaginalis. **B.** Features of the testis, epididymis, and distal spermatic cord are shown. A quarter-section of the testis has been removed.

Inguinal Hernias

An **inguinal hernia** (rupture) is a protrusion of parietal peritoneum and viscera, such as the small intestine, through a normal or abnormal opening from the cavity in which they belong. Most hernias are reducible, meaning that they can be returned to their normal place in the peritoneal cavity by appropriate manipulation. Between 80% and 90% of abdominal hernias are in the inguinal region; the two main types are *direct* and *indirect inguinal hernias*. More than two thirds are indirect hernias. Characteristics of direct and indirect inguinal hernias are listed and illustrated in Table B2.1, with related anatomy illustrated in Fig. B2.3*A–C*.

Normally, most of the processus vaginalis obliterates before birth, except for the distal part that forms the tunica vaginalis of the testis (Table 2.6). The peritoneal part of the hernial sac of an indirect inguinal hernia is formed by the persisting processus vaginalis. If the entire stalk of the processus vaginalis persists, the hernia extends into the scrotum superior to the testis, forming a complete indirect inguinal hernia (Table B2.1).

The superficial inguinal ring is palpable superolateral to the pubic tubercle by invaginating the skin of the upper scrotum with the index finger (Fig. B2.3*D*). The examiner's finger follows the spermatic cord superolaterally to the superficial inguinal ring. If the ring is dilated, it may admit the finger without causing pain. Should a hernia be present, a sudden impulse is felt against either the tip or pad of the examining finger when the patient is asked to cough (Swartz, 2001). However, because both inguinal hernia types exit the superficial ring, palpation of an impulse at this site does not discriminate type. With the palmar surface of the finger against the anterior abdominal wall, the *deep inguinal ring* may be felt as a skin depression superior to the inguinal ligament, 2–4 cm superolateral to the pubic tubercle. Detection of an impulse at the superficial ring and a mass at the site of the deep ring suggests an indirect hernia. Palpation of a direct inguinal hernia is performed by placing the palmar surface of the index and/or middle finger over the inguinal triangle and asking the person to cough or bear down (strain). If a hernia is present, a forceful impulse is felt against the pad of the ▶

Table B2.1. Characteristics of Inguinal Hernias

Peritoneum
Transversalis fascia
Transverse abdominal muscle
Internal oblique muscle
External oblique muscle
Testicular vessels entering spermatic cord
Ductus deferens
Deep inguinal ring

Direct (acquired) inguinal hernia

Lateral umbilical fold
Inguinal triangle
Medial umbilical fold
Median umbilical fold

Indirect (congenital) inguinal hernia

Ductus deferens

Herniating bowel passes MEDIAL to inferior epigastric vessels, pushing through peritoneum and transversalis fascia in inguinal triangle to enter inguinal canal.

Herniating bowel passes LATERAL to inferior epigastric vessels to enter deep inguinal ring.

Femoral artery and vein
Superficial inguinal ring
Hernial sac (parallels spermatic cord)
Spermatic cord

Loop of bowel inside cord
Hernial sac (within spermatic cord)

Characteristic	Direct (Acquired)	Indirect (Congenital)
Predisposing factors	Weakness of anterior abdominal wall in inguinal triangle (e.g., owing to distended superficial ring, narrow inguinal falx, or attenuation of aponeurosis in males >40 years of age)	Patency of processus vaginalis (complete or at least superior part) in younger persons, the great majority of which are males
Frequency	Less common (one third to one quarter of inguinal hernias)	More common (two thirds to three quarters) of inguinal hernias
Exit from abdominal cavity (Fig. B2.3A & B)	Peritoneum plus transversalis fascia (lies outside inner one or two fascial coverings of cord)	Peritoneum of persistent processus vaginalis plus all three fascial coverings of cord/round ligament
Course (Fig. B2.3C)	Passes through or around inguinal canal, usually traversing only medial third of canal, external and parallel to vestige of processus vaginalis	Traverses inguinal canal (entire canal if it is of sufficient size) within processus vaginalis
Exit from anterior abdominal wall	Via superficial ring, lateral to cord; rarely enters scrotum	Via superficial ring inside cord, commonly passing into scrotum/labium majus

(A) Anterior view

- Lateral margin of rectus abdominis muscle
- Inferior epigastric artery
- Site of deep inguinal ring
- Inguinal (Hesselbach) triangle
- Superficial inguinal ring

(B) Posterior view of right anterior abdominal wall

- Inferior epigastric artery and vein
- Rectus abdominis
- Inguinal triangle
- Iliopubic tract
- Ductus deferens

(C) Anterior view

- Direct inguinal hernia
- Indirect inguinal hernia
- Anterior superior iliac spine
- Inguinal ligament
- Deep inguinal ring
- Inguinal canal
- Superficial inguinal ring
- Scrotum

(D) Anterior view

- Anterior superior iliac spine
- Inguinal ligament
- Superficial inguinal ring

Figure B2.3.

finger. The finger can also be placed in the superficial inguinal ring; if a direct hernia is present, a sudden impulse is felt medial to the finger when the person coughs or bears down.

Cremasteric Reflex

Contraction of the cremaster muscle is elicited by lightly stroking the skin on the medial aspect of the superior part of the thigh with an applicator stick or tongue depressor. The ilioinguinal nerve supplies this area of skin. The rapid elevation of the testis on the same side is the **cremasteric reflex.** This reflex is extremely active in children; consequently, hyperactive cremasteric reflexes may simulate undescended testes. A hyperactive reflex can be abolished by having the child sit in a cross-legged, squatting position; if the testes are descended, they can then be palpated in the scrotum.

Cysts and Hernias of the Canal of Nuck

Indirect inguinal hernias can occur in women; however, they are approximately 20 times more common in men. If the processes vaginalis persists in females, it forms a small peritoneal pouch, known as the *canal of Nuck,* in the inguinal canal that may extend to the labium majus. In female infants, such remnants can enlarge and form cysts in the inguinal canal. The cysts may produce a bulge in the anterior part of the labium majus and have the potential to develop into an indirect inguinal hernia.

Hydrocele

A **hydrocele** is the presence of excess fluid in a *persistent processus vaginalis.* This congenital anomaly may be associated with an indirect inguinal hernia. The fluid ▶

(A) Hydrocele of testis   (B) Hydrocele of cord   (C) Hematocele of testis

Figure B2.4.

accumulation results from secretion of an abnormal amount of serous fluid from the visceral layer of the tunica vaginalis. The size of the hydrocele depends on how much of the processus vaginalis persists. A *hydrocele of the testis* is confined to the scrotum and distends the tunica vaginalis (Fig. B2.4*A*). A *hydrocele of the cord* is confined to the spermatic cord and distends the persistent part of the stalk of the processus vaginalis (Fig. B2.4*B*). A congenital hydrocele of the cord and testis may communicate with the peritoneal cavity.

Detection of a hydrocele requires **transillumination,** a procedure during which a bright light is applied to the side of the scrotal enlargement in a darkened room. The transmission of light as a red glow indicates excess serous fluid in the scrotum.

Newborn male infants often have residual peritoneal fluid in their tunica vaginalis; however, this fluid is usually absorbed during the 1st year of life. Certain pathological conditions, such as injury and/or inflammation of the epididymis, may also produce a hydrocele in adults—a collection of serous fluid in the tunica vaginalis of the testis.

Hematocele

A **hematocele of the testis** is a collection of blood in the tunica vaginalis that results, for example, from rupture of branches of the testicular artery by trauma to the testis (Fig. B2.4*C*). Trauma may produce a scrotal and/or testicular **hematoma** (accumulation of blood, usually clotted, in any extravascular location). Blood does not transilluminate; therefore, transillumination can differentiate a hematocele or hematoma from a hydrocele. A hematocele of the testis may be associated with a *scrotal hematocele,* resulting from effusion of blood into the scrotal tissues.

Torsion of the Spermatic Cord

Torsion (twisting) **of the spermatic cord** is a surgical emergency because the testicle may die. The torsion obstructs the venous drainage, with resultant edema and hemorrhage, and subsequent arterial obstruction. If not untwisted promptly, necrosis of the entire testicle is likely. Testicular torsion may occur at any age, but it is most common during adolescence. The twisting usually occurs just above the superior pole of the testis (Fig. B2.5). A high scrotal incision is made to approach the cord, and the testis and/or cord is rotated as necessary to reduce the torsion. To prevent recurrence or occurrence on the contralateral side, which is likely, both testes are surgically fixed to the scrotal septum. ☉

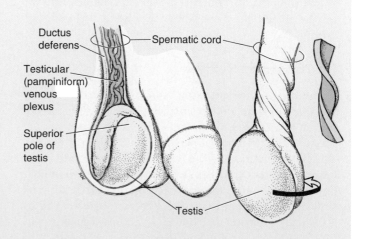

Figure B2.5.

THE BOTTOM LINE: In their passage through the inguinal canal, the processus vaginalis, testis, ductus deferens, and neurovascular structures of the testis (or processus vaginalis and lower ovarian gubernaculum of the female) become engulfed by fascial extensions derived from most (three of four) of the layers traversed. This results in a trilaminar covering. The transversalis fascia, internal oblique, and external oblique layers contribute the internal spermatic fascia, cremasteric muscle and fascia, and external spermatic fascia, respectively, to the spermatic cord. Although the portion of the processus vaginalis within the spermatic cord occludes, that adjacent to the testis remains patent as the tunica vaginalis testis. The contents of the spermatic cord are the duct and neurovascular structures, which trailed the testis as it descended from the posterior abdominal wall during development.

Scrotum

The **scrotum** is a cutaneous sac consisting of two layers: heavily pigmented skin and the closely related **dartos fascia**, a fat-free fascial layer including smooth muscle fibers (dartos muscle) responsible for the rugose (wrinkled) appearance of the scrotum (Fig. 2.8B; Table 2.6). Because the dartos muscle attaches to the skin, its contraction causes the scrotum to wrinkle when cold, thickening the integumentary layer while reducing scrotal surface area and assisting the cremaster muscles in holding the testes (testicles) closer to the body, all of which reduces heat loss.

The scrotum is divided internally by a continuation of the dartos fascia, the *septum of the scrotum*, into right and left compartments. The septum is demarcated externally by the *scrotal raphe* (see Chapter 3), a cutaneous ridge marking the line of fusion of the embryonic *labioscrotal swellings* (Moore and Persaud, 2003). The superficial dartos fascia of the scrotum is devoid of fat and is continuous anteriorly with the *membranous layer of subcutaneous tissue of the abdomen* (Scarpa fascia) and posteriorly with the *membranous layer of subcutaneous tissue of the perineum* (Colles fascia) (Fig. 2.8B).

The development of the scrotum is closely related to the formation of the inguinal canals. The scrotum develops from the *labioscrotal swellings*, two cutaneous outpouchings of the anterior abdominal wall that fuse to form a pendulous cutaneous pouch. Later in the fetal period, the testes and spermatic cords enter the scrotum.

The arterial supply of the scrotum (Fig. 2.15) is from the:

- **Posterior scrotal branches of the perineal artery:** a branch of the internal pudendal artery.

- **Anterior scrotal branches of the deep external pudendal artery:** a branch of the femoral artery.

- **Cremasteric artery:** a branch of the inferior epigastric artery.

Scrotal veins accompany the arteries. The lymphatic vessels of the scrotum drain into the superficial inguinal lymph nodes.

The nerves of the scrotum (Fig. 2.15) include branches of the lumbar plexus to the anterior surface:

- *Genital branch of the genitofemoral nerve* (L1, L2): supplying the anterolateral surface.

- **Anterior scrotal nerves:** branches of the ilioinguinal nerve (L1) supplying the anterior surface.

The nerves also include branches of the sacral plexus to the posterior and inferior surfaces:

- **Posterior scrotal nerves:** branches of the perineal branch of the **pudendal nerve** (S2–S4) supplying the posterior surface.

- **Perineal branches of the posterior femoral cutaneous nerve** (S2, S3): supplying the inferior surface.

Anesthetizing the Scrotum

The anterior third of the scrotum is supplied by the L1 segment of the spinal cord through the ilioinguinal nerve, and the posterior two thirds of the scrotum are supplied mainly by the S3 spinal segment through the perineal and posterior femoral cutaneous nerves. Therefore, when a spinal anesthetic agent is administered, it must be injected more superiorly to anesthetize the anterior surface of the scrotum than is necessary to anesthetize the posterior surface. ✪

THE BOTTOM LINE: The scrotum is the integumentary bag formed from the labioscrotal swellings of the male to house the testes after their descent. The fatty layer of subcutaneous tissue of the abdominal wall is replaced in the scrotum by the smooth dartos muscle, whereas the membranous layer is continued as the dartos fascia and scrotal septum. The scrotum receives anterior scrotal arteries from the thigh (via the external pudendal artery), posterior scrotal arteries from the perineum (internal pudendal artery), and internally cremasteric arteries from the abdomen (inferior epigastric artery). Anterior scrotal nerves are derived from the lumbar plexus (via the genitofemoral and ilioinguinal nerves) and posterior scrotal nerves from the sacral plexus (via the pudendal nerve).

Testis

The **testes** (G. *orchis*) are the male gonads—paired ovoid male reproductive glands that produce the male germ cells (**sperms, or spermatozoa**) and male hormones, primarily testosterone (Fig. 2.16). The testes are suspended in the scrotum by the spermatic cord, with the left testis (testicle) usually suspended (hanging) more inferiorly than the right testis. The testes have a tough fibrous outer surface, the **tunica albuginea,** that thickens into a ridge on its internal, posterior aspect as the **mediastinum of the testis** (Fig. 2.16*B*). From this internal ridge, fibrous septa extend inward between lobules of minute but long and highly coiled **seminiferous tubules** in which the sperms are produced. The seminiferous tubules are joined by **straight tubules** to the **rete testis** (L. *rete*, a net), a network of canals in the mediastinum of the testis.

The surface of each testis is covered by the **visceral layer of the tunica vaginalis**, except where the testis attaches to the epididymis and spermatic cord (Fig. 2.16*A*). The tunica vaginalis is a closed peritoneal sac partially surrounding the testis, which represents the closed-off distal part of the embryonic processus vaginalis. The visceral layer of the tunica vaginalis is closely applied to the testis, epididymis, and inferior part of the ductus deferens. The slit-like recess of the tunica vaginalis, the **sinus of the epididymis**, is between the body of the epididymis and the posterolateral surface of the testis. The **parietal layer of the tunica vaginalis**, adjacent to the internal spermatic fascia, is more extensive than the visceral layer and extends superiorly for a short distance into the distal part of the spermatic cord. The small amount of fluid in the cavity of the tunica vaginalis separates the visceral and parietal layers, allowing the testis to move freely in the scrotum.

The long and slender **testicular arteries** arise from the anterolateral aspect of the *abdominal aorta* just inferior to the *renal arteries* (Figs. 2.15 and 2.16*B*). They pass retroperitoneally (posterior to the peritoneum) in an oblique direction, crossing over the ureters and the inferior parts of the external iliac arteries to reach the deep inguinal rings. They enter the inguinal canals through the deep rings, pass through the canals, exit them through the superficial inguinal rings, and enter the spermatic cords to supply the testes. The testicular artery or one of its branches anastomoses with the *artery of the ductus deferens*.

The veins emerging from the testis and epididymis form the **pampiniform venous plexus**, a network of 8–12 veins lying anterior to the ductus deferens and surrounding the testicular artery in the spermatic cord. The pampiniform plexus is part of the thermoregulatory system of the testis (along with the cremasteric and dartos muscles) helping keep this gland at a constant temperature. The veins of each pampiniform plexus converge superiorly, forming a **right testicular vein**, which enters the inferior vena cava (IVC), and a **left testicular vein**, which enters the left renal vein.

The lymphatic drainage of the testis follows the testicular artery and vein to the **right** and **left lumbar** (**caval/aortic**) and **preaortic lymph nodes** (Fig. 2.15). The autonomic nerves of the testis arise as the **testicular plexus of nerves** on the testicular artery, which contains vagal parasympathetic and visceral afferent fibers and sympathetic fibers from the T7 segment of the spinal cord.

Epididymis

The **epididymis** is an elongated structure on the posterior surface of the testis (Fig. 2.16). **Efferent ductules** of the testis transport newly developed sperms to the epididymis from the rete testis. The epididymis is formed by minute convolutions of the **duct of the epididymis**, so tightly compacted that they appear solid (Fig. 2.16*B*). The duct becomes progressively smaller as it passes from the head of the epididymis on the superior part of the testis to its tail. At the tail of the epididymis, the ductus deferens begins as the continuation of the epididymal duct. In the lengthy course of this convoluted duct, the sperms are stored and continue to mature. The epididymis consists of the:

- **Head of the epididymis:** the superior expanded part that is composed of lobules formed by the coiled ends of 12–14 *efferent ductules.*

- **Body of the epididymis:** consists of the convoluted duct of the epididymis.

- **Tail of the epididymis:** continuous with the ductus deferens, the duct that transports the sperm from the epididymis to the ejaculatory duct for expulsion via the urethra during ejaculation (see Chapter 3).

Spermatocele and Epididymal Cyst

A **spermatocele** is a retention cyst (collection of fluid) in the epididymis (Fig. B2.6*A*), usually near its head. Spermatoceles contain a milky fluid and are generally asymptomatic. An **epididymal cyst** is a collection of fluid anywhere in the epididymis (Fig. B2.6*B*).

Vestigial Remnants of Embryonic Genital Ducts

When the tunica vaginalis is opened, rudimentary structures may be observed at the superior extremities of the testes and epididymis (Fig. B2.7). These structures are small remnants of genital ducts in the embryo (Moore and Persaud, 2003). They are rarely observed unless pathological changes occur. The *appendix of the testis* is a vesicular remnant of the cranial end of the paramesonephric duct, the embryonic genital duct that in the female forms half of the uterus. It is attached to the superior pole of the testis. The *appendices of the epididymis* are remnants of the cranial end of the mesonephric duct, the embryonic genital duct that in the male forms part of the ductus deferens, which are attached to the head of the epididymis. This part of the duct, together with the mesonephric tubules associated with it, normally forms the efferent ductules and epididymis.

Varicocele

The vine-like pampiniform plexus of veins may become dilated (varicose) and tortuous, producing a **varicocele,** which is usually visible only when the man is ▶

Spermatocele

Head of epididymis

Epididymal cyst

Head of epididymis

Testis covered by visceral layer of tunica vaginalis

Tootio

(A)

(B)

Lateral views

Figure B2.6. A. Spermatocele. **B.** Epididymal cyst.

standing or straining (the enlargement usually disappears when the person lies down, particularly if the scrotum is elevated while supine, allowing gravity to empty the veins). Palpating a varicocele can be likened to feeling a bag of worms. Varicoceles may result from defective valves in the testicular vein, but kidney or renal vein problems can also result in distension of the pampiniform veins. Consequently, it is necessary to rule out kidney or other abdominal causes of varicocele.

Varicocele occurs predominantly (99%) on the left side, probably because the acute angle at which the right vein enters the IVC is more favorable to flow than the nearly right angle at which the left testicular vein enters the left renal vein, making it more susceptible to obstruction or reversal of flow. Patients with the sudden onset of a varicocele, a right-sided varicocele, or a varicocele that does not reduce in size in the supine position should be suspected of having a retroperitoneal neoplasm in the region of termination of the testicular vein.

Cancer of the Testis and Scrotum

Lymphogenous metastasis is common to all testicular tumors, so a knowledge of lymphatic drainage is helpful in treatment (Cotran et al., 1999). Because the testes descend from the posterior abdominal wall to the scrotum during fetal development, their lymphatic drainage differs from that of the scrotum, which is an outpouching of anterolateral abdominal skin (Fig. 2.15). Consequently:

• **Cancer of the testis:** metastasizes initially to the retroperitoneal *lumbar lymph nodes,* which lie just inferior to the renal veins; subsequent spread may be to mediastinal and supraclavicular nodes.

• **Cancer of the scrotum:** metastasizes to the *superficial inguinal lymph nodes,* which lie in the subcutaneous tissue inferior to the inguinal ligament and along the terminal part of the great saphenous vein.

However, metastasis of testicular cancer may also occur by hematogenous spread to the lungs, liver, brain, and bone. ☉

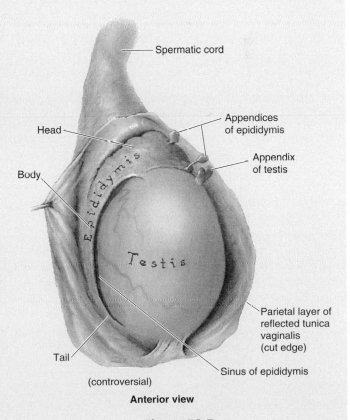

Spermatic cord

Appendices of epididymis

Head

Appendix of testis

Body

Epididymis

Testis

Parietal layer of reflected tunica vaginalis (cut edge)

Tail

Sinus of epididymis

(controversial)

Anterior view

Figure B2.7.

THE BOTTOM LINE: The mature testis is the male gonad, shaped and sized like a large olive or small plum, that produces sperms and male hormones. It is engulfed, except posteriorly and superiorly, by a double-layered serous sac, derived developmentally from the peritoneum, the tunica vaginalis. The outer surface is covered with the fibrous tunica albuginea, which is thickened internally and posteriorly as the mediastinum of the testis from which septa radiate. Between the septa are the loops of fine seminiferous tubules in which the sperms develop. The tubules converge and empty into the rete testis in the mediastinum, which is connected in turn to the epididymis by the efferent ductules. The innervation, blood vasculature, and lymphatic drainage all reflect the posterior abdominal origin of the testis and are, for the main part, independent of the surrounding scrotal sac.

The epididymis is formed of the highly convoluted and compacted epididymal duct leading from the efferent ductules to the ductus deferens. It is the site of sperm storage and maturation. The epididymis clings to the more protected superior and posterior aspects of the testis.

Surface Anatomy of the Anterolateral Abdominal Wall

The **umbilicus** is an obvious feature of the anterolateral abdominal wall and is the reference point for the **transumbilical plane** (Fig. SA2.1). This puckered indentation of skin in the center of the anterior abdominal wall is typically at the level of the IV disc between the L3 and L4 vertebrae; however, its position varies with the amount of subcutaneous fat present. It indicates the level of the T10 dermatome. The **epigastric fossa** (pit of the stomach) is a slight depression in the epigastric region, just inferior to the **xiphoid process.** This fossa is particularly noticeable when a person is in the supine position because the abdominal organs spread out, drawing the anterolateral abdominal wall posteriorly in this region. The pain caused by pyrosis ("heartburn," resulting from reflux of gastric acid into the esophagus) is often felt at this site. The 7th–10th costal cartilages unite on each side of the epigastric fossa, their medial borders forming the *costal margin.* Although the abdominal cavity extends higher, the costal margin is the demarcation between the thoracic and abdominal portions of the body wall. When a person is in the supine position, observe the rise and fall of the abdominal wall with respiration: superiorly with inspiration and inferiorly with expiration. The rectus abdominis muscles can be palpated and observed when a supine person is asked to raise the head and shoulders against resistance.

The location of the **linea alba** is visible because of the vertical skin groove superficial to this raphe. The groove is usually obvious because the linea alba is approximately 1 cm wide between the two parts of the rectus abdominis superior to the umbilicus. Inferior to the umbilicus, the linea ▶

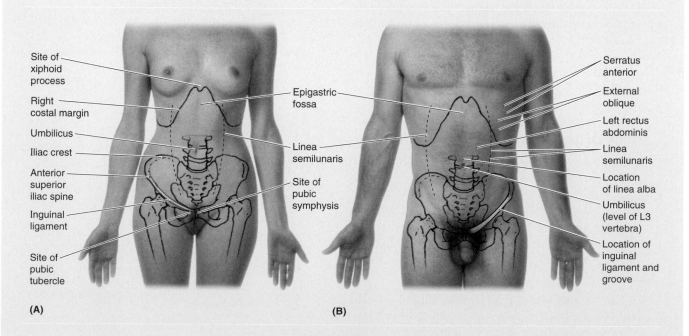

(A)

(B)

Figure SA2.1.

alba is not indicated by a groove. Some pregnant women, especially those with dark hair and a dark complexion, have a heavily pigmented line, the **linea nigra,** in the midline skin external to the linea alba. After pregnancy, the color of this line fades.

The upper margins of the pubic bones (**pubic crest**) and the cartilaginous joint that unite them (**pubic symphysis**) can be felt at the inferior end of the linea alba. The inguinal folds are shallow oblique grooves overlying the inguinal ligaments as they extend between the **anterior superior iliac spines** (ASIS) and the **pubic tubercles.** The bony **iliac crest** at the level of L4 vertebra can be easily palpated as it extends posteriorly from the ASIS. The pubic crest, inguinal folds, and iliac crests demarcate the inferior limit of the anterior abdominal wall, distinguishing it from the perineum centrally and the lower limbs (thigh) laterally.

The **semilunar lines** (L. *lineae semilunares*) are slightly curved, linear impressions in the skin that extend from the inferior costal margin near the 9th costal cartilages to the pubic tubercles. These semilunar skin grooves (5–8 cm from the midline) are clinically important because they are parallel with the lateral edges of the rectus sheath. Skin grooves also overlie the **tendinous intersections** of the rectus abdominis, which are clearly visible in persons with well-developed rectus muscles. The interdigitating bellies of the *serratus anterior* and *external oblique* muscles are also visible. The site of the inguinal ligament is indicated by the **inguinal groove,** a skin crease that is parallel and just inferior to the inguinal ligament, which is readily visualized by having the person drop one leg to the floor while lying supine on an examining table. The inguinal groove marks the division between the anterolateral abdominal wall and the thigh. ○

Peritoneum and Peritoneal Cavity

The **peritoneum** is a continuous, glistening and slippery transparent serous membrane. It lines the abdominopelvic cavity and invests the viscera (Fig. 2.17). The peritoneum consists of two continuous layers: the **parietal peritoneum,** which lines the internal surface of the abdominopelvic wall, and the **visceral peritoneum,** which invests viscera such as the stomach and intestines. Both layers of peritoneum consist of *mesothelium,* a layer of simple squamous epithelial cells.

The *parietal peritoneum* is served by the same blood and lymphatic vasculature and the same somatic nerve supply as is the region of the wall it lines. Like the overlying skin, the peritoneum lining the interior of the body wall is sensitive to pressure, pain, heat and cold, and laceration. Pain from the parietal peritoneum is generally well localized, except for that on the inferior surface of the central part of the diaphragm, where innervation is provided by the phrenic nerve (discussed later in this chapter); irritation here is often referred to the C3–C5 dermatomes over the shoulder.

The *visceral peritoneum* and the organs it covers are served by the same blood and lymphatic vasculature and visceral nerve supply. The visceral peritoneum is insensitive to touch, heat and cold, and laceration; it is stimulated primarily by stretching and chemical irritation. The pain produced is poorly localized, being referred to the dermatomes of the spinal ganglia providing the sensory fibers, particularly to midline portions of these dermatomes. Consequently, pain from foregut derivatives is usually experienced in the epigastric region, that from midgut derivatives in the umbilical region, and that from hindgut derivatives in the pubic region.

The peritoneum and viscera are in the abdominopelvic cavity. The relationship of the viscera to the peritoneum is as follows:

- *Intraperitoneal organs* are almost completely covered with visceral peritoneum (e.g., the stomach and spleen). *Intraperitoneal* in this case does *not* mean inside the peritoneal cavity (although the term is used clinically for substances injected into this cavity). Intraperitoneal organs have conceptually, if not literally, invaginated into the closed sac, like pressing your fist into an inflated balloon (see the discussion of potential spaces in the Introduction).

- *Extraperitoneal, retroperitoneal,* and *subperitoneal organs* are also outside the peritoneal cavity—external, posterior, or inferior to the parietal peritoneum—and are only partially covered with peritoneum (usually on just one surface). Organs such as the kidneys are between the parietal peritoneum and the posterior abdominal wall and have parietal peritoneum only on their anterior surfaces (unless fat intervenes). Similarly, the urinary bladder has parietal peritoneum only on its superior surface.

The **peritoneal cavity** is within the abdominal cavity and continues inferiorly into the pelvic cavity. The peritoneal cavity is a potential space of capillary thinness between the parietal and visceral layers of peritoneum. It contains no organs but contains a thin film of **peritoneal fluid,** which is composed of water, electrolytes, and other substances derived from interstitial fluid in adjacent tissues. Peritoneal fluid lubricates the peritoneal surfaces, enabling the viscera to move over each other without friction and allowing the movements of digestion. In addition to lubricating the surfaces of the viscera, the peritoneal fluid contains leukocytes and antibodies that resist infection. Lymphatic vessels, particularly on the inferior

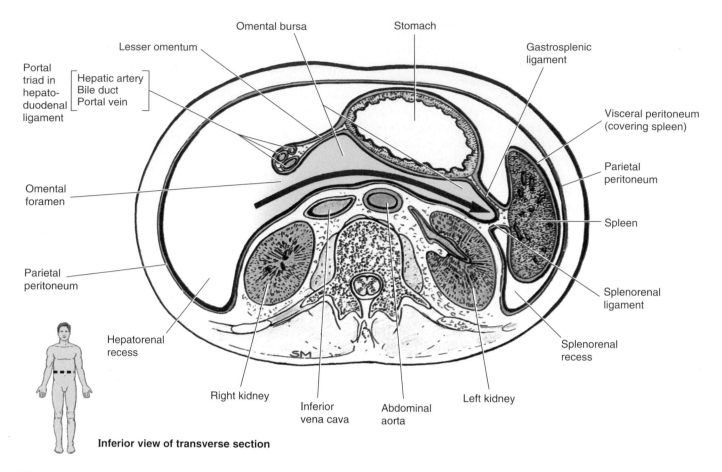

Figure 2.17. Transverse section of abdomen at level of omental bursa. The orientation figure indicates the level of the section superficially. The *dark arrow* passes from the greater sac of the peritoneal cavity through the omental (epiploic) foramen and across the full extent of the omental bursa (lesser sac).

surface of the unceasingly active diaphragm, absorb the peritoneal fluid. The peritoneal cavity is completely closed in males; however, there is a communication pathway in females to the exterior of the body through the uterine tubes, uterine cavity, and vagina. This communication constitutes a potential pathway of infection from the exterior.

Patency and Blockage of the Uterine Tubes

While theoretically it is possible for organisms to enter the female peritoneal cavity directly via the uterine tubes, such primary peritonitis is rare, bearing testimony to the effectiveness of the protective mechanisms of the female reproductive tract. A primary mechanism in preventing such infection is a *mucous plug* that effectively (but not literally) blocks the external opening of the uterus. However, for fertilization to occur, the pathway from the peritoneal cavity to the vaginal orifice must be patent. The patency of the uterine tubes can be tested clinically by means of a technique in which air or radiopaque dye is injected into the uterine cavity, from which it normally flows through the uterine tubes and into the peritoneal cavity (*hysterosalpingography;* see Chapter 3).

The Peritoneum and Surgical Procedures

Because the peritoneum is well innervated, patients undergoing abdominal surgery experience more pain with large, invasive, open incisions of the peritoneum (*laparotomy*) than they do with small, laparoscopic incisions or vaginal operations.

It is the covering of peritoneum (often referred to clinically as the *serosa*) that makes watertight end-to-end anastomoses of intraperitoneal organs, such as the small intestine, relatively easy to achieve. It is more difficult to achieve watertight anastomoses of extraperitoneal structures that have an outer adventitial layer, such as the thoracic esophagus.

Because of the high incidence of complications such as peritonitis and adhesions (see clinical correlation [blue] ▶

box "Peritoneal Adhesions and Adhesiotomy," on this page) after operations in which the peritoneal cavity is opened, efforts are made to remain outside the peritoneal cavity whenever possible (e.g., translumbar or extraperitoneal anterior approach to the kidneys). When opening the peritoneal cavity is necessary, great effort is made to avoid contamination of the cavity.

Peritonitis and Ascites

When bacterial contamination occurs during laparotomy or when the gut is traumatically penetrated or ruptured as the result of infection and inflammation (as in appendicitis), allowing gas, fecal matter, and bacteria to enter the peritoneal cavity, the result is infection and inflammation of the peritoneum, called **peritonitis**. Exudation of serum, fibrin, cells, and pus into the peritoneal cavity occurs, accompanied by pain in the overlying skin and an increase in the tone of the anterolateral abdominal muscles. Given the extent of the peritoneal surfaces and the rapid absorption of material, including bacterial toxins, from the peritoneal cavity, when a peritonitis becomes *generalized* (widespread in the peritoneal cavity), the condition is dangerous and perhaps lethal. In addition to the severe abdominal pain, tenderness, nausea and/or vomiting, fever, and constipation are present.

General peritonitis occurs not only as a result of infection but also when an ulcer perforates the wall of the stomach or duodenum, spilling acid content into the peritoneal cavity. Excess fluid in the peritoneal cavity is called **ascitic fluid**. The clinical condition in which one has ascitic fluid is referred to as *ascites*. Ascites may also occur as a result of mechanical injury (which may also produce internal bleeding) or other pathological conditions, such as portal hypertension (venous congestion), widespread metastasis of cancer cells to the abdominal viscera, and starvation (when plasma proteins fail to be produced, altering concentration gradients and producing a paradoxically protuberant abdomen). In all these cases, the peritoneal cavity may be distended with several liters of abnormal fluid, interfering with movements of the viscera.

Rhythmic movements of the anterolateral abdominal wall normally accompany respirations. If the abdomen is drawn in as the chest expands (*paradoxical abdominothoracic rhythm*) and muscle rigidity is present, either peritonitis or pneumonitis (inflammation of the lungs) may be present. Because the intense pain worsens with movement, people with peritonitis commonly lie with their knees flexed to relax their anterolateral abdominal muscles and breath shallowly (and hence more rapidly) reducing the intra-abdominal pressure and pain.

Peritoneal Adhesions and Adhesiotomy

If the peritoneum is damaged, by a stab wound for example, or infected, the peritoneal surfaces become inflamed, making them sticky with *fibrin*. As healing occurs, the fibrin may be replaced with fibrous tissue, forming abnormal attachments between the visceral peritoneum of adjacent viscera or between the visceral peritoneum of a viscus and the parietal peritoneum of the adjacent abdominal wall. **Adhesions** (scar tissue) may also form after an abdominal operation (e.g., owing to a ruptured appendix) and limit the normal movements of the viscera. This tethering may cause chronic pain or emergency complications such as intestinal obstruction when the gut becomes twisted around an adhesion (*volvulus*). *Adhesiotomy* refers to the surgical separation of adhesions. Adhesions are often found during dissection of cadavers (see the adhesion binding the spleen to the diaphragm in Fig. 2.31B, for example).

Abdominal Paracentesis

Treatment of generalized peritonitis includes removal of the ascitic fluid and, in the presence of infection, administration of large doses of antibiotics. Occasionally, more localized accumulations of fluid may have to be removed for analysis. Surgical puncture of the peritoneal cavity for the aspiration or drainage of fluid is called **paracentesis**. After injection of a local anesthetic agent, a needle or trocar and a cannula are inserted through the anterolateral abdominal wall into the peritoneal cavity through the linea alba, for example. The needle is inserted superior to the empty urinary bladder and in a location that avoids the inferior epigastric artery.

Intraperitoneal Injection and Peritoneal Dialysis

The peritoneum is a semipermeable membrane with an extensive surface area, much of which (the subdiaphragmatic portions in particular) overlies blood and lymphatic capillary beds; therefore, fluid injected into the peritoneal cavity is absorbed rapidly. For this reason, certain anesthetic agents, such as solutions of barbiturate compounds, may be injected into the peritoneal cavity by **intraperitoneal (I.P.) injection**. In renal failure, waste products such as urea accumulate in the blood and tissues and ultimately reach fatal levels. Peritoneal dialysis may be performed in which soluble substances and excess water are removed from the system by transfer across the peritoneum, using a dilute sterile solution that is introduced into the peritoneal cavity on one side and then drained from the other side. Diffusible solutes and water are transferred between the blood and ▶

the peritoneal cavity as a result of concentration gradients between the two fluid compartments. Peritoneal dialysis is usually employed only temporarily, however, because changes in the mesothelial cells of the peritoneum and in the underlying connective tissue cause it to become progressively ineffective. For the long term it is preferable to use direct blood flow through a renal dialysis machine. ⊕

Embryology of the Peritoneal Cavity

When it is initially formed, the gut is the same length as the developing body. It undergoes exuberant growth, however, to provide the large absorptive surface required by nutrition, and by the end of the 10th week of development, it is much longer than the body that contains it. For this increase in length to occur, the gut must gain freedom of movement relative to the body wall at an early stage, while still maintaining the connection with it necessary for innervation and blood supply. This growth (and later, the activity of the gut) is accommodated by the development of a serous cavity within the trunk that houses the increasingly lengthy and convoluted gut in a relatively compact space. The rate of growth of the gut initially outpaces the development of adequate space within the trunk, and for a time the rapidly lengthening gut extends outside the developing body wall (see "Brief Review of the Embryological Rotation of the Midgut," in this chapter).

Early in its development, the embryonic body cavity (*intraembryonic coelom*) is lined with *mesoderm*, the primordium of the peritoneum (Moore and Persaud, 2003). At a slightly later stage, the primordial abdominal cavity is lined with *parietal peritoneum* derived from mesoderm, which forms a closed sac. The lumen of the peritoneal sac is the *peritoneal cavity*. As the organs develop, they invaginate (protrude) to varying degrees into the peritoneal sac, acquiring a peritoneal covering, the *visceral peritoneum*. A viscus such as the kidney protrudes only partially into the peritoneal cavity; hence, it is primarily retroperitoneal, always remaining external to the peritoneal cavity and posterior to the peritoneum lining the abdominal cavity. Other viscera, such as the stomach and spleen, protrude completely into the peritoneal sac and are almost completely invested by visceral peritoneum—that is, they are *intraperitoneal*. These viscera are connected to the abdominal wall by a *mesentery* of variable length, which is composed of two layers of peritoneum with a thin layer of loose connective tissue between them. Generally, viscera that vary relatively little in size and shape, such as the kidneys, are retroperitoneal, whereas viscera that undergo marked changes in shape owing to filling, emptying and peristalsis, such as the stomach, are invested with visceral pleura. Intraperitoneal viscera with a mesentery, such as most of the small intestine, are mobile, the degree of which varies with the length of the mesentery. Although the liver and spleen do not change shape as a result of intrinsic activity (although they may slowly change in size

when engorged with blood), their need for a covering of visceral peritoneum is dictated by the need to accommodate passive changes in position imposed by the adjacent, highly active diaphragm.

As organs protrude into the peritoneal sac, their vessels, nerves, and lymphatics remain connected to their extraperitoneal (usually retroperitoneal) sources or destinations so that these connecting structures lie between the layers of the peritoneum forming their mesenteries. Initially, the entire primordial gut is suspended in the center of the peritoneal cavity by a posterior mesentery attached to the midline of the posterior body wall. As the organs grow, they gradually reduce the size of the peritoneal cavity until it is only a potential space between the parietal and the visceral layers of peritoneum. As a consequence, several parts of the gut come to lie against the posterior abdominal wall, and their posterior mesenteries become gradually reduced because of pressure from overlying organs (Fig. 2.18). For example, during development, the growing coiled mass of small intestine pushes the part of the gut that will become the descending colon to the left side and presses its mesentery against the posterior abdominal wall. The mesentery is held there until the layer of peritoneum that formed the left side of the mesentery, and the part of the visceral peritoneum of the colon lying against the body wall, fuse with the parietal peritoneum of the body wall. As a result, the colon becomes fixed to the posterior abdominal wall on the left side with peritoneum covering only its anterior aspect. The descending colon (as well as the ascending colon on the right side) has thus become *secondarily retroperitoneal*, having once been intraperitoneal.

The layers of peritoneum that fused now form a **fusion fascia,** a connective tissue plane in which the nerves and vessels of the descending colon continue to lie. Thus the descending colon of the adult can be freed from the posterior body wall (surgically mobilized) by incising the peritoneum along the lateral border of the descending colon and then bluntly dissecting along the plane of the fusion fascia, elevating the neurovascular structures from the posterior body wall until the midline is reached. The ascending colon can be similarly mobilized on the right side.

Several parts of the digestive tract and associated organs become secondarily retroperitoneal (e.g., most of the duodenum and pancreas as well as the ascending and descending parts of the colon). They are covered with peritoneum only on their anterior surface. Other parts of the viscera (e.g., the sigmoid colon and spleen) retain a short mesentery. However, the roots of the short mesenteries do not remain attached to the midline but shift to the left or right by a fusion process like that described for the descending colon.

THE BOTTOM LINE: The peritoneum is a continuous, serous membrane that lines the abdominopelvic cavity (the parietal peritoneum) and the contained viscera (the visceral peritoneum). The collapsed peritoneal cavity between these layers normally contains only enough peritoneal fluid (about 50 mL) to lubricate the inner surface of the

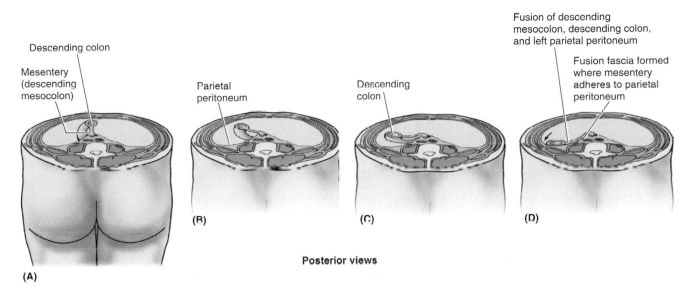

Figure 2.18. Migration and fusion of descending mesocolon. Starting from the primordial position, suspended from the midline of the posterior abdominal wall (**A**), the mesocolon shifts to the left (**B**) and gradually fuses with the left posterior parietal peritoneum (**C**). **D.** The descending colon has become secondarily retroperitoneal. The arrow indicates the left paracolic gutter, the site where an incision is made during mobilization of the colon during surgery. Sometimes the descending colon retains a short mesentery, similar to the stage shown in part **C**, especially where the colon is in the iliac fossa.

membrane. This arrangement allows the gut the freedom of movement required for alimentation. Adhesions formed as a result of infection or injury interfere with these movements. The parietal pleura is a sensitive, semipermeable membrane, with blood and lymphatic capillary beds especially abundant deep to its subdiaphragmatic surface.

Peritoneal Formations

The peritoneal cavity has a complex shape. Some of the facts relating to this include the following:

- The peritoneal cavity houses a great length of gut, most of which is covered with peritoneum.

- Extensive continuities are required between the parietal and visceral peritoneum to convey the necessary neurovascular structures from the body wall to the viscera.

- Although the volume of the abdominal cavity is a fraction of the body's volume, the parietal and visceral peritoneum lining the peritoneal cavity within it have a much greater surface area than the body's outer surface (skin); therefore, the peritoneum must be highly convoluted.

Various terms are used to describe the parts of the peritoneum that connect organs with other organs or to the abdominal wall, and the compartments and recesses that are formed as a consequence.

A **mesentery** is a double layer of peritoneum that occurs as a result of the invagination of the peritoneum by an organ and constitutes a continuity of the visceral and parietal peritoneum. It provides a means for neurovascular communica-

tion between the organ and the body wall (Fig. 2.19A & E). A mesentery connects an intraperitoneal organ to the body wall—usually the posterior abdominal wall (e.g., the mesentery of the small intestine). The small intestine mesentery is usually referred to simply as "the mesentery"; however, mesenteries related to other specific parts of the alimentary tract are named accordingly—for example, the *transverse* and *sigmoid mesocolons* (Fig. 2.19B), *mesoesophagus*, *mesogastrium*, and *mesoappendix*. Mesenteries have a core of connective tissue containing blood and lymphatic vessels, nerves, lymph nodes, and fat (Table 2.9, fig. *A*).

An **omentum** is a double-layered extension or fold of peritoneum that passes from the stomach and proximal part of the duodenum to adjacent organs in the abdominal cavity (Fig. 2.19).

- The **greater omentum** is a prominent peritoneal fold that hangs down like an apron from the greater curvature of the stomach and the proximal part of the duodenum (Fig. 2.19A, C, & E). After descending, it folds back and attaches to the anterior surface of the transverse colon and its mesentery.

- The **lesser omentum** connects the lesser curvature of the stomach and the proximal part of the duodenum to the liver (Fig. 2.19B & D); it also connects the stomach to a triad of structures that run between the duodenum and liver in the free edge of the lesser omentum (Fig. 2.17).

A **peritoneal ligament** consists of a double layer of peritoneum that connects an organ with another organ or to the abdominal wall.

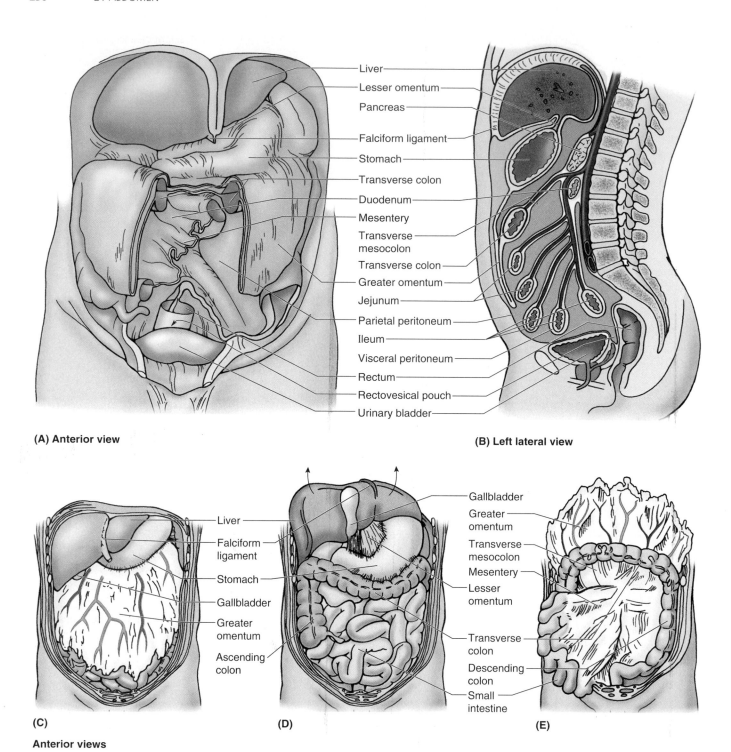

(A) Anterior view

Liver
Lesser omentum
Pancreas
Falciform ligament
Stomach
Transverse colon
Duodenum
Mesentery
Transverse mesocolon
Transverse colon
Greater omentum
Jejunum
Parietal peritoneum
Ileum
Visceral peritoneum
Rectum
Rectovesical pouch
Urinary bladder

(B) Left lateral view

Liver
Falciform ligament
Stomach
Gallbladder
Greater omentum
Ascending colon

Gallbladder
Greater omentum
Transverse mesocolon
Mesentery
Lesser omentum
Transverse colon
Descending colon
Small intestine

(C)   **(D)**   **(E)**

Anterior views

Figure 2.19. Principal formations of peritoneum. A. In this anterior view of the opened peritoneal cavity, parts of the greater omentum, transverse colon, and the small intestine and its mesentery have been cut away to reveal deep structures and the layers of the mesenteric structures. The mesentery of the jejunum and ileum (small intestine) and sigmoid mesocolon have been cut close to their parietal attachments. **B.** The median section of the abdominopelvic cavity of a male shows the relationships of the peritoneal attachments. **C.** The greater omentum is shown in its "normal" position, covering most of the abdominal viscera. **D.** The lesser omentum, attaching the liver to the lesser curvature of the stomach, is shown by reflecting the liver and gallbladder superiorly. The greater omentum has been removed from the greater curvature of the stomach and transverse colon to reveal the intestines. **E.** The greater omentum has been reflected superiorly and the small intestine has been retracted to the right side to reveal the mesentery of the small intestine and the mesentery of the transverse colon (transverse mesocolon).

The liver is connected to the:

- Anterior abdominal wall by the *falciform ligament* (Fig. 2.20).

- Stomach by the **hepatogastric ligament,** the membranous portion of the lesser omentum.

- Duodenum by the **hepatoduodenal ligament,** the thickened free edge of the lesser omentum, which conducts

the *portal triad*: portal vein, hepatic artery, and bile duct (Fig. 2.17).

The hepatogastric and hepatoduodenal ligaments are continuous parts of the lesser omentum and are separated only for descriptive convenience (Fig. 2.20).

The stomach is connected to the:

- Inferior surface of the diaphragm by the **gastrophrenic ligament.**

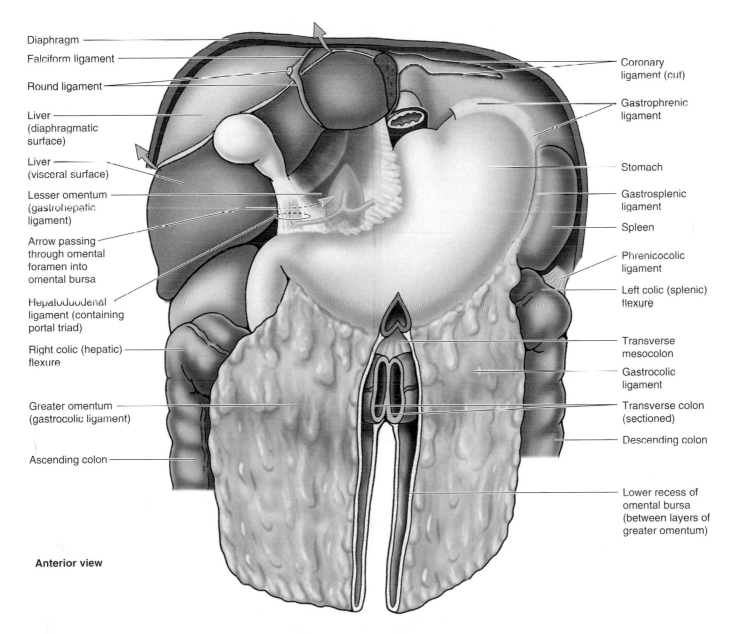

Anterior view

Figure 2.20. Parts of greater and lesser omenta. The *blue arrows* indicate that the liver and gallbladder have been reflected superiorly. The central part of the greater omentum has been cut out to show its relation to the transverse colon and mesocolon. The term *greater omentum* is often used as a synonym for the gastrocolic ligament, but it actually also includes the gastrosplenic and gastrophrenic ligaments, all of which have a continuous attachment to the greater curvature of the stomach. The hepatoduodenal ligament (free edge of the lesser omentum) conveys the portal triad: hepatic artery, bile duct, and portal vein.

- Spleen by the **gastrosplenic ligament** (gastrolienal ligament), which reflects to the hilum of the spleen.

- Transverse colon by the **gastrocolic ligament**, the apron-like part of the greater omentum, which descends from the greater curvature, turns under, and then ascends to the transverse colon.

These structures have a continuous attachment along the greater curvature, and are all part of the greater omentum, separated only for descriptive purposes.

Although intraperitoneal organs may be almost entirely covered with visceral peritoneum, every organ must have an area that is not covered to allow the entrance or exit of neurovascular structures. Such areas are called **bare areas,** formed in relation to the attachments of the peritoneal formations to the organs, including mesenteries, omenta, and ligaments that convey the neurovascular structures.

A **peritoneal fold** is a reflection of peritoneum that is raised from the body wall by underlying blood vessels, ducts, and obliterated fetal vessels (e.g., the medial and lateral *umbilical folds* on the internal surface of the anterolateral abdominal wall). Some peritoneal folds contain blood vessels and bleed if cut, such as the lateral umbilical folds, which contain the inferior epigastric arteries (see "Vessels of the Anterolateral Abdominal Wall," in this chapter).

A **peritoneal recess,** or fossa, is a pouch of peritoneum that is formed by a peritoneal fold (e.g., the inferior recess of the omental bursa between the layers of the greater omentum and the supravesical and umbilical fossae between the umbilical folds).

Functions of the Greater Omentum

The greater omentum, large and fat laden, prevents the visceral peritoneum from adhering to the parietal peritoneum. It has considerable mobility and moves around the peritoneal cavity with peristaltic movements of the viscera. It often forms adhesions adjacent to an inflamed organ such as the appendix, sometimes walling it off and thereby protecting other viscera from it. Thus it is common when entering the abdominal cavity, in either dissection or surgery, to find the omentum markedly displaced from the "normal" position in which it is almost always depicted in anatomical illustrations. The greater omentum also cushions the abdominal organs against injury and forms insulation against loss of body heat.

Abscess Formation

Perforation of a duodenal ulcer, rupture of the gallbladder, or perforation of the appendix may lead to the formation of a *circumscribed collection of purulent exudate* in the subphrenic recess. The abscess may be walled inferiorly by adhesions (see clinical correlation [blue] box "Subphrenic Abscesses," in this chapter). ▶

Spread of Pathological Fluids

Peritoneal recesses are of clinical importance in connection with the spread of pathological fluids such as pus, a product of inflammation. The recesses determine the extent and direction of the spread of fluids that may enter the peritoneal cavity when an organ is diseased or injured (see also other clinical correlation [blue] boxes in this chapter). ✪

Subdivisions of the Peritoneal Cavity

After the rotation and development of the greater curvature of the stomach during development (see clinical correlation [blue] box "Brief Review of the Embryological Rotation of the Midgut," in this chapter), the peritoneal cavity is divided into the greater and lesser peritoneal sacs (Fig. 2.21*A*). The *greater sac* is the main and larger part of the peritoneal cavity. A surgical incision through the anterolateral abdominal wall enters the greater sac. The *omental bursa* (*lesser sac*) lies posterior to the stomach and lesser omentum.

The **transverse mesocolon** (mesentery of the transverse colon) divides the abdominal cavity into a **supracolic compartment,** containing the stomach, liver, and spleen, and an **infracolic compartment,** containing the small intestine and ascending and descending colon. The infracolic compartment lies posterior to the greater omentum and is divided into *right* and *left infracolic spaces* by the *mesentery* of the small intestine (Fig. 2.21*B*). Free communication occurs between the supracolic and the infracolic compartments through the **paracolic gutters,** the grooves between the lateral aspect of the ascending or descending colon and the posterolateral abdominal wall.

Flow of Ascitic Fluid and Pus

The paracolic gutters are of considerable clinical importance because they provide pathways for the flow of ascitic fluid and the spread of intraperitoneal infections (Fig. 2.21*B*). Purulent material (consisting of or containing pus) in the abdomen can be transported along the paracolic gutters into the pelvis, especially when the person is upright. Thus, to facilitate the flow of exudate into the pelvic cavity where absorption of toxins is slow, patients with peritonitis are often placed in the sitting position (at least a 45° angle). Conversely, infections in the pelvis may extend superiorly to a subphrenic recess situated under the diaphragm (see clinical correlation [blue] box "Subphrenic Abscesses," in this chapter), especially when the person is supine. Similarly, the paracolic gutters provide pathways for the spread of tumor cells that have sloughed from the ulcerated surface of a tumor and entered the peritoneal cavity. ✪

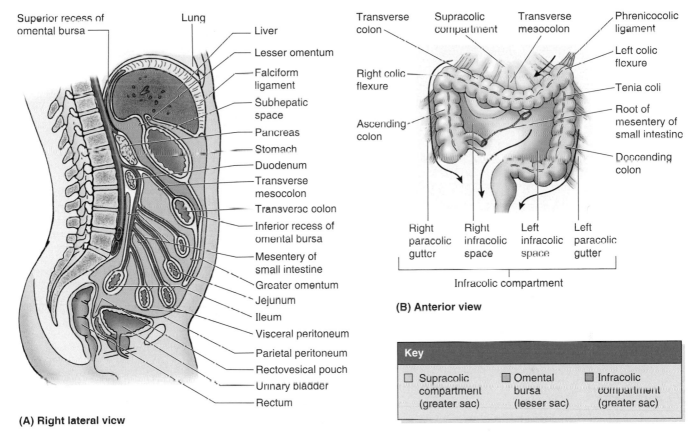

Superior recess of omental bursa — Lung — Liver — Lesser omentum — Falciform ligament — Subhepatic space — Pancreas — Stomach — Duodenum — Transverse mesocolon — Transverse colon — Inferior recess of omental bursa — Mesentery of small intestine — Greater omentum — Jejunum — Ileum — Visceral peritoneum — Parietal peritoneum — Rectovesical pouch — Urinary bladder — Rectum

(A) Right lateral view

Transverse colon — Supracolic compartment — Transverse mesocolon — Phrenicocolic ligament — Left colic flexure — Right colic flexure — Tenia coli — Ascending colon — Root of mesentery of small intestine — Descending colon — Right paracolic gutter — Right infracolic space — Left infracolic space — Left paracolic gutter — Infracolic compartment

(B) Anterior view

Key
| □ Supracolic compartment (greater sac) | □ Omental bursa (lesser sac) | ■ Infracolic compartment (greater sac) |

Figure 2.21. Subdivisions of peritoneal cavity. A. This median section of the abdominopelvic cavity shows the subdivisions of the peritoneal cavity. **B.** The supracolic and infracolic compartments of the greater sac are shown after removal of the greater omentum. The infracolic spaces and paracolic gutters determine the flow of ascitic fluid (*arrows*) when inclined or upright.

The **omental bursa** is an extensive sac-like cavity that lies posterior to the stomach, lesser omentum, and adjacent structures (Figs. 2.21*A*, 2.22*B*, and 2.23). The omental bursa has a *superior recess,* limited superiorly by the diaphragm and the posterior layers of the coronary ligament of the liver, and an *inferior recess* between the superior parts of the layers of the greater omentum (Fig. 2.23*A*). The omental bursa permits free movement of the stomach on the structures posterior and inferior to it because the anterior and posterior walls of the omental bursa slide smoothly over each other. Most of the inferior recess of the bursa becomes sealed off from the main part posterior to the stomach after adhesion of the anterior and posterior layers of the greater omentum (Fig. 2.23*B*).

The omental bursa communicates with the greater peritoneal sac through the **omental foramen** (epiploic foramen), an opening situated posterior to the free edge of the lesser omentum (hepatoduodenal ligament). The omental foramen can be located by running a finger along the gallbladder to the free edge of the lesser omentum (Fig. 2.22*A*). The omental foramen usually admits two fingers. The boundaries of the omental foramen are

• *Anteriorly:* the hepatoduodenal ligament (free edge of the lesser omentum), containing the portal vein, hepatic artery, and bile duct (Fig. 2.22*B*).

• *Posteriorly:* the IVC and right crus of the diaphragm, covered anteriorly with parietal peritoneum (they are retroperitoneal).

• *Superiorly:* the liver, covered with visceral peritoneum (Fig. 2.23).

• *Inferiorly:* the superior or first part of the duodenum.

Fluid in the Omental Bursa

Perforation of the posterior wall of the stomach results in the passage of its fluid contents into the omental bursa. An inflamed or injured pancreas can also result in the passage of pancreatic fluid into the bursa, forming a *pancreatic pseudo-cyst.*

Intestine in the Omental Bursa

Although uncommon, a loop of small intestine may pass through the omental foramen into the omental bursa and be strangulated by the edges of the foramen. As none of the boundaries of the foramen can be incised ▶

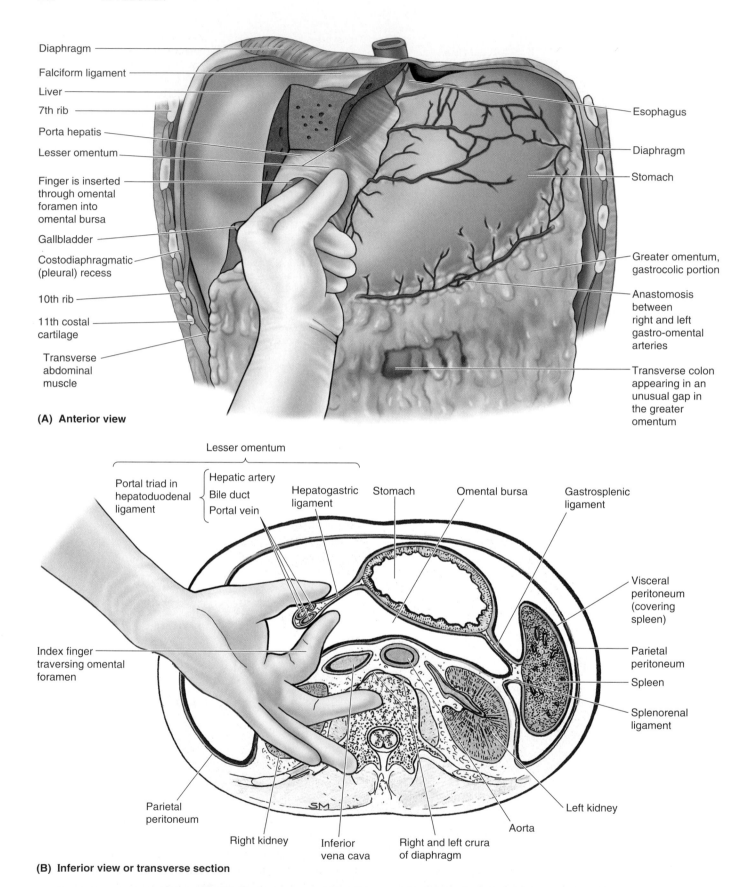

(A) Anterior view

Diaphragm
Falciform ligament
Liver
7th rib
Porta hepatis
Lesser omentum
Finger is inserted through omental foramen into omental bursa
Gallbladder
Costodiaphragmatic (pleural) recess
10th rib
11th costal cartilage
Transverse abdominal muscle

Esophagus
Diaphragm
Stomach
Greater omentum, gastrocolic portion
Anastomosis between right and left gastro-omental arteries
Transverse colon appearing in an unusual gap in the greater omentum

(B) Inferior view or transverse section

Lesser omentum
Portal triad in hepatoduodenal ligament
Hepatic artery
Bile duct
Portal vein
Hepatogastric ligament
Stomach
Omental bursa
Gastrosplenic ligament
Visceral peritoneum (covering spleen)
Parietal peritoneum
Spleen
Splenorenal ligament
Index finger traversing omental foramen
Parietal peritoneum
Right kidney
Inferior vena cava
Right and left crura of diaphragm
Aorta
Left kidney

Figure 2.22. Omental (epiploic) foramen and omental bursa. A. The index finger is passing from the greater sac through the omental foramen into the omental bursa (lesser sac). **B.** The hepatic artery is being compressed between the index finger (passing through the omental foramen into the omental bursa) and the thumb (on the anterior wall of the foramen).

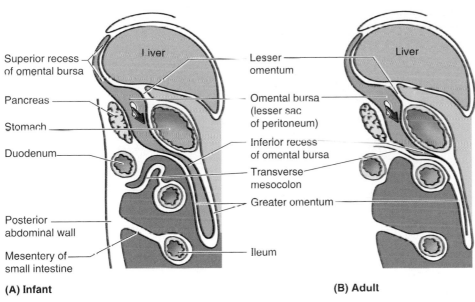

Superior recess
of omental bursa

Pancreas

Stomach

Duodenum

Posterior
abdominal wall

Mesentery of
small intestine

Liver

Lesser
omentum

Omental bursa
(lesser sac
of peritoneum)

Inferior recess
of omental bursa

Transverse
mesocolon

Greater omentum

Ileum

Liver

(A) Infant   **(B) Adult**

Schematic sagittal sections, lateral view

Figure 2.23. Walls and recesses of omental bursa. A. This section of the abdomen of an infant shows that the omental bursa (lesser sac) is an isolated part of the peritoneal cavity, lying dorsal to the stomach and extending superiorly to the liver and diaphragm (superior recess of the omental bursa) and inferiorly between the layers of the greater omentum (inferior recess of the omental bursa). **B.** This section shows the abdomen of an adult after fusion of the layers of the greater omentum. The inferior recess of the omental bursa now extends inferiorly only as far as the transverse colon because of the fused layers of the greater omentum. The red arrows pass from the greater sac through the omental (epiploic) foramen into the omental bursa.

because each contains blood vessels, the swollen intestine must be decompressed using a needle so it can be returned to the greater peritoneal sac through the omental foramen.

Severance of the Cystic Artery

The cystic artery must be ligated or clamped and then severed during *cholecystectomy,* removal of the gallbladder. Sometimes, however, it is accidentally severed before it has been adequately ligated. The surgeon can control the hemorrhage by compressing the hepatic artery as it traverses the hepatoduodenal ligament. The index finger is placed in the omental foramen and the thumb on its anterior wall (Fig. 2.22). Alternate compression and release of pressure on the hepatic artery allows the surgeon to identify the bleeding artery and clamp it. ○

THE BOTTOM LINE: Continuities and connections between the visceral and the parietal peritoneum occur where the gut enters and exits the abdominopelvic cavity. They also occur as double folds (mesenteries and omenta, and subdivisions called ligaments) that convey neurovascular structures and the ducts of accessory organs to and from the viscera. Peritoneal ligaments are named for the particular

structures connected by them. As a result of the rotation and exuberant growth of the gut during development, the disposition of the peritoneal cavity becomes complex. The main part of the peritoneal cavity (the greater sac) is divided by the transverse mesocolon into supracolic and intracolic compartments. A smaller part of the cavity, the omental bursa (lesser sac) lies posterior to the stomach, separating it from retroperitoneal viscera on the posterior wall. It communicates with the greater sac via the omental foramen. The complex disposition of the peritoneal cavity determines the flow and pooling of excess (ascitic) fluid occupying the peritoneal cavity during pathological conditions.

Abdominal Viscera

The principal viscera of the abdomen are the terminal part of the esophagus and the stomach, intestines, spleen, pancreas, liver, gallbladder, kidneys, and suprarenal (adrenal) glands (Figs. 2.24 and 2.25). When the abdominal cavity is opened to study these organs, it becomes evident that the liver, stomach, and spleen almost fill the domes of the diaphragm. By thus indenting the thoracic cavity, they receive protection from the lower thoracic cage. It is also seen that the *falciform ligament* normally attaches along a continuous line to the anterior abdominal wall as far inferiorly as the umbilicus and divides the liver superficially into right and left lobes. The fat-laden *greater omentum,* when in its typical position, conceals almost all of the intestine. The

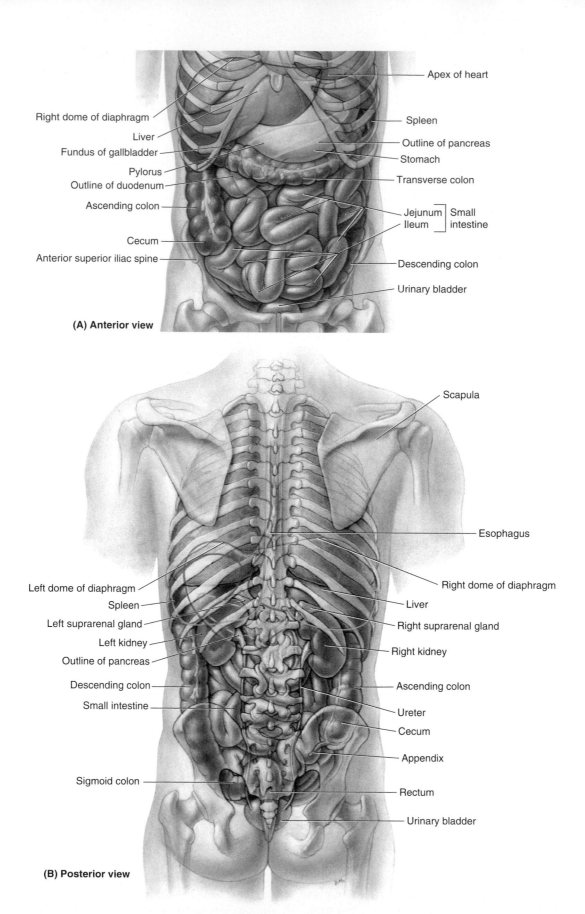

Figure 2.24. Overview of thoracic and abdominal viscera. A and B. Some abdominal organs extend superiorly into the thoracic cage (rib cage) and are protected by it. A large part of the small intestine is in the pelvis, and the right kidney is lower than the left kidney, owing to the mass of the liver on the right side. The appendix projects posteriorly and inferomedially toward the pelvic brim; consequently, it is visible only in the posterior view.

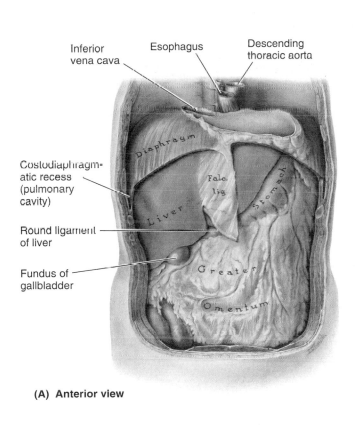

Inferior vena cava
Esophagus
Descending thoracic aorta
Costodiaphragm-atic recess (pulmonary cavity)
Round ligament of liver
Fundus of gallbladder

Diaphragm
Falc. lig
Stomach
Liver
Greater
Omentum

(A) Anterior view

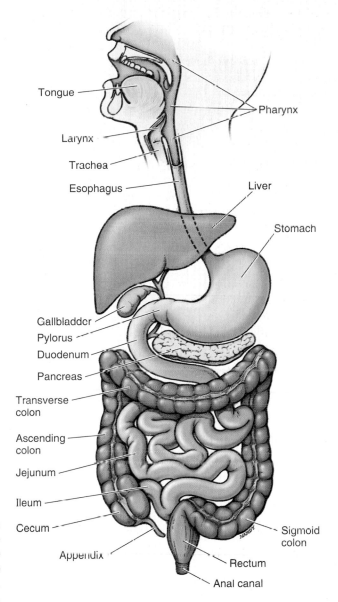

Tongue
Pharynx
Larynx
Trachea
Esophagus
Liver
Stomach
Gallbladder
Pylorus
Duodenum
Pancreas
Transverse colon
Ascending colon
Jejunum
Ileum
Cecum
Sigmoid colon
Appendix
Rectum
Anal canal

(B) Diagrammatic anterior view; medial view of bisected head

Figure 2.25. Abdominal contents in situ and in relation to alimentary system. A. The undisturbed abdominal contents are shown. The anterior abdominal and thoracic walls are cut away. The fundus of the gallbladder projects inferior to the sharp, inferior border of the liver. The falciform ligament (*Falc. lig.*) is severed at its attachment to the anterior abdominal wall. **B.** An overview of the alimentary system (gastrointestinal tract and accessory glands, the liver, and the pancreas) is presented.

gallbladder projects inferior to the sharp border of the liver (Fig. 2.25*A*).

Food passes from the mouth and pharynx through the *esophagus* to the *stomach*, where it mixes with gastric secretions (Fig. 2.25*B*). Digestion mostly occurs in the stomach and duodenum. *Peristalsis,* a series of ring-like contraction waves that begin around the middle of the stomach and move slowly toward the *pylorus,* is responsible for mixing the masticated (chewed) food mass with gastric juices and for emptying the contents of the stomach into the duodenum.

Absorption of chemical compounds occurs principally in the *small intestine,* a coiled 5- to 6-m-long tube (shorter in life, when tonus is present, than in the cadaver) consisting of the *duodenum, jejunum, and ileum.* Peristalsis also occurs in the jejunum and ileum; however, it is not forceful unless an obstruction is present. The stomach is continuous with the duodenum, which receives the openings of the ducts from the *pancreas* and *liver* (major glands of the digestive tract).

The *large intestine* consists of the *cecum* (which receives the terminal part of the ileum), *appendix, colon* (ascending, transverse, descending, and sigmoid), *rectum,* and *anal canal* (which ends at the *anus*). Most reabsorption of water occurs in the ascending colon. Feces form in the descending and sigmoid colon and accumulate in the rectum before defecation. The esophagus, stomach, and intestine constitute the **alimentary (digestive) tract** and are derived from the *primordial foregut, midgut,* and *hindgut.*

The arterial supply to the alimentary tract is from the *ab-*

dominal aorta. The three major branches of the aorta supplying the gut are the *celiac trunk* and the *superior* and *inferior mesenteric arteries* (Fig. 2.26*A*).

The *portal vein* (Fig. 2.26*B*), formed by the union of the *superior mesenteric* and *splenic veins,* is the main channel of the *portal venous system,* which collects blood from the abdominal part of the alimentary tract, pancreas, spleen, and most of the gallbladder and carries it to the liver.

Esophagus

The **esophagus** is a muscular tube (approximately 25 cm [10 in.] long) with an average diameter of 2 cm that conveys food from the pharynx to the stomach (Fig. 2.27*A*). As seen under fluoroscopy after a barium swallow, the esophagus normally has three constrictions where adjacent structures produce impressions (see "Medical Imaging of the Abdomen," in this chapter):

- **Cervical constriction:** at its beginning at the **pharyngoesophageal junction,** approximately 15 cm from the incisor teeth; caused by the **cricopharyngeus muscle** (see Chapter 8); referred to clinically as the *upper esophageal sphincter.*

- **Thoracic (broncho-aortic) constriction:** a compound constriction where it is first crossed by the arch of the aorta, 22.5 cm from the incisor teeth, and then where it is crossed by the left main bronchus, 27.5 cm from the incisor teeth; the former is seen in anteroposterior views, the latter in lateral views.

- **Diaphragmatic constriction:** where it passes through the esophageal hiatus of the diaphragm, approximately 40 cm from the incisor teeth.

Awareness of these constrictions is important when passing instruments through the esophagus into the stomach (Williams et al., 1995) and when viewing radiographs of patients who are experiencing *dysphagia* (difficulty in swallowing).

The esophagus:

- Follows the curve of the vertebral column as it descends through the neck and mediastinum—the median partition of the thoracic cavity (Fig. 2.27*A*).

- Has internal *circular* and external *longitudinal layers of muscle* (Fig. 2.27*B*). In its superior third, the external layer consists of voluntary striated muscle; the inferior third is composed of smooth muscle, and the middle third is made up of both types of muscle.

- Passes through the elliptical *esophageal hiatus* in the muscular *right crus of the diaphragm,* just to the left of the median plane at the level of the T10 vertebra.

- Terminates by entering the stomach at the cardial orifice of the stomach (Fig. 2.27*C*) to the left of the midline at the level of the 7th left costal cartilage and T11 vertebra.

- Is encircled by the esophageal nerve plexus distally (Fig. 2.28).

Food passes through the esophagus rapidly because of the peristaltic action of its musculature, aided by but not dependent on gravity (one can still swallow if inverted). The esophagus is attached to the margins of the esophageal hiatus in the diaphragm by the **phrenicoesophageal ligament** (Fig. 2.27*C*), an extension of inferior diaphragmatic fascia. This ligament permits independent movement of the diaphragm and esophagus during respiration and swallowing.

The trumpet-shaped abdominal part of the esophagus, only 1.25 cm long, passes from the esophageal hiatus in the right crus of the diaphragm to the *cardial (cardiac) orifice of the stomach,* widening as it approaches, passing anteriorly and to the left as it descends inferiorly. Its anterior surface is covered with peritoneum of the greater sac, continuous with that covering the anterior surface of the stomach. It fits into a groove on the posterior (visceral) surface of the liver. The posterior surface of the esophagus is covered with peritoneum of the omental bursa, continuous with that covering the posterior surface of the stomach. The right border of the esophagus is continuous with the lesser curvature of the stomach; however, its left border is separated from the fundus of the stomach by the cardial notch.

The **esophagogastric junction** lies to the left of the T11 vertebra on the horizontal plane that passes through the tip of the xiphoid process. Surgeons and endoscopists designate the **Z-line,** a jagged line where the mucosa abruptly changes from esophageal to gastric mucosa, as the junction. Immediately superior to this junction, the diaphragmatic musculature forming the esophageal hiatus functions as a physiological *inferior esophageal sphincter* that contracts and relaxes. Radiological studies show that food stops here momentarily and that the sphincter mechanism is normally efficient in preventing reflux of gastric contents into the esophagus. When one is not eating, the lumen of the esophagus is normally collapsed superior to this level to prevent food or stomach juices from regurgitating into the esophagus.

Details concerning the neurovasculature of the cervical and thoracic portions of the esophagus are provided in Chapters 1 and 8. The arterial supply of the abdominal part of the esophagus is from the *left gastric artery,* a branch of the celiac trunk, and the *left inferior phrenic artery* (Fig. 2.26*A*). The venous drainage from the *submucosal veins* of this part of the esophagus is both to the *portal venous system* through the *left gastric vein* (Fig. 2.26*B*) and into the *systemic venous system* through **esophageal veins** entering the *azygos vein.*

The lymphatic drainage of the abdominal part of the esophagus is into the **left gastric lymph nodes** (Fig. 2.28); efferent lymphatic vessels from these nodes drain mainly to **celiac lymph nodes.**

The esophagus is innervated by the **esophageal nerve plexus,** formed by the *vagal trunks* (becoming anterior and posterior gastric branches) and the *thoracic sympathetic trunks* via the *greater (abdominopelvic) splanchnic nerves* and *periarterial plexuses* around the left gastric and inferior phrenic arteries. (For an overview of the innervation of the abdominal organs, see "Summary of the Innervation of the Abdominal Viscera," in this chapter.)

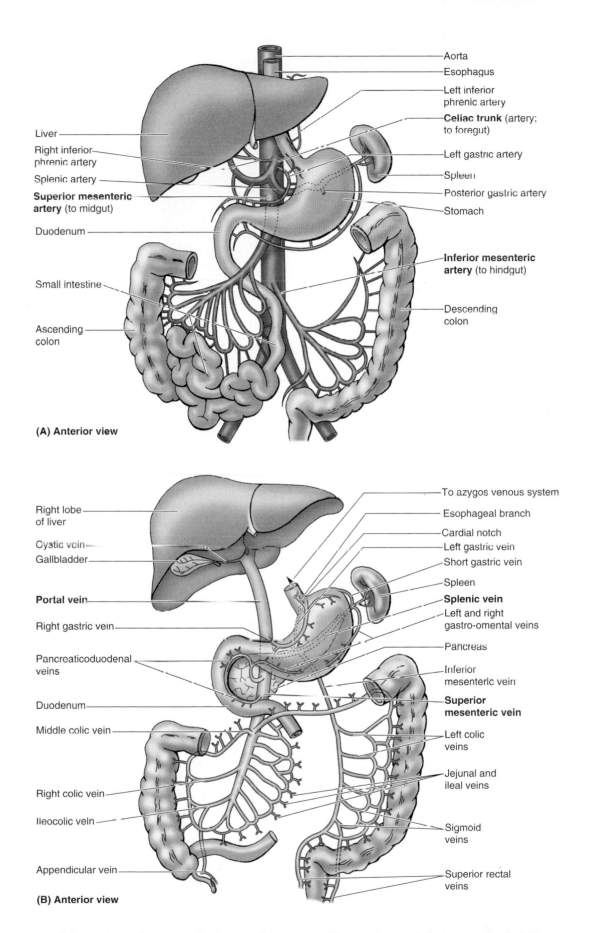

Figure 2.26. Arterial supply and venous drainage of GI tract. A. The arterial supply is demonstrated. **B.** The venous drainage is shown. The portal vein drains poorly oxygenated, nutrient-rich blood from the gastrointestinal tract, spleen, pancreas, and gallbladder to the liver. The *black arrow* indicates the communication of the esophageal vein with the azygos (systemic) venous system.

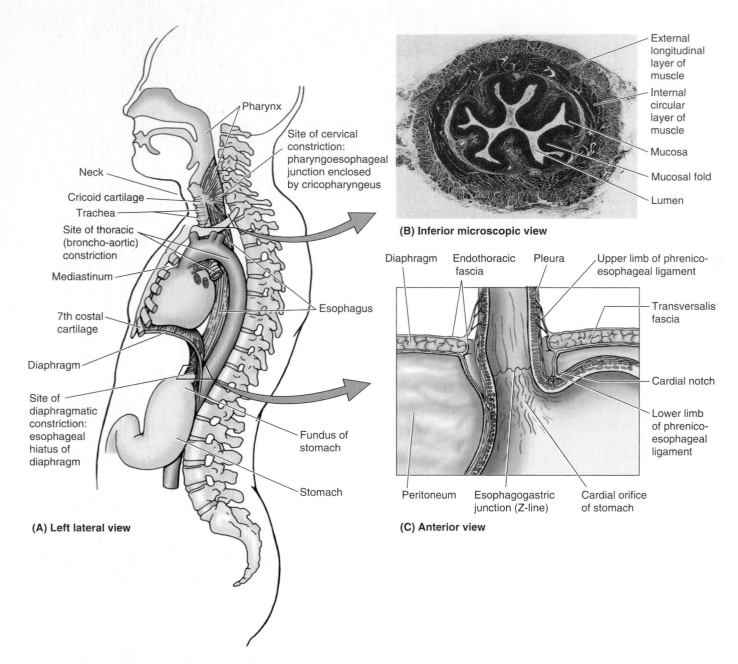

(A) Left lateral view

Pharynx

Site of cervical constriction: pharyngoesophageal junction enclosed by cricopharyngeus

Neck

Cricoid cartilage

Trachea

Site of thoracic (broncho-aortic) constriction

Mediastinum

7th costal cartilage

Diaphragm

Site of diaphragmatic constriction: esophageal hiatus of diaphragm

Esophagus

Fundus of stomach

Stomach

(B) Inferior microscopic view

External longitudinal layer of muscle

Internal circular layer of muscle

Mucosa

Mucosal fold

Lumen

(C) Anterior view

Diaphragm   Endothoracic fascia   Pleura   Upper limb of phrenico-esophageal ligament

Transversalis fascia

Cardial notch

Lower limb of phrenico-esophageal ligament

Peritoneum   Esophagogastric junction (Z-line)   Cardial orifice of stomach

Figure 2.27. The esophagus and its relationships. A. The lateral view shows the esophagus and related structures (trachea, vertebral column, descending aorta, and stomach). The esophagus begins at the level of the palpable cricoid cartilage and descends posterior to the trachea. It leaves the thorax through the esophageal hiatus of the diaphragm. **B.** The transverse section of the esophagus shows the muscular and mucosal layers of its wall. **C.** A coronal section of the inferior esophagus, diaphragm, and superior stomach is shown. The phrenicoesophageal ligament connects the esophagus flexibly to the diaphragm; it limits upward movement of the esophagus while permitting some movement during swallowing and respiration.

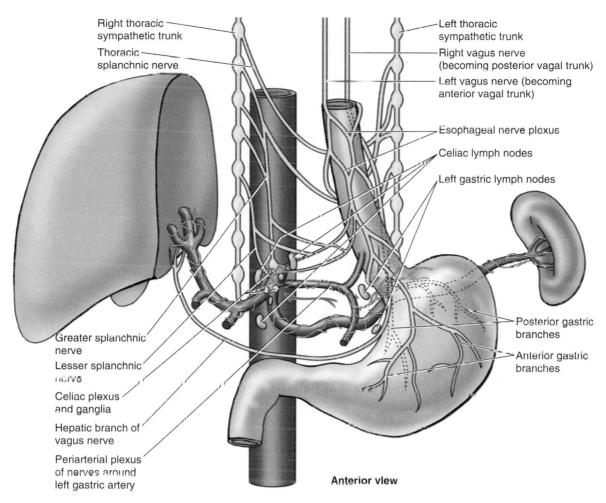

Right thoracic sympathetic trunk

Thoracic splanchnic nerve

Left thoracic sympathetic trunk

Right vagus nerve (becoming posterior vagal trunk)

Left vagus nerve (becoming anterior vagal trunk)

Esophageal nerve plexus

Celiac lymph nodes

Left gastric lymph nodes

Greater splanchnic nerve

Lesser splanchnic nerve

Celiac plexus and ganglia

Hepatic branch of vagus nerve

Periarterial plexus of nerves around left gastric artery

Posterior gastric branches

Anterior gastric branches

Anterior view

Figure 2.28. Nerves and lymphatics of abdominal esophagus and stomach. The right and left vagus nerves (CN X) divide into branches that form the esophageal plexus around the inferior esophagus. Anterior and posterior gastric branches of the plexus accompany the esophagus through the esophageal hiatus for distribution to the anterior and posterior aspects of the stomach. The anterior branches also extend to the pylorus and liver. Postsynaptic sympathetic nerve fibers from the celiac plexus are distributed to these organs through periarterial plexuses. The lymphatic vessels of the stomach follow a pattern similar to that of the arteries, although the flow is in the opposite direction. Thus, lymph from the stomach and abdominal part of the esophagus drains to the gastric and then celiac lymph nodes.

Esophageal Varices

Because the submucosal veins of the inferior esophagus drain to both the portal and the systemic venous systems, they constitute a portosystemic anastomosis. In *portal hypertension* (an abnormally increased blood pressure in the portal venous system), blood is unable to pass through the liver via the portal vein, causing a reversal of flow in the esophageal tributary. The large volume of blood causes the submucosal veins to enlarge markedly, forming **esophageal varices** (Fig. B2.8). These distended collateral channels may rupture and cause severe hemorrhage that is life-threatening and difficult to control surgically. Esophageal varices commonly develop in alcoholics who have developed *cirrhosis* (fibrous scarring) *of the liver* (see

clinical correlation [blue] box "Cirrhosis of the Liver," in this chapter). ▶

View through esophagoscope of esophageal varices

Figure B2.8.

Pyrosis

Pyrosis, or heartburn, is the most common type of esophageal discomfort or substernal pain. This burning sensation in the abdominal part of the esophagus is usually the result of regurgitation of small amounts of food or gastric fluid into the lower esophagus (*gastroesophageal reflux disorder; GERD*). Pyrosis (G. burning) may also be associated with *hiatal (hiatus) hernia* (see clinical correlation [blue] box "Hiatal Hernia," in this chapter). As indicated by its common name, heartburn, pyrosis is commonly perceived as a "chest" (vs. abdominal) sensation. As mentioned in Chapter 1, determining the nature and source of chest pains can be one of the more challenging aspects of physical diagnosis. ⊙

THE BOTTOM LINE: The esophagus is a tubular conveyer of food, delivering it from the pharynx to the stomach. It penetrates the diaphragm at the T10 vertebral level, passing through its right crus, which decussates around it to form the physiological inferior esophageal sphincter. The trumpet-shaped abdominal part, composed entirely of smooth muscle innervated by the esophageal nerve plexus, enters the cardial part of the stomach. It receives blood from esophageal branches of the left gastric artery (from the celiac trunk). Its submucosal veins drain to both the systemic and the portal venous systems and thus constitute portocaval anastomoses that may become varicose in the presence of portal hypertension. Internally, in the living, the esophagus is demarcated from the stomach by an abrupt mucosal transition, the Z-line.

Stomach

The **stomach** is the expanded part of the alimentary tract between the esophagus and the small intestine (Fig. 2.25*B*). It is specialized for the accumulation of ingested food, which it chemically and mechanically prepares for digestion and passage into the duodenum. In most people, the shape of the stomach resembles the letter J; however, the shape and position of the stomach can vary markedly in persons of different body types (bodily habitus) and even in the same individual as a result of diaphragmatic movements during respiration, the stomach's contents, and the position of the person (i.e., whether lying down or standing) (Fig. 2.29). The stomach acts as a food blender and reservoir; its chief function is enzymatic digestion. The *gastric juice* gradually converts a mass of food into a semiliquid mixture, *chyme* (G. juice), which passes fairly quickly into the duodenum. An empty stomach is only of slightly larger caliber than the large intestine; however, it is capable of considerable expansion and can hold 2–3 L of food. A newborn infant's stomach, approximately the size of a lemon, can expand to hold up to 30 mL of milk.

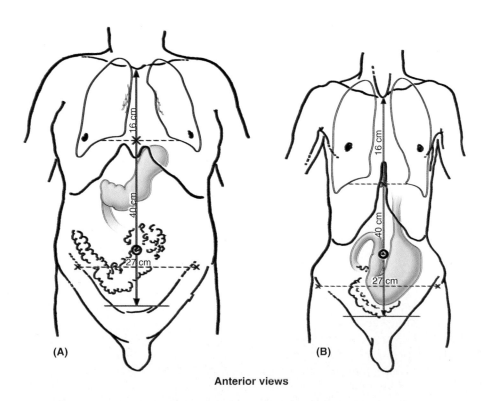

Anterior views

Figure 2.29. Effect of body type (bodily habitus) on disposition and shape of stomach. A. A heavily built hypersthenic individual with short thorax and long abdomen is likely to have a stomach that is placed high and more transversely disposed. **B.** In those with a slender asthenic physique, the stomach is low and vertical.

Parts of the Stomach

The stomach has four parts (Fig. 2.30*A*):

- **Cardia:** the part surrounding the cardial orifice.

- **Fundus:** the dilated superior part that is related to the left dome of the diaphragm and is limited inferiorly by the horizontal plane of the **cardial orifice.** The superior part of

the fundus usually reaches the level of the left 5th intercostal space. The **cardial notch** is between the esophagus and the fundus. The fundus may be dilated by gas, fluid, food, or any combination of these.

- **Body:** the major part of the stomach between the fundus and the pyloric antrum.

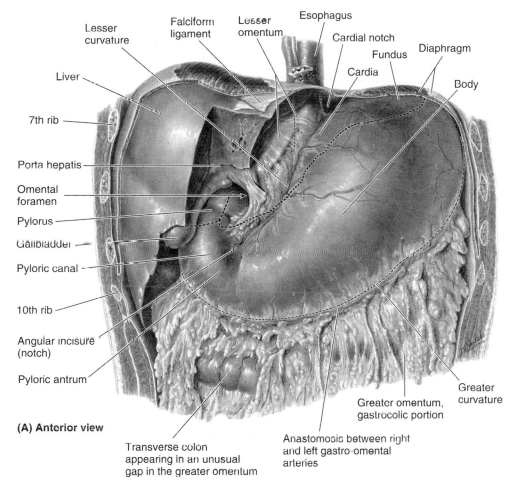

(A) Anterior view

Figure 2.30. Abdominal part of esophagus and stomach. A. The stomach and the greater and lesser omenta are shown. The left part of the liver is cut away so that the lesser omentum and the omental foramen (entrance to omental bursa) can be seen. The extent of the intact liver is indicated by a *dotted line*. The stomach is inflated with air. **B.** The internal surface (mucous membrane) is demonstrated. The longitudinal gastric folds, or rugae, disappear on distension. Along the lesser curvature, several longitudinal mucosal folds extend from the esophagus to the pylorus, making up the gastric canal along which ingested liquids pass. **C.** The pylorus is the significantly constricted terminal part of the stomach. The pyloric orifice is the distal opening of the pyloric canal into the duodenum.

(B) Anterior view

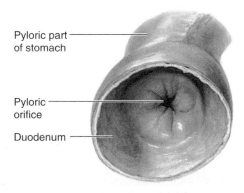

(C) Internal (lateral) view from duodenum

- **Pyloric part:** the funnel-shaped outflow region of the stomach; its wide part, the **pyloric antrum,** leads into the **pyloric canal,** its narrow part (Fig. 2.30*A* & *B*). The **pylorus** (G. gatekeeper), the distal, sphincteric region of the pyloric part, is a marked thickening of the circular layer of smooth muscle (Fig. 2.30*B* & *C*), which controls discharge of the stomach contents through the **pyloric orifice** into the duodenum.

The stomach also has two curvatures:

- **Lesser curvature:** forms the shorter concave border of the stomach; the **angular incisure** (notch) is the sharp indentation approximately two thirds the distance along the lesser curvature that indicates the junction of the body and the pyloric part of the stomach (Fig. 2.30*A*).

- **Greater curvature:** forms the longer convex border of the stomach.

Intermittent emptying of the stomach occurs when intragastric pressure overcomes the resistance of the pylorus (Fig. 2.30*C*). It is normally tonically contracted so that the pyloric orifice is reduced, except when emitting chyme. At irregular intervals, *gastric peristalsis* passes the chyme through the pyloric canal and orifice into the small intestine for further mixing, digestion, and absorption.

Interior of the Stomach

The smooth surface of the gastric mucosa is reddish brown during life, except in the pyloric part, where it is pink. In life, it is covered by a continuous mucous layer that protects its surface from the gastric acid the stomach's glands secrete. When contracted, the gastric mucosa is thrown into longitudinal ridges called **gastric folds,** or **gastric rugae** (Fig. 2.30*B*); they are most marked toward the pyloric part and along the greater curvature. A **gastric canal** (furrow) forms temporarily during swallowing between the longitudinal gastric folds of the mucosa along the lesser curvature. It can be observed radiographically and endoscopically. The gastric canal forms because of the firm attachment of the gastric mucosa to the muscular layer, which does not have an oblique layer at this site. Saliva and small quantities of masticated food and other fluids pass through the gastric canal to the pyloric canal when the stomach is mostly empty. The gastric folds diminish and obliterate as the stomach is distended (fills).

Relations of the Stomach

The stomach is covered by peritoneum, except where blood vessels run along its curvatures and in a small area posterior to the cardial orifice. The two layers of the lesser omentum extend around the stomach and leave its greater curvature as the greater omentum (Figs. 2.23, 2.25, and 2.30A). Anteriorly, the stomach is related to the diaphragm, the left lobe of liver, and the anterior abdominal wall. Posteriorly, the stomach is related to the omental bursa and the pancreas; the posterior surface of the stomach forms most of the anterior wall of the omental bursa (Fig. 2.31*A*).

The **bed of the stomach,** on which the stomach rests in the supine position, is formed by the structures forming the posterior wall of the omental bursa. From superior to inferior, the stomach bed is formed by the left dome of the diaphragm, spleen, left kidney and suprarenal gland, splenic artery, pancreas, and transverse mesocolon and colon (Fig. 2.31*B*).

Displacement of the Stomach

Pancreatic pseudo-cysts and abscesses in the omental bursa may push the stomach anteriorly. This displacement is usually visible in lateral radiographs of the stomach and other diagnostic images, such as CT studies. Following *pancreatitis* (inflammation of the pancreas), the posterior wall of the stomach may adhere to the part of the posterior wall of the omental bursa that covers the pancreas. This adhesion occurs because of the close relationship of the posterior wall of the stomach to the pancreas.

Hiatal Hernia

A **hiatal,** or **hiatus, hernia** is a protrusion of a part of the stomach into the mediastinum through the esophageal hiatus of the diaphragm. The hernias occur most often in people after middle age, possibly because of weakening of the muscular part of the diaphragm and widening of the esophageal hiatus. The hernias are often distressful and cause pain. Although clinically there are several types of hiatal hernias (Skandalakis et al., 1996), the two main types are paraesophageal hiatal hernia and sliding hiatal hernia.

In the less common **paraesophageal hiatal hernia,** the cardia remains in its normal position (Fig. B2.9*A*). However, a pouch of peritoneum, often containing part of the fundus, extends through the esophageal hiatus anterior to the esophagus. In these cases, usually no regurgitation of gastric contents occurs because the cardial orifice is in its normal position.

In **sliding hiatal hernia,** the abdominal part of the esophagus, the cardia, and parts of the fundus of the stomach slide superiorly through the esophageal hiatus into the thorax, especially when the person lies down or bends over (Fig. B2.9*B*). Some regurgitation of stomach contents into the esophagus is possible because the ▶

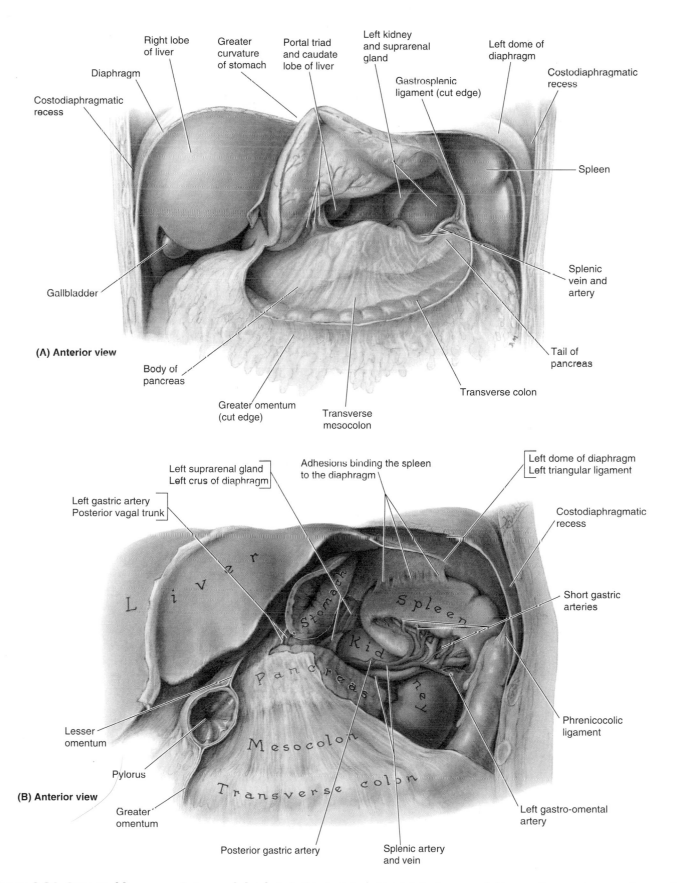

(A) Anterior view

Diaphragm

Costodiaphragmatic recess

Right lobe of liver

Greater curvature of stomach

Portal triad and caudate lobe of liver

Left kidney and suprarenal gland

Gastrosplenic ligament (cut edge)

Left dome of diaphragm

Costodiaphragmatic recess

Spleen

Splenic vein and artery

Tail of pancreas

Transverse colon

Gallbladder

Body of pancreas

Greater omentum (cut edge)

Transverse mesocolon

(B) Anterior view

Left gastric artery
Posterior vagal trunk

Left suprarenal gland
Left crus of diaphragm

Adhesions binding the spleen to the diaphragm

Left dome of diaphragm
Left triangular ligament

Costodiaphragmatic recess

Short gastric arteries

Phrenicocolic ligament

Lesser omentum

Pylorus

Greater omentum

Posterior gastric artery

Splenic artery and vein

Left gastro-omental artery

Liver

Stomach

Spleen

Kidney

Pancreas

Mesocolon

Transverse colon

Figure 2.31. Omental bursa and stomach bed. A. In this anterior approach to the omental bursa, the greater omentum and gastrosplenic ligament have been cut along the greater curvature of the stomach, and the stomach has been reflected superiorly to open the bursa anteriorly. At the right end of the bursa, two of the boundaries of the omental foramen can be seen: the inferior root of the hepatoduodenal ligament (containing the portal triad) and the caudate lobe of the liver. **B.** The stomach and most of the lesser omentum have been excised, and the peritoneum of the posterior wall of the omental bursa covering the stomach bed is largely removed to reveal the organs in the bed. Although adhesions, such as those binding the spleen to the diaphragm here, are common postmortem findings, they are not normal anatomy.

Barium swallow radiograph of
sliding hiatal hernia

(A) Paraesophageal hiatal hernia

(B) Sliding hiatal hernia

Figure B2.9.

clamping action of the right crus of the diaphragm on the inferior end of the esophagus is weak.

Congenital Diaphragmatic Hernia

In **congenital diaphragmatic hernia** (CDH), part of the stomach and intestine herniate through a large posterolateral defect (foramen of Bochdalek) in the diaphragm. This type of hernia is found in approximately 1 of every 2200 newborn infants. CDH results from the complex development of the diaphragm (Moore and Persaud, 2003). With abdominal viscera in the limited space of the prenatal pulmonary cavity, the lungs (especially the left lung) does not have room to develop. Because of the consequent *pulmonary hypoplasia,* the mortality rate in these infants is high (approximately 76%). ☉

Vessels and Nerves of the Stomach

The stomach has a rich arterial supply arising from the celiac trunk and its branches. The origin, course, and distribution of the arteries of the stomach are described in Table 2.7. Most blood is supplied by anastomoses formed along the lesser curvature by the **right** and **left gastric arteries,** and along the greater curvature by the **right** and **left gastro-omental arteries.** The fundus and upper body receive blood from the **short** and **posterior gastric arteries.**

Table 2.7. Arterial Supply to Abdominal Foregut Derivatives: Esophagus, Stomach, Liver, Gallbladder, Pancreas, and Spleen

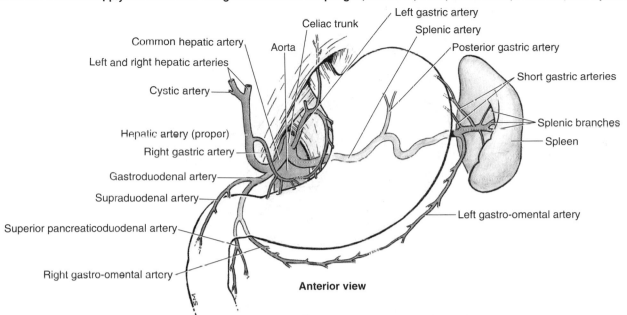

Anterior view

Artery	Origin	Course	Distribution
Celiac trunk	Initial abdominal aorta (within aortic hiatus)	After short anteroinferior course, bifurcates into splenic and common mesenteric arteries	Esophagus, stomach, proximal duodenum, liver/biliary apparatus, pancreas
Left gastric	Celiac trunk	Ascends retroperitoneally to esophageal hiatus, giving rise to an esophageal branch; then descending along lesser curvature to anatomose with right gastric artery	Distal (mostly abdominal) part of esophagus and lesser curvature of stomach
Splenic	Celiac trunk	Runs retroperitoneally along superior border of pancreas; traverses spenorenal ligament to hilum of spleen	Body of pancreas, spleen, and greater curvature and posterior stomach body
Posterior gastric	Splenic artery posterior to stomach	Ascends retroperitoneally along posterior wall of lesser omental bursa to enter gastrophrenic ligament	Posterior wall and fundus of stomach
Left gastro-omental (left gastroepiploic)	Splenic artery in hilum of spleen	Passes between layers of gastrosplenic ligament to stomach, then along greater curvature in greater omentum to anastomose with right gastro-omental artery	Left portion of greater curvature of stomach
Short gastric ($n = 4–5$)	Splenic artery in hilum of spleen	Passes between layers of gastrosplenic ligament to fundus of stomach	Fundus of stomach
Hepatic[a]	Celiac trunk	Passes retroperitoneally to reach hepatoduodenal ligament; passing between layers to porta hepatis; bifurcates into right and left hepatic arteries	Liver, gallbladder and biliary ducts, stomach, duodenum, pancreas and respective lobes of liver
Cystic	Right hepatic artery	Arises within hepatiduodenal ligament in triangle of Calot	Gallbladder and cystic duct
Right gastric	Hepatic artery	Runs along lesser curvature of stomach to anastomose with left gastric artery	Right portion of lesser curvature of stomach
Gastroduodenal	Hepatic artery	Descends retroperitoneally, posterior to gastroduodenal junction	Stomach, pancreas, first part of duodenum, and distal part of bile duct
Right gastro-omental (right gastroepiploic)	Gastroduodenal artery	Passes between layers of greater omentum along greater curvature of stomach to anastomose with left gastro-omental artery	Right portion of greater curvature of stomach
Superior pancreaticoduodenal	Gastroduodenal artery	Divides into anterior and posterior arteries that descend on each side of pancreatic head, anastomosing with similar branches of inferior pancreaticoduodenal artery	Proximal portion of duodenum and superior part of head of pancreas
Inferior pancreaticoduodenal	Superior mesenteric artery	Divides into anterior and posterior arteries that ascend on each side of pancreatic head, anastomosing with similar branches of superior pancreaticoduodenal artery	Distal portion of duodenum and head of pancreas

[a]For descriptive purposes, the hepatic artery is often divided into the *common hepatic artery*, from its origin to the origin of the gastroduodenal artery, and *hepatic artery proper*, made up of the remainder of the vessel.

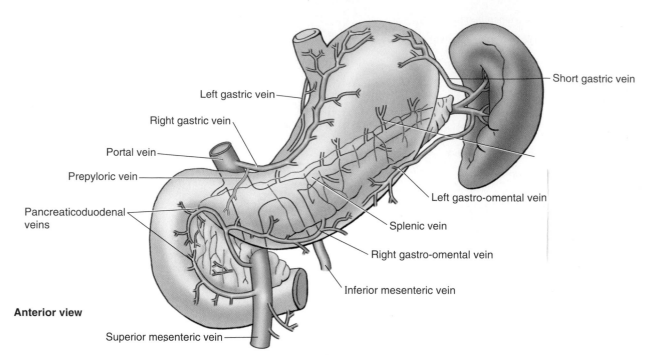

Short gastric vein

Left gastric vein

Right gastric vein

Portal vein

Prepyloric vein

Pancreaticoduodenal veins

Left gastro-omental vein

Splenic vein

Right gastro-omental vein

Inferior mesenteric vein

Anterior view

Superior mesenteric vein

Figure 2.32. Veins of stomach, duodenum, and spleen. Venous drainage from the stomach and duodenum is into the portal vein, either directly or indirectly via the splenic or superior mesenteric vein (SMV). The splenic vein usually receives the inferior mesenteric vein and then unites with the SMV to form the portal vein, as shown here.

The gastric veins parallel the arteries in position and course (Fig. 2.32). The **right** and **left gastric veins** drain into the *portal vein*; the **short gastric veins** and **left gastro-omental veins** drain into the *splenic vein,* which joins the superior mesenteric vein (SMV) to form the portal vein. The **right gastro-omental vein** empties in the SMV. A **prepyloric vein** ascends over the pylorus to the right gastric vein. Because this vein is obvious in living persons, surgeons use it for identifying the pylorus.

The **gastric lymphatic vessels** (Fig. 2.33*A*) accompany the arteries along the greater and lesser curvatures of the stomach. They drain lymph from its anterior and posterior surfaces toward its curvatures, where the **gastric** and **gastro-omental lymph nodes** are located. The efferent vessels from these nodes accompany the large arteries to the *celiac lymph nodes.* The following is a summary of the lymphatic drainage of the stomach:

- Lymph from the superior two thirds of the stomach drains along the right and left gastric vessels to the **gastric lymph nodes;** lymph from the fundus and superior part of the body of the stomach also drains along the short gastric arteries and left gastro-omental vessels to the **pancreaticosplenic lymph nodes.**

- Lymph from the right two thirds of the inferior third of the stomach drains along the right gastro-omental vessels to the **pyloric lymph nodes.**

- Lymph from the left one third of the greater curvature drains along the short gastric and splenic vessels to the **pancreaticoduodenal lymph nodes.**

The *parasympathetic nerve supply of the stomach* (Fig. 2.33*B*) is from the anterior and posterior vagal trunks and their branches, which enter the abdomen through the esophageal

Key for (A)

- ■ Celiac
- □ Pancreaticosplenic
- ■ Gastro-omental
- ■ Gastric
- □ Mesenteric
- ■ Pyloric
- □ Pancreaticoduodenal

Gastric lymph nodes

Celiac lymph nodes

Superior mesenteric lymph nodes

Superior and inferior pyloric lymph nodes

Pancreatico-duodenal lymph nodes

Mesenteric lymph nodes

Pancreaticosplenic lymph nodes

Splenic artery

Splenic lymph nodes

Gastro-omental lymph nodes

⬈ = Initial drainage

⬈ = Secondary (subsequent) drainage

(A) Anterior view

Anterior and posterior vagal trunks

Thoracic splanchnic nerves (greater, lesser, least)

Celiac ganglion and plexus

Sympathetic trunk and ganglia (lumbar portion)

Lumbar splanchnic nerves

Duodenum

Stomach

Superior mesenteric ganglion and plexus

Duodenojejunal junction

Jejunum

Ileum

Key for (B)

- □ Sympathetic nerves and ganglia
- ■ Parasympathetic nerves
- ■ Plexuses (sympathetic and parasympathetic)

(B) Anterior view

Figure 2.33. Lymphatic drainage and innervation of stomach and small intestine. A. The lymphatic drainage is demonstrated. The arrows indicate the direction of lymph flow to the lymph nodes. **B.** Innervation of the stomach is both parasympathetic, from the vagus nerves (CN X) via the esophageal plexus, and sympathetic, via the greater (abdominopelvic) splanchnic, the celiac plexus, and peri-arterial plexuses.

hiatus. The **anterior vagal trunk,** derived mainly from the left vagus nerve (CN X), usually enters the abdomen as a single branch that lies on the anterior surface of the esophagus. It runs toward the lesser curvature of the stomach, where it gives off hepatic and duodenal branches, which leave the stomach in the hepatoduodenal ligament. The rest of the anterior vagal trunk continues along the lesser curvature, giving rise to anterior gastric branches. The larger **posterior vagal trunk,** derived mainly from the right vagus nerve, enters the abdomen on the posterior surface of the esophagus and passes toward the lesser curvature of the stomach. The posterior vagal trunk supplies branches to the anterior and posterior surfaces of the stomach. It gives off a celiac branch, which runs to the **celiac plexus,** and then continues along the lesser curvature, giving rise to posterior gastric branches.

The *sympathetic nerve supply of the stomach* from the T6 through T9 segments of the spinal cord passes to the celiac plexus through the **greater splanchnic nerve** and is distributed through the plexuses around the gastric and gastro-omental arteries (see also "Summary of the Innervation of the Abdominal Viscera," in this chapter.)

Pylorospasm

Spasmodic contraction of the pylorus sometimes occurs in infants, usually between 2 and 12 weeks of age. **Pylorospasm** is characterized by failure of the smooth muscle fibers encircling the pyloric canal to relax normally. As a result, food does not pass easily from the stomach into the duodenum and the stomach becomes overly full, usually resulting in vomiting.

Congenital Hypertrophic Pyloric Stenosis

Congenital hypertrophic pyloric stenosis is a marked thickening of the smooth muscle in the pylorus that affects approximately 1 of every 150 male infants and 1 of every 750 female infants (Moore and Persaud, 2003). Normally, gastric peristalsis pushes chyme through the pyloric canal and orifice into the small intestine at irregular intervals (Fig. B2.10*A*). In these babies, however, the elongated overgrown pylorus is hard, and severe stenosis (narrowing) of the pyloric canal is present (Fig. B2.10*B*), resisting gastric emptying. The proximal part of the stomach becomes secondarily dilated because of the pyloric obstruction. Although the cause of congenital hypertrophic pyloric stenosis is unknown, genetic factors appear to be involved because of this condition's high incidence in infants of monozygotic twins.

Carcinoma of the Stomach

When the body or pyloric part of the stomach contains a malignant tumor, the mass may be palpable. Using *gastroscopy,* physicians can inspect the mucosa of the air-inflated stomach, enabling them to observe gastric lesions and take biopsies. The extensive lymphatic drainage of the stomach and the impossibility of removing all the lymph nodes create a surgical problem. The nodes along the splenic vessels can be excised by removing the spleen, gastrosplenic and splenorenal ligaments, and the body and tail of the pancreas. Involved nodes along the gastro-omental vessels can be removed by resecting the greater omentum;

Figure B2.10. Congenital hypertrophic pyloric stenosis. A. Normal passage through the pyloric sphincter is shown. **B.** Stoppage of flow owing to stenosis is demonstrated.

however, removal of the aortic and celiac nodes and those around the head of the pancreas is difficult.

Gastrectomy

Total gastrectomy (removal of the entire stomach) is uncommon. **Partial gastrectomy** (removal of part of the stomach) may be performed to remove a region of the stomach involved by a carcinoma, for example. Because the anastomoses of the arteries supplying the stomach provide good collateral circulation, one or more arteries may be ligated during this procedure without seriously affecting the blood supply to the part of the stomach remaining in place. When removing the pyloric antrum, for example, the greater omentum is incised parallel and inferior to the right gastro-omental artery, requiring ligation of all the omental branches of this artery. The omentum does not degenerate, however, because of anastomoses with other arteries, such as the omental branches of the left gastro-omental artery, which are still intact. Partial gastrectomy ▶

to remove a carcinoma usually also requires removal of all involved regional lymph nodes. Because cancer frequently occurs in the pyloric region, removal of the *pyloric lymph nodes* as well as the right *gastro-omental lymph nodes* also receiving lymph drainage from this region is especially important. As stomach cancer becomes more advanced, the lymphogenous dissemination of malignant cells involves the *celiac lymph nodes,* to which all gastric nodes drain.

Gastric Ulcers, *Helicobacter pylori*, and Vagotomy

An *ulcer* is an open sore. *Gastric ulcers* are open lesions of the mucosa of the stomach, whereas the term *peptic ulcers* is applied to lesions of the mucosa of the pyloric canal or, more often, the duodenum. Most ulcers (9 of 10) of the stomach and duodenum are associated with an infection of a specific bacterium, *Helicobacter pylori* (*H. pylori*). People experiencing severe chronic anxiety are most prone to the development of peptic ulcers. They often have gastric acid secretion rates that are as much as 15 times higher than normal between meals. It is thought that the high acid in the stomach and duodenum overwhelms the bicarbonate normally produced by the duodenum and reduces the effectiveness of the mucous lining, leaving it vulnerable to *H. pylori*. The bacteria erode the protective mucous lining of the stomach, inflaming the mucosa and making it vulnerable to the effects of the gastric acid and digestive enzymes (pepsin) produced by the stomach.

If the ulcer erodes into the gastric arteries, it can cause life-threatening bleeding. Most ulcers are eradicated, with low rates of recurrence, after antibiotic therapy combined with use of antacids. Because the secretion of acid by parietal cells of the stomach is largely controlled by the vagus nerves, *vagotomy* (surgical section of the vagus nerves) is performed in some people with chronic or recurring ulcers to reduce the production of acid. Vagotomy may also be performed in conjunction with resection of the ulcerated area (*antrectomy,* or resection of the pyloric antrum) to reduce acid secretion. A *truncal vagotomy* (surgical section of the vagal trunks) is rarely performed because the innervation of other abdominal structures is also sacrificed (Fig. B2.11*A*). In *selective gastric vagotomy,* the stomach is denervated but the vagal branches to the pylorus, liver and biliary ducts, intestines, and celiac plexus are preserved (Fig. B2.11*B*). A *selective proximal vagotomy* attempts to denervate even more specifically the area in which the parietal cells are located, hoping to affect the acid-producing cells while sparing other gastric function (motility) stimulated by the vagus nerve (Fig. B2.11*C*).

A *posterior gastric ulcer* may erode through the stomach wall into the pancreas, resulting in referred pain to the back. In such cases, *erosion of the splenic artery* results in se-

Anterior views

Figure B2.11. Vagotomy. Truncal (**A**), selective gastric (**B**), and selective proximal (**C**) vagotomy are shown.

vere hemorrhage into the peritoneal cavity. Pain impulses from the stomach are carried by visceral afferent fibers that accompany sympathetic nerves. This fact is evident because the pain of a recurrent peptic ulcer may persist after complete vagotomy, whereas patients who have had a bilateral sympathectomy may have a perforated peptic ulcer and experience no pain.

Visceral Referred Pain

Pain is an unpleasant sensation associated with actual or potential tissue damage and mediated by specific nerve fibers to the brain, where its conscious appreciation may be modified. *Organic pain* arising from an organ such as the stomach varies from dull to severe; however, the pain is poorly localized. It radiates to the dermatome level, which receives visceral afferent fibers from the organ concerned. *Visceral referred pain* from a gastric ulcer, for example, is referred to the epigastric region because the stomach is supplied by pain afferents that reach the T7 and T8 spinal sensory ganglia and spinal cord segments through the greater splanchnic nerve (Fig. B2.12). The brain interprets the pain as though the irritation occurred in the skin of the epigastric region, which is also supplied by the same sensory ganglia and spinal cord segments.

Pain arising from the parietal peritoneum is of the somatic type and is usually severe. The site of its origin can be localized. The anatomical basis for this localization of pain is that the parietal peritoneum is supplied by somatic sensory fibers through thoracic nerves, whereas a viscus such as the appendix is supplied by visceral afferent fibers in the ▶

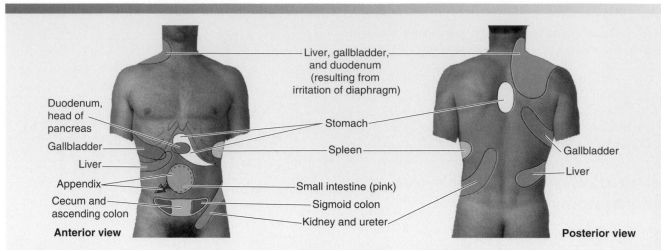

Figure B2.12.

lesser splanchnic nerve. Inflamed parietal peritoneum is extremely sensitive to stretching. When digital pressure is applied to the anterolateral abdominal wall over the site of inflammation, the parietal peritoneum is stretched. When the fingers are suddenly removed, extreme localized pain is usually felt, known as *rebound tenderness.* ○

Surface Anatomy of the Stomach

The surface markings of the **stomach** vary because its size and position change under various circumstances (e.g., after a heavy meal). In the supine position, the stomach commonly lies in the right and left upper quadrants, or epigastric, umbilical, and left hypochondriac and lumbar regions (Fig. SA2.2). In the erect position, the stomach moves inferiorly. In asthenic (thin, weak) individuals, the body of the stomach may extend into the pelvis (Fig. 2.29). The stomach is usually partially overlain by the **transverse colon** near the left colic ▶

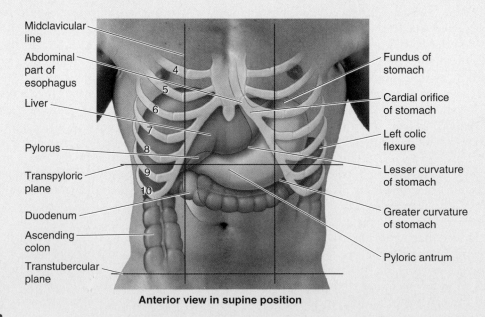

Anterior view in supine position

Figure SA2.2.

flexure. The surface markings of the stomach in the supine position include (Fig. SA2.2) the:

- **Cardial orifice:** which usually lies posterior to the 6th left costal cartilage, 2–4 cm from the median plane at the level of the T11 vertebra.
- **Fundus:** which usually lies posterior to the left 6th rib in the plane of the MCL.
- **Greater curvature:** which passes inferiorly to the left as far as the 10th left cartilage before turning medially to reach the pyloric antrum.

- **Lesser curvature:** which passes from the right side of the cardia to the pyloric antrum; the most inferior part of the curvature is marked by the **angular incisure**, which lies just to the left of the midline.
- **Pyloric part of the stomach** in the supine position: which usually lies at the level of the 9th costal cartilages at the level of L1 vertebra; the pyloric orifice is approximately 1.25 cm left of the midline.
- **Pylorus** in the erect position: which usually lies on the right side; its location varies from the L2 through L4 vertebra. ⊙

THE BOTTOM LINE: The stomach is the dilated portion of the alimentary tract between the esophagus and the duodenum, specialized to accumulate ingested food and prepare it chemically and mechanically for digestion. The stomach lies asymmetrically in the abdominal cavity, to the left of the midline and usually in the upper left quadrant. The abdominal portion of the esophagus enters its cardial portion, and its pyloric part leads to the exit to the duodenum. Gastric emptying is controlled by the pylorus. In life, its internal surface is covered with a protective layer of mucus, overlying gastritic folds that disappear with distension. The stomach is intraperitoneal, with the lesser omentum (enclosing the anastomoses between right and left gastric vessels) attached to its lesser curvature, and the greater omentum (enclosing the anastomoses between right and left gastro-omental vessels) attached to its greater curvature. The vessels of its curvatures serve the body and pyloric antrum of the stomach. The upper body and fundus are served by short and posterior gastric vessels. The trilaminar smooth muscle of the stomach and gastric glands receive parasympathetic innervation from the vagus; sympathetic innervation to the stomach is vasoconstrictive and antiperistaltic.

Small Intestine

The **small intestine,** consisting of the duodenum, jejunum, and ileum (Fig. 2.34), is the primary site for absorption of nutrients from ingested materials, and extends from the pylorus to the ileocecal junction where the ileum joins the cecum (the first part of the large intestine). The pyloric part of the stomach empties into the duodenum, duodenal admission being regulated by the pylorus.

Duodenum

The **duodenum** (L. the breadth of 12 fingers), the first and shortest (25 cm) part of the small intestine, is also the widest and most fixed part. The duodenum pursues a C-shaped course around the head of the pancreas (Fig. 2.35C). The duodenum begins at the pylorus on the right side and ends at the **duodenojejunal junction** on the left side (Fig. 2.35B & C).

This junction occurs approximately at the level of the L2 vertebra, 2–3 cm to the left of the midline. The junction usually takes the form of an acute angle, the **duodenojejunal flexure.** Most of the duodenum is fixed by peritoneum to structures on the posterior abdominal wall and is considered partially retroperitoneal. The duodenum is divisible into four parts (Fig. 2.35C; Table 2.8):

- *Superior* (first) *part:* short (approximately 5 cm) and lies anterolateral to the body of the L1 vertebra.
- *Descending* (second) *part:* longer (7–10 cm) and descends along the right sides of the L1–L3 vertebrae.
- *Horizontal* (third) *part:* 6–8 cm long and crosses the L3 vertebra.
- *Ascending* (fourth) *part:* short (5 cm) and begins at the left of the L3 vertebra and rises superiorly as far as the superior border of the L2 vertebra.

The first 2 cm of the superior part of the duodenum, immediately distal to the pylorus, has a mesentery and is mobile. This free part, called the **ampulla** (duodenal cap), has an appearance distinct from the remainder of the duodenum when observed radiographically using contrast medium. The distal 3 cm of the superior part and the other three parts of the duodenum have no mesentery and are immobile because they are retroperitoneal. The principal relationships of the duodenum are outlined in Table 2.8 and illustrated in Figure 2.35.

The **superior part of the duodenum** ascends from the pylorus and is overlapped by the liver and gallbladder. Peritoneum covers its anterior aspect, but it is bare of peritoneum posteriorly, except for the ampulla. The proximal part has the *hepatoduodenal ligament* (part of the lesser omentum) attached superiorly and the greater omentum attached inferiorly (see Fig. 2.20).

The **descending part of the duodenum** runs inferiorly, curving around the head of the pancreas (Fig. 2.35; Table 2.8). Initially, it lies to the right of and parallel to the IVC. The *bile* and *main pancreatic ducts* enter its posteromedial

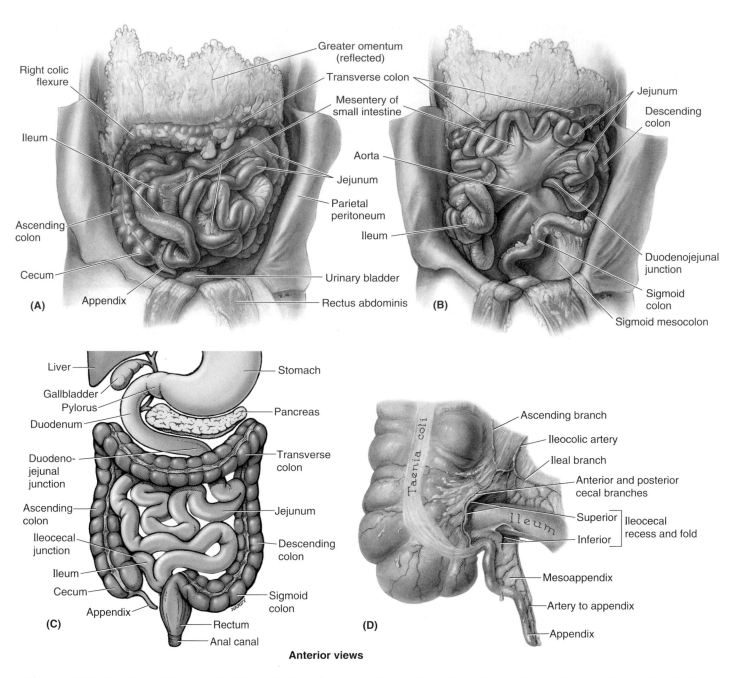

Anterior views

Figure 2.34. Small and large intestines. A. Note the convolutions of small intestine in situ, encircled on three sides by the large intestine and revealed by elevating greater omentum. **B.** The convolutions of small intestine have been retracted superiorly to demonstrate the mesentery. **C.** This orientation drawing of the alimentary system indicates the general position and relationships of the intestines. **D.** The blood supply of the ileocecal region is shown.

wall. These ducts usually unite to form the **hepatopancreatic ampulla**, which opens on the summit of an eminence, called the **major duodenal papilla**, located posteromedially in the descending duodenum. The descending part of the duodenum is entirely retroperitoneal. The anterior surface of its proximal and distal thirds is covered with peritoneum; however, the peritoneum reflects from its middle third to form the double-layered mesentery of the transverse colon, the transverse mesocolon.

The **inferior or horizontal part of the duodenum** runs transversely to the left, passing over the IVC, aorta, and L3 vertebra. It is crossed by the superior mesenteric artery and vein and the root of the mesentery of the jejunum and ileum. Superior to it is the head of the pancreas and its uncinate process. The anterior surface of the horizontal part is covered with peritoneum, except where it is crossed by the superior mesenteric vessels and the root of the mesentery. Posteriorly it is separated from the vertebral column by the

(cont'd on page 263)

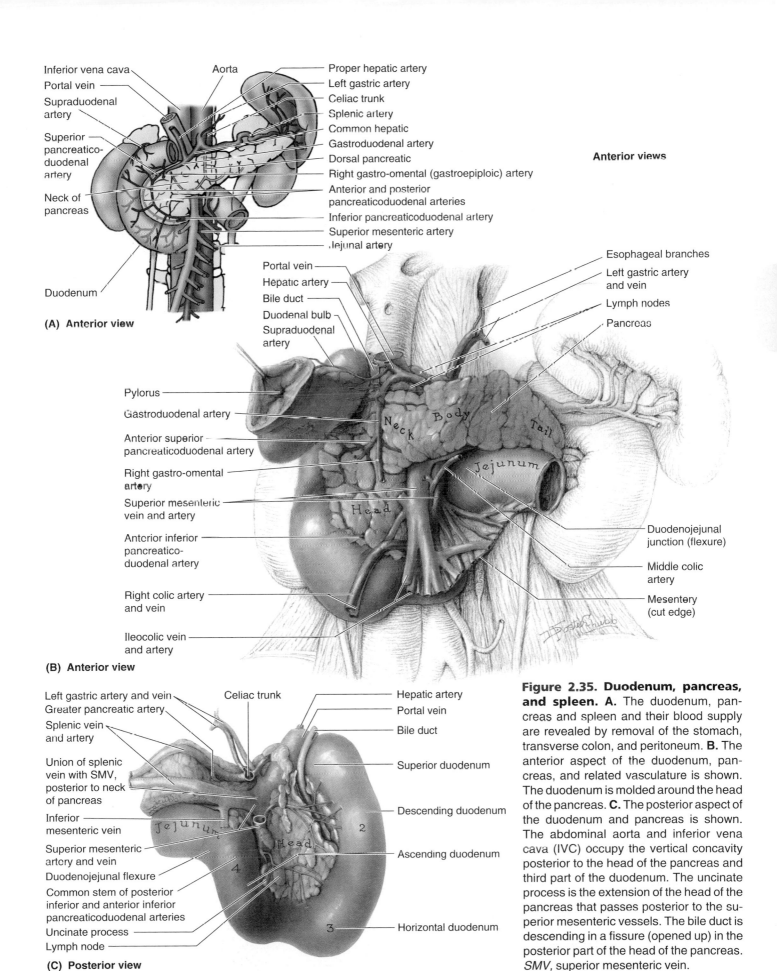

(A) Anterior view

Inferior vena cava
Portal vein
Supraduodenal artery
Superior pancreatico-duodenal artery
Neck of pancreas
Duodenum

Aorta
Proper hepatic artery
Left gastric artery
Celiac trunk
Splenic artery
Common hepatic
Gastroduodenal artery
Dorsal pancreatic
Right gastro-omental (gastroepiploic) artery
Anterior and posterior pancreaticoduodenal arteries
Inferior pancreaticoduodenal artery
Superior mesenteric artery
Jejunal artery

Anterior views

(B) Anterior view

Portal vein
Hepatic artery
Bile duct
Duodenal bulb
Supraduodenal artery

Esophageal branches
Left gastric artery and vein
Lymph nodes
Pancreas

Pylorus
Gastroduodenal artery
Anterior superior pancreaticoduodenal artery
Right gastro-omental artery
Superior mesenteric vein and artery
Anterior inferior pancreatico-duodenal artery
Right colic artery and vein
Ileocolic vein and artery

Neck   Body   Tail
Jejunum
Head

Duodenojejunal junction (flexure)
Middle colic artery
Mesentery (cut edge)

(C) Posterior view

Left gastric artery and vein
Greater pancreatic artery
Splenic vein and artery
Union of splenic vein with SMV, posterior to neck of pancreas
Inferior mesenteric vein
Superior mesenteric artery and vein
Duodenojejunal flexure
Common stem of posterior inferior and anterior inferior pancreaticoduodenal arteries
Uncinate process
Lymph node

Celiac trunk
Hepatic artery
Portal vein
Bile duct
Superior duodenum
Descending duodenum
Ascending duodenum
Horizontal duodenum

Jejunum   Head   2   4   3

Figure 2.35. Duodenum, pancreas, and spleen. A. The duodenum, pancreas and spleen and their blood supply are revealed by removal of the stomach, transverse colon, and peritoneum. **B.** The anterior aspect of the duodenum, pancreas, and related vasculature is shown. The duodenum is molded around the head of the pancreas. **C.** The posterior aspect of the duodenum and pancreas is shown. The abdominal aorta and inferior vena cava (IVC) occupy the vertical concavity posterior to the head of the pancreas and third part of the duodenum. The uncinate process is the extension of the head of the pancreas that passes posterior to the superior mesenteric vessels. The bile duct is descending in a fissure (opened up) in the posterior part of the head of the pancreas. *SMV,* superior mesenteric vein.

Table 2.8. Relationships of the Duodenum

Part of Duodenum	Anterior	Posterior	Medial	Superior	Inferior	Vertebral Level
Superior (1st part) **(A & B)**	Peritoneum Gallbladder Quadrate lobe of liver	Bile duct Gastroduodenal artery Portal vein IVC		Neck of gallbladder	Neck of pancreas	Anterolateral to L1 vertebra
Descending (2nd part) **(C)**	Transverse colon Transverse mesocolon Coils of small intestine	Hilum of right kidney Renal vessels Ureter Psoas major	Head of pancreas Pancreatic duct Bile duct			Right of L2–L3 vertebrae
Horizontal or Inferior (3rd part) **(D)**	SMA SMV Coils of small intestine	Right psoas major IVC Aorta Right ureter		Head and uncinate process of pancreas Superior mesenteric vessels		Anterior to L3 vertebra
Ascending (4th part) **(E)**	Beginning of root of mesentery Coils of jejunum	Left psoas major Left margin of aorta	Head of pancreas	Body of pancreas		Left of L3 vertebra

A = Intraperitoneal part ⎫ of superior part of duodenum
B = Retroperitoneal part ⎭

right psoas major, IVC, aorta, and the right testicular or ovarian vessels.

The **ascending part of the duodenum** runs superiorly and along the left side of the aorta to reach the inferior border of the body of the pancreas. Here it curves anteriorly to join the jejunum at the duodenojejunal junction, supported by the attachment of a **suspensory muscle of the duodenum** (ligament of Treitz). This muscle is composed of a slip of skeletal muscle from the diaphragm and a fibromuscular band of smooth muscle from the third and fourth parts of the duodenum. Contraction of this muscle widens the angle of the duodenojejunal flexure, facilitating movement of the intestinal contents. The suspensory muscle passes posterior to the pancreas and splenic vein and anterior to the left renal vein.

The *arteries of the duodenum* arise from the celiac trunk and the superior mesenteric artery (Fig. 2.35). The celiac trunk, via the **gastroduodenal artery** and its branch, the **superior pancreaticoduodenal artery**, supplies the duodenum proximal to the entry of the bile duct into the descending part of the duodenum. The superior mesenteric artery, through its branch, the **inferior pancreaticoduodenal artery**, supplies the duodenum distal to the entry of the bile duct. The pancreaticoduodenal arteries lie in the curve between the duodenum and the

head of the pancreas and supply both structures. The anastomosis of the superior and inferior pancreaticoduodenal arteries, which occurs approximately at the level of entry of the bile duct (or, according to some authors, at the junction of the descending and horizontal parts of the duodenum) is formed between the celiac and the superior mesenteric arteries. An important transition in the blood supply of the digestive tract occurs here: proximally, extending *orad* (toward the mouth) to and including the abdominal part of the esophagus, the blood is supplied to the alimentary tract by the celiac trunk; distally, extending *aborad* (away from the mouth) to the left colic flexure, the blood is supplied by the SMA. The basis of this transition in blood supply is embryological; this is the junction of the foregut and midgut (Moore and Persaud, 2003).

The *veins of the duodenum* follow the arteries and drain into the *portal vein*, some directly and others indirectly, through the superior mesenteric and splenic veins (Fig. 2.32).

The *lymphatic vessels of the duodenum* follow the arteries. The *anterior lymphatic vessels* of the duodenum drain into the *pancreaticoduodenal lymph nodes*, located along the superior and inferior pancreaticoduodenal arteries, and into the *pyloric lymph nodes*, which lie along the gastroduodenal artery (Fig. 2.36). The *posterior lymphatic vessels* pass posterior to the head

Vagal trunks

Abdominopelvic (greater and lesser) splanchnic nerves

Inferior vena cava

Celiac ganglia and plexus

Portal vein

Superior mesenteric ganglion and plexus

Pyloric lymph nodes

Pancreatico-duodenal lymph nodes

Periarterial plexuses

Superior mesenteric lymph nodes

Pancreaticosplenic lymph nodes (posterior to stomach)

Stomach

Spleen

Splenic lymph nodes

Celiac lymph nodes

Anterior view

Figure 2.36. Lymphatic drainage and innervation of duodenum, pancreas, and spleen. The close positional relationship of these organs results in sharing of blood vessels, lymphatic vessels, and nerve pathways, in whole or in part.

of the pancreas and drain into the **superior mesenteric lymph nodes.** Efferent lymphatic vessels from the duodenal lymph nodes drain into the *celiac lymph nodes.*

The *nerves of the duodenum* derive from the *vagus* and *greater* and *lesser (abdominopelvic) splanchnic nerves* by way of the celiac and superior mesenteric plexuses, from which they are conveyed to the duodenum via periarterial plexuses extending to the pancreaticoduodenal arteries (see also "Summary of the Innervation of the Abdominal Viscera," in this chapter).

Duodenal Ulcers

Duodenal (*peptic*) **ulcers** are inflammatory erosions of the duodenal mucosa. Most (65%) duodenal ulcers occur in the posterior wall of the superior part of the duodenum within 3 cm of the pylorus. Occasionally, an ulcer perforates the duodenal wall, permitting the contents to enter the peritoneal cavity and causing *peritonitis.* Because the superior part of the duodenum closely relates to the liver, gallbladder, and pancreas, any of these structures may become adherent to the inflamed duodenum and also become ulcerated as the lesion continues to the tissue that surrounds it. Although bleeding from gastric or duodenal ulcers commonly occurs, *erosion of the gastroduodenal artery* (a posterior relation of the superior part of the duodenum) by a duodenal ulcer results in severe hemorrhage into the peritoneal cavity and subsequent peritonitis.

Developmental Changes in the Mesoduodenum

During the early fetal period, the entire duodenum has a mesentery; however, most of it fuses with the posterior abdominal wall because of pressure from the overlying transverse colon. Because the attachment of the mesoduodenum to the wall is secondary (has occurred through formation of a *fusion fascia;* discussed under "Embryology of the Peritoneal Cavity," in this chapter), the duodenum and the closely associated pancreas can be separated (surgically mobilized) from the underlying retroperitoneal viscera during surgical operations involving the duodenum without endangering the blood supply to the kidney or the ureter.

Paraduodenal Hernias

There are two or three inconstant folds and fossae (recesses) around the duodenojejunal junction (Fig. B2.13). The *paraduodenal fold and fossa* are large and lie to the left of the ascending part of the duodenum. If a loop of intestine enters this fossa, it may strangulate. During repair of a **paraduodenal hernia,** care must be taken not to injure the branches of the inferior mesenteric artery and vein or the ascending branches of the left colic artery, which are related to the paraduodenal fold and fossa. ✪

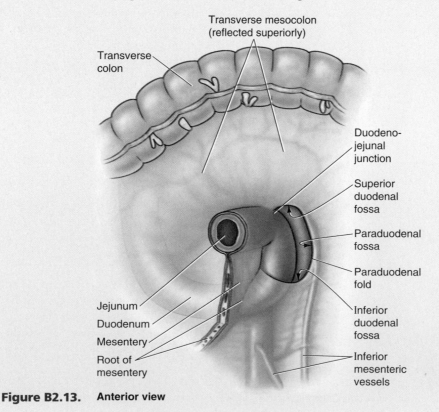

Transverse mesocolon (reflected superiorly)

Transverse colon

Duodenojejunal junction

Superior duodenal fossa

Paraduodenal fossa

Paraduodenal fold

Inferior duodenal fossa

Inferior mesenteric vessels

Jejunum

Duodenum

Mesentery

Root of mesentery

Figure B2.13.   Anterior view

THE BOTTOM LINE: The duodenum is the first part of the small intestine, receiving chyme mixed with gastric acid and pepsin directly from the stomach via the pylorus. It follows a mostly secondarily retroperitoneal, C-shaped course around the head of the pancreas. Its descending part receives both the bile and the pancreatic ducts. At or just distal to this level, a transition occurs in the blood supply of the abdominal part of the alimentary tract. Proximal to this point it is supplied by branches of the celiac trunk; distal to this point, it is supplied by branches of the superior mesenteric artery.

Jejunum and Ileum

The second part of the small intestine, the **jejunum**, begins at the duodenojejunal flexure where the alimentary tract resumes an intraperitoneal course. The third part of the small intestine, the **ileum**, ends at the **ileocecal junction**, the union of the terminal ileum and the cecum (Figs. 2.34D and 2.37). Together, the jejunum and ileum are 6–7 m long, the jejunum constituting approximately two fifths and the ileum approximately three fifths of the intraperitoneal section of the small intestine. Most of the jejunum lies in the left upper quadrant of the infracolic compartment,

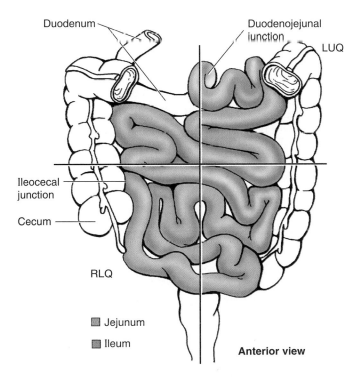

Figure 2.37. Jejunum and ileum. The jejunum begins at the duodenojejunal flexure and the ileum ends at the cecum. The combined term *jejunoileum* is sometimes used as an expression of the fact that there is no clear external line of demarcation between the jejunum and the ileum. *LUQ*, left upper quadrant; *RLQ*, right lower quadrant.

whereas most of the ileum lies in the right lower quadrant. The terminal ileum usually lies in the pelvis from which it ascends, ending in the medial aspect of the cecum. Although no clear line of demarcation between the jejunum and ileum exists, they have distinctive characteristics that are surgically important (Table 2.9).

The **mesentery** is a fan-shaped fold of peritoneum that attaches the jejunum and ileum to the posterior abdominal wall (Fig. 2.34B; Table 2.9A). The **root (origin) of the mesentery** (approximately 15 cm long) is directed obliquely, inferiorly, and to the right (Fig. 2.38A). It extends from the duodenojejunal junction on the left side of vertebra L2 to the ileocolic junction and the right sacroiliac joint. The average breadth of the mesentery from its root to the intestinal border is 20 cm. The root of the mesentery crosses (successively) the ascending and horizontal parts of the duodenum, abdominal aorta, IVC, right ureter, right psoas major, and right testicular or ovarian vessels. Between the two layers of the mesentery are the superior mesenteric vessels, lymph nodes, a variable amount of fat, and autonomic nerves.

The **superior mesenteric artery** supplies the jejunum and ileum (Fig. 2.38). The SMA usually arises from the abdominal aorta at the level of the L1 vertebra, approximately 1 cm inferior to the celiac trunk, and runs between the layers of the mesentery, sending 15–18 branches to the jejunum and ileum. The arteries unite to form loops or arches, called **arterial arcades,** which give rise to straight arteries, called **vasa recta** (Fig. 2.38B; Table 2.9C).

The **superior mesenteric vein** drains the jejunum and ileum (Fig. 2.38B). It lies anterior and to the right of the SMA in the root of the mesentery (Fig. 2.38A). The SMV ends posterior to the neck of the pancreas, where it unites with the splenic vein to form the portal vein (Fig. 2.35).

Specialized lymphatic vessels in the **intestinal villi** (tiny projections of the mucous membrane) that absorb fat are called **lacteals.** They empty their milk-like fluid into the lymphatic plexuses in the walls of the jejunum and ileum. The lacteals drain in turn into lymphatic vessels between the layers of the mesentery. Within the mesentery, the lymph passes sequentially through three groups of lymph nodes (Fig. 2.39):

- **Juxta-intestinal lymph nodes:** located close to the intestinal wall.

- **Mesenteric lymph nodes:** scattered among the arterial arcades.

- **Superior central nodes:** located along the proximal part of the SMA.

Efferent lymphatic vessels from the mesenteric lymph nodes drain to the *superior mesenteric lymph nodes.* Lymphatic vessels from the terminal ileum follow the ileal branch of the ileocolic artery to the **ileocolic lymph nodes.**

The SMA and its branches are surrounded by a *perivascular nerve plexus* through which the nerves are conducted to the parts of the intestine supplied by this artery (Fig. 2.40). The sympathetic fibers in the nerves to the jejunum and ileum

(cont'd on page 268)

Table 2.9. Distinguishing Characteristics of the Jejunum and Ileum in the Living Body

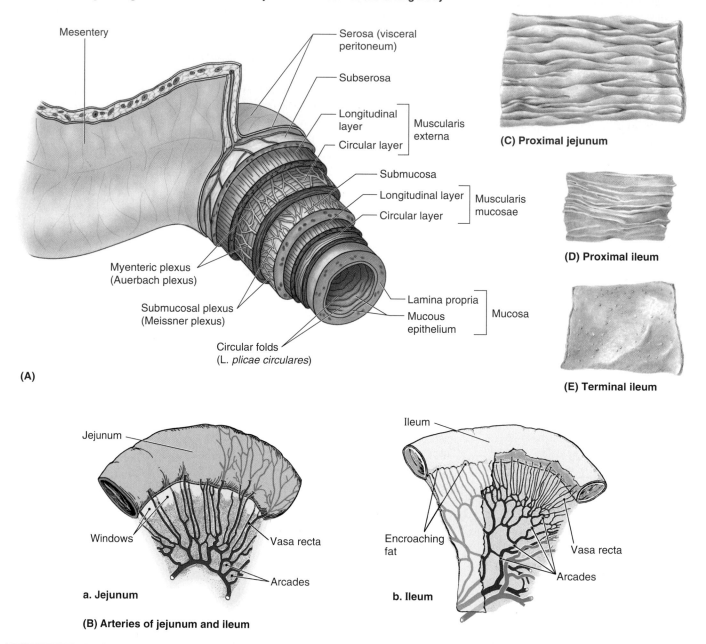

(C) Proximal jejunum

(D) Proximal ileum

(E) Terminal ileum

(A)

(B) Arteries of jejunum and ileum

a. Jejunum

b. Ileum

Characteristic	Jejunum (Ba, & C)		Ileum (Bb, D, & E)	
Color	Deeper red		Paler pink	
Caliber	2–4 cm		2–3 cm	
Wall	Thick and heavy		Thin and light	
Vascularity	Greater		Less	
Vasa recta	Long	Ba	Short	Bb
Arcades	A few large loops		Many short loops	
Fat in mesentery	Less		More	
Circular folds (L. *plicae circulares*)	Large, tall, and closely packed (C)		Low and sparse (D); absent in distal part (E)	
Lymphoid nodules (Peyer patches)	Few		Many (E)	

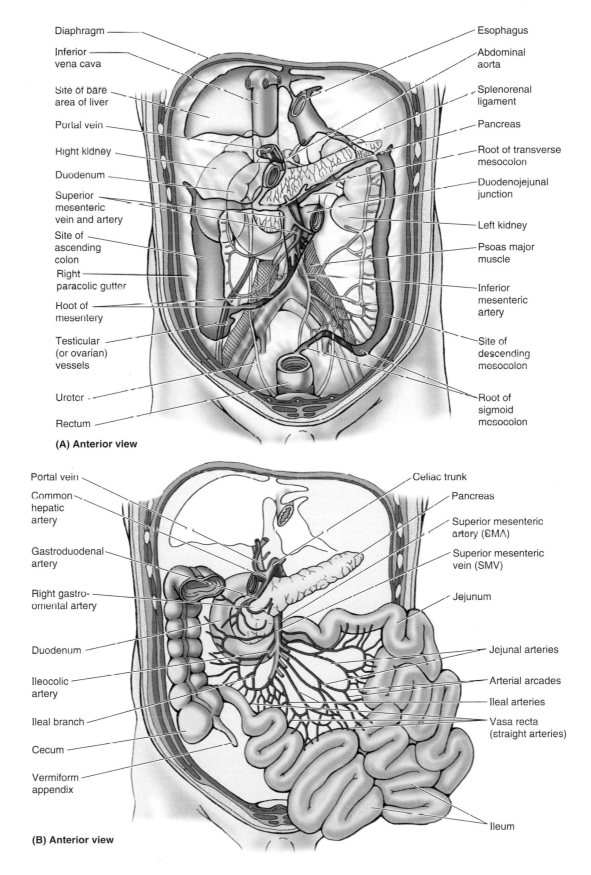

Figure 2.38. Arterial supply and mesenteries of intestines. A. The arteries supplying the large intestine are shown. The transverse and sigmoid mesocolons and the mesentery of the jejunum and ileum have been cut at their roots. The ileocolic and right colic arteries on the right side and the left colic and sigmoid arteries on the left side originally coursed within mesenteries (ascending and descending mesocolons) that became fused to the posterior wall; they can be re-established surgically. **B.** Arterial supply and venous drainage of the small intestine. The superior mesenteric artery supplies the jejunoileum, the ascending, and most of the transverse colon (not shown). The superior mesenteric vein drains blood from the intestine into the portal vein.

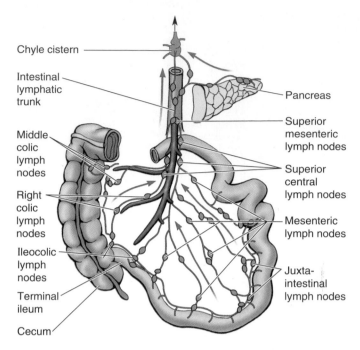

Figure 2.39. Mesenteric lymph nodes. The superior mesenteric lymph nodes form a system in which the central nodes, at the root of the superior mesenteric artery, receive lymph from the mesenteric, ileocolic, right colic, and middle colic lymph nodes. The nodes are more numerous adjacent to the intestine (juxta-intestinal lymph nodes) and less numerous along the arteries. The efferent vessels of the celiac and superior mesenteric lymph nodes form the intestinal lymphatic trunk, which usually ends in the left lumbar trunk but ends in the chyle cistern in 25% of people.

originate in the T8–T10 segments of the spinal cord and reach the **superior mesenteric nerve plexus** through the *sympathetic trunks* and *thoracic abdominopelvic (greater, lesser, and least) splanchnic nerves.* The presynaptic sympathetic fibers synapse on cell bodies of postsynaptic sympathetic neurons in the *celiac* and *superior mesenteric (prevertebral) ganglia.* The parasympathetic fibers in the nerves to the jejunum and ileum derive from the *posterior vagal trunks.* The presynaptic parasympathetic fibers synapse with postsynaptic parasympathetic neurons in the *myenteric* and *submucosal plexuses* in the intestinal wall (see also "Summary of the Innervation of the Abdominal Viscera," in this chapter).

In general, sympathetic stimulation reduces motility of the intestine and secretion and acts as a vasoconstrictor, reducing or stopping digestion and making blood (and energy) available for "fleeing or fighting." Parasympathetic stimulation increases motility of the intestine and secretion, restoring digestive activity following a sympathetic reaction. The small intestine also has sensory (visceral afferent) fibers. The intestine is insensitive to most pain stimuli, including cutting and burning; however, it is sensitive to distension that is perceived as *colic* (spasmodic abdominal pains).

Brief Review of the Embryological Rotation of the Midgut

An understanding of the rotation of the midgut clarifies the adult arrangement of the intestines. The primordial gut comprises the foregut, midgut, and hindgut (Moore and Persaud, 2003). Pain arising from foregut derivatives—esophagus, stomach, pancreas, duodenum, liver, and biliary ducts—localizes in the epigastric region. Pain arising from midgut derivatives—the small intestine distal to bile duct, cecum, appendix, ascending colon, and most of the transverse colon—localizes in the periumbilical region. Pain arising from hindgut derivatives—the distal part of the transverse colon, descending colon, sigmoid colon, and rectum—localizes in the hypogastric region.

For 4 weeks, the rapidly growing midgut, supplied by the SMA, is physiologically herniated into the proximal part of the umbilical cord (Fig. B2.14*A*). It is attached to the yolk sac by the yolk stalk. As it returns to the abdominal cavity, the midgut rotates 270° around the axis of the SMA (Fig. B2.14*B–C*). As the relative size of the liver and kidneys decreases, the midgut returns to the abdominal cavity as increased space becomes available. As the parts of the intestine reach their definitive positions, their mesenteric attachments undergo modification (Fig. B2.14*D–E*). Some mesenteries shorten and others disappear (e.g., most of duodenal mesentery). Malrotation of the midgut results in several congenital anomalies such as volvulus (twisting) of the intestine.

Navigating the Small Intestine

When portions of the small intestine have been delivered through a surgical wound, the proximal (orad) and distal (aborad) ends of a loop of bowel are not apparent. If you are trying to follow the intestine in a particular direction (e.g., attempting to follow the ileum to the ileocecal junction), it is important to know which end is which. Normal peristalsis may not be present to provide a clue. Place your hands on each side of the intestine and its mesentery, and then follow the mesentery with your fingers to its root (its attachment to the posterior abdominal wall), untwisting the loop of intestine as necessary. Once the mesentery and intestine are straightened to match the direction of the root, the cranial end must be the orad end, and the caudal end the aborad end.

Ischemia of the Intestine

Occlusion of the vasa recta by emboli results in *ischemia* of the part of the intestine concerned. If the ischemia is severe, *necrosis* of the involved segment results and **ileus** ▶

Rotation of the Midgut

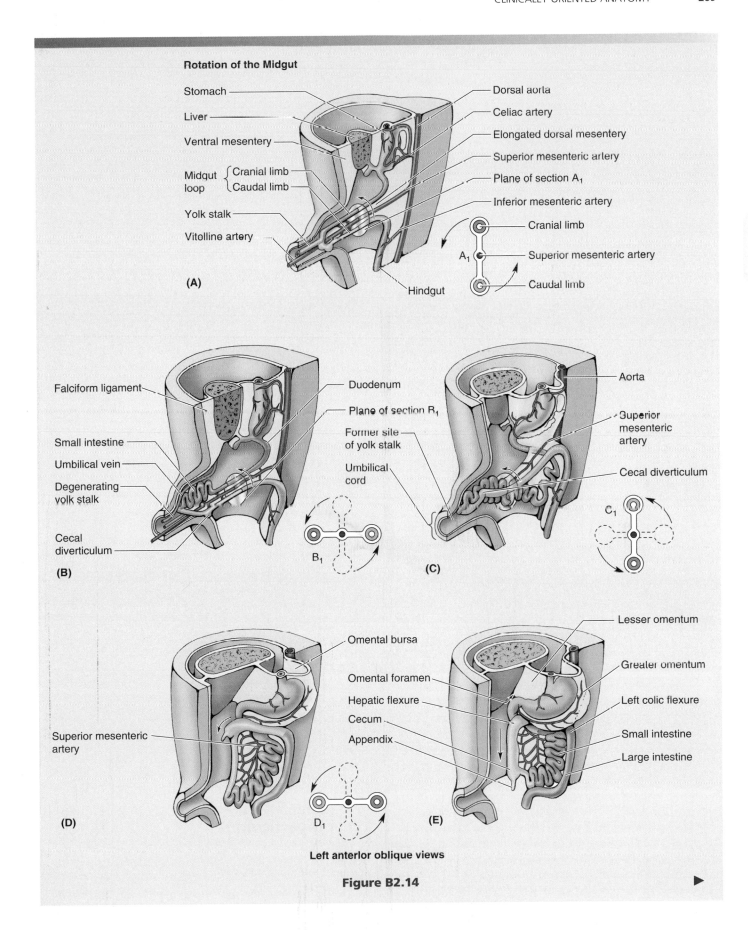

(A)
Stomach
Liver
Ventral mesentery
Midgut loop { Cranial limb / Caudal limb }
Yolk stalk
Vitelline artery
Dorsal aorta
Celiac artery
Elongated dorsal mesentery
Superior mesenteric artery
Plane of section A_1
Inferior mesenteric artery
Cranial limb
Superior mesenteric artery
Caudal limb
A_1
Hindgut

(B)
Falciform ligament
Small intestine
Umbilical vein
Degenerating yolk stalk
Cecal diverticulum
Duodenum
Plane of section B_1
Former site of yolk stalk
Umbilical cord
B_1

(C)
Aorta
Superior mesenteric artery
Cecal diverticulum
C_1

(D)
Superior mesenteric artery
Omental bursa
Omental foramen
Hepatic flexure
Cecum
Appendix
D_1

(E)
Lesser omentum
Greater omentum
Left colic flexure
Small intestine
Large intestine

Left anterior oblique views

Figure B2.14

Components of vagus nerve in medulla

Brainstem slice (medulla)

Sympathetic trunk

Sympathetic trunk ganglion

Spinal ganglion

Spinal nerve to vessels and glands of skin

White ramus communicans

Gray ramus communicans

Sympathetic trunk ganglion

Posterior root

Thoracic part of spinal cord (T8–T10)

Sensory cell body in sensory (nodose) ganglion of vagus

Motor fiber

Right vagus nerve

Anterior root

Abdominopelvic splanchnic nerve

Pain fiber

Posterior vagal trunk

Celiac ganglion in celiac plexus

Superior mesenteric ganglion

Pariarterial plexus around SMA and branches

Key

Sympathetic fibers	Parasympathetic fibers	
—— Presynaptic	—— Presynaptic	—— Visceral afferent fibers
- - - Postsynaptic	- - - Postsynaptic	—— Somatic afferent fibers

Figure 2.40. Innervation of small intestine. Presynaptic sympathetic nerve fibers originate in T8 or T9 through T10 or T11 segments of the spinal cord and reach the celiac plexus through the sympathetic trunks and greater and lesser (abdominopelvic) splanchnic nerves. After synapsing in the celiac and superior mesenteric ganglia, postsynaptic nerve fibers accompany the arteries to the intestine. Afferent fibers are concerned with reflexes and pain. Presynaptic parasympathetic (vagus) nerves originate in the medulla (oblongata) and pass to the intestine via the posterior vagal trunk. They synapse with intrinsic postsynaptic neurons located in the intestinal wall. *SMA,* superior mesenteric artery.

(obstruction of the intestine) of the paralytic type occurs. Ileus is accompanied by a severe colicky pain, along with abdominal distension, vomiting, and often fever and dehydration. If the condition is diagnosed early (e.g., using a *superior mesenteric arteriogram*), the obstructed part of the vessel may be cleared surgically.

Ileal Diverticulum

An **ileal diverticulum** (of Meckel) is a congenital anomaly that occurs in 1–2% of the population. A remnant of the proximal part of the embryonic yolk stalk, the diverticulum usually appears as a finger-like pouch ▶

(Fig. B2.15*A*). It is always at the site of attachment of the yolk stalk on the antimesenteric border (border opposite the mesenteric attachment) of the ileum. The diverticulum is usually located 30–60 cm from the ileocecal junction in infants and 50 cm in adults. It may be free (74%) or attached to the umbilicus (26%) (Fig. B2.15*B*). Although its mucosa is mostly ileal in type, it may also include areas of acid-producing gastric tissue, pancreatic tissue, or jejunal or colonic mucosa. An ileal diverticulum may become inflamed and produce pain mimicking that produced by appendicitis. If gastric tissue is included, a peptic ulcer may occur here. For discussion and illustrations of the various types of ileal diverticula, see Moore et al. (2000) and Moore and Persaud (2003). ✛

Figure B2.15

THE BOTTOM LINE: The jejunum and ileum make up the convolutions of the small intestine occupying most of the infracolic division of the greater sac of the peritoneal cavity. The jejunum is mostly to the upper right, and the ileum to the lower left. Together they are 3–4 m in length (in the cadaver; less in living people owing to the structures' tonicity). The orad two fifths is jejunum and the aborad three fifths is ileum, although there is no clear line of transition.

The diameter of the small intestine becomes increasingly smaller as the semifluid chyme progresses through it. Its blood vessels also become smaller, but the number of tiers of arcades increases while the length of the vasa recta decreases. However, the fat in which the vessels are embedded within the mesentery increases, making these features more difficult to see. The ileum is characterized by an abundance of lymphoid tissue, aggregated into nodules (Peyer patches). As the intraperitoneal portion of the small intestine, the jejunum and ileum are suspended by the mesentery, the root of which extends from the duodenojejunal junction to the left of the midline at the L2 level, to the ileocecal junction in the right iliac fossa. An ileal diverticulum is a congenital anomaly present in 1–2% of the population, is 3–6 cm in length, and is typically located 50 cm from the ileocecal junction.

Large Intestine

The **large intestine** is the site where water is absorbed from the indigestible residues of the liquid chyme, converting it into semisolid stool or feces that is stored temporarily and allowed to accumulate until defecation occurs. The large intestine consists of the *cecum;* the *appendix;* the *ascending, transverse, descending,* and *sigmoid colon;* the *rectum;* and the *anal canal* (Fig. 2.41). The large intestine can be distinguished from the small intestine by:

- **Omental appendices:** small, fatty, omentum-like projections.

- Three *teniae coli:* (1) *mesocolic,* to which the transverse and sigmoid mesocolons attach; (2) *omental,* to which the omental appendices attach; and (3) *free* (L. *libera*), to which neither mesocolons nor omental appendices are attached.

- **Haustra:** sacculations of the wall of the colon between the teniae

- A much greater caliber (internal diameter).

The **teniae coli** (thickened bands of smooth muscle representing most of the longitudinal coat) begin at the base of the appendix as the thick longitudinal layer of the appendix splits to form three bands. The teniae run the length of the large intestine, merging again at the rectosigmoid junction into a continuous longitudinal layer around the rectum. Because the teniae are shorter than the intestine, the colon becomes sacculated between the teniae, forming the haustra.

Cecum and Appendix

The **cecum** is the first part of the large intestine that is continuous with the ascending colon. It is a blind intestinal pouch, approximately 7.5 cm in both length and breadth, located in the right lower quadrant, where it lies in the iliac fossa inferior to the junction of the terminal ileum and cecum (Figs. 2.41 and 2.42). If distended with feces or gas, the cecum may be palpable through the anterolateral abdominal wall. The cecum usually lies within 2.5 cm of the

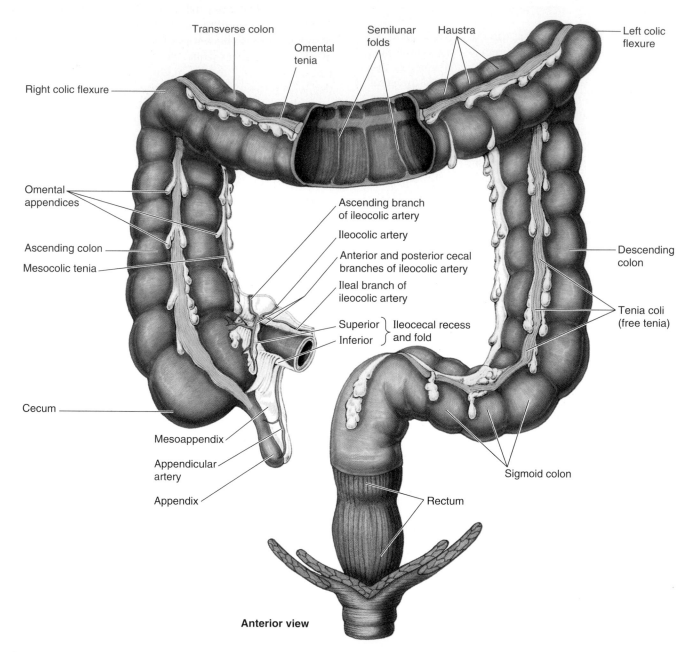

Figure 2.41. Terminal ileum and large intestine (including appendix). The mucosa, musculature (teniae), haustra, and omental (fatty) appendices of the colon are demonstrated. There are no teniae coli (thickened bands of longitudinal muscle) or omental appendices associated with the rectum.

inguinal ligament, is almost entirely enveloped by peritoneum, and can be lifted freely. However, the cecum has no mesentery. Because of its relative freedom, it may be displaced from the iliac fossa, but it is commonly bound to the lateral abdominal wall by one or more **cecal folds** of peritoneum (Fig. 2.42B). The terminal ileum enters the cecum obliquely and partly invaginates into it.

Traditionally, based on cadaveric studies, this manner of entrance produces **ileocolic lips** (superior and inferior) at the

ileal orifice, which form the **ileal papilla** (Fig. 2.42A). The folds meet laterally to form ridges, called the **frenula** of the valve. When the cecum is distended or when it contracts, the frenula tighten, closing the valve to prevent reflux from the cecum into the ileum. However, direct observation by endoscopy in living persons does not support this description. The circular muscle is poorly developed around the orifice; therefore, the valve is unlikely to have any sphincteric action that controls passage of the intestinal contents from the

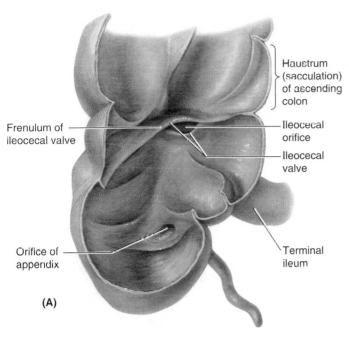

Figure 2.42. Terminal ileum, cecum, and appendix. A. The cecum was filled with air until dry, and then opened. Observe the ileocecal valve and ileal orifice. The frenulum is a fold (more evident in cadavers) that runs from the ileocecal valve along the wall at the junction of the cecum and ascending colon. **B.** The interior of the cecum showing the endoscopic (living) appearance of the ileocecal valve. **C.** The approximate incidences of various locations of the appendix, based on an analysis of 10,000 cases, are shown.

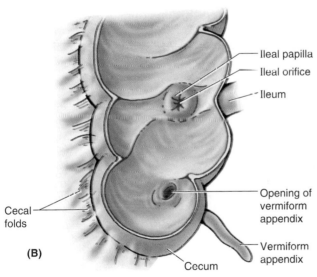

Anterior views

ileum into the cecum. The orifice is usually closed by tonic contraction, however, making it appear as the ileal papilla on the cecal side (Fig. 2.42B). The valve probably does prevent reflux from the cecum into the ileum as contractions occur to propel contents up the ascending colon and into the transverse colon (Magee and Dalley, 1986).

The **appendix** (traditionally, vermiform appendix; L. *vermis*, worm-like) is a blind intestinal diverticulum (6–10 cm in length) that contains masses of lymphoid tissue. It arises from the posteromedial aspect of the cecum inferior to the ileocecal junction. The appendix has a short triangular mesentery, the **mesoappendix**, which derives from the posterior side of

the mesentery of the terminal ileum (Fig. 2.41). The mesoappendix attaches to the cecum and the proximal part of the appendix. The position of the appendix is variable, but it is usually retrocecal (Fig. 2.42C).

The cecum is supplied by the **ileocolic artery,** the terminal branch of the SMA (Table 2.10). The **appendicular artery,** a branch of the ileocolic artery, supplies the appendix. A tributary of the SMV, the **ileocolic vein,** drains blood from the cecum and appendix (Fig. 2.43A).

The lymphatic vessels from the cecum and appendix pass to lymph nodes in the mesoappendix and to the *ileocolic lymph nodes* that lie along the ileocolic artery (Fig. 2.43B). Ef-

Table 2.10. Arterial Supply to the Intestines

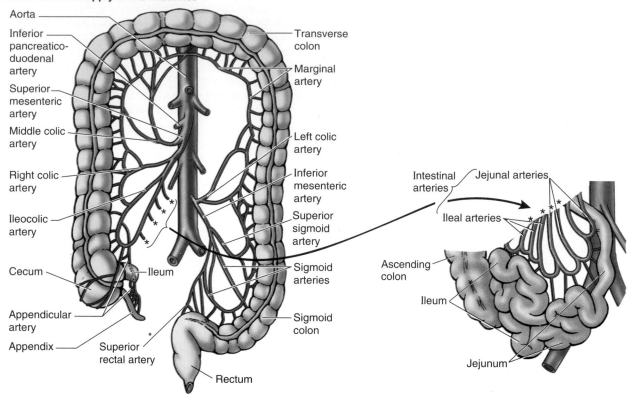

Artery	Origin	Course	Distribution
Superior mesenteric	Abdominal aorta	Runs in root of mesentery to ileocecal junction	Part of gastrointestinal tract derived from midgut
Intestinal (jejunal and ileal) (*n* = 15–18)	Superior mesenteric artery	Passes between two layers of mesentery	Jejunum and ileum
Middle colic	Superior mesenteric artery	Ascends retroperitoneally and passes between layers of transverse mesocolon	Transverse colon
Right colic	Superior mesenteric artery	Passes retroperitoneally to reach ascending colon	Ascending colon
Ileocolic	Terminal branch of superior mesenteric artery	Runs along root of mesentery and divides into ileal and colic branches	Ileum, cecum, and ascending colon
Appendicular	Ileocolic artery	Passes between layers of mesoappendix	Appendix
Inferior mesenteric	Abdominal aorta	Descends retroperitoneally to left of abdominal aorta	Supplies part of gastrointestinal tract derived from hindgut
Left colic	Inferior mesenteric artery	Passes retroperitoneally toward left to descending colon	Descending colon
Sigmoid (*n* = 3–4)	Inferior mesenteric artery	Passes retroperitoneally toward left to descending colon	Descending and sigmoid colon
Superior rectal	Terminal branch of inferior mesenteric artery	Descends retroperitoneally to rectum	Proximal part of rectum
Middle rectal	Internal iliac artery	Passes retroperitoneally to rectum	Midpart of rectum
Inferior rectal	Internal pudendal artery	Crosses ischioanal fossa to reach rectum	Distal part of rectum and anal canal

ferent lymphatic vessels pass to the *superior mesenteric lymph nodes.*

The nerve supply to the cecum and appendix derives from the sympathetic and parasympathetic nerves from the *superior mesenteric plexus* (Fig. 2.43C). The *sympathetic nerve fibers* orig-inate in the lower thoracic part of the spinal cord, and the *parasympathetic nerve fibers* derive from the vagus nerves. Affer-ent nerve fibers from the appendix accompany the sympathetic nerves to the T10 segment of the spinal cord (see also "Summary of the Innervation of the Abdominal Viscera," in this chapter).

Position of the Appendix

A *retrocecal appendix* extends superiorly toward the right colic flexure and is usually free (Fig. 2.42C). It occasion-ally lies beneath the peritoneal covering of the cecum, where it is often fused to the cecum or the posterior ab dominal wall. The appendix may project inferiorly to-ward or across the pelvic brim. The anatomical position of the appendix determines the symptoms and the site of muscular spasm and tenderness when the appendix is in-flamed. The base of the appendix lies deep to a point that is one third of the way along the oblique line joining the right ASIS to the umbilicus (the *McBurney point* on the *spinoumbilical line*).

Appendicitis

Acute inflammation of the appendix is a common cause of an *acute abdomen* (severe abdominal pain arising sud-denly). Usually, digital pressure over the McBurney point registers maximum abdominal tenderness. **Appendicitis** in young people is usually caused by hyperplasia of lym-phatic follicles in the appendix that occludes the lumen. In older people, the obstruction usually results from a *fe-calith* (*coprolith*), a concretion that forms around a center of fecal matter. When secretions from the appendix can-not escape, the appendix swells, stretching the visceral peritoneum. The pain of appendicitis usually commences as a vague pain in the periumbilical region because affer-ent pain fibers enter the spinal cord at the T10 level. Later, severe pain in the right lower quadrant results from irritation of the parietal peritoneum lining the posterior abdominal wall. Extending the thigh at the hip joint elic-its pain.

Acute infection of the appendix may result in *thrombo-sis* (clotting of blood) in the appendicular artery, which often results in ischemia, gangrene (death of tissue), and perforation of an acutely inflamed appendix. *Rupture of the appendix* results in infection of the peritoneum (*peritoni-tis*), increased abdominal pain, nausea and/or vomiting, and *abdominal rigidity* (stiffness of the abdominal mus-cles). Flexion of the right thigh ameliorates the pain be-cause it causes relaxation of the right psoas muscle, a flexor of the thigh.

Appendectomy

Surgical removal of the appendix (**appendectomy**) is usu-ally performed through a transverse or gridiron (muscle-splitting) incision centered at the McBurney point in the right lower quadrant (see clinical correlation [blue] box "Abdominal Surgical Incisions," in this chapter). Tradi-tionally, a gridiron incision is made perpendicular to the spinoumbilical line, but a transverse incision is also com-monly used. The choice of incision site and type is at the surgeon's discretion. While typically the inflamed ap-pendix is deep to the McBurney point, the site of maximal pain and tenderness indicates the actual location. The fol-lowing description outlines the clinical anatomy of an appendectomy—not the technique.

Following incision of the skin and subcutaneous tissue, the external oblique aponeurosis is incised along the lines of its fibers. An opening is then made in the same way in the internal oblique and transverse abdominal muscles, thus avoiding their nerve supply. The iliohypogastric nerve is identified between the fleshy muscle layers and re-tracted. The transversalis fascia and peritoneum are in-cised, and the cecum is delivered into the surgical wound. The appendix arises from the convergence of the three teniae coli. Thus, if the appendix is not obvious, one of the teniae coli is traced to its base. The mesoappendix con-taining the appendicular vessels is firmly ligated and divided. The base of the appendix is tied, the appendix is excised, and its stump is usually cauterized and invagi-nated into the cecum. The incision is then closed in layers. Because each muscle layer runs in a different direction, the incision is well protected when the retracted layers are re-turned to their normal position.

In unusual cases of *malrotation of the intestine,* or failure of descent of the cecum, the appendix is not in the lower right quadrant (Moore and Persaud, 2003). When the ce-cum is high (*subhepatic cecum*), the appendix is in the right hypochondriac region and the pain localizes there, not in the lower right quadrant.

Laparoscopy

When the diagnosis is unclear, examination of the ab-dominal contents with a *laparoscope* passed through a ▶

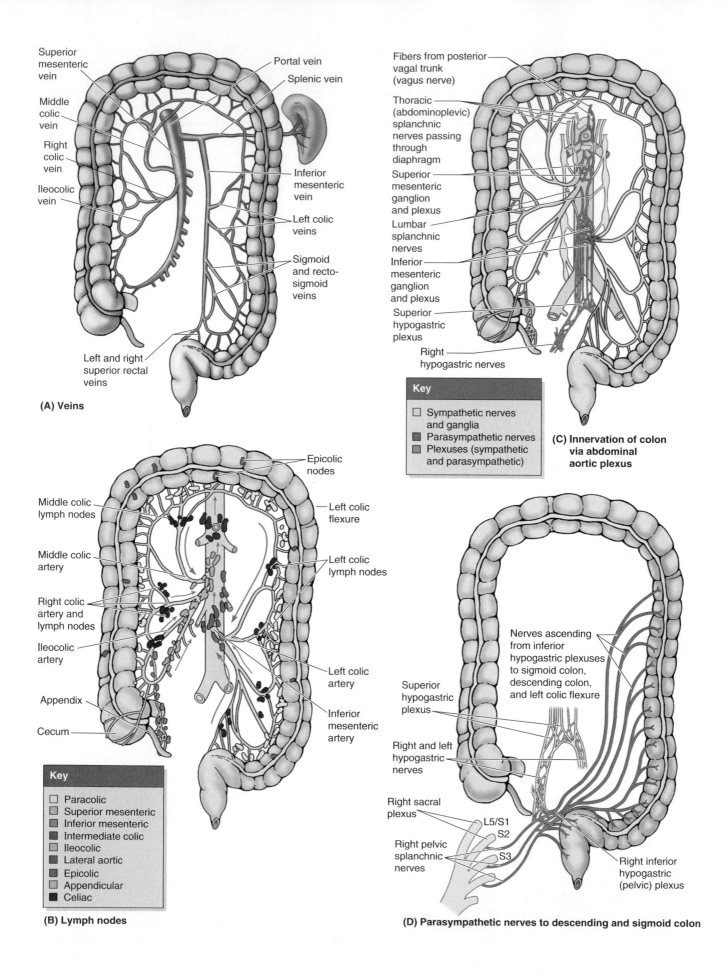

(A) Veins

Superior mesenteric vein
Middle colic vein
Right colic vein
Ileocolic vein
Portal vein
Splenic vein
Inferior mesenteric vein
Left colic veins
Sigmoid and recto-sigmoid veins
Left and right superior rectal veins

(C) Innervation of colon via abdominal aortic plexus

Fibers from posterior vagal trunk (vagus nerve)
Thoracic (abdominoplevic) splanchnic nerves passing through diaphragm
Superior mesenteric ganglion and plexus
Lumbar splanchnic nerves
Inferior mesenteric ganglion and plexus
Superior hypogastric plexus
Right hypogastric nerves

Key
☐ Sympathetic nerves and ganglia
■ Parasympathetic nerves
■ Plexuses (sympathetic and parasympathetic)

(B) Lymph nodes

Middle colic lymph nodes
Middle colic artery
Right colic artery and lymph nodes
Ileocolic artery
Appendix
Cecum
Epicolic nodes
Left colic flexure
Left colic lymph nodes
Left colic artery
Inferior mesenteric artery

Key
☐ Paracolic
☐ Superior mesenteric
■ Inferior mesenteric
■ Intermediate colic
☐ Ileocolic
■ Lateral aortic
■ Epicolic
☐ Appendicular
■ Celiac

(D) Parasympathetic nerves to descending and sigmoid colon

Nerves ascending from inferior hypogastric plexuses to sigmoid colon, descending colon, and left colic flexure
Superior hypogastric plexus
Right and left hypogastric nerves
Right sacral plexus
Right pelvic splanchnic nerves
L5/S1
S2
S3
Right inferior hypogastric (pelvic) plexus

small incision in the anterolateral abdominal wall is useful in differentiating acute appendicitis from other causes of abdominal pain, including inflammatory pelvic disease. Laparoscopy has been used for many years by gynecologists in evaluating women with lower abdominal pain (Soper, 2000). In addition, laparoscopy is used for removing the gallbladder and appendix and for treating abdominal obstruction. ☉

THE BOTTOM LINE: The large intestine consists of the cecum; appendix; ascending, transverse, descending, and sigmoid colon; rectum; and anal canal. The large intestine is characterized by teniae coli, haustra, omental appendices, and a large caliber. The large intestine begins at the ileocecal valve; but its first part, the cecum, is a pocket that hangs inferior to the valve. The pouch-like cecum, the widest part of the large intestine, is completely intraperitoneal and lacking a mesentery, so that it is mobile within the right iliac fossa. The ileocecal valve is a combination valve and weak sphincter, actively opening periodically to allow entry of ileal contents and forming a largely passive one-way valve between the ileum and the cecum, preventing reflux. The appendix is an intestinal diverticulum, rich in lymphoid tissue, that enters the medial aspect of the cecum, usually deep to the junction of the lateral third and medial two thirds of the spinoumbilical line. Most commonly, the appendix is retrocecal in position, but 32% of the time it descends into the lesser pelvis. The cecum and appendix are supplied by branches of the ileocecal vessels.

Colon

The **colon** is described as having four parts—ascending, transverse, descending, and sigmoid—that succeed one another in an arch (Fig. 2.41). The colon lies first to the right of the small intestine, then successively superior and anterior to it, to the left of it, and eventually inferior to it.

The **ascending colon** is the second part of the large intestine. It passes superiorly on the right side of the abdominal cavity from the cecum to the right lobe of the liver, where it turns to the left at the **right colic flexure** (*hepatic flexure*). The ascending colon is narrower than the cecum and is secondarily retroperitoneal along the right side of the posterior abdominal wall. The ascending colon is covered by peritoneum anteriorly and on its sides; however, in approximately 25% of people it has a short mesentery. The ascending colon is separated from the anterolateral abdominal wall by the greater omentum. A deep vertical groove lined with parietal peritoneum, the *right paracolic gutter*, lies between the lateral aspect of the ascending colon and the adjacent abdominal wall (Fig. 2.38A).

The arterial supply to the ascending colon and right colic flexure is from branches of the SMA, the *ileocolic* and **right colic arteries** (Table 2.10). These arteries anastomose with each other and with the *right branch of the middle colic artery*, the first of a series of anastomotic arcades that is continued by the left colic and sigmoid arteries to form a continuous arterial channel, the **marginal artery** (*juxtacolic artery*), that parallels and extends the length of the colon close to its mesenteric border. Tributaries of the SMV, the *ileocolic* and **right colic veins**, drain blood from the ascending colon (Fig. 2.43A). The lymphatic vessels pass first to the **epicolic** and **paracolic lymph nodes**, next to the *ileocolic* and intermediate **right colic lymph nodes**, and from them to the *superior mesenteric lymph nodes* (Fig. 2.43B). The nerves to the ascending colon derive from the *superior mesenteric nerve plexus* (Fig. 2.43C).

Mobile Ascending Colon

When the inferior part of the ascending colon has a mesentery, the cecum and proximal part of the colon are abnormally mobile. This condition, present in approximately 11% of individuals, may cause *volvulus of the colon* (L. *volvo*, to roll), an obstruction of intestine resulting from twisting. *Cecopexy* may avoid volvulus and possible obstruction of the colon. In this anchoring procedure, a tenia coli of the cecum and proximal ascending colon is sutured to the abdominal wall. ☉

Figure 2.43. Veins, lymphatics, and innervation of large intestine and appendix. A. The venous drainage by the superior and inferior mesenteric veins corresponds to the pattern of the arteries they accompany. The IMV is most commonly a tributary of the splenic vein (as shown here), which then merges with the SMV to form the portal vein. **B.** From any part of the large intestine, the lymph flows sequentially to (1) epicolic nodes directly on the gut; (2) paracolic nodes along the mesenteric border; (3) intermediate (meso-) colic nodes, along the colic arteries (ileo-, right, middle, and left); and then (4) to the superior or inferior mesenteric nodes, which usually drain by intestinal trunks to the chyle cistern. **C.** Presynaptic sympathetic fibers from T10 through L2 spinal cord levels pass through thoracic and lumbar splanchnic nerves to postsynaptic neurons in the superior and inferior (prevertebral) ganglia. Postsynaptic sympathetic fibers travel along the colic arteries to reach the large intestine. Presynaptic parasympathetic fibers from the vagus (CN X) nerves also pass along the colic arteries to the cecum, ascending colon, and most of the transverse colon. **D.** Presynaptic parasympathetic fibers from S2 through S4 spinal cord levels pass through pelvic splanchnic nerves to the inferior hypogastric (pelvic) plexuses and continue by way of nerves ascending from both right and left plexuses (left plexus not shown) to reach the sigmoid colon, descending colon, and most of the distal transverse colon. Pain fibers from most of the large intestine follow the sympathetic fibers retrograde to sensory ganglia of spinal nerves T10–L2; pain fibers from the distal sigmoid colon and rectum follow the parasympathetic fibers retrograde to sensory ganglia of spinal nerves S2–S4.

The **transverse colon** (approximately 45 cm long) is the third, longest, and most mobile part of the large intestine (Fig. 2.41). It crosses the abdomen from the *right colic flexure* to the *left colic flexure,* where it bends inferiorly to become the descending colon. The **left colic flexure** (splenic flexure) is usually more superior, more acute, and less mobile than the right colic flexure. It lies anterior to the inferior part of the left kidney and attaches to the diaphragm through the *phrenicocolic ligament* (Fig. 2.20). The mesentery of the transverse colon, the *transverse mesocolon,* loops down, often inferior to the level of the iliac crests, and is adherent to or fused with the posterior wall of the omental bursa. The **root of the transverse mesocolon** (Fig. 2.38A) lies along the inferior border of the pancreas and is continuous with the parietal peritoneum posteriorly. Being freely movable, the transverse colon is variable in position, usually hanging to the level of the umbilicus (L3 vertebral level) (Fig. 2.44A). However, in tall thin people, the transverse colon may extend into the pelvis (Fig. 2.44B).

(A) Anteroposterior view

(B) Anteroposterior view

Figure 2.44. Effect of body type (bodily habitus) on disposition of transverse colon. A. A heavily built hypersthenic individual with a short thorax and long abdomen is likely to have a transverse colon that is placed high. **B.** Individuals with a slender asthenic physique are likely to have a transverse colon that dips down toward or into the pelvis.

The arterial supply of the transverse colon is mainly from the **middle colic artery** (Table 2.10), a branch of the SMA. However, the transverse colon may also receive arterial blood from the *right* and *left colic arteries* via anastomoses, part of the series of anastomotic arcades that collectively form the *marginal artery* (juxtacolic artery). Venous drainage of the transverse colon is through the SMV (Fig. 2.43A). The lymphatic drainage of the transverse colon is to the **middle colic lymph nodes,** which in turn drain to the *superior mesenteric lymph nodes* (Fig. 2.43B).

The nerves of the transverse colon pass from the *superior mesenteric nerve plexus* via the periarterial plexuses of the right and middle colic arteries (Fig. 2.43C). These nerves transmit sympathetic, parasympathetic (vagal), and visceral afferent nerve fibers (see also "Summary of the Innervation of the Abdominal Viscera," in this chapter).

The **descending colon** occupies a secondarily retroperitoneal position between the left colic flexure and the left iliac fossa, where it is continuous with the sigmoid colon (Fig. 2.41). Thus peritoneum covers the colon anteriorly and laterally and binds it to the posterior abdominal wall. Although retroperitoneal, the descending colon, especially in the iliac fossa, has a short mesentery in approximately 33% of people; however, it is usually not long enough to cause volvulus of the colon. As it descends, the colon passes anterior to the lateral border of the left kidney. As with the ascending colon, the descending colon has a *paracolic gutter* (the left) on its lateral aspect (Fig. 2.38A).

The **sigmoid colon,** characterized by its S-shaped loop of variable length (usually approximately 40 cm), links the descending colon and the rectum (Fig. 2.41). The sigmoid colon extends from the iliac fossa to the S3 segment, where it joins the rectum. The termination of the teniae coli, approximately 15 cm from the anus, indicates the *rectosigmoid junction.* The sigmoid colon usually has a long mesentery and, therefore, has considerable freedom of movement, especially its middle part. The **root of the sigmoid mesocolon** has an inverted V-shaped attachment, extending first medially and superiorly along the external iliac vessels and then medially and inferiorly from the bifurcation of the common iliac vessels to the anterior aspect of the sacrum. The *left ureter* and the division of the left common iliac artery lie retroperitoneally, posterior to the apex of the root of the sigmoid mesocolon. The *omental appendices* of the sigmoid colon are long; they disappear when the sigmoid mesentery terminates. The teniae coli also disappear as the longitudinal muscle in the wall of the colon broadens to form a complete layer in the rectum.

The arterial supply of the descending and sigmoid colon is from the *left colic* and **sigmoid arteries,** branches of the inferior mesenteric artery (Table 2.10). Thus, at approximately the left colic flexure, a second transition occurs in the blood supply of the abdominal part of the alimentary tract: the superior mesenteric artery supplying blood to that part orad to the flexure (the embryonic midgut), and the inferior mesenteric artery supplying blood to that part aborad to the flexure (the embryonic hindgut). The sigmoid arteries descend obliquely to the left, where they divide into ascending and descending branches. The superior branch of the most superior sigmoid artery anastomoses with the descending branch of the left colic artery, thereby forming a part of the *marginal artery*. The *inferior mesenteric vein* returns blood from the descending colon and sigmoid colon, flowing usually into the splenic vein and then the portal vein on its way to the liver (Figs. 2.43A and 2.88).

The lymphatic vessels from the descending colon and sigmoid colon pass to the epicolic and paracolic nodes and then through the **intermediate colic lymph nodes** along the left colic artery (Fig. 2.43B). Lymph from these nodes passes to the **inferior mesenteric lymph nodes** that lie around the inferior mesenteric artery. However, lymph from the left colic flexure may also drain to the *superior mesenteric lymph nodes*.

Orad to the left colic flexure, sympathetic and parasympathetic fibers travel together from the abdominal aortic plexus via periarterial plexuses to reach the abdominal part of the alimentary tract (Fig. 2.43C); however, aborad to the flexure, they follow separate routes. The sympathetic nerve supply of the descending and sigmoid colon is from the lumbar part of the sympathetic trunk via lumbar (abdominopelvic) splanchnic nerves, the superior mesenteric plexus, and the periarterial plexuses following the inferior mesenteric artery and its branches. The parasympathetic nerve supply is from the *pelvic splanchnic nerves* via the inferior hypogastric (pelvic) plexus and nerves, which ascend retroperitoneally from the plexus, independent of the arterial supply to this part of the alimentary tract (Fig. 2.43D). Orad to the middle of the sigmoid colon, visceral afferents conveying pain sensation pass retrogradely with sympathetic fibers to thoracolumbar spinal sensory ganglia, whereas those carrying reflex information travel with the parasympathetic fibers to vagal sensory ganglia. Aborad to the middle of the sigmoid colon, all visceral afferents follow the parasympathetic fibers retrogradely to the sensory ganglia of spinal nerves S2–S4 (see also "Summary of the Innervation of the Abdominal Viscera," in this chapter).

Rectum and Anal Canal

The **rectum** is the fixed (primarily retroperitoneal and subperitoneal) terminal part of the large intestine. It is continuous with the sigmoid colon at the level of S3 vertebra. The junction is at the inferior end of the mesentery of the sigmoid colon (Fig. 2.41). The rectum is continuous inferiorly with the anal canal. These parts of the large intestine are described with the pelvis in Chapter 3.

Colitis, Colectomy, Ileostomy, and Colostomy

Chronic inflammation of the colon (*ulcerative colitis, Crohn disease*) is characterized by severe inflammation and ulceration of the colon and rectum. In some cases a *colectomy* is performed, during which the terminal ileum and colon, as well as the rectum and anal canal, are removed. An *ileostomy* is then constructed to establish an opening between the ileum and the skin of the anterolateral abdominal wall (Fig. B2.16A). Sometimes a *colostomy* is performed to create an artificial cutaneous opening into the colon (Fig. B2.16B). A *sigmoidostomy* establishes an artificial anus by creating a cutaneous opening into the sigmoid colon.

Colonoscopy

The interior of the colon can be observed and photographed in a procedure called **colonoscopy** or *coloscopy* (Fig. B2.17A), using an elongated endoscope, usually a fiberoptic *colonoscope* (Fig. B2.17B). The endoscope is ▶

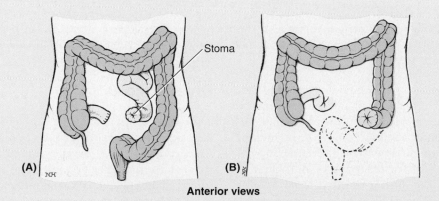

Stoma

(A)   (B)

Anterior views

Figure B2.16. A. Ileostomy. **B.** Colostomy.

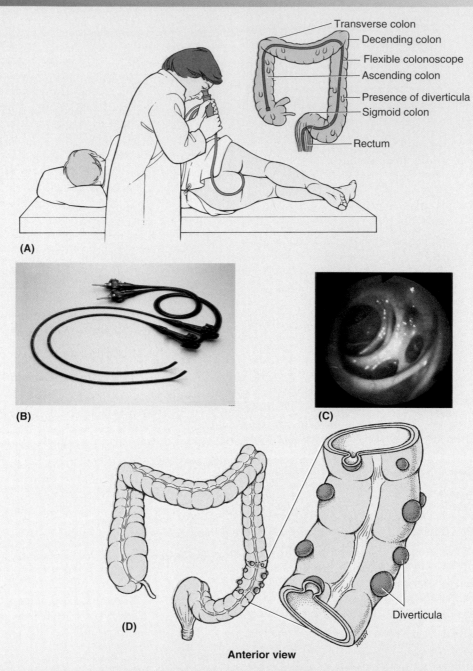

Transverse colon
Decending colon
Flexible colonoscope
Ascending colon
Presence of diverticula
Sigmoid colon
Rectum

(A)

(B)

(C)

(D)

Diverticula

Anterior view

Figure B2.17. Examination of large intestine. A. The colonoscopic procedure is shown. **B.** The parts of a colonoscope are shown. **C.** Diverticulosis of the colon can be photographed through a colonoscope. **D.** Diverticula in the sigmoid colon are shown.

a flexible tube that inserts into the colon through the anus and rectum (Fig. B2.17*A*). Small instruments can be passed through the colonoscope and used to facilitate minor operative procedures, such as biopsies or removal of polyps. Most tumors of the large intestine occur in the rectum; approximately 12% of them appear near the rectosigmoid junction. The interior of the sigmoid colon is observed with a *sigmoidoscope* (*sigmoscope*), a shorter endoscope, in a procedure called *sigmoidoscopy*.

Diverticulosis

Diverticulosis is a disorder in which multiple false **diverticula** (external evaginations or out-pocketings of the mucosa of the colon) develop along the intestine. It primarily affects middle-aged and elderly people. Diverticulosis is commonly (60%) found in the sigmoid colon (Fig. B2.17*C* & *D*). *Colonic diverticula* are not true diverticula because they are formed from protrusions of mucous ▶

membrane only, evaginated through weak points (separations) developed between muscle fibers rather than involving the whole wall of the colon. They occur most commonly on the mesenteric side of the two nonmesenteric teniae coli, where nutrient arteries perforate the muscle coat to reach the submucosa. Diverticula are subject to infection and rupture, leading to diverticulitis, and they can distort and erode the nutrient arteries, leading to hemorrhage. Diverticulosis is less likely to develop in individuals adhering to a diet high in fiber. ☉

THE BOTTOM LINE: The colon is described as having four parts: ascending, transverse, descending, and sigmoid. The ascending colon is a superior, secondarily retroperitoneal continuation of the cecum, extending between the level of the ileocecal valve and the right colic flexure. The transverse colon, suspended by the transverse mesocolon between the right and the left flexures, is the longest and most mobile part of the large intestine. The level to which it descends depends largely on body type (habitus). The descending colon occupies a secondarily retroperitoneal position between the left colic flexure and the left iliac fossa, where it is continuous with the sigmoid colon. The typically S-shaped sigmoid colon, suspended by the sigmoid mesocolon, is highly variable in length and disposition, ending at the rectosigmoid junction. The teniae, haustra, and omental appendices cease at the junction, located anterior to the third sacral segment.

Proximal (orad) to the left colic flexure, the large intestine (cecum, appendix, and ascending and transverse colons) is supplied by branches of the superior mesenteric vessels; distal (aborad) to the flexure, the colon (descending and sigmoid colons and superior rectum) is supplied by the inferior mesenteric vessels. The left colic flexure also marks the divide between cranial (vagal) and sacral (pelvic splanchnic) parasympathetic innervation of the alimentary tract. Sympathetic fibers are conveyed to the large intestine via abdominopelvic (lesser and lumbar) splanchnic nerves via the prevertebral (superior and inferior mesenteric) ganglia and periarterial plexuses. The middle of the sigmoid colon marks a divide in the sensory innervation of the abdominal alimentary tract. Orad, visceral afferents for pain travel retrogradely with sympathetic fibers to spinal sensory ganglia, whereas those conveying reflex information travel with parasympathetic fibers to vagal sensory ganglia. Aborad, both types of visceral afferent fibers travel with parasympathetic fibers to spinal sensory ganglia.

Spleen

The **spleen** is an ovoid, usually purplish, pulpy mass about the size and shape of one's fist. It is relatively delicate and considered the most vulnerable abdominal organ. The spleen is located in the left upper abdominal quadrant or hypochondrium, where it receives the protection of the lower thoracic cage (Figs. 2.45A and 2.46). As the largest of the lymphatic organs, it participates in the body's defense system as a site of lymphocyte (white blood cell) proliferation and of immune surveillance and response. Prenatally, it is a hematopoietic (blood-forming) organ, but after birth is involved primarily in identifying, removing, and destroying expended red blood cells (RBCs) and broken-down platelets, and in recycling iron and globin. It serves as a blood reservoir, storing RBCs and platelets, and, to a limited degree, can provide a sort of "self-transfusion" as a response to the stress imposed by hemorrhage. In spite of its size and the many useful and important functions it provides, it is not a vital organ (not necessary to sustain life).

To accommodate these functions, the spleen is a soft, vascular (sinusoidal) mass with a relatively delicate fibroelastic capsule, entirely surrounded by peritoneum except at the **splenic hilum**, where the splenic branches of the splenic artery and vein enter and leave (Fig. 2.45B). Consequently, it is capable of marked expansion and some relatively rapid contraction. It is a mobile organ although it normally does not descend inferior to the costal (rib) region; it rests on the left colic flexure. It is associated posteriorly with the left 9th–11th ribs and separated from them by the diaphragm and the *costodiaphragmatic recess*—the cleft-like extension of the pleural cavity between the diaphragm and the lower part of the thoracic cage (see Chapter 1). The **relations of the spleen** are

- Anteriorly, the stomach.
- Posteriorly, the left part of the diaphragm, which separates it from the pleura, lung, and ribs 9–11.
- Inferiorly, the left colic flexure.
- Medially, the left kidney.

The spleen varies considerably in size, weight, and shape; however, it is usually approximately 12 cm long and 7 cm wide. (A nonmetric memory device exploits odd numbers: the spleen is 1 inch thick, 3 inches wide, 5 inches long, and weighs 7 ounces.) The **diaphragmatic surface of the spleen** is convexly curved to fit the concavity of the diaphragm. The **anterior** and **superior borders of the spleen** are sharp and often notched, whereas its **posterior (medial) end** and **inferior border** are rounded.

The spleen normally contains a large quantity of blood that is expelled periodically into the circulation by the action of the smooth muscle in its capsule and trabeculae. The large size of the splenic artery (or vein) indicates the volume of blood that passes through the spleen's capillaries and sinuses. The thin **fibrous capsule of the spleen** is composed of dense, irregular, fibroelastic connective tissue (Fig. 2.45C). The

(cont'd on page 284)

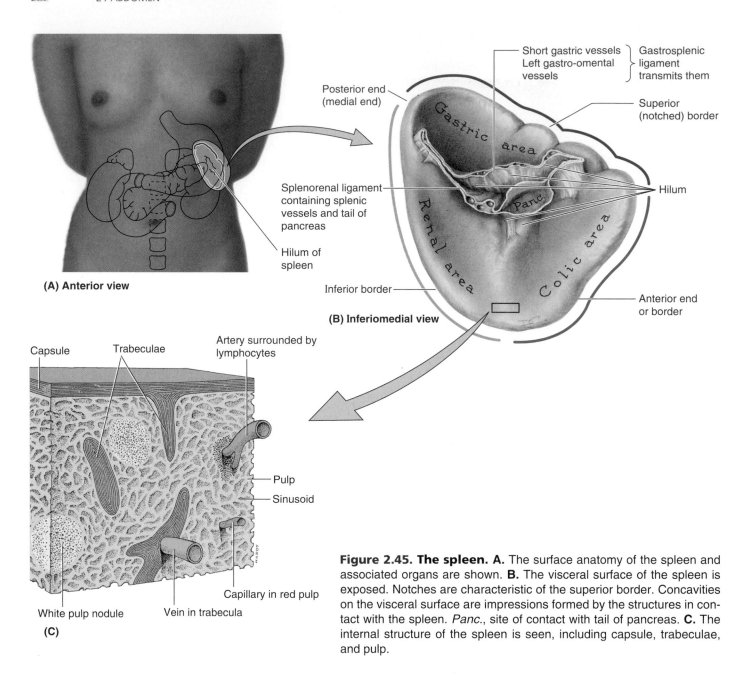

(A) Anterior view

Posterior end
(medial end)

Short gastric vessels
Left gastro-omental
vessels

Gastrosplenic
ligament
transmits them

Superior
(notched) border

Splenorenal ligament
containing splenic
vessels and tail of
pancreas

Gastric area

Panc.

Renal area

Colic area

Hilum

Hilum of
spleen

Inferior border

Anterior end
or border

(B) Inferiomedial view

Capsule

Trabeculae

Artery surrounded by
lymphocytes

Pulp

Sinusoid

White pulp nodule

Vein in trabecula

Capillary in red pulp

(C)

Figure 2.45. The spleen. A. The surface anatomy of the spleen and associated organs are shown. **B.** The visceral surface of the spleen is exposed. Notches are characteristic of the superior border. Concavities on the visceral surface are impressions formed by the structures in contact with the spleen. *Panc.*, site of contact with tail of pancreas. **C.** The internal structure of the spleen is seen, including capsule, trabeculae, and pulp.

Figure 2.46. Pancreas, duodenum, biliary ducts, and spleen. A. The pancreas, extrahepatic bile passages, pancreatic ducts, and duodenum are shown. **B.** The entry of the bile duct and pancreatic duct into the duodenum through the hepatopancreatic ampulla—the dilation within the major duodenal papilla that normally receives the bile duct and the main pancreatic duct—is shown. Smooth muscle sphincters encircle the bile and pancreatic ducts and the hepatopancreatic ampulla. **C.** The interior of the descending part of the duodenum reveals the major and minor duodenal papillae. There is a hood over the larger papilla onto which the hepatopancreatic ampulla is opening. The bile duct and main pancreatic duct open separately on the papilla in approximately 5% of people. The accessory pancreatic duct opens on the minor duodenal papilla. **D.** The structure of the acinar (enzyme-producing) tissue is demonstrated. The photomicrograph of the pancreas displays secretory acini and a pancreatic islet.

(A)

Neck of gallbladder

Common hepatic duct

Gallbladder

Bile duct (common bile duct)

Portal vein

Common hepatic artery

Right suprarenal gland

Superior part of duodenum

Gastroduodenal artery

Accessory pancreatic duct

Right kidney

Descending part of duodenum

Pancreas

Main pancreatic duct

Hepatopancreatic ampulla

Hepatopancreatic sphincter

Cystic duct

Cystohepatic (Calot's) triangle with cystic artery

Liver

Splenorenal ligament

Left suprarenal gland

Tail

Spleen

Splenic artery

Splenic vein

Left kidney

Left renal vein

Superior mesenteric artery

Bile duct

Main pancreatic duct

Neck

Body

Head

Sphincter of bile duct

Bile duct

Descending part of duodenum

Main pancreatic duct

Sphincter of pancreatic duct

Hepato-pancreatic ampulla

Major duodenal papilla

(B) Anterior view

Aorta

Inferior vena cava

Inferior mesenteric artery

Lumen of intralobular duct

Pancreatic islet

Acinar cells

(D)

Minor duodenal papilla

Hood

Major duodenal papilla

Longitudinal fold

(C)

fibrous capsule is thickened at the splenic hilum. Internally the **trabeculae,** arising from the deep aspect of the capsule, carry blood vessels to and from the parenchyma or splenic **pulp,** the substance of the spleen (Fig. 2.45*C*).

The spleen contacts the posterior wall of the stomach and is connected to its greater curvature by the *gastrosplenic ligament* and to the left kidney by the **splenorenal ligament** (Fig. 2.22). These ligaments, containing splenic vessels, are attached to the hilum of the spleen on its medial aspect (Fig. 2.45*B*). The splenic hilum is often in contact with the tail of the pancreas and constitutes the left boundary of the omental bursa.

The **splenic artery** is the largest branch of the celiac trunk and follows a tortuous course posterior to the omental bursa, anterior to the left kidney, and along the superior border of the pancreas (Figs. 2.47*A* and 2.48*A*). Between the layers of the splenorenal ligament, the splenic artery divides into five or more branches that enter the hilum. The lack of anastomosis of the arterial vessels in the spleen results in the formation of vascular segments of the spleen: two in 84% of spleens and three in the others, with relatively avascular planes between them, enabling subtotal splenectomy (see clinical correlation [blue] box, "Splenectomy and Splenomegaly," in this chapter).

The **splenic vein** is formed by several tributaries that emerge from the hilum (Figs. 2.46*A* and 2.47*B*). It is joined by the IMV and runs posterior to the body and tail of the pancreas throughout most of its course. The splenic vein unites with the SMV posterior to the neck of the pancreas to form the *portal vein.*

The splenic lymphatic vessels leave the lymph nodes in the splenic hilum and pass along the splenic vessels to the *pancreaticosplenic lymph nodes* (Fig. 2.48*A*). These nodes relate to the posterior surface and superior border of the pancreas. The nerves of the spleen, derived from the *celiac nerve plexus* (Fig. 2.48*B*), are distributed mainly along branches of the splenic artery, and are vasomotor in function.

Rupture of the Spleen

Although well protected by the 9th–12th ribs, the spleen is the most frequently injured organ in the abdomen. Severe blows on the left side may fracture one or more of these ribs, resulting in sharp bone fragments that can lacerate the spleen. In addition, blunt trauma to other regions of the abdomen that cause a sudden, marked increase in intra-abdominal pressure (e.g., by impalement on the steering wheel of a car or the handlebars of a motor cycle) can cause the thin capsule and overlying peritoneum of the spleen to burst, disrupting its soft parenchyma or pulp (*ruptured spleen*). If ruptured, there is profuse bleeding (*intraperitoneal hemorrhage*) and shock. ▶

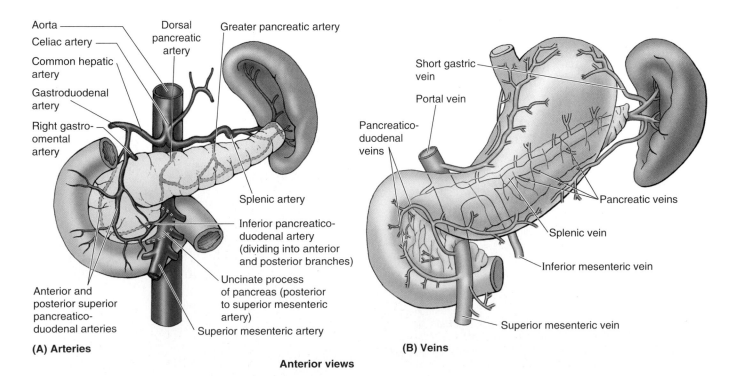

(A) Arteries

Aorta
Celiac artery
Common hepatic artery
Gastroduodenal artery
Right gastro-omental artery
Dorsal pancreatic artery
Greater pancreatic artery
Splenic artery
Inferior pancreatico-duodenal artery (dividing into anterior and posterior branches)
Anterior and posterior superior pancreatico-duodenal arteries
Uncinate process of pancreas (posterior to superior mesenteric artery)
Superior mesenteric artery

(B) Veins

Short gastric vein
Portal vein
Pancreatico-duodenal veins
Pancreatic veins
Splenic vein
Inferior mesenteric vein
Superior mesenteric vein

Anterior views

Figure 2.47. Arterial supply and venous drainage of pancreas. Because of the close relationship of the pancreas and duodenum, their blood vessels are the same in whole or in part.

(A) Lymph nodes

Key	
☐	Pancreaticosplenic nodes
■	Celiac nodes
☐	Superior mesenteric nodes
■	Pyloric nodes
☐	Hepatic nodes

Vagus nerve — Esophagus

Abdominopelvic (greater, lesser, least) splanchnic nerves

Spleen

Celiac ganglion, trunk, and plexus

Sympathetic trunk and ganglion (lumbar portion)

Superior mesenteric ganglion, plexus, and artery

Sympathetic trunk and ganglion

Pancreas

Aorta

(B) Nerves

Anterior views

Key	
☐	Sympathetic nerves
■	Parasympathetic nerves
■	Plexuses (sympathetic and parasympathetic)

Figure 2.48. Lymphatic drainage and innervation of pancreas and spleen. A. The *arrows* indicate lymph flow to the lymph nodes. **B.** The nerves of the pancreas are autonomic nerves from the celiac and superior mesenteric plexuses. A dense network of nerve fibers passes from the celiac plexus along the splenic artery to the spleen. Most are postsynaptic sympathetic fibers to smooth muscle of the splenic capsule, trabeculae, and intrasplenic vessels.

Splenectomy and Splenomegaly

Repair of a ruptured spleen is difficult; consequently, **splenectomy** (removal of the spleen) is often performed to prevent the person from bleeding to death. *Sub-total* (*partial*) *splenectomy*, when possible, is followed by rapid regeneration. Even *total splenectomy* usually does not produce serious effects, especially in adults, because most of its functions are assumed by other reticuloendothelial organs (e.g., the liver and bone marrow), but there is a greater susceptibility to certain bacterial infections. When the spleen is diseased, resulting from, for example, granulocytic leukemia (high leukocyte and white blood cell count), it may enlarge to 10 or more times its normal size and average a weight of 100–250 g (**splenomegaly**). Spleen engorgement sometimes accompanies hypertension (high blood pressure). The spleen is not usually palpable in the adult; generally, if its lower edge can be detected when palpating below the left costal margin at the end of inspiration (Fig. B2.18*A*), it is enlarged about three times its "normal" size. Splenomegaly also occurs in some forms of hemolytic or granulocytic anemias, in which RBCs or white blood cells (WBCs), respectively, are destroyed at abnormally high rates (Fig. B2.18*B*). In such cases, a splenectomy may be life-saving.

(A)

Rib cage
Enlarged spleen
Colon

(B)

Figure B2.18. Examination of spleen. A. Palpation of the spleen is demonstrated. **B.** This 4200 g spleen was seen at autopsy.

Accessory Spleen(s)

One or more small **accessory spleens** may form near the splenic hilum; they may be embedded partly or wholly in the tail of the pancreas, between the layers of the ▶

Tail of pancreas

Hilum of spleen

Gastrosplenic ligament

Greater omentum (left)

Mesentery

Uterine tube/ovary (female)

Course of testicular descent

Left scrotal sac

Figure B2.19. Potential sites of accessory spleens. The dots indicate where small accessory spleens may be located.

gastrosplenic ligament, in the infracolic compartment in the mesentery, or in close proximity to the ovary or testis (Fig. B2.19). In most affected individuals, only one accessory spleen is present. Accessory spleens are common (10%), are usually small (approximately 1 cm in diameter, but range from 0.2 to 10 cm), and often resemble a lymph node. Awareness of the possible presence of an accessory spleen is important because if not removed during splenectomy, the symptoms that indicated removal of the spleen (e.g., *splenic anemia*) may persist.

Splenic Needle Biopsy and Splenoportography

The relationship of the costodiaphragmatic recess of the pleural cavity to the spleen is clinically important (see Fig. 2.31*B*). This potential space descends to the level of the 10th rib in the midaxillary line. Its existence must be kept in mind when doing a *splenic needle biopsy,* or when injecting radiopaque material into the spleen for visualization of the portal vein (*splenoportography*). If care is not exercised, this material may enter the pleural cavity, causing *pleuritis* (inflammation of the pleura). ○

THE BOTTOM LINE: The spleen is highly vascular (sinusoidal), pulpy mass surrounded by a delicate fibroelastic capsule. It is completely covered by peritoneum, except at the splenic hilum, where the splenorenal ligament (conveying splenic vessels to the spleen) and gastrosplenic ligament (conveying the short gastric and left gastroomental vessels to the stomach) attach. Its average size is about that of one's fist, within a considerable range of normal variation. It is the largest of the lymphoid organs, but is not vital. As a blood reservoir, it is normally capable of considerable temporary expansion and contraction, but may undergo much more marked, chronic enlargement in disease. Although it receives protection from the overlying left 9th–11th ribs, the relatively delicate spleen is the abdominal organ most vulnerable to indirect trauma. Strong blows to the abdomen can cause a sudden increase in intra-abdominal pressure that may rupture the organ, resulting in profuse intraperitoneal hemorrhage.

Pancreas

The **pancreas** is an elongated, accessory digestive gland that lies retroperitoneally and transversely across the posterior abdominal wall, posterior to the stomach between the duodenum on the right and the spleen on the left (Fig. 2.46*A*). The

transverse mesocolon attaches to its anterior margin. The pancreas produces

- An exocrine secretion (*pancreatic juice* from the acinar cells) that enters the duodenum through the main and accessory pancreatic ducts.

- Endocrine secretions (*glucagon* and *insulin* from the pancreatic islets [of Langerhans]) that enter the blood (Fig. 2.46*D*).

For descriptive purposes the pancreas is divided into four parts: *head, neck, body,* and *tail.* The **head of the pancreas** is the expanded part of the gland that is embraced by the C-shaped curve of the duodenum to the right of the superior mesenteric vessels. It firmly attaches to the medial aspect of the descending and horizontal parts of the duodenum. The **uncinate process,** a projection from the inferior part of the pancreatic head, extends medially to the left, posterior to the SMA (Fig. 2.47*A*). The head of the pancreas rests posteriorly on the IVC, right renal artery and vein, and the left renal vein. On its way to opening into the descending part of the duodenum, the *bile duct* lies in a groove on the posterosuperior surface of the head or is embedded in its substance (Fig. 2.46*A* & *B*).

The **neck of the pancreas** is short (1.5–2 cm) and overlies the superior mesenteric vessels (Fig. 2.46*A*), which form a groove in its posterior aspect (Fig. 2.35*B* & *C*). The anterior surface of the neck, covered with peritoneum, is adjacent to the *pylorus of the stomach.* The SMV joins the splenic vein posterior to the neck to form the portal vein.

The **body of the pancreas** continues from the neck and lies to the left of the superior mesenteric vessels, passing over the aorta and L2 vertebra, posterior to the omental bursa. The anterior surface of the body of the pancreas is covered with peritoneum and lies in the floor of the omental bursa and forms part of the stomach bed. The posterior surface of the pancreatic body is devoid of peritoneum and is in contact with the aorta, SMA, left suprarenal gland, and left kidney and renal vessels (Fig. 2.46A).

The **tail of the pancreas** lies anterior to the left kidney, where it is closely related to the splenic hilum and the left colic flexure. The tail is relatively mobile and passes between the layers of the splenorenal ligament with the splenic vessels (Figs. 2.46A and 2.47A). The tip of the tail is usually blunted and turned superiorly.

The **main pancreatic duct** begins in the tail of the pancreas and runs through the parenchyma of the gland to the pancreatic head: here it turns inferiorly and is closely related to the bile duct (Fig. 2.46A & B). Most of the time, the main pancreatic duct and the bile duct unite to form the short, dilated **hepatopancreatic ampulla** (of Vater), which opens into the descending part of the duodenum at the summit of the *major duodenal papilla* (Fig. 2.46B & C). At least 25% of the time, the ducts open into the duodenum separately. The **sphincter of the pancreatic duct** (around the terminal part of the pancreatic duct), the **sphincter of the bile duct** (around the termination of the bile duct), and the **hepatopancreatic sphincter** (of Oddi)—around the hepatopancreatic ampulla—are smooth muscle sphincters that control the flow of bile and pancreatic juice into the duodenum.

An **accessory pancreatic duct** (Fig. 2.46A) opens into the duodenum at the summit of the *minor duodenal papilla* (Fig. 2.46C). Usually (60%), the accessory duct communicates with the main pancreatic duct. In some cases, the main pancreatic duct is smaller than the accessory pancreatic duct and the two are not connected. In such people, the accessory duct carries most of the pancreatic juice. These variations of the pancreatic ducts are explainable from their fusion or lack of fusion during pancreatic development (Moore and Persaud, 2003).

The **pancreatic arteries** derive mainly from the branches of the markedly tortuous *splenic artery*, which form several arcades with pancreatic branches of the *gastroduodenal* and *superior mesenteric arteries* (Fig. 2.47A). Up to 10 branches of the splenic artery supply the body and tail of the pancreas. The *anterior* and *posterior superior pancreaticoduodenal arteries*, branches of the gastroduodenal artery, and the *anterior* and *posterior inferior pancreaticoduodenal arteries*, branches of the SMA, supply the head. The corresponding *pancreatic veins* are tributaries of the splenic and superior mesenteric parts of the portal vein; however, most of them empty into the *splenic vein* (Fig. 2.47B).

The pancreatic lymphatic vessels follow the blood vessels (Fig. 2.48A). Most vessels end in the *pancreaticosplenic lymph nodes,* that lie along the splenic artery. Some vessels end in the *pyloric lymph nodes.* Efferent vessels from these nodes drain to the *superior mesenteric lymph nodes* or to the *celiac lymph nodes* via the *hepatic lymph nodes.*

The nerves of the pancreas are derived from the *vagus* and *abdominopelvic splanchnic nerves* passing through the diaphragm (Fig. 2.48B). The parasympathetic and sympathetic fibers reach the pancreas by passing along the arteries from the *celiac plexus* and **superior mesenteric plexus** (see also "Summary of the Innervation of the Abdominal Viscera," in this chapter). In addition to sympathetic fibers that pass to blood vessels, sympathetic and parasympathetic fibers are distributed to pancreatic acinar cells and islets. The parasympathetic fibers are secretomotor, but pancreatic secretion is primarily mediated by secretin and cholecystokinin, hormones formed by the epithelial cells of the duodenum and upper intestinal mucosa under the stimulus of acid contents from the stomach.

Blockage of the Hepatopancreatic Ampulla and Pancreatitis

Because the main pancreatic duct joins the bile duct to form the hepatopancreatic ampulla and pierces the duodenal wall, a *gallstone* passing along the extrahepatic bile passages may lodge in the constricted distal end of the ampulla, where it opens at the summit of the major duodenal papilla (Fig. 2.46A & B). In this case, both the biliary and pancreatic duct systems are blocked and neither bile nor pancreatic juice can enter the duodenum. However, bile may back up and enter the pancreatic duct, usually resulting in *pancreatitis* (inflammation of the pancreas). A similar reflux of bile sometimes results from *spasms of the hepatopancreatic sphincter*. Normally, the sphincter of the pancreatic duct prevents reflux of bile into the pancreatic duct; however, if the hepatopancreatic ampulla is obstructed, the weak pancreatic duct sphincter may be unable to withstand the excessive pressure of the bile in the hepatopancreatic ampulla. If the accessory pancreatic duct connects with the main pancreatic duct and opens into the duodenum, it may compensate for an obstructed main pancreatic duct or spasm of the hepatopancreatic sphincter.

Accessory Pancreatic Tissue

It is not unusual for *accessory pancreatic tissue* to develop in the stomach, duodenum, ileum, or an ileal diverticulum; however, the stomach and duodenum are the most common sites. The accessory pancreatic tissue may contain pancreatic islet cells that produce glucagon and insulin. ▶

Pancreatectomies

In the treatment of some people with chronic pancreatitis, most of the pancreas is removed, a procedure called **pancreatectomy.** The anatomical relationships and the blood supply of the head of the pancreas, bile duct, and duodenum make it impossible to remove the entire head of the pancreas (Skandalakis et al., 1995). Usually a rim of the pancreas is retained along the medial border of the duodenum to preserve the duodenal blood supply.

Rupture of the Pancreas

The pancreas is centrally located within the body and thus is well protected from all but the most severe penetrating trauma. The duodenum, into which its duct opens, is normally sterile. The pancreas, like the liver, has a considerable functional reserve. For all these reasons, the pancreas, as an exocrine organ, is not commonly a primary cause of clinical problems (discounting *diabetes,* an endocrine disorder of the islet cells); most exocrine pancreatic problems are secondary to biliary problems. Pancreatic injury can result, however, from sudden, severe, forceful compression of the abdomen, such as the force of impalement on a steering wheel in an automobile accident. Because the pancreas lies transversely, the vertebral column acts as an anvil, and the traumatic force may rupture the friable pancreas. Rupture of the pancreas frequently tears its duct system, allowing pancreatic juice to enter the parenchyma of the gland and to invade adjacent tissues. Digestion of pancreatic and other tissues by pancreatic juice is quite painful.

Pancreatic Cancer

Cancer involving the pancreatic head accounts for most cases of extrahepatic obstruction of the biliary ducts. Because of the posterior relationships of the pancreas, cancer of the head often compresses and obstructs the bile duct and/or the hepatopancreatic ampulla. This condition causes obstruction, resulting in the retention of bile pigments, enlargement of the gallbladder, and *jaundice* (*obstructive jaundice*). Jaundice (Fr. *jaune,* yellow) is the yellow staining of most body tissues, skin, mucous membranes, and conjunctiva by circulating bile pigments. Approximately 90% of people with pancreatic cancer have *ductular adenocarcinoma.* Severe pain in the back is frequently present. Cancer of the neck and body of the pancreas may cause portal or inferior vena caval obstruction because the pancreas overlies these large veins (Fig. 2.46*B*). The pancreas's extensive drainage to relatively inaccessible lymph nodes and the fact that pancreatic cancer typically metastasizes to the liver early, via the portal vein, make surgical resection of the cancerous pancreas nearly futile (median survival time, regardless of therapy, is 2–3 months after diagnosis; Cotran et al., 1999). ✷

THE BOTTOM LINE: The pancreas is both an exocrine gland, producing pancreatic juice that is secreted into the duodenum for digestion, and an endocrine gland, producing insulin and glucagon that are released as hormones into the blood. The secondarily retroperitoneal pancreas consists of a head and uncinate process, neck, body, and tail. The head, to the right of the SMA, is embraced by the C-shaped duodenum and penetrated by the termination of the bile duct, whereas its extension, the uncinate process, passes posterior to the SMA. The neck passes anterior to the SMA and SMV, the latter merging there with the splenic vein to form the portal vein. The body lies to the left of the SMA, running transversely across the posterior wall of the omental bursa and crossing anteriorly over the L2 vertebral body and abdominal aorta. The tail enters the splenorenal ligament as it approaches the splenic hilum. The splenic vein runs parallel and posterior to the tail and body as it runs from the spleen to the portal vein. The main pancreatic duct runs a similar course within the pancreas, continuing transversely through the head to merge with the bile duct to form the hepatopancreatic ampulla, which enters the descending part of the duodenum. As an endocrine gland, the pancreas receives an abundant blood supply from the pancreaticoduodenal and splenic arteries. Although it receives vasomotor sympathetic and secretomotor parasympathetic nerve fibers, regulation of pancreatic secretion is primarily hormonal. The pancreas is well protected by its central location in the abdomen. The exocrine pancreas is seldom the cause of clinical problems; although diabetes, involving the endocrine pancreas, has become increasingly common.

Surface Anatomy of the Spleen and Pancreas

The **spleen** lies superficially in the left hypochondrium between the 9th and 11th ribs; its costal surface is convex to fit the inferior surface of the **diaphragm** and the curved bodies of these adjacent bones (Fig. SA2.3*A*). In the supine position, the long axis of the spleen is roughly parallel to the long axis of ▶

Figure SA2.3.

the 10th rib (Fig. SA2.3*B*). The close relationship of the spleen to the ribs that normally protect it can be a detrimental one in the presence of rib fractures. Normally, the spleen does not extend inferior to the left costal margin; thus it is seldom palpable through the anterolateral abdominal wall unless it is enlarged. When it is hardened and enlarged to approximately three times its normal size, it moves inferior to the left costal margin, and its **notched superior border** lies inferomedially. The notched

border is helpful when palpating an enlarged spleen because when the person takes a deep breath, the notches can often be palpated.

The **neck of the pancreas** overlies the L1 and L2 vertebrae in the transpyloric plane (Fig. SA2.3*A*). Its head is to the right and inferior to this plane, and its body and tail are to the left and superior to this level. Because the pancreas is deep in the abdominal cavity, posterior to the stomach and omental bursa, it is usually not palpable. ⊘

Liver

The **liver** is the largest gland in the body and, after the skin, the largest single organ. It weighs approximately 1500 g and accounts for approximately 2.5% of adult body weight. In the late fetus—in which it also serves as a hematopoietic organ—it is proportionately twice as large (5% of body weight). From early childhood onward, it occupies almost all of the right hypochondrium and epigastrium. It extends into the left hypochondrium, inferior to the diaphragm, which separates it from the pleura, lungs, pericardium, and heart (Fig. 2.49*A*). Except for fat, all nutrients absorbed from the gastrointestinal tract are initially conveyed first to the liver by the portal venous system. In addition to its many metabolic activities, the liver stores glycogen and secretes *bile*. **Bile** passes from the liver via the *biliary ducts—right* and *left hepatic ducts* that join to form the *common hepatic duct*, which unites with the *cystic duct* to form the *bile duct*. The liver produces bile continuously; however, between meals it accumulates and is stored in the gallbladder, which also concentrates the bile by absorbing

water and salts. When food arrives in the duodenum, the gallbladder sends concentrated biliary through the bile ducts to the duodenum.

Surfaces, Peritoneal Reflections, and Relationships of the Liver

The liver has a convex *diaphragmatic surface* (anterior, superior, and some posterior) and a relatively flat or even concave *visceral surface* (posteroinferior), which are separated anteriorly by its sharp *inferior border* (Fig. 2.49*A*).

The **diaphragmatic surface of the liver** is smooth and dome shaped, where it is related to the concavity of the inferior surface of the diaphragm (Fig. 2.49*A* & *C*). **Subphrenic recesses**—superior extensions of the peritoneal cavity (greater sac)—exist between diaphragm and the anterior and superior aspects of the diaphragmatic surface of the liver. The subphrenic recesses are separated into right and left recesses by the *falciform ligament,* which extends between the liver and the anterior abdominal wall. The portion of the supracolic compartment of the peritoneal cavity immediately inferior to

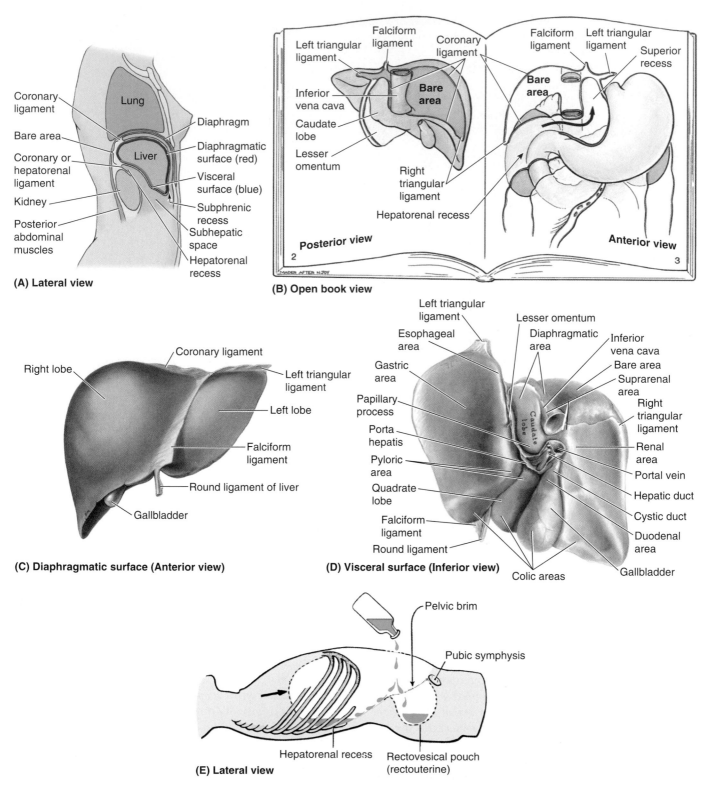

(A) Lateral view

(B) Open book view

(C) Diaphragmatic surface (Anterior view)

(D) Visceral surface (Inferior view)

(E) Lateral view

Figure 2.49. Surfaces and peritoneal relationships of liver. A. This sagittal section through the diaphragm, liver, and right kidney demonstrates the two surfaces of the liver and related peritoneal recesses. **B.** The peritoneal reflections (ligaments) and cavity related to the liver are shown. The attachments of the liver are cut through and the liver is turned to the right and posteriorly, as when turning the page of a book. **C.** The anterior part of the domed diaphragmatic surface of the liver conforms to the inferior surface of the diaphragm. This extensive surface of the liver is divided into superior, anterior (shown here), right, and posterior parts. **D.** In the anatomical position, the visceral surface of the liver is directed inferiorly, posteriorly, and to the left. In embalmed specimens, impressions remain where this surface is contacted by adjacent structures. **E.** In the supine position, the hepatorenal recess is gravity dependent, receiving drainage from the omental bursa and upper abdominal (supracolic) portions of the greater sac.

the liver is the **subhepatic space** (Figs. 2.49*A* and 2.21*A*). The **hepatorenal recess** (hepatorenal pouch; Morison pouch) is the posterosuperior extension of the subhepatic space, lying between the right part of the visceral surface of the liver and the right kidney and suprarenal gland (Fig. 2.49*A & B*). The hepatorenal recess is a gravity-dependent part of the peritoneal cavity in the supine position; fluid draining from the omental bursa flows into this recess (Figs. 2.49*E* and 2.17). The hepatorenal recess communicates anteriorly with the right subphrenic recess (Fig. 2.49*A*). Recall that normally all recesses of the peritoneal cavity are potential spaces only, containing only enough peritoneal fluid to lubricate the adjacent peritoneal membranes.

The diaphragmatic surface of the liver is covered with visceral peritoneum, except posteriorly in the **bare area of the liver** (Fig. 2.49*A, B, & D*), where it lies in direct contact with the diaphragm. The bare area is demarcated by the reflection of peritoneum from the diaphragm to it as the anterior (upper) and posterior (lower) layers of the **coronary ligament.** These layers meet on the right to form the **right triangular ligament** and diverge toward the left to enclose the triangular bare area. The anterior layer of the coronary ligament is continuous on the left with the right layer of the falciform ligament, and the posterior layer is continuous with the right layer of the lesser omentum. Near the apex (the left extremity) of the wedge-shaped liver, the anterior and posterior layers of the left part of the coronary ligament meet to form the **left triangular ligament** (Fig. 2.49*C & D*). The inferior vena cava traverses a deep **groove for the vena cava** within the bare area of the liver.

The **visceral surface of the liver** is covered with peritoneum (Fig. 2.49*D*), except at the **fossa for the gallbladder** and the **porta hepatis**—a transverse fissure where the vessels (portal vein, hepatic artery, and lymphatic vessels), the hepatic nerve plexus, and hepatic ducts that supply and drain the liver enter and leave it. In contrast to the smooth diaphragmatic surface, the visceral surface bears multiple fissures and impressions from contact with other organs. Two sagittal fissures, linked centrally by the transverse porta hepatis, form the letter *H* on the visceral surface (Fig. 2.50*A*). The **right sagittal fissure** is the continuous groove formed anteriorly by the fossa for the gallbladder and posteriorly by the groove for the vena cava; the **left sagittal fissure** is the continuous groove formed anteriorly by the **fissure for the ligamentum teres** or *round ligament,* and posteriorly by the **fissure for the ligamentum venosum.** The **round ligament of the liver** is the fibrous remnant of the *umbilical vein,* which carried well-oxygenated and nutrient-rich blood from the placenta to the fetus; the round ligament and small *paraumbilical veins* course in the free edge of the falciform ligament. The **ligamentum venosum** is the fibrous remnant of the fetal *ductus venosus,* which shunted blood from the umbilical vein to the IVC, short-circuiting the liver (Moore and Persaud, 2003).

The *lesser omentum,* enclosing the **portal triad** (bile duct, hepatic artery, and portal vein) passes from the liver to the

(A) Posteroinferior view

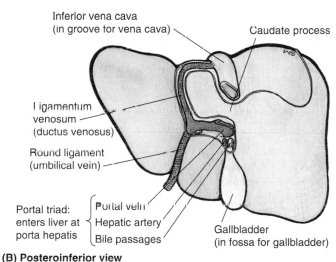

(B) Posteroinferior view

Figure 2.50. Visceral surface of the liver. A. The four anatomical lobes of the liver are defined by external features (peritoneal reflections and fissures). The left sagittal fissure (and the falciform ligament on the diaphragmatic surface) demarcate right and left lobes. The right and left sagittal fissures and the porta hepatis connecting them form an H on the visceral surface, demarcating the quadrate and caudate lobes. **B.** Structures forming the fissures of the visceral surface are shown. The round ligament of the liver is the occluded remains of the fetal umbilical vein. The ligamentum venosum is the fibrous remnant of the ductus venosus that shunted blood from the umbilical vein to the IVC.

lesser curvature of the stomach and the first 2 cm of the superior part of the duodenum (Fig. 2.51). The thick, free edge of the lesser omentum extends between the porta hepatis and the duodenum (the *hepatoduodenal ligament*) and encloses the structures that pass through the porta hepatis. The sheet-like remainder of the lesser omentum, the *hepatogastric ligament,*

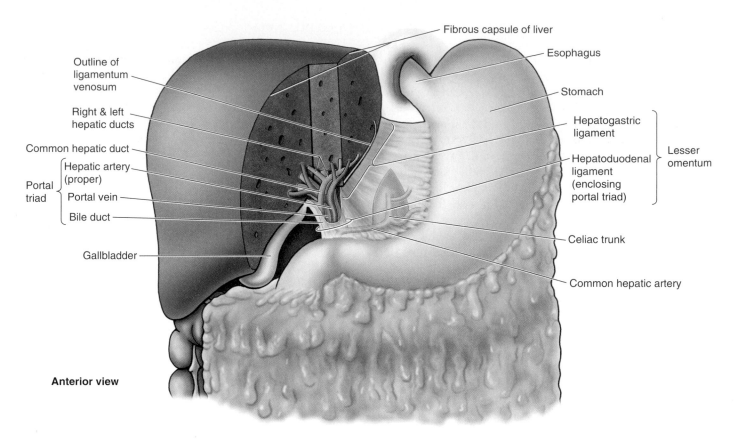

Figure 2.51. Lesser omentum and portal triad. The anterior sagittal cut is made in the plane of the fossa for the gallbladder, and the posterior sagittal cut is in the plane of the fissure for the ligamentum venosum. These cuts have been joined by a narrow coronal cut in the plane of the porta hepatis. The portal triad passes between the layers of the hepatoduodenal ligament to enter the liver at the porta hepatis. The common hepatic artery passes between the layers of the hepatogastric ligament.

extends between the groove for the ligamentum venosum of the liver and the lesser curvature of the stomach.

In addition to the fissures, impressions on (areas of) the visceral surface reflect the liver's relationship to the:

- Right side of the anterior aspect of the stomach (the *gastric* and *pyloric areas*).

- Superior part of the duodenum (the *duodenal area*).

- Lesser omentum (extends into the fissure for the ligamentum venosum).

- Gallbladder (fossa for gallbladder).

- Right colic flexure and right transverse colon (the *colic area*).

- Right kidney and suprarenal gland (the *renal* and *suprarenal areas*).

Subphrenic Abscesses

Peritonitis may result in the formation of localized abscesses in various parts of the peritoneal cavity. A common site for pus to collect is in a subphrenic recess or space. These *subphrenic abscesses* are more common on the right side because of the frequency of ruptured appendices and perforated duodenal ulcers. Because the right and left subphrenic recesses are continuous with the hepatorenal recess (the lowest [most gravity dependent] parts of the peritoneal cavity when supine), pus from a subphrenic abscess may drain into one of the hepatorenal recesses, especially when patients are bedridden. A subphrenic abscess is often drained by an incision inferior to, or through, the bed of the 12th rib (Ellis, 1992), obviating the formation of an opening in the pleura or peritoneum. An anterior subphrenic abscess is often drained through a subcostal incision located inferior and parallel to the right costal margin. ○

Anatomical Lobes of the Liver

Externally, the liver is divided into two topographical (anatomical) lobes and two accessory lobes by the reflections of peritoneum from its surface, the fissures formed in relation to those reflections, and the vessels serving the liver and gallbladder. These superficial "lobes" are not true lobes as the term is generally used in relation to glands and are only secondarily related to the liver's internal architecture. The essentially midline plane defined by the attachment of the falciform ligament and the left sagittal fissure separates a large **right lobe** from a much smaller **left lobe** (Figs. 2.49C & D and 2.50). On the slanted visceral surface, the right and left sagittal fissures surround and the transverse porta hepatis demarcates two accessory lobes (parts of the anatomic right lobe): the **quadrate lobe** anteriorly and inferiorly and the **caudate lobe** posteriorly and superiorly. The caudate lobe is so-named not because it is caudal in position (it is not) but because it often gives rise to a "tail" in the form of an elongated **papillary process** (Fig. 2.49D). A **caudate process** extends to the right, between the IVC and the portal hepatis, connecting the caudate and right lobes (Fig. 2.50B).

Functional Subdivision of the Liver

Although not distinctly demarcated internally, where the parenchyma appears continuous, the liver has functionally independent **right** and **left livers** (parts or portal lobes) that are much more equal in size than the anatomical lobes; however, the right liver is still somewhat larger (Fig. 2.52; Table 2.11). Each part receives its own *primary branch* of the hepatic artery and portal vein and is drained by its own hepatic duct. The *caudate lobe* may in fact be considered a third liver; its vascularization is independent of the bifurcation of the portal triad (it receives vessels from both bundles) and is drained by one or two small hepatic veins, which enter directly into the IVC distal to the main hepatic veins. The liver can be further subdivided into four *divisions* and then into eight surgically resectable **hepatic segments**, each served independently by a *secondary* or *tertiary branch* of the portal triad (Fig. 2.52; see legend for details).

Blood Vessels of the Liver

The liver, like the lungs, has a dual blood supply (afferent vessels): a dominant venous source and a lesser arterial one (Fig. 2.51). The *portal vein* brings 75–80% of the blood to the liver. Portal blood, containing about 40% more oxygen than blood returning to the heart from the systemic circuit, sustains the liver parenchyma (liver cells or *hepatocytes*). The portal vein carries virtually all of the nutrients absorbed by the alimentary tract (except lipids, which bypass the liver in the lymphatic system) to the sinusoids of the liver (Fig. 2.53). Arterial blood from the *hepatic artery,* accounting for only 20–25% of blood received by the liver, is distributed initially to non-parenchymal structures, particularly the intrahepatic bile ducts.

The *portal vein,* a short, wide vein, is formed by the superior mesenteric and splenic veins posterior to the neck of the pancreas and ascends anterior to the IVC as part of the portal triad in the hepatoduodenal ligament (Fig. 2.51). The **hepatic artery,** a branch of the celiac trunk, may be divided into the **common hepatic artery,** from the celiac trunk to the origin of the gastroduodenal artery, and the **hepatic artery proper,** from the origin of the gastroduodenal artery to the bifurcation of the hepatic artery. At or close to the porta hepatis, the hepatic artery and portal vein terminate by dividing into right and left branches, these primary branches supply the right and left livers, respectively. Within each part, the simultaneous secondary branchings of the portal vein and hepatic artery (portal pedicles) are consistent enough to supply the medial and lateral divisions of the right and left liver, with three of the four secondary branches undergoing further (tertiary) branchings to supply independently seven of the eight hepatic segments (Fig. 2.52). Between the divisions are the **right, intermediate (middle),** and **left hepatic veins,** which are intersegmental in their distribution and function, draining parts of adjacent segments. The hepatic veins, formed by the union of *collecting veins* that in turn drain the *central veins* of the hepatic parenchyma (Fig. 2.53), open into the IVC just inferior to the diaphragm. The attachment of these veins to the IVC helps hold the liver in position.

Hepatic Lobectomies and Segmentectomy

When it was discovered that the right and left hepatic arteries and ducts, as well as branches of the right and left portal veins, do not communicate, it became possible to perform **hepatic lobectomies,** removal of the right or left (part of the) liver, without excessive bleeding. Most injuries to the liver involve the right liver. More recently, especially since the advent of the cauterizing scalpel and laser surgery, it has become possible to perform **hepatic segmentectomies.** This procedure makes it possible to remove (resect) only those segments that have sustained a severe injury or are affected by a tumor. The intersegmental hepatic veins serve as guides to the planes between the hepatic divisions; however, they also provide a major source of bleeding with which the surgeon must contend. While the pattern of branching described here is the most common pattern, the segments vary considerably in size and shape as a result of individual variation in the branching of the hepatic and portal vessels, so that each hepatic resection is empirical, requiring ultrasonography, injection of dye, or balloon catheter occlusion to establish the patient's segmental pattern. (Cheng et al., 1997) A more extensive ▶

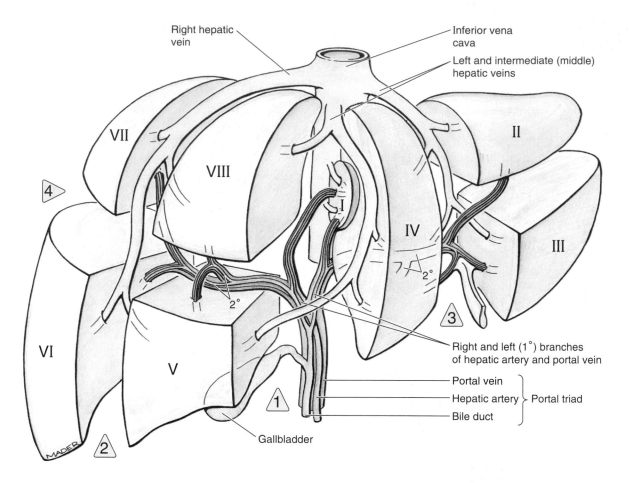

Figure 2.52. Hepatic segmentation. Except for the caudate lobe (segment I), the liver is divided into right and left livers based on the primary (1°) division of the portal triad into right and left branches, the plane between the right and the left livers being the main portal fissure (1) in which the middle hepatic vein lies. On the visceral surface, this plane is demarcated by the right sagittal fissure. The plane is demarcated on the diaphragmatic surface by an imaginary line—the Cantlie line (Cantlie, 1898)—running from the notch for the fundus of the gallbladder to the IVC (Table 2.11). The right and left livers are subdivided vertically into medial and lateral divisions by the right portal (2) and left portal (umbilical) (3) fissures, in which the right and left hepatic veins lie. The left portal fissure is demarcated externally by the falciform ligament and the left sagittal fissure. The right portal fissure has no external demarcation. Each division receives a secondary (2°) branch of the portal triad (a portal pedicle). (Note: the medial division of the left liver is part of the right anatomical lobe; the lateral division of the left liver is the same as the left anatomical lobe.) A transverse plane at the level of the horizontal parts of the right and left branches of the portal triad (4) subdivides three of the four divisions (all but the left medial division), creating six hepatic segments receiving tertiary branches. The left medial division is also counted as a hepatic segment, so that the main part of the liver has seven segments (segments II–VIII, numbered clockwise). The caudate lobe (segment I, bringing the total number of segments to eight) is supplied by branches of both divisions and is drained by its own minor hepatic veins. Each segment thus has its own blood supply and biliary drainage. The hepatic veins are intersegmental, draining the portions of the multiple segments adjacent to them.

injury that is likely to leave large areas of the liver devascularized may still require lobectomy.

Rupture of the Liver

The liver is easily injured because it is large, fixed in position, and friable (easily crumbled). Often a fractured rib that perforates the diaphragm tears the liver. Because of the liver's great vascularity and friability, liver lacerations often cause considerable hemorrhage and right upper quadrant pain. In such cases, the surgeon must decide whether to remove foreign material and the contaminated or devitalized tissue by dissection or to perform a segmentectomy. ▶

Table 2.11. Terminology for subdivisions of the Liver

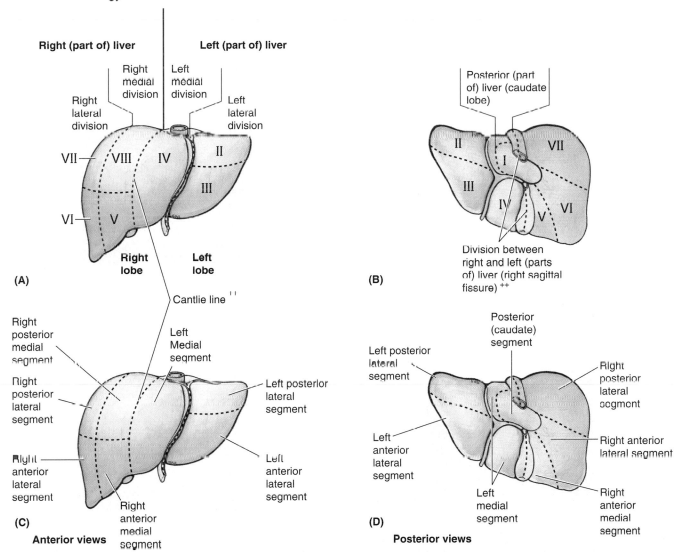

Anatomical Term	Right Lobe			Left Lobe	Caudate Lobe	
	Right (part of) Liver [Right portal lobe*]			Left (part of) Liver [Left portal lobe+]	Posterior (part of) Liver	
	Right lateral division	Right medial division	Left medial division	Left lateral division	[Right caudate lobe*]	[Left caudate lobe+]
Functional/ Surgical Term**	Posterior lateral segment **Segment VII** [Posterior superior area]	Posterior medial segment **Segment VIII** [Anterior superior area]	[Medial superior area] Left medial segment **Segment IV** [Medial inferior area = quadrate lobe]	Lateral segment **Segment II** [Lateral superior area] Left lateral anterior segment **Segment III** [Lateral inferior area]	Posterior segment **Segment I**	
	Right anterior lateral segment **Segment VI** [Posterior inferior area]	Anterior medial segment **Segment V** [Anterior inferior area]				

** The labels in the table and figure above reflect the new *Terminologia Anatomica: International Anatomical Terminology.* Previous terminology is in brackets.
*+ Under the schema of the previous terminology, the caudate lobe was divided into right and left halves, and
 * the right half of the caudate lobe was considered a subdivision of the right portal lobe;
 + the left half of the caudate lobe was considered a subdivision of the left portal lobe.
++ Cantlie line and the right sagittal fissure are surface markings defining the main portal fissure.

Figure 2.53. Flow of blood and bile in the liver. A. This view of a small part of a liver lobule illustrates the components of the interlobular portal triad and the positioning of the sinusoids and bile canaliculi. The enlarged view of the surface of a block of parenchyma removed from the liver in part B shows the hexagonal pattern of lobes and the place of part A within that pattern. **B.** Extrahepatic bile passages, gallbladder, and pancreatic ducts are demonstrated. **C.** The bile duct and pancreatic duct enter into the hepatopancreatic ampulla, which opens into the descending part of the duodenum.

Aberrant Hepatic Arteries

A more common variety of right or left hepatic artery that arises as a terminal branch of the hepatic artery proper may be replaced in part or entirely by an aberrant (accessory or replaced) artery arising from another source. The most common source of an *aberrant right hepatic artery* is the SMA (Fig. B2.20*A*). The most common source of an *aberrant left hepatic artery* is the left gastric artery (Fig. B2.20*B*).

Variations in the Relationships of the Hepatic Arteries

In most people, the right hepatic artery crosses anterior to the portal vein (Fig. B2.20*C*); however, in some people, the artery crosses posterior to the portal vein (Fig. B2.20*D*). In most people, the right hepatic artery runs posterior to the common hepatic duct (Fig. B2.20*F*). In some individuals the right hepatic artery crosses anterior to the common hepatic duct (Fig. B2.20*E*), or the right hepatic artery arises from the IVC and so does not cross the common hepatic duct at all (Fig. B2.20*G*). ▶

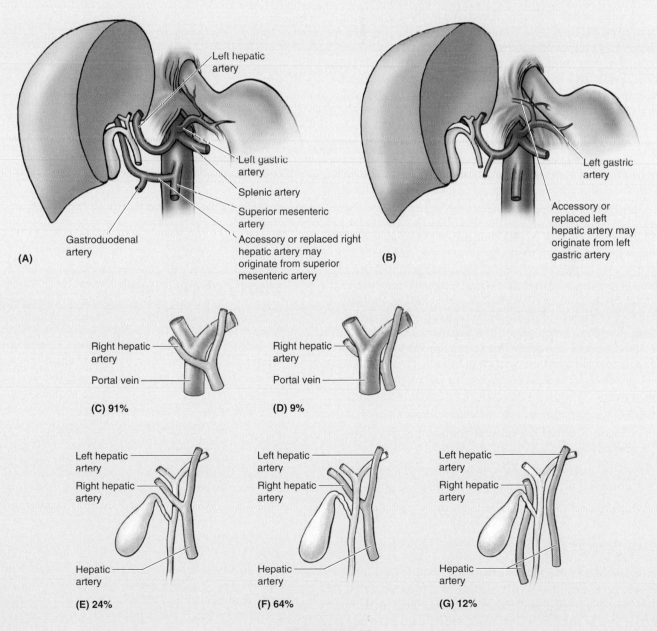

Figure B2.20.

Unusual Formation of the Portal Vein

Usually, the portal vein forms posterior to the neck of the pancreas by the union of the superior mesenteric and splenic veins and ascends anterior to the IVC. In approximately one third of individuals, the IMV joins the confluence of the superior mesenteric and splenic veins; hence, all three veins form the portal vein. In most people, the IMV enters the splenic vein (60%) or the SMV (40%). ⊕

Lymphatic Drainage and Innervation of the Liver

The liver is a major lymph-producing organ. Between one quarter and one half of the lymph received by the thoracic duct comes from the liver. The lymphatic vessels of the liver occur as *superficial lymphatics* in the subperitoneal **fibrous capsule of the liver** (Glisson capsule), which forms its outer surface (Fig. 2.51), and as *deep lymphatics* in the connective tissue, which accompany the ramifications of the portal triad and hepatic veins (Fig. 2.53*A*). Most of the lymph is formed in the **perisinusoidal spaces** (of Disse) and drains to the deep lymphatics in the surrounding **intralobular portal triads**. Superficial lymphatics from the anterior aspects of the diaphragmatic and visceral surfaces and the deep lymphatic vessels accompanying the portal triads converge toward the porta hepatis. They drain to the **hepatic lymph nodes** scattered along the hepatic vessels and ducts in the lesser omentum (Fig. 2.54*A*). Efferent lymphatic vessels from the hepatic nodes drain into *celiac lymph nodes,* which in turn drain into the *chyle cistern,* a dilated sac at the inferior end of the thoracic duct. Superficial lymphatics from the posterior aspects of the diaphragmatic and visceral surfaces of the liver drain toward the bare area of the liver. Here they drain into **phrenic lymph nodes,** or join deep lymphatics that have accompanied the hepatic veins converging on the IVC, and pass with this large vein through the diaphragm to drain into the **posterior mediastinal lymph nodes.** Efferent vessels from these nodes join the right lymphatic and thoracic ducts. A few lymphatic vessels follow different routes:

- From the posterior surface of the left lobe toward the esophageal hiatus of the diaphragm to end in the *left gastric lymph nodes* (Fig. 2.54*A*).

- From the anterior central diaphragmatic surface along the falciform ligament to the *parasternal lymph nodes.*

- Along the round ligament of the liver to the umbilicus and lymphatics of the anterior abdominal wall.

The nerves of the liver are derived from the **hepatic plexus** (Fig. 2.54*B*), the largest derivative of the celiac plexus. The hepatic plexus accompanies the branches of the hepatic artery and portal vein to the liver. It consists of sympathetic fibers from the celiac plexus and parasympathetic fibers from the anterior and posterior vagal trunks. Nerve fibers accompany the vessels and biliary ducts of the portal triad. Other than vasoconstriction, their function is unclear.

Hepatomegaly

The liver is a soft and highly vascular organ that receives a large amount of blood immediately before it enters the heart. Both the inferior vena cava and hepatic veins lack valves. Any rise in central venous pressure is directly transmitted to the liver, which enlarges as it becomes engorged with blood. Marked temporary engorgement stretches the fibrous capsule of the liver, producing pain around the lower ribs, particularly in the right hypochondrium. This engorgement, particularly in conjunction with increased or sustained diaphragmatic activity, has been proposed as an underlying cause of "runner's stitch," perhaps explaining why it is a right-sided phenomenon. In addition to diseases that produce hepatic engorgement such as congestive heart failure, bacterial and viral diseases such as hepatitis cause liver enlargement, or **hepatomegaly.** When the liver is massively enlarged, its inferior edge may be readily palpated below the right costal margin and may even reach the pelvic brim in the right lower quadrant of the abdomen. Tumors also enlarge the liver. The liver is a common site of *metastatic carcinoma* (secondary cancers spreading from organs drained by the portal system of veins). Cancer cells may also pass to the liver from the thorax, especially from the right breast, because of the communications between thoracic lymph nodes and the lymphatic vessels draining the bare area of the liver. Metastatic tumors form hard, rounded nodules within the hepatic parenchyma. In view of the great functional reserve of the liver, signs of liver failure may be absent in a liver loaded with metastatic tumors.

Cirrhosis of the Liver

The liver is the primary site for detoxification of substances absorbed by the digestive system, and so it is vulnerable to cellular damage and consequent scarring, accompanied by regenerative nodules. There is progressive destruction of hepatocytes (parenchymal liver cells) in *hepatic cirrhosis* and replacement of them by fat and fibrous tissue. Although many industrial solvents, such as carbon tetrachloride, produce cirrhosis, the condition develops most frequently in persons suffering from chronic alcoholism. *Alcoholic cirrhosis,* the most common of many causes of *portal hypertension,* is characterized by enlargement of the liver resulting from fatty changes and fibrosis. The liver has great functional reserve, and so the metabolic evidence of liver failure is late to appear. Fibrous tissue surrounds the intrahepatic blood vessels and biliary ducts, making the liver firm, and impeding the circulation of blood through it (*portal hypertension*). The treatment of advanced cirrhosis may include the surgical creation of a *portosystemic* or *portocaval shunt,* anastomosing the portal and systemic venous systems (see clinical correlation [blue] box "Portosystemic Shunts," in this chapter). ⊕

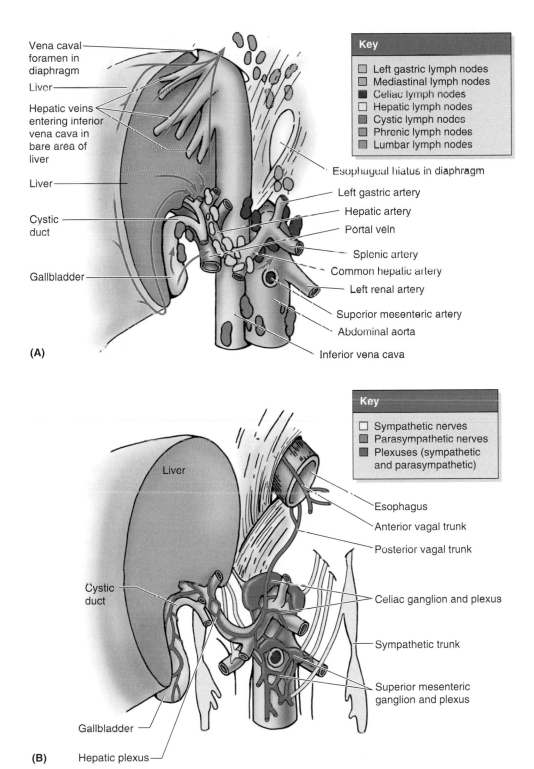

Key
- ☐ Left gastric lymph nodes
- ☐ Mediastinal lymph nodes
- ☐ Celiac lymph nodes
- ☐ Hepatic lymph nodes
- ☐ Cystic lymph nodes
- ☐ Phrenic lymph nodes
- ☐ Lumbar lymph nodes

Vena caval foramen in diaphragm

Liver

Hepatic veins entering inferior vena cava in bare area of liver

Liver

Cystic duct

Gallbladder

Esophageal hiatus in diaphragm

Left gastric artery

Hepatic artery

Portal vein

Splenic artery

Common hepatic artery

Left renal artery

Superior mesenteric artery

Abdominal aorta

Inferior vena cava

(A)

Key
- ☐ Sympathetic nerves
- ☐ Parasympathetic nerves
- ☐ Plexuses (sympathetic and parasympathetic)

Liver

Cystic duct

Gallbladder

Hepatic plexus

Esophagus

Anterior vagal trunk

Posterior vagal trunk

Celiac ganglion and plexus

Sympathetic trunk

Superior mesenteric ganglion and plexus

(B)

Figure 2.54. Lymphatic drainage and innervation of liver. A. Lymph from the posterior aspect of the liver (superficial and deep) flows toward the bare area to enter the phrenic lymph nodes, or pass with the IVC through the caval foramen in the diaphragm to enter mediastinal lymph nodes. Lymph from the anterior and inferior aspects (superficial and deep) flows toward the porta hepatis to enter hepatic lymph nodes in the lesser omentum. **B.** The nerves of the liver derive from the hepatic plexus, the largest derivative of the celiac plexus. The hepatic plexus accompanies the branches of the hepatic artery and portal vein to the liver. It consists of sympathetic fibers from the celiac plexus and parasympathetic fibers from the anterior and posterior vagal trunks.

Surface Anatomy of the Liver

The **liver** lies mainly in the right upper quadrant of the abdomen where it is hidden and protected by the **thoracic cage** and **diaphragm**. The normal liver lies deep to ribs 7–11 on the right side and crosses the midline toward the left nipple. Consequently, the liver occupies most of the right hypochondrium, the upper epigastrium, and extends into the left hypochondrium. The liver is located more inferiorly when one is erect because of gravity. Its sharp inferior border follows the right costal margin. When a person in the supine position is asked to inspire deeply, the liver may be palpated because of the inferior movement of the diaphragm and liver (Fig. SA2.4*A*). One method of palpating the liver is to place the left hand posteriorly behind the **lower rib cage**. Then, put the right hand on the person's right upper quadrant, lateral to the **rectus abdominis** and inferior to the **costal margin** (Fig. SA2.4*B*). The person is asked to take a deep breath as the examiner presses posterosuperiorly with the right hand and pulls anteriorly with the left hand (Bickley and Szilagyi, 2003). ☻

Full expiration

Neutral respiratory position

4–8 cm in midline

6–12 cm in right midclavicular line

Inspiration

(A) Vertical dimensions and range of movement of liver

(B) Palpation of inferior margin of liver

Figure SA2.4.

Liver Biopsy

Hepatic tissue may be obtained for diagnostic purposes by *liver biopsy*. Because the liver is located in the right hypochondriac region where it receives protection from the overlying thoracic cage, the needle is commonly directed through the right 10th intercostal space in the midaxillary line. Before the physician takes the biopsy, the person is asked to hold his or her breath in full expiration to reduce the costodiaphragmatic recess and to lessen the possibility of damaging the lung and contaminating the pleural cavity. ☻

THE BOTTOM LINE: The liver has multiple functions. It is our greatest metabolic organ, initially receiving all absorbed foodstuffs, except fats. It is also our largest gland, functioning as an extrinsic intestinal gland in producing bile. The liver occupies essentially all of the right dome of the diaphragm and extends to the apex of the left dome. Consequently, it enjoys protection from the lower thoracic cage, and moves with respiratory excursions. It is divided superficially by the falciform ligament and groove for the ligamentum venosum into a large anatomical right lobe and a much smaller left one; formations on its visceral surface demarcate caudate and quadrate lobes. It is covered with peritoneum except for a sizable bare area, demarcated by peritoneal reflections comprising the coronary ligaments. Based on interdigitated branchings of the portal triad (portal vein, hepatic artery and intrahepatic bile ducts) and hepatic veins, its continuous parenchyma can be divided into right and left livers (plus the caudate lobe). It can be further subdivided into four divisions and then eight surgically resectable hepatic segments. The liver, like the lungs, receives a dual blood supply, with 75–80% of the blood arriving via the portal vein, meeting the nutritional needs of the hepatic parenchyma; 20–25% arrives via the hepatic artery, delivered primarily to the non-parenchymal elements. These vessels enter the liver via the porta hepatis, where the hepatic ducts exit. Three large hepatic veins drain directly to the IVC as it is embedded in the liver's bare area. The liver is also the body's largest lymph-producing organ. Its visceral aspect drains via an abdominal route and its diaphragmatic aspect drains via a thoracic route.

Biliary Ducts and Gallbladder

The **biliary ducts** convey bile from the liver to the duodenum. Bile is produced continuously by the liver and stored and concentrated in the gallbladder, which releases it intermittently when fat enters the duodenum. Bile emulsifies the fat, so that it can be absorbed in the distal intestine.

Normal hepatic tissue, when sectioned, is traditionally described as demonstrating a pattern of hexagonal-shaped *liver lobules* (Fig. 2.53*A*) when viewed under low magnification. Each lobule has a **central vein** running through its center from which **sinusoids** (large capillaries) and plates of *hepatocytes* (liver cells) radiate toward an imaginary perimeter extrapolated from surrounding **interlobular portal triads** (terminal branches of the portal vein and hepatic artery, and initial branches of the biliary ducts). Although commonly said to be the anatomical units of the liver, hepatic "lobules" are not structural entities; instead, the lobular pattern is a physiological consequence of pressure gradients and is altered by disease. Because the bile duct is not central, the hepatic lobule does not represent a functional unit like acini of other glands. However, the hepatic lobule is a firmly established concept and is useful for descriptive purposes. The hepatocytes secrete bile into the **bile canaliculi** formed between them. The canaliculi drain into the small *interlobular biliary ducts* and then into large *collecting bile ducts* of the intrahepatic portal triad, which merges to form the right and left hepatic ducts (Fig. 2.53*B*). The **right** and **left hepatic ducts** drain the right and left (parts of the) liver, respectively. Shortly after leaving the porta hepatis, the right and left hepatic ducts unite to form the **common hepatic duct**, which is joined on the right side by the *cystic duct* to form the *bile duct* (part of the extrahepatic portal triad of the lesser omentum), which conveys the bile to the duodenum.

Bile Duct

The **bile duct** (formerly, common bile duct) forms in the free edge of the lesser omentum by the union of the *cystic duct* and the *common hepatic duct* (Figs. 2.51 and 2.53*B*). The length of the bile duct varies from 5 to 15 cm, depending on where the cystic duct joins the common hepatic duct. The bile duct descends posterior to the superior part of the duodenum and lies in a groove on the posterior surface of the head of the pancreas. On the left side of the descending part of the duodenum, the bile duct comes into contact with the *main pancreatic duct*. These ducts run obliquely through the wall of this part of the duodenum, where they unite to form the *hepatopancreatic ampulla*, the dilation within the major duodenal papilla. The distal end of the ampulla opens into the duodenum through the *major duodenal papilla* (Fig. 2.47). The circular muscle around the distal end of the bile duct is thickened to form the *sphincter of the bile duct*. When this sphincter contracts, bile cannot enter the ampulla and the duodenum; hence bile backs up and passes along the cystic duct to the gallbladder for concentration and storage.

The arteries supplying the bile duct include (Fig. 2.55) the:

- *Cystic artery:* supplying the proximal part of the duct.

- *Right hepatic artery:* supplying the middle part of the duct.

- *Posterior superior pancreaticoduodenal artery* and *gastroduodenal artery:* supplying the retroduodenal part of the duct.

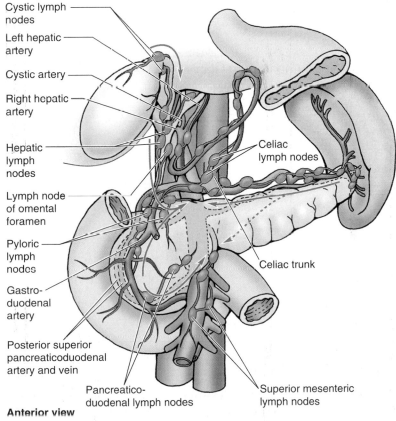

Cystic lymph nodes
Left hepatic artery
Cystic artery
Right hepatic artery
Hepatic lymph nodes
Lymph node of omental foramen
Pyloric lymph nodes
Gastroduodenal artery
Posterior superior pancreaticoduodenal artery and vein
Pancreaticoduodenal lymph nodes
Celiac lymph nodes
Celiac trunk
Superior mesenteric lymph nodes

Anterior view

Figure 2.55. Lymphatic drainage of gallbladder and bile duct. Lymph passes from the cystic and hepatic lymph nodes and the node of the omental foramen to the celiac lymph nodes surrounding the celiac trunk. The lymphatic vessels of the gallbladder and biliary passages anastomose superiorly with those of the liver and inferiorly with those of the pancreas.

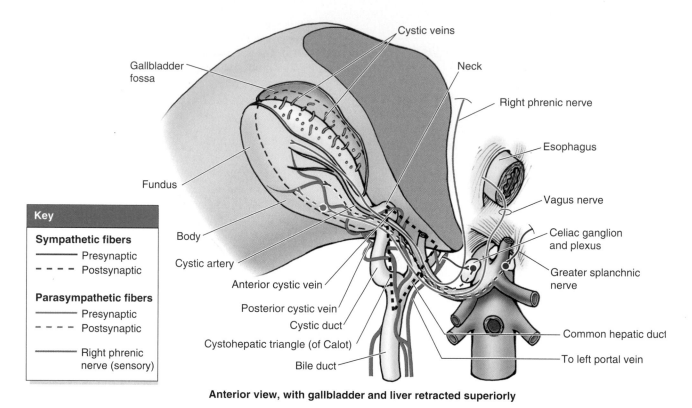

Cystic veins

Gallbladder fossa

Neck

Right phrenic nerve

Esophagus

Vagus nerve

Celiac ganglion and plexus

Greater splanchnic nerve

Fundus

Body

Cystic artery

Anterior cystic vein

Posterior cystic vein

Cystic duct

Cystohepatic triangle (of Calot)

Bile duct

Common hepatic duct

To left portal vein

Key

Sympathetic fibers
———— Presynaptic
- - - - Postsynaptic

Parasympathetic fibers
———— Presynaptic
- - - - Postsynaptic

———— Right phrenic nerve (sensory)

Anterior view, with gallbladder and liver retracted superiorly

Figure 2.56. Nerves and veins of liver and biliary system. Nerves are prominent along the hepatic artery, portal vein, and bile duct. The sympathetic nerve supply is vasomotor in the liver and biliary system. The veins of the gallbladder neck communicate with veins along the cystic and biliary ducts. Small cystic veins pass from the gallbladder into the liver.

The veins from the proximal part of the bile duct and the hepatic ducts usually enter the liver directly. The *posterior superior pancreaticoduodenal vein* drains the distal part of the bile duct and empties into the portal vein or one of its tributaries.

The lymphatic vessels from the bile duct pass to the **cystic lymph nodes** near the neck of the gallbladder, the **node of the omental foramen**, and the *hepatic lymph nodes*. Efferent lymphatic vessels from the bile duct pass to the *celiac lymph nodes*.

Gallbladder

The **gallbladder** (7–10 cm long) lies in the fossa for the gallbladder on the visceral surface of the liver (Figs. 2.49*D* and 2.56). This shallow fossa lies at the junction of the right and left (parts of the) liver. The relationship of the gallbladder to the duodenum is so intimate that the superior part of the duodenum is usually stained with bile in the cadaver (Fig. 2.57). Because the liver and gallbladder must be retracted superiorly to expose the gallbladder during an anterior approach (and atlases often depict it in this position), it is easy to forget that in its natural position the body of the gallbladder lies anterior to the duodenum, and its neck and the cystic duct are immediately superior to the duodenum. The pear-shaped gallbladder can hold up to 50 mL of bile. Peritoneum completely surrounds the fundus of the gallbladder and binds its body and neck to the liver. The hepatic surface of the gallbladder attaches to the liver by connective tissue of the fibrous capsule of the liver.

The gallbladder has three parts (Figs. 2.53*B* and 2.56) the:

- **Fundus:** the wide end of the organ, projects from the inferior border of the liver and is usually located at the tip of the right 9th costal cartilage in the MCL (Fig. 2.24*A*).

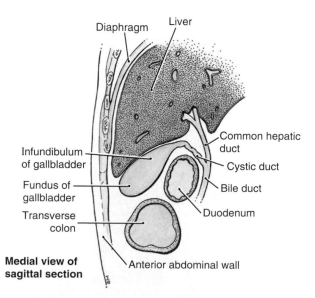

Diaphragm

Liver

Infundibulum of gallbladder

Fundus of gallbladder

Transverse colon

Common hepatic duct

Cystic duct

Bile duct

Duodenum

Anterior abdominal wall

Medial view of sagittal section

Figure 2.57. Normal relationship of gallbladder to superior part of the duodenum.

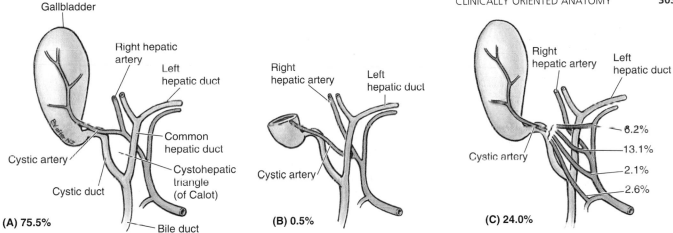

Figure 2.58. Variation in origin and course of cystic artery. A. The cystic artery usually arises from the right hepatic artery in the cystohepatic triangle (of Calot), bounded by the cystic duct, common hepatic duct, and visceral surface of the right liver. **B and C.** Variations in the origin and course of the cystic artery occur in 24.5% of people (Daseler et al., 1947), which is of clinical significance during cholecystectomy (surgical removal of the gallbladder).

- **Body:** contacts the visceral surface of the liver, the transverse colon, and the superior part of the duodenum.

- **Neck:** narrow and tapered; directed toward the porta hepatis; it makes an S-shaped bend and joins the cystic duct.

The **cystic duct** (3–4 cm long) connects the neck of the gallbladder to the common hepatic duct (Figs. 2.53B and 2.56). The mucosa of the neck spirals into the **spiral fold** (spiral valve) (Fig. 2.53B). The spiral fold helps keep the cystic duct open; thus bile can easily be diverted into the gallbladder when the distal end of the bile duct is closed by the sphincter of the bile duct and/or hepatopancreatic sphincter, or bile can pass to the duodenum as the gallbladder contracts. The spiral fold also offers additional resistance to sudden dumping of bile when the sphincters are closed, and intra-abdominal pressure is suddenly increased, as during a sneeze or cough. The cystic duct passes between the layers of the lesser omentum, usually parallel to the common hepatic duct, which it joins to form the bile duct.

The **cystic artery**, supplying the gallbladder and cystic duct (Figs. 2.56 and 2.58A), commonly arises from the *right hepatic artery* in the angle between the common hepatic duct and the cystic duct (cystohepatic triangle). Variations occur in the origin and course of the cystic artery (Fig. 2.58B & C).

The **cystic veins**, draining the neck of the gallbladder and cystic duct, enter the liver directly or drain through the portal vein to the liver, after joining the veins draining the hepatic ducts and upper bile duct (Fig. 2.56). The veins from the fundus and body of the gallbladder pass directly into the visceral surface of the liver and drain into the hepatic sinusoids. Because this is drainage from one capillary (sinusoidal) bed to another, it constitutes an addition (parallel) portal system.

The lymphatic drainage of the gallbladder is to the *hepatic lymph nodes* (Fig. 2.55), often through *cystic lymph nodes* located near the neck of the gallbladder. Efferent lymphatic vessels from these nodes pass to the *celiac lymph nodes*.

The nerves to the gallbladder and cystic duct (Fig. 2.56) pass along the cystic artery from the *celiac nerve plexus* (sympathetic and visceral afferent [pain] fibers), the *vagus nerve* (parasympathetic), and the *right phrenic nerve* (actually *somatic* afferent fibers). Parasympathetic stimulation causes contractions of the gallbladder and relaxation of the sphincters at the hepatopancreatic ampulla. However, these responses are generally stimulated by the hormone cholecystokinin (CCK), produced by the duodenal walls (in response to the arrival of a fatty meal) and circulated through the bloodstream.

Infundibulum of the Gallbladder

In diseased states of the gallbladder, a dilation or pouch appears at the junction of the neck of the gallbladder and the cystic duct. This pouch is called the *infundibulum of the gallbladder* (Hartmann pouch). When this pouch is large, the cystic duct arises from its upper left aspect, not from what appears to be the apex of the gallbladder. Gallstones commonly collect in the infundibulum. If a peptic duodenal ulcer ruptures, a false passage may form between the infundibulum and the superior part of the duodenum, allowing gallstones to enter the duodenum (see the clinical correlation [blue] box "Gallstones in the Duodenum," in this chapter).

Mobile Gallbladder

The gallbladder has a short mesentery in approximately 4% of people. Such gallbladders are subject to vascular torsion and infarction (sudden insufficiency of arterial or venous blood supply).

Variations in the Cystic and Hepatic Ducts

Occasionally, the cystic duct runs alongside the common hepatic duct and adheres closely to it. The cystic duct may be short or even absent. In some people, there is low union of the cystic and common hepatic ducts (Fig. B2.21A). ▶

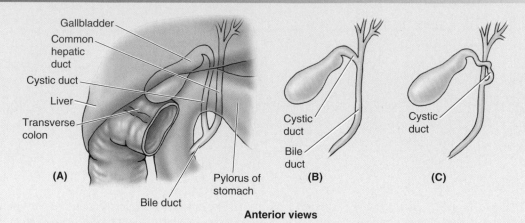

Anterior views

Figure B2.21. Union of cystic and common hepatic ducts. A. Low union. **B.** High union. **C.** Swerving course.

As a result, the bile duct is short and lies posterior to the superior part of the duodenum, or even inferior to it. When there is low union, the two ducts may be joined by fibrous tissue, making clamping the cystic duct difficult without injuring the common hepatic duct. Occasionally, there is high union of the cystic and common hepatic ducts near the porta hepatis (Fig. B2.21*B*). In other cases, the cystic duct spirals anteriorly over the common hepatic duct before joining it on the left side (Fig. B2.21*C*). Understanding the variations in arteries and bile duct formation is important for surgeons when they ligate the cystic duct during *cholecystectomy,* the surgical removal of the gallbladder.

Accessory Hepatic Ducts

Accessory (**aberrant**) **hepatic ducts** are common and are in positions of danger during cholecystectomy. An accessory duct is a normal segmental duct that joins the biliary system outside the liver instead of within it (Fig. B2.22). Because it drains a normal segment of the liver, it leaks bile if inadvertently cut during surgery (Skandalakis et al., 1995). Of 95 gallbladders and biliary ducts studied, 7 had accessory ducts, 4 joined the common hepatic duct near the cystic ducts, 2 joined the cystic duct, and 1 was an anasto-

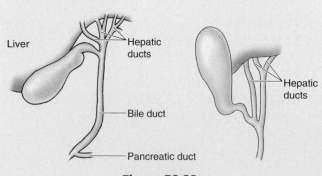

Figure B2.22.

mosing duct connecting the cystic duct with the common hepatic duct (Agur and Dalley, 2005).

Gallstones

A **gallstone** is a concretion in the gallbladder, cystic duct, or bile duct composed chiefly of cholesterol crystals. Gallstones are much more common in females, and incidence increases with age. However, in approximately 50% of persons, gallstones are "silent" (asymptomatic). Over a 20-year period, two thirds of asymptomatic people with gallstones remain symptom free. The longer stones remain quiescent, the less likely symptoms are to develop. For gallstones to cause clinical symptoms, they must obtain a size sufficient to produce mechanical injury to the gallbladder or obstruction of the biliary tract (Townsend, 2001).

The distal end of the hepatopancreatic ampulla is the narrowest part of the biliary passages and is the common site for impaction of gallstones. The **infundibulum of the gallbladder** is another common site for impaction. Gallstones may also lodge in the hepatic and cystic ducts. A stone lodged in the cystic duct causes *biliary colic* (intense, spasmodic pain). When the gallbladder relaxes, the stone may pass back into the gallbladder. If the stone blocks the cystic duct, *cholecystitis* (inflammation of the gallbladder) occurs because of bile accumulation, causing enlargement of the gallbladder. Pain develops in the epigastric region and later shifts to the right hypochondriac region at the junction of the 9th costal cartilage and the lateral border of the rectus sheath, indicated by the linea semilunaris. Inflammation of the gallbladder may cause pain in the posterior thoracic wall or right shoulder owing to irritation of the diaphragm. If bile cannot leave the gallbladder, it enters the blood and causes *jaundice* (see clinical correlation [blue] box "Pancreatic Cancer," in this chapter). Ultrasound and CT scans are common non-invasive techniques for locating stones. ▶

Gallstones in the Duodenum

Normal anatomy may be distorted by disease processes. A gallbladder that is dilated and inflamed owing to an impacted gallstone in its duct may develop adhesions with adjacent viscera. Continued inflammation may break down (ulcerate) the tissue boundaries between the gall bladder and a part of the alimentary tract adherent to it, resulting in a *cholecystenteric fistula*. Because of their proximity to the gallbladder, the superior part of the duodenum and the transverse colon are most likely to develop a fistula of this type (Fig. 2.24A). The fistula would enable a large gallstone, incapable of passing though the cystic duct, to enter the alimentary tract (Fig. B2.23). A large gallstone

Left lateral view

Figure B2.23.

entering the small intestine in this way may become trapped at the ileocecal valve, producing a bowel obstruction (*gallstone ileus*). A cholecystenteric fistula also permits gas from the alimentary tract to enter the gallbladder, providing a diagnostic radiographic sign.

Cholecystectomy

People with severe *biliary colic* usually have their gallbladders removed. *Laparoscopic cholecystectomy* often replaces the open surgical method (for details of this technique, see Skandalakis et al., 1995). The cystic artery most commonly arises from the right hepatic artery in the **cystohepatic triangle** (Calot triangle) (Fig. 2.56). In current clinical use, the cystohepatic triangle is defined inferiorly by the cystic duct, medially by the common hepatic duct, and superiorly by the inferior surface of the liver (Calot originally described the cystic artery itself as the superior boundary) (Fig. 2.58A). Careful dissection of the cystohepatic triangle early during cholecystectomy safeguards these important structures should there be anatomical variations. Errors during gallbladder surgery commonly result from failure to appreciate the common variations in the anatomy of the biliary system, especially its blood supply. Before dividing any structure and removing the gallbladder, surgeons identify all three biliary ducts, as well as the cystic and hepatic arteries. It is usually the right hepatic artery that is in danger during surgery and must be located before ligating the cystic artery. Bile duct injury is a serious complication of cholecystectomy, which is estimated to occur in 1 per 600 cases, and the risk appears to be modestly higher for laparoscopic cholecystectomy (Sabiston and Lyerly, 1994). ☉

THE BOTTOM LINE: Right and left hepatic ducts drain the bile produced by the right and left livers into the common hepatic duct, which thus carries all bile from the liver. The common hepatic duct merges with the cystic duct to form the bile duct, which conveys the bile to the duodenum. When the sphincter of the bile duct is closed, bile backs up in the bile and cystic ducts, filling the gallbladder, where bile is stored and concentrated between meals. Although parasympathetic innervation can open the sphincter of the bile duct (and the weaker sphincter of the hepatopancreatic ampulla) and contract the gallbladder, typically these are hormonally regulated responses to fat entering the duodenum, emptying the accumulated bile into the duodenum. The pear-shaped gallbladder is attached to the visceral surface of the liver, with its fundus projecting from the liver's inferior border against the anterior abdominal wall at the intersection of the transpyloric plane and the right MCL. The gallbladder, cystic duct, and uppermost bile duct are sup-

plied by the cystic artery, a branch arising from the right hepatic artery within the cystohepatic triangle. In addition to drainage via cystic veins that accompany the cystic artery and enter the portal vein, veins from the fundus and body make up a mini-portal system that drains directly into the hepatic sinusoids deep to the visceral surface of the liver.

Portal Vein and Portal–Systemic Anastomoses

The **portal vein** is the main channel of the **portal venous system** (Figs. 2.51 and 2.59). It is formed anterior to the IVC and posterior to the neck of the pancreas (close to the level of the L1 vertebra and the transpyloric plane) by the union of the superior mesenteric and splenic veins. Although it is a large vessel, it runs a short course (7–8 cm), most of which is contained within the hepatoduodenal ligament. As it approaches the porta hepatis, the portal vein divides into right and left branches. The portal vein collects blood of reduced oxygenation but rich in nutrients from the abdominal part of

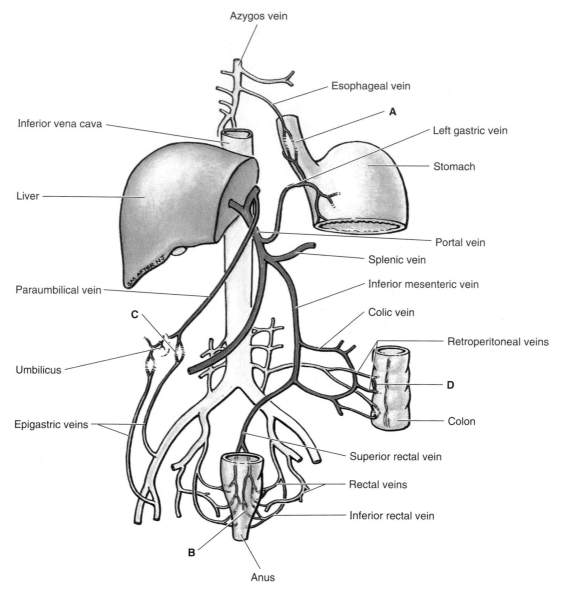

Figure 2.59. Portal–systemic anastomoses. Anastomoses provide a collateral circulation in cases of obstruction in the liver or portal vein. Here, the portal tributaries are darker blue and systemic tributaries are lighter blue. **A–D** indicate sites of anastomoses. **A** is between the submucosal esophageal veins draining into either the azygos vein (systemic) or the left gastric vein (portal); when dilated these are esophageal varices. **B** is between the inferior and middle rectal veins draining into the inferior vena cava (systemic) and the superior rectal vein, continuing as the inferior mesenteric vein (portal). The submucosal veins involved are normally dilated (varicose in appearance), even in newborns. When the mucosa containing them prolapses, they form *hemorrhoids.* (The varicose appearance of the veins and the occurrence of hemorrhoids are not typically related to portal hypertension, as is commonly stated.) **C** shows paraumbilical veins (portal) anastomosing with small epigastric veins of the anterior abdominal wall (systemic); this may produce the "caput medusae" (Fig. B2.24). **D** is on the posterior aspects (bare areas) of secondarily retroperitoneal viscera, or the liver, where twigs of visceral veins—for example, the colic vein, splenic veins, or the portal vein itself (portal system)—anastomose with retroperitoneal veins of the posterior abdominal wall or diaphragm (systemic system).

the alimentary tract, including the gallbladder, pancreas, and spleen, and carries it to the liver. Streaming of the blood flow is said to occur in which blood from the splenic vein, carrying the products of RBC breakdown from the spleen, passes mostly to the left liver. Blood from the SMV, rich in absorbed nutrients from the intestines, passes mostly to the right liver. Within the liver, its branches are distributed in a segmental pattern (see "Blood Vessels of the Liver," in this chapter) and end in expanded capillaries, the *venous sinusoids of the liver* (Fig. 2.53*A*).

Portal–systemic anastomoses, in which the portal venous system communicates with the systemic venous system, are formed in the submucosa of the inferior esophagus, in the submucosa of the anal canal, in the paraumbilical region, and on the posterior aspects (bare areas) of secondarily retroperitoneal viscera, or the liver (Fig. 2.59; see legend for details). When portal circulation through the liver is dimin- ished or obstructed because of liver disease or physical pressure from a tumor, for example, blood from the alimentary tract can still reach the right side of the heart through the IVC by way of these collateral routes. These alternate routes are available because the portal vein and its tributaries have no valves; hence blood can flow in a reverse direction to the IVC.

Anterior views

Figure B2.24.

Portosystemic Shunts

A common method for reducing portal hypertension is to divert blood from the portal venous system to the systemic venous system by creating a communication between the portal vein and the IVC. This *portacaval anastomosis* or *portosystemic shunt* may be done where these vessels lie close to each other posterior to the liver (Fig. B2.24*A–C*). Another way of reducing portal pressure is to join the splenic vein to the left renal vein, after splenectomy (*splenorenal anastomosis* or *shunt*) (Fig. B2.24*D*) (Skandalakis et al., 1995).

Portal Hypertension

When scarring and fibrosis from cirrhosis obstruct the portal vein in the liver, pressure rises in the portal vein and its tributaries, producing **portal hypertension**. The large volume of blood flowing from the portal system to the systemic system at the sites of portal–systemic anastomoses produces *varicose veins,* especially in the lower esophagus. The veins may become so dilated that their walls rupture, resulting in hemorrhage (see Fig. B2.8).

Bleeding from esophageal varices (abnormally dilated veins) at the distal end of the esophagus is often severe and may be fatal. In severe cases of portal obstruction, the veins of the anterior abdominal wall (normally caval tributaries) that anastomose with the paraumbilical veins (normally portal tributaries) may become varicose and look somewhat like small snakes radiating under the skin around the umbilicus. This condition is referred to as *caput medusae* because of its resemblance to the serpents on the head of Medusa, a character in Greek mythology. Figure B2.25 shows the more typical variation seen in relation to portal hypertension; a more unusual variation, occurring as a result of caval obstruction, is shown in Figure B2.2. ▶

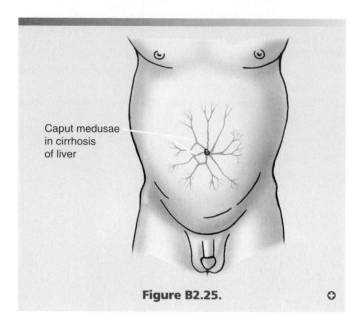

Caput medusae
in cirrhosis
of liver

Figure B2.25.

THE BOTTOM LINE: The large but short portal vein, formed posterior to the neck of the pancreas by the merger of the SMV and splenic vein, conveys all venous blood and bloodborne nutrients from the GI tract to the liver. The portal vein terminates at the porta hepatis, bifurcating into the right and left portal vein, distributed in a segmental pattern to the right and left livers. The portal vein traverses the hepatoduodenal ligament (free edge of the lesser omentum and anterior boundary of the omental foramen) as part of an extrahepatic portal triad (portal vein, hepatic artery, bile duct). Portal–systemic anastomoses provide a potential collateral pathway by which blood can return to the heart when there is an obstruction of the portal vein or disease of the liver. However, when the collateral pathways must convey large volumes, potentially lethal esophageal varices may develop.

Kidneys, Ureters, and Suprarenal Glands

The superior urinary organs (kidneys and ureters) and their vessels are primary retroperitoneal structures on the posterior abdominal wall (Fig. 2.60)—that is, they were originally formed as and remain retroperitoneal viscera. The *kidneys* produce urine that is conveyed by the *ureters* to the *urinary bladder* in the pelvis. The superomedial aspect of each kidney normally contacts a *suprarenal gland* enclosed in a fibrous capsule and a cushion of pararenal fat (Fig. 2.61). A weak fascial septum separates the glands from the kidneys so that they are not actually attached to each other. The suprarenal glands function as part of the endocrine system, completely separate in function from the kidneys.

Perinephric fat (the **perirenal fat capsule**) surrounds the kidneys and their vessels as it extends into their hollow centers, the renal sinuses (Fig. 2.61*B*). The kidneys, suprarenal glands, and the fat surrounding them are enclosed (except inferiorly) by a condensed, membranous layer of **renal fascia**, which continues medially to ensheath the renal vessels, blending with the vascular sheaths of the latter. Inferomedially, a delicate extension of the renal fascia is prolonged along the ureter as the **periureteric fascia.** External to the renal fascia is **paranephric fat** (or the **pararenal fat body**), the extraperitoneal fat of the lumbar region that is most obvious posterior to the kidney. The renal fascia sends collagen bundles through the paranephric fat.

The collagen bundles, renal fascia, and perinephric and paranephric fat, along with the tethering provided by the renal vessels and ureter, hold the kidneys in a relatively fixed position. However, movement of the kidneys occurs during respiration and when changing from the supine to the erect position, and vice versa. Normal renal mobility is approximately 3 cm, approximately the height of one vertebral body. Superiorly, the renal fascia is continuous with the fascia on the inferior surface of the diaphragm (diaphragmatic fascia); thus the primary attachment of the suprarenal glands is to the diaphragm. Inferiorly, the anterior and posterior layers of renal fascia are only loosely united, if attached at all.

Perinephric Abscess

The attachments of the renal fascia determine the path of extension of a *perinephric abscess.* For example, fascia at the renal hilum attaches to the renal vessels and ureter, usually preventing the spread of pus to the contralateral side. However, pus from an abscess (or blood from an injured kidney) may force its way into the pelvis between the loosely attached anterior and posterior layers of the pelvic fascia.

Nephroptosis

Because the layers of renal fascia do not fuse firmly inferiorly to offer resistance, abnormally mobile kidneys may descend more than the normal 3 cm when the body is erect. When kidneys descend, the suprarenal glands remain in place because they lie in a separate fascial compartment and are firmly attached to the diaphragm. **Nephroptosis** (dropped kidney) is distinguished from an **ectopic kidney** (congenital misplaced kidney) by a ureter of normal length that has loose coiling or kinks because the distance to the bladder has been reduced. The kinks do not seem to be of significance. Symptoms of intermittent pain in the renal region, relieved by lying down, appear to result from ▶

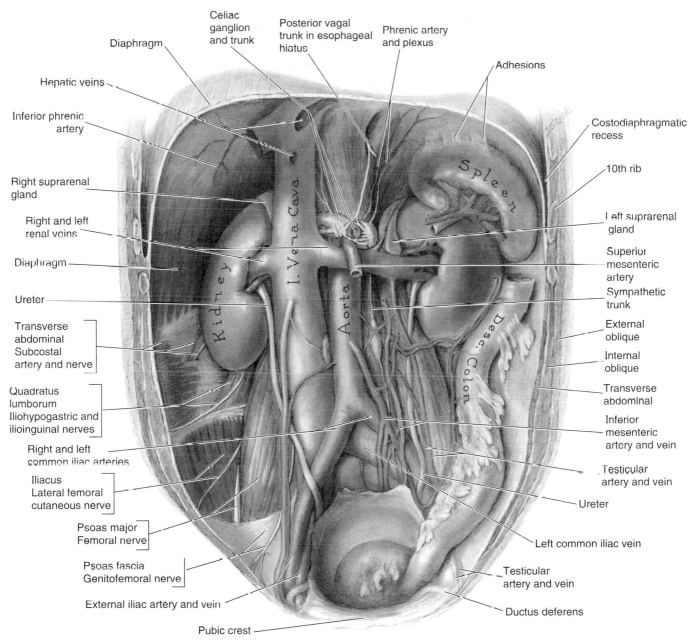

Figure 2.60. Posterior abdominal wall showing great vessels, kidneys, and suprarenal glands. Most of the fascia has been removed in this view. The ureter crosses the external iliac artery just beyond the common iliac bifurcation. In males, the testicular vessels cross anterior to the ureter and join the ductus deferens to enter the inguinal canal. The renal arteries are not seen because they lie posterior to the renal veins. The left renal vein is compressed between the aorta posteriorly and the superior mesenteric artery anteriorly, the latter being pulled inferiorly by the weight of the intestine.

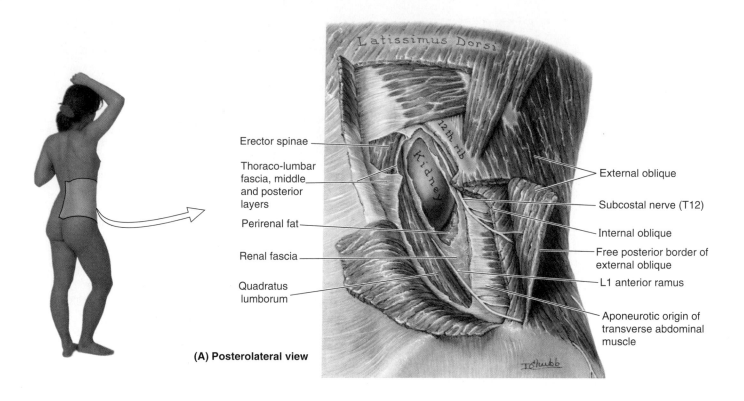

Erector spinae

Thoraco-lumbar fascia, middle and posterior layers

Perirenal fat

Renal fascia

Quadratus lumborum

External oblique

Subcostal nerve (T12)

Internal oblique

Free posterior border of external oblique

L1 anterior ramus

Aponeurotic origin of transverse abdominal muscle

(A) Posterolateral view

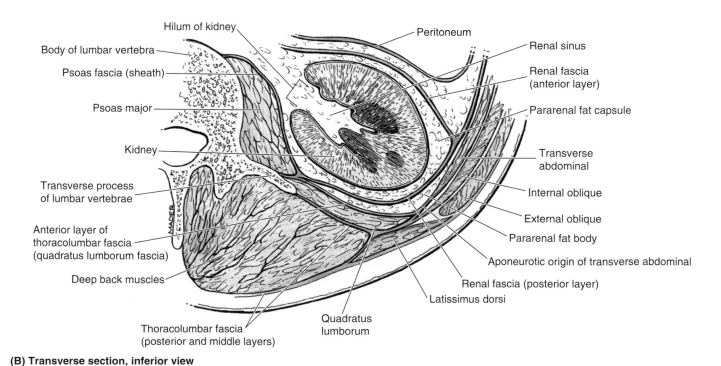

Hilum of kidney

Body of lumbar vertebra

Psoas fascia (sheath)

Psoas major

Kidney

Transverse process of lumbar vertebrae

Anterior layer of thoracolumbar fascia (quadratus lumborum fascia)

Deep back muscles

Thoracolumbar fascia (posterior and middle layers)

Quadratus lumborum

Peritoneum

Renal sinus

Renal fascia (anterior layer)

Pararenal fat capsule

Transverse abdominal

Internal oblique

External oblique

Pararenal fat body

Aponeurotic origin of transverse abdominal

Renal fascia (posterior layer)

Latissimus dorsi

(B) Transverse section, inferior view

Figure 2.61. Lumbar approach to kidney and relationships of kidney to muscles and fascia. A. The external aspect of the right posterior abdominal wall is shown. On dividing the posterior aponeurosis of the transverse abdominal muscle between the subcostal and the iliohypogastric nerves, and lateral to the oblique lateral border of the quadratus lumborum, the retroperitoneal fat surrounding the kidney is exposed. The renal fascia is within this fat. The fat inside the renal fascia is termed the perirenal fat capsule (perinephric fat); the fat outside the capsule is the pararenal fat body (paranephric fat). See Figure. 2.76A for an earlier stage of this dissection. **B.** This transverse section of the kidney shows the relationships of the muscles and fascia. Because the renal fascia surrounds the kidney as a separate sheath, it must be incised in any surgical operation on the kidney, whether from an anterior or a posterior approach.

traction on the renal vessels. The lack of inferior support for the kidneys in the lumbar region is one of the reasons transplanted kidneys are placed in the iliac fossa of the greater pelvis. Other reasons for this placement are the availability of major blood vessels and convenient access to the nearby bladder. ✪

Kidneys

The ovoid **kidneys** remove excess water, salts, and wastes of protein metabolism from the blood while returning nutrients and chemicals to the blood. They lie retroperitoneally on the posterior abdominal wall, one on each side of the vertebral column at the level of the T12–L3 vertebrae (Figs. 2.60 and 2.62). The right kidney usually lies slightly inferior to the left kidney, probably owing to its relationship to the liver. During life, the kidneys are reddish brown and measure approximately 10 cm in length, 5 cm in width, and 2.5 cm in thickness. Superiorly, the kidneys are associated with the diaphragm, which separates them from the pleural cavities and the 12th pair of ribs. More inferiorly, the posterior surfaces of the kidney are related to the quadratus lumborum muscle (Figs. 2.60 and 2.61). The subcostal nerve and vessels and the iliohypogastric and ilioinguinal nerves descend diagonally across the posterior surfaces of the kidneys. The liver, duodenum, and ascending colon are anterior to the right kidney (Fig. 2.63). The right kidney is separated from the liver by the *hepatorenal recess*. The left kidney is related to the stomach, spleen, pancreas, jejunum, and descending colon.

At the concave medial margin of each kidney is a vertical cleft, the **renal hilum,** where the renal artery enters and the renal vein and renal pelvis leave the renal sinus (Fig. 2.64A). At the hilum, the *renal vein* is anterior to the *renal artery,* which is anterior to the renal pelvis. The renal hilum is the entrance to a space within the kidney, the **renal sinus** (Fig. 2.64B), which is occupied by the renal pelvis, calices, vessels, and nerves and a variable amount of fat (Fig. 2.64C & D). Each kidney has anterior and posterior surfaces, medial and lateral margins, and superior and inferior poles. However, because of the protrusion of the lumbar vertebral column into the abdominal cavity, the kidneys are obliquely placed, lying at an angle to each other (Fig. 2.61B). Consequently, the transverse diameter of the kidneys is foreshortened in anteroposterior (AP) radiographs. The lateral margin of each kidney is convex, and the medial margin is concave where the renal sinus and renal pelvis are located. The indented medial margin gives the kidney a somewhat bean-shaped appearance.

The **renal pelvis** is the flattened, funnel-shaped expansion of the superior end of the ureter (Fig. 2.64B–D). The apex of the renal pelvis is continuous with the ureter. The renal pelvis receives two or three **major calices** (calyces), each of which divides into two or three **minor calices.** Each minor calyx is indented by the **renal papilla,** the apex of the *renal pyramid,* from which the urine is excreted. In living persons, the renal pelvis and its calices are usually collapsed (empty). The pyramids and their associated cortex form the lobes of the kidney. The lobes are visible on the external surfaces of the kidneys in fetuses, and evidence of the lobes may persist for some time after birth (Moore and Persaud, 2003).

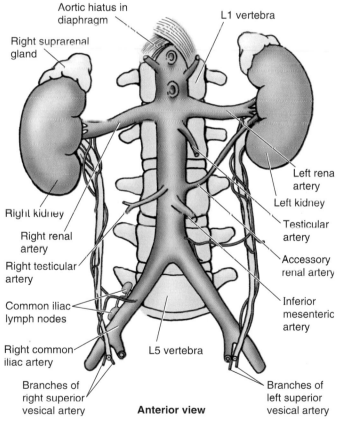

Figure 2.62. Arterial supply of kidneys and ureters.
The abdominal aorta lies anterior to the L1–L4 vertebral bodies, usually immediately to the left of the midline. An accessory left renal artery is present. Multiple renal arteries are common and usually enter the hilum of the kidney, as shown here. Extrahilar renal arteries from the renal artery or aorta may enter the external surface of the kidney, commonly at their poles. Their presence presents a hazard during operations on the kidney.

Renal Transplantation

Renal transplantation is now an established operation for the treatment of selected cases of chronic renal failure. The kidney can be removed from the donor without damaging the suprarenal gland because of the weak septum of renal fascia that separates the kidney from this gland. The site for transplanting a kidney is in the iliac fossa of the greater pelvis. This site supports the transplanted kidney, so that traction is not placed on the ▶

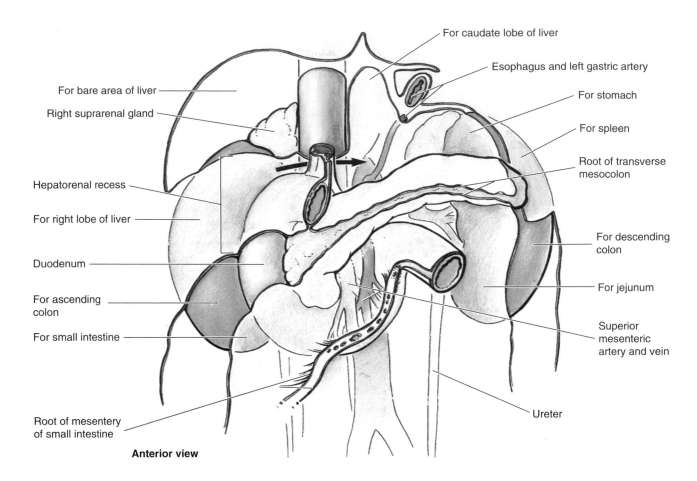

For caudate lobe of liver

Esophagus and left gastric artery

For stomach

For spleen

Root of transverse mesocolon

For descending colon

For jejunum

Superior mesenteric artery and vein

Ureter

For bare area of liver

Right suprarenal gland

Hepatorenal recess

For right lobe of liver

Duodenum

For ascending colon

For small intestine

Root of mesentery of small intestine

Anterior view

Figure 2.63. Relationships of kidneys, suprarenal glands, pancreas, and duodenum. The right suprarenal gland is at the level of the omental foramen, indicated by the black arrow.

surgically anastomosed vessels. The renal artery and vein are joined to the external iliac artery and vein, respectively, and the ureter is sutured into the urinary bladder.

Renal Cysts

Cysts in the kidney, multiple or solitary, are common findings during ultrasound examinations and dissection of cadavers. Adult *polycystic disease of the kidneys* is an important cause of renal failure; it is inherited as an autosomal dominant trait. The kidneys are markedly enlarged and distorted by cysts as large as 5 cm.

Pain in the Pararenal Region

The close relationship of the kidneys to the psoas major muscles explains why extension of the hip joints may increase pain resulting from inflammation in the pararenal areas. These muscles flex the thighs at the hip joints. ☉

THE BOTTOM LINE: The abdominal urinary organs and the suprarenal glands are primary retroperitoneal structures, embedded within perinephric fat (perirenal fat capsule) that is separated from the surrounding extraperitoneal paranephric fat by a membranous condensation, the renal fascia. The kidneys are bean-shaped structures located between the T12 and the L3 vertebral levels, deep (anterior) to the 12th ribs. Closely related to the diaphragm, the kidneys move with its excursions. The suprarenal glands are located superomedially to the kidneys but are not attached to them. The kidneys are hollow. The central renal sinus is occupied by the renal calices and renal pelvis, segmental arteries and renal veins that are embedded in perinephric fat. The papillae of the renal pyramids, from which urine is excreted, evaginate into and are surrounded by minor calices. The minor calices merge to form major calices that in turn merge to form the renal pelvis. The vascular structures and renal pelvis exit the renal sinus at the medially directed hilum.

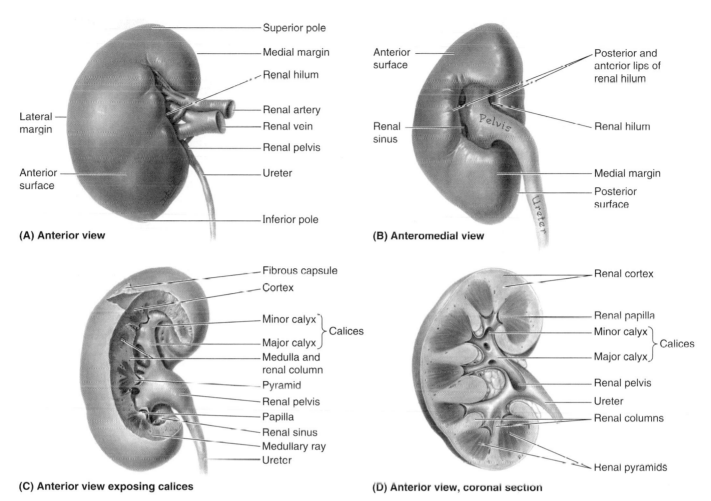

(A) Anterior view

- Superior pole
- Medial margin
- Renal hilum
- Renal artery
- Renal vein
- Renal pelvis
- Ureter
- Inferior pole
- Lateral margin
- Anterior surface

(B) Anteromedial view

- Anterior surface
- Posterior and anterior lips of renal hilum
- Renal hilum
- Renal sinus
- Medial margin
- Posterior surface
- Pelvis
- Ureter

(C) Anterior view exposing calices

- Fibrous capsule
- Cortex
- Minor calyx ⎫
- Major calyx ⎬ Calices
- Medulla and renal column
- Pyramid
- Renal pelvis
- Papilla
- Renal sinus
- Medullary ray
- Ureter

(D) Anterior view, coronal section

- Renal cortex
- Renal papilla
- Minor calyx ⎫
- Major calyx ⎬ Calices
- Renal pelvis
- Ureter
- Renal columns
- Renal pyramids

Figure 2.64. External and internal appearance of kidneys. A. The right kidney is shown. **B.** Renal sinus, as seen through the renal hilum, is demonstrated. As shown here and in part A, the renal sinus contains the renal pelvis and renal vessels. **C.** The anterior lip of the renal hilum has been cut away to expose the renal pelvis and calices within the renal sinus. **D.** This coronal section of the kidney shows the organ's internal structure. The renal pyramids contain the collecting tubules and form the medulla of the kidney. The renal cortex contains the renal corpuscles. The renal papillae (the blunted apices of the pyramids) project into the minor calices, into which they discharge urine, which then passes into the major calices and renal pelvis.

Ureters

The **ureters** are muscular ducts (25–30 cm long) with narrow lumina that carry urine from the kidneys to the urinary bladder (Figs. 2.60 and 2.64). They run inferiorly from the apex of the renal pelves at the hila of the kidneys, passing over the pelvic brim at the bifurcation of the common iliac arteries. They then run along the lateral wall of the pelvis and enter the urinary bladder. The abdominal parts of the ureters adhere closely to the parietal peritoneum and are retroperitoneal throughout their course. As demonstrated radiographically using contrast medium (Fig. 2.89), the ureters are normally constricted to a variable degree in three places: (1) at the junction of the ureters and renal pelves, (2) where the ureters cross the brim of the pelvic inlet, and (3) during their passage through the wall of the urinary bladder (Fig. 2.65). These constricted areas are potential sites of obstruction by ureteric (kidney) stones.

Arterial branches to the abdominal portion of the ureter arise consistently from the *renal arteries*, with less constant branches arising from the *testicular* or *ovarian arteries*, the *abdominal aorta*, and the *common iliac arteries* (Fig. 2.62). The branches approach the ureters medially and divide into ascending and descending branches, forming a longitudinal anastomosis on the ureteric wall. However, ureteric branches are small and relatively delicate, and disruption may lead to ischemia in spite of the continuous anastomotic channel formed. In operations in the posterior abdominal region, surgeons pay special attention to the location of ureters and are careful not to retract them laterally or unnecessarily. The arteries supplying the pelvic portion of the ureter are discussed in Chapter 3.

Veins draining the abdominal part of the ureters drain into the renal and gonadal (testicular or ovarian) veins (Fig. 2.66). The lymphatic vessels of the ureters join the renal collecting vessels or pass directly to **right** or **left lumbar** (**caval** or **aortic**) **lymph nodes** and the **common iliac lymph nodes** (Fig. 2.65). Lymph drainage from the pelvic parts of the ureters is into the common, external, and **internal iliac lymph nodes.**

Figure 2.65. Lymphatics of kidneys and suprarenal glands. The lymphatic vessels of the kidneys form three plexuses: one in the substance of the kidney, one under the fibrous capsule, and one in the perirenal fat. Four or five lymphatic trunks leave the renal hilum and are joined by vessels from the capsule (arrows). The lymphatic vessels follow the renal vein to the lumbar (caval and aortic) lymph nodes. Lymph from the suprarenal glands also drains to the lumbar nodes. Lymphatic drainage of the ureters is also illustrated. The lumbar lymph nodes drain through the lumbar lymphatic trunks to the chyle cistern. Also demonstrated are the three sites at which the ureter is normally relatively constricted: ① the junction of pelvis and ureter, as it crosses the ② external iliac vessels and pelvic brim, and ③ as it penetrates the wall of the urinary bladder.

Accessory Renal Vessels

During their "ascent" to their final site, the embryonic kidneys receive their blood supply and venous drainage from successively more superior vessels (Moore and Persaud, 2003). Usually the inferior vessels degenerate as superior ones take over the blood supply and venous drainage. Failure of these vessels to degenerate results in *accessory renal arteries* (Fig. 2.62) and *veins* (known as "polar arteries and veins" when they enter/exit the poles of the kidneys). Variations in the number and position of these vessels occur in approximately 25% of people.

Congenital Anomalies of the Kidneys and Ureters

Bifid renal pelvis and ureter are fairly common (Fig. B2.26*A* & *B*). These anomalies result from division of the *metanephric diverticulum* (ureteric bud), the primordium of the renal pelvis and ureter (Moore and Persaud, 2003). The extent of ureteral duplication depends on the completeness of embryonic division of the metanephric diverticulum. The bifid renal pelvis and/or ureter may be unilateral or bilateral; however, separate openings into the bladder are uncommon. Incomplete division of the metanephric diverticulum results in a bifid ureter; complete division results in a *supernumerary kidney*.

(A) Bifid renal pelvis

Figure B2.26.

An uncommon anomaly is a *retrocaval ureter* (Fig. B2.26*C*), which leaves the kidney and passes posterior to the IVC.

The embryonic kidneys are close together in the pelvis. In approximately 1 in 600 fetuses, the inferior poles ▶

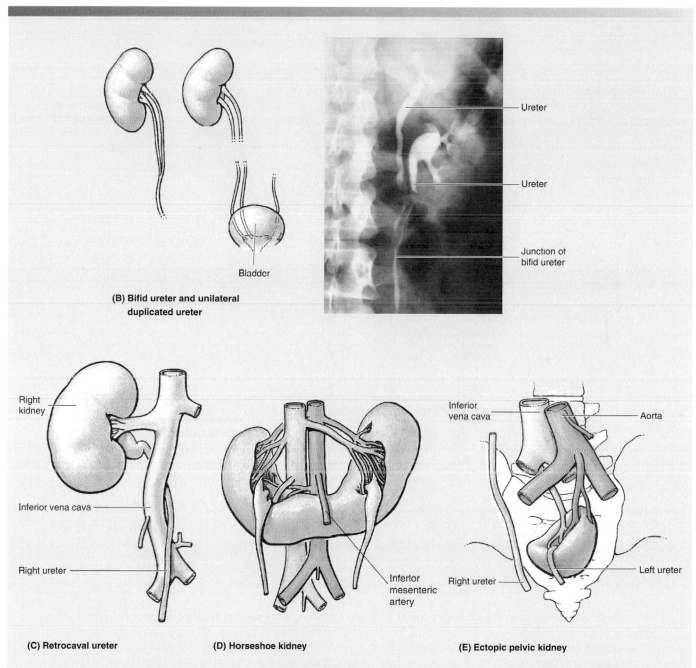

(B) Bifid ureter and unilateral duplicated ureter

Ureter

Ureter

Junction of bifid ureter

Bladder

Right kidney

Inferior vena cava

Right ureter

(C) Retrocaval ureter

Inferior mesenteric artery

(D) Horseshoe kidney

Inferior vena cava

Aorta

Right ureter

Left ureter

(E) Ectopic pelvic kidney

Figure B2.26. *(Continued)*

(rarely, the superior poles) of the kidneys fuse to form a *horseshoe kidney* (Fig. B2.26D). This U-shaped kidney usually lies at the level of L3–L5 vertebrae because the root of the *inferior mesenteric artery* prevented normal ascent of the abnormal kidney. Horseshoe kidney usually produces no symptoms; however, associated abnormalities of the kidney and renal pelvis may be present, obstructing the ureter.

Sometimes the embryonic kidney on one or both sides fails to ascend to the abdomen and lies anterior to the sacrum. Although uncommon, awareness of the possibility of an *ectopic pelvic kidney* (Fig. B2.26E) should prevent it from being mistaken for a pelvic tumor and removed. A pelvic kidney in a woman also can be injured by or cause obstruction during childbirth. Pelvic kidneys usually receive their blood supply from the common iliac arteries. ✪

Inferior vena cava

Right and left inferior phrenic arteries

Celiac trunk

Right superior suprarenal arteries

Right middle suprarenal artery

Right suprarenal gland

Superior pole

Esophagus
Left crus of diaphragm
Left inferior phrenic vein

Left superior suprarenal arteries

Cross section of suprarenal gland

Capsule

Cortex

Medulla

Superior pole of kidney
Left suprarenal gland
Left middle suprarenal artery
Left suprarenal vein
Left inferior suprarenal artery
Segmental arteries

Right inferior suprarenal artery

Ureteric branch of right renal artery

Right renal artery and vein

Right testicular (ovarian) artery and vein

Inferior vena cava

Ureteric branch of left renal artery
Inferior pole of kidney
Left renal artery and vein
Left 2nd lumbar vein and communication to ascending lumbar and/or hemiazygos veins

Superior mesenteric artery

Left testicular (ovarian) artery and vein

Inferior mesenteric artery

Abdominal aorta

Anterior view

Figure 2.66. Blood vessels of suprarenal glands, kidneys, and superior part of ureters. The celiac plexus of nerves and ganglia that surrounds the celiac trunk has been removed. The IVC has been transected, and its superior part has been elevated from its normal position to reveal the arteries that pass posterior to it. The renal veins have been cut so that the kidneys could be moved laterally. For the normal relationships of the kidneys and suprarenal glands with the great vessels, see Figure 2.60. Observe the gross structure of the suprarenal glands and their rich arterial supply. The cross section of the suprarenal gland (inset) shows that it is composed of two distinct parts: the cortex and medulla, which are two separate endocrine glands that became closely related during embryonic development. Multiple suprarenal arteries arise from the inferior phrenic artery; one or more inferior suprarenal arteries often arise from the renal artery, and a middle suprarenal artery arises from the abdominal artery. The number and patterns of arrangement of the suprarenal arteries are very variable. The endocrine function of the suprarenal glands make their abundant blood supply necessary.

Surface Anatomy of the Kidneys and Ureters

The **hilum of the left kidney** lies near the transpyloric plane, approximately 5 cm from the median plane (Fig. SA2.5). The **transpyloric plane** passes through the superior pole of the right kidney, which is approximately 2.5 cm lower than the left pole. Posteriorly, the superior parts of the kidneys lie deep to the 11th and 12th ribs. The levels of the kidneys change during respiration and with changes in posture. Each kidney moves 2–3 cm in a vertical direction during the movement of the diaphragm that occurs with deep breathing. Because the usual surgical approach to the kidneys is through the posterior abdominal wall, it is helpful to know that the inferior pole of the right kidney is approximately a finger's breadth superior to the **iliac crest**.

The kidneys may be impalpable. In lean adults, the inferior pole of the right kidney is palpable by bimanual examination as a firm, smooth, somewhat rounded mass that descends during inspiration. Palpation of the right kidney is possible because it is 1–2 cm inferior to the left one. To palpate the kidneys, press the **flank** (the side of the trunk between the 11th and 12th ribs and the iliac crest) anteriorly with one hand while palpating deeply at the **costal margin** with the other. The left kidney is usually not palpable unless it is enlarged or a retroperitoneal mass has displaced it inferiorly.

From the back, the surface marking of the ureter is a line joining a point 5 cm lateral to the L1 spinous process and the posterior superior iliac spine. The ureters occupy a sagittal plane that intersects the tips of the transverse processes of the lumbar vertebrae. ✪

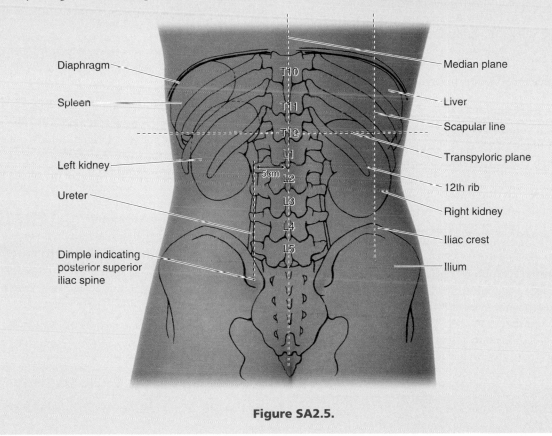

Diaphragm
Spleen
Left kidney
Ureter
Dimple indicating posterior superior iliac spine

T10
T11
T12
L1
5cm L2
L3
L4
L5

Median plane
Liver
Scapular line
Transpyloric plane
12th rib
Right kidney
Iliac crest
Ilium

Figure SA2.5.

THE BOTTOM LINE: The abdominal portions of the ureters descend on the anterior surface of the psoas muscles from the apex of the renal pelvis to the pelvic brim. The ureters normally have three sites of relative constriction, where kidney stones may lodge: the uteropelvic junction, the pelvic brim, and the bladder wall. The abdominal portions of the ureters receive multiple, relatively delicate ureteric branches from the renal, testicular or ovarian, and common iliac arteries and from the abdominal aorta, which ap-

proach the ureters medially. A vertical line 5 cm lateral to the lumbar spinous processes, intersecting the posterior superior iliac spine, approximates the position of the ureter.

Suprarenal Glands

The **suprarenal (adrenal) glands,** yellowish in living persons, are located between the superomedial aspects of the kidneys and the diaphragm (Fig. 2.66), where they are surrounded by connective tissue containing considerable perinephric fat.

The glands are enclosed by renal fascia by which they are attached to the *crura of the diaphragm*. Despite their name, this is the primary relationship of the suprarenal glands. They are separated from the kidneys by a thin septum (part of the renal fascia). The shape and relations of the suprarenal glands differ on the two sides. The pyramidal right gland is more apical (situated over the superior pole) relative to the right kidney, lies anterolateral to the right crus of the diaphragm, and makes contact with the IVC anteromedially (Fig. 2.63) and the liver anterolaterally. The crescent-shaped left gland is medial to the superior half of the left kidney and is related to the spleen, stomach, pancreas, and the left crus of the diaphragm. Each gland has a *hilum,* where the veins and lymphatic vessels exit the gland; whereas arteries and nerves enter the glands at multiple sites. The medial borders of the suprarenal glands are 4–5 cm apart. In this area, from right to left, are the IVC, right crus of the diaphragm, celiac ganglion, celiac trunk, SMA, and the left crus of the diaphragm.

Each suprarenal gland has two parts: the suprarenal cortex and suprarenal medulla Fig. 2.66, *inset*); these parts have different embryological origins and different functions (Moore and Persaud, 2003).

The **suprarenal cortex** derives from mesoderm and secretes corticosteroids and androgens. These hormones cause the kidneys to retain sodium and water in response to stress, increasing the blood volume and blood pressure. They also affect muscles and organs such as the heart and lungs.

The **suprarenal medulla** is a mass of nervous tissue permeated with capillaries and sinusoids that derives from neural crest cells associated with the sympathetic nervous system. The *chromaffin cells* of the medulla are related to sympathetic ganglion (postsynaptic) neurons in both derivation (neural crest cells) and function. These cells secrete catecholamines (mostly epinephrine) into the bloodstream in response to signals from presynaptic neurons (Naftel and Hardy, 2002). The powerful medullary hormones epinephrine (adrenaline) and norepinephrine (noradrenaline) activate the body to a flight-or-fight status in response to traumatic stress. They also increase heart rate and blood pressure, dilate the bronchioles, and change blood flow patterns, preparing for physical exertion.

THE BOTTOM LINE: The suprarenal glands are located superomedially to the kidneys but are attached primarily to the diaphragmatic crura by the surrounding renal fascia. Each suprarenal gland is actually two endocrine glands of different origin and function: suprarenal cortex and suprarenal medulla (the latter surrounded by the former). The adrenal cortex derives from mesoderm and secretes corticosteroids and androgens; the adrenal medulla derives from neural crest cells and secretes catecholamines (mostly epinephrine). The right suprarenal gland is more pyramidal in shape and apical in position relative to the right kidney, whereas the left gland is more crescentic and lies more medial to the superior half of the kidney.

Vessels and Nerves of the Kidneys and Suprarenal Glands

The Renal Arteries and Veins. The renal arteries arise at the level of the IV disc between the L1 and the L2 vertebrae (Figs. 2.62 and 2.66). The longer **right renal artery** passes posterior to the IVC. Typically, each artery divides close to the hilum into five segmental arteries that are end arteries (i.e., they do not anastomose significantly with other segmental arteries, so that the area supplied by each segmental artery is an independent, surgically resectable unit or **renal segment**). Segmental arteries are distributed to the renal segments as follows (Fig. 2.67):

- The superior (apical) segment is supplied by the **superior (apical) segmental artery**; the anterosuperior and anteroinferior segments are supplied by the **anterosuperior segmental** and **anteroinferior segmental arteries**; and the inferior segment is supplied by the **inferior segmental artery.** These arteries originate from the anterior branch of the renal artery.

- The **posterior segmental artery,** which originates from a continuation of the posterior branch of the renal artery, supplies the posterior segment of the kidney.

Several *renal veins* drain each kidney and unite in a variable fashion to form the **right** and **left renal veins.** The right and left renal veins lie anterior to the right and left renal arteries. The longer left renal vein receives the *left suprarenal vein,* the *left gonadal* (*testicular* or *ovarian*) *vein,* and a communication with the *ascending lumbar vein,* then passes anterior to the aorta. Each renal vein drains into the IVC.

The Suprarenal Arteries and Veins. The endocrine function of the suprarenal glands makes their abundant blood supply necessary. The suprarenal arteries branch freely before entering each gland so that 50–60 arteries penetrate the capsule covering the entire surface of the glands (Fig. 2.66). Suprarenal arteries arise from three sources:

- **Superior suprarenal arteries** (6–8) from the *inferior phrenic arteries.*

- **Middle suprarenal arteries** (≤ 1) from the *abdominal aorta* near the level of origin of the SMA.

- **Inferior suprarenal arteries** (≤ 1) from the renal arteries.

The venous drainage of the suprarenal gland is into a large suprarenal vein (Fig. 2.66). The short **right suprarenal vein** drains into the IVC, whereas the longer **left suprarenal vein,** often joined by the *inferior phrenic vein,* empties into the left renal vein.

Lymphatics of the Kidneys, Ureters, and Suprarenal Glands. The *renal lymphatic vessels* follow the renal veins and drain into the *right* and *left lumbar* (*caval* and *aortic*) *lymph nodes* (Fig. 2.65). Lymphatic vessels from the superior part of the ureter may join those from the kidney or pass directly to the lumbar nodes. Lymphatic vessels from the middle part of the ureter usually drain into the *common iliac lymph nodes,*

Figure 2.67. Renal segments and segmental arteries A. According to its arterial supply, the kidney has five segments: superior (apical), anterosuperior, anteroinferior, inferior, and posterior. **B.** Only the superior and inferior arteries supply the whole thickness of the kidney. The posterior artery crosses superior to the renal pelvis to reach its segment. **C.** Typically, the renal artery divides into five branches, each supplying a segment of the kidney, as seen in this renal arteriogram. Although the veins of the kidney anastomose freely, segmental arteries are end arteries. (Courtesy of Dr. E. L. Lansdown, Professor of Medical Imaging, University of Toronto, Toronto, ON, Canada.)

(C) Anteroposterior view of right kidney

whereas vessels from its inferior part drain into the common, external, or internal **iliac lymph nodes.** The *suprarenal lymphatic vessels* arise from a plexus deep to the capsule of the gland and from one in its medulla. The lymph passes to the *lumbar lymph nodes.* Many lymphatic vessels leave the suprarenal glands.

Nerves of the Kidneys, Ureters, and Suprarenal Glands. Nerves to the kidneys arise from the renal nerve plexus and consist of sympathetic and parasympathetic fibers (Fig. 2.68*B*). The **renal nerve plexus** is supplied by fibers from the abdominopelvic (especially the least) splanchnic nerves. The nerves of the abdominal part of the ureters derive from the renal, abdominal aortic, and superior hypogastric plexuses (Fig. 2.68*A*). Visceral afferent fibers conveying pain sensation (e.g., resulting from obstruction and consequent distension) follow the sympathetic fibers retrograde to spinal ganglia and cord segments T11–L2. Ureteric pain is usually referred to the ipsilateral lower quadrant of the anterior abdominal wall and especially to the groin (see the adjacent clinical correlation [blue] box "Renal and Ureteric Calculi").

The suprarenal glands have a rich nerve supply from the celiac plexus and abdominopelvic (greater, lesser and least)

splanchnic nerves. Myelinated presynaptic sympathetic fibers—mainly derived from the Intermediolateral cell column (IML), or lateral horn, of gray matter of the spinal cord segments T10–L1—traverse both the paravertebral and the prevertebral ganglia, without synapse, to be distributed to the chromaffin cells in the suprarenal medulla (Fig. 2.68*B*).

Renal and Ureteric Calculi

Calculi (L. pebbles) are composed of salts of inorganic or organic acids or of other materials. They may form and become located in the calices of the kidneys, ureters, or urinary bladder. A **renal calculus** (kidney stone) may pass from the kidney into the renal pelvis and then into the ureter. If the stone is sharp, or it is larger than the normal lumen of the ureter (approximately 3 mm) causing excessive distension of this muscular tube, the **ureteric calculus** will cause severe ▶

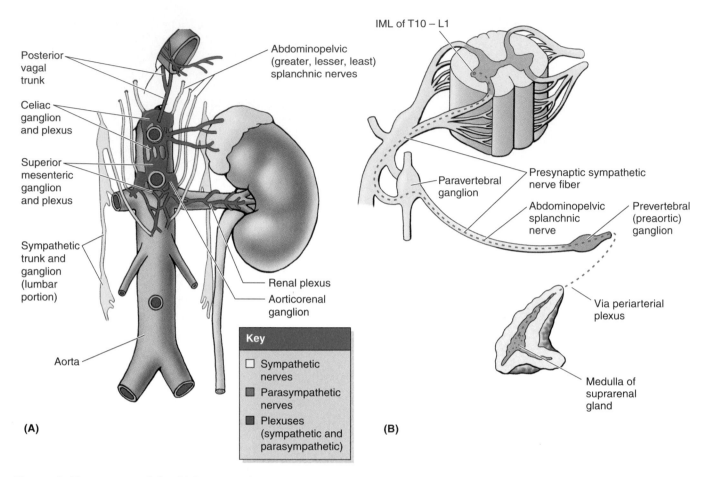

Figure 2.68. Nerves of the kidneys and suprarenal glands. A. The nerves of the kidneys and suprarenal glands are derived from the celiac plexus, abdominopelvic (lesser and least) splanchnic nerves, and the aorticorenal ganglion. Most of the fibers conveyed by the abdominopelvic splanchnic nerves to the prevertebral ganglia are presynaptic sympathetic fibers that passed through the paravertebral ganglia without synapsing. The main efferent innervation of the kidney is vasomotor, autonomic nerves supplying the afferent and efferent arterioles. **B.** Exclusively in the case of the suprarenal medulla, the presynaptic sympathetic fibers pass through both the paravertebral and prevertebral ganglia without synapsing to end directly on the secretory cells of the suprarenal medulla.

intermittent pain (*ureteric colic*) as it is gradually forced down the ureter by waves of contraction. The calculus may cause complete or intermittent obstruction of urinary flow. Depending on the level of obstruction, which changes, the pain may be referred to the lumbar or inguinal regions, or the external genitalia and/or testis.

The pain is referred to the cutaneous areas innervated by spinal cord segments and sensory ganglia, which also receive visceral afferents from the ureter, mainly T11–L2. The pain passes inferoanteriorly "from the loin to the groin" as the stone progresses through the ureter. (The loin is the lumbar region, and the groin is the inguinal region.)

The pain may extend into the proximal anterior aspect of the thigh by projection through the genitofemoral nerve (L1, L2), the scrotum in males and the labia majora in females. The extreme pain may be accompanied by marked alimentary upset (nausea, vomiting, cramping, and diarrhea) and a generalized sympathetic response that may to various degrees mask the more specific symptoms.

Ureteric calculi can be observed and removed with a *nephroscope,* an instrument that is inserted through a small incision. Another technique, *lithotripsy,* focuses a shockwave through the body that breaks the stone into small fragments that pass with the urine. ✚

THE BOTTOM LINE: The renal arteries arise from the abdominal aorta at the level of the L1–L2 IV disc. They lie anterior to the renal veins, with the right renal artery being longer than the left, and the left renal vein being longer than the right. Both renal veins receive renal and superior ureteric veins and drain into the IVC, but the long left vein also receives the left suprarenal vein, the left gonadal vein, and a communication with the left ascending lumbar vein. Near the hilum, the renal arteries divide into anterior and posterior branches, the anterior branches giving rise to four segmental renal arteries, whereas the posterior branch makes up a fifth. The segmental renal arteries are end arteries, so that each supplies an independent, surgically resectable segment of the kidney (renal segment).

Suprarenal arteries arise from three sources: superior suprarenal arteries from the inferior phrenic arteries, middle suprarenal arteries from the abdominal aorta, and inferior suprarenal arteries from the renal arteries. The suprarenal glands drain via one large suprarenal vein, the right entering the IVC and the left entering the left renal vein.

Lymphatics from the suprarenal glands, kidneys, and upper ureters follow the venous drainage to the right or left lumbar (caval or aortic) lymph nodes.

Visceral afferent fibers (accompanying the sympathetic fibers) conduct pain sensation from the ureters to spinal cord segments T11–L2, with sensation referred to the corresponding dermatomes overlying the loin and groin.

The suprarenal glands receive a rich nerve supply via presynpatic sympathetic fibers originating in the IML of the T10–L1 spinal cord segments. These fibers traverse both the paravertebral (sympathetic trunks) and prevertebral (celiac) ganglia without synapsing. They terminate directly on the chromaffin cells of the suprarenal medulla.

Summary of the Innervation of the Abdominal Viscera

For autonomic innervation of the abdominal viscera, several different splanchnic nerves and one cranial nerve (the vagus, CN X) deliver presynaptic sympathetic and parasympathetic fibers, respectively, to the abdominal aortic plexus and its associated sympathetic ganglia (Fig. 2.69; Table 2.12). The periarterial extensions of these plexuses deliver postsynaptic sympathetic and the continuations of the parasympathetic fibers to the abdominal viscera, where intrinsic parasympathetic ganglia occur.

Sympathetic Innervation

The sympathetic part of the autonomic innervation of the abdominal viscera consists of the:

- Abdominopelvic splanchnic nerves from the thoracic and abdominal sympathetic trunks.

- Prevertebral sympathetic ganglia.

- Abdominal aortic plexus and its extensions, the periarterial plexuses.

The plexuses are mixed, shared with the parasympathetic nervous system and visceral afferent fibers.

The **abdominopelvic splanchnic nerves** (Fig. 2.69*B*; Table 2.12) convey presynaptic sympathetic fibers to the abdominopelvic cavity. The fibers arise from cell bodies in the IML (or lateral horn) of the gray matter of spinal cord segments T5–L2 or L3. The fibers pass successively through the anterior roots, anterior rami, and white communicating branches of thoracic and upper lumbar spinal nerves to reach the sympathetic trunks. They pass through the paravertebral ganglia of the trunks without synapsing to enter the abdominopelvic splanchnic nerves, which convey them to the prevertebral ganglia of the abdominal cavity. The abdominopelvic splanchnic nerves include the:

- *Lower thoracic splanchnic nerves* (greater, lesser, and least): from the thoracic part of the sympathetic trunks.

- *Lumbar splanchnic nerves:* from the lumbar part of the sympathetic trunks.

The **lower thoracic splanchnic nerves** are the main source of presynaptic sympathetic fibers serving abdominal viscera. The **greater** (from the sympathetic trunk at T5 through T9 or T10 vertebral levels), **lesser** (from T10 and T11 levels), and **least** (from the T12 level) **splanchnic nerves** are the specific abdominopelvic splanchnic nerves that arise from the thoracic part of the sympathetic trunks and pierce the corresponding crus of the diaphragm to convey the presynaptic sympathetic fibers to the celiac, superior mesenteric, and aorticorenal (prevertebral) sympathetic ganglia, respectively.

The **lumbar splanchnic nerves** arise from the abdominal part of the sympathetic trunks. Medially, the lumbar sympathetic trunks give off three to four lumbar splanchnic nerves, which pass to the **intermesenteric, inferior mesenteric**, and **superior hypogastric plexuses**, conveying presynaptic sympathetic fibers to the associated prevertebral ganglia of those plexuses.

The cell bodies of postsynaptic sympathetic neurons constitute the major prevertebral ganglia that cluster around the roots of the major branches of the abdominal aorta: the *celiac, aorticorenal, superior mesenteric*, and *inferior mesenteric ganglia*. Minor, unnamed prevertebral ganglia occur within the intermesenteric and superior hypogastric plexuses. With the exception of the innervation of the suprarenal medulla (discussed earlier in this chapter), the synapse between presynaptic and postsynaptic sympathetic neurons occurs in the prevertebral ganglia. Postsynaptic sympathetic nerve fibers pass from the prevertebral ganglia to the abdominal viscera by means of the periarterial plexuses associated with the branches of the abdominal aorta. Sympathetic innervation in the abdomen, as elsewhere, is primarily involved in producing vasoconstriction. With regard to the alimentary tract, it acts to inhibit (slow down or stop) peristalsis.

Visceral afferent fibers conveying pain sensations accompany the sympathetic (visceral motor) fibers; the pain impulses pass retrogradely to those of the motor fibers along

(cont'd on page 324)

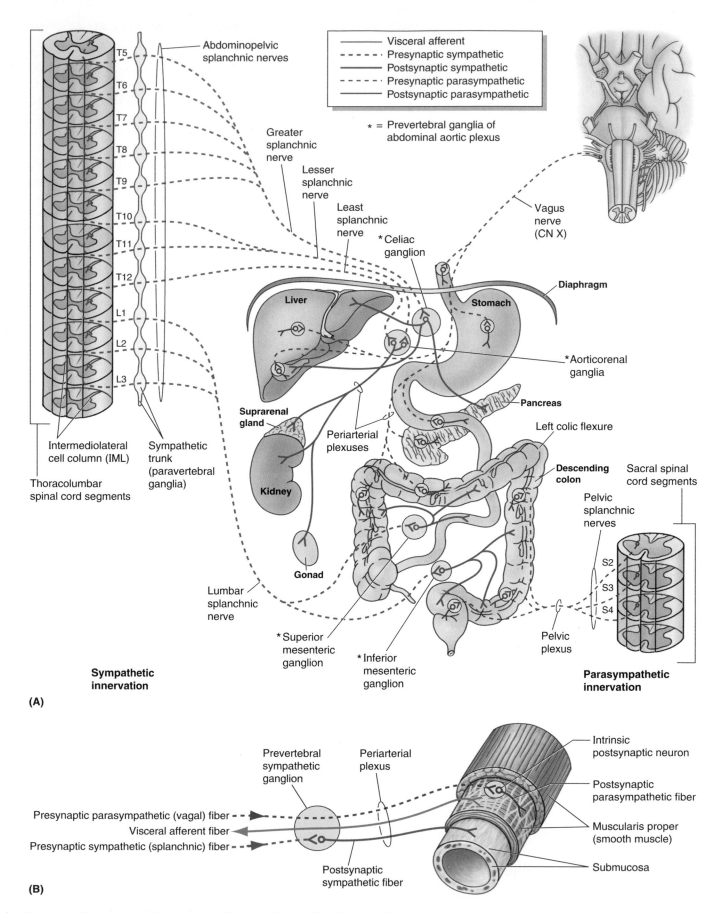

Figure 2.69. Autonomic nerves of posterior abdominal wall. A. Origin and distribution of presynapatic and postsynapatic sympathetic and parasympathetic fibers, and the ganglia involved in supplying abdominal viscera are shown. **B.** The fibers supplying the intrinsic plexuses of abdominal viscera are demonstrated.

Table 2.12. Autonomic Innervation of the Abdominal Viscera (Splanchnic Nerves)

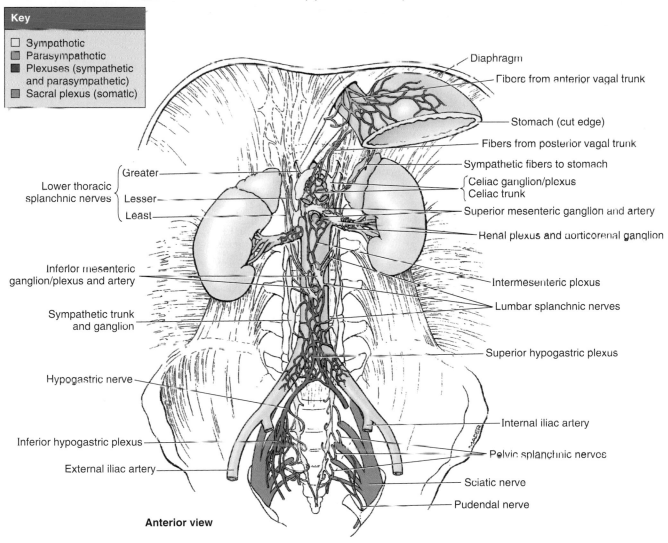

Key
- ☐ Sympathetic
- ☐ Parasympathetic
- ■ Plexuses (sympathetic and parasympathetic)
- ■ Sacral plexus (somatic)

Labels (clockwise):
Diaphragm · Fibers from anterior vagal trunk · Stomach (cut edge) · Fibers from posterior vagal trunk · Sympathetic fibers to stomach · Celiac ganglion/plexus · Celiac trunk · Superior mesenteric ganglion and artery · Renal plexus and aorticorenal ganglion · Intermesenteric plexus · Lumbar splanchnic nerves · Superior hypogastric plexus · Internal iliac artery · Pelvic splanchnic nerves · Sciatic nerve · Pudendal nerve

Lower thoracic splanchnic nerves { Greater, Lesser, Least } · Inferior mesenteric ganglion/plexus and artery · Sympathetic trunk and ganglion · Hypogastric nerve · Inferior hypogastric plexus · External iliac artery

Anterior view

Splanchnic Nerves	Autonomic Fiber Type[a]	System	Origin	Destination
A. **Cardiopulmonary** (Cervical and upper thoracic)	Postsynaptic		Cervical and upper thoracic sympathetic trunk	Thoracic cavity (viscera superior to level of diaphragm)
B. **Abdominopelvic**			Lower thoracic and abdomino-pelvic sympathetic trunk:	Abdominopelvic cavity (prevertebral ganglia serving viscera and suprarenal glands inferior to level of diaphragm)
1. Lower thoracic a. Greater b. Lesser c. Least 2. Lumbar	Presynaptic	Sympathetic	1. Thoracic sympathetic trunk: a. T5–T9 or T10 level b. T10–T11 level c. T12 level 2. Abdominal sympathetic trunk	1. Abdominal prevertebral ganglia: a. Celia ganglia b. Aorticorenal ganglia c. & 2. Other abdominal prevertebral ganglia (superior and inferior mesenteric, and of inter-mesenteric/hypogastric plexuses)
3. Sacral			3. Pelvic (sacral) sympathetic trunk	3. Pelvic prevertebral ganglia
C. **Pelvic**	Presynaptic	Parasympathetic	Anterior rami of S2–S4 spinal nerves	Intrinsic ganglia of descending and sigmoid colon, rectum, and pelvic viscera

[a]Splanchnic nerves also convey visceral afferent fibers, which are not part of the autonomic nervous system.

the splanchnic nerves to the sympathetic trunk, through white communicating branches to the anterior rami of the spinal nerves. Then they pass into the posterior root to the spinal sensory ganglia and spinal cord. Progressively lower spinal sensory ganglia and spinal cord segments are involved in innervating the abdominal viscera as the tract proceeds caudally. The stomach (foregut) receives innervation from the T6 to T9 levels, small intestine through transverse colon (midgut) from the T8 to 12 levels, and descending colon (hindgut) from the T12 to L2 levels (Fig. 2.70). Starting from the midpoint of the sigmoid colon, visceral pain fibers run with parasympathetic fibers, the sensory impulses being conducted to S2–S4 sensory ganglia and spinal cord levels. These are the same spinal cord segments involved in the sympathetic innervation of those portions of alimentary tract.

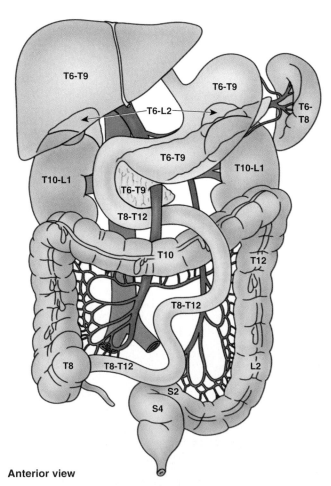

Anterior view

Figure 2.70. Approximate spinal cord segments and spinal sensory ganglia involved in sympathetic and visceral afferent (pain) innervation of abdominal viscera.

Parasympathetic Innervation

The parasympathetic part of the autonomic innervation of the abdominal viscera (Fig. 2.69; Table 2.12, figure) consists of the following:

- *Anterior* and *posterior vagal trunks.*

- *Pelvic splanchnic nerves.*

- *Abdominal* (para-aortic) *autonomic plexuses* and their extensions, the periarterial plexuses.

- *Intrinsic* (enteric) *parasympathetic ganglia.*

The nerve plexuses are mixed, shared with the sympathetic nervous system and visceral afferent fibers.

The *anterior* and *posterior vagal trunks* are the continuation of the left and right vagus nerves that emerge from the esophageal plexus and pass through the esophageal hiatus on the anterior and posterior aspects of the esophagus and stomach (Figs. 2.28 and 2.69A; Table 2.12). The vagus nerves convey presynaptic parasympathetic and visceral afferent fibers (mainly for unconscious sensations associated with reflexes) to the abdominal aortic plexuses and the periarterial plexuses, which extend along the branches of the aorta.

The **pelvic splanchnic nerves** are distinct from other splanchnic nerves (Table 2.12) in that they:

- Have nothing to do with the sympathetic trunks.

- Derive directly from anterior rami of spinal nerves S2–S4.

- Convey presynaptic parasympathetic fibers to the inferior hypogastric (pelvic) plexus.

Presynaptic fibers terminate on the isolated and widely scattered cell bodies of postsynaptic neurons lying on or within the abdominal viscera, constituting intrinsic ganglia (Fig. 2.69B).

The presynaptic parasympathetic and visceral afferent reflex fibers conveyed by the vagus nerves extend to intrinsic ganglia of the lower esophagus, stomach, small intestine, including the duodenum, ascending colon, and most of the transverse colon (Fig. 2.69A). Those conveyed by the pelvic splanchnic nerves supply the descending and sigmoid parts of the colon, rectum, and pelvic organs. Thus, in terms of the alimentary tract, the vagus nerves provide parasympathetic innervation of the smooth muscle and glands of the gut as far as the left colic flexure; the pelvic splanchnic nerves provide the remainder.

The **abdominal autonomic plexuses** are nerve networks consisting of both sympathetic and parasympathetic fibers, which surround the abdominal aorta and its major branches (Table 2.12). The celiac, superior mesenteric, and inferior mesenteric plexuses are interconnected. The **prevertebral sympathetic ganglia** are scattered among the celiac and mesenteric plexuses. The **intrinsic parasympathetic ganglia,** such as the **myenteric plexus** (Auerbach plexus) in the muscular coat of the stomach and intestine, are in the walls of the viscera (Fig. 2.69B; Table 2.9A).

The *celiac plexus,* surrounding the root of the celiac (arterial) trunk, contains irregular right and left *celiac ganglia* (approximately 2 cm long) that unite superior and inferior to the celiac trunk (Fig. 2.69A; Table 2.12). The *parasympathetic root* of the celiac plexus is a branch of the *posterior vagal trunk,* which contains fibers from the right and left vagus nerves. The *sympathetic roots* of the plexus are the greater and lesser splanchnic nerves.

The *superior mesenteric plexus* and ganglion or ganglia surround the origin of the SMA. The plexus has one median and two lateral roots. The median root is a branch of the celiac plexus, and the lateral roots arise from the lesser and least splanchnic nerves, sometimes with a contribution from the first lumbar ganglion of the sympathetic trunk.

The **inferior mesenteric plexus** surrounds the inferior mesenteric artery and gives offshoots to its branches. It receives a medial root from the intermesenteric plexus and lateral roots from the lumbar ganglia of the sympathetic trunks. An *inferior mesenteric ganglion* may also appear just inferior to the root of the inferior mesenteric artery.

The **intermesenteric plexus** is part of the aortic plexus of nerves between the superior and the inferior mesenteric arteries. It gives rise to renal, testicular or ovarian, and ureteric plexuses.

The **superior hypogastric plexus** is continuous with the intermesenteric plexus and the inferior mesenteric plexus and lies anterior to the inferior part of the abdominal aorta at its bifurcation (Table 2.12). Right and left **hypogastric nerves** join the superior hypogastric plexus to the inferior hypogastric plexus. The superior hypogastric plexus supplies *ureteric* and *testicular plexuses* and a plexus on each common iliac artery.

The **inferior hypogastric plexus** is formed on each side by a hypogastric nerve from the superior hypogastric plexus. The right and left plexuses are situated on the sides of the rectum, uterine cervix, and urinary bladder. The plexuses receive small branches from the superior sacral sympathetic ganglia and the sacral parasympathetic outflow from S2 through S4 sacral spinal nerves (*pelvic [parasympathetic] splanchnic nerves*). Extensions of the inferior hypogastric plexus send autonomic fibers along the blood vessels, which form visceral plexuses on the walls of the pelvic viscera (e.g., the *rectal* and *vesical plexuses*).

THE BOTTOM LINE: Presynaptic sympathetic nerve fibers involved in innervating abdominal viscera arise from cell bodies in the lower two thirds of the IML, (T5–T6 to L2–L3 spinal cord levels) and travel via spinal nerves, anterior rami, and white communicating branches to the sympathetic trunks. The fibers traverse the paravertebral ganglia of the trunks without synapsing, continuing as components of abdominopelvic splanchnic nerves. These nerves convey them to the abdominal aortic plexus, where they are joined by presynaptic parasympathetic fibers delivered by the vagus nerve. The sympathetic fibers pass to prevertebral ganglia, most of which are clustered around the major branches of the abdominal aorta. After synapsing within the ganglia, the postsynaptic sympathetic fibers join the presynaptic parasympathetic fibers, traveling via periarterial plexuses around the branches of the abdominal aorta to reach the viscera. A continuation of the abdominal aortic plexus inferior to the aortic bifurcation (the superior and inferior hypogastric plexuses) convey sympathetic innervation to most of the pelvic viscera. The sympathetic fibers mainly innervate the blood vessels of abdominal viscera and are inhibitory to the parasympathetic stimulation. The parasympathetic fibers synapse on or in the walls of the viscera with intrinsic postsynaptic parasympathetic neurons, which terminate on the smooth muscle or glands of the viscera.

The vagus nerve supplies parasympathetic fibers to the alimentary tract from the esophagus through the transverse colon. Pelvic splanchnic nerves supply the descending and sigmoid colon and rectum. Parasympathetic stimulation promotes peristalsis and secretion (although much of the latter is usually hormonally regulated). Visceral afferent fibers follow the autonomic fibers retrograde to sensory ganglia. Afferent fibers conveying pain sensation from abdominal viscera orad to the middle of the sigmoid colon run with the sympathetic fibers to thoracolumbar spinal sensory ganglia; all other visceral afferent fibers run with the parasympathetic fibers. Thus visceral afferent fibers conveying reflex information from the gut orad to the middle of the sigmoid colon pass to vagal sensory ganglia; fibers conveying both pain and reflex information from the gut aborad to the middle of the sigmoid colon pass to spinal sensory ganglia S2–S4.

Diaphragm

The **diaphragm** is a double-domed, musculotendinous partition separating the thoracic and abdominal cavities. Its mainly convex superior surface faces the thoracic cavity, and its concave inferior surface faces the abdominal cavity (Fig. 2.71). The diaphragm is the chief muscle of inspiration (actually, of respiration altogether, because expiration is largely passive). It descends during inspiration; however, only its central part moves because its periphery, as the fixed origin of the muscle, attaches to the inferior margin of the thoracic cage and the superior lumbar vertebrae. The *pericardium,* containing the heart, lies on the central part of the diaphragm, depressing it slightly (Fig. 2.72A). The diaphragm curves superiorly into *right* and *left domes;* normally the right dome is higher than the left owing to the presence of the liver. During expiration, the right dome reaches as high as the 5th rib and the left dome ascends to the 5th intercostal space. The level of the domes of the diaphragm varies according to the:

- Phase of respiration (inspiration or expiration).
- Posture (e.g., supine or standing).
- Size and degree of distension of the abdominal viscera.

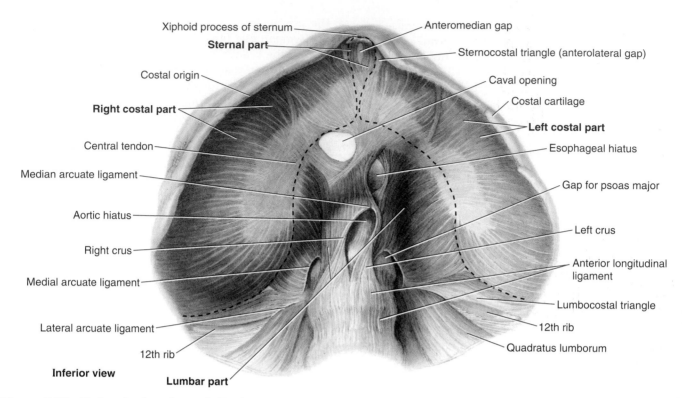

Xiphoid process of sternum
Sternal part
Costal origin
Right costal part
Central tendon
Median arcuate ligament
Aortic hiatus
Right crus
Medial arcuate ligament
Lateral arcuate ligament
12th rib
Inferior view
Lumbar part

Anteromedian gap
Sternocostal triangle (anterolateral gap)
Caval opening
Costal cartilage
Left costal part
Esophageal hiatus
Gap for psoas major
Left crus
Anterior longitudinal ligament
Lumbocostal triangle
12th rib
Quadratus lumborum

Figure 2.71. Abdominal surface of diaphragm and its attachments. The fleshy sternal, costal, and lumbar origins of the diaphragm attach centrally to the trefoil-shaped central tendon, the aponeurotic insertion of the diaphragmatic muscle fibers.

The muscular part of the diaphragm is situated peripherally with fibers that converge radially on the trifoliate central aponeurotic part, the **central tendon** (Fig. 2.71). The central tendon has no bony attachments and is incompletely divided into three leaves, resembling a wide cloverleaf. Although it lies near the center of the diaphragm, the central tendon is closer to the anterior part of the thorax. The *caval opening* (vena caval foramen), through which the terminal part of the IVC passes to enter the heart, perforates the central tendon. The surrounding muscular part of the diaphragm forms a continuous sheet; however, for descriptive purposes it is divided into three parts, based on the peripheral attachments:

- **Sternal part:** consisting of two muscular slips that attach to the posterior aspect of the xiphoid process; this part is not always present.

- **Costal part:** consisting of wide muscular slips that attach to the internal surfaces of the inferior six costal cartilages and their adjoining ribs on each side; the costal parts form the right and left domes.

- **Lumbar part:** arising from two aponeurotic arches, the *medial* and *lateral arcuate ligaments,* and the three superior lumbar vertebrae; the lumbar part forms right and left muscular crura that ascend to the central tendon.

The **crura of the diaphragm** are musculotendinous bundles that arise from the anterior surfaces of the bodies of the supe-

rior three lumbar vertebrae, the anterior longitudinal ligament, and the IV discs. The **right crus,** larger and longer than the left crus, arises from the first three or four lumbar vertebrae. The **left crus** arises from the first two or three. Because it lies to the left of the midline, it is surprising to find that the *esophageal hiatus* is a formation in the right crus; however, if the muscular fibers bounding each side of the hiatus are traced inferiorly, it will be seen that they pass to the right of the aortic hiatus. The right and left crura and the fibrous **median arcuate ligament,** which unites them as it arches over the anterior aspect of the aorta, form the *aortic hiatus.* The diaphragm is also attached on each side to the **medial** and **lateral arcuate ligaments**. These are thickenings of the fascia covering the psoas major (and spanning between lumbar vertebral bodies and the tip of the transverse process of L1) and the quadratus lumborum muscles (continuing from the L12 transverse process to the tip of the 12th rib), respectively. The superior aspect of the central tendon of the diaphragm (the thin, strong aponeurotic tendon of all the muscular fibers of the diaphragm) is fused with the inferior surface of the fibrous pericardium, the strong, external part of the fibroserous *pericardial sac* that encloses the heart.

Vessels and Nerves of the Diaphragm

The arteries of the diaphragm form a branch-like pattern on both its superior and inferior surfaces. The arteries supplying

(A) Arteries and veins of superior surface of diaphragm, posterior view

Labels (A):
Right and left internal thoracic arteries
Right internal thoracic vein
Pericardiacophrenic artery and vein
Thoracic aorta
Internal thoracic artery and vein
Heart inside pericardium
Superior phrenic artery
Right and left domes of diaphragm
Right and left superior epigastric arteries and veins
Right and left musculophrenic arteries and veins

(B) Arteries and veins of inferior surface of diaphragm, anterior view

Labels (B):
Superior phrenic arteries
Inferior vena cava
Thoracic aorta
Left inferior phrenic artery and vein
Suprarenal artery and vein
Abdominal aorta

Figure 2.72. Blood vessels of diaphragm. A. The arteries and veins of the superior surface of the diaphragm are derived from the pericardiacophrenic and musculophrenic arteries and veins (branches of the internal thoracic artery and vein) and from the superior phrenic arteries. **B.** The inferior phrenic arteries and veins supply and drain blood from the inferior surface of the diaphragm. The inferior phrenic arteries are usually the first branches of the abdominal aorta, but they may arise as branches of the celiac trunk. The right inferior phrenic vein drains to the IVC; the left inferior phrenic vein is often double, with one (anterior) branch ending in the IVC and the other (posterior) branch ending in the left renal or suprarenal vein. The two veins may anastomose with each other, as shown here.

the superior surface of the diaphragm (Fig. 2.72; Table 2.13) are the **pericardiacophrenic** and **musculophrenic arteries,** branches of the internal thoracic artery, and the **superior phrenic arteries,** arising from the thoracic aorta. The arteries supplying the inferior surface of the diaphragm are the **inferior phrenic arteries,** which typically are the first branches of the *abdominal aorta;* however, they may arise from the celiac trunk.

The veins draining the superior surface of the diaphragm are the **pericardiacophrenic** and **musculophrenic veins,** which empty into the *internal thoracic veins* and, on the right side, a **superior phrenic vein,** which drains into the IVC. Some veins from the posterior curvature of the diaphragm drain into the *azygos and hemiazygos veins* (see Chapter 1). The inferior phrenic veins drain blood from the inferior surface of the diaphragm. The **right inferior phrenic vein** usually opens into the IVC, whereas the **left inferior phrenic vein** is usually double, with one branch passing anterior to the esophageal hiatus to end in the IVC and the other, more posterior branch usually joining the left suprarenal vein.

The lymphatic plexuses on the thoracic and abdominal surfaces of the diaphragm communicate freely (Fig. 2.73*A*). The **anterior** and **posterior diaphragmatic lymph nodes** are on the thoracic surface of the diaphragm. Lymph from these nodes drains into the *parasternal, posterior mediastinal,* and *phrenic lymph nodes.* Lymphatic vessels from the abdominal surface of the diaphragm drain into the anterior diaphragmatic, phrenic, and superior *lumbar (caval/aortic) lymph nodes.* Lymphatic capillaries are dense on the inferior surface of the diaphragm, constituting the primary means for absorption of peritoneal fluid and substances introduced by I.P. injection.

The entire motor supply to the diaphragm is from the **right** and **left phrenic nerves,** each of which arises from the anterior rami of C3–C5 segments of the spinal cord and is distributed to ipsilateral half of the diaphragm from its inferior surface (Fig. 2.73*B*). The phrenic nerves also supply sensory fibers (pain and proprioception) to most of the diaphragm. Peripheral parts of the diaphragm receive their sensory nerve supply from the **intercostal nerves** (lower six or seven) and the **subcostal nerves.**

Table 2.13. Neurovascular Structures of the Diaphragm

Vessels and Nerves	Superior Surface of Diaphragm	Inferior Surface of Diaphragm
Arterial supply	Superior phrenic arteries from thoracic aorta Musculophrenic and pericardiophrenic arteries from internal thoracic arteries	Inferior phrenic arteries from abdominal aorta
Venous drainage	Musculophrenic and pericardiacophrenic veins drain into internal thoracic veins; superior phrenic vein (right side) drains into IVC	Inferior phrenic veins; right vein drains into IVC; left vein is doubled and drains into IVC and suprarenal vein
Lymphatic drainage	Diaphragmatic lymph nodes to phrenic nodes, then to parasternal and posterior mediastinal nodes	Superior lumbar lymph nodes; lymphatic plexuses on superior and inferior surfaces communicate freely
Innervation	Motor supply: phrenic nerves (C3–C5) Sensory supply: centrally by phrenic nerves (C3–C5), peripherally by intercostal nerves (T5–T11), and subcostal nerves (T12)	

Hiccups

Hiccups (hiccoughs) are involuntary, spasmodic contractions of the diaphragm, causing sudden inhalations that are rapidly interrupted by spasmodic closure of the glottis (aperture of the larynx) which checks the inflow of air and produces a characteristic sound. Hiccups result from irritation of afferent or efferent nerve endings or of medullary centers in the brainstem that control the muscles of respiration, particularly the diaphragm. Hiccups have many causes, such as indigestion, diaphragm irritation, alcoholism, cerebral lesions, and thoracic and abdominal lesions, all which disturb the phrenic nerves. ⊕

Diaphragmatic Apertures

The **diaphragmatic apertures** (openings, hiatuses) permit structures (vessels, nerves, and lymphatics) to pass between the thorax and the abdomen (Figs. 2.71, 2.72, and 2.74). There are three large apertures for the IVC, esophagus, and aorta and a number of small ones.

Caval Opening
The **caval opening** (vena caval aperture) is an opening in the central tendon primarily for the IVC. Also passing through the caval opening are terminal branches of the right phrenic nerve and a few lymphatic vessels on their way from the liver to the middle phrenic and mediastinal lymph nodes. The caval opening is located to the right of the median plane at the junction of the tendon's right and middle leaves. The most superior of the three large diaphragmatic apertures, the caval opening lies at the level of the IV disc between the T8 and T9 vertebrae. The IVC is adherent to the margin of the opening; consequently, when the diaphragm contracts during inspiration, it widens the opening and dilates the IVC.

These changes facilitate blood flow through this large vein to the heart.

Esophageal Hiatus
The **esophageal hiatus** (aperture) is an oval opening for the esophagus in the muscle of the right crus of the diaphragm at the level of the T10 vertebra. The esophageal hiatus also transmits the anterior and posterior vagal trunks, esophageal branches of the left gastric vessels, and a few lymphatic vessels. The fibers of the right crus of the diaphragm decussate (cross one another) inferior to the hiatus, forming a muscular sphincter for the esophagus that constricts it when the diaphragm contracts. The esophageal hiatus is superior to and to the left of the aortic hiatus. In most individuals (70%), both margins of the hiatus are formed by muscular bundles of the right crus. In others (30%), a superficial muscular bundle from the left crus contributes to the formation of the right margin of the hiatus.

Aortic Hiatus
The **aortic hiatus** (aperture) is the opening posterior to the diaphragm for the aorta. Because the aorta does not pierce the diaphragm, movements of the diaphragm do not affect blood flow through it during respiration. The aorta passes between the crura of the diaphragm posterior to the median arcuate ligament, which is at the level of the inferior border of the T12 vertebra. The aortic hiatus also transmits the thoracic duct and sometimes the azygos and hemiazygos veins.

Small Apertures in the Diaphragm
In addition to the three main apertures, there is a small opening, the **sternocostal triangle** (**foramen**), between the sternal and the costal attachments of the diaphragm. This triangle transmits lymphatic vessels from the diaphragmatic surface of the liver and the superior epigastric vessels. The sympathetic trunks pass deep to the medial arcuate ligament, accompanied by the least splanchnic nerves. There are two small apertures in each crus of the diaphragm; one transmits the greater splanchnic nerve and the other the lesser splanchnic nerve.

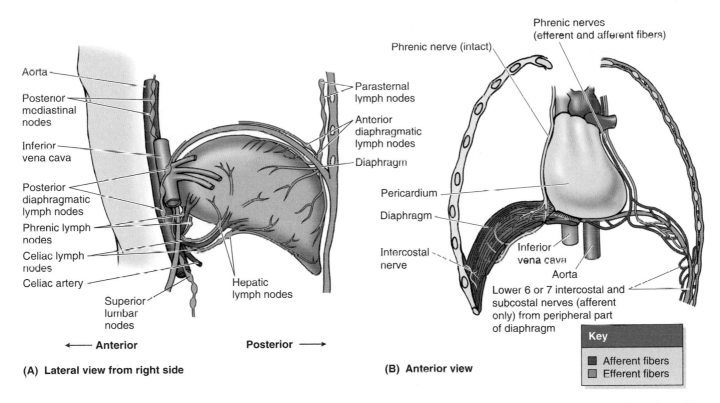

(A) Lateral view from right side

(B) Anterior view

Figure 2.73. Lymphatics and nerves of diaphragm. A. Lymphatics are formed in two plexuses, one on the thoracic surface of the diaphragm and the other on its abdominal surface; they communicate freely. Lymph from the thoracic surface of the diaphragm passes to the anterior and posterior diaphragmatic nodes; the anterior drainage continues to the parasternal lymph nodes, and posterior drainage passes to phrenic and posterior mediastinal nodes. Lymph drainage from the abdominal surface of the diaphragm drains into anterior diaphragmatic, phrenic, and superior lumbar (caval/aortic) nodes. **B.** Each phrenic nerve (from spinal nerves C3–C5) is the sole motor nerve to the ipsilateral half of the diaphragm; it also carries sensory fibers to the central part of that half, including the pleura superiorly and the peritoneum inferiorly. The lower six or seven intercostal and subcostal nerves carry sensory fibers from the peripheral part of the diaphragm.

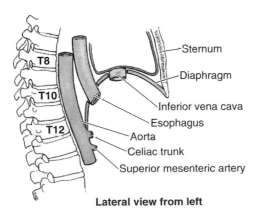

Lateral view from left

Figure 2.74. Apertures of diaphragm. There are three large apertures in the diaphragm for major structures to pass to and from the thorax into the abdomen. The caval opening for the IVC, most anterior, is at the T8 level and to the right of the midline; the esophageal hiatus, intermediate, is at T10 and to the left of the midline; the aortic hiatus for the aorta passes posterior to the vertebral attachment of the diaphragm in the midline at T12 (see also Fig. 2.71).

Actions of the Diaphragm

When the diaphragm contracts, its domes are pulled inferiorly so that the convexity of the diaphragm is somewhat flattened. Although this movement is often described as the "descent of the diaphragm," only the domes of the diaphragm descend. Its periphery remains attached to the ribs and cartilages of the inferior six ribs. As the diaphragm descends, it pushes the abdominal viscera inferiorly. This increases the volume of the thoracic cavity and decreases the intrathoracic pressure, resulting in air being taken into the lungs. In addition, the volume of the abdominal cavity decreases slightly and intra-abdominal pressure increases somewhat. Movements of the diaphragm are also important in circulation because the increased intra-abdominal pressure and decreased intrathoracic pressure help return venous blood to the heart. When the diaphragm contracts, compressing the abdominal viscera, blood in the IVC is forced superiorly into the heart.

The diaphragm is at its most superior level when a person is supine (with the upper body lowered, the *Trendelenburg position).* In this position, the abdominal viscera push the diaphragm superiorly in the thoracic cavity. When a person lies on one side, the hemidiaphragm rises to a more superior level because of the greater push of the viscera on that side. Conversely, the diaphragm assumes an inferior level when a person is sitting or standing. For this reason, people with *dyspnea* (difficult breathing) prefer to sit up, not lie down; non-tidal (reserve) lung volume is increased, and the diaphragm is working with gravity rather than opposing it).

Section of a Phrenic Nerve

Section of a phrenic nerve in the neck results in complete paralysis and eventual atrophy of the muscular part of the corresponding half of the diaphragm, except in persons who have an accessory phrenic nerve (see Chapter 8). *Paralysis of a hemidiaphragm* can be recognized radiographically by its permanent elevation and paradoxical movement (Fig. B2.27). Instead of descending on inspiration, it is forced superiorly by the increased intra-abdominal pressure secondary to descent of the opposite unparalyzed hemidiaphragm.

Referred Pain from the Diaphragm

Pain from the diaphragm radiates to two different areas because of the difference in the sensory nerve supply of the diaphragm (Table 2.12). Pain resulting from irritation of the diaphragmatic pleura or the diaphragmatic peritoneum is referred to the shoulder region, the area of skin supplied by the C3–C5 segments of the spinal cord (see clinical correlation [blue] box "Visceral Referred Pain," in this chapter). These segments also contribute anterior rami to the phrenic nerves. Irritation of peripheral regions of the diaphragm, innervated by the inferior intercostal nerves, is more localized, being referred to the skin over the costal margins of the anterolateral abdominal wall.

Rupture of the Diaphragm and Herniation of Viscera

Rupture of the diaphragm and herniation of viscera can result from a sudden large increase in either the intrathoracic or intra-abdominal pressure. The common cause of this injury is severe trauma to the thorax or abdomen during a motor vehicle accident. Most diaphragmatic ruptures are on the left side (95%) because the right side of the diaphragm receives reinforcement from its close association with the liver. A non-muscular area of variable size called the *lumbocostal triangle* usually occurs between the costal and the lumbar parts of the diaphragm (Figs. 2.71 and 2.75B). This part of the diaphragm is normally formed only by fusion of the superior and inferior fascias of the diaphragm. When a *traumatic diaphragmatic hernia* occurs, the stomach, small intestine and mesentery, transverse colon, and spleen may herniate through this area into the thorax. *Hiatal or hiatus hernia,* a protrusion of part of the stomach into the thorax through the esophageal hiatus, was discussed earlier in this chapter. The structures that pass through the esophageal hiatus (vagal trunks, left inferior phrenic vessels, esophageal branches of the left gastric vessels) may be injured in surgical procedures on the esophageal hiatus (e.g., repair of a hiatus hernia).

Congenital Diaphragmatic Hernia

Posterolateral defect of the diaphragm is the only relatively common congenital anomaly of the diaphragm (Moore and Persaud, 2003). Herniation almost always occurs on the left owing to the presence of the liver on the right. This defect occurs approximately once in 2200 newborn infants and is associated with *congenital diaphragmatic hernia* (prenatal herniation of abdominal contents into the thoracic cavity). Life-threatening breathing difficulties may be associated with this anomaly because of the compromised space available for the development and inflation of lungs. ☉

Normal inspiration   **Paralysis of right hemidiaphragm**

Resting
Normal inspiration
Paralyzed inspiration

■ Inspiration   ■ Resting (normal expiration)

Figure B2.27.

THE BOTTOM LINE: The diaphragm is the double-domed, musculotendinous partition separating the thoracic and abdominal cavities and is the chief muscle of inspiration. Its muscular portion arises from the ring-like inferior thoracic aperture from which the diaphragm rises steeply, invaginating the thoracic cage and forming a common central tendon. The right dome (higher because of the underlying liver) rises nearly to the level of the nipple, whereas the left dome is slightly lower. The central portion is slightly depressed by the heart within the pericardium and is fused to the mediastinal surface of the central tendon. In the neutral respiratory position, the central tendon lies at the level of the T8–T9 IV disc and the xiphisternal joint. When stimulated by the phrenic nerves, the domes are pulled downward (descend), compressing the abdominal viscera. When stimulation ceases and the diaphragm relaxes, the diaphragm is pushed upward (ascends) by the combined decompression of the viscera and tonus of the muscles of the anterolateral abdominal wall. The diaphragm is perforated by the IVC and phrenic nerves at the T8 vertebral level. The fibers of the right crus form a sphincteric hiatus for the esophagus at the T10 vertebral level. The descending aorta and thoracic duct pass posterior to the diaphragm at the T12 vertebral level, in the midline between the crura, overlapped by the median arcuate ligament connecting them. Superior and inferior phrenic arteries and veins supply most of the diaphragm, with additional drainage occurring via the musculophrenic and azygos/hemiazygos veins. In addition to exclusive motor innervation, the phrenic nerves supply most of the pleura and peritoneum covering the diaphragm. Peripheral parts of the diaphragm receive sensory innervation from the lower intercostal and subcostal nerves. The left lumbocostal triangle and the esophageal hiatus are potential sites of acquired hernias through the diaphragm. Developmental defects in the left lumbocostal region account for most congenital diaphragmatic hernias.

Posterior Abdominal Wall

The posterior abdominal wall (Figs. 2.75 and 2.76) is mainly composed of the:

- Five lumbar vertebrae and associated IV discs (centrally).

- Posterior abdominal wall muscles, including the psoas, quadratus lumborum, iliacus, transverse abdominal, and oblique muscles (laterally).

- Diaphragm, which contributes to the superior part of the posterior wall.

- Fascia, including the thoracolumbar fascia.

- Lumbar plexus, composed of the anterior rami of lumbar spinal nerves.

- Fat, nerves, vessels (e.g., aorta and IVC), and lymph nodes.

If observing the anatomy of the posterior abdominal wall in only two-dimensional diagrams, such as Figure 2.76B, it would be easy to suppose that it is flat. In observing a dissected cadaver, or a transverse cross section such as that in Figures 2.61B and 2.75, it is apparent that the lumbar vertebral column is a marked central prominence in the posterior wall, creating two paravertebral "gutters" on each side. The deepest (most posterior) part of these gutters is occupied by the kidneys and their surrounding fat. The abdominal aorta lies on the anterior aspect of the anteriorly protruding vertebral column. It is usually surprising to find how close the lower abdominal aorta lies to the anterior abdominal wall in lean individuals (see Fig. B2.28C). Of course, many structures lie anterior to the aorta (SMA, parts of the duodenum, pancreas and left renal vein, etc.) and so these "posterior abdominal structures" may approach the anterior abdominal wall closer than might be expected in thin persons, especially when they are in the supine position.

Fascia of the Posterior Abdominal Wall

The posterior abdominal wall is covered with a continuous layer of endoabdominal fascia that lies between the parietal peritoneum and the muscles (Figs. 2.61B and 2.75). The fascia lining the posterior abdominal wall is continuous with the transversalis fascia that lines the transverse abdominal muscle. It is customary to name the fascia according to the structure it covers.

The **psoas fascia** covering the psoas major (**psoas sheath**) is attached medially to the lumbar vertebrae and pelvic brim (Fig. 2.75). The psoas fascia (sheath) is thickened superiorly to form the *medial arcuate ligament* (Fig. 2.71). The psoas fascia fuses laterally with the *quadratus lumborum* and *thoracolumbar fascias*. Inferior to the iliac crest, the psoas fascia is continuous with the part of the iliac fascia covering the iliacus. The psoas fascia also blends with the fascia covering the quadratus lumborum.

The **thoracolumbar fascia** is an extensive fascial complex attached to the vertebral column medially that, in the lumbar region, has posterior, middle and anterior layers with muscles enclosed between them (Figs. 2.61B and 2.75). It is thin and transparent where it covers the thoracic parts of the deep muscles but is thick and strong in the lumbar region (Fig. 2.75C). The enclosure of the vertical deep back muscles (erector spinae) by the **posterior** and **middle layers of the thoracolumbar fascia** on the posterior aspect of the trunk is comparable to the enclosure of the rectus abdominis by the rectus sheath on the anterior aspect (Fig. 2.75A). This posterior sheath is even more formidable than the rectus sheath, however, because of the thickness of its posterior layer and the central attachment to the lumbar vertebrae, as opposed to the rectus sheaths, which lack bony support where they fuse to each other at the linea alba. The lumbar part of this posterior sheath, extending between the 12th rib and the iliac crest, attaches laterally to the internal oblique and transverse abdominal muscles, as does the rectus sheath. However, in contrast

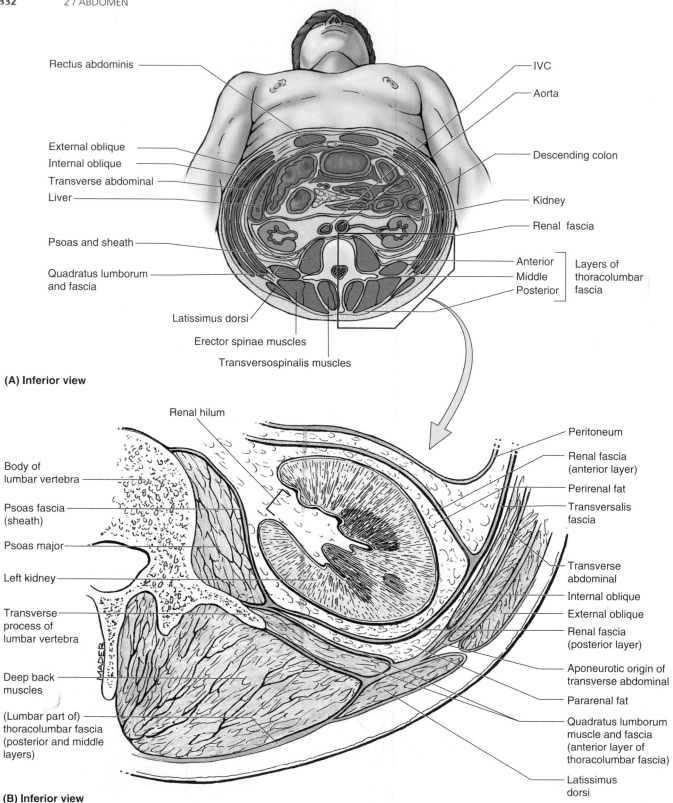

(A) Inferior view

(B) Inferior view

Figure 2.75. Fascia and aponeuroses of the abdominal wall at the level of the renal hilum. A. The relationships of the muscles, aponeurotic muscle sheaths, and fascia of the abdominal wall are demonstrated in transverse section. The three flat abdominal muscles forming the lateral walls span between complex anterior and posterior aponeurotic formations that ensheath vertically disposed muscles. The thin anterolateral walls (appearing disproportionately thick here) are distensible. Although flexible, the posterior abdominal wall is weight bearing and so is reinforced by the vertebral column and muscles that act on it; thus it is not distensible. **B.** Details of the disposition of the aponeurotic and fascial layers of the posterior abdominal wall. For details concerning those of the anterior abdominal wall, see Figure 2.5B. **C.** Dimensional view of the region demonstrated in section in **B.** Note the free posterior border of the external oblique muscle.

(C) Posterolateral view

Figure 2.75. (continued)

to the rectus sheath, the thoracolumbar fascia is not attached to the external oblique; it is attached to the latissimus dorsi (Figs. 2.61*B* and 2.75*C*)

The **anterior layer of the thoracolumbar fascia** (**quadratus lumborum fascia**), covering the quadratus lumborum, a thinner, more transparent layer than the other two layers, attaches to the anterior surfaces of the transverse processes of the lumbar vertebrae, the iliac crest, and the 12th rib. The anterior layer is continuous laterally with the aponeurotic origin of the transverse abdominal muscle (Fig. 2.61*A*). It thickens superiorly to form the *lateral arcuate ligament* and is adherent inferiorly to the **iliolumbar ligaments** (Fig. 2.76).

Muscles of the Posterior Abdominal Wall

The main paired muscles in the posterior abdominal wall (Table 2.14) are the:

- *Psoas major:* passing inferolaterally.

- *Iliacus:* lying along the lateral sides of the inferior part of the psoas major.

- *Quadratus lumborum:* lying adjacent to the transverse processes of the lumbar vertebrae and lateral to superior parts of the psoas major.

The attachments, nerve supply, and main actions of these muscles are summarized in Table 2.14.

Psoas Abscess

Although the prevalence of *tuberculosis* (TB) has been greatly reduced, there is currently a resurgence of TB, especially in Africa and Asia, sometimes in pandemic proportions, owing to AIDS and drug resistance. TB of the vertebral column is quite common. An infection may spread through the blood to the vertebrae (*hematogenous spread*), particularly during childhood. An abscess resulting from tuberculosis in the lumbar region tends to spread from the vertebrae into the psoas sheath, where it produces a *psoas abscess*. As a consequence, the psoas fascia thickens to form a strong stocking-like tube. Pus from the psoas abscess passes inferiorly along the psoas muscle within this fascial tube over the pelvic brim and deep to the inguinal ligament. The pus usually surfaces in the superior part of the thigh. Pus can also reach the psoas sheath by passing from the posterior mediastinum when the thoracic vertebrae are diseased.

The inferior part of the *iliac fascia* is often tense and raises a fold that passes to the internal aspect of the iliac crest. The superior part of this fascia is loose and may form a pocket, the *iliacosubfascial fossa,* posterior to the above-mentioned fold. Part of the large intestine, such as the cecum and/or appendix on the right side and the sigmoid colon on the left side, may become trapped in this fossa, causing considerable pain. ☉

Table 2.14. Muscles of Posterior Abdominal Wall

Anterior view

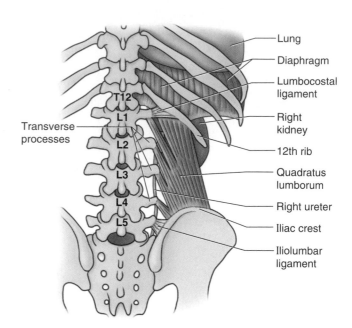

Posterior view

Muscle	Superior Attachment	Inferior Attachment	Innervation	Main Action
Psoas major	Transverse processes of lumbar vertebrae; sides of bodies of T12–L5 vertebrae and intervening intervertebral discs	By a strong tendon to lesser trochanter of femur	Lumbar plexus via anterior branches of L2–L4 nerves	Acting inferiorly with iliacus, it flexes thigh; acting superiorly it flexes vertebral column laterally; it is used to balance the trunk; when sitting it acts inferiorly with iliacus to flex trunk
Iliacus	Superior two thirds of iliac fossa, ala of sacrum, and anterior sacroiliac ligaments	Lesser trochanter of femur and shaft inferior to it, and to psoas major tendon	Femoral nerve (L2–L4)	Flexes thigh and stabilizes hip joint; acts with psoas major
Quadratus lumborum	Medial half of inferior border of 12th ribs and tips of lumbar transverse processes	Iliolumbar ligament and internal lip of iliac crest	Anterior branches of T12 and L1–L4 nerves	Extends and laterally flexes vertebral column; fixes 12th rib during inspiration

Psoas Major

The long, thick, fusiform **psoas major** lies lateral to the lumbar vertebrae (Fig. 2.76). *Psoas* is a Greek word meaning "muscle of the loin." (Butchers refer to the psoas of animals as the *tenderloin.*) The psoas passes inferolaterally, deep to the inguinal ligament to reach the lesser trochanter of the femur (see Chapter 4). The lumbar plexus of nerves is embedded in the posterior part of the psoas, anterior to the lumbar transverse processes.

Iliacus

The **iliacus** is a large triangular muscle that lies along the lateral side of the inferior part of the psoas major. This muscle extends across the sacroiliac joint and attaches to the superior two thirds of the iliac fossa. Most of its fibers join the tendon of the psoas major. Together the psoas and iliacus form the **iliopsoas,** the chief flexor of the thigh. It is also a stabilizer of the hip joint and helps maintain the erect posture at this joint. The psoas and iliacus share in hip flexion; however, only the psoas can produce movement (flexion or lateral bending) of the lumbar spine.

Quadratus Lumborum

The quadrilateral **quadratus lumborum** forms a thick muscular sheet in the posterior abdominal wall (Figs. 2.75 and 2.76). It lies adjacent to the lumbar transverse processes and is broader inferiorly. Close to the 12th rib, the *lateral arcuate ligament* crosses the quadratus lumborum. The *subcostal nerve* passes posterior to this ligament and runs inferolaterally on the quadratus lumborum. Branches of the *lumbar nerve plexus* run inferiorly on the anterior surface of this muscle.

Posterior Abdominal Pain

The iliopsoas has extensive and clinically important relations to the kidneys, ureters, cecum, appendix, sigmoid colon, pancreas, lumbar lymph nodes, and nerves of the posterior abdominal wall. When any of these structures is diseased, movement of the iliopsoas usually causes pain. When intra-abdominal inflammation is suspected, the *iliopsoas test* is performed. The person is asked to lie on the unaffected side and to extend the thigh on the affected side against the resistance of the examiner's hand (Bickley and Szilagyi, 2003). The elicitation of pain with this maneuver is a *positive psoas sign.* An acutely inflamed appendix, for example, will produce a *positive right psoas sign.* Because the psoas lies along the vertebral column and the iliacus crosses the sacroiliac joint, disease of the intervertebral and sacroiliac joints may cause *spasm of the iliopsoas,* a protective reflex. *Adenocarcinoma of the pancreas* in advanced stages invades the muscles and nerves of the posterior abdominal wall, producing excruciating pain because of the close relationship of the pancreas to the posterior abdominal wall. ☉

THE BOTTOM LINE: Large, complex aponeurotic formations cover the central parts of the trunk both anteriorly and posteriorly, forming dense sheaths centrally that house vertical muscles and attach laterally to the flat muscles of the anterolateral abdominal wall. The thoracolumbar fascia is the posterior aponeurotic formation. In addition to ensheathing the erector spinae between its posterior and middle layers, it encloses the quadratus lumborum between its middle and anterior layers. The anterior layer, part of the endoabdominal fascia, is continuous medially with the psoas fascia (enclosing the psoas) and laterally with the transversalis fascia (lining the transverse abdominal). The tube-like psoas fascia provides a potential pathway for the spread of infections between the vertebral column and hip joint. The endoabdominal fascia covering the anterior aspects of both the quadratus lumborum and psoas is thickened over the superiormost aspects of the muscles, forming the lateral and medial arcuate ligaments, respectively. A highly variable layer of extraperitoneal fat intervenes between the endoabdominal fascia and the peritoneum. It is especially thick in the paravertebral gutters of the lumbar region, comprising the paranephric fat (pararenal fat body).

Nerves of the Posterior Abdominal Wall

Components of both the somatic and the autonomic (visceral) nervous systems are associated with the posterior abdominal wall.

The *subcostal nerves* (anterior rami of T12) arise in the thorax, pass posterior to the lateral arcuate ligaments into the abdomen, and run inferolaterally on the anterior surface of the quadratus lumborum (Fig. 2.76). They pass through the transverse abdominal and internal oblique muscles to supply the external oblique and skin of the anterolateral abdominal wall.

The **lumbar spinal nerves** (L1–L5) pass from the spinal cord through the IV foramina inferior to the corresponding vertebrae, where they divide into posterior and anterior rami. Each ramus contains sensory and motor fibers. The posterior rami pass posteriorly to supply the muscles of the back and overlying skin, whereas the anterior rami pass laterally and inferiorly, to supply the skin and muscles of the inferiormost trunk and lower limb. The initial portions of the anterior rami of the L1, L2, and occasionally L3 spinal nerves give rise to *white communicating branches* (L. *rami communicantes*), which convey presynaptic sympathetic fibers to the lumbar sympathetic trunks.

The *abdominal part of the sympathetic trunks* (*lumbar sympathetic trunks*), consisting of four lumbar *paravertebral sympathetic ganglia* and the *interganglionic branches* that connect them, are continuous with the thoracic part of the trunks deep to the medial arcuate ligaments of the diaphragm. The lumbar trunks descend on the anterolateral aspects of the bodies of the lumbar vertebrae in a groove formed by the adjacent psoas major. Inferiorly, they cross the sacral promontory and continue inferiorly into the pelvis as the sacral part of the trunks. For the innervation of the abdominal wall and lower limbs, synapses between the presynaptic and postsynaptic fibers occur in the sympathetic trunks. Postsynaptic sympathetic fibers travel from the lateral aspect of the trunks via *gray communicating branches* to the anterior rami. They become the thoracoabdominal and subcostal nerves, and the lumbar plexus (somatic nerves) that stimulate vasomotion, sudomotion and pilomotion in the lowermost trunk and lower limb. *Lumbar splanchnic nerves* arising from the medial aspect of the lumbar sympathetic trunks convey presynaptic sympathetic fibers for the innervation of pelvic viscera.

The **lumbar plexus of nerves** is formed anterior to the lumbar transverse processes, within the proximal attachment of the psoas major. This nerve network is composed of the anterior rami of L1 through L4 nerves. The following nerves are branches of the lumbar plexus; the three largest are listed first:

- The **femoral nerve** (L2–L4) emerges from the lateral border of the psoas major and innervates the iliacus and passes deep to the inguinal ligament/iliopubic tract to the anterior thigh, supplying the flexors of the hip and extensors of the knee.

- The **obturator nerve** (L2–L4) emerges from the medial border of the psoas major and passes into the lesser pelvis, passing inferior to the superior pubic ramus (through the obturator foramen) to the medial thigh, supplying the adductor muscles.

- The **lumbosacral trunk** (L4, L5) passes over the ala (wing) of the sacrum and descends into the pelvis to participate in the formation of the sacral plexus with the anterior rami of S1–S4 nerves.

- The **ilioinguinal** and **iliohypogastric nerves** (L1) arise from the anterior ramus of L1, entering the abdomen posterior to the medial arcuate ligament and passing inferolaterally, anterior to the quadratus lumborum. They run superior and parallel to the iliac crest, piercing the transverse abdominal near the ASIS. They then pass through the internal and external obliques to supply the abdominal muscles and skin of the inguinal and pubic regions. The division of the L1 anterior ramus may occur as far distally as the ASIS, so that often only one nerve (L1) crosses the posterior abdominal wall instead of two.

- The **genitofemoral nerve** (L1, L2) pierces the psoas major and runs inferiorly on its anterior surface, deep to the psoas

fascia; it divides lateral to the common and external iliac arteries into femoral and genital branches.

- The **lateral cutaneous nerve of the thigh,** or lateral femoral cutaneous nerve (L2, L3) runs inferolaterally on the iliacus and enters the thigh deep to the inguinal ligament/iliopubic tract, just medial to the ASIS; it supplies skin on the anterolateral surface of the thigh.

- An **accessory obturator nerve** (L3, L4) is present almost 10% of the time. It parallels the medial border of the psoas, anterior to the obturator nerve, crossing superior to the superior pubic ramus in close proximity to the femoral vein.

Although the larger branches (femoral, obturator, and lumbosacral trunk) are consistent in their placement, variation should be anticipated in the disposition of the smaller branches of the lumbar plexus.

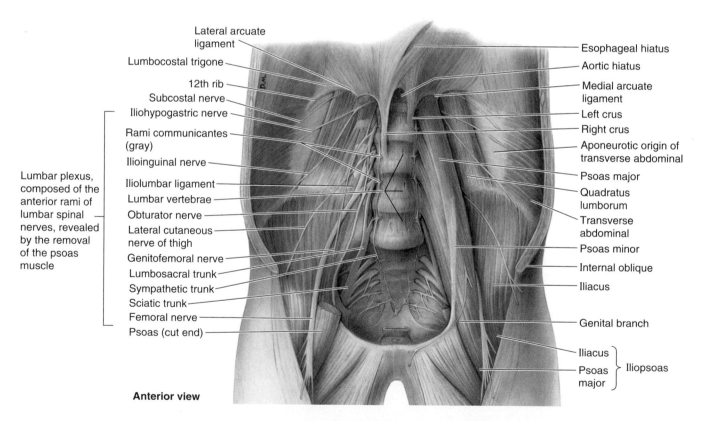

Anterior view

Figure 2.76. Muscles and nerves of posterior abdominal wall. Most of the right psoas major has been removed to show that the lumbar plexus of nerves is formed by the anterior rami of the first four lumbar spinal nerves, and that it lies in the substance of the psoas major.

Partial Lumbar Sympathectomy

The treatment of some patients with arterial disease in the lower limbs may include a **partial lumbar sympathectomy**, the surgical removal of two or more lumbar sympathetic ganglia by division of their rami communicantes. Surgical access to the sympathetic trunks is commonly through a lateral extraperitoneal approach because the sympathetic trunks lie retroperitoneally in the extraperitoneal fatty tissue (Fig. 2.76*B*). The surgeon splits the muscles of the anterior abdominal wall and moves the peritoneum medially and anteriorly to expose the medial edge of the psoas major, along which the sympathetic trunk lies. The left trunk is often overlapped slightly by the aorta. The right sympathetic trunk is covered by the IVC. The intimate relationship of the sympathetic trunks to the aorta and IVC also makes these large vessels vulnerable to injury during lumbar sympathectomy. Consequently, the surgeon carefully retracts them to expose the sympathetic trunks that usually lie in the groove between the psoas major laterally and the lumbar vertebral bodies medially. These trunks are often obscured by fat and lymphatic tissue. Knowing that identification of the sympathetic trunks is not easy, great care is taken not to remove inadvertently part of the genitofemoral nerve, lumbar lymphatics, or ureter. ✪

THE BOTTOM LINE: The lumbar sympathetic trunks deliver postsynaptic sympathetic fibers to the lumbar plexus for distribution with somatic nerves, and presynaptic parasympathetic fibers to the abdominal aortic plexus, the latter ultimately innervating pelvic viscera. With the exception of the subcostal nerve (T12) and lumbosacral trunk (L4–L5), the somatic nerves of the posterior abdominal wall are products of the lumbar plexus, formed by the anterior rami of L1–L4 deep to the psoas. Only the subcostal nerve and the derivatives of the anterior ramus of L1 (iliohypogastric and ilioinguinal nerves) have an abdominal distribution—to the muscles and skin of the inguinal and pubic regions. All other nerves pass to the muscles and skin of the lower limb.

Vessels of the Posterior Abdominal Wall

The major neurovascular bundle of the inferior trunk, including the abdominal aorta, the inferior vena cava, and the aortic periarterial nerve plexus, courses in the midline of the posterior abdominal wall, anterior to the bodies of the lumbar vertebrae (Figs. 2.60 and 2.75).

Abdominal Aorta

Most arteries supplying the posterior abdominal wall arise from the **abdominal aorta** (Table 2.15*A*). The **subcostal arteries** arise from the thoracic aorta and distribute inferior to the 12th rib. The abdominal aorta is approximately 13 cm in length. It begins at the *aortic hiatus* in the diaphragm at the level of the T12 vertebra and ends at the level of the L4 vertebra by dividing into the right and left common iliac arteries. The level of the aortic bifurcation is 2–3 cm inferior and to the left of the umbilicus at the level of the iliac crests. The **common iliac arteries** diverge and run inferolaterally, following the medial border of the psoas muscles to the pelvic brim. Here each common iliac artery divides into the **internal** and **external iliac arteries**. The internal iliac artery enters the pelvis (its course and branches are described in Chapter 3). The external iliac artery follows the iliopsoas muscle. Just before leaving the abdomen, the external iliac artery gives rise to the **inferior epigastric** and **deep circumflex iliac** arteries, which supply the anterolateral abdominal wall.

Relations of the Abdominal Aorta. From superior to inferior, the important anterior relations of the abdominal aorta are the:

- *Celiac plexus* and *ganglion* (Figs. 2.54 and 2.60).
- Body of the *pancreas* and *splenic vein* (Fig. 2.55).
- *Left renal vein* (Figs. 2.66 and 2.72*B*).
- Horizontal part of the *duodenum*.
- Coils of the *small intestine*.

The abdominal aorta descends anterior to the bodies of the T12–L4 vertebrae. The left lumbar veins pass posterior to the aorta to reach the IVC (Fig. 2.77). On the right, the aorta is related to the azygos vein, chyle cistern, thoracic duct, right crus of the diaphragm, and right celiac ganglion. On the left, the aorta is related to the left crus of the diaphragm and the left celiac ganglion.

Branches of the Abdominal Aorta. The branches of the descending (thoracic and abdominal) aorta may be described as arising and coursing in three "vascular planes," and can be classified as being visceral or parietal and paired or unpaired (Table 2.15). *Paired parietal branches* of the aorta serve the diaphragm and posterior abdominal wall.

The **median sacral artery**, an *unpaired parietal branch*, may be said to occupy a fourth (posterior) plane because it arises from the posterior aspect of the aorta just proximal to its bifurcation. Although markedly smaller, it could also be considered a midline "continuation" of the aorta, in which case its lateral branches, the **small lumbar arteries** (L. *arteriae lumbales imae*) and **lateral sacral branches**, would also be included as part of the paired parietal branches.

Pulsations of the Aorta and Abdominal Aortic Aneurysm

Because the aorta lies posterior to the pancreas and stomach, a tumor of these organs may transmit pulsations of the aorta that could be mistaken for an *abdominal aortic aneurysm,* a localized enlargement of the aorta (Fig. B2.28*A* & *B*). Deep palpation of the midabdomen can detect an aneurysm, which usually results from a congenital or acquired weakness of the arterial wall (Fig. B2.28*C* & *D*). Pulsations of a large aneurysm can be detected to the left of the midline; the pulsatile mass can be moved easily from side to side. Medical imaging can confirm the diagnosis in doubtful cases.

Acute rupture of an abdominal aortic aneurysm is associated with severe pain in the abdomen or back. If un-recognized, such an aneurysm has a mortality rate of nearly 90% because of heavy blood loss (Swartz, 2001). Surgeons can repair an aneurysm by opening it, inserting a prosthetic graft (such as one made of Dacron), and sewing the wall of the aneurysmal aorta over the graft to protect it. Many vascular problems formerly treated with open repair, including aneurysm repair, are now being treated by means of endovascular catheterization procedures

When the anterior abdominal wall is relaxed, particularly in children and thin adults, the inferior part of the abdominal aorta may be compressed against the body of the L4 vertebra by firm pressure on the anterior abdominal wall, over the umbilicus (Fig. B2.28*C* & *D*). This pressure may be applied to control bleeding in the pelvis or lower limbs. ✚

Renal arteries

Aorta

Renal veins

Inferior mesenteric artery

Common iliac arteries

(A)

(B)

Anterior views

L4 vertebra   Level of umbilicus

(C) Medial view (from left)

(D) Anterior view

Figure B2.28.

Table 2.15. Branches of the Abdominal Aorta

(A)

(B)

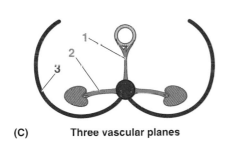

(C)   **Three vascular planes**

	Vascular plane	Class	Distribution	Abdominal Branches (Arteries)	Vertebral Level
1	Anterior midline	Unpaired visceral	Alimentary tract	Celiac	T12
				Superior mesenteric (SMA)	L1
				Inferior mesenteric (IMA)	L3
2	Lateral	Paired visceral	Urogenital and endocrine organs	Suprarenal	L1
				Renal	L1
				Gonadal (testicular or ovarian)	L2
3	Postero-lateral	Paired parietal (segmental)	Diaphragm Body Wall	Subcostal	L2
				Inferior phrenic	T12
				Lumbar	L1–L4

THE BOTTOM LINE: Except for the subcostal arteries, the arteries supplying the posterior abdominal wall arise from the abdominal aorta. The abdominal aorta descends from the aortic hiatus, coursing on the anterior aspects of the T12–L4 vertebra, immediately left of the midline, and bifurcates into the common iliac arteries at the level of the supracristal plane. Branches of the aorta arise and course in three vascular planes: anterior (unpaired visceral branches), lateral (paired visceral branches), and posterolateral (paired parietal). The median sacral may be considered a diminutive continuation of the aorta, which continues to give rise to paired parietal branches.

Veins of the Posterior Abdominal Wall

The veins of the posterior abdominal wall are tributaries of the IVC, except for the *left testicular* or *ovarian vein*, which enters the left renal vein instead of entering the IVC (Fig. 2.77). The IVC, the largest vein in the body, has no valves except for a variable, non-functional one at its orifice in the right atrium of the heart. The IVC returns poorly oxygenated blood from the lower limbs, most of the back, the abdominal walls, and the abdominopelvic viscera. Blood from the abdominal viscera passes through the *portal venous system* and the liver before entering the IVC through the *hepatic veins.*

Surface Anatomy of the Abdominal Aorta

The **abdominal aorta** may be represented on the anterior abdominal wall by a band (approximately 2 cm wide) extending from a median point, approximately 2.5 cm superior to the transpyloric plane to a point slightly inferior to and to the left of the **umbilicus** (Fig. SA2.6). This point indicates the level of bifurcation of the aorta into the common iliac arteries. The site of the aortic bifurcation is also indicated just to the left of the midpoint of a line joining the highest points of the **iliac crests.** This line is helpful when examining obese persons in whom the umbilicus is not a reliable surface landmark. ◐

Transpyloric plane

Highest point of iliac crest

Internal iliac artery

Abdominal aorta

Bifurcation of aorta

Common iliac arteries

External iliac artery

Figure SA2.6.

The IVC begins anterior to the L5 vertebra by the union of the common iliac veins. This union occurs approximately 2.5 cm to the right of the median plane, inferior to the bifurcation of the aorta and posterior to the proximal part of the right common iliac artery (Fig. 2.60). The IVC ascends on the right sides of the bodies of the L3–L5 vertebrae and on the right psoas major to the right of the aorta. The IVC leaves the abdomen by passing through the *caval opening* in the diaphragm to enter the thorax at the T8 vertebral level. Because it is formed one vertebral level inferior to the bifurcation of the aorta, and traverses the diaphragm four vertebral levels superior to the aortic hiatus, the overall length of the IVC is 7 cm greater than that of the abdominal aorta, although most of the additional length is intrahepatic. The IVC collects poorly oxygenated blood from the lower limbs and non-portal blood from the abdomen and pelvis. Almost all the blood from the digestive tract is collected by the portal system and passes through the hepatic veins to the IVC.

The tributaries of the IVC correspond to the paired visceral and parietal branches of the abdominal aorta. The veins that correspond to the unpaired visceral branches of the aorta are instead tributaries of the portal vein. The blood they carry does ultimately enter the IVC via the hepatic veins, after traversing the liver. The branches corresponding to the paired viscera branches of the abdominal aorta include the right suprarenal vein, the right and left renal veins, and the right gonadal (testicular or ovarian) vein. The left suprarenal and gonadal veins drain indirectly into the IVC because they are tributaries of the left renal vein. Paired parietal branches of the IVC include the inferior phrenic veins, the 3rd (L3) and 4th (L4) lumbar veins, and the common iliac veins, formed by union of the external and internal iliac veins. The ascending lumbar and azygos veins connect the IVC and superior vena cava, either directly or indirectly (see Chapter 1).

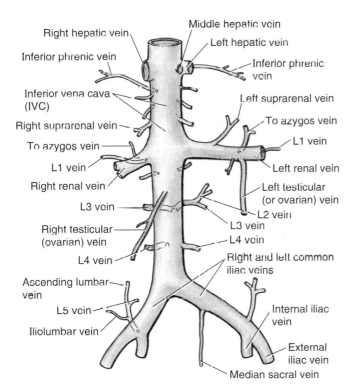

Figure 2.77. Inferior vena cava and its tributaries. The asymmetry in the renal and common iliac veins reflects the placement of the IVC to the right of the midline.

THE BOTTOM LINE: The veins of the posterior abdominal wall are mostly direct tributaries of the IVC, although some enter indirectly via the left renal vein. The IVC is the largest vein and lacks valves. The IVC is formed at the L5 vertebral level by the union of the common iliac veins. It ascends to the T8 vertebral level, passing through the diaphragm and entering the heart almost simultaneously. It drains poorly oxygenated blood from the body inferior to the diaphragm. The IVC receives the drainage of the abdominal viscera indirectly via the portal vein, liver, and hepatic veins. Except for the hepatic veins, the tributaries of the IVC mostly correspond to the lateral paired visceral and posterolateral paired parietal branches of the abdominal aorta. Three collateral routes (two involving the anterior abdominal wall, and one involving the vertebral canal) are available to return blood to the heart when the IVC is obstructed.

Lymphatics of the Posterior Abdominal Wall

Lymphatic vessels and lymph nodes lie along the aorta, IVC, and iliac vessels (Fig. 2.78*A*). The *common iliac lymph nodes* receive lymph from the external and internal iliac lymph nodes. Lymph from the common iliac lymph nodes passes to the right and left *lumbar lymph nodes*. Lymph from the alimentary tract, liver, spleen, and pancreas passes along the celiac and superior and inferior mesenteric arteries to the *preaortic lymph nodes* (*celiac* and *superior* and *inferior mesen*

Collateral Routes for Abdominopelvic Venous Blood

Three collateral routes, formed by valveless veins of the trunk, are available for venous blood to return to the heart when the IVC is obstructed or ligated. Two of these routes (one involving the superior and inferior epigastric veins, and another involving the thoracoepigastric vein) were discussed earlier in this chapter with the anterior abdominal wall. The third collateral route involves the *epidural venous plexus* inside the vertebral column (illustrated and discussed in Chapter 3), which communicates with the *lumbar veins* of the inferior caval system, and the tributaries of the *azygos system of veins*, which is part of the superior caval system.

The inferior part of the IVC has a complicated developmental history because it forms from parts of three sets of embryonic veins (Moore and Persaud, 2003). Therefore, IVC anomalies are relatively common and most of them, such as a *persisting left IVC*, occur inferior to the renal veins (Fig. B2.29). These anomalies result from the persistence of embryonic veins on the left side, which normally disappear. If a left IVC is present, it may cross to the right side at the level of the kidneys. ✪

Figure B2.29.

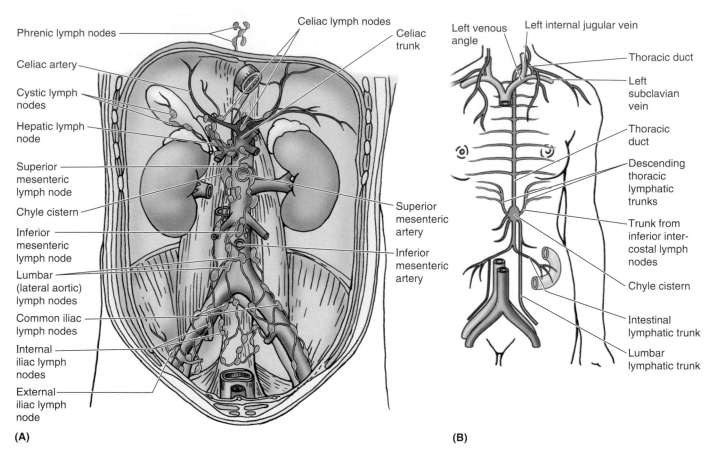

Phrenic lymph nodes

Celiac artery

Cystic lymph nodes

Hepatic lymph node

Superior mesenteric lymph node

Chyle cistern

Inferior mesenteric lymph node

Lumbar (lateral aortic) lymph nodes

Common iliac lymph nodes

Internal iliac lymph nodes

External iliac lymph node

Celiac lymph nodes

Celiac trunk

Superior mesenteric artery

Inferior mesenteric artery

(A)

Left venous angle

Left internal jugular vein

Thoracic duct

Left subclavian vein

Thoracic duct

Descending thoracic lymphatic trunks

Trunk from inferior intercostal lymph nodes

Chyle cistern

Intestinal lymphatic trunk

Lumbar lymphatic trunk

(B)

Figure 2.78. Lymphatic drainage of posterior abdominal wall and lymphatic trunks of abdomen. A. The parietal lymph nodes are shown. The external iliac, common iliac, and lumbar (aortic) lymph nodes lie in a continuous chain along the abdominal aorta and its terminal branches, receiving lymph from the posterior abdominal wall as well as the efferent drainage of lymph nodes of the abdominal viscera and lower limbs. **B.** The abdominal lymphatic trunks are shown. The thoracic duct begins posterior to the aorta at the aortic hiatus as a convergence of lymphatic trunks that may or may not take the form of a chyle cistern. The converging lymphatic trunks include the paired lumbar lymph trunks, the intestinal lymphatic trunk(s), and a pair of descending thoracic lymphatic trunks. All lymphatic drainage from the lower half of the body converges in the abdomen to enter the beginning of the thoracic duct. The thoracic duct conducts it to the convergence of the left internal jugular and subclavian veins (left venous angle) where the lymph enters the venous system.

teric nodes) scattered around the origins of these arteries from the aorta. Efferent vessels from these nodes form the **intestinal lymphatic trunks,** which may be single or multiple, and participate in the confluence of lymphatic trunks that gives rise to the thoracic duct (Fig. 2.78*B*).

The *right* and *left lumbar* (*caval* and *aortic*) *lymph nodes* lie on both sides of the IVC and aorta. These nodes receive lymph directly from the posterior abdominal wall, kidneys, ureters, testes or ovaries, uterus, and uterine tubes. They also receive lymph from the descending colon, pelvis, and lower limbs through the *inferior mesenteric* and **common iliac lymph nodes.** Efferent lymphatic vessels from the large lumbar lymph nodes form the right and left **lumbar lymphatic trunks.**

The inferior end of the **thoracic duct** lies anterior to the bodies of the L1 and L2 vertebrae between the right crus of the diaphragm and the aorta. The thoracic duct begins with the convergence of the main lymphatic ducts of the abdomen, which in only a small proportion of individuals takes the form

of the commonly depicted, thin-walled sac or dilation, the **chyle cistern** (L. *cisterna chyli*) (Fig. 2.78). Chyle cisterns vary greatly in size and shape. More often there is merely a simple or plexiform convergence at this level of the right and left lumbar lymphatic trunks, the intestinal lymph trunk(s), and a pair of **descending thoracic lymphatic trunks,** which carry lymph from the lower six intercostal spaces on each side. Consequently, essentially all the lymphatic drainage from the lower half of the body (deep lymphatic drainage inferior to the level of the diaphragm, and all superficial drainage inferior to the level of the umbilicus) converges in the abdomen to enter the beginning of the thoracic duct. The thoracic duct ascends through the aortic hiatus in the diaphragm into the posterior mediastinum, where it collects more parietal and visceral drainage, particularly from the left upper quadrant of the body. The duct ultimately ends by entering the venous system at the junction of the **left subclavian** and **internal jugular veins** (the **left venous angle**).

THE BOTTOM LINE: Lymphatic drainage from the abdominal viscera courses retrograde along the ramifications of the three unpaired visceral branches of the abdominal aorta. Lymphatic drainage from the abdominal wall merges with that from the lower limbs, both pathways following the arterial supply retrograde from those parts. Ul-

timately, all lymphatic drainage from structures inferior to the diaphragm, plus that draining from the lower six intercostal spaces via the descending thoracic lymphatic trunks, enters the beginning of the thoracic duct at the T12 level, posterior to the aorta. The origin of the thoracic duct may take the form of a saccular chyle cistern.

Medical Imaging of the Abdomen

Radiographs of the abdomen demonstrate abnormal anatomical relationships of organs such as those resulting from tumors. Radiographs also demonstrate gas and calcifications in the intestine. Abnormal intestinal gas patterns indicate a dilated large intestine and intestinal perforation. The anatomy of the esophagus and alimentary tract can be demonstrated radiographically after the swallowing of **barium meal**, a contrast medium composed of a mixture of barium sulfate and water. Examinations of the alimentary tract are performed with fluoroscopic guidance, supplemented by cineradiography or videotape and radiographs. These procedures enable the radiologist to detect abnormalities of the esophagus, stomach, and intestines as well as lesions in adjacent structures that displace these organs. Most early knowledge concerning the shape, position, and movements of the esophagus, stomach, and intestines came from barium studies.

Peristaltic waves in the esophagus appear as ring-like contractions that propel the barium toward the stomach (Fig. 2.79). Once the stomach is distended, circular peristaltic waves begin in the body of the stomach and sweep toward the pyloric canal, where they stop. Gas in the fundus of the stomach is clearly visible superior to the barium shadow (Fig. 2.80A). When the pyloric sphincter opens and closes, the proximal part of the duodenum expands to form the *ampulla* (duodenal cap). The outline of the barium in the superior part of the duodenum is smooth; in other parts, the outline has a feathery appearance because of the circular folds in the duodenum (Fig. 2.80B & C).

To examine the colon, a **barium enema** is given after the bowel is cleared of fecal material by a cleansing enema. Radiographs show the typical *haustra* (Fig. 2.81). The single-contrast examinations of the colon show its various parts; the dilated *rectum* is well illustrated. In chronic stages of *colitis* (inflammation of the colon), the mucosa atrophies and the typical pattern of the haustra disappears. The outline of the haustra is accentuated by the double-contrast method: the patient evacuates the barium and air is injected through the anal canal to distend the colon that is still lined with a thin layer of barium (Fig. 2.81B). MRI can also be used to study the intestines. This imaging procedure is particularly effective after double-contrast radiographic studies when the structures are still distended with air (Fig. 2.81C).

A wide variety of radiographic methods are available for studying the structure and function of the bile passages and

gallbladder clinically, each with its own criteria, advantages, and disadvantages. Radiographic examination of the biliary ducts at the time of surgery (**preoperative cholangiography**) is an important procedure for all patients undergoing *cholecystectomy* to determine the presence and location of stones in the biliary tract, that all calculi have been removed, and that no other obstructions are present (Fig. 2.82A). A tube is implanted directly into the biliary duct system to inject radiopaque dye.

Endoscopic retrograde cholangiopancreatography (ERCP) has become a standard procedure for the diagnosis of both pancreatic and biliary disease (Fig. 2.82B). First, a fiberoptic endoscope is passed through the mouth, esophagus, and stomach. Then the duodenum is entered and a cannula is inserted into the major duodenal papilla and advanced under fluoroscopic control into the duct of ▶

Figure 2.79. Radiograph of esophagus after swallowing barium meal. In this left posterior oblique (LPO) view, note the normal "constrictions" (impressions) caused by the arch of the aorta and left main bronchus. The phrenic ampulla, which is seen only radiographically, is the distensible part of the esophagus, lying just superior to the diaphragm. (Courtesy of Dr. E. L. Lansdown, Professor of Medical Imaging, University of Toronto, Toronto, ON, Canada.)

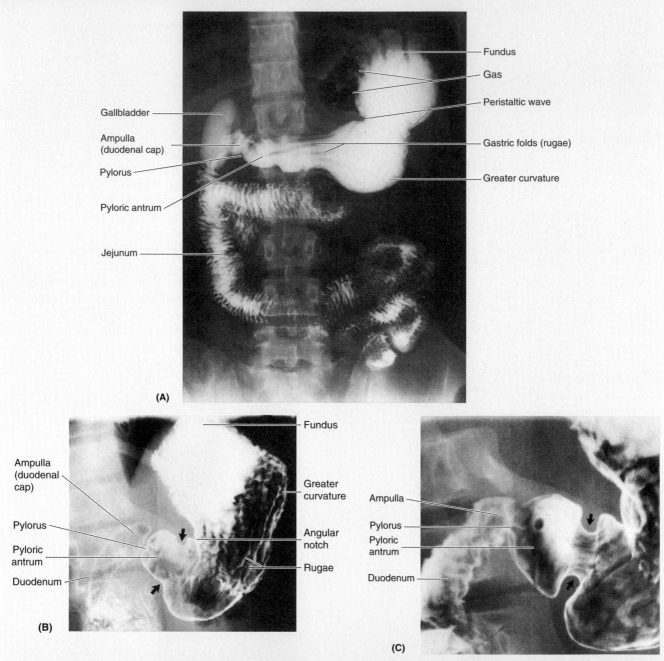

Figure 2.80. Radiographs of stomach, small intestine, and gallbladder. A. Observe the peristaltic wave in the stomach and the longitudinal gastric folds (rugae) of mucous membrane. (A, Courtesy of Dr. J. Helsin, Toronto, ON, Canada.) **B.** The stomach and small intestine were imaged after a barium meal. Observe the peristaltic wave (arrowheads), pylorus, ampulla (duodenal cap), and the feathery appearance of the barium in the small intestine. Also observe the relationship of the gallbladder to the ampulla in the superior part of the duodenum. **C.** This radiograph demonstrates the pyloric region of the stomach and the superior part of the duodenum. (B and C, Courtesy of Dr. E. L. Lansdown, Professor of Medical Imaging, University of Toronto, Toronto, ON, Canada.)

choice (bile duct or pancreatic duct) for injection of radiographic contrast medium. One radiographic method of studying the anatomy and function of the gallbladder has been used for more than 8 decades (Fig. 2.82C). This procedure, **oral or intravenous cholecystography,** is a test of gallbladder function and also demonstrates its location and shape. This procedure has largely been replaced by *ultrasonography* and **cholescintigraphy.** The latter is a dynamic function test, in many ways similar to cholecystography; however, radioactive tracer and marker compounds are used. ▶

(cont'd on page 347)

(A) Anteroposterior view

(B) Anteroposterior view

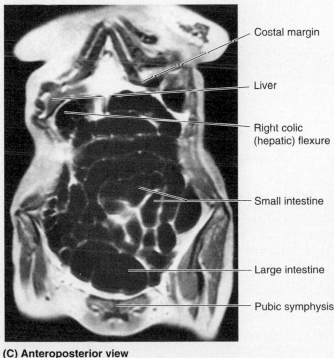

(C) Anteroposterior view

Costal margin

Liver

Right colic
(hepatic) flexure

Small intestine

Large intestine

Pubic symphysis

Figure 2.81. Barium enema examination of colon and MRI study of intestine. A. In this single-contrast study, barium can be seen coating the walls of the colon distended with air, giving a vivid view of the mucosa and haustra. A, ascending colon; C, cecum; D, descending colon; G, sigmoid colon; H, hepatic or right colic flexure; R, rectum; S, splenic or left colic flexure; T, transverse colon; U, haustra. (Courtesy of Dr. C. S. Ho, Professor of Medical Imaging, University of Toronto, Toronto, ON, Canada.) **B.** In this double-contrast study, barium has filled the colon. Observe the level of the right colic flexure. (Courtesy of Dr. E. L. Lansdown, Professor of Medical Imaging, University of Toronto, Toronto, ON, Canada.) **C.** A coronal MRI of the lower thoracic cage and abdomen is shown. (Courtesy of Dr. W. Kucharczyk, Professor and Chair of Medical Imaging, University of Toronto, and Clinical Director of Tri-Hospital Resonance Centre, Toronto, ON, Canada.)

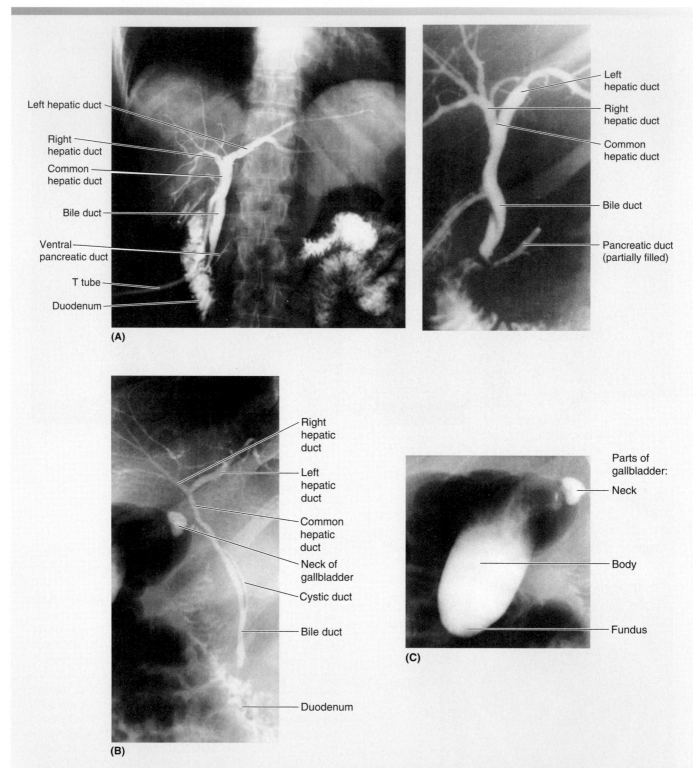

Left hepatic duct

Right hepatic duct

Common hepatic duct

Bile duct

Ventral pancreatic duct

T tube

Duodenum

(A)

Left hepatic duct

Right hepatic duct

Common hepatic duct

Bile duct

Pancreatic duct (partially filled)

Right hepatic duct

Left hepatic duct

Common hepatic duct

Neck of gallbladder

Cystic duct

Bile duct

Duodenum

(B)

Parts of gallbladder:

Neck

Body

Fundus

(C)

Figure 2.82. Radiographs of bile passages and gallbladder. A. After an open-incision cholecystectomy, contrast medium was injected through a T tube inserted into the bile passages. (Courtesy of Dr. J. Helsin, Toronto, ON, Canada.) **B and C.** Endoscopic retrograde cholangiography studies of the gallbladder and bile passages are shown. The cystic duct usually lies on the right side of the common hepatic duct and joins it just superior to the superior part of the duodenum. (Courtesy of Dr. G. B. Haber, Assistant Professor of Medicine, University of Toronto, Toronto, ON, Canada.)

Psoas major

Superior pole of right kidney

Renal pelvis
Major calyx

Dilated segment of abdominal part of ureter

Dilated segment of pelvic part of ureter

12th rib

Minor calyx

Constricted segment of abdominal part of ureter

Crest of ilium

Ilium

Constricted segment of pelvic part of ureter

Urinary bladder

Figure 2.83. Intravenous urogram (pyelogram). The contrast medium was injected intravenously and was concentrated and excreted by the kidneys. This AP projection shows the calices, renal pelves, and ureters outlined by the contrast medium filling their lumina. Note the difference in shape and level of the renal pelves and the constrictions and dilations in the ureter resulting from peristaltic contractions of their smooth muscle walls. The arrows indicate narrowing of the lumen resulting from peristaltic contractions. (Courtesy of Dr. John Campbell, Department of Medical Imaging, Sunnybrook Medical Centre, University of Toronto, Toronto, ON, Canada.)

The radiological anatomy of the kidneys and ureters can be examined by **intravenous urography,** or **pyelography** (Fig. 2.83). The kidneys excrete an intravenously injected contrast medium. In **retrograde pyelography,** the contrast medium is injected into the ureters and ascends to fill the pelves and calices of the kidneys.

Ultrasound, CT scans, and **MRIs** are also used to examine the abdominal viscera (Figs. 2.84–2.88). Because MRIs provide better differentiation between soft tissues, its images are more revealing. An image in virtually any plane can be reconstructed after scanning is completed.

Abdominal arteriography, radiography after the injection of radiopaque material directly into the bloodstream, detects abnormalities of the abdominal arteries, such as blood clots (Fig. 2.89*A*). Angiographic studies may also now be performed using MRA (magnetic resonance angiography) (Fig. 2.89*B* & *C*). **Nuclear scanning** is useful for detection of lower GI hemorrhage. A positive nuclear scan may be followed by arteriography.⊕

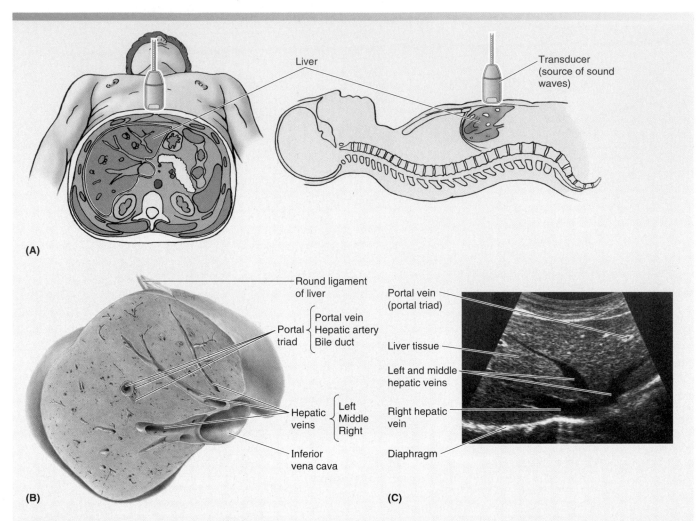

(A)

(B)

(C)

Figure 2.84. Ultrasound scan of abdomen. A. The orientation drawings demonstrate the placement of the transducer on the anterior abdominal wall. The transverse anatomical section **(B)** and ultrasound scan **(C)** of the liver demonstrate the hepatic veins. (Courtesy of Dr. A. M. Arenson, Assistant Professor of Medical Imaging, University of Toronto, Toronto, ON, Canada.)

Ao	Aorta	**LGA**	Left gastric artery
BD	Bile duct	**LRV**	Left renal vein
CA	Celiac artery	**P**	Pancreas
Cr	Crus of diaphragm	**Pu**	Uncinate process of pancreas
CT	Celiac trunk		
D	Duodenum	**PV**	Portal vein
FL	Falciform ligament	**PVC**	Portal venous confluence
GDA	Gastroduodenal artery	**SA**	Splenic artery
GE	Gastroesophageal junction	**SMA**	Superior mesenteric artery
HA	Hepatic artery	**SMV**	Superior mesenteric vein
IVC	Inferior vena cava	**SV**	Splenic vein
L	Liver	**V**	Vertebra

Figure 2.85. Ultrasound scans of abdomen. A. A transverse scan through the celiac trunk is shown. **B.** A transverse scan through the pancreas is shown. **C.** A sagittal scan through the aorta is shown. (Courtesy of Dr. A.M. Arenson, Assistant Professor of Medical Imaging, University of Toronto, Toronto, ON, Canada.)

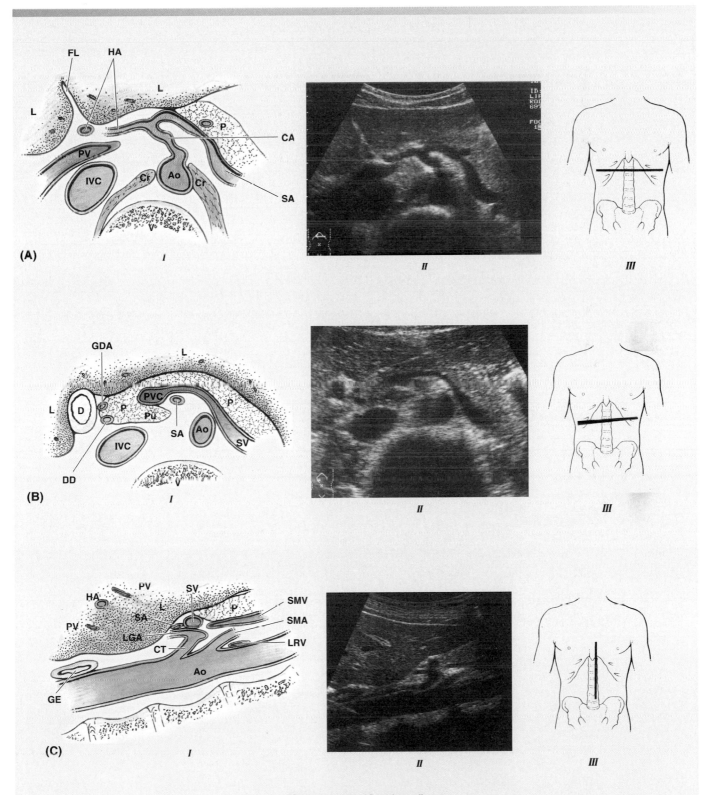

Figure 2.85. *(Continued)*

Figure 2.86. Transverse MRIs of abdomen. (Courtesy of Dr. W. Kucharczyk, Professor and Chair of Medical Imaging, University of Toronto, and Clinical Director of Tri-Hospital Resonance Centre, Toronto, ON, Canada.)

(A)

(B)

(C)

Ao	Aorta
BAo	Bifurcation of aorta
CC	Costal cartilage
CO	Cardiac orifice of stomach
D	Duodenum
DBM	Deep back muscles
F	Fat
FS	Fundus of stomach
GB	Gallbladder
GM	Gluteus medius muscle
I	Intestine
Il	Ilium
IM	Iliacus muscle
IVC	Inferior vena cava
L	Liver
LC	Left crus
LHV	Left hepatic vein
LK	Left kidney
LPC	Left pleural cavity
LRA	Inferior vena cava
LRV	Left renal vein
P	Pancreas
PC	Portal confluence
PF	Perirenal fat
PS	Psoas muscle
PV	Portal vein (triad)
R	Rib
RHV	Right hepatic vein
RK	Right kidney
RLL	Right lobe of liver
RPC	Right pleural cavity
RRV	Right renal vein
SC	Spinal cord
Sp	Spleen
SpV	Spinous process of vertebra
Sv	Splenic vein
SV	Splenic vessels
TC	Transverse colon
VB	Vertebral body
VC	Vertebral canal
XP	Xiphoid process

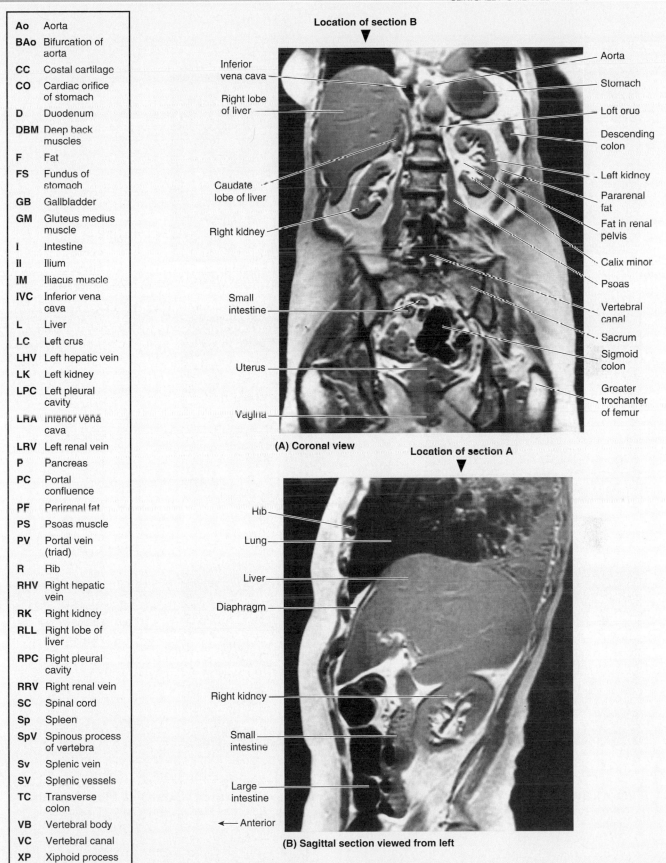

Figure 2.87. MRI studies of abdomen and pelvis. Both coronal **(A)** sagittal **(B)** scans are shown. Note that the location of the plane of section B is shown in part A, and vice versa. (Courtesy of Dr. W. Kucharczyk, Professor and Chair of Medical Imaging, University of Toronto, and Clinical Director of Tri-Hospital Resonance Centre, Toronto, ON, Canada.)

Figure 2.88. CT scans of abdomen at progressively lower levels showing viscera and blood vessels. (Courtesy of Dr. Tom White, Department of Radiology, The Health Sciences Center, University of Tennessee, Memphis, TN.)

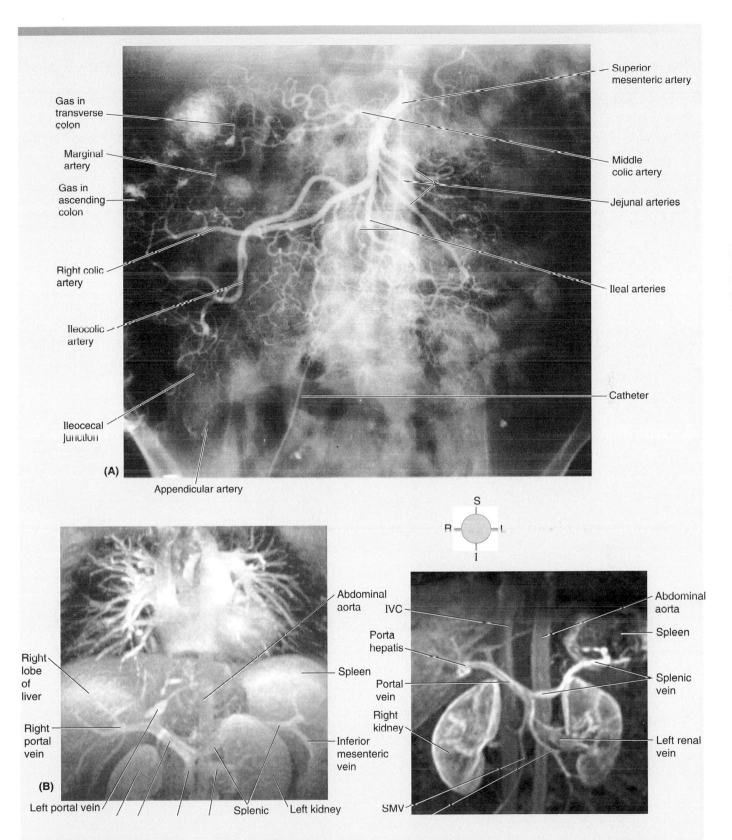

Figure 2.89. Arteriogram and angiograms. A. For this conventional (radiographic) superior mesenteric arteriogram, radiopaque dye was injected into the artery by means of the catheter introduced into the femoral artery and advanced through the iliac arteries and aorta to the opening of the SMA. (Courtesy of Dr. E. L. Lansdown, Professor of Medical Imaging, University of Toronto, Toronto, ON, Canada.) **B and C.** These coronal MR angiograms demonstrate abdominal venous anatomy. Both show the formation of the portal vein from the superior mesenteric vein (*SMV*) and splenic vein. In part B, the inferior mesenteric vein (*IMV*) is a tributary of the splenic vein, close to the spleen. In part **C,** the inferior mesenteric vein enters the junction of the superior mesenteric and splenic veins.

References and Suggested Readings

Agur AMR, Dalley AF: *Grant's Atlas of Anatomy,* 11th ed. Baltimore, Lippincott Williams & Wilkins, 2005.

Behrman RE, Kliegman RM, Jenson HB (eds): *Nelson Textbook of Pediatrics,* 16th ed. Philadelphia, Saunders, 2000.

Bickley LS, Szilagyi PG: *Bates' Guide to Physical Examination and History Taking,* 8th ed. Baltimore, Lippincott Williams & Wilkins, 2003.

Cantlie J: On a new arrangement of the right and left lobes of the liver. J Anat Physiol [Lond] 32:iv, 1898.

Cheng YF, Huang TL, Chen CL, Chen TY, Huang CC, Ko SF, Yand BY, Lee TY: Variations of the middle and inferior right hepatic vein: Application in hepatectomy. J Clin Ultrasound 25:175, 1997.

Cotran RS, Kumar V, Collins T: *Robbins Pathological Basis of Disease,* 6th ed. Philadelphia, Saunders, 1999.

Daseler EH, Anson BJ, Hambley WC, Reimann AF: The cystic artery and constituents of the hepatic pedicle. Surg Gynecol Obstet 85:47, 1947.

Ellis H: *Clinical Anatomy: A Revision and Applied Anatomy for Clinical Students.* 8th ed. Oxford, Blackwell Scientific, 1992.

Fruchaud H: Anatomie chirurgicales des hernies de l'aine. Paris, Doin, 1956. [Cited in Skandalakis LJ, Gadacz TR, Mansberger AR Jr, Mitchell WE Jr, Colborn GL, Skandalakis JE: *Modern Hernia Repair: The Embryological and Anatomical Basis of Surgery.* New York, Parthenon, 1996.]

Magee DF, Dalley AF: *Digestion and the Structure and Function of the Gut* [Karger Continuing Education Series, Vol. 8]. Basel, Karger, 1986.

Moore KL, Persaud TVN: *The Developing Human. Clinically Oriented Embryology,* 7th ed. Philadelphia, WB Saunders, 2003.

Moore KL, Persaud TVN, Shiota K: *Color Atlas of Clinical Embryology,* 2nd ed. Philadelphia, Saunders, 2000.

Naftel JP, Hardy SGP: Visceral motor pathways. *In* Haines DE (ed): *Fundamental Neuroscience,* 2nd ed. New York, Churchill Livingstone, 2002.

Rosse C, Gaddum-Rosse P: *Hollinshead's Textbook of Anatomy,* 5th ed. Philadelphia, Lippincott-Raven, 1997.

Sabiston DC Jr, Lyerly H (eds): *Sabiston Essentials of Surgery,* 2nd ed. Philadelphia, Saunders, 1994.

Skandalakis JE, Skandalakis PN, Skandalakis JL: *Surgical Anatomy and Technique. A Pocket Manual.* New York, Springer-Verlag, 1995.

Skandalakis LJ, Gadacz TR, Mansberger AR Jr, Mitchell WE Jr, Colborn GL, Skandalakis JE: *Modern Hernia Repair. The embryology of anatomical basis of surgery.* New York, Parthenon, 1996.

Soper DF: Upper genital tract infections. *In* Copeland LJ (ed): *Textbook of Gynecology,* 2nd ed. Philadelphia, Saunders, 2000.

Swartz MH: *Textbook of Physical Diagnosis, History and Examination,* 4th ed. Philadelphia, Saunders, 2001.

Townsend CM, Beauchamp RD, Evers BM, Mattox KL: *Sabiston Textbook of Surgery,* 16th ed. Philadelphia, Saunders, 2001.

Williams PL, Bannister LH, Berry MM, Collins P, Dyson M, Dussek JE, Ferguson MWJ (eds): *Gray's Anatomy, The Anatomical Basis of Medicine and Surgery,* 38th British ed. New York, Churchill Livingstone, 1995.

Pelvis and Perineum

Introduction to the Pelvis and Perineum

The term *pelvis* (L. basin) is used to denote a variety of structures: a region, the pelvic girdle, and the pelvic cavity.

In common usage, the pelvis is the part of the trunk infero-posterior to the abdomen and is the area of transition between the trunk and the lower limbs. Anatomically, the pelvis is the space or compartment surrounded by the pelvic girdle (bony pelvis), part of the appendicular skeleton of the lower limb (Fig. 3.1). The pelvis is subdivided into *greater* and *lesser pelves*. The greater pelvis affords protection to inferior abdominal viscera similar to the way the inferior thoracic cage protects superior abdominal viscera. The lesser pelvis provides the skeletal framework for both the *pelvic cavity* and the *perineum*—compartments of the trunk separated by the musculofascial *pelvic diaphragm*. Externally, the pelvis is covered or overlapped by the inferior anterolateral abdominal wall anteriorly, the gluteal region of the lower limb posterolaterally, and the perineum inferiorly.

The *perineum*[1] refers both to the *area* of the surface of the trunk between the thighs and the buttocks, extending from

---

[1] The term *perineum* has been used different ways, in different languages, and in different circumstances. In its most restricted sense, and in obstetrics, it has been used to refer to the area superficial to the perineal body, between the vulva or scrotum and the anus or to the perineal body itself. In an intermediate sense, it has included only the superficial (surface) area of the pelvis bounded by the thighs laterally, the mons pubis anteriorly, and the coccyx posteriorly. In its widest sense, as used in *Terminologia Anatomica* (the international anatomical terminology) and in this book, it refers the region of the body that includes all structures of the anal and urogenital triangles, superficial and deep, extending as far superiorly as the inferior fascia of the pelvic diaphragm.

the coccyx to the pubis, and to the shallow *compartment* lying deep (superior) to this area and inferior to the pelvic diaphragm. The perineum includes the anus and external genitalia: the penis and scrotum of the male and the vulva of the female. Anatomically, "regions" are defined by an area of the surface of the body, so there is no external "pelvic region" per se; although commonly used, it is not a term recognized by *Terminologia Anatomica* (FICAT, 1998).

THE BOTTOM LINE: The pelvis is the space enclosed by the pelvic girdle, which is subdivided into the greater pelvis (the inferior part of the abdominal cavity, which receives the protection of the alae of the ilia) and the lesser pelvis (the space inside the bony ring of pelvis inferior to the pelvic brim). The lesser pelvis provides the skeletal framework for both the pelvic cavity and the perineum, which are separated by the musculofascial pelvic diaphragm. The term *perineum* refers to both the region that includes the anus and external genitalia and to a shallow compartment deep to that area. The inferior anterolateral abdominal wall, gluteal region, and perineum overlap the pelvis.

Pelvic Girdle

The **pelvic girdle** is a basin-shaped ring of bones that connects the vertebral column to the two femurs. The *primary* functions of the pelvic girdle are to:

- Bear the weight of the upper body when sitting and standing.

- Transfer that weight from the axial to the lower appendicular skeleton for standing and walking.

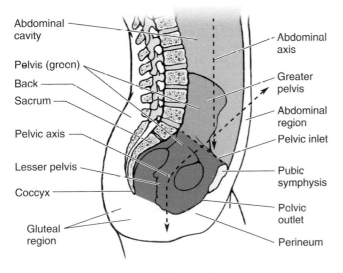

(A) Medial view of left half of bisected trunk

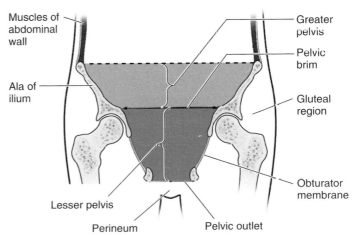

(B) Anterior view of coronal section

Figure 3.1. Pelvis and perineum. A and B. The pelvis (green) is the space (compartment) within the pelvic girdle, overlapped externally by the abdominal and gluteal (lower limb) regions and the perineum. Thus the pelvis has no external surface area. The greater pelvis (light green) is pelvic by virtue of its bony boundaries, but abdominal in terms of its contents. The lesser pelvis (dark green) provides the bony framework for the pelvic cavity and deep perineum.

- Provide attachment for the powerful muscles of locomotion and posture, as well as those of the abdominal wall, withstanding the forces generated by their actions.

Consequently, the pelvic girdle is quite strong and rigid, especially compared to the pectoral (shoulder) girdle. These aspects of the pelvic girdle will be discussed more thoroughly elsewhere (Chapter 2, in relation to the abdominal wall; Chapter 4, in relation to the vertebral column; and Chapter 6, in relation to the lower limb).

The *secondary* functions of the pelvic girdle, discussed here, are to:

- Contain and protect the pelvic viscera (inferior parts of the urinary tracts and the internal reproductive organs) especially but also the inferior abdominal viscera (intestines), while permitting passage of their terminal parts (and, in females, a full-term fetus) via the perineum.

- Provide support for the abdominopelvic viscera and gravid (pregnant) uterus.

- Provide attachment for the erectile bodies of the external genitalia.

- Provide attachment for the muscles and membranes that assist in these functions by forming the pelvic floor and filling gaps that exist in or around it.

Bones and Features of the Pelvic Girdle

In the mature individual, the pelvic girdle is formed by three bones (Fig. 3.2*A*):

- Right and left **hip bones** (coxal bones; pelvic bones): large, irregularly shaped bones, each of which develops from the fusion of three bones, the *ilium, ischium,* and *pubis.*

- **Sacrum:** formed by the fusion of five, originally separate, sacral vertebrae.

The internal (medial or pelvic) aspects of the hip bones bound the pelvis, forming its lateral walls; these aspects of the bones are emphasized here. Their external aspects, primarily involved in providing attachment for the lower limb muscles, are discussed in Chapter 5. As they are part of the vertebral column, the sacrum and coccyx are discussed in detail in Chapter 4.

In infants and children, the hip bones consist of three separate bones that are united by a **triradiate** (i.e., radiating in three directions) **cartilage** at the **acetabulum** (Fig. 3.2*B*), the cup-like depression in the lateral surface of the hip bone, which articulates with the head of the femur. After puberty, the ilium, ischium, and pubis fuse to form the hip bone. The two hip bones are joined anteriorly at the **pubic symphysis** (L. *symphysis pubis*) and articulate posteriorly with the sacrum at the *sacroiliac joints* to form the pelvic girdle.

The **ilium** is the superior, fan-shaped part of the hip bone (Fig. 3.2*B* & *C*). The **ala,** or **wing of the ilium,** represents the spread of the fan; and the **body of the ilium,** the handle of the fan. On its external aspect, the body participates in formation of the acetabulum. The **iliac crest,** the rim of the fan, has a curve that follows the contour of the ala between the **anterior** and the **posterior superior iliac spines.** The anteromedial concave surface of the ala forms the iliac fossa. Posteriorly, the **sacropelvic surface of the ilium** features an **auricular surface** and an **iliac tuberosity,** for synovial and syndesmotic articulation with the sacrum, respectively.

The **ischium** has a body and ramus (L. branch). The **body of the ischium** helps form the acetabulum and the **ramus of the ischium** forms part of the **obturator foramen.** The large posteroinferior protuberance of the ischium is the **ischial tuberosity;** the small pointed posteromedial projection near the junction of the ramus and body is the **ischial spine.** The concavity between the ischial spine and the ischial tuberosity is the **lesser sciatic notch.** The larger concavity, the **greater sciatic notch,** is superior to the ischial spine and is formed in part by the ilium.

The **pubis** is an angulated bone with a **superior pubic ramus,** which helps form the acetabulum, and an **inferior pubic ramus,** which helps form the obturator foramen. A thickening on the anterior part of the **body of the pubis** is the **pubic crest,** which ends laterally as a prominent knob or swelling, the **pubic tubercle.** The lateral part of the superior pubic ramus has an oblique ridge, the **pecten pubis** (pectineal line of pubis).

The pelvis is divided into *greater* (*false*) and *lesser* (*true*) *pelves* by the oblique plane of the **pelvic inlet** (superior pelvic aperture) (Figs. 3.1 and 3.2*A*). The bony edge (rim) surrounding and defining the pelvic inlet is the **pelvic brim,** formed by the:

- *Promontory* and *ala of the sacrum* (superior surface of its lateral part, adjacent to the body).

- A **right** and **left linea terminalis** (terminal line) together form a continuous oblique ridge consisting of the:

  - **Arcuate line** on the inner surface of the ilium.

  - *Pecten pubis* (pectineal line) and *pubic crest,* forming the superior border of the superior pubic ramus and body.

The **pubic arch** is formed by the **ischiopubic rami** (conjoined inferior rami of the pubis and ischium) of the two sides (Fig. 3.2*A* & *C*). These rami meet at the *pubic symphysis,* their inferior borders defining the **subpubic angle.** The width of the subpubic angle is determined by the distance between the right and the left ischial tuberosities, which can be measured with the fingers in the vagina during a pelvic examination. The **pelvic outlet** (inferior pelvic aperture) is bounded by the (Fig. 3.3*C*):

- *Pubic arch* anteriorly.

- *Ischial tuberosities* laterally.

- Inferior margin of the *sacrotuberous ligament* (running between the coccyx and the ischial tuberosity) *posterolaterally.*

- *Tip* of the coccyx posteriorly.

(A) Anterior view of pelvic girdle

Iliac crest

Greater pelvis — Iliac fossa / Ala

Ilium

Hip bone — Pubis

Ischium

Key
☐ Greater (false) pelvis
■ Lesser (true) pelvis

Posterior superior iliac spine
Sacroiliac joint
Ala of sacrum
Sacral promontory
Sacrum
Anterior superior iliac spine
Coccyx
Pelvic inlet (outlined by superior pelvic aperture or pelvic brim)
Acetabulum
Pubic tubercle
Pubic symphysis
Subpubic angle
Pubic arch

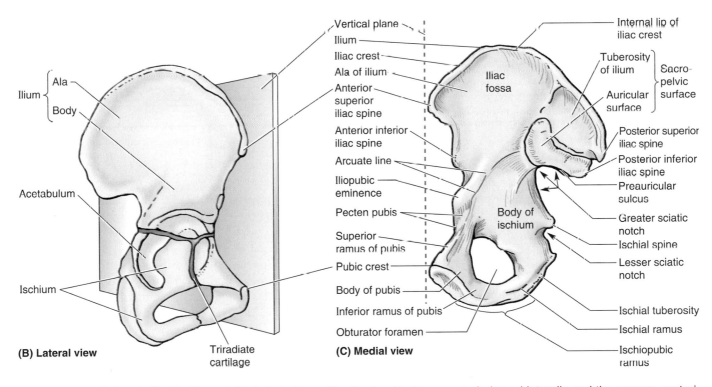

(B) Lateral view

Ilium — Ala / Body

Acetabulum

Ischium

Triradiate cartilage

Vertical plane
Ilium
Iliac crest
Ala of ilium
Anterior superior iliac spine
Anterior interior iliac spine
Arcuate line
Iliopubic eminence
Pecten pubis
Superior ramus of pubis
Pubic crest
Body of pubis
Inferior ramus of pubis
Obturator foramen

(C) Medial view

Iliac fossa
Iliac fossa
Body of ischium

Internal lip of iliac crest
Tuberosity of ilium — Sacro-pelvic surface
Auricular surface
Posterior superior iliac spine
Posterior inferior iliac spine
Preauricular sulcus
Greater sciatic notch
Ischial spine
Lesser sciatic notch
Ischial tuberosity
Ischial ramus
Ischiopubic ramus

Figure 3.2. Pelvic girdle. A. The pelvic girdle is formed by the two hip bones anteriorly and laterally and the sacrum posteriorly. The sacrum is also part of the vertebral column, in continuity with the lumbar vertebrae superiorly and the coccyx inferiorly. **B.** When a child's hip bone is in the anatomical position, the anterior superior iliac spine (ASIS) and the anterior aspect of the pubis lie in the same vertical plane. The hip bone at this stage is composed of three bones—ilium, ischium, and pubis—that meet in the cup-shaped acetabulum. The bones are not fused at this age but are united by a triradiate cartilage along a Y-shaped line (*blue*). **C.** An adult's right hip bone in the anatomical position shows the bones when fused.

Sacroiliac joint

Lumbosacral joint

Acetabulum

Head of femur

Sacrococcygeal joint

Pubic symphysis

(A) Anterior view—joints of pelvic girdle

Transverse process of L5 vertebra

Iliac crest

Anterior superior iliac spine (ASIS)

Greater sciatic foramen

Sacrotuberous and sacrospinous ligaments

Head of femur (joint capsule removed)

Obturator membrane

Pubic symphysis

Anterior longitudinal ligament

Iliolumbar ligament

Anterior sacroiliac ligament

Anterior inferior iliac spine

Iliofemoral ligament

Pubofemoral ligament

Anterior sacrococcygeal ligament

(B) Anterior view—ligaments

Supraspinous ligament

Posterior superior iliac spine

Greater sciatic foramen

Ischiofemoral ligament

Sacrotuberous ligament

Pelvic outlet*

Tip of coccyx

Pubic arch

Iliolumbar ligament

Posterior sacroiliac ligament

Posterior sacrococcygeal ligaments

Sacrospinous ligament and ischial spine

Lesser sciatic foramen

Ischial tuberosity

(C) Posterior view—ligaments

*Inferior pelvic aperture

Figure 3.3. Joints and ligaments of pelvis. A. The joints of the adult pelvic girdle include the sacroiliac joints and the pubic symphysis. The lumbosacral and sacrococcygeal are joints of the axial skeleton directly related to the pelvic girdle. **B and C.** The ligaments of the pelvis are shown.

The boundaries of the pelvic outlet are also the deep boundaries of the perineum.

The **greater pelvis** (false pelvis, pelvis major) is the part of the pelvis (Fig. 3.2A):

- Superior to the pelvic inlet.

- Bounded by the iliac alae posterolaterally and the anterosuperior aspect of the S1 vertebra posteriorly.

- Occupied by abdominal viscera (e.g., the ileum and sigmoid colon).

The **lesser pelvis** (true pelvis, pelvis minor) is the part of the pelvis:

- Between the *pelvic inlet* and the *pelvic outlet*.

- Bounded by the pelvic surfaces of the hip bones, sacrum, and coccyx.

- That includes the true *pelvic cavity* and the deep parts of the *perineum* (perineal compartment), specifically the ischioanal fossae.

- Of major obstetrical and gynecological significance.

The concave superior surface of the musculofascial pelvic diaphragm forms the floor of the true pelvic cavity, which is thus deepest centrally. The convex inferior surface of the pelvic diaphragm forms the roof of the perineum, which is therefore shallow centrally and deep peripherally. Its lateral parts (ischioanal fossae) extending well up into the lesser pelvis. The terms *pelvis, lesser pelvis,* and *pelvic cavity* are commonly used incorrectly, as if they were synonymous terms.

Orientation of the Pelvic Girdle

When a person is in the anatomical position, the right and left ASISs and the anterior aspect of the pubic symphysis lie in the same vertical plane (Fig. 3.2B). When a pelvic girdle in this position is viewed anteriorly (Fig. 3.2A; Table 3.1A & B), the tip of the coccyx appears close to the center of the pelvic inlet, and the pubic bones and pubic symphysis constitute more of a weight-bearing floor than an anterior wall. In the median view (Fig. 3.1A), the sacral promontory is located directly superior to the center of the pelvic outlet (site of the perineal body). Consequently, the curved axis of the pelvis intersects the axis of the abdominal cavity at an oblique angle.

Table 3.1. Comparison of Male and Female Bony Pelves

(A)   (B)

Bony Pelvis	Male (♂)	Female (♀)
General structure	Thick and heavy	Thin and light
Greater pelvis (pelvis major)	Deep	Shallow
Lesser pelvis (pelvis minor)	Narrow and deep, tapering	Wide and shallow, cylindrical
Pelvic inlet (superior pelvic aperture)	Heartshaped, narrow	Oval and rounded; wide
Pelvic outlet (inferior pelvic aperture)	Comparatively small	Comparatively large
Pubic arch and subpubic angle	Narrow (< 70°)	Wide (> 80°)
Obturator foramen	Round	Oval
Acetabulum	Large	Small
Greater sciatic notch	Narrow (~ 70°); inverted V	Almost 90°

The pelvic girdles of males and females differ in several respects (Table 3.1). These sexual differences are related mainly to the heavier build and larger muscles of most men and to the adaptation of the pelvis (particularly the lesser pelvis) in women for parturition (childbearing). The *male pelvic girdle* is heavier and thicker than the female girdle and usually has more prominent bone markings. The *female pelvic girdle* is wider, shallower, and has a larger pelvic inlet and outlet. The *subpubic angle* is nearly a right angle in females; it is considerably less in males (approximately 60°).

Variations in the Male and Female Pelves

Although anatomical differences between male and female pelves are usually clear cut, the pelvis of any person may have some features of the opposite sex. The pelvic types shown in Figure B3.1*A* and *C* are most common in males, *B* and *A* in white females, *B* and *C* in black females, whereas *D* is uncommon in both sexes. The **gynecoid pelvis** is the normal female type (Fig. B3.1*B*); its pelvic inlet typically has a rounded oval shape and a wide transverse diameter. An **android** (masculine or funnel-shaped) **pelvis** in a woman may present hazards to successful vaginal delivery of a fetus (Fig. B3.1*A*).

In **forensic medicine** (the application of medical and anatomical knowledge for the purposes of law), identification of human skeletal remains usually involves the diagnosis of sex. A prime focus of attention is the pelvic girdle because sexual differences usually are clearly visible. Even fragments of the pelvic girdle are useful in determining sex.

Pelvic Diameters (Conjugates)

The size of the lesser pelvis is particularly important in obstetrics because it is the bony canal through which the fetus passes during a vaginal birth. To determine the capacity of the female pelvis for childbearing, the diameters of the lesser pelvis are noted radiographically or manually during a pelvic examination. The minimum anteroposterior (AP) diameter of the lesser pelvis, the **true** (obstetrical) **conjugate** from the middle of the sacral promontory to the posterosuperior margin (closest point) of the pubic symphysis (Fig. B3.2*A* & *B*), is the narrowest *fixed* distance through which the baby's head must pass in a vaginal delivery. This distance, however, cannot be measured directly during a pelvic examination because of the presence of the bladder. Consequently, the **diagonal conjugate** (Fig. B3.2*B*) is measured by palpating the sacral promontory with the tip of the *middle* finger, using the other hand to mark the level of the inferior margin of the pubic symphysis on the examining hand (Fig. B3.2*C*). After the examining hand is withdrawn, the distance between the tip of the *index* finger (1.5 cm shorter than the middle finger) and the marked level of the pubic symphysis is measured to estimate the true conjugate, which should be 11.0 cm or greater.

In all pelvic girdles, the ischial spines extend toward each other, and the **interspinous distance** between them is normally the narrowest part of the **pelvic canal** (the passageway through the pelvic inlet, lesser pelvis and pelvic outlet, through which a baby's head must pass at birth; ▶

(A) Android (C) Anthropoid (B) Gynecoid (D) Platypelloid

Superior views

Figure B3.1

(A) Superior view

Oblique diameter

Obstetrical conjugate > 10 cm

Interspinous distance, 10 cm
Transverse diameter, 13.5 cm

Sacral promontory

Anatomical conjugate

True (obstetric) conjugate

Diagonal conjugate

Pubic symphysis

(B) Medial view (from left)

Plane of least pelvic dimension

Obstetric conjugate (11.5 cm)

(C) Medial view (from right)

Diagonal conjugate (13 cm)

Distance measured after hand is withdrawn (11.5 cm)

Figure D3.2

Fig. B3.2B), but it is not a fixed distance (see clinical correlation [blue] box "Relaxation of Pelvic Ligaments and Increased Joint mobility during Pregnancy," in this chapter). During a pelvic examination, if the ischial tuberosities are far enough apart to permit three fingers to enter the vagina side by side, the subpubic angle is considered sufficiently wide to permit passage of an average fetal head at full term.

Pelvic Fractures

Anteroposterior compression of the pelvis occurs during crush accidents (e.g., when a heavy object falls on the pelvis) (Fig. B3.3A). This type of trauma commonly produces fractures of the pubic rami. When the pelvis is compressed laterally, the acetabula and ilia are squeezed toward each other and may be broken. Fractures of the bony pelvic ring are almost always multiple fractures or a fracture combined with a joint dislocation. To illustrate this, try breaking a pretzel ring at just one point. Some pelvic fractures result from the tearing away of bone by the strong ligaments associated with the sacroiliac joints (these ligaments are shown in Figs 3.3 and 3.4A). Pelvic fractures can result from direct trauma to the pelvic bones, such as occurs during an automobile accident (Fig. B3.3A), or be caused by forces transmitted to these bones from the lower limbs during falls on the feet (Fig. B3.3B). Weak areas of the pelvis, where fractures often occur, are the pubic rami, the acetabula (or the area immediately surrounding them), the region of the sacroiliac joints, and the alae of the ilium.

Pelvic fractures may cause injury to pelvic soft tissues, blood vessels, nerves, and organs. Fractures in the pubo-obturator area are relatively common and are often complicated because of their relationship to the urinary bladder and urethra, which may be ruptured or torn. Falls on the feet or buttocks from a high ladder may drive the head of the femur through the acetabulum into the pelvic cavity, injuring pelvic viscera, nerves, and vessels. In individuals < 17 years of age, the acetabulum may fracture through the triradiate cartilage into its three developmental parts (Fig. 3.2B) or the bony acetabular margins may be torn away. ▶

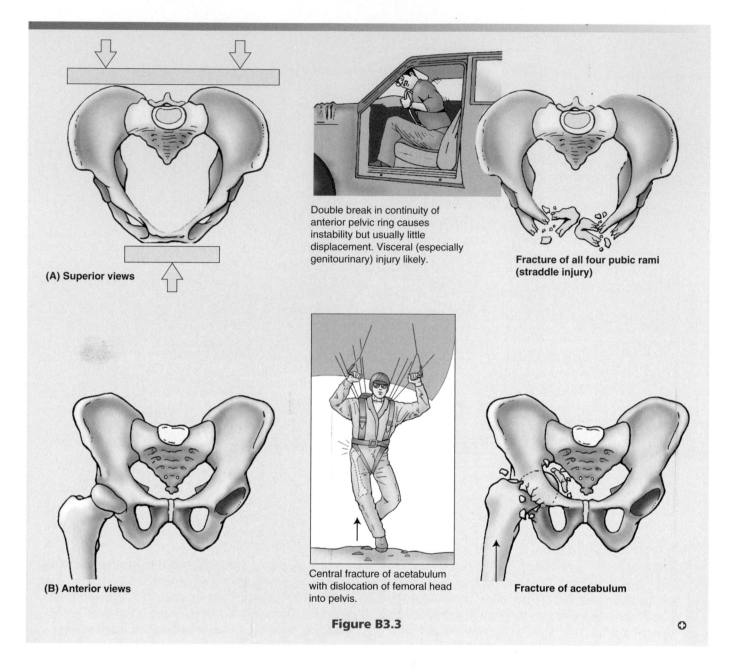

Double break in continuity of anterior pelvic ring causes instability but usually little displacement. Visceral (especially genitourinary) injury likely.

(A) Superior views

Fracture of all four pubic rami (straddle injury)

Central fracture of acetabulum with dislocation of femoral head into pelvis.

(B) Anterior views

Fracture of acetabulum

Figure B3.3

THE BOTTOM LINE: The pelvic girdle is an articulated bony ring composed of the sacrum and two hip bones. Whereas the pelvic girdle is part of the appendicular skeleton of the lower limb, the sacrum is also part of the axial skeleton, continuous with the lumbar vertebrae superiorly and coccyx inferiorly. The hips bones are formed by the fusion of the ilium, ischium, and pubis. The primary functions of the pelvic girdle are weight bearing and transfer; secondary functions include protection and support of abdominopelvic viscera and housing and attachment for structures of the genital and urinary systems. The pelvic girdle is in the anatomical position when its three anterior-most points (right and left ASISs and anterior aspect of pubic symphysis) lie in the same vertical plane. Male and female pelves are distinct; the characteristic features of the normal (gynecoid) female pelvis reflect the fact that the fetus must traverse the pelvic canal during childbirth. Because atypical female pelves may not be conducive to a vaginal birth, determination of the pelvic diameters is of clinical importance.

Joints and Ligaments of the Pelvic Girdle

The primary joints of the pelvic girdle are the *sacroiliac joints* and the *pubic symphysis* (Fig. 3.3*A*). The sacroiliac joints link the **axial skeleton** (the skeleton of the trunk, composed of the vertebral column at this level) and the **inferior appendicular skeleton** (skeleton of the lower limb). The lumbosacral and sacrococcygeal joints, although joints of the axial skeleton, are directly related to the pelvic girdle. Strong ligaments support and strengthen these joints.

Sacroiliac Joints

The **sacroiliac joints** are strong, weight-bearing compound joints, consisting of an anterior synovial joint (between the ear-shaped *auricular surfaces* of the sacrum and ilium, covered with articular cartilage) and a posterior syndesmosis (between the *tuberosities* of the same bones) (Figs. 3.3 and 3.4). The articular (auricular) surfaces of the synovial joint have irregular but congruent elevations and depressions that interlock. The

sacroiliac joints differ from most synovial joints in that limited mobility is allowed, a consequence of their role in transmitting the weight of most of the body to the hip bones. Weight is transferred from the axial skeleton to the ilia and then to the femurs during standing (Fig. 3.3A & B) and to the ischial tuberosities during sitting. As long as tight apposition is maintained between the articular surfaces, the sacroiliac joints remain stable.

Unlike a keystone at the top of an arch, the sacrum is actually suspended between the iliac bones and is firmly attached to them by posterior and interosseous sacroiliac

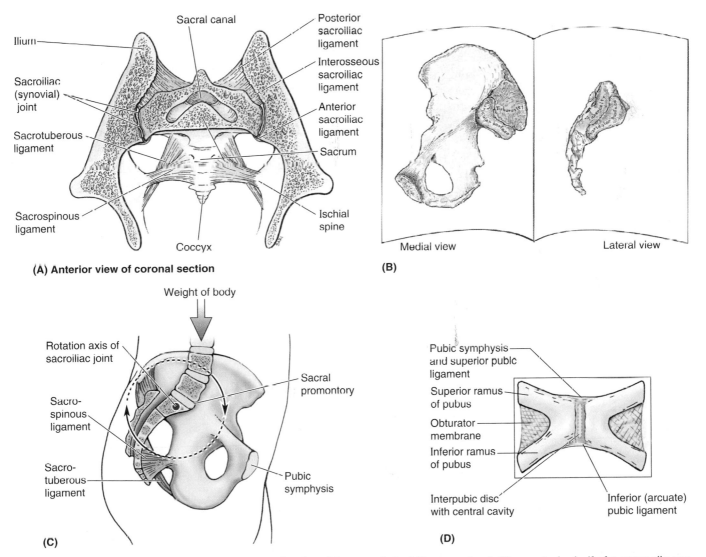

(A) Anterior view of coronal section

(B)   Medial view   Lateral view

(C)   **(D)**

Figure 3.4. Sacroiliac joints and pubic symphysis with associated ligaments. A. The posterior half of a coronally sectioned pelvic girdle and its sacroiliac joints are shown. The strong interosseous sacroiliac ligaments lie deep (anteroinferior) to the posterior sacroiliac ligaments and consist of shorter fibers connecting the tuberosity of the sacrum to the tuberosity of the ilium, suspending the sacrum. **B.** The auricular surfaces and tuberosities of the ilium and sacrum are demonstrated. **C.** The weight of the body is transmitted to the sacrum anterior to the axis of rotation at the sacroiliac joint. The tendency for increased weight or force to rotate the upper sacrum anteriorly and inferiorly is resisted by the strong sacrotuberous and sacrospinous ligaments anchoring the inferior sacrum and coccyx to the ischium. **D.** The pubic symphysis is a secondary cartilaginous joint between the bodies of the pubic bones (Fig. 3.3).

ligaments (Figs. 3.3*B* and 3.4*A*). The thin **anterior sacroiliac ligaments** are merely the anterior part of the fibrous capsule of the synovial part of the joint. The abundant **interosseous sacroiliac ligaments** (lying deep between the tuberosities of the sacrum and ilium and occupying an area of approximately 10 cm²) are the primary structures involved in transferring the weight of the upper body from the axial skeleton to the two ilia of the appendicular skeleton. The **posterior sacroiliac ligaments** are the posterior external continuation of the same mass of fibrous tissue. Because the fibers of the interosseous and posterior sacroiliac ligaments run obliquely upward and outward from the sacrum, the axial weight pushing down on the sacrum actually pulls the ilia inward (medially) so that they compress the sacrum between them, locking the irregular but congruent surfaces of the sacroiliac joints together. The iliolumbar ligaments are accessory ligaments to this mechanism.

Inferiorly, the posterior sacroiliac ligaments are joined by fibers extending from the posterior margin of the ilium (between the posterior superior and posterior inferior iliac spines) and the base of the coccyx to form the **sacrotuberous ligament**. This massive ligament thus passes from the posterior ilium and lateral sacrum and coccyx to the ischial tuberosity, transforming the sciatic notch of the hip bone into a large sciatic foramen. The **sacrospinous ligament**, passing from lateral sacrum and coccyx to the ischial spine, further subdivides this foramen into **greater** and **lesser sciatic foramina.**

Most of the time, movement at the sacroiliac joint is limited by the interlocking of the articulating bones and the sacroiliac ligaments to slight gliding and rotary movements (Fig. 3.4*C*). When landing after a high jump or when weightlifting in the standing position, exceptional force is transmitted through the bodies of the lumbar vertebrae to the superior end of the sacrum. Because this transfer of weight occurs anterior to the axis of the sacroiliac joints, the superior end of the sacrum is pushed inferiorly and anteriorly. However, rotation of the superior sacrum is counter-balanced by the strong sacrotuberous and sacrospinous ligaments that anchor the inferior end of the sacrum to the ischium, preventing its superior and posterior rotation (Figs. 3.3*B* & *C* and 3.4*A–C*). By allowing only slight upward movement of the inferior end of the sacrum relative to the hip bones, resilience is provided to the sacroiliac region when the vertebral column sustains sudden increases in force or weight.

Pubic Symphysis

This secondary cartilaginous joint consists of a fibrocartilaginous interpubic disc and surrounding ligaments uniting the bodies of the pubic bones in the median plane (Figs. 3.3 and 3.4*D*). The **interpubic disc** is generally wider in women. The ligaments joining the bones are thickened at the superior and inferior margins of the symphysis, forming superior and inferior pubic ligaments. The **superior pubic ligament** connects the superior aspects of the pubic bodies and interpubic disc, extending as far laterally as the pubic tubercles. The **inferior (arcuate) pubic ligament** (Fig. 3.4*D*) is a thick arch of fibers that connects the inferior aspects of the joint components, rounding off the *subpubic angle* as it forms the apex of the *pubic arch* (Fig. 3.2*A*; Table 3.1). The decussating, fibers of the tendinous attachments of the rectus abdominis and external oblique muscles also strengthen the pubic symphysis anteriorly (see Chapter 2).

Lumbosacral Joints

L5 and S1 vertebrae articulate at the anterior **intervertebral (IV) joint** formed by the **IV disc** between their bodies (Fig. 3.3*A*) and at two posterior **zygapophysial joints** (facet joints) between the articular processes of these vertebrae. The facets on the S1 vertebra face posteromedially, interlocking with the anterolaterally facing inferior articular facets of the L5 vertebra, preventing the lumbar vertebra from sliding anteriorly down the incline of the sacrum. These joints are further strengthened by fan-like **iliolumbar ligaments** radiating from the transverse processes of the L5 vertebra to the ilia (Fig. 3.3*B* & *C*).

Spondylolysis and Spondylolisthesis

Spondylolysis is a defect allowing part of a *vertebral arch* (the posterior projection from the vertebral body that surrounds the spinal canal and bears the articular, transverse, and spinal processes) to be separated from its body. Spondylolysis of vertebra L5 results in the separation of the vertebral body from the part of its vertebral arch bearing the inferior articular processes. The inferior articular processes of L5 normally interlock with the articular processes of the sacrum. When the defect is bilateral, the body of the L5 vertebrae may slide anteriorly on the sacrum (**spondylolisthe**-sis) so that it overlaps the sacral promontory (Fig. B3.4*A*). The intrusion of the L5 body into the pelvic inlet reduces the AP diameter of the pelvic inlet, which may interfere with parturition. It may also compress spinal nerves, causing low back or lower limb pain (see Chapter 4). Obstetricians test for spondylolisthesis by running their fingers along the lumbar spinous processes. An abnormally prominent L5 process indicates that the anterior part of L5 vertebra and the vertebral column superior to it may have moved anteriorly relative to the sacrum and the vertebral arch of L5. Medical images, such as sagittal MRI, are taken to confirm the diagnosis and to measure the AP diameter of the pelvic inlet. ▶

(A) Normal

Spondylolysis (A)
Spondylolisthesis (B)

Defect separating L5
vertebra into two parts
(spondylolysis)

L4

L5

5

S1

S2

S3

Anterior displacement
of L5 vertebral body
(spondylolisthesis)

(B)

Anterior
displacement
of L5 vertebra
(Spondylo-
listhesis)

Defect
(spondylolysis)

Sacral
canal

Acetabular rim

Head of femur

Dotted line follows posterior vertebral
margins of L5 and the sacrum

(C) Left lateral views

Figure B3.4. A. Comparison of a normal L5 vertebra with intact articular processes that prevent spondylolisthesis and an L5 vertebra with spondylolysis (A) resulting in spondylolisthesis (B). **B.** Interpretive figure of radiograph (**C**) demonstrating spondylolysis and spondylolisthesis. ✚

Sacrococcygeal Joint

The **sacrococcygeal joint** is a secondary cartilaginous joint (Fig. 3.3*A*) with an IV disc. Fibrocartilage and ligaments join the apex of the sacrum to the base of the coccyx. The anterior and posterior **sacrococcygeal ligaments** are long strands that reinforce the joint, much like the anterior and posterior longitudinal ligaments do for the superior vertebrae (Fig. 3.3*B* & *C*).

Relaxation of Pelvic Ligaments and Increased Joint Mobility during Pregnancy

The larger cavity of the interpubic disc of females increases in size during pregnancy. This change in size increases the circumference of the lesser pelvis and contributes to increased flexibility of the pubic symphysis. Increased levels of sex hormones and the presence of the hormone *relaxin* cause the pelvic ligaments to relax during the latter half of pregnancy, allowing increased movement at the pelvic joints. Relaxation of sacroiliac joints and the pubic symphysis permits as much as a 10–15% increase in diameters (mostly transverse, including the interspinous distance), facilitating passage of the fetus through the pelvic canal. The coccyx is also allowed to move posteriorly.

The one diameter that remains unaffected is the true (conjugate) diameter between the sacral promontory and the posterosuperior aspect of the pubic symphysis. Relaxation of sacroiliac ligaments causes the interlocking mechanism of the sacroiliac joint to become less effective, permitting greater rotation of the pelvis and ▶

contributing to the lordotic ("swayback") posture often assumed during pregnancy with the change in the center of gravity. Relaxation of ligaments is not limited to the pelvis, and the possibility of joint dislocation increases during late pregnancy. ⊙

THE BOTTOM LINE: The sacroiliac joints are specialized compound synovial and syndesmotic joints, the structures of which reflect both the primary (weightbearing/weight transfer and stability) and the secondary (parturition) functions of the pelvis. Strong interosseous and posterior sacroiliac ligaments suspend the sacrum between the ilia, transferring weight and stabilizing the bony ring of the pelvis. The synovial joints allow slight but significant movement during childbirth, when the pubic symphysis and the

ligaments are softened by hormones. To counterbalance the weight of the upper body and additional forces generated by activities such as jumping and load bearing, which are received by the superior sacrum anterior to the rotatory axis of the sacroiliac joints, the inferior end of the sacrum is anchored to the ischium by the substantial sacrotuberous and sacrospinous ligaments.

Pelvic Cavity

The *abdominopelvic cavity* extends superiorly into the thoracic cage and inferiorly into the pelvis, so that its superior and inferior parts are relatively protected (Fig. 3.5*A*). Perforating wounds in either the thorax or the pelvis may therefore involve the abdominopelvic cavity and its contents. The funnel-shaped **pelvic cavity**—the space bounded peripherally by the bony, ligamentous, muscular pelvic walls and floor—is the inferoposterior part of the abdominopelvic cavity, continuous

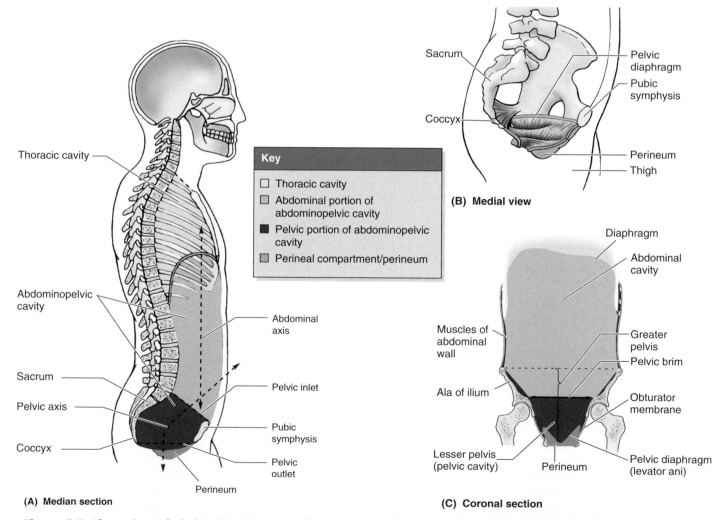

Key

☐ Thoracic cavity
☐ Abdominal portion of abdominopelvic cavity
■ Pelvic portion of abdominopelvic cavity
☐ Perineal compartment/perineum

(A) Median section

(B) Medial view

(C) Coronal section

Figure 3.5. Thoracic and abdominopelvic cavities. A and C. These sections of the trunk show the relationship of the thoracic and abdominopelvic cavities. Although the greater pelvis and lesser pelvis (pelvic cavity) are actually continuous, they are demarcated by the plane of the pelvic inlet (defined by the pelvic brim). **B.** The pelvic diaphragm is a dynamic barrier separating the lesser pelvis and the perineum, forming the floor of the former and roof of the latter.

with the abdominal cavity at the *pelvic inlet* but angulated posteriorly from it (Fig. 3.5A & C). Although continuous, the abdominal and pelvic cavities are described separately for descriptive purposes, facilitating the regional approach.

The pelvic cavity contains the terminal parts of the ureters and the urinary bladder, rectum, pelvic genital organs, blood vessels, lymphatics, and nerves. In addition to these distinctly pelvic viscera, it also contains what might be considered an overflow of abdominal viscera: loops of small intestine (mainly ileum) and, frequently, large intestine (appendix and transverse and/or sigmoid colon). The pelvic cavity is limited inferiorly by the musculofascial *pelvic diaphragm*, which is suspended above (but descends centrally to the level of) the *pelvic outlet*, forming a bowl like *pelvic floor*. The pelvic cavity is bounded posteriorly by the coccyx and inferiormost sacrum, with the superior part of the sacrum forming a roof over the posterior half of the cavity (Fig. 3.5A & B). The bodies of the pubic bones and the pubic symphysis uniting them form an anteroinferior wall that is much shallower (shorter) than the posterosuperior wall and ceiling formed by sacrum and coccyx. Consequently, the **axis of the pelvis** (a line in the median plane defined by the center point of the pelvic cavity at every level) is curved, pivoting around the pubic symphysis. The curving form of the axis and the disparity in depth between the anterior and the posterior walls of the cavity are important factors in the mechanism of fetal passage through the pelvic canal.

Walls and Floor of the Pelvic Cavity

The pelvic cavity has an anteroinferior wall, two lateral walls, a posterior wall (or posterolateral wall and a roof), and a floor (Fig. 3.6; Table 3.2).

Anteroinferior Pelvic Wall

The anteroinferior pelvic wall (more of a weight-bearing floor than an anterior wall in the anatomical position) is formed primarily by the bodies and rami of the pubic bones and the pubic symphysis (Figs. 3.4D and 3.6B–D). It participates in bearing the weight of the urinary bladder.

Lateral Pelvic Walls

Figure 3.6B & C shows the lateral pelvic wall being constructed as layers are added in a "reversed-dissection" sequence. The lateral pelvic walls are formed by the right and left hip bones, each of which includes an obturator foramen closed by an **obturator membrane** (Fig. 3.6A). The fleshy attachments of the **obturator internus muscles** cover and thus pad most of the lateral pelvic walls (Figs. 3.6C). The fleshy fibers of each obturator internus converge posteriorly, become tendinous, and turn sharply laterally to pass from the lesser pelvis through the *lesser sciatic foramen* to attach to the greater trochanter of the femur. The medial surfaces of these muscles are covered by **obturator fascia**, thickened centrally as a *tendinous arch* that provides attachment for the pelvic diaphragm (Fig. 3.6D). Because this diaphragm is the boundary between the pelvis and the perineum, forming the floor of the pelvic cavity and the roof of the perineum (Fig. 3.7A), this attachment divides the muscle into a superior pelvic portion and an inferior perineal portion (Fig. 3.7B). Medial to the pelvic portions of these muscles are the obturator nerves and vessels and other branches of the internal iliac vessels.

Posterior Wall (Posterolateral Wall and Roof)

In the anatomical position, the posterior pelvic wall consists of a bony wall and roof in the midline (formed by the sacrum and coccyx) and musculoligamentous posterolateral walls, formed by the ligaments associated with the sacroiliac joints and **piriformis muscles** (Fig. 3.6A–C). The ligaments include the anterior sacroiliac, sacrospinous, and sacrotuberous ligaments. The piriformis muscles arise from the superior sacrum, lateral to its pelvic foramina (Fig. 3.6A; Table 3.2A). The muscles pass laterally, leaving the lesser pelvis through the *greater sciatic foramen* to attach to the superior border of the greater trochanter of the femur (Table 3.2B). These muscles occupy much of the greater sciatic foramen, forming the posterolateral walls of the pelvic cavity (Fig. 3.6A). Immediately deep (anteromedial) to these muscles (often embedded in the fleshy fibers) are the nerves of the *sacral plexus* (Fig. 3.6D). A gap at the inferior border of the piriformis allows passage of neurovascular structures between the pelvis and the lower limb (gluteal region).

Pelvic Floor

The pelvic floor is formed by the bowl- or funnel-shaped **pelvic diaphragm**, which consists of the coccygeus and levator ani muscles and the fascias (L. *fasciae*) covering the superior and inferior aspects of these muscles (Figs. 3.6A and 3.7; Table 3.2). The pelvic diaphragm separates the pelvic cavity from the perineum within the lesser pelvis.

The **coccygeus muscles** arise from the lateral aspects of the inferior sacrum and coccyx, their fleshy fibers underlying the deep surface of the sacrospinous ligament (Fig. 3.6B & C). The **levator ani** (a broad muscular sheet) is the larger and more important part of the pelvic floor. It is attached to the bodies of the pubic bones anteriorly, to the ischial spines posteriorly, and to a thickening in the obturator fascia (the **tendinous arch of the levator ani**) between the two bony sites on each side. The pelvic diaphragm thus stretches between the anterior, the lateral, and the posterior walls of the lesser pelvis, giving it the appearance of a hammock suspended from these attachments, closing much of the ring of the pelvic girdle. An anterior gap between the medial borders of the levator ani muscles of each side—the **urogenital hiatus**—gives passage to the urethra and, in females, the vagina.

The levator ani consists of three parts, designated according to the attachment and course of its fibers (Figs. 3.6A & D and 3.7; Table 3.2):

- **Puborectalis:** the thicker, narrower, medial part of the levator ani, consisting of muscle fibers that are continuous between the posterior aspects of the right and left pubic

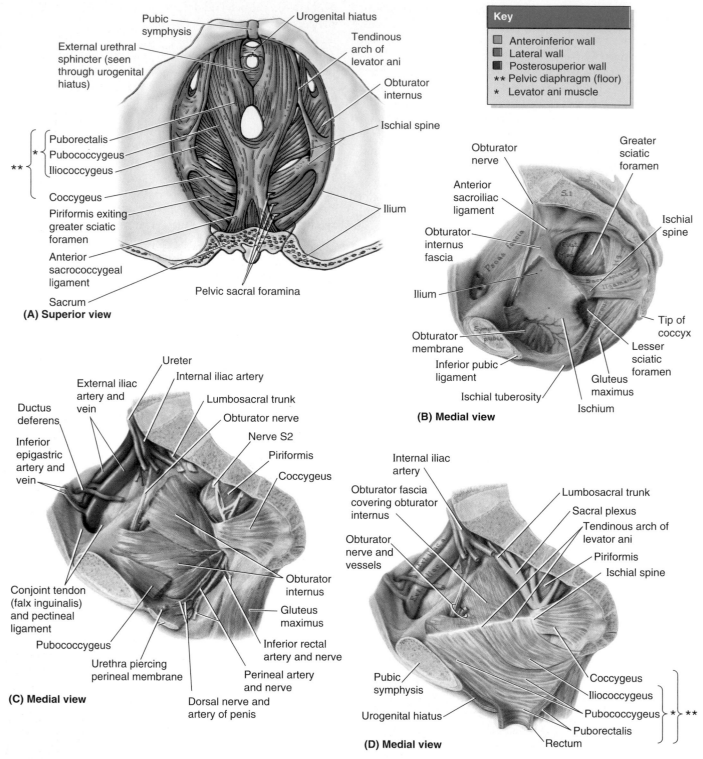

Key
- ☐ Anteroinferior wall
- ☐ Lateral wall
- ■ Posterosuperior wall
- ** Pelvic diaphragm (floor)
- * Levator ani muscle

(A) Superior view

Pubic symphysis
Urogenital hiatus
External urethral sphincter (seen through urogenital hiatus)
Tendinous arch of levator ani
Obturator internus
Puborectalis
Pubococcygeus
Iliococcygeus
Ischial spine
Coccygeus
Piriformis exiting greater sciatic foramen
Anterior sacrococcygeal ligament
Sacrum
Ilium
Pelvic sacral foramina

(B) Medial view

Obturator nerve
Greater sciatic foramen
Anterior sacroiliac ligament
Obturator internus fascia
Ischial spine
Ilium
Obturator membrane
Inferior pubic ligament
Ischial tuberosity
Tip of coccyx
Lesser sciatic foramen
Gluteus maximus
Ischium

(C) Medial view

Ureter
Internal iliac artery
External iliac artery and vein
Lumbosacral trunk
Ductus deferens
Obturator nerve
Inferior epigastric artery and vein
Nerve S2
Piriformis
Coccygeus
Conjoint tendon (falx inguinalis) and pectineal ligament
Obturator internus
Pubococcygeus
Gluteus maximus
Urethra piercing perineal membrane
Inferior rectal artery and nerve
Perineal artery and nerve
Dorsal nerve and artery of penis

(D) Medial view

Internal iliac artery
Obturator fascia covering obturator internus
Lumbosacral trunk
Sacral plexus
Tendinous arch of levator ani
Obturator nerve and vessels
Piriformis
Ischial spine
Pubic symphysis
Urogenital hiatus
Coccygeus
Iliococcygeus
Pubococcygeus
Puborectalis
Rectum

Figure 3.6. Floor and walls of pelvis. A. The floor of the pelvis is formed by the pelvic diaphragm, encircled by and suspended in part from the pubic symphysis and pubic bones anteriorly, the ilia laterally, and the sacrum and coccyx posteriorly. Parts **B** through **D** show the staged reconstruction of the parietal structures of the right hemipelvis. **B.** Posterolaterally, the coccyx and inferior part of the sacrum are attached to the ischial tuberosity by the sacrotuberous ligament and to the ischial spine by the sacrospinous ligament. The obturator membrane, composed of strong interlacing fibers, fills the obturator foramen. **C.** The muscles of the lesser pelvis are added. The obturator internus pads the lateral wall of the pelvis, its fibers converging to escape posteriorly through the lesser sciatic foramen (see part **B**). **D.** The levator ani is added, suspended from a thickening in the obturator fascia (the tendinous arch), which extends from the pubic body to the ischial spine.

Table 3.2. Muscles of the Pelvic Walls and Floor

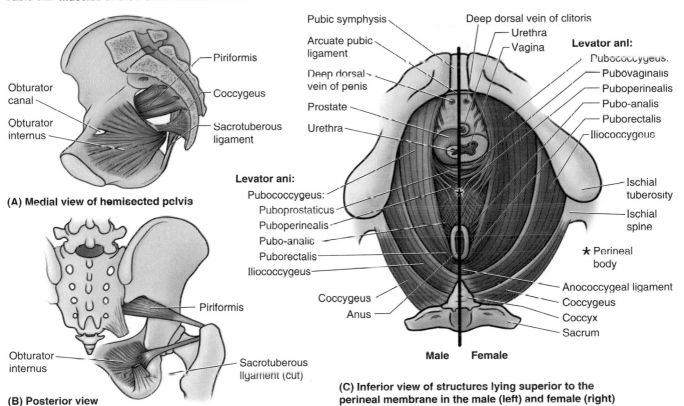

(A) Medial view of hemisected pelvis

(B) Posterior view

(C) Inferior view of structures lying superior to the perineal membrane in the male (left) and female (right)

Boundary	Muscle	Proximal Attachment	Distal Attachment	Innervation	Main Action
Lateral wall	Obturator internus	Pelvic surfaces of ilium and ischium; obturator membrane	Greater trochanter of femur	Nerve to obturator internus (L5, S1, S2)	Rotates thigh laterally; assists in holding head of femur in acetabulum
Posterolateral wall	Piriformis	Pelvic surface of S2–S4 segments; superior margin of greater sciatic notch and sacrotuberous ligament	Greater trochanter of femur	Anterior rami of S1 and S2	Rotates thigh laterally; abducts thigh; assists in holding head of femur in acetabulum
Floor	Coccygeus (ischio-coccygeus)	Ischial spine	Inferior end of sacrum	Branches of S4 and S5 spinal nerves	Forms small part of pelvic diaphragm that supports pelvic viscera; flexes coccyx
	Levator ani (pubococcygeus and iliococcygeus)	Body of pubis; tendinous arch of obturator fascia; ischial spine	Perineal body; coccyx; anococcygeal ligament; walls of prostate or vagina, rectum, and anal canal	Nerve to levator ani (branches of S4), inferior anal (rectal) nerve, and coccygeal plexus	Helps support pelvic viscera and resists increases in intra-abdominal pressure

bodies. It forms a U-shaped muscular sling (puborectal sling) that passes posterior to the anorectal junction (Fig. 3.8), bounding the urogenital hiatus. This part plays a major role in maintaining fecal continence.

- **Pubococcygeus:** the wider but thinner intermediate part of the levator ani, which arises lateral to the puborectalis from the posterior aspect of the body of the pubis and anterior tendinous arch (Figs. 3.6A & D and 3.7; Table 3.2). It passes posteriorly in a nearly horizontal plane; its lateral fibers attach to the coccyx and its medial fibers merge with those of the contralateral muscle to form a fibrous raphe or tendinous plate, part of the **anococcygeal body** or **ligament** between the anus and the coccyx (often referred to clinically as the "levator plate").

- **Iliococcygeus:** the posterolateral part of the levator ani, which arises from the posterior tendinous arch and ischial spine. It is thin and often poorly developed (aponeurotic) and also blends with the anococcygeal body posteriorly.

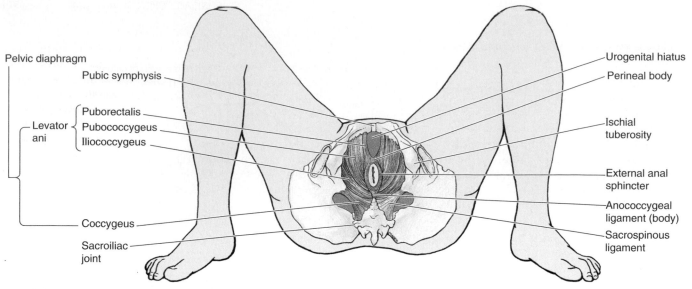

(A) Inferior view of perineum, lithotomy position

Pelvic diaphragm

Pubic symphysis

Levator ani — Puborectalis
Pubococcygeus
Iliococcygeus

Coccygeus

Sacroiliac joint

Urogenital hiatus

Perineal body

Ischial tuberosity

External anal sphincter

Anococcygeal ligament (body)

Sacrospinous ligament

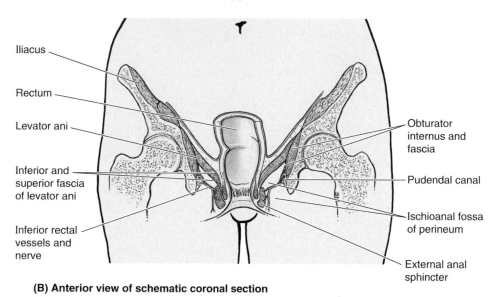

Iliacus

Rectum

Levator ani

Inferior and superior fascia of levator ani

Inferior rectal vessels and nerve

Obturator internus and fascia

Pudendal canal

Ischioanal fossa of perineum

External anal sphincter

(B) Anterior view of schematic coronal section

Figure 3.7. Pelvic diaphragm and anorectum in situ. A and B. The components of the pelvic diaphragm (levator ani and coccygeus) form the floor of the pelvic cavity and the roof of the perineum. **B.** The basin-like nature for which the pelvis was named is evident in this cross-section. The fat-filled ischioanal fossae of the perineum also lie within the bony ring of the lesser pelvis.

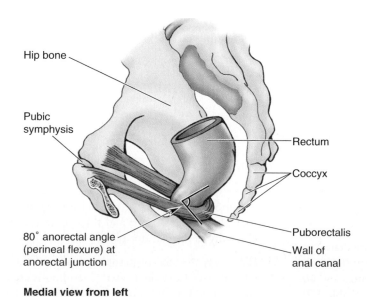

Hip bone

Pubic symphysis

80° anorectal angle (perineal flexure) at anorectal junction

Rectum

Coccyx

Puborectalis

Wall of anal canal

Medial view from left

Figure 3.8. Puborectalis muscle. Most of left hip bone has been removed to demonstrate that this part of the levator ani is formed by continuous muscle fibers following a U-shaped course around the anorectal junction. The puborectalis thus forms a puborectal sling, the tonus of which is responsible for maintaining the anorectal angle (perineal flexure).

The levator ani forms a dynamic floor for supporting the abdominopelvic viscera. It is tonically contracted most of the time to support the abdominopelvic viscera and to assist in maintaining urinary and fecal continence. It is actively contracted during activities such as forced expiration, coughing, sneezing, vomiting, and fixation of the trunk during strong movements of the upper limbs (e.g., when lifting heavy objects), primarily to increase support of the viscera during periods of increased intra-abdominal pressure (resisting forces that would push it through the pelvic outlet), and perhaps secondarily to contribute to the increased pressure (to aid expulsion). Penetrated centrally by the anal canal, the levator ani is funnel shaped, with the U-shaped puborectalis

looping around the "funnel spout," its tonic contraction bends it anteriorly. Active contraction of the (voluntary) puborectalis portion is important in maintaining fecal continence immediately after rectal filling or during peristalsis when the rectum is full and the involuntary sphincter muscle is inhibited (relaxed). The levator ani must relax to allow urination and defecation. The increased intra-abdominal pressure for defecation is provided by contraction of the (thoracic) diaphragm and muscles of the anterolateral abdominal wall. Acting together, the parts of the levator ani elevate the pelvic floor after their relaxation and the consequent descent of the pelvic diaphragm that occurs during urination and defecation.

Injury to the Pelvic Floor

During childbirth, the pelvic floor supports the fetal head while the cervix of the uterus is dilating to permit delivery of the fetus. The perineum, levator ani, and pelvic fascia may be injured during childbirth (Fig. B3.5*A*); the pubococcygeus, the main and most medial part of the levator ani, is torn most often (Fig. B3.5*B*). This part of the muscle is important because it encircles and supports the urethra, vagina, and anal canal. Weakening of the levator ani and pelvic fascia, resulting from stretching or tearing during childbirth, may alter the position of the neck of the bladder and the urethra. These

changes may cause *urinary stress incontinence,* characterized by dribbling of urine when intra-abdominal pressure is raised during coughing and lifting, for instance.

Prenatal "Relaxation" Training for Participatory Childbirth

Parents wishing to participate actively in the birth of their baby may take prenatal training (e.g., Lamaze classes) that, among other things, attempts to train women to learn how to relax voluntarily the muscles of the pelvic floor while simultaneously increasing intra-abdominal pressure through contraction of the diaphragm and anterolateral ▶

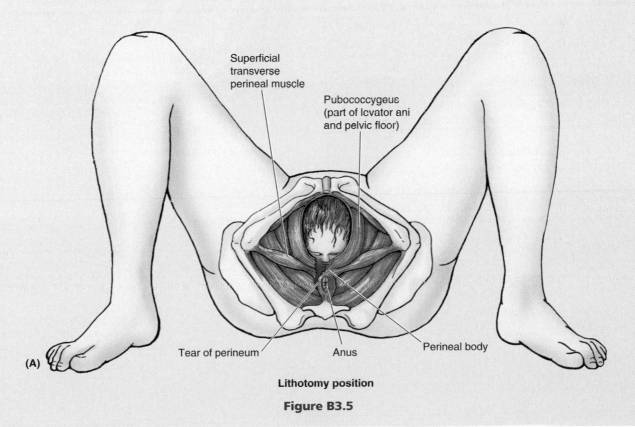

Superficial transverse perineal muscle

Pubococcygeus (part of levator ani and pelvic floor)

Tear of perineum   Anus   Perineal body

(A)

Lithotomy position

Figure B3.5

Table 3.3. Peritoneal Reflections in the Pelvis[a]

(A) Anterior view of female

(B) Right lateral view of male

(C) Right lateral view of female

Male (Fig. *B*)	Female (Fig. *A* & *C*)
1. Descends anterior abdominal wall (loose attachment allows insertion of bladder as it fills)	1. Descends anterior abdominal wall (loose attachment allows insertion of bladder as it fills)
2. Reflects onto superior surface of bladder, creating supravesical fossa	2. Reflects onto superior surface of bladder, creating supravesical fossa
3. Covers convex superior surface (roof) of bladder and slopes down sides of roof to ascend lateral wall of pelvis, creating paravesical fossae on each side	3. Covers convex superior surface (roof) of bladder and slopes down sides of roof to ascend lateral wall of pelvis, creating paravesical fossae on each side
4. Descends posterior surface of bladder as much as 2 cm	4. Reflects from bladder roof onto body of uterus forming vesicouterine pouch
5. Laterally, forms fold over ureters (ureteric fold), ductus deferens, and superior ends of seminal glands	5. Covers body and fundus of uterus and posterior fornix of vagina; extends laterally from uterus as double fold or mesentery—broad ligament that engulfs uterine tubes, ovaries, and round ligaments of uterus

(continues)

Tear of pubococcygeus

Figure B3.5 *(Continued)*

abdominal wall muscles. The aim of this method is to facilitate passage of the fetus through the birth canal, actively pushing ("bearing down") to aid the uterine contractions that expel the baby without providing resistance (and perhaps minimizing obstetrical tearing) caused by contraction of the pelvic muscles. Except when defecating or urinating, the natural reflex is to contract pelvic musculature in response to increased intra-abdominal pressure. ⊙

THE BOTTOM LINE: The pelvic cavity, between the pelvic inlet superiorly and the pelvic diaphragm inferiorly, contains the terminal parts of the urinary and alimentary systems, the internal genital organs, the associated vascular structures, and the nerves supplying both the pelvis and lower limbs. The pubic symphysis and bones of the lesser pelvis bound the cavity; they do so directly in the region of the midline anteriorly and posterosuperiorly. The lateral walls are padded by the obturator internus muscles. The sacrotuberous and sacrospinous ligaments form the greater sciatic foramen in the posterolateral walls. This foramen is filled by the structures that traverse it, including the piriformis muscles. The dynamic floor of the pelvic cavity is the hammock-like pelvic diaphragm, composed of the levator ani and coccygeus muscles. The levator ani is a tripartite, funnel-shaped muscular sheet formed by the puborectalis, pubococcygeus, and iliococcygeus muscles. In addition to the levator's general role of supporting abdominopelvic viscera as part of the pelvic diaphragm, the puborectalis is particularly involved in maintaining fecal continence. The ability of the musculofascial pelvic floor to relax and distend is critical to the functions of defecation and parturition.

Table 3.3. Peritoneal Reflections in the Pelvis *(Continued)*

Male (Fig. *B*)	Female (Fig. *A & C*)
6. Reflects from bladder and seminal glands onto rectum, forming rectovesical pouch	6. Reflects from vagina onto rectum, forming rectouterine pouch
7. Rectovesical pouch extends laterally and posteriorly to form pararectal fossae on each side of rectum	7. Rectouterine pouch extends laterally and posteriorly to form pararectal fossae on each side of rectum
8. Ascends rectum; from inferior to superior, rectum is subperitoneal and then retroperitoneal	8. Ascends rectum; from inferior to superior, rectum is subperitoneal and then retroperitoneal
9. Engulfs sigmoid colon beginning at rectosigmoid junction	9. Engulfs sigmoid colon beginning at rectosigmoid junction

[a]Numbers refer to table figures.

Peritoneum and Peritoneal Cavity of the Pelvis

The parietal peritoneum lining the abdominal cavity continues inferiorly into the pelvic cavity but does not reach the pelvic floor, from which it is separated by the pelvic viscera—onto which it is reflected—and the pelvic fascia in which the viscera are embedded (Table 3.3). Except for the ovaries and uterine tubes, the pelvic viscera are not completely ensheathed by the peritoneum, lying inferior to it for the main part; only their superior and superolateral surfaces are covered. Only the uterine tubes (except for their ostia, which are open) are intraperitoneal and suspended by a mesentery. The ovaries, although suspended in the peritoneal cavity by a mesentery, are not covered with glistening peritoneum; instead a special, relatively-dull epithelium of cuboidal cells covers them.

A loose areolar layer between the transversalis fascia and the parietal peritoneum of the inferior part of the anterior abdominal wall allows the bladder to expand between these layers as it becomes distended with urine. The region superior to the bladder (*1* in Table 3.3) is the only site where the parietal peritoneum is not firmly bound to the underlying structures. Consequently, the level at which the peritoneum reflects onto the superior surface of the bladder, creating the **supravesical fossa** (*2* in Table 3.3) is variable, depending on the fullness of the bladder. When the peritoneum reflects from the abdominopelvic wall onto the pelvic viscera and fascia, a series of folds and fossae are created (*2–7* in Table 3.3).

In the female, as the peritoneum at or near the midline reaches the posterior border of the roof of the bladder, it reflects onto the anterior aspect of the uterus at the uterine neck or isthmus (see "Female Internal Genital Organs," in this chapter); thus it is not related to the anterior vaginal fornix, which is subperitoneal in location. The peritoneum passes over the fundus and descends the entire posterior aspect of the uterus onto the posterior vaginal wall before reflecting superiorly onto the anterior wall of the inferior rectum (rectal ampulla). The "pocket" thus formed between the uterus and the rectum is the **rectouterine pouch** (or cul-de-sac, of Douglas) (*6* in Table 3.3*C*). The median rectouterine pouch is often described as the being inferiormost extent of the peritoneal cavity in the female, but often its lateral extensions on each side of the rectum, the **pararectal fossae**, are deeper.

Prominent peritoneal ridges, the **rectouterine folds**, formed by underlying fascial ligaments demarcate the lateral boundaries of the pararectal fossae (Table 3.3*A*). As the peritoneum passes up and over the uterus in the middle of the pelvic cavity, a double peritoneal fold, the *broad ligament of the uterus,* extends between the uterus and the lateral pelvic wall on each side, forming a partition that separates the paravesical fossae and pararectal fossae of each side. The uterine tubes, ovaries, ligaments of the ovaries, and round ligaments of the uterus are enclosed within the broad liga-

ments. Subdivisions of the broad ligament related to these structures will be discussed with the uterus later in this chapter. Recall that in the female the pelvic peritoneal cavity communicates with the external environment via the uterine tubes, uterus, and vagina.

In males and in women who have had their uterus removed (a *hysterectomy*), the central peritoneum descends a short distance (as much as 2 cm) down the posterior surface (base) of the bladder and then reflects superiorly onto the anterior surface of the inferior rectum, forming the **rectovesical pouch,** often described as the inferiormost extent of the peritoneal cavity in those lacking a uterus. Once again, however, the lateral continuities of the rectovesical pouch to each side of the rectum, the pararectal fossae, are often deeper than the median portion. The female rectouterine pouch is normally deeper (extends farther caudally) than the male rectovesical pouch. In the male, a gentle peritoneal fold or ridge, the **ureteric fold,** is formed as the peritoneum passes up and over the ureter and *ductus (vas) deferens* (the secretory duct of the testis) on each side of the posterior bladder, separating the paravesical and pararectal fossae; in this regard, it is the male equivalent of the broad ligament. Posterior to the ureteric folds and lateral to the central rectovesical pouch, the peritoneum often descends far enough caudally to cover the superior ends or superior posterior surfaces of the *seminal glands (vesicles)* and *ampullae of the ductus deferens.* Except for these sites (and the testis in its tunica vaginalis, which is derived from peritoneum), the male reproductive organs are not in contact with the peritoneum.

In both sexes, the inferior third of the rectum is below the inferior limits of the peritoneum (i.e., it is subperitoneal), the middle third is covered with peritoneum only on its anterior surface, and the superior third is covered on both its anterior and its lateral surfaces. The rectosigmoid junction, near the pelvic brim, is intraperitoneal.

THE BOTTOM LINE: The peritoneum lining the abdominal cavity continues into the pelvic cavity, reflecting onto the superior aspects of most pelvic viscera (only the lengths of the uterine tubes, but not their free ends, are fully intraperitoneal and have a mesentery). In so doing, the peritoneum creates a number of folds and fossae. Because the peritoneum is not firmly bound to the suprapubic abdominal wall, the bladder is able to expand between the peritoneum and the anterior abdominal wall as it fills, elevating the supravesical fossae. The rectovesical pouch and its lateral extensions, the pararectal fossae, are the inferiormost extents of the peritoneal cavity in males. In females, the uterus is located between the bladder and rectum, creating uterovesical and rectouterine pouches. The lateral extensions of the peritoneal fold engulfing the uterine fundus form the broad ligament, a transverse duplication of peritoneum separating the paravesical and pararectal fossae. The rectouterine fossa and its lateral extensions, the pararectal fossae, are the inferiormost extents of the peritoneal cavity in females.

Pelvic Fascia

The **pelvic fascia** is connective tissue that occupies the space between the membranous peritoneum and the muscular pelvic walls and floor not occupied by the pelvic viscera. This "layer" is a continuation of the comparatively thin (except around kidneys) endoabdominal fascia that lies between the muscular abdominal walls and the peritoneum superiorly. Traditionally, the pelvic fascia has been described as having parietal and visceral components (Fig. 3.9).

Membranous Pelvic Fascia: Parietal and Visceral
The **parietal pelvic fascia** is a membranous layer of variable thickness that lines the inner (deep or pelvic) aspect of the muscles forming the walls and floor of the pelvis (Fig. 3.9). The parietal pelvic fascia therefore covers the pelvic surfaces of the obturator internus, piriformis, coccygeus, levator ani, and part of the urethral sphincter muscles. Specific parts of the parietal fascia are named for the muscle they cover (e.g., obturator fascia). This layer is continuous superiorly with the transversalis and iliopsoas fascias.

The **visceral pelvic fascia** includes the membranous fascia that directly ensheathes the pelvic organs, forming the adventitial layer of each. The membranous parietal and visceral layers become continuous where the organs penetrate the pelvic floor (Fig. 3.9A & C). Here the parietal fascia thickens, forming the **tendinous arch of pelvic fascia,** a continuous bilateral band running from the pubis to the sacrum along the pelvic floor adjacent to the viscera (Fig. 3.9B, D, & E). The anteriormost part of this tendinous arch (**puboprostatic ligament** in males; **pubovesical ligament** in females) connects the prostate to the pubis in the male or the fundus (base) of the bladder to the pubis in the female. The posteriormost part of the band runs as the **sacrogenital ligaments** from the sacrum around the side of the rectum to attach to the prostate in the male or the vagina in the female.

Endopelvic Fascia: Loose and Condensed
Usually, the abundant connective tissue remaining between the parietal and the visceral membranous layers is considered part of the visceral fascia, but various authors label parts of it as parietal. It is probably more realistic to consider this remaining fascia simply as extraperitoneal or *subperitoneal endopelvic fascia* (Fig. 3.9A & C), which is continuous with both the parietal and the visceral membranous fascias. This fascia forms a connective tissue matrix or packing material for the pelvic viscera (Fig. 3.9B & D). It varies markedly in density and content. Some of it is extremely loose **areolar** (fatty) **tissue,** relatively devoid of all but minor lymphatics and nutrient vessels. In dissection or surgery, the fingers can be pushed into this loose tissue with ease, creating actual spaces by blunt dissection; for example, between the pubis and the bladder anteriorly and between the sacrum and the rectum posteriorly. These *potential spaces,* normally consisting only of a layer of loose fatty tissue, are the **retropubic** (or *prevesical,* extended posterolaterally as *paravesical*) and **retrorectal** (or *presacral*) **spaces,** respectively. The presence of loose connective tissue here accommodates the expansion of the urinary bladder and rectal ampulla as they fill.

Although these types of endopelvic fascia do not differ much in their gross appearance, other parts of the endopelvic fascia have a much more fibrous consistency, containing an abundance of collagen and elastic fibers and, according to some authors, a scattering of smooth muscle fibers. These parts are often described as "fascial condensations" or pelvic "ligaments." For example, during dissection, if you insert the fingers of one hand into the retropubic space and the fingers of the other hand into the presacral space and attempt to bring them together along the lateral pelvic wall, you will find that they do not meet or pass from one space to the other. They encounter the so-called **hypogastric sheath,** a thick band of condensed pelvic fascia. This fascial condensation is not merely a barrier separating the two potential spaces; it gives passage to essentially all the vessels and nerves passing from the lateral wall of the pelvis to the pelvic viscera, along with the ureters and, in the male, the ductus deferens. As it extends medially from the lateral wall, the hypogastric sheath divides into three laminae (leaflets or wings) that pass to or between the pelvic organs, conveying neurovascular structures and providing support. Because of the latter function, they are also referred to as ligaments. The anteriormost lamina, the **lateral ligament of the bladder,** passes to the bladder, conveying the superior vesical arteries and veins. The posteriormost lamina passes to the rectum, conveying the middle rectal artery and vein.

In the male, the middle lamina forms a relatively thin fascial partition, the **rectovesical septum** (Fig. 3.9D), between the posterior surface of the bladder and the prostate anteriorly and the rectum posteriorly. In the female, the middle lamina is markedly more substantial than the other two, passing medially to the uterine cervix and vagina as the **transverse cervical (cardinal) ligament,** also known clinically as the *lateral cervical* or *Mackenrodt ligament* (Fig. 3.9B). In its superiormost portion, at the base of the peritoneal broad ligament, the uterine artery runs transversely toward the cervix while the ureters pass immediately inferior to them as they pass on each side of the cervix heading anteriorly toward the bladder. This relationship ("water passing under the bridge") is an especially important one for surgeons (see clinical correlation [blue] boxes "Iatrogenic Injury of the Ureters during Ligation of Uterine Artery" and "Iatrogenic Injury of the Ureters during Ligation of Ovarian Artery," in this chapter). The transverse cervical ligament, and the way in which the uterus normally "rests" on top of the bladder, provide the main passive support for the uterus. The perineal muscles provide dynamic support

(A)+(B) Female (endo-) pelvic fascia

(C)+(D) Male (endo-) pelvic fascia

(A) Anterior view of coronal section

Peritoneum
Obturator fascia
Obturator internus
Cervix
Visceral fascia
Uterine artery
Ureter
Levator ani
Superior and inferior fascia of pelvic diaphragm
External urethral sphincter
Periosteum
Iliacus
Pelvic brim
Planes of section for (B) and (D)
Subperitoneal endopelvic fascia
Tendinous arch of pelvic fascia

(C) Anterior view of coronal section

Peritoneum
Ileum
Obturator fascia
Obturator internus
Visceral fascia
Tendinous arch of levator ani
Levator ani
Superior and inferior fascia of pelvic diaphragm
Ischioanal fossa
Perineal membrane
External urethral sphincter

(B) Superior view of transverse section

Pubic bone
Bladder
Visceral fascia of bladder
Paravesical space
Obturator internus
Obturator fascia
Plane of (A)
Cervix
Tendinous arch of pelvic fascia (green)
Sacrogenital (uterosacral or rectouterine) ligament—part of tendinous arch of pelvic fascia (green)
Rectum
Retrorectal (presacral) space
Retropubic (prevesical) space
Pubovesical ligament (below) (green)
Obturator membrane
Lateral ligament of bladder
Ureter
Paravesical space
Rectovesical septum
Transverse (cardinal) ligament
Hypogastric sheath
Lateral rectal ligaments
Visceral fascia of rectum
Piriformis
Sacrum

(D) Superior view of transverse section

Prostate (below bladder)
Visceral fascia of bladder
Pubic symphysis
Retropubic (prevesical) space
Puboprostatic ligament (below) (green)
Pubovesical ligament (higher level) (green)
Plane of (C)
Ampulla of ductus deferens
Seminal gland
Lateral ligament of bladder
Pelvirectal space
Sacrogenital (rectoprostatic) ligament—part of tendinous arch of pelvic fascia (green)

(E) Male pelvic floor, superior view

Tendinous arch of pelvic fascia
Obturator fascia
*Levator ani
Parietal pelvic fascia (cut edges)
External urethral sphincter
Puboprostatic ligament
Obturator internus
Tendinous arch of levator ani (thickening of obturator fascia)
Root of hypogastric sheath
Coccygeus*
Piriformis
Sacrogenital (rectoprostatic) ligament

*pelvic diaphragm

Key

☐ Loose areolar fascia	} Endopelvic
☐ Ligamentous fascia	} fascia
── Visceral fascia	
── Parietal fascia	
── Peritoneum	

Figure 3.9. Pelvic fascia: endopelvic fascia and fascial ligaments. Sections of female (**A and B**) and male (**C and D**) pelves demonstrating the parietal and visceral pelvic fascia and the endopelvic fascia between them, with its ligamentous and loose areolar components. **E.** The pelvic fascial ligaments adjacent to the male pelvic floor are shown (viscera, visceral fascia, and loose areolar endopelvic fascia removed). The tendinous arch of the levator ani is a thickening of the obturator (parietal) fascia, providing the anterolateral attachment (origin) of the levator ani. The tendinous arch of the pelvic fascia is a thickening at the point of reflection of parietal fascia onto the pelvic viscera, where it becomes visceral fascia.

for the uterus by contracting during moments of increased intra-abdominal pressure (sneezing, coughing, etc.). Passive and dynamic supports together resist the tendency for the uterus to fall or be pushed through the hollow tube formed by the vagina (uterine prolapse). The transverse cervical ligament has enough fibrous content to anchor wide loops of suture during surgical repairs.

In addition to the ischioanal fossae inferior to the pelvic diaphragm (i.e., in the perineum) (Fig. 3.9*A* & *C*), there is a surgically important potential **pelvirectal space** in the loose extraperitoneal connective tissue superior to the pelvic diaphragm (Fig. 3.9*D*). It is divided into anterior and posterior regions by the **lateral rectal ligaments** (rectal stalks), which are the posterior laminae of the hypogastric sheaths. These ligaments connect the rectum to the parietal pelvic fascia at the S2–S4 levels (Fig. 3.9*B* & *D*). The middle rectal arteries and rectal nerve plexuses are embedded in the lateral rectal ligaments.

THE BOTTOM LINE: Membranous parietal pelvic fascia, continuous with the fascia lining the abdominal cavity, lines the pelvic walls and reflects onto the pelvic viscera as pelvic visceral fascia. The right and left lines of reflection are thickened into paramedian fascial bands extending from pubis to coccyx, the tendinous arches of the pelvic fascia. The subperitoneal space between the parietal and visceral pelvic fascias is occupied with fatty endopelvic fascia. This endopelvic fascial matrix has loose areolar portions, occupying potential spaces, and condensed fibrous tissue, surrounding neurovascular structures in transit to the viscera while also tethering (supporting) the viscera. The two portions of endopelvic fascia are indistinct in appearance but have distinctly different textures. The primary fascial condensations form the hypogastric sheaths along the posterolateral pelvic walls. As these fascial sheaths extend toward the viscera, three laminae are formed, including the lateral ligament of the bladder anteriorly and the lateral rectal ligaments posteriorly. In females, the middle lamina is the transverse cervical or cardinal ligament that passively supports the vagina and uterine cervix, while conveying their neurovasculature. In males, the middle lamina is the rectovesical septum.

Neurovascular Structures of the Pelvis

The major neurovascular structures of the pelvis lie extraperitoneally against the posterolateral walls. The nerves lie most external or superficial (adjacent to the walls), with the vascular structures internal or deep (medial) to them. Generally, the veins are external (lateral) to the arteries (Fig. 3.11*A–C*).

Pelvic Nerves

The pelvis is innervated mainly by the **sacral** and **coccygeal spinal nerves** and the *pelvic part of the autonomic nervous system.* The piriformis and coccygeus muscles form a bed for the sacral and coccygeal nerve plexuses (Fig. 3.10*A*). The anterior rami of the S2 and S3 nerves emerge between the digitations of these muscles. At or immediately superior to the pelvic brim, the descending part of the L4 nerve unites with the anterior ramus of the L5 nerve to form the thick, cord-like **lumbosacral trunk** (Figs. 3.6*D* and 3.10*A*; Table 3.4). The trunk passes inferiorly, on the anterior surface of the ala of the sacrum, and joins the sacral plexus.

Sacral Plexus

The **sacral plexus** is located on the posterolateral wall of the lesser pelvis, where it is closely related to the anterior surface of the piriformis muscle. The two main nerves arising from the sacral plexus, the *sciatic* and *pudendal nerves,* lie external to the parietal pelvic fascia. Most branches of the sacral plexus leave the pelvis through the *greater sciatic foramen.*

The **sciatic nerve** is the largest nerve in the body. It is formed by the anterior rami of spinal nerves L4–S3, which converge on the anterior surface of the piriformis (Fig. 3.10*A*; Table 3.4). Most commonly, the sciatic nerve passes through the greater sciatic foramen inferior to the piriformis to enter the gluteal region (Fig. 3.10*B*). It then descends along the posterior aspect of the thigh to supply the posterior aspect of the lower limb (see Chapter 5).

The **pudendal nerve** is the main nerve of the perineum and the chief sensory nerve of the external genitalia. It is derived from the anterior rami of spinal nerves S2–S4 (Table 3.4). Accompanied by the internal pudendal artery, it leaves the pelvis through the greater sciatic foramen between the piriformis and the coccygeus muscles. It then hooks around the ischial spine and sacrospinous ligament and enters the perineum through the lesser sciatic foramen (Fig. 3.10*B*). It supplies the skin and muscles of the perineum.

The **superior gluteal nerve** arises from the anterior rami of spinal nerves L4–S1 and leaves the pelvis through the greater sciatic foramen, superior to the piriformis (Fig. 3.10*A*; Table 3.4). It supplies three muscles in the gluteal region: the gluteus medius and minimus and the tensor of the fascia lata (see Chapter 5).

The **inferior gluteal nerve** arises from the anterior rami of spinal nerves L5–S2 and leaves the pelvis through the greater sciatic foramen (Table 3.4), inferior to the piriformis and superficial to the sciatic nerve. It accompanies the inferior gluteal artery and breaks up into several branches, which supply the overlying gluteus maximus muscle (see Chapter 5).

Obturator Nerve

The **obturator nerve** arises from the anterior rami of spinal nerves L2–L4 of the *lumbar plexus* in the abdomen (greater pelvis) and enters the lesser pelvis (Fig. 3.10*A*). It runs in the extraperitoneal fat along the lateral wall of the pelvis to the *obturator canal,* an opening in the obturator membrane that otherwise fills the obturator foramen. Here it divides into anterior and posterior parts, which leave the pelvis through this canal and supply the medial thigh muscles (see Chapter 5). No pelvic structures are supplied by the obturator nerve.

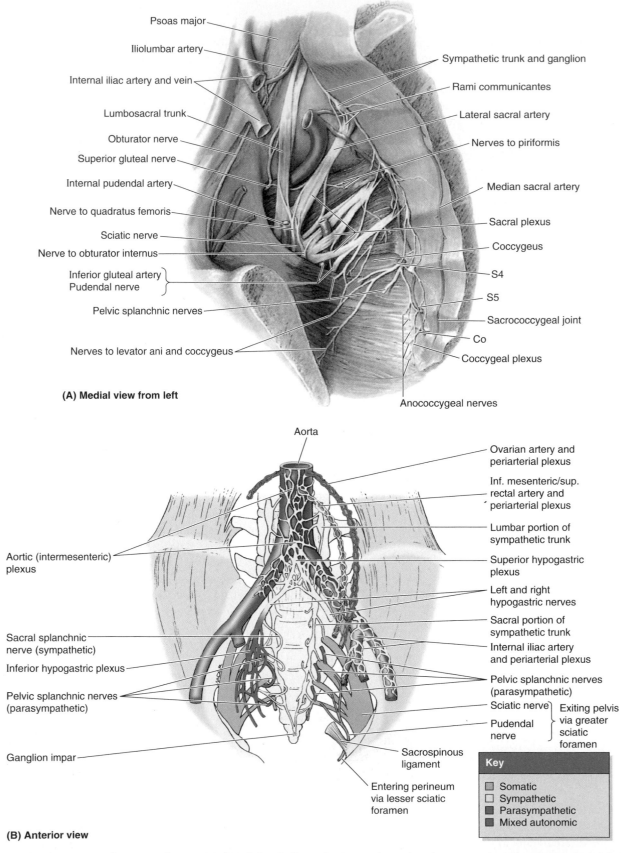

(A) Medial view from left

Psoas major

Iliolumbar artery

Internal iliac artery and vein

Lumbosacral trunk

Obturator nerve

Superior gluteal nerve

Internal pudendal artery

Nerve to quadratus femoris

Sciatic nerve

Nerve to obturator internus

Inferior gluteal artery
Pudendal nerve

Pelvic splanchnic nerves

Nerves to levator ani and coccygeus

Sympathetic trunk and ganglion

Rami communicantes

Lateral sacral artery

Nerves to piriformis

Median sacral artery

Sacral plexus

Coccygeus

S4

S5

Sacrococcygeal joint

Co

Coccygeal plexus

Anococcygeal nerves

(B) Anterior view

Aorta

Ovarian artery and
periarterial plexus

Inf. mesenteric/sup.
rectal artery and
periarterial plexus

Lumbar portion of
sympathetic trunk

Superior hypogastric
plexus

Left and right
hypogastric nerves

Sacral portion of
sympathetic trunk

Internal iliac artery
and periarterial plexus

Pelvic splanchnic nerves
(parasympathetic)

Sciatic nerve

Pudendal
nerve

Exiting pelvis
via greater
sciatic
foramen

Sacrospinous
ligament

Entering perineum
via lesser sciatic
foramen

Aortic (intermesenteric)
plexus

Sacral splanchnic
nerve (sympathetic)

Inferior hypogastric plexus

Pelvic splanchnic nerves
(parasympathetic)

Ganglion impar

Key

☐ Somatic
☐ Sympathetic
☐ Parasympathetic
☐ Mixed autonomic

Figure 3.10. Nerves and nerve plexuses of pelvis. A. Somatic nerves (sacral and coccygeal nerve plexuses) and the pelvic (sacral) part of the sympathetic trunk are shown. Although located in the pelvis, most of the nerves seen here are involved with the innervation of the lower limb rather than the pelvic structures. **B.** Autonomic nerves are demonstrated. The superior hypogastric plexus is a continuation of the aortic (intermesenteric) plexus. It divides into left and right hypogastric nerves as it enters the pelvis. The hypogastric and pelvic splanchnic nerves merge to form the inferior hypogastric plexuses, which thus consist of both sympathetic and parasympathetic fibers. Autonomic (sympathetic) fibers also enter the pelvis via the sympathetic trunks and periarterial plexuses.

Table 3.4. Somatic Nerves of the Pelvis

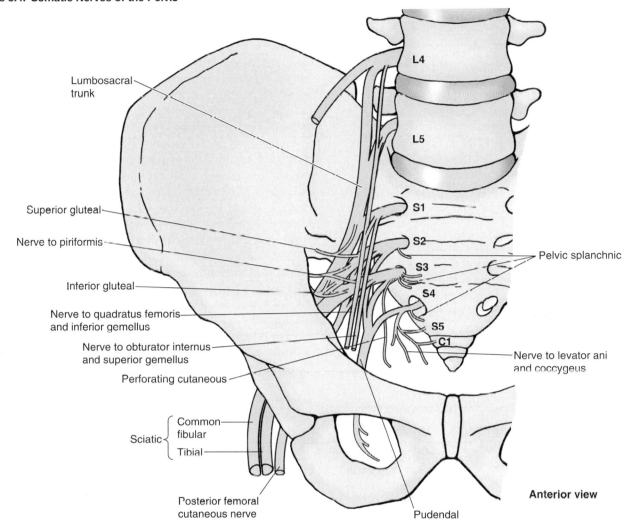

Nerve	Origin	Distribution
Sciatic	L4, L5, S1, S2, S3	Articular branches to hip joint and muscular branches to flexors of knee in thigh and all muscles in leg and foot
Superior gluteal	L4, L5, S1	Gluteus medius and gluteus minimus muscles
Nerve to quadratus femoris and inferior gemellus	L4, L5, S1	Quadratus femoris and inferior gemellus muscles
Inferior gluteal	L5, S1, S2	Gluteus maximus
Nerve to obturator internus and superior gemellus	L5, S1, S2	Obturator internus and superior gemellus muscles
Nerve to piriformis	S1, S2	Piriformis muscle
Posterior femoral cutaneous	S2, S3	Cutaneous branches to buttock and uppermost medial and posterior surfaces of thigh
Perforating cutaneous	S2, S3	Cutaneous branches to medial part of buttock
Pudendal	S2, S3, S4	Structures in perineum: sensory to genitalia; muscular branches to perineal muscles, external urethral sphincter, and external anal sphincter
Pelvic splanchnic	S2, S3, S4	Pelvic viscera via inferior hypogastric and pelvic plexuses
Nerves to levator ani and coccygeus	S3, S4	Levator ani and coccygeus muscles

Injury to the Pelvic Nerves

During childbirth, the fetal head may compress the nerves of the mother's sacral plexus, producing pain in the lower limbs. The *obturator nerve* is vulnerable to injury during surgery (e.g., during removal of cancerous lymph nodes from the lateral pelvic wall). Injury to this nerve may cause painful spasms of the adductor muscles of the thigh and sensory deficits in the medial thigh region (see Chapter 5). ⊙

Coccygeal Plexus

The **coccygeal plexus** is a small network of nerve fibers formed by the anterior rami of S4 and S5 and the **coccygeal nerves** (Fig. 3.10*A*). It lies on the pelvic surface of the coccygeus and supplies this muscle, part of the levator ani, and the sacrococcygeal joint. The **anococcygeal nerves** arising from this plexus pierce the coccygeus and anococcygeal ligament to supply a small area of skin between the tip of the coccyx and the anus.

Pelvic Autonomic Nerves

Autonomic nerves enter the pelvic cavity via four routes (Fig. 3.10*B*):

- *Sacral sympathetic trunks:* primarily provide sympathetic innervation to the lower limbs.

- *Periarterial plexuses* of superior rectal, ovarian, and internal iliac arteries: postsynaptic, sympathetic, vasomotor fibers to involved artery and its derivative branches.

- *Hypogastric plexuses:* most important route by which sympathetic fibers are conveyed to the pelvic viscera.

- *Pelvic splanchnic nerves:* pathway for parasympathetic innervation of pelvic viscera and descending and sigmoid colon.

The hypogastric plexuses and pelvic splanchnic nerves merge within the pelvis.

The **sacral sympathetic trunks** are the inferior continuation of the lumbar sympathetic trunks (Fig. 3.10*A* & *B*). Each of the sacral trunks is diminished in size from that of the lumbar trunks and usually has four sympathetic ganglia. The sacral trunks descend on the pelvic surface of the sacrum just medial to the pelvic sacral foramina and converge to form the small median **ganglion impar** (coccygeal ganglion) anterior to the coccyx. The sacral sympathetic trunks descend posterior to the rectum in the extraperitoneal connective tissue and send communicating branches (gray rami communicantes) to each of the anterior rami of the sacral and coccygeal nerves. They also send small branches to the median sacral artery and the inferior hypogastric plexus. The primary function of the sacral

sympathetic trunks is to provide postsynaptic fibers to the sacral plexus for sympathetic (vasomotor, pilomotor, and sudomotor) innervation of the lower limb.

The **periarterial plexuses** of the ovarian, superior rectal, and internal iliac arteries are minor routes by which sympathetic fibers enter the pelvis. Their primary function is vasomotion of the arteries they accompany.

The *hypogastric plexuses* (superior and inferior) are networks of sympathetic and visceral afferent nerve fibers. The main part of the **superior hypogastric plexus** is a prolongation of the **intermesenteric plexus** (see Chapter 2), which lies inferior to the bifurcation of the aorta (Fig. 3.10*B*). It carries fibers conveyed to and from the intermesenteric plexus by the L3 and L4 splanchnic nerves. The superior hypogastric plexus enters the pelvis, dividing into right and left **hypogastric nerves**, which descend on the anterior surface of the sacrum. These nerves descend lateral to the rectum within the *hypogastric sheaths* and then spread in a fan-like fashion as they merge with the pelvic splanchnic nerves to form the right and left *inferior hypogastric plexuses*.

The **inferior hypogastric plexuses** thus contain both sympathetic and the parasympathetic fibers as well as visceral afferent fibers, which continue through the lamina of the hypogastric sheath to the pelvic viscera, upon which they form sub-plexuses collectively referred to as the **pelvic plexuses**. In both sexes, sub-plexuses are associated with the lateral aspects of the rectum and inferolateral surfaces of the bladder. In addition, in the male, sub-plexuses are also associated with the prostate and seminal glands; in females, sub-plexuses are also associated with the cervix of the uterus and the lateral fornices of the vagina.

Pelvic splanchnic nerves arise in the pelvis from the anterior rami of spinal nerves S2–S4 of the sacral plexus (Fig. 3.10; Table 3.4). They convey presynaptic parasympathetic fibers derived from the S2–S4 spinal cord segments, which make up the sacral outflow of the parasympathetic (craniosacral) nervous system, and visceral afferent fibers from cell bodies in the spinal ganglia of the corresponding spinal nerves. The greatest contribution of these fibers is usually from the S3 nerve.

The hypogastric/pelvic system of plexuses, receiving sympathetic fibers via lumbar splanchnic nerves and parasympathetic fibers via pelvic splanchnic nerves, innervate the pelvic viscera. Although the sympathetic component largely produces vasomotion as elsewhere, here it also inhibits peristaltic contraction of the rectum and stimulates contraction of the internal genital organs during orgasm, producing ejaculation in the male. Because the pelvis does not include a cutaneous area, pelvic sympathetic fibers do not produce pilomotion or vasomotion functions. The parasympathetic fibers distributed within the pelvis stimulate contraction of the rectum and bladder for defecation and urination, respectively. Parasympathetic fibers in the prostatic plexus penetrate the pelvic floor to reach the erectile bodies of the external genitalia, producing erection.

Visceral Afferent Innervation in the Pelvis

Visceral afferent fibers travel with autonomic nerve fibers, although the sensory impulses are conducted centrally, retrograde to the efferent impulses conveyed by the autonomic fibers. All visceral afferent fibers conducting reflexive sensation (information that does not reach consciousness) travel with parasympathetic fibers. Thus, in the case of the pelvis, they travel through the pelvic and inferior hypogastric plexuses and the pelvic splanchnic nerves to the spinal sensory ganglia of spinal nerves S2–S4.

The paths followed by visceral afferent fibers conducting pain from the pelvic viscera differ in terms of course and destination, depending on whether the viscus or part of the viscus from which the pain is emanating is located superior or inferior to the **pelvic pain line**. Except in the case of the alimentary canal, the pelvic pain line corresponds to the inferior limit of the peritoneum (Table 3.3*A*–*C*). Intraperitoneal abdominopelvic viscera, or aspects of visceral structures that are in contact with the peritoneum, are superior to the pain line; subperitoneal pelvic viscera or portions of viscera are inferior to the pain line. In the case of the alimentary tract (large intestine), the pain line does not correlate with the peritoneum; the pain line occurs in the middle of the sigmoid colon.

Visceral afferent fibers conducting pain impulses from abdominopelvic viscera superior to the pain line follow sympathetic fibers retrograde, ascending through hypogastric/aortic plexuses, abdominopelvic splanchnic nerves, lumbar sympathetic trunks, and white rami communicantes to reach cell bodies in the inferior thoracic/upper lumbar spinal ganglia. Afferent fibers conducting pain impulses from the viscera or portions of viscera inferior to the pain line follow the parasympathetic fibers retrograde through the pelvic and inferior hypogastric plexuses and pelvic splanchnic nerves to reach cell bodies in the spinal sensory ganglia of S2–S4.

THE BOTTOM LINE: Progressing from the pelvic cavity outward, as when dissecting the pelvis, the retroperitoneal hypogastric/pelvic autonomic nerve plexuses are encountered first (nearest the viscera), then pelvic arteries, pelvic veins, and finally the pelvic somatic nerves and sympathetic trunks, the latter two being adjacent to the pelvic walls. Somatic nerves within the pelvis form the sacral plexus, primarily concerned with innervation of the lower limbs and perineum. The pelvic portions of the sympathetic trunks are also primarily concerned with innervation of the lower limbs. Autonomic nerves are primarily brought to the pelvis via the superior hypogastric plexus (sympathetic fibers) and pelvic splanchnic nerves (parasympathetic fibers), the two merging to form the inferior hypogastric and pelvic plexuses. Sympathetic fibers to the pelvis produce vasomotion and contraction of internal genital organs during orgasm; they also inhibit rectal peristalsis. Pelvic parasympathetic fibers stimulate bladder and rectal emptying and extend to the erectile bodies of the external genitalia to produce erection. Visceral afferent fibers travel retrogradely along the autonomic nerve fibers. Visceral afferents conveying unconscious reflex sensation follow the course of the parasympathetic fibers to the spinal sensory ganglia of S2–S4, as do those transmitting pain sensations from the viscera inferior to the pelvic pain line (structures that do not contact the peritoneum plus the distal sigmoid colon and rectum). Visceral afferent fibers conducting pain from structures superior to the pelvic pain line (structures in contact with the peritoneum, except for the distal sigmoid colon and rectum) follow the sympathetic fibers retrogradely to inferior thoracic and superior lumbar spinal ganglia.

Pelvic Arteries

The pelvis is richly supplied with arteries, among which multiple anastomoses occur, providing an extensive collateral circulation. Details concerning the origin, course, distribution, and anastomoses of the arteries of both the greater and lesser pelves are summarized in Table 3.5 and Figure 3.11. Six main arteries enter the lesser pelvis of females, whereas four main arteries enter the lesser pelvis of males: the internal iliac and ovarian arteries (females only) are paired, and the median sacral and superior rectal arteries are unpaired.

Internal Iliac Artery

Each **internal iliac artery**, approximately 4 cm long, begins as the **common iliac artery** and bifurcates into the internal and external iliac arteries at the level of the IV disc between the L5 and the S1 vertebrae. The ureter crosses the common iliac artery or its terminal branches at or immediately distal to the bifurcation (Fig. 3.11*C*; Table 3.5). The internal iliac artery is separated from the sacroiliac joint by the internal iliac vein and the lumbosacral trunk. It descends posteromedially into the lesser pelvis, medial to the external iliac vein and obturator nerve and lateral to the peritoneum. The internal iliac artery is the principal artery of the pelvis, supplying most of the blood to the pelvic viscera and some to the musculoskeletal part of the pelvis (Fig. 3.11; Table 3.5); however, it also supplies branches to the gluteal region, medial thigh regions, and the perineum.

Although variations are common, the internal iliac artery usually ends at the superior edge of the greater sciatic foramen by dividing into anterior and posterior divisions (trunks). The branches of the **anterior division of the internal iliac artery** are mainly visceral (i.e., they supply the bladder, rectum, and reproductive organs), but they also include parietal branches that pass to the buttock and thigh. The arrangement of the visceral branches is variable. The following arteries discussed next commonly arise as branches of the anterior division of the internal iliac artery.

Umbilical Artery. Before birth, the umbilical arteries are the main continuation of the internal iliac arteries, passing along the lateral pelvic wall and then ascending the anterior abdominal wall to and through the umbilical ring into the umbilical cord.

(cont'd on page 387)

Table 3.5. Arteries of the Pelvis

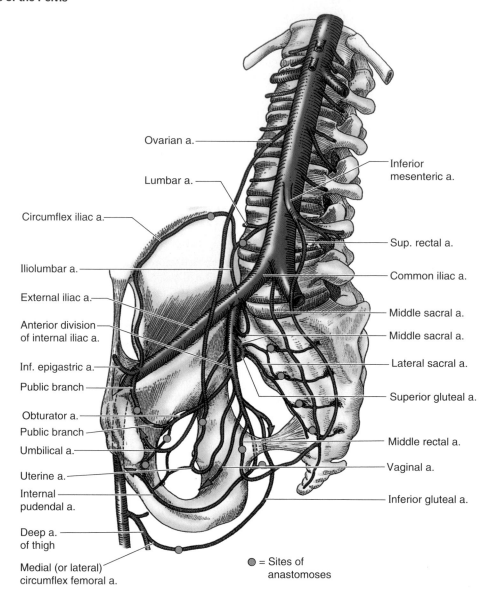

Ovarian a.

Lumbar a.

Circumflex iliac a.

Iliolumbar a.

External iliac a.

Anterior division of internal iliac a.

Inf. epigastric a.

Public branch

Obturator a.

Public branch

Umbilical a.

Uterine a.

Internal pudendal a.

Deep a. of thigh

Medial (or lateral) circumflex femoral a.

Inferior mesenteric a.

Sup. rectal a.

Common iliac a.

Middle sacral a.

Middle sacral a.

Lateral sacral a.

Superior gluteal a.

Middle rectal a.

Vaginal a.

Inferior gluteal a.

● = Sites of anastomoses

Artery	Origin	Course	Distribution	Anastomoses
Gonadal:		Descends retroperitoneally;		
testicular (♂)	Abdominal aorta	traverses inguinal canal and enters scrotum	Abdominal ureter, testis, and epididymis	Cremasteric artery, artery of ductus deferens
ovarian (♀)		crosses pelvic brim, descends in suspensory ligament of ovary	Abdominal and/or pelvic ureter, ovary, and ampullary end of uterine tube	Uterine artery via tubal and ovarian branches
Superior rectal	Continuation of inferior mesenteric artery	Crosses left common iliac vessels and descends into pelvis between layers of sigmoid mesocolon	Superior part of rectum	Middle rectal artery; inferior rectal (internal pudendal) artery
Median sacral	Posterior aspect of abdominal aorta	Descends close to midline over (L4,) L5 vertebrae and sacrum and coccyx	Inferior lumbar vertebrae, sacrum, and coccyx	Lateral sacral artery (via medial sacral branches)
Internal iliac	Common iliac artery	Passes medially over pelvic brim and descends into pelvic cavity; often forms anterior and posterior divisions	Main blood supply to pelvic organs, gluteal muscles, and perineum	

(continues)

Table 3.5. Arteries of the Pelvis *(Continued)*

Artery	Origin	Course	Distribution	Anatomoses
Anterior divisioin of internal iliac	Internal iliac artery	Passes anteriorly along lateral wall of pelvis, dividing into visceral, obturator, and internal pudendal arteries	Pelvic viscera, muscles of superior medial thigh, and perineum	
Umbilical	Anterior division of internal iliac artery	Runs a short pelvic course, gives off superior vesical arteries, then obliterates, becoming medial umbilical ligament	Superior aspect of urinary bladder and, in some males, ductus deferens (via superior vesical arteries and artery to ductus deferens)	(Occasionally the patent part of the umbilical artery)
Superior vesical	(Patent proximal umbilical artery)	Usually multiple; pass to superior aspect of urinary bladder	Superior aspect of urinary bladder; in some males, ductus deferens (via artery to ductus deferens)	Inferior vesical (♂); vaginal artery (♀)
Obturator		Runs anteroinferiorly on obturator fascia of lateral pelvic wall, exiting pelvis via obturator canal	Pelvic muscles, nutrient artery to ilium, head of femur, and muscles of medial compartment of the thigh	Inferior epigastric (via pubic branch); umbilical artery
Inferior vesical (♂)	(Superior or inferior vesical artery) (Inferior vesical artery)	Passes subperitoneally in lateral ligament of bladder, giving rise to prostatic artery (♂) and occasionally the artery to the ductus deferens	Inferior aspect of male urinary bladder, prostate, and seminal glands; occasionally ductus deferens	Superior vesical artery
Artery to ductus deferens (♂)		Runs subperitoneally to ductus deferens	Ductus deferens	Testicular artery; cremasteric artery
Prostatic branches (♂)		Descends on posterolateral aspects of prostate	Prostate and prostatic urethra	Deep perineal (internal pudendal)
Uterine (♀)		Runs anteromedially in base of broad ligament/superior cardinal ligament, gives rise to vaginal branch, then crosses ureter superiorly to reach lateral aspect of uterine cervix	Uterus, ligaments of uterus, medial parts of uterine tube and ovary, and superior vagina	Ovarian artery (via tubal and ovarian branches); vaginal artery
Vaginal (♀)		Divides into vaginal and inferior vesical branches, the former descending on the vagina, the latter passing to the urinary bladder	Vaginal branch: lower vagina, vestibular bulb, and adjacent rectum; inferior vesical branch: fundus of urinary bladder	Vaginal branch of uterine artery, superior vesical artery
Internal pudendal		Exits pelvis via infrapiriform part of greater sciatic foramen, enters perineum (ischioanal fossa) via lesser sciatic foramen, passes via pudendal canal to UG triangle	Main artery of perineum, including muscles and skin of anal and urogenital triangles, erectile bodies	(Umbilical artery; prostatic branches of inferior vesical artery in males)
Middle rectal		Descends in pelvis to inferior part of rectum	Seminal glands and inferior part of rectum	Superior and inferior rectal arteries
Inferior gluteal		Exits pelvis via infrapiriform part of greater sciatic foramen	Pelvic diaphragm (coccygeus and levator ani) piriformis, quadratus femoris, superiormost hamstrings, gluteus maximus, and sciatic nerve	Deep femoral artery (via medial and lateral femoral circumflex arteries)
Posterior division of internal iliac	Internal iliac artery	Passes posteriorly and gives rise to parietal branches	Pelvic wall and gluteal region	
Illiolumbar		Ascends anterior to sacroiliac joint and posterior to common iliac vessels and psoas major, dividing into iliac and lumbar branches	Psoas major, iliacus, and quadratus lumborum muscles; cauda equina in vertebral canal	Circumflex iliac artery and 4th (and lowest) lumbar artery
Lateral sacral (superior and inferior)	Posterior division of internal iliac artery	Runs on anteromedial aspect of piriformis to send branches into pelvic sacral foramina	Piriformis, structures in sacral canal, erector spinae, and overlying skin	Medial sacral arteries (from median sacral artery)
Superior gluteal		Exits pelvis via suprapiriform portion of greater sciatic foramen	Piriformis, all three gluteal muscles, and tensor of fascia lata	Lateral sacral, inferior gluteal, internal pudendal, deep circumflex femoral, lateral circumflex femoral

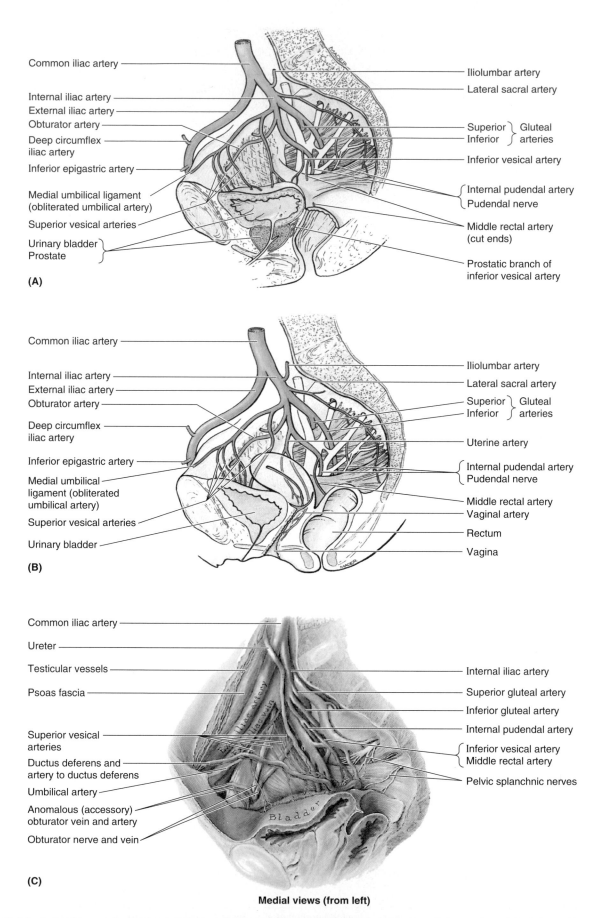

(A)

Common iliac artery

Internal iliac artery
External iliac artery
Obturator artery
Deep circumflex iliac artery

Inferior epigastric artery

Medial umbilical ligament (obliterated umbilical artery)

Superior vesical arteries

Urinary bladder
Prostate

Iliolumbar artery
Lateral sacral artery

Superior ⎱ Gluteal
Inferior ⎰ arteries

Inferior vesical artery

Internal pudendal artery
Pudendal nerve

Middle rectal artery (cut ends)

Prostatic branch of inferior vesical artery

(B)

Common iliac artery

Internal iliac artery
External iliac artery
Obturator artery

Deep circumflex iliac artery

Inferior epigastric artery

Medial umbilical ligament (obliterated umbilical artery)

Superior vesical arteries

Urinary bladder

Iliolumbar artery
Lateral sacral artery

Superior ⎱ Gluteal
Inferior ⎰ arteries

Uterine artery

Internal pudendal artery
Pudendal nerve

Middle rectal artery
Vaginal artery

Rectum

Vagina

(C)

Common iliac artery

Ureter

Testicular vessels

Psoas fascia

Superior vesical arteries

Ductus deferens and artery to ductus deferens

Umbilical artery

Anomalous (accessory) obturator vein and artery

Obturator nerve and vein

Internal iliac artery

Superior gluteal artery

Inferior gluteal artery

Internal pudendal artery

Inferior vesical artery
Middle rectal artery

Pelvic splanchnic nerves

Bladder

Medial views (from left)

Figure 3.11. Arteries and neurovascular relationships of pelvis. The arteries of the male pelvis (**A**) and female pelvis (**B**) are shown. Anterior divisions of the internal iliac arteries usually supply most of the blood to pelvic structures. The arteries are internal (lie medial) to the nerves making up the sacral plexus. **C.** The neurovascular structures of the male pelvis are shown. Generally, the pelvic veins lie between the pelvic arteries (which lie medially or internally) and the somatic nerves (which lie laterally or externally).

At this stage of life, the **umbilical arteries** conduct oxygen- and nutrient-deficient blood to the placenta for replenishment. When the umbilical cord is cut, the distal parts of these vessels no longer function and become occluded distal to branches that pass to the bladder. The *occluded parts* form fibrous cords called the **medial umbilical ligaments** or cords of the umbilical arteries (Figs. 3.11*A* & *B* and 3.14*B;* Table 3.5). The ligaments raise folds of peritoneum (the *medial umbilical folds*) on the deep surface of the anterior abdominal wall (see Chapter 2). Postnatally, the *patent part of the umbilical artery* runs anteroinferiorly between the urinary bladder and the lateral wall of the pelvis, giving off the **superior vesical artery** (or arteries) that supplies (or arise as) numerous branches to the fundus of the urinary bladder (Fig. 3.11; Table 3.5). In males, the **artery to the ductus deferens** usually arises as a branch of the superior vesical artery.

Obturator Artery. The origin of the **obturator artery** is variable; usually it arises close to the origin of the umbilical artery, where it is crossed by the ureter. It runs anteroinferiorly on the obturator fascia on the lateral wall of the pelvis and passes between the obturator nerve and vein. It then leaves the pelvis through the *obturator canal* and supplies the muscles of the medial thigh. Within the pelvis, the obturator artery gives off muscular branches, a nutrient artery to the ilium, and a pubic branch. The **pubic branch** arises just before the obturator artery leaves the pelvis. It ascends on the pelvic surface of the pubis to anastomose with its fellow of the opposite side and the pubic branch of the *inferior epigastric artery,* a branch of the external iliac artery. In a common variation (20%), an **aberrant** or **accessory obturator artery** arises from the inferior epigastric artery and descends into the pelvis along the usual route of the pubic branch (Fig. 3.11*C;* Table 3.5). Surgeons performing hernia repairs must keep this common variation in mind. The extrapelvic distribution of the obturator artery is described with the lower limb (see Chapter 5).

Inferior Vesical Artery. The **inferior vesical artery** occurs only in males, being replaced by the vaginal artery in females (Fig. 3.11*A;* Table 3.5). It passes to the fundus of the urinary bladder, where it supplies the seminal glands, prostate, fundus of the bladder, and inferior part of the ureter. The branches to the ductus deferens and prostate are the *artery to the ductus deferens* and the *prostatic artery.* The artery to the ductus deferens may arise from the superior vesical artery.

Middle Rectal Artery. The **middle rectal artery** may arise independently from the internal iliac artery, or it may arise in common with the inferior vesical artery or the internal pudendal artery (Fig. 3.11; Table 3.5). The middle rectal artery supplies the inferior part of the rectum, anastomosing with the superior and inferior rectal arteries, supplying the seminal glands and prostate (or the vagina).

Vaginal Artery. The **vaginal artery** is the homolog to the inferior vesical artery in males. It runs anteriorly and then passes along the side of the vagina, where it supplies numerous branches to the anterior and posterior surfaces of the vagina, posteroinferior parts of the urinary bladder, and the pelvic part of the urethra (Figs 3.11*B* and 3.12; Table 3.5). It anastomoses with the vaginal branch of the uterine artery.

Uterine Artery. The **uterine artery** usually arises separately and directly from the internal iliac artery, but it may arise from the umbilical artery. It is the homolog to the artery to the ductus deferens in the male. It descends on the lateral wall of the pelvis, anterior to the internal iliac artery, and enters the root of the broad ligament. Here it passes medially to reach the lateral margin of the uterus immediately superior to the lateral part of the fornix of the vagina (Fig. 3.12). As it passes medially in the broad ligament, the uterine artery passes directly superior to the ureter near the lateral part of the fornix of the vagina. The relationship of ureter to artery is often remembered by the phrase *Water* (urine) *passes under the bridge* (uterine artery). On reaching the side of the cervix, the uterine artery divides into a smaller descending **vaginal branch,** which supplies the cervix and vagina, and a larger **ascending branch,** which runs along the lateral margin of the uterus, supplying the body and fundus of the uterus. The ascending branch bifurcates into **ovarian** and **tubal branches,** which continue within the broad ligament to supply the medial ends of the ovary and uterine tube and anastomose with the ovarian and tubal branches of the ovarian artery.

Iatrogenic Injury of the Ureters during Ligation of Uterine Artery

The fact that the ureter passes immediately inferior to the uterine artery near the lateral part of the fornix of the vagina is clinically important. The ureter is in danger of being inadvertently clamped (crushed), ligated, or transected during a **hysterectomy** (excision of uterus) when the uterine artery is ligated and severed to remove the uterus. The point at which the uterine artery and ureter cross lies approximately 2 cm superior to the ischial spine. ☉

Internal Pudendal Artery. The **internal pudendal artery**, larger in males than in females, passes inferolaterally, anterior to the piriformis muscle and sacral plexus (Fig. 3.11; Table 3.5). It leaves the pelvis between the piriformis and the coccygeus muscles by passing through the inferior part of the *greater sciatic foramen.* The internal pudendal artery then passes around the posterior aspect of the ischial spine or the sacrospinous ligament and enters the *ischioanal fossa* through the *lesser sciatic foramen.* The internal pudendal artery, along with the internal pudendal veins and branches of the pudendal nerve, passes through the pudendal canal in the lateral wall of the ischioanal fossa (Fig. 3.7*B*). As it exits the pudendal canal, medial to the ischial tuberosity, the internal pudendal artery divides into its terminal branches, the *deep and dorsal arteries of the penis or clitoris.*

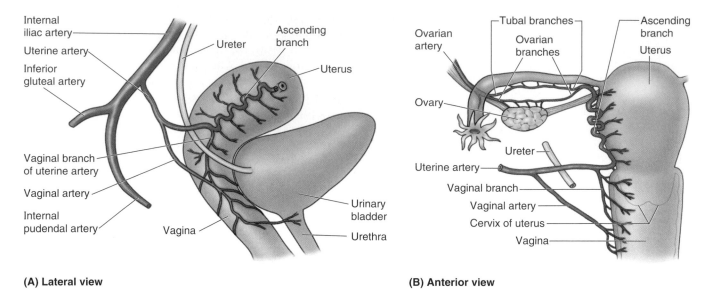

(A) Lateral view

(B) Anterior view

Figure 3.12. Uterine and vaginal arteries. A. The origin of the arteries from the anterior division of the internal iliac artery and distribution to the uterus and vagina are shown. **B.** The anastomoses between the ovarian and tubal branches of the ovarian and uterine arteries and between the vaginal branch of the uterine artery and the vaginal artery provide potential pathways of collateral circulation. These communications occur, and the ascending branch courses, between the layers of the broad ligament.

Inferior Gluteal Artery. The **inferior gluteal artery** passes posteriorly between the sacral nerves (usually S2 and S3) and leaves the pelvis through the inferior part of the *greater sciatic foramen,* inferior to the piriformis muscle (Fig. 3.11; Table 3.5). It supplies the muscles and skin of the buttock and the posterior surface of the thigh.

Posterior Division of the Internal Iliac Artery. The following three arteries are branches of the posterior division of the internal iliac artery:

- **Superior gluteal artery:** This artery passes posteriorly and runs between the lumbosacral trunk and the anterior ramus of the S1 nerve. It leaves the pelvis through the superior part of the *greater sciatic foramen,* superior to the piriformis muscle, to supply the gluteal muscles in the buttocks.

- **Iliolumbar artery:** This artery runs superolaterally in a *recurrent fashion* (turning sharply backward relative to its source) to the iliac fossa. Within the fossa, the artery divides into an *iliac branch,* which supplies the iliacus muscle and ilium, and a *lumbar branch,* which supplies the psoas major and quadratus lumborum muscles.

- **Lateral sacral arteries:** These arteries, usually made up of superior and inferior arteries on each side, may arise from a common trunk. The lateral sacral arteries pass medially and descend anterior to the sacral anterior rami, giving off spinal branches, which pass through the anterior sacral foramina and supply the spinal meninges enclosing the roots of the sacral nerves. Some branches of these arteries pass from the sacral canal through the posterior sacral foramina and supply the erector spinae muscles of the back and skin overlying the sacrum.

Ligation of the Internal Iliac Artery and Collateral Circulation in the Pelvis

Occasionally the internal iliac artery is ligated to control pelvic hemorrhage. Because of the numerous anastomoses between the artery's branches and adjacent arteries (Table 3.5), ligation does not stop blood flow but it does reduce blood pressure, allowing *hemostasis* (arrest of bleeding) to occur. Examples of collateral pathways to the internal iliac artery include the following pairs of anastomosing arteries: lumbar and iliolumbar, median sacral and lateral sacral, superior rectal and middle rectal, and inferior gluteal and deep artery of the thigh. Blood flow in the artery is maintained, although it may be reversed in the anastomotic branch. The collateral pathways may maintain the blood supply to the pelvic viscera, gluteal region, and genital organs. ⊙

Ovarian Artery

The **ovarian artery** arises from the abdominal aorta inferior to the renal artery but considerably superior to the inferior mesenteric artery (Table 3.5). As it passes inferiorly, the ovarian artery adheres to the parietal peritoneum and runs anterior to the ureter on the posterior abdominal wall, usually giving branches to it (Fig. 3.12). As it enters the lesser pelvis, it crosses the origin of the external iliac vessels. It then runs medially in the suspensory ligament of the ovary and enters the superolateral part of the broad ligament, dividing into an **ovarian branch** and a **tubal branch**, which supply the ovary and uterine tube, respectively (Fig. 3.12*B*). These branches anastomose with the corresponding branches of the uterine artery.

Iatrogenic Injury of the Ureters during Ligation of Ovarian Artery

The ureters are vulnerable to injury when the ovarian vessels are ligated during an **ovariectomy** (excision of ovary) because these structures are close to each other as they cross the pelvic brim. ⊙

Median Sacral Artery

The **median sacral artery** is a small unpaired artery that usually arises from the posterior surface of the abdominal aorta, just superior to its bifurcation, but it may arise from its anterior surface (Table 3.5). This vessel runs anterior to the bodies of the last one or two lumbar vertebrae, the sacrum, and the coccyx and ends in a series of anastomotic loops. Before the median sacral artery enters the lesser pelvis, it sometimes gives rise to a pair of *L5 arteries*. As it descends over the sacrum, the median sacral artery gives off small parietal (lateral sacral) branches that anastomose with the lateral sacral arteries. It also gives rise to small visceral branches to the posterior part of the rectum, which anastomose with the superior and middle rectal arteries. The median sacral artery represents the caudal end of the embryonic dorsal aorta, which reduced in size as the tail-like caudal eminence of the embryo disappeared.

Superior Rectal Artery

The **superior rectal artery** is the direct continuation of the inferior mesenteric artery (Table 3.5). It crosses the left common iliac vessels and descends in the sigmoid mesocolon to the lesser pelvis. At the level of the S3 vertebra, the superior rectal artery divides into two branches, which descend on each side of the rectum and supply it as far inferiorly as the internal anal sphincter. The superior rectal artery anastomoses with branches of the middle rectal artery (a branch of the internal iliac artery) and with the inferior rectal artery (a branch of the internal pudendal artery).

Pelvic Veins

Pelvic venous plexuses are formed by the interjoining veins surrounding the pelvic viscera (Fig. 3.13*B* & *C*). These intercommunicating networks of veins are clinically important. The various plexuses within the lesser pelvis (rectal, vesical, prostatic, uterine, and vaginal) unite and are drained mainly by the **internal iliac veins**, but some of them drain through the superior rectal vein into the inferior mesenteric vein or through lateral sacral veins into the *internal vertebral venous plexus* (see Chapter 4). Additional paths of venous drainage from the lesser pelvis include the parietal **median sacral vein**, the **superior rectal vein** (to the portal system) (Fig. 3.13*A*) and, in females, the ovarian veins.

The internal iliac veins merge with the external iliac veins to form the **common iliac veins**, which unite at the level of vertebra L4 or L5 to form the **inferior vena cava** (Fig. 3.13*A*). The internal iliac veins lie posteroinferior to the internal iliac arteries; their tributaries are similar to the branches of the arteries, except that there are no veins accompanying the umbilical arteries between the pelvis and the umbilicus.

The **iliolumbar veins** from the iliac fossae of the greater pelvis usually drain into the common iliac veins. The **superior gluteal veins**, the accompanying veins (L. *venae comitantes*) of the superior gluteal arteries of the gluteal region, are the largest tributaries of the internal iliac veins except during pregnancy, when the uterine veins become larger. Testicular veins traverse the greater pelvis as they pass from the deep inguinal ring toward their posterior abdominal terminations, but do not usually drain pelvic structures.

THE BOTTOM LINE: Multiple anastomosing arteries provide a collateral circulatory system that helps ensure an adequate blood supply to the greater and lesser pelves. Most arterial blood is delivered to the lesser pelvis by the internal iliac arteries, which commonly bifurcate into an anterior division (providing all the visceral branches) and a posterior division (usually exclusively parietal). Postnatally, the umbilical arteries become occluded distal to the origin of the superior vesical arteries and, in the male, the artery to the ductus deferens. The inferior vesical (males) and vaginal arteries (females) supply the inferior bladder and pelvic urethra. The inferior vesical artery also supplies the prostate; the vaginal artery supplies the superior vagina. The uterine artery is exclusively female, but both sexes have middle rectal arteries.

Parietal branches of the anterior trunk in both sexes include the obturator, inferior gluteal, and internal pudendal arteries, the main branches of which arise outside of the lesser pelvis. A clinically significant aberrant obturator artery arises from the inferior epigastric vessels in approximately 20% of the population. The iliolumbar, superior gluteal, and lateral sacral arteries are parietal branches of the posterior division of the internal iliac artery, distributed outside of the lesser pelvis. The iliolumbar is a major supply to structures of the iliac fossae (greater pelvis). The gonadal arteries of both sexes descend into the greater pelvis from the abdominal aorta, but only the ovarian arteries enter the lesser pelvis.

The venous plexuses associated with and named for the various pelvic viscera intercommunicate with each other and the internal vertebral (epidural) venous plexuses of the vertebral canal. However, most venous blood exits the pelvis via the internal iliac veins.

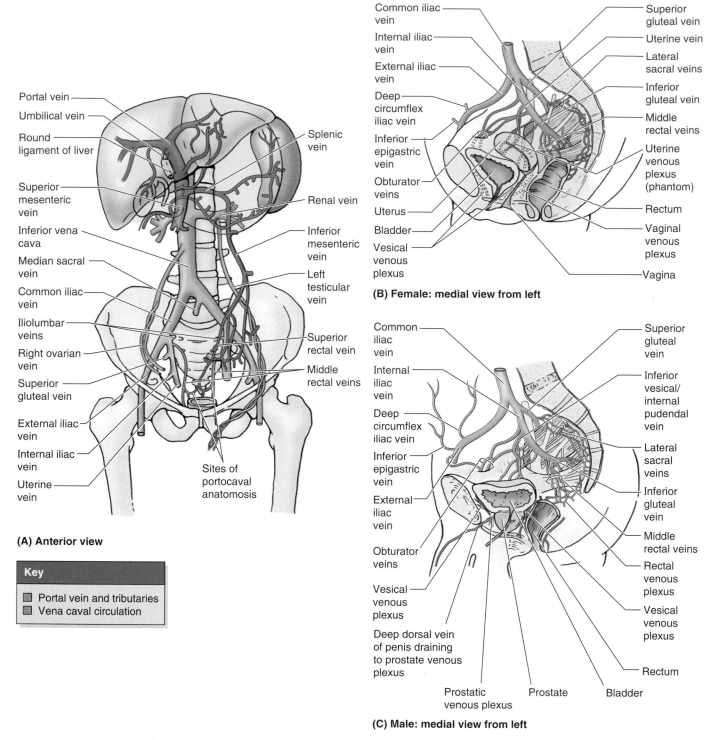

(A) Anterior view

Portal vein
Umbilical vein
Round ligament of liver
Superior mesenteric vein
Inferior vena cava
Median sacral vein
Common iliac vein
Iliolumbar veins
Right ovarian vein
Superior gluteal vein
External iliac vein
Internal iliac vein
Uterine vein

Splenic vein
Renal vein
Inferior mesenteric vein
Left testicular vein
Superior rectal vein
Middle rectal veins
Sites of portocaval anatomosis

Key

▢ Portal vein and tributaries
▢ Vena caval circulation

(B) Female: medial view from left

Common iliac vein
Internal iliac vein
External iliac vein
Deep circumflex iliac vein
Inferior epigastric vein
Obturator veins
Uterus
Bladder
Vesical venous plexus

Superior gluteal vein
Uterine vein
Lateral sacral veins
Inferior gluteal vein
Middle rectal veins
Uterine venous plexus (phantom)
Rectum
Vaginal venous plexus
Vagina

(C) Male: medial view from left

Common iliac vein
Internal iliac vein
Deep circumflex iliac vein
Inferior epigastric vein
External iliac vein
Obturator veins
Vesical venous plexus
Deep dorsal vein of penis draining to prostate venous plexus

Superior gluteal vein
Inferior vesical/internal pudendal vein
Lateral sacral veins
Inferior gluteal vein
Middle rectal veins
Rectal venous plexus
Vesical venous plexus
Rectum

Prostatic venous plexus   Prostate   Bladder

Figure 3.13. Pelvic veins. A. The female (*right*) and male (*left*) patterns of portal and systemic (vena caval) venous systems of the abdominopelvic cavity are shown. Venous drainage from pelvic organs flows mainly to the caval system via the internal iliac veins. The upper rectum normally drains into the portal system, although the superior rectal veins anastomose with the middle and inferior rectal veins, which are tributaries of the internal iliac veins. The female (**B**) and male (**C**) pelvic veins and venous plexuses are demonstrated.

Lymph Nodes of the Pelvis

The lymph nodes receiving lymph drainage from pelvic organs are variable in number, size, and location and division into definite groups is often somewhat arbitrary. Four primary groups of nodes are located in or adjacent to the pelvis, named for the blood vessels with which they are associated (Table 3.6):

- **External iliac lymph nodes:** lie above the pelvic brim, along the external iliac vessels. They receive lymph mainly from the inguinal lymph nodes; however, they receive lymph from pelvic viscera, especially the superior parts of the middle to anterior pelvic organs. Whereas most of the lymphatic drainage from the pelvis tends to parallel routes of venous drainage, the lymphatic drainage to the external iliac nodes does not. These nodes drain into the common iliac nodes.

- **Internal iliac lymph nodes:** clustered around the anterior and posterior divisions of the internal iliac artery and the origins of the gluteal arteries. They receive drainage from the inferior pelvic viscera, deep perineum, and gluteal region and drain into the common iliac nodes.

- **Sacral lymph nodes:** lie in the concavity of the sacrum, adjacent to the median sacral vessels. They receive lymph from posteroinferior pelvic viscera and drain either to internal or common iliac nodes.

- **Common iliac lymph nodes:** lie superior to the pelvis and receive drainage from the three main groups listed above, beginning a common route for drainage from the pelvis that passes next to the lumbar (caval/aortic) nodes. Inconstant direct drainage to the common iliac nodes occurs from some pelvic organs (e.g., from the neck of the bladder and inferior vagina).

Additional minor groups of nodes (e.g., the **pararectal nodes**) occupy the connective tissue along the branches of the internal iliac vessels. In females, lymphatic drainage from the ovaries and uterine tubes follows the ovarian veins to the lumbar (caval/aortic) nodes; in males the testis and epididymis also drain to the lumbar nodes, but these structures lie outside the pelvis. Both primary and minor groups of pelvic nodes are highly interconnected, so that many nodes can be removed without disturbing drainage. The interconnections also allow cancer to spread in virtually any direction, to any pelvic or abdominal viscus. While the lymphatic drainage tends to parallel the venous drainage (except for that to the external iliac nodes, where proximity provides a rough guide), the pattern is not sufficiently predictable to allow the progress of metastatic cancer from pelvic organs to be anticipated or staged in a manner comparable to that of breast cancer progressing though the axillary nodes.

THE BOTTOM LINE: Lymphatic drainage from the pelvis follows a pattern that generally, but not reliably, follows the pattern of venous drainage through variable minor and major sets of lymph nodes, the latter including the sacral,

internal, external, and common iliac nodes. Aspects of the anterior to middle pelvic organs, approximately at the level of (and including) the roof of the undistended urinary bladder, drain to the external iliac nodes, independent of the venous drainage. The pelvic lymph nodes are highly interconnected, so that lymphatic drainage (and metastatic cancer) can pass in almost any direction, to any pelvic or abdominal organ.

Pelvic Viscera

The **pelvic viscera** include the urinary bladder and parts of the ureters, the reproductive system, and the distal part of the alimentary tract (rectum). Although the sigmoid colon and parts of the small bowel extend into the pelvic cavity, they are abdominal rather than pelvic viscera. The sigmoid colon is continuous with the rectum anterior to S3 vertebra.

Urinary Organs

The pelvic urinary organs (Fig. 3.14) are the:

- Ureters, which carry urine from the kidneys.

- Urinary bladder, which temporarily stores urine.

- Urethra, which conducts urine from the bladder to the exterior.

Ureters

The **ureters** are muscular tubes, 25–30 cm long, that connect the kidneys to the urinary bladder. The ureters are retroperitoneal; their superior halves are in the abdomen (see Chapter 2) and their inferior halves lie in the pelvis. As the ureters cross the bifurcation of the common iliac artery or the beginning of the external iliac artery (Fig. 3.14A) they pass over the pelvic brim, thus leaving the abdomen and entering the lesser pelvis. The pelvic parts of the ureters run on the lateral walls of the pelvis, parallel to the anterior margin of the greater sciatic notch, between the parietal pelvic peritoneum and the internal iliac arteries. Opposite the ischial spine, they curve anteromedially, superior to the levator ani, to enter the urinary bladder. The inferior ends of the ureters are surrounded by the **vesical venous plexus** (Fig. 3.13B & C). The ureters pass obliquely through the muscular wall of the urinary bladder in an inferomedial direction, entering the outer surface of the bladder approximately 5 cm apart, but their internal openings into the lumen of the empty bladder are separated by only half that distance. This oblique passage through the bladder wall forms a one-way "flap valve," the internal pressure of the filling bladder causing the intramural passage to collapse. In addition, contractions of the bladder musculature act as a sphincter preventing the reflux of urine into the ureters when the bladder contracts, increasing internal pressure during micturition. Urine is transported down the ureters by means of peristaltic contractions, a few drops being transported at intervals of 12–20 sec.

Table 3.6. Lymphatic Drainage of the Structures of the Pelvis and Perineum

Lymph nodes:
- Lumbar (caval/aortic)
- Inferior mesenteric
- Common iliac
- Internal iliac
- External iliac
- Superficial inguinal
- Deep inguinal
- Sacral
- Pararectal

(A)

(B)

(C)

Lymph Node Group		Structures Typically Draining to Lymph Node Group	
Lumbar	*Female:* along ovarian vessels	Gonads and associated structures; common iliac nodes	*Female:* ovary; uterine tube (except isthmus and intrauterine parts); fundus of uterus
	Male: along testicular vessels		*Male urethra:* testis; epididymis
Inferior mesenteric		Superiormost rectum; sigmoid colon; descending colon; pararectal nodes	
Common iliac		External and internal iliac lymph nodes	
Internal iliac		Inferior pelvic structures; deep perineal structures; sacral nodes	*Female:* base of bladder; inferior pelvic ureter; anal canal (above pectinate line); inferior rectum; middle and upper vagina; cervix; body of uterus
			Male: prostatic urethra; prostate; base of bladder; inferior pelvic ureter; inferior seminal glands; cavernous bodies; anal canal (above pectinate line); inferior rectum
External iliac		Anterosuperior pelvic structures; deep inguinal nodes	*Female:* superior bladder; superior pelvic ureter; upper vagina; cervix; lower body of uterus
			Male: superior bladder; superior pelvic ureter; upper seminal gland; pelvic part of ductus deferens; intermediate and spongy urethra (secondary)

(continues)

Table 3.6. Lymphatic Drainage of the Structures of the Pelvis and Perineum *(continued)*

Lymph Node Group	Structures Typically Draining to Lymph Node Group	
Superficial inguinal	Lower limb; superficial drainage of inferolateral quadrant of trunk, including anterior abdominal wall inferior to umbilicus, gluteal region, and superficial perineal structures	*Female:* superolateral uterus (near attachment of round ligament); skin of perineum including vulva; ostium of vagina (inferior to hymen); prepuce of clitoris; perianal skin; anal canal inferior to pectinate line
		Male: skin of perineum including skin and prepuce of penis; scrotum; perianal skin; anal canal inferior to pectinate line
Deep inguinal	Glans of clitoris or penis; superficial inguinal nodes	*Female:* glans of clitoris
		Male: glans of penis; distal spongy urethra
Sacral	Posteroinferior pelvic structures: inferior rectum; inferior vagina	
Pararectal	Superior rectum	

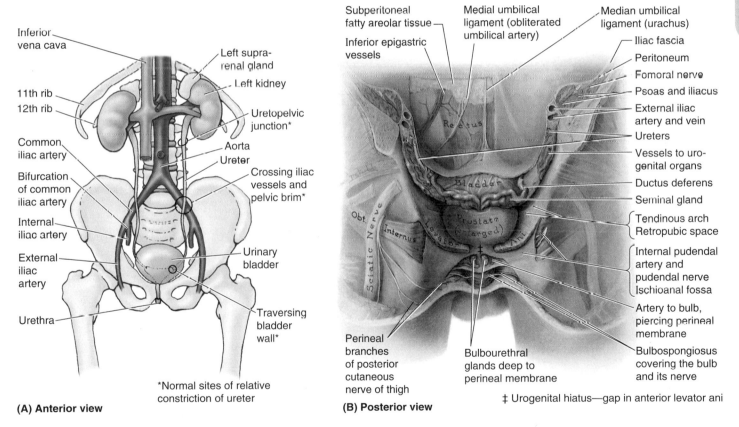

(A) Anterior view

*Normal sites of relative constriction of ureter

(B) Posterior view

‡ Urogenital hiatus—gap in anterior levator ani

Figure 3.14. Genitourinary viscera. A. This view of the urinary apparatus demonstrates the course and normal sites of relative constriction of the ureters. **B.** In this posterior dissection approach to the anterior male pelvis, the posterior pelvic wall and rectum have been removed. The medial umbilical ligament (occluded part of umbilical artery) and the median umbilical ligament (remnant of fetal urachus), like the urinary bladder, lie in the subperitoneal loose areolar tissue. The levator ani (pelvic floor) supports the pelvic viscera and separates the pelvic retropubic space from the perineal ischioanal fossae. The free medial (anterior) borders of the levator ani are separated by a gap, the *urogenital hiatus,* through which the urethra (and, in the female, the vagina) passes.

In males, the only structure that passes between the ureter and the peritoneum is the *ductus deferens* (Fig. 3.14B); it crosses the ureter within the ureteric fold of peritoneum. The ureter lies posterolateral to the ductus deferens and enters the posterosuperior angle of the bladder, just superior to the seminal gland.

In females, the ureter passes medial to the origin of the uterine artery and continues to the level of the ischial spine, where it is crossed superiorly by the uterine artery (see clinical correlation [blue] boxes "Iatrogenic Injury of the Ureters during Ligation of Uterine Artery" and "Iatrogenic Injury of the Ureters during Ligation of Ovarian Artery," in this chapter"). It then passes close to the lateral part of the fornix of the vagina and enters the posterosuperior angle of the bladder.

Arterial Supply of the Ureters. Variable branches from the common iliac, internal iliac, and ovarian arteries extend to and supply the pelvic parts of the ureters, anastomosing along the length of the ureter to form a continuous blood supply (Fig. 3.15; Table 3.5). The most constant arteries supplying the terminal parts of the ureter in females are branches of the *uterine arteries.* The source of similar branches in males are the *inferior vesical arteries.*

Venous and Lymphatic Drainage of the Ureters. Veins from the ureters accompany the arteries and have corresponding names. Lymph drains sequentially, from superior to inferior, into the lumbar (caval/ aortic) and common iliac nodes (abdominal part) and the external and internal iliac nodes (pelvic part) (Fig. 3.16A).

Innervation of the Ureters. The nerves to the ureters derive from adjacent autonomic plexuses (renal, aortic, superior and inferior hypogastric). The ureters are superior to the pelvic pain line. Afferent (pain) fibers from the ureters follow sympathetic fibers in a retrograde direction to reach the spinal ganglia and spinal cord segments of T11–L1 or L2 (Fig. 3.16B). *Ureteric pain* is usually referred to the ipsilateral lower quadrant of the abdomen, especially to the groin (inguinal region).

Iatrogenic Compromise of the Ureteric Blood Supply

The ureters may be injured during abdominal, retroperitoneal, pelvic, or gynecological operations as a result of inadvertently interrupting their blood supply. Identification of the ureters during their full course through the pelvis is an important preventive measure. The longitudinal anastomoses between arterial branches to the ureter are usually adequate to maintain the blood supply along the length of the ureters, but occasionally they are not. Traction on the ureter during surgery may lead to delayed rupture of the ureter. The denuded ureteral segment becomes gangrenous and leaks or ruptures 7–10 days after surgery. When traction is necessary, it should be applied with great care. It is useful to realize that, although the blood supply to the abdominal segment of the ureter approaches from a medial direction, that of the pelvic segment approaches from a lateral direction (Fig. 3.15); the ureters should be retracted accordingly.

Ureteric Calculi

The ureters are expansile muscular tubes that dilate if obstructed. Acute obstruction usually results from a ureteric calculus (L. pebble). The symptoms and severity depend on the location, type, and size of the calculus and on whether it is smooth or spiky. Although passage of small calculi usually causes little or no pain, larger ones produce severe pain. The pain caused by a calculus is a *colicky pain* (resembling colonic pain), which results from hyperperistalsis in the ureter superior to the level of the obstruction. Ureteric calculi may cause complete or intermittent obstruction of urinary flow. The obstruction may occur anywhere along the ureter but it occurs most often at the three sites where the ureters are normally relatively constricted (Fig. 3.14A): (1) at the junction of the ureters and renal pelves, (2) where they cross the external iliac artery and pelvic brim, and (3) during their passage through the wall of the urinary bladder. The presence of calculi can often be confirmed by abdominal radiographs or an intravenous urogram (see Chapter 2). Ureteric calculi may be removed by open surgery, by endoscopy (**endourology**), or lithotripsy. **Lithotripsy** uses shock waves to break up a stone into small fragments that can be passed in the urine. ✛

THE BOTTOM LINE: The ureters carry urine from the renal pelves to the urinary bladder. They descend subperitoneally into the pelvis, passing inferior to the ductus deferens of the male or the uterine artery of the female, the latter relationship being of particular surgical importance. They penetrate the bladder wall obliquely from its posteroinferior angle, creating a one-way valve. The pelvic portion of each ureter is served by the inferior vesical (male) or vaginal (female) artery, the vesical venous plexus and internal iliac veins, and the external (superior part) and inferior iliac (lower part) lymph nodes. Calculi, likely to become entrapped where the ureter crosses the pelvic brim or enters the bladder, produce severe groin pain.

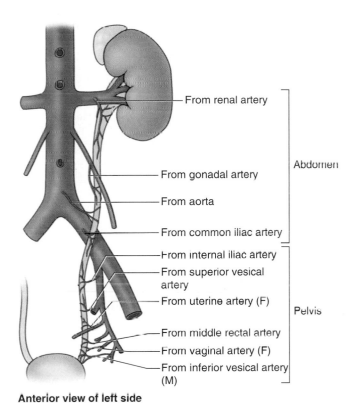

From renal artery

Abdomen

From gonadal artery

From aorta

From common iliac artery

From internal iliac artery

From superior vesical artery

From uterine artery (F)

Pelvis

From middle rectal artery

From vaginal artery (F)

From inferior vesical artery (M)

Anterior view of left side

Figure 3.15. Blood supply of ureter. Branches supplying the abdominal half of the ureter approach medially, while those supplying the pelvic half approach laterally. During surgery, the ureters are avoided and left undisturbed when possible; if necessary, traction of the ureters should be applied gently and only toward the blood supply to avoid disruption of the small (delicate) branches.

Urinary Bladder

The **urinary bladder,** a hollow viscus with strong muscular walls, is characterized by its distensibility (Fig. 3.17A). The urinary bladder is a temporary reservoir for urine and varies in size, shape, position, and relationships according to its content and the state of neighboring viscera. When empty, the adult urinary bladder is located in the lesser pelvis, lying partially superior to and partially posterior to the pubic bones (Fig. 3.17B). It is separated from these bones by the potential *retropubic space* (of Retzius) and lies mostly inferior to the peritoneum, resting on the pubic bones and pubic symphysis anteriorly and the pelvic floor posteriorly (Fig. 3.17). The bladder is relatively free within the extraperitoneal subcutaneous fatty tissue, except for its neck, which is held firmly by the lateral ligaments of bladder and the tendinous arch of the pelvic fascia—especially its anterior components, the *puboprostatic ligament* in males and the *pubovesical ligament* in females (Figs. 3.9 and 3.17).

In infants and young children, the urinary bladder is in the abdomen even when empty (Fig. 3.18A). The bladder usually enters the greater pelvis by 6 years of age; however, it is not located entirely within the lesser pelvis until after puberty. An empty bladder in an adult lies almost entirely in the lesser pelvis, its superior surface level with the superior margin of the pubic symphysis (Fig. 3.18B). As the bladder fills, it enters the greater pelvis as it ascends in the extraperitoneal fatty tissue of the anterior abdominal wall (Fig. 3.17A). In some individuals, a full bladder may ascend to the level of the umbilicus.

At the end of micturition (urination) the bladder of a normal adult contains virtually no urine. When empty, the bladder is somewhat tetrahedral (Fig. 3.18B) and externally has an apex, body, fundus, and neck. The bladder's four surfaces (superior, two inferolateral, and posterior) are most apparent when viewing an empty, contracted bladder that has been removed from a cadaver, when the bladder appears rather boat shaped.

The **apex of the bladder** points toward the superior edge of the pubic symphysis when the bladder is empty. The **fundus of the bladder** is opposite the apex, formed by the somewhat convex posterior wall. The **body of the bladder** is the major portion of the bladder between the apex and the fundus. The fundus and *inferolateral surfaces* meet inferiorly at the **neck of the bladder.**

The **bladder bed** is formed by the structures that directly contact it. On each side, the pubic bones and the fascia covering the levator ani and the superior obturator internus lie in contact with the inferolateral surfaces of the bladder (Fig. 3.18C). Only the superior surface is covered by peritoneum. Consequently, in males the fundus is separated from the rectum centrally by only the fascial rectovesical septum and laterally by the seminal glands and ampullae of the ductus deferentes (Fig. 3.17A); in females the fundus is directly related to the superior anterior wall of the vagina (Fig. 3.17B). The bladder is enveloped by a loose connective tissue visceral fascia.

The walls of the bladder are composed chiefly of the **detrusor muscle.** Toward the neck of the male bladder, the muscle fibers form the involuntary **internal urethral sphincter.** This sphincter contracts during ejaculation to prevent *retrograde ejaculation* (*ejaculatory reflux*) of semen into the bladder. Some fibers run radially and assist in opening the **internal urethral orifice.** In males, the muscle fibers in the neck of the bladder are continuous with the fibromuscular tissue of the prostate, whereas in females these fibers are continuous with muscle fibers in the wall of the urethra. The **ureteric orifices** and the internal urethral orifice are at the angles of the **trigone of the bladder** (Fig. 3.18C). The ureteric orifices are encircled by loops of detrusor musculature that tighten when the bladder contracts to assist in preventing reflux of urine into the ureter. The **uvula of the bladder** is a slight elevation of the trigone; it is usually more prominent in older men owing to enlargement of the posterior lobe of the prostate (see Fig. 3.20A).

Arterial Supply of the Bladder. The main arteries supplying the bladder are branches of the internal iliac arteries (Table 3.5). The *superior vesical arteries* supply anterosuperior parts of the bladder. In males, *inferior vesical arteries*

Key

- ☐ Lumbar (caval/aortic)
- ■ Inferior mesenteric
- ☐ Common iliac
- ■ Internal iliac
- ☐ External iliac
- ■ Deep inguinal

(A) Anterior view

Key

- ☐ Sympathetic nerves
- ■ Parasympathetic nerves
- ■ Mixed sympathetic and parasympathetic nerves
- ■ Somatic nerves

(B) Anterior view

Figure 3.16. Lymphatic drainage of lower urinary system and innervation of ureter. A. The lymphatic drainage of the ureters, urinary bladder, and urethra in the male is shown. The *arrows* indicate the direction of lymph flow to the lymph nodes. The same routes are followed from the urinary systems of females. **B.** Nerve fibers from the renal, aortic, and superior and inferior hypogastric plexuses extend to the ureter, carrying visceral afferent and sympathetic fibers to the T10–L1 spinal sensory ganglia and cord segments and parasympathetic fibers primarily from the S2–S4 spinal cord segments.

supply the fundus and neck of the bladder. In females, the *vaginal arteries* replace the inferior vesical arteries and send small branches to posteroinferior parts of the bladder (Fig. 3.11*B*). The obturator and inferior gluteal arteries also supply small branches to the bladder.

Venous and Lymphatic Drainage of the Bladder. The names of the veins correspond to the arteries and are tributaries of the internal iliac veins. In males, the *vesical venous plexus* is continuous with the *prostatic venous plexus* (Fig. 3.13*C*) and the combined plexus complex envelops the fundus of the bladder and prostate, the seminal glands, the ductus deferentes,

and the inferior ends of the ureters. It also receives blood from the deep dorsal vein of the penis, which drains into the prostatic venous plexus. The *vesical venous plexus* is the part of the plexus complex that is most directly associated with the bladder itself. It mainly drains through the inferior vesical veins into the internal iliac veins; however, it may drain through the sacral veins into the *internal vertebral venous plexuses* (see Chapter 4). In females, the vesical venous plexus envelops the pelvic part of the urethra and the neck of the bladder, receives blood from the *dorsal vein of the clitoris,* and communicates with the *vaginal or uterovaginal venous plexus* (Fig. 3.13*B*).

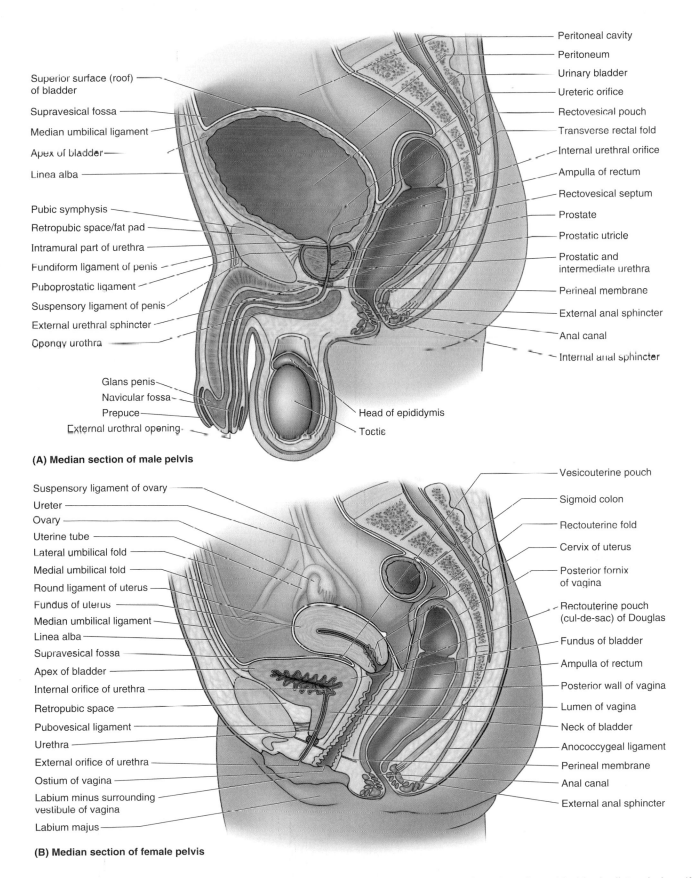

(A) Median section of male pelvis

Superior surface (roof) of bladder
Supravesical fossa
Median umbilical ligament
Apex of bladder
Linea alba
Pubic symphysis
Retropubic space/fat pad
Intramural part of urethra
Fundiform ligament of penis
Puboprostatic ligament
Suspensory ligament of penis
External urethral sphincter
Spongy urethra
Glans penis
Navicular fossa
Prepuce
External urethral opening

Peritoneal cavity
Peritoneum
Urinary bladder
Ureteric orifice
Rectovesical pouch
Transverse rectal fold
Internal urethral orifice
Ampulla of rectum
Rectovesical septum
Prostate
Prostatic utricle
Prostatic and intermediate urethra
Perineal membrane
External anal sphincter
Anal canal
Internal anal sphincter
Head of epididymis
Testis

(B) Median section of female pelvis

Suspensory ligament of ovary
Ureter
Ovary
Uterine tube
Lateral umbilical fold
Medial umbilical fold
Round ligament of uterus
Fundus of uterus
Median umbilical ligament
Linea alba
Supravesical fossa
Apex of bladder
Internal orifice of urethra
Retropubic space
Pubovesical ligament
Urethra
External orifice of urethra
Ostium of vagina
Labium minus surrounding vestibule of vagina
Labium majus

Vesicouterine pouch
Sigmoid colon
Rectouterine fold
Cervix of uterus
Posterior fornix of vagina
Rectouterine pouch (cul-de-sac) of Douglas
Fundus of bladder
Ampulla of rectum
Posterior wall of vagina
Lumen of vagina
Neck of bladder
Anococcygeal ligament
Perineal membrane
Anal canal
External anal sphincter

Figure 3.17. Viscera in hemisected male and female pelves. A. In this male pelvis, the urinary bladder is distended, as if full. Compare its relation to the anterior abdominal wall, pubic symphysis, and level of the supravesical fossa to that of the non-distended (empty) bladder in part **B. B.** In this female pelvis, the uterus was sectioned in its own median plane and is depicted as though it coincided with the median plane of the body, which is seldom the case. With the bladder empty, the normal disposition of the uterus shown here—bent on itself (anteflexed) at the junction of the body and cervix and tipped anteriorly (anteverted)—causes its weight to be borne mainly by the bladder. The urethra lies anterior and parallel to the lower half of the vagina.

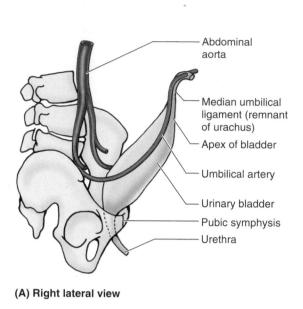

(A) Right lateral view

- Abdominal aorta
- Median umbilical ligament (remnant of urachus)
- Apex of bladder
- Umbilical artery
- Urinary bladder
- Pubic symphysis
- Urethra

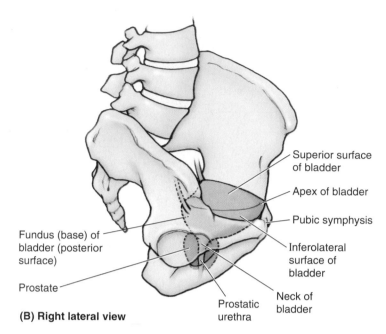

(B) Right lateral view

- Superior surface of bladder
- Apex of bladder
- Pubic symphysis
- Inferolateral surface of bladder
- Neck of bladder
- Prostatic urethra
- Prostate
- Fundus (base) of bladder (posterior surface)

Figure 3.18. Urinary bladder and prostatic urethra. A. The bladder of an infant has a fusiform shape and lies almost entirely in the abdominal cavity, above the pelvic inlet (superior pelvic aperture). **B.** This view of an adult bladder and prostate demonstrates their pelvic location and the surfaces of the bladder. **C.** In this view of the posterior part of a male pelvis sectioned coronally in the plane of the prostatic urethra, the obturator internus forms the pelvic walls and the levator ani muscles support the prostate and bladder.

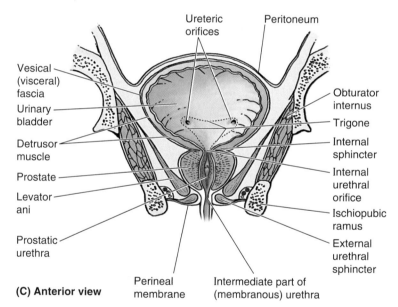

(C) Anterior view

- Ureteric orifices
- Peritoneum
- Vesical (visceral) fascia
- Urinary bladder
- Detrusor muscle
- Prostate
- Levator ani
- Prostatic urethra
- Obturator internus
- Trigone
- Internal sphincter
- Internal urethral orifice
- Ischiopubic ramus
- External urethral sphincter
- Perineal membrane
- Intermediate part of (membranous) urethra

In both sexes, **lymphatic vessels** from the superolateral aspects of the bladder pass to the *external iliac lymph nodes* (Fig. 3.16*A;* Table 3.6), whereas those from the fundus and neck pass to the *internal iliac lymph nodes*. Some vessels from the neck of the bladder drain into the sacral or common iliac lymph nodes.

Innervation of the Bladder. Sympathetic fibers are conveyed from inferior thoracic and upper lumbar spinal cord levels to the vesical (pelvic) plexuses primarily through the hypogastric plexuses and nerves, whereas parasympathetic fibers from sacral spinal cord levels are conveyed by the

pelvic splanchnic nerves and the inferior hypogastric plexus (Fig. 3.19). The parasympathetic fibers are motor to the detrusor muscle and inhibitory to the internal urethral sphincter of the male bladder. Hence, when visceral afferent fibers are stimulated by stretching, the bladder contracts reflexively, the internal urethral sphincter relaxes (in males), and urine flows into the urethra. With toilet training, we learn to suppress this reflex when we do not wish to void. The sympathetic innervation that stimulates ejaculation simultaneously causes contraction of the internal urethral sphincter, to prevent reflux of semen into the bladder. A sympathetic

Figure 3.19. Innervation of bladder and urethra. Presynaptic sympathetic fibers from the T11–L2 or L3 spinal cord levels involved in innervation of the bladder, prostate, and proximal urethra pass via lumbar splanchnic nerves to the aortic/hypogastric system of plexuses, synapsing in the plexuses en route to the pelvic viscera. Presynaptic parasympathetic fibers to the bladder arise from neurons in the S2–S4 spinal cord segments and pass from the anterior rami of spinal nerves S2–S4 via the pelvic splanchnic nerves and inferior hypogastric and vesical (pelvic) plexuses to the bladder. They synapse with postsynaptic neurons located on or near the bladder wall. Visceral afferent fibers conveying reflex information and pain sensation from subperitoneal viscera (inferior to the pelvic pain line) follow parasympathetic fibers retrogradely to the S2–S4 spinal ganglia, whereas those conducting pain from the bladder roof (superior to the pelvic pain line) follow sympathetic fibers retrogradely to the T11–L2 or L3 spinal ganglia. The pelvic (sacral) sympathetic trunk primarily serves the lower limb. The somatic nerves shown here are distributed to the perineum.

response at moments other than ejaculation (e.g., self-consciousness when standing at the urinal in front of a waiting line) can cause the internal sphincter to contract, hampering the ability to urinate until parasympathetic inhibition of the sphincter occurs.

Sensory fibers from the bladder are visceral; reflex afferents follow the course of the parasympathetic fibers, as do those transmitting pain sensations (such as results from overdistension) from the inferior part of the bladder. The superior surface (roof) of the bladder is covered with peritoneum and is therefore superior to the *pelvic pain line;* thus pain fibers from the superior bladder follow the sympathetic fibers retrogradely to the inferior thoracic and upper lumbar spinal ganglia (T11–L2 or L3).

Cystocele—Hernia of the Bladder

Loss of bladder support in females by damage to the perineal muscles or their associated fascia can result in herniation of the bladder into the vaginal wall (Fig. B3.6A). A cystocele may also result from prolapse of pelvic viscera secondary to injury to the pelvic floor during childbirth.

Suprapubic Cystotomy

Although the superior surface of the empty bladder lies at the level of the superior margin of the pubic symphysis (Fig. B3.6B), as the bladder fills it extends superiorly above the symphysis into the loose areolar tissue between the parietal peritoneum and anterior abdominal wall (Fig. B3.6C). The bladder then lies adjacent to this wall without the intervention of peritoneum. Consequently, the distended bladder may be punctured (*suprapubic cystotomy*) or approached surgically superior to the pubic

symphysis for the introduction of in-dwelling catheters or instruments without traversing the peritoneum and entering the peritoneal cavity (Fig. B3.6D). Urinary calculi, foreign bodies, and small tumors may also be removed from the bladder through a suprapubic extraperitoneal incision.

Rupture of the Bladder

Because of the superior position of the distended bladder, it may be ruptured by injuries to the inferior part of the anterior abdominal wall or by fractures of the pelvis. The rupture may result in the escape of urine extraperitoneally or intraperitoneally. Rupture of the superior part of the bladder frequently tears the peritoneum, resulting in *extravasation (passage) of urine into the peritoneal cavity*. Posterior rupture of the bladder usually results in passage of urine extraperitoneally into the perineum. ▶

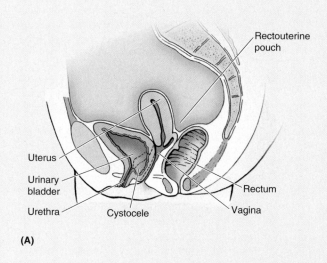

Rectouterine pouch

Uterus

Urinary bladder

Urethra

Cystocele

Rectum

Vagina

(A)

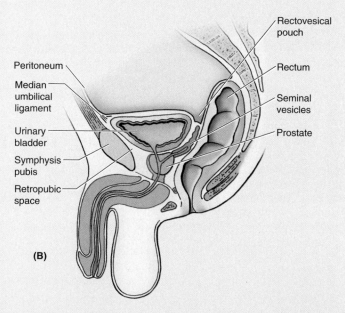

Peritoneum

Median umbilical ligament

Urinary bladder

Symphysis pubis

Retropubic space

Rectovesical pouch

Rectum

Seminal vesicles

Prostate

(B)

Figure B3.6

0–10 cm

(C)

Supra-
pubic
catheter

Bladder

(D)

Urethral
catheter

Figure B3.6. *(Continued)*

Cystoscopy

The interior of the bladder and its three orifices can be examined with a *cystoscope* (see clinical correlation [blue] box "Ureteric Calculi," in this chapter). During *transurethral resection of a tumor*, the instrument is passed into the bladder through the urethra (Fig. B3.7). Using a high-frequency electrical current, the tumor is removed in small fragments that are washed from the bladder with water. ○

Urinary bladder

Cystoscope

Medial view (from left)

Figure B3.7

THE BOTTOM LINE: The superior and inferior portions of the urinary bladder are quite distinct anatomically and functionally. The body is highly distensible, embedded in loose extraperitoneal fat, and covered on its superior aspect with peritoneum, all of which allow expansion with filling. In contrast, the relatively indistensible neck is anchored in place by pelvic ligaments and the floor of the bladder overlying it (which includes the trigone of the bladder) and remains relatively unchanged with filling. Most of the bladder body is served by superior vesical arteries and veins and lymphatic vessels that drain to external iliac lymph nodes. The neck and adjacent inferior body are served by inferior vesical arteries, the vesical venous plexus, and lymphatic vessels that drain to internal iliac nodes. Sympathetic fibers from inferior thoracic and superior lumbar spinal cord segments maintain the tonus of the bladder neck and, in males during ejaculation, stimulate contraction of the internal urethra sphincter to prevent reflux of semen. Parasympathetic fibers conveyed by pelvic splanchnic nerves from the S2–S4 spinal cord segments inhibit the neck musculature and stimulate increased tonus of the detrusor muscle of the bladder walls for urination. Visceral afferent fibers conducting pain sensation from the roof of the bladder (superior to the pelvic pain line) follow the sympathetic fibers retrogradely to spinal sensory ganglia; the remaining visceral afferent fibers follow the parasympathetic fibers.

Proximal Male Urethra

The **male urethra** is a muscular tube (18–22 cm long) that conveys urine from the *internal urethral orifice* of the urinary bladder to the *external urethral orifice,* located at the tip of the glans penis in males (Fig. 3.17*A*). The urethra also provides an exit for semen (sperms and glandular secretions). In the *flaccid* (non-erect) state, the urethra has a double curvature. For descriptive purposes, the urethra is divided into four parts, described in Table 3.7 and demonstrated in Figures 3.17*A* and 3.20. The distal *intermediate part* and *spongy urethra* will be described further with the perineum (later in this chapter).

The **intramural part of the urethra (preprostatic urethra)** varies in diameter and length, depending on whether the bladder is filling (bladder neck is tonically contracted so the internal urethral orifice is small and high; the *filling internal urethral orifice*) or emptying (the neck is relaxed so the orifice is wide and low; the *emptying internal urethral orifice*). The most prominent feature of the **prostatic urethra** is the **urethral crest,** a median ridge between bilateral grooves, the **prostatic sinuses** (Fig. 3.20). The secretory ducts of the prostate, the *prostatic ducts,* open into the prostatic sinuses. The **seminal colliculus** is a rounded eminence in the middle of the urethral crest with a slit-like orifice that opens into a small cul-de-sac, the **prostatic utricle** (Figs. 3.20 and 3.21). The prostatic utricle is the vestigial remnant of the embryonic uterovaginal canal, the surrounding walls of which, in the female, constitute the primordium of the uterus and a part of the vagina (Moore and Persaud, 2003). The *ejaculatory ducts* open into the prostatic urethra via minute, slit-like openings located adjacent to and occasionally just within the orifice of the prostatic utricle. Thus urinary and reproductive tracts merge at this point.

Arterial Supply of the Proximal Male Urethra. The proximal two parts of the urethra are supplied by *prostatic branches* of the *inferior vesical* and *middle rectal arteries* (Figs. 3.11*A* & *C* and 3.22; Table 3.5).

Venous and Lymphatic Drainage of the Proximal Male Urethra. The veins from the proximal two parts of the urethra drain into the *prostatic venous plexus* (Fig. 3.22). The lymphatic vessels pass mainly to the *internal iliac lymph nodes;* a few vessels drain into the *external iliac lymph nodes* (Fig. 3.16*A;* Table 3.6).

Innervation of the Proximal Male Urethra. The nerves are derived from the prostatic plexus (mixed sympathetic, parasympathetic, and visceral afferent fibers) (Fig. 3.19). The **prostatic plexus** is one of the pelvic plexuses (an inferior extension of the vesical plexus) arising as organ-specific extensions of the inferior hypogastric plexus.

Female Urethra

The **female urethra** (approximately 4 cm long and 6 mm in diameter) passes anteroinferiorly from the *internal urethral orifice* of the urinary bladder (Fig. 3.17*B*), posterior and then inferior to the pubic symphysis, to the *external urethral orifice.* The musculature surrounding the internal urethral orifice of the female bladder is not organized into an internal sphincter. In females, the **external urethral orifice** is located in the vestibule, directly anterior to the *vaginal orifice.* The urethra lies anterior to the vagina (forming an elevation in the anterior vaginal wall) (Fig. 3.27*C*); its axis is parallel to that of the vagina. The urethra passes with the vagina through the pelvic diaphragm, external urethral sphincter, and perineal membrane. Urethral glands are present, particularly in the superior part of the urethra. One group of glands on each side, the *paraurethral glands,* are homologues to the prostate. These glands have a common paraurethral duct, which opens (one on each side) near the external urethral orifice. The inferior half of the urethra is located in the perineum and is discussed in that section.

Table 3.7. Parts of the Male Urethra

Part	Length	Location/Disposition	Features
Intramural (preprostatic) part	0.5–1.5 cm	Extends almost vertically through neck of bladder	Surrounded by internal urethral sphincter; diameter and length vary, depending on whether bladder is filling or emptying
Prostatic urethra	3.0–4.0 cm	Descends through anterior prostate, forming a gentle, anteriorly concave curve; is bounded anteriorly by a vertical trough-like part (rhabdosphincter) of external urethral sphincter	Widest and most dilatable part; features urethral crest with seminal colliculus, flanked by prostatic sinuses into which prostatic ducts open; ejaculatory ducts open onto colliculus, hence urinary and reproductive tracts merge in this part
Intermediate (membranous) part	1.0–1.5 cm	Passes through deep perineal pouch, surrounded by circular fibers of external urethral sphincter; penetrates perineal membrane	Narrowest and least distensible part (except for external urethral orifice)
Spongy urethra	~ 15 cm	Courses through corpus spongiosum; initial widening occurs in bulb of penis; widens again distally as navicular fossa (in glans penis)	Longest and most mobile part; bulbourethral glands open into bulbous part; distally, urethral glands open into small urethral lacunae entering lumen of this part

Arterial Supply of the Female Urethra. Blood is supplied to the female urethra by the *internal pudendal* and *vaginal arteries* (Figs. 3.11*B* and 3.12*A*; Table 3.5).

Venous and Lymphatic Drainage of the Female Urethra. The veins follow the arteries and have similar names (Fig. 3.13*B*). Most lymphatic vessels from the urethra pass to the *sacral* and *internal iliac lymph nodes* (Table 3.6), but a few vessels from the distal urethra drain into the *inguinal lymph nodes*.

Innervation of the Female Urethra. The nerves to the urethra arise from the *vesical (nerve) plexus* and the *pudendal nerve*. The pattern is similar to that in the male (Fig. 3.19), given the absence of a prostatic plexus and an internal urethra sphincter. Visceral afferents from most of the urethra run in the pelvic splanchnic nerves, but the termination receives somatic afferents from the pudendal nerve. Both the visceral and the somatic afferent fibers extend from cell bodies in the S2–S4 spinal ganglia.

(A) Anterior view

(B) Diagrammatic enlargement of (A)

Figure 3.20. Interior of male bladder and urethra. A. The anterior parts of the bladder, prostate, and urethra are cut away. A portion of the posterior wall of the bladder has been removed to reveal the intramural ureter and the ductus deferens posterior to the bladder. The interureteric fold runs between the entrances of the ureters into the bladder lumen, demarcating the superior limit of the trigone of the bladder. The prominence of the posterior wall of the internal urethral orifice (at the tip of the leader line indicating this orifice), when exaggerated, becomes the uvula of the bladder. This small projection is produced by the middle (median) lobe of the prostate. The prostatic utricle opens via an oval mouth on the summit of the seminal colliculus, with orifices of an ejaculatory duct on each side. The prostatic fascia encloses the prostatic venous plexus. **B.** This enlarged detail of the boxed area in **A** demonstrates the bulbourethral glands embedded in the substance of the external urethral sphincter.

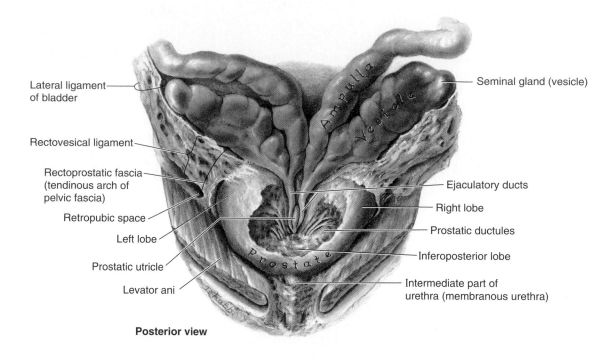

Lateral ligament of bladder

Rectovesical ligament

Rectoprostatic fascia (tendinous arch of pelvic fascia)

Retropubic space

Left lobe

Prostatic utricle

Levator ani

Seminal gland (vesicle)

Ampulla

Vesicle

Ejaculatory ducts

Right lobe

Prostatic ductules

Inferoposterior lobe

Intermediate part of urethra (membranous urethra)

Prostate

Posterior view

Figure 3.21. Dissection of posterior part of prostate, lateral ligament of bladder, and rectoprostatic fascia. The ejaculatory ducts are formed by the merger of the duct of the seminal gland and the ductus deferens. The vestigial prostatic utricle, usually seen as an invagination in an anterior view, appears in this posterior dissection as an evagination lying between the ejaculatory ducts.

Ureter

Ureteric artery

Deferential artery (artery to ductus deferens)

Inferior vesicle artery

Ampulla of ductus deferens

Arteries to seminal gland

Ejaculatory duct

Prostatic artery

Prostatic ducts

Levator ani muscle (cut)

Bulbourethral gland

Intermediate (membranous) part of the urethra

Corpus cavernosum (cut)

Cut edge of peritoneum

Ductus deferens

Urinary bladder

Seminal gland

Prostate

Prostatic venous plexus

External urethral sphincter

Compressor urethrae muscle (cut)

Perineal membrane

Spongy urethra

Bulb of penis covered by bulbospongiosus muscle

Posterior view

Figure 3.22. Urinary bladder, seminal glands, terminal parts of ductus deferens, and prostate. The left seminal gland and ampulla of the ductus deferens are dissected free and sliced open. Part of the prostate is also cut away to expose the ejaculatory duct. The perineal membrane lies between the external genitalia and the deep part of the perineum (anterior recess of ischioanal fossa). It is pierced by the urethra, ducts of the bulbourethral glands, dorsal and deep arteries of the penis, cavernous nerves, and the dorsal nerve of the penis.

Clinically Significant Differences between Male and Female Urethrae

The female urethra is distensible because it contains considerable elastic tissue, as well as smooth muscle. It can be easily dilated without injury; consequently, the passage of catheters or cystoscopes is easier in females than in males. Infections of the urethra, and especially the bladder, are more common in women because the female urethra is short, more distensible, and is open to the exterior through the vestibule of the vagina. ○

THE BOTTOM LINE: The male urethra consists of four parts, two of which are the intramural and prostatic parts. The intramural part varies in length and caliber, depending on whether the bladder is filling or emptying. The prostatic urethra is distinguished both by its surroundings and the structures that open into it. It is surrounded by the prostate, the muscular anterior "lobe" that includes the trough-like superior extension of the external urethral sphincter anteriorly, and by the glandular lobes posteriorly. Opening into the prostatic sinuses on each side of the urethral crest are the prostatic ducts. The vestigial utricle is a relatively large opening in the center of the seminal colliculus, flanked by the tiny openings of the ejaculatory ducts. Thus the reproductive and urinary tracts merge within the prostatic urethra.

The female urethra runs parallel to the vagina. It is firmly attached to and indents the anterior vaginal wall centrally and distally.

Male Internal Genital Organs

The male internal genital organs include the testes, epididymides (singular = epididymis), ductus deferentes (singular = ductus deferens), seminal glands, ejaculatory ducts, prostate, and bulbourethral glands (Figs. 3.22 and 3.23). Although external in position postnatally, the testes and epididymides (described in Chapter 2) are considered internal genital organs on the basis of their developmental position and homology with the internal female gonads (ovaries).

Ductus Deferens

The **ductus deferens** (deferent duct, vas deferens) is the continuation of the duct of the epididymis. The ductus deferens:

- Has relatively thick muscular walls and a minute lumen, giving it a cord-like firmness.

- Begins in the tail of the epididymis, at the inferior pole of the testis.

- Ascends posterior to testis, medial to the epididymis.

- Is the primary component of the spermatic cord.

- Penetrates the anterior abdominal wall via the inguinal canal.

- Crosses over the external iliac vessels and enters the pelvis.

- Passes along the lateral wall of the pelvis, where it lies external to the parietal peritoneum.

- Ends by joining the duct of the seminal gland to form the *ejaculatory duct.*

During the pelvic part of its course, the ductus deferens maintains direct contact with the peritoneum; no other structure intervenes between them. The ductus crosses superior to the ureter near the posterolateral angle of the bladder, running between the ureter and the peritoneum of the ureteric fold to reach the fundus of the bladder. The relationship of the ductus deferens to the ureter in the male is similar, although of lesser clinical importance, to that of the uterine artery to the ureter in the female. The developmental basis of this relationship is shown in Figure 3.24. Posterior to the bladder, the ductus deferens at first lies superior to the seminal gland, then descends medial to the ureter and the gland. Here the ductus deferens enlarges to form the **ampulla of the ductus deferens** before its termination (Fig. 3.22).

Arterial Supply of the Ductus Deferens. The tiny *artery to the ductus deferens* usually arises from a superior (sometimes inferior) vesical artery (Figs. 3.22 and 3.23; Table 3.5) and terminates by anastomosing with the testicular artery, posterior to the testis.

Venous and Lymphatic Drainage of the Ductus Deferens. Veins from most of the ductus drain into the testicular vein, including the distal pampiniform plexus. Its terminal portion drains into the vesicular/prostatic venous plexus. Lymphatic vessels from the ductus deferens end in the *external iliac lymph nodes* (Fig. 3.25; Table 3.6).

Male Sterilization

The common method of male sterilization is a **deferentectomy,** popularly called a *vasectomy.* During this procedure, part of the ductus deferens is ligated and/or excised through an incision in the superior part of the scrotum (Fig. B3.8). Hence, the subsequent ejaculated fluid from the seminal glands, prostate, and bulbourethral glands contains no sperms. The unexpelled sperms degenerate in the epididymis and the proximal part of the ductus deferens. *Reversal of a deferentectomy* is successful in favorable cases (patients < 30 years of age and ▶

< 7 years postoperation) in most instances. The ends of the sectioned ductus deferentes are reattached under an operating microscope. ✪

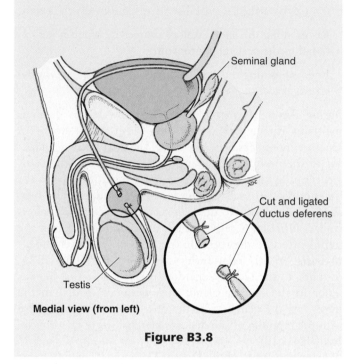

Figure B3.8

Labels in figure: Seminal gland; Cut and ligated ductus deferens; Testis; Medial view (from left)

THE BOTTOM LINE: The cord-like ductus deferens is the primary component of the spermatic cord, conducting sperms from the epididymis to the ejaculatory duct. Its distal portion is superficial within the scrotum (and, therefore, easily accessible for deferentectomy) before it penetrates the anterior abdominal wall via the inguinal canal. Its pelvic portion lies immediately external to the peritoneum, with its terminal portion enlarging externally as its lumen becomes tortuous internally, forming the ampulla of the ductus deferens.

Seminal Glands

Each **seminal gland** (vesicle) is an elongated structure (typically approximately 5 cm long but sometimes much shorter) that lies between the fundus of the bladder and the rectum (Figs. 3.21 and 3.23). The seminal glands are obliquely placed glands superior to the prostate and do not store sperms, as their name implies. They secrete a thick alkaline fluid with fructose (an energy source for the sperms) and a coagulating agent that mixes with the sperms as they pass into the ejaculatory ducts and urethra. The superior ends of the seminal glands are covered with peritoneum and lie posterior to the ureters, where the peritoneum of the *rectovesical pouch* separates them from the rectum. The inferior ends of the seminal glands are closely related to the rectum and are separated from it only by the rectovesical septum (Fig. 3.23). The duct of the seminal gland joins the ductus deferens to form the *ejaculatory duct.*

Arterial Supply of the Seminal Glands. The arteries to the seminal glands derive from the *inferior vesical* and *middle rectal arteries* (Fig. 3.22; Table 3.5).

Venous and Lymphatic Drainage of the Seminal Glands. The veins accompany the arteries and have similar names (Fig. 3.13C). The iliac lymph nodes receive lymph from the seminal glands: the *external iliac nodes* from the superior part, and the *internal iliac nodes* from the inferior part (Fig. 3.25; Table 3.6).

Abscesses in the Seminal Glands

Localized collections of pus (abscesses) in the seminal glands may rupture, allowing pus to enter the peritoneal cavity. Seminal glands can be palpated during a rectal examination, especially if enlarged or full. They are palpated most easily when the bladder is moderately full. They can also be massaged to release their secretions for microscopic examination to detect *gonococci,* for example (the organisms that cause gonorrhea). ✪

Ejaculatory Ducts

The **ejaculatory ducts** are slender tubes that arise by the union of the ducts of a seminal glands with the ductus deferentes (Figs. 3.21–3.23). The ejaculatory ducts (approximately 2.5 cm long) arise near the neck of the bladder and run close together as they pass anteroinferiorly through the posterior part of the prostate and along the sides of the prostatic utricle. The ejaculatory ducts converge to open on the seminal colliculus by tiny, slit-like apertures on, or just within, the opening of the prostatic utricle (Fig. 3.19). Although the ejaculatory ducts traverse the glandular prostate, prostatic secretions join the seminal fluid in the prostatic urethra after the ejaculatory ducts have terminated.

Arterial Supply of the Ejaculatory Ducts. The *arteries to the ductus deferens,* usually branches of the superior (but frequently inferior) vesical arteries, supply the ejaculatory ducts (Figs. 3.22–3.23).

Venous and Lymphatic Drainage of the Ejaculatory Ducts. The veins join the *prostatic* and *vesical venous plexuses* (Fig. 3.13C). The lymphatic vessels drain into the *external iliac lymph nodes* (Fig. 3.25).

Prostate

The **prostate** (approximately 3 cm long, 4 cm wide, and 2 cm in AP depth) is the largest accessory gland of the male reproductive system (Figs. 3.19 and 3.21–3.23). The glandular part makes up approximately two thirds of the prostate; the other third is fibromuscular. The firm, walnut-size prostate surrounds the *prostatic urethra.* The **fibrous capsule of the prostate** is dense and neurovascular, incorporating the prostatic plexuses of veins and nerves. All this is surrounded in turn by the *visceral layer of the pelvic fascia,* forming a fibrous *prostatic sheath* that is thin anteriorly, continuous anterolaterally with the *puboprostatic ligaments,* and

Common iliac artery and vein

Internal iliac artery and vein

External iliac artery and vein

Ureter

Cut edge of peritoneum

Sciatic nerve

Inferior vesical artery

Ductus deferens and artery to ductus deferens

Rectovesical pouch

Urinary bladder

Rectovesical septum

Retropubic space

Seminal gland

Prostate (middle lobe)

Coccyx

Prostatic utricle

Rectum (ampulla)

Puboprostatic ligament

Ampulla of ductus deferens

Prostatic urethra

Internal urethral orifice

Ejaculatory duct

Deep dorsal vein of penis

Prostate (inferoposterior lobe)

Isthmus of prostate

Levator ani

External urethral sphincter

Bulbourethral gland

Spongy urethra

Deep transverse perineal muscle

Corpus cavernosum

External anal sphincter

Corpus spongiosum

Internal anal sphincter

Bulb of penis

Spermatic cord

Testicular artery

Pampiniform venous plexus

Epididymis

Glans penis

Testis

Scrotum

External urethral orifice

Medial view

Figure 3.23. Hemisected male pelvis and perineum (right half). The genital organs are demonstrated: testis, epididymis, ductus deferens, ejaculatory duct, and penis, with the accessory glandular structures (seminal gland, prostate, and bulbourethral gland). The spermatic cord connects the testis to the abdominal cavity, and the testis lies externally in a musculocutaneous pouch, the scrotum.

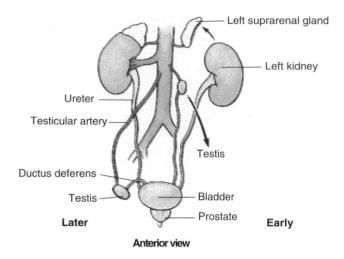

Left suprarenal gland

Left kidney

Ureter

Testicular artery

Testis

Ductus deferens

Testis

Bladder

Prostate

Later   **Early**

Anterior view

Figure 3.24. Structures crossing male ureter in abdomen and pelvis. During development, as the testis descends inferiorly and laterally from its original position (medial to the site of the kidneys on the posterior abdominal wall) to and then through the inguinal canal, the ureter is crossed by testicular vessels in the abdomen and by the ductus deferens in the pelvis. This relationship is retained throughout life.

Key	
☐ Lumbar (caval/aortic)	☐ Internal iliac
■ Inferior mesenteric	☐ External iliac
☐ Common iliac	■ Sacral

Figure 3.25 Lymphatic drainage of male internal genital organs. Lymphatic drainage of the testis, ductus deferens, seminal glands, and prostate is shown. The *arrows* indicate the direction of lymph flow to the lymph nodes.

dense posteriorly where it blends with the *rectovesical septum*. The prostate has

- A base closely related to the neck of the bladder.

- An apex that is in contact with fascia on the superior aspect of the urethral sphincter and deep perineal muscles.

- A muscular anterior surface, featuring mostly transversely oriented muscle fibers forming a vertical, trough-like hemisphincter (rhabdosphincter), which is part of the urethral sphincter, separated from the pubic symphysis by retroperitoneal fat in the retropubic space.

- A posterior surface that is related to the ampulla of the rectum.

- Inferolateral surfaces that are related to the levator ani.

Although not clearly distinct anatomically, the following lobes of the prostate are traditionally described (Figs. 3.21 and 3.23):

- The **isthmus of the prostate** (commissure of prostate; historically, the anterior "lobe") lies anterior to the urethra. It is fibromuscular, the muscle fibers representing a superior continuation of the urethral sphincter muscle, and contains little, if any, glandular tissue.

- The **inferoposterior** (posterior) **lobe** lies posterior to the urethra and inferior to the ejaculatory ducts; it is readily palpable by digital rectal examination.

- The **right** and **left** (lateral) **lobes** on either side of the urethra form the major part of the prostate.

- The **middle** (median) **lobe** lies between the urethra and the ejaculatory ducts and is closely related to the neck of the bladder. Enlargement of the middle lobe is believed to be at least partially responsible for the formation of the *uvula* that may project into the internal urethral orifice (Fig. 3.20).

Some authors, especially urologists and sonographers, divide the prostate into peripheral and central (internal) zones. The central zone is comparable to the middle lobe. Within each lobe are four lobules, which are defined by the arrangement of the ducts and connective tissue.

The **prostatic ducts** (20–30) open chiefly into the grooves, the *prostatic sinuses,* that lie on either side of the seminal colliculus on the posterior wall of the prostatic urethra. Prostatic fluid, a thin, milky fluid, provides approximately 20% of the volume of semen (a mixture of secretions produced by the testes, seminal glands, prostate, and bulbourethral glands) and plays a role in activating the sperms.

Arterial Supply of the Prostate. The prostatic arteries are mainly branches of the internal iliac artery (Fig. 3.11*A* & *C;* Table 3.5), especially the *inferior vesical arteries* but also the internal pudendal and middle rectal arteries.

Venous and Lymphatic Drainage of the Prostate. The veins join to form a plexus around the sides and base of the prostate (Figs. 3.13*C* and 3.22). This **prostatic venous**

plexus, between the fibrous capsule of the prostate and the prostatic sheath, drains into the *internal iliac veins.* The prostatic venous plexus is continuous superiorly with the *vesical venous plexus* and communicates posteriorly with the *internal vertebral venous plexus.* The lymphatic vessels terminate chiefly in the *internal iliac lymph nodes,* but some drainage may pass to the *sacral nodes* (Fig. 3.25; Table 3.6).

Bulbourethral Glands

The two pea-size **bulbourethral glands** (Cowper glands) lie posterolateral to the intermediate part of the urethra, largely embedded within the external urethral sphincter (Figs. 3.20*B* and 3.22–3.23). The **ducts of the bulbourethral glands** pass through the perineal membrane with the intermediate urethra and open through minute apertures into the proximal part of the spongy urethra in the bulb of the penis. Their mucus-like secretion enters the urethra during sexual arousal.

Innervation of the Internal Genital Organs of the Male Pelvis

The ductus deferens, seminal glands, ejaculatory ducts, and prostate are richly innervated by sympathetic nerve fibers. Presynaptic sympathetic fibers originate from cell bodies in the intermediolateral cell column of the T12–L2 (or L3) spinal cord segments. They traverse the paravertebral ganglia of the sympathetic trunks to become components of lumbar (abdominopelvic) splanchnic nerves and the hypogastric and pelvic plexuses. Presynaptic parasympathetic fibers from S2 and S3 spinal cord segments traverse *pelvic splanchnic nerves,* which also join the inferior hypo-gastric/pelvic plexuses. Synapses with postsynaptic sympathetic and parasympathetic neurons occur within the plexuses, en route to or near the pelvic viscera. As part of an orgasm, the sympathetic system stimulates rapid peristaltic-like contractions of the ductus deferens, and the combined contraction of and secretion from the seminal and prostate glands provides the vehicle (semen) and the expulsive force to discharge the sperms (L. *spermatozoa*) during ejaculation. The function of the parasympathetic innervation of the internal genital organs is unclear. However, parasympathetic fibers traversing the prostatic nerve plexus form the *cavernous nerves* that pass to the erectile bodies of the penis, which are responsible for producing penile erection.

Hypertrophy of the Prostate

The prostate is of considerable medical interest because enlargement or **benign hypertrophy of the prostate (BHP),** is common after middle age, affecting virtually every male who lives long enough. An enlarged prostate projects into the urinary bladder and impedes urination by distorting the prostatic urethra. The middle lobe usually enlarges the most and obstructs the internal urethral orifice; the more the person strains, the more the valve-like prostatic mass occludes the urethra. BHP is a common cause of urethral obstruction, leading to **nocturia** (need to void during the night), **dysuria** (difficulty and/or pain during urination), and **urgency** (sudden desire to void). BHP also increases the risk of bladder infections (cystitis) as well as kidney damage.

The prostate is examined for enlargement and tumors (focal masses or asymmetry) by *digital rectal examination* (Fig. B3.9). The palpability of the prostate depends on the fullness of the bladder. A full bladder offers resistance, holding the gland in place and making it more readily palpable. The malignant prostate feels hard and often irregular. In advanced stages, cancer cells metastasize both via lymphatic routes (initially to the internal iliac and sacral lymph nodes and later to distant nodes) and via venous routes (by way of the internal vertebral venous plexus, to the vertebrae and brain).

Because of the close relationship of the prostate to the prostatic urethra, obstructions may be relieved endoscopically. The instrument is inserted transurethrally through the external urethral orifice and spongy urethra into the prostatic urethra. All or part of the prostate, or just

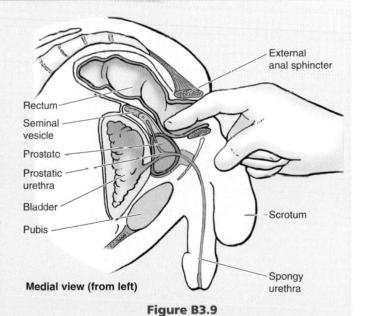

Medial view (from left)

External anal sphincter
Rectum
Seminal vesicle
Prostate
Prostatic urethra
Bladder
Pubis
Scrotum
Spongy urethra

Figure B3.9

the hypertrophied part, is removed (*transurethral resection of the prostate; TURP*). In more serious cases, the entire prostate is removed along with the seminal glands, ejaculatory ducts, and the terminal parts of the deferent ducts (**radical prostatectomy**). TURP and improved open operative techniques attempt to preserve the nerves and blood vessels associated with the capsule of the prostate that pass to and from the penis, increasing the possibility for patients to retain sexual function after surgery as well as restoring normal urinary control. ✪

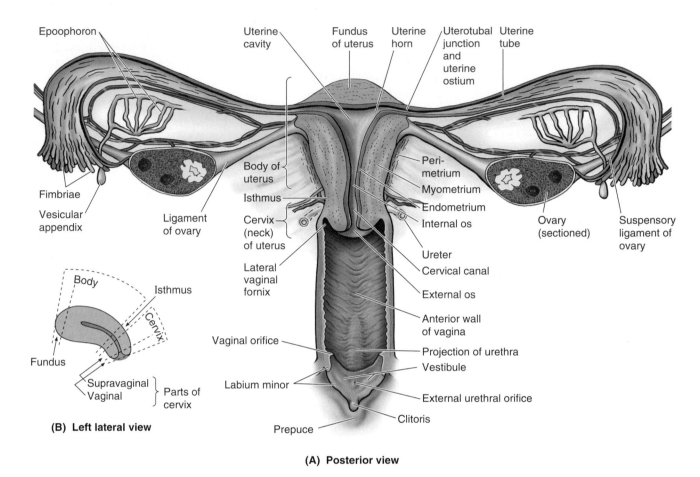

Epoophoron
Uterine cavity
Fundus of uterus
Uterine horn
Uterotubal junction and uterine ostium
Uterine tube
Fimbriae
Vesicular appendix
Ligament of ovary
Body of uterus
Isthmus
Cervix (neck) of uterus
Lateral vaginal fornix
Vaginal orifice
Labium minor
Prepuce
Peri-metrium
Myometrium
Endometrium
Internal os
Ureter
Cervical canal
External os
Anterior wall of vagina
Projection of urethra
Vestibule
External urethral orifice
Clitoris
Ovary (sectioned)
Suspensory ligament of ovary

(B) Left lateral view
Body
Isthmus
Cervix
Fundus
Supravaginal
Vaginal
Parts of cervix

(A) Posterior view

Figure 3.26. Internal female genital organs. A. In this coronal section, the parts of the uterus are demonstrated, including the uterine walls, cervix, and uterine cavity. The uterine tube and ovarian ligament are attached, close together, to the lateral wall of the uterus. The epoophoron is a collection of rudimentary tubules in the mesosalpinx (mesentery of uterine tube). The epoophoron and vesicular appendage are vestiges of the embryonic mesonephros. **B.** This median section of the uterus demonstrates the parts of the body and cervix, which are separated by the isthmus.

THE BOTTOM LINE: Obliquely placed seminal glands converge at the base of the bladder, where each gland merges with the ipsilateral ductus deferens to form an ejaculatory duct. The two ejaculatory ducts immediately enter the posterior aspect of the prostate, running closely parallel through the gland to open on the seminal colliculus. Prostatic ducts open into prostatic sinuses, adjacent to the seminal colliculus. Thus the major secretions and sperms are delivered to the prostatic urethra. The seminal glands and prostate produce by far the greatest portion of the seminal fluid, indispensable for transport and delivery of sperms. These internal genital organs, located within the anterior male pelvis, receive blood from the inferior vesicle and middle rectal arteries, which drain into the continuous prostatic/vesicle venous plexus. Their lymphatic vessels drain to internal and external iliac nodes. Sympathetic fibers from lumbar levels stimulate the contraction and secretion resulting in ejaculation. The function of parasympathetic fibers from S2–S4 to the internal genital organs is unclear, but those traversing the prostatic nerve plexus to form the cavernous nerves produce erection.

Female Internal Genital Organs

The female internal genital organs include the vagina, uterus, uterine tubes, and ovaries.

Vagina

The **vagina**, a musculomembranous tube (7–9 cm long), extends from the cervix of the uterus to the *vestibule*, the cleft between the labia minora. It contains the vaginal and external urethral orifices and the openings of the two greater vestibular glands (Figs. 3.26 and 3.27A–C). The superior end of the vagina surrounds the cervix.

The vagina:

- Serves as a canal for menstrual fluid.

- Forms the inferior part of the pelvic (birth) canal.

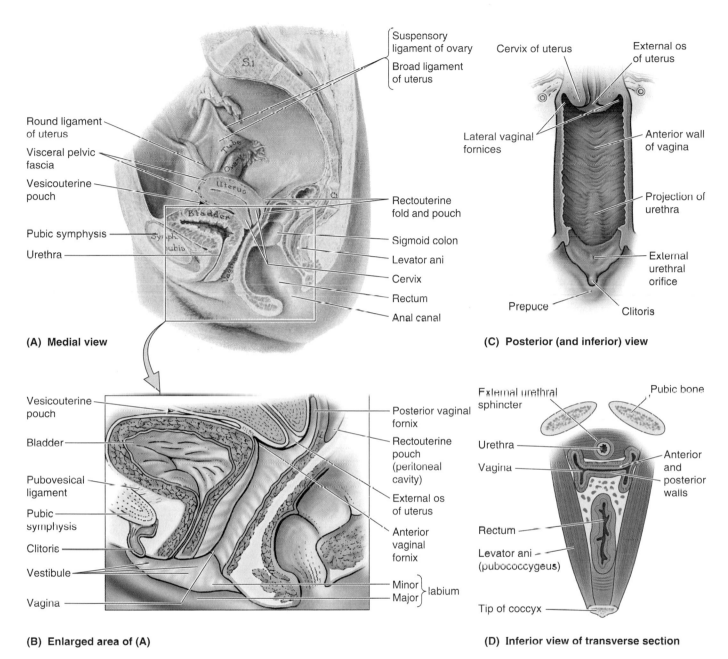

(A) Medial view

(C) Posterior (and inferior) view

(B) Enlarged area of (A)

(D) Inferior view of transverse section

Figure 3.27. Vagina. A and B. The axes of the urethra and vagina are parallel, and the urethra is adherent to the anterior vaginal wall. Placing a finger in the vagina can help direct the insertion of a catheter through the urethra into the bladder. **C.** This view of the anterior wall of the vagina demonstrates the projection of the cervix (superiorly) and urethra (inferior and anteriorly) into the vagina. **D.** A transverse section through the inferior female pelvic organs as they penetrate the pelvic floor through the urogenital hiatus (the gap between the right and the left sides of the levator ani) demonstrates the disposition of the non-distended lumina.

- Receives the penis and ejaculate during sexual intercourse.

- Communicates superiorly with the **cervical canal** (a fusiform canal extending from the isthmus of the uterus to the external os of the uterus) and inferiorly with the vestibule.

The vagina is usually collapsed (H-shaped in cross section) so that its anterior and posterior walls are in contact (Fig. 3.27D), except at its superior end where the cervix holds

them apart. The vagina lies posterior to the urethra, which projects into its inferior anterior wall, and urinary bladder, and it lies anterior to the rectum, passing between the medial margins of the levator ani muscles. The **vaginal fornix**, the recess around the cervix, has *anterior, posterior*, and *lateral parts* (Figs. 3.26A and 3.27B). The **posterior vaginal fornix** is the deepest part and is closely related to the rectouterine pouch. Four muscles compress the vagina and act as sphincters: **pubovaginalis, external urethral sphinc-**

ter, **urethrovaginal sphincter**, and **bulbospongiosus** (Fig. 3.28). The relations of the vagina are (Fig. 3.27) as follows:

- Anteriorly: the fundus of the urinary bladder and urethra.

- Laterally: the levator ani, visceral pelvic fascia, and ureters.

- Posteriorly (inferior to superior): the anal canal, rectum, and rectouterine pouch.

Arterial Supply of the Vagina

The arteries supplying the superior part of the vagina derive from the *uterine arteries;* the arteries supplying the middle and inferior parts of the vagina derive from the *vaginal* and *internal pudendal arteries* (Figs. 3.12 and 3.29).

Venous and Lymphatic Drainage of the Vagina

The vaginal veins form **vaginal venous plexuses** along the sides of the vagina and within the vaginal mucosa (Fig. 3.29). These veins are continuous with the *uterine venous plexus* as the **uterovaginal venous plexus** and drain into the internal iliac veins through the uterine vein. This plexus also communicates with the vesical and rectal venous plexuses.

The vaginal lymphatic vessels drain from the parts of the vagina as follows (Fig. 3.30; Table 3.6):

- Superior part: to the internal and external iliac lymph nodes.

- Middle part: to the internal iliac lymph nodes.

- Inferior part: to the sacral and common iliac nodes.

- External orifice: to the superficial inguinal lymph nodes.

Distension of the Vagina

The vagina can be markedly distended, particularly in the region of the posterior part of the fornix. For example, distension of this part allows palpation of the sacral promontory during a pelvic examination (see clinical correlation [blue] box "Pelvic Diameters (Conjugates)," in this chapter) and accommodates the erect penis during intercourse. The vagina is especially distended by the fetus during parturition, particularly in an AP direction when the fetus's shoulders are delivered. Lateral distension is limited by the ischial spines, which project posteromedially, and the sacrospinous ligaments extending from these spines to the lateral margins of the sacrum and coccyx. The birth canal is thus deep anteroposteriorly and narrow transversely at this point, causing the fetus's shoulders to rotate into the AP plane (Fig. B3.10). ▶

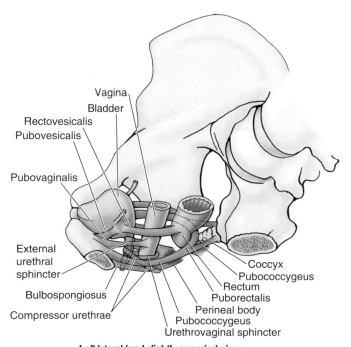

Left lateral (and slightly superior) view

Figure 3.28. Muscles compressing urethra and vagina. Muscles that compress the vagina and act as sphincters include the pubovaginalis, external urethral sphincter (especially its urethrovaginal sphincter part), and bulbospongiosus. The compressor urethrae and external urethral sphincter compress the urethra.

Delivery of right shoulder

Delivery of left shoulder

Figure B3.10

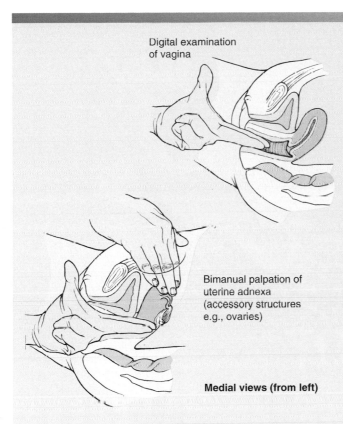

Digital examination of vagina

Bimanual palpation of uterine adnexa (accessory structures e.g., ovaries)

Medial views (from left)

Figure B3.11

Speculum

Rectouterine pouch

Culdoscope

Vagina

Medial view (from left)

Figure B3.13

vagina and/or rectum (**manual pelvic examination**). Pulsations of the uterine arteries may also be felt through the lateral parts of the fornix, as may irregularities of the ovaries, such as cysts (Fig. B3.11),

Vaginal Fistulae

Because of the close relationship of the vagina to adjacent pelvic organs, obstetrical trauma during long and difficult labor may result in weaknesses, necrosis, or tears in the vaginal wall and sometimes beyond. These may form or subsequently develop into open communications (**fistulas**) between the vaginal lumen and that of the adjacent bladder, urethra, rectum, or perineum (Fig. B3.12). Urine enters the vagina from both *vesicovaginal* and *urethrovaginal fistulas,* but the flow is continuous from the former and occurs only during micturition from the latter. Fecal matter may be discharged from the vagina when there is a *rectovaginal fistula*.

Culdoscopy and Culdocentesis

An endoscopic instrument (*culdoscope*) can be inserted through the posterior part of the vaginal fornix (Fig. B3.13) to examine the ovaries or uterine tubes (e.g., for the presence of a tubal pregnancy). Because it involves less disruption of tissue, *culdoscopy* has been largely replaced by *laparoscopy*, which, however, provides greater flexibility for operative procedures and better visualization of pelvic organs (see clinical correlation [blue] box "Laparoscopic Examination of Pelvic Viscera," in this chapter). There is also less risk of bacterial contamination of the peritoneal cavity. A pelvic abscess in the rectouterine pouch can be drained through an incision made in the posterior part of the vaginal fornix (*culdocentesis*). Similarly, fluid in the peritoneal cavity (e.g., blood) can be aspirated by this technique. ○

Digital Examination through the Vagina

Because of its relatively thin, distensible walls and central location within the pelvis, the cervix, ischial spines, and sacral promontory can be palpated with the digits in the

Vesicovaginal fistula

Rectovaginal fistula

Urethrovaginal fistula

Vaginoperineal fistula

Medial view (from left)

Figure B3.12

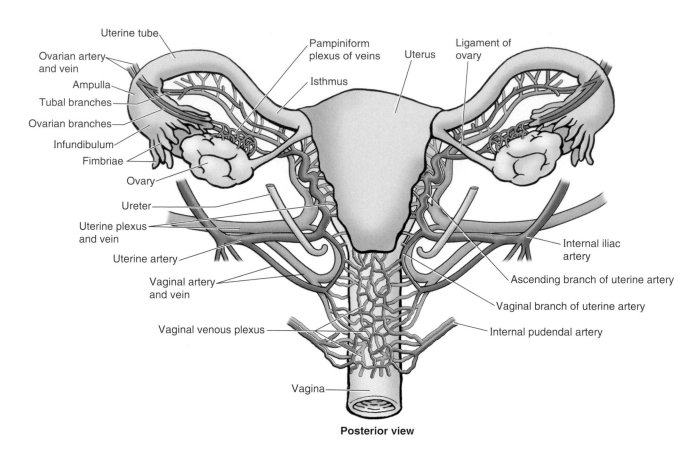

Posterior view

Figure 3.29. Blood supply and venous drainage of uterus, vagina, and ovaries. The broad ligament of the uterus is removed to show the anastomosing branches of the ovarian artery from the aorta and the uterine artery from the internal iliac artery supplying the ovary, uterine tube, and uterus. The veins follow a similar pattern, flowing retrograde to the arteries, but are more plexiform, including a pampiniform plexus related to the ovary and continuous uterine and vaginal plexuses (collectively, the uterovaginal plexus).

A = Body and fundus of uterus, uterine tubes and ovaries
B = Cervix of uterus and vaginal fornices
C = Middle part of vagina
D = Inferior part of vagina
E = Vestibule of vagina

Lymphatic drainage

Key		
☐ Lumbar (caval/aortic)	☐ Internal iliac	☐ Deep inguinal
■ Inferior mesenteric	☐ External iliac	☐ Sacral
☐ Common iliac	☐ Superficial inguinal	

Figure 3.30. Lymphatic drainage of female internal genital organs.
The *arrows* indicate the direction of lymph flow to the lymph nodes.

THE BOTTOM LINE: The vagina is a musculomembranous passage connecting the uterine cavity to the exterior, allowing the entrance/insertion of the penis, ejaculate, tampons, or examining digits and the exit of a fetus or menstrual fluid. The vagina lies between and is closely related to the urethra anteriorly and rectum posteriorly but is separated from the latter by the peritoneal rectouterine pouch superiorly and the fascial rectovaginal septum inferiorly. It is indented (invaginated) anterosuperiorly by the uterine cervix so that an encircling pocket or vaginal fornix is formed around it. Most of the vagina is located within the pelvis, receiving blood via pelvic branches of the internal iliac artery (uterine and vaginal arteries) and draining directly into the uterovaginal venous plexus and, via deep (pelvic) routes, to the internal and external iliac and sacral lymph nodes. The inferiormost part of the vagina is located within the perineum, receiving blood from the internal pudendal artery and draining via superficial (perineal) routes into superficial inguinal nodes. The vagina is capable of remarkable distension, enabling manual examination (palpation) of pelvic landmarks and viscera (especially the ovaries) as well as of pathology (e.g., ovarian cysts).

Uterus

The **uterus** (womb) is a thick-walled, pear-shaped, hollow muscular organ. The embryo and fetus develop in the uterus, its muscular walls adapting to the growth of the fetus and then providing the power for its expulsion during childbirth. The non-gravid (non-pregnant) uterus usually lies in the lesser pelvis, with its body lying on the urinary bladder and its cervix between the urinary bladder and the rectum (Figs. 3.27A & B and 3.31A). The adult uterus is usually *anteverted* (tipped anterosuperiorly relative to the axis of the vagina) and *anteflexed* (flexed or bent anteriorly relative to the cervix) so that its mass lies over the bladder. The position of the uterus changes with the degree of fullness of the bladder and rectum. Although its size varies considerably, the uterus is approximately 7.5 cm long, 5 cm wide, and 2 cm thick and weighs approximately 90 g. The uterus is divisible into two main parts (Fig. 3.26): the body and cervix.

The **body of the uterus,** forming the superior two thirds of the organ, includes the **fundus of the uterus,** the rounded part that lies superior to the orifices of the uterine tubes. The body lies between the layers of the broad ligament and is freely movable (Fig. 3.31B). It has two surfaces: vesical (related to the bladder) and intestinal. The body is demarcated from the cervix by the **isthmus of the uterus,** a relatively constricted segment, approximately 1 cm long (Figs. 3.26 and 3.31B).

The **cervix of the uterus** is the cylindrical, relatively narrow inferior third of the uterus, approximately 2.5 cm long in an adult non-pregnant woman. For descriptive purposes, two parts are described: a *supravaginal part* between the isthmus and the vagina, and a *vaginal part,* which protrudes into the vagina. The rounded vaginal part surrounds the *external os of the uterus* and is surrounded in turn by a narrow space, the *vaginal fornix* (Fig. 3.27). The supravaginal part is separated from the bladder anteriorly by loose connective tissue and from the rectum posteriorly by the *rectouterine pouch.*

The slit-like uterine cavity is approximately 6 cm in length from the external os to the wall of the fundus. The uterine horns (L. *cornua*) are the superolateral regions of the uterine cavity, where the uterine tubes enter (Fig. 3.26A). Incomplete fusion of the embryonic paramesonephric ducts from which the uterus is formed results in a variety of congenital anomalies (e.g., double or bicornate uterus; see "Medical Imaging of the Pelvis and Perineum," in this chapter). The uterine cavity continues inferiorly as the fusiform *cervical canal.* The canal extends from a narrowing inside the isthmus of the uterine body, the **anatomical internal os,** through the supravaginal and vaginal parts of the cervix, communicating with the lumen of the vagina through the external os (Figs. 3.26 and 3.31B). The uterine cavity (in particular, the cervical canal) and the lumen of the vagina together constitute the birth canal through which the fetus passes at the end of gestation.

The wall of the body of the uterus consists of three coats, or layers (Fig. 3.26):

- **Perimetrium**—the serosa or outer serous coat—consists of peritoneum supported by a thin layer of connective tissue.

- **Myometrium**—the middle coat of smooth muscle—becomes greatly distended (more extensive but much thinner) during pregnancy. The main branches of the blood vessels and nerves of the uterus are located in this coat. During childbirth, contraction of the myometrium is hormonally stimulated at intervals of decreasing length to dilate the cervical os and expel the fetus and placenta. During the menses, myometrial contraction may produce cramping.

- **Endometrium**—the inner mucous coat—is firmly adhered to the underlying myometrium. The endometrium is actively involved in the menstrual cycle, differing in structure with each stage of the cycle. If conception occurs, the blastocyst becomes implanted in this layer; if conception does not occur, the inner surface of this coat is shed through menstruation.

The amount of muscular tissue in the cervix is markedly less than in the body of the uterus. The cervix is mostly fibrous and is composed mainly of collagen with a small amount of smooth muscle and elastin.

Ligaments of the Uterus. Externally, the **ligament of the ovary** attaches to the uterus posteroinferior to the uterotubal junction (Figs. 3.26 and 3.31B). The **round ligament of the uterus** (L. *ligamentum teres uteri*) attaches anteroinferiorly to this junction (Fig. 3.31A & B). These two ligaments are vestiges of the *ovarian gubernaculum,* related to the descent of the gonad from its developmental position on the posterior abdominal wall (see Chapter 2).

(A) Anterior view

Inferior vena cava

Psoas major

Right ureter

Internal iliac artery

External iliac artery

Round ligament of uterus

Uterine artery

Vaginal arteries

Pubic bone

Crura of clitoris (cut ends)

Aorta

Ovarian artery

Sigmoid colon

Sigmoid mesocolon

Suspensory ligament of ovary

Uterine tube
Ovary

Broad ligament of uterus

Fundus of uterus

Round ligament of uterus

Trigone of urinary bladder

Obturator externus

Vestibule

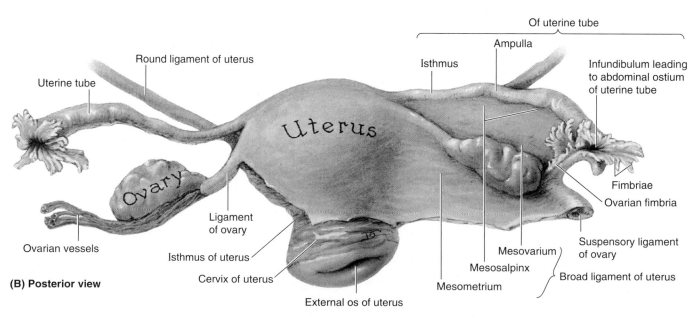

(B) Posterior view

Uterine tube

Round ligament of uterus

Ovary

Ovarian vessels

Ligament of ovary

Isthmus of uterus

Cervix of uterus

External os of uterus

Mesometrium

Mesosalpinx

Mesovarium

Of uterine tube

Isthmus

Ampulla

Infundibulum leading to abdominal ostium of uterine tube

Fimbriae

Ovarian fimbria

Suspensory ligament of ovary

Broad ligament of uterus

Figure 3.31. Female pelvic viscera. A. In this dissection of the female genital organs, the bladder and adjacent anterior pelvis (superior ramus and bodies of pubic bones) have been coronally sectioned and the anterior segment has been removed. On the right side, the uterine tube, ovary, broad ligament, and peritoneum covering the lateral wall of the pelvis have been removed to display the ureter and branches of the internal iliac artery. **B.** This dissection reveals the uterus, ovaries, uterine tubes, and related structures. The broad ligament is removed on the right side.

The **broad ligament of the uterus** is a double layer of peritoneum (mesentery) that extends from the sides of the uterus to the lateral walls and floor of the pelvis. This ligament assists in keeping the uterus in position. The two layers of the broad ligament are continuous with each other at a free edge that surrounds the uterine tube. Laterally, the peritoneum of the broad ligament is prolonged superiorly over the vessels as the **suspensory ligament of the ovary**. Between the layers of the broad ligament on each side of the uterus, the ligament of the ovary lies posterosuperiorly and the round ligament of the uterus lies anteroinferiorly. The uterine tube lies in the anterosuperior free border of the broad ligament, within a small mesentery called the **mesosalpinx**. Similarly, the ovary lies within a small mesentery called the **mesovarium** on the posterior aspect of the broad ligament. The largest part of the broad ligament, inferior to the mesosalpinx and mesovarium, which serves as a mesentery for the uterus itself, is the mesometrium.

The uterus is a dense structure located in the center of the pelvic cavity. The principal supports of the uterus holding it in this position are both passive and active or dynamic. Dynamic support of the uterus is provided by the pelvic diaphragm. Its tone during sitting and standing and active contraction during periods of increased intra-abdominal pressure (sneezing, coughing, etc.) is transmitted through the surrounding pelvic organs and the endopelvic fascia in which they are embedded. Passive support of the uterus is provided by its position—the way in which the normally *anteverted* and *anteflexed* uterus rests on top of the bladder. When intra-abdominal pressure is increased, the uterus is pressed against the bladder. The cervix is the least mobile part of the uterus because of the passive support provided by attached condensations of endopelvic fascia (ligaments), which may also contain smooth muscle (Fig. 3.9*B*):

- *Transverse cervical* (cardinal) *ligaments* extend from the cervix and lateral parts of the fornix of the vagina to the lateral walls of the pelvis.

- *Uterosacral ligaments* pass superiorly and slightly posteriorly from the sides of the cervix to the middle of the sacrum; they are palpable during a rectal examination.

Together these passive and active supports keep the uterus centered in the pelvic cavity and resist the tendency for the uterus to fall or be pushed through the vagina (see clinical correlation [blue] box "Disposition of the Uterus and Uterine Prolapse," in this chapter).

Relations of the Uterus. Peritoneum covers the uterus anteriorly and superiorly (Figs. 3.27*A* & *B* and 3.31*B*), except for the cervix. The peritoneum is reflected anteriorly from the uterus onto the bladder and posteriorly over the posterior part of the fornix of the vagina to the rectum.

Anteriorly, the uterine body is separated from the urinary bladder by the **vesicouterine pouch**, where the peritoneum is reflected from the uterus onto the posterior margin of the superior surface of the bladder. Posteriorly, the uterine body and supravaginal part of the cervix are separated from the sigmoid colon by a layer of peritoneum and the peritoneal cavity and from the rectum by the *rectouterine pouch*. Laterally, the uterine artery crosses the ureter superiorly, near the cervix (Fig. 3.29).

Summary of the relations of the uterus:

- *Anteriorly* (anteroinferiorly in its normal anteverted position): the vesicouterine pouch and superior surface of the bladder; the supravaginal part of the cervix is related to the bladder and is separated from it by only fibrous connective tissue.

- *Posteriorly:* the rectouterine pouch containing loops of small intestine and the anterior surface of rectum; only the visceral pelvic fascia uniting the rectum and uterus here resists increased intra-abdominal pressure

- *Laterally:* the peritoneal broad ligament flanking the uterine body and the fascial transverse cervical ligaments on each side of the cervix and vagina; in the transition between the two ligaments, the ureters run anteriorly slightly superior to the lateral part of the vaginal fornix and inferior to the uterine arteries, usually approximately 2 cm lateral to the supravaginal part of the cervix.

Arterial Supply of the Uterus. The blood supply of the uterus derives mainly from the *uterine arteries,* with potential collateral supply from the ovarian arteries (Fig. 3.29).

Venous and Lymphatic Drainage of the Uterus. The *uterine veins* enter the broad ligaments with the arteries and form a **uterine venous plexus** on each side of the cervix. Veins from the uterine plexus drain into the internal iliac veins.

Lymphatic vessels from the uterus drain in many directions, coursing along the blood vessels that supply it as well as the ligaments attached to it (Fig. 3.30; Table 3.6):

- Most lymphatic vessels from the fundus and superior uterine body pass along the ovarian vessels to the *lumbar (caval/aortic) lymph nodes;* but some vessels from the fundus, particularly those near the entrance of the uterine tubes and attachments of the round ligaments, run along the round ligament of the uterus to the *superficial inguinal lymph nodes.*

- Vessels from most of the uterine body and some from the cervix pass within the broad ligament to the *external iliac lymph nodes.*

- Vessels from the uterine cervix also pass along the uterine vessels, within the transverse cervical ligaments, to the *internal iliac lymph nodes,* and along uterosacral (sacrogenital) ligaments to the *sacral lymph nodes.*

Cervical Cancer, Cervical Examination, and Pap Smear

Until 1940, cervical cancer was the leading cause of death in North American women (Krebs, 2000). The decline in the incidence and number of women dying from cervical cancer is related to the accessibility of the cervix to direct visualization and to cell and tissue study by means of Pap (Papanicolaou) smears, leading to the detection of premalignant cervical conditions (Copeland, 2000; Morris and Burke, 2000). The vagina can be distended with a *vaginal speculum* to enable inspection of the cervix (Fig. B3.14*A* & *B*). To prepare a Pap smear, a spatula is placed on the external os of the uterus (Fig. B3.14*A*). The spatula is rotated to scrape cellular material from the mucosa of the vaginal cervix (Fig. B3.14*C*), followed by a insertion of a cytobrush into the cervical canal that is rotated to gather cellular material from the supravaginal cervical mucosa. The cellular material is then placed on glass slides for microscopic examination (Fig. B3.14*D* & *E*).

Examination of the Uterus

The size and disposition of the uterus may be examined by *bimanual palpation* (Fig. B3.15*A*). Two fingers of the right hand are passed superiorly in the vagina, while the other hand is pressed inferoposteriorly on the pubic region of the anterior abdominal wall. The size and other characteristics of the uterus can be determined in this way (e.g., whether the uterus is in its normal anteverted position). When softening of the uterine isthmus occurs (*Hegar sign*), the cervix feels as though it were separated from the body. Softening of the isthmus is an early sign of pregnancy. The uterus can be further stabilized through rectovaginal examination, which is used if examination via the vagina alone does not yield clear findings (Fig. B3.15*B*)

Lifetime Changes in the Normal Anatomy of the Uterus

The uterus is possibly the most dynamic structure in human anatomy (Fig. B3.16). At birth, the uterus is relatively large and has adult proportions (body to cervical ratio = 2:1) due to the prepartum (before childbirth) influence of the adult maternal hormones (Fig. B3.16*A*). Several weeks **postpartum** (after childbirth), childhood dimensions and proportions are obtained: the body and cervix are approximately of equal length (body to cervical ratio = 1:1), with the cervix being of greater diameter (thickness) (Fig. B3.16*B*). Because of the small size of the pelvic cavity during infancy, the uterus is mainly an abdominal organ. The cervix remains relatively large (approximately 50% of total uterus) throughout childhood. During puberty, the uterus (especially its body) grows rapidly in size, once again assuming adult proportions (Fig. B3.16*C*). In the ▶

Figure B3.14

(A)   Bimanual palpation; uterus
       anteverted and anteflexed

Medial view
(from left)

(B)

Rectovaginal examination;
uterus retroverted and retroflexed

Figure B3.15

postpubertal, premenopausal, non-pregnant woman, the body is pear shaped; the thick-walled superior two thirds of the uterus lies within the pelvic cavity (Fig. B3.16D). During this phase of life, the uterus undergoes monthly changes in size, weight, and density in relation to the menstrual cycle.

Over the 9 months of pregnancy, the uterus expands greatly to accommodate the fetus, becoming larger and increasingly thin walled (Fig. B3.16G). At the end of pregnancy (B3.16G, line 10), the fetus "drops," as the head becomes engaged in the lesser pelvis. The uterus becomes nearly membranous, with the fundus dropping below its highest level (achieved in the 9th month), at which time it extends superiorly to the costal margin, occupying most of the abdominopelvic cavity (Fig. B3.16H). Immediately after delivery, the large uterus becomes thick walled and edematous (Fig. B3.16I), but its size reduces rapidly. The multiparous non-gravid uterus has a large and nodular body and usually extends into the greater pelvis, often causing a slight protrusion of the inferior abdominal wall in lean women (Figs. B3.16E & J and 3.64).

During menopause (46–52 years of age), the uterus (again, especially the body) decreases in size. Postmenopause, the uterus is involuted and regresses to a markedly smaller size, once again assuming childhood

proportions (Fig. B3.16F). All these stages represent *normal anatomy* for the particular age and reproductive status of the woman.

Disposition of the Uterus and Uterine Prolapse

When intra-abdominal pressure is increased, the normally anteverted and anteflexed uterus is pressed against the bladder (Fig. B3.17A). However, the uterus may assume other dispositions, including excessive anteflexion (Fig. B3.17B), anteflexion with retroversion (Fig. B3.17C), and retroflexion with retroversion (Fig. B3.17D). Instead of pressing the uterus against the bladder, increased intra-abdominal pressure tends to push the retroverted uterus, a solid mass positioned upright over the vagina (a flexible, hollow tube), into or even through the vagina (Fig. B3.17E–G). A retroverted uterus will not necessarily prolapse but is more likely to do so, and pregnancies involving a retroverted uterus are considered to be higher risk pregnancies. The situation is exacerbated in the presence of a disrupted perineal body or with atrophic ("relaxed") pelvic floor ligaments and muscles (see clinical correlation [blue] box "Disruption of Perineal Body," in this chapter). ▶

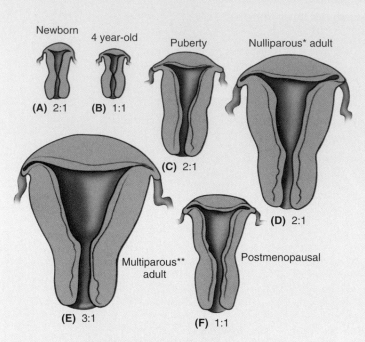

Newborn 4 year-old Puberty Nulliparous* adult

(A) 2:1 (B) 1:1 (C) 2:1 (D) 2:1

Multiparous**
adult

Postmenopausal

(E) 3:1 (F) 1:1

(A-F) Anterior views

Placenta

Umbilical
cord

Uterus

Cervix

(H) Uterus at end of pregnancy

(I) Postpartum uterus
(immediately following childbirth)

9
10
8
7
6
5
4
3

(G) Monthly changes in size
of uterus during pregnancy

*Never having borne an infant
**Having given birth to an infant
two or more times

(J) Multiparous** uterus

Figure B3.16 ▶

(A) Normal (anteverted, anteflexed)

(B) Excessive anteflexion

(C) Retroverted

(D) Retroverted and retroflexed

(E) First degree prolapse

(F) Second degree prolapse

(G) Third degree prolapse

Figure B3.17

(A) Abdominal hysterectomy

(B) Vaginal hysterectomy

Figure B3.18

Hysterectomy

Owing to the frequency of uterine and cervical cancer, **hysterectomy**, excision of the uterus (G. *hystera*), is a relatively common procedure. The uterus may be surgically approached and removed through the anterior abdominal wall or through the vagina (Fig. B3.18). ○

THE BOTTOM LINE: Shaped like an inverted pear, the uterus is the organ in which the blastocyst (early embryo) implants and develops into a mature embryo and then a fetus. Although its size and proportions change during the various phases of life, the non-gravid uterus consists of a body and cervix, demarcated by a relatively narrow isthmus. The uterus has a trilaminar wall consisting of (1) an inner vascular and secretory endometrium, which undergoes cyclical changes to prepare for implantation to occur and sheds with menstrual flow if it does not; (2) a hormonally stimulated intermediate smooth muscle myometrium, which dilates the cervical canal (exit) and expels the fetus during childbirth; and (3) visceral peritoneum (perimetrium), which covers most of the fundus and body (except for a bare area abutting the bladder) and continues bilaterally as the broad ligament (mesometrium).

The uterus is normally anteverted and anteflexed so that its weight is borne largely by the urinary bladder, although it also receives significant passive support from the transverse cervical ligaments and active support from the muscles of the pelvic floor. The uterine artery supplies the uterus and, during pregnancy, the placenta. The uterus drains to the uterovaginal venous plexus and to all major groups of pelvic lymph nodes, with parts near the attachments of the round ligaments draining to superficial inguinal nodes.

Innervation of the Vagina and Uterus

Only the inferior one fifth to one quarter of the vagina is somatic in terms of innervation. Innervation of this part of the vagina is from the *deep perineal nerve,* a branch of the *pudendal nerve,* which conveys sympathetic and visceral afferent fibers but no parasympathetic fibers (Fig. 3.32). Only this somatically innervated part is sensitive to touch and temperature, even though the somatic and visceral afferent fibers have their cell bodies in the same (S2–S4) spinal ganglia.

Most of the vagina (superior three quarters to four fifths) is visceral in terms of its innervation. Nerves to this part of the vagina and to the uterus are derived from the **uterovaginal nerve plexus,** which travels with the uterine artery at the junction of the base of the (peritoneal) broad ligament and the superior part of the (fascial) transverse cervical ligament. The uterovaginal nerve plexus is one of the pelvic plexuses that extends to the pelvic viscera from the inferior hypogastric plexus. Sympathetic, parasympathetic, and visceral afferent fibers pass through this plexus.

Sympathetic innervation originates in the inferior thoracic spinal cord segments and passes through *lumbar splanchnic nerves* and the intermesenteric-hypogastric-pelvic series of plexuses. Parasympathetic innervation originates in the S2–S4 spinal cord segments and passes through the *pelvic splanchnic nerves* to the inferior hypogastric-uterovaginal plexus. The visceral afferent innervations of the superior (intraperitoneal; fundus and body) and inferior (subperitoneal; cervical) parts of the uterus and vagina differ in terms of course and destination. Visceral afferent fibers conducting pain impulses from the intraperitoneal uterine fundus and body (superior to the *pelvic pain line*) follow the sympathetic innervation retrograde to reach cell bodies in the inferior thoracic-superior lumbar spinal ganglia. Afferent fibers conducting pain impulses from the subperitoneal uterine cervix and vagina (inferior to the pelvic pain line) follow the parasympathetic fibers retrograde through the uterovaginal and inferior hypogastric plexuses and pelvic splanchnic nerves to reach cell bodies in the spinal sensory ganglia of S2–S4. All visceral afferent fibers from the uterus and vagina not concerned with pain (those conveying unconscious sensations) also follow the latter route.

Anesthesia for Childbirth

Several options are available to women to reduce the pain and discomfort experienced during childbirth. *General anesthesia* has advantages for emergency procedures and for women who choose it over regional anesthesia. General anesthesia renders the mother unconscious; she is unaware of the labor and delivery. Clinicians monitor and regulate maternal respiration and both maternal and fetal cardiac function. Childbirth occurs passively under the control of maternal hormones with the assistance of an obstetrician. The mother is spared pain and discomfort but is unaware of the earliest moments of her baby's life.

Women who choose *regional anesthesia,* such as a spinal, pudendal nerve, or caudal epidural block, often wish to participate actively (e.g., using the Lamaze method) and be conscious of their uterine contractions to "bear down," or push, to assist the contractions and expel the fetus, yet do not wish to experience all the pain of labor.

A **spinal block,** in which the anesthetic agent is introduced with a needle into the spinal subarachnoid space at the L3–L4 vertebral level (A in Fig. B3.19), produces complete anesthesia inferior to approximately the waist level. The perineum, pelvic floor, and birth canal are anesthetized, and motor and sensory functions of the entire lower limbs, as well as sensation of uterine contractions, are temporarily eliminated. The mother is conscious, but she must depend on electronic monitoring of uterine contractions. If labor is extended or the level of anesthesia is inadequate, it may be difficult or impossible to re-administer the anesthesia. Because the anesthetic agent is heavier than cerebrospinal fluid, it remains in the inferior spinal ▶

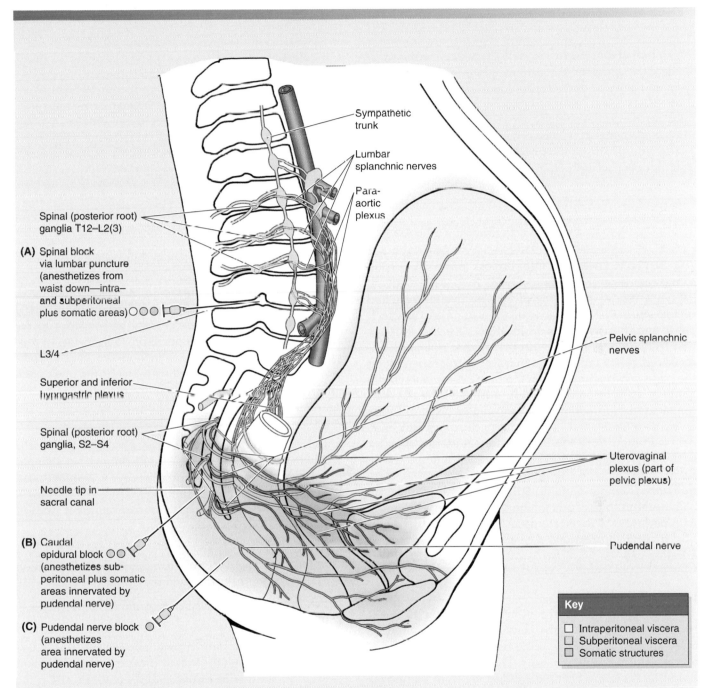

Sympathetic trunk

Lumbar splanchnic nerves

Para-aortic plexus

Spinal (posterior root) ganglia T12–L2(3)

(A) Spinal block via lumbar puncture (anesthetizes from waist down—intra– and subperitoneal plus somatic areas) ○○○ ⌐□

L3/4

Pelvic splanchnic nerves

Superior and inferior hypogastric plexus

Spinal (posterior root) ganglia, S2–S4

Uterovaginal plexus (part of pelvic plexus)

Needle tip in sacral canal

(B) Caudal epidural block ○○ (anesthetizes sub-peritoneal plus somatic areas innervated by pudendal nerve)

Pudendal nerve

(C) Pudendal nerve block ○ (anesthetizes area innervated by pudendal nerve)

Key

☐ Intraperitoneal viscera
☐ Subperitoneal viscera
☐ Somatic structures

Figure B3.19

subarachnoid space while the patient is inclined. The anesthetic agent circulates into the cerebral subarachnoid space in the cranial cavity when the patient lies flat following the delivery. A severe headache is a common sequel to spinal anesthesia.

A **pudendal nerve block** is a peripheral nerve block that provides local anesthesia over the S2–S4 dermatomes (the majority of the perineum) and the inferior quarter of the vagina (C in Fig. B3.19). It does not block pain from the superior birth canal (uterine cervix and superior vagina), so

the mother is able to feel uterine contractions. It can be re-administered, but to do so may be disruptive and involve the use of a sharp instrument in close proximity to the infant's head. The anatomical basis of the administration of a pudendal block is provided in the clinical correlation (blue) box "Administration of Pudendal and Ilioinguinal Nerve Blocks," in this chapter.

The **caudal epidural block** is a popular choice for participatory childbirth (B in Fig. B3.19). It must be administered in advance of the actual delivery, which is not ▶

possible with a precipitous birth. The anesthetic agent is administered using an in-dwelling catheter in the *sacral canal* (see Chapter 4), enabling administration of more anesthetic agent for a deeper or more prolonged anesthesia, if necessary. Within the sacral canal, the anesthesia bathes the S2–S4 spinal nerve roots, including the pain fibers from the uterine cervix and superior vagina, and the afferent fibers from the pudendal nerve. Thus the entire birth canal, pelvic floor, and majority of the perineum are anesthetized, but the lower limbs are not usually affected. The pain fibers from the uterine body (superior to the pelvic pain line) ascend to the inferior thoracic-superior lumbar levels; these and the fibers superior to them are not affected by the anesthetic, so the mother is aware of her uterine contractions. With epidural anesthesia, no "spinal headache" occurs because the vertebral epidural space is not continuous with the cranial epidural space (see Chapter 4). ○

THE BOTTOM LINE: The inferiormost (perineal) portion of the vagina receives somatic innervation via the pudendal nerve (S2–S4) and is, therefore, sensitive to touch and temperature. The remainder of the vagina and uterus is pelvic and thus visceral in its location, receiving innervation from autonomic and visceral afferent fibers. All unconscious, reflex-type sensation travels retrogradely along the parasympathetic pathways to the S2–S4 spinal sensory ganglia, as does pain sensation arising in the subperitoneal uterus (primarily cervix) and vagina (inferior to the pelvic pain line)—that is, from the birth canal. However, pain sensation from the intraperitoneal uterus (superior to the pelvic pain line) travels retrogradely along the sympathetic pathway to the inferiormost thoracic and superior lumbar spinal ganglia. Epidural anesthesia may be administered to take advantage of the discrepancy in the pain pathways to facilitate participatory childbirth methods; uterine contractions are felt, but the birth canal is anesthetized.

Uterine Tubes

The **uterine tubes** (oviducts; formerly called fallopian tubes) conduct the oocyte (ovum), discharged monthly from an ovary during child-bearing years, from the periovarian peritoneal cavity to the uterine cavity. They also provide the usual site of fertilization. They extend laterally from the *uterine horns* and open into the peritoneal cavity near the ovaries (Figs. 3.26 and 3.31). The uterine tubes (approximately 10 cm long) lie in the *mesosalpinx* in the free edges of the broad ligaments. In the "ideal" disposition, as typically illustrated, the tubes extend symmetrically posterolaterally to the lateral pelvic walls, where they arch anterior and superior to the ovaries in the horizontally disposed broad ligament. In reality, as seen in an ultrasound examination, the tubes are commonly asymmetrically arranged with one or the other often lying superior and even posterior to the uterus.

The uterine tubes are divisible into four parts, from lateral to medial (Fig. 3.31*B*):

- **Infundibulum:** the funnel-shaped distal end of the tube that opens into the peritoneal cavity through the **abdominal ostium;** the finger-like processes of the fimbriated end of the infundibulum (the **fimbriae**) spread over the medial surface of the ovary; one large **ovarian fimbria** is attached to the superior pole of the ovary.

- **Ampulla:** the widest and longest part of the tube, which begins at the medial end of the infundibulum; fertilization of the oocyte usually occurs in the ampulla.

- **Isthmus:** the thick-walled part of the tube, which enters the uterine horn.

- **Uterine part:** the short intramural segment of the tube that passes through the wall of the uterus (Fig. 3.26) and opens via the **uterine ostium** into the uterine cavity at the uterine horn.

Figure 3.32. Innervation of female internal genital organs. Pelvic splanchnic nerves, arising from the S2–S4 anterior rami, supply parasympathetic motor fibers to the uterus and vagina (and vasodilator fibers to the erectile tissue of the clitoris and bulb of the vestibule; not shown). Presynaptic sympathetic fibers traverse the sympathetic trunk and pass through the lumbar splanchnic nerves to synapse in prevertebral ganglia with postsynaptic fibers; the latter fibers travel through the superior and inferior hypogastric plexuses to reach the pelvic viscera. Visceral afferent fibers conducting pain from intraperitoneal structures (such as the uterine body) travel with the sympathetic fibers to the T12–L2 spinal ganglia. Visceral afferent fibers conducting pain from subperitoneal structures, such as the cervix and vagina (i.e., the birth canal), travel with parasympathetic fibers to the S2–S4 spinal ganglia. Somatic sensation from the opening of the vagina also passes to the S2–S4 spinal ganglia via the pudendal nerve. In addition, muscular contractions of the uterus are hormonally induced.

Key

——————	Visceral afferents running with parasympathetic fibers
- - - - - Presynaptic	} Parasympathetic
—————— Postsynaptic	
- - - - - Presynaptic	} Sympathetic
—————— Postsynaptic	
——————	Visceral afferents running with sympathetic fibers
- - - - -	Somatic motor
——————	Somatic afferent

Innervation of female pelvic viscera

Upper lumbar sympathetic trunk

Spinal ganglia (posterior root ganglia)

T12
L1
L2
L3
L4
L5
S1
S2
S3
S4
S5

Lumbar splanchnic nerves

Spinal ganglia

Pelvic splanchnic nerves

Pelvic plexus

Sacral plexus

Prevertebal ganglia

Para-aortic plexus

Superior hypogastric plexus

Inferior hypogastric plexuses

Uterine plexus

Pudendal nerve

Pelvic intra-peritoneal viscera

Ovarian plexus

Lower limit of peritoneum

Pelvic plexus

Pelvic plexus

Pelvic sub-peritoneal viscera

Uterovaginal plexus

Anterior view

Pudendal nerve

Perineum

Infections of the Female Genital Tract

Because the female genital tract communicates with the peritoneal cavity through the abdominal ostia of the uterine tubes, infections of the vagina, uterus, and tubes may result in *peritonitis*. Conversely, inflammation of the tube (**salpingitis**) may result from infections that spread from the peritoneal cavity. A major cause of infertility in women is blockage of the uterine tubes, often the result of salpingitis.

Patency of the Uterine Tubes

Hysterosalpingography

Patency of the uterine tubes may be determined by a radiographic procedure involving injection of a water-soluble radiopaque material into the uterus and tubes (**hysterosalpingography**). See "Medical Imaging of the Pelvis and Perineum," later in this chapter.

Endoscopy

Patency of the uterine tubes can also be determined by **hysteroscopy**, examination of the interior of the tubes using an endoscopic instrument (*hysteroscope*), which is introduced through the vagina and uterus.

Ligation of the Uterine Tubes

Ligation of the uterine tubes is a surgical method of birth control. Oocytes discharged from the ovaries that enter the tubes of these patients degenerate and are soon absorbed. Most surgical sterilizations are done by either abdominal tubal ligation or laparoscopic tubal ligation. **Abdominal tubal ligation** is usually performed through a short suprapubic incision made at the pubic hairline (Fig. B3.20A). **Laparoscopic tubal ligation** is done with a laparoscope, which is similar to a small telescope with a powerful light (Fig. B3.20B). It is inserted through a small incision, usually near the umbilicus.

Ectopic Tubal Pregnancy

In some women, collections of pus may develop in the uterine tube (**pyosalpinx**) and the tube may be partly occluded by adhesions. In these cases, the blastocyst may not be able to pass along the tube to the uterus, although sperms have obviously done so. The blastocyst may implant in the mucosa of the uterine tube, producing an **ectopic tubal pregnancy**. Although implantation may occur in any part of the tube, the common site is in the ampulla (Fig. B3.21). ▶

Irving

Pomeroy

Uchida

Kroener
fimbriectomy

(A)

Cautery

Falope
ring

Hulka clip

(B)

Figure B3.20

Posterior view

Figure B3.21

Tubal pregnancy is the most common type of ectopic gestation; it occurs in approximately 1 of every 250 pregnancies in North America (Moore and Persaud, 2003). If not diagnosed early, ectopic tubal pregnancies may result in rupture of the uterine tube and severe hemorrhage into the abdominopelvic cavity during the first 8 weeks of gestation. Tubal rupture and the associated hemorrhage constitute a threat to the mother's life and result in death of the embryo.

On the right side, the appendix often lies close to the ovary and uterine tube. This close relationship explains why a *ruptured tubal pregnancy* and the resulting peritonitis may be misdiagnosed as acute appendicitis. In both cases, the parietal peritoneum is inflamed in the same general area, and the pain is referred to the right lower quadrant of the abdomen.

Remnants of the Embryonic Ducts

Occasionally the mesosalpinx between the uterine tube and the ovary contains embryonic remnants (Fig. 3.26). The *epoophoron* forms from remnants of the mesonephric tubules of the *mesonephros*, the transitory embryonic kidney. There may also be a persistent *duct of the epoophoron* (duct of Gartner), a remnant of the mesonephric duct that forms the ductus deferens and ejaculatory duct in the male. It lies between layers of the broad ligament along each side of the uterus and/or vagina. A *vesicular appendage* is sometimes attached to the infundibulum of the uterine tube. It is the remains of the cranial end of the mesonephric duct that forms the *ductus epididymis* (Moore and Persaud, 2003). Although these vestigial structures are mostly of embryological and morphological interest, they occasionally accumulate fluid and form cysts (e.g., Gartner duct cysts). ⊙

THE BOTTOM LINE: The uterine tubes are the conduits and the site of fertilization for oocytes discharged into the peritoneal cavity. Coursing in a peritoneal fold (mesosalpinx) that makes up the superior margin of the broad ligament, each uterine tube has a fimbriated, funnel-like infundibulum, a wide ampulla, a narrow isthmus, and a short uterine part that traverses the uterine wall to enter the cavity.

Ovaries

The **ovaries** are almond-shaped and -sized female gonads in which the ova develop. They are also endocrine glands that produce reproductive hormones. The ovaries are typically located near the attachment of the broad ligament to the lateral pelvic walls, suspended from both by peritoneal folds: from the posterosuperior aspect of the broad ligament by

the mesovarium and from the lateral pelvic walls by the suspensory ligaments of the ovaries (Fig. 3.31). In prepubertal females, the surface of the ovary is covered by a smooth layer of ovarian surface epithelium, a single layer of cuboidal cells that gives the surface a dull, grayish appearance, contrasting with the shiny surface of the adjacent peritoneal mesovarium with which it is continuous. After puberty, the surface becomes progressively scarred and distorted because of the repeated rupture of ovarian follicles and discharge of oocytes that are part of ovulation. The scarring is less in women who have been taking oral contraceptives that inhibit ovulation.

The ovarian vessels, lymphatics, and nerves pass to and from the superolateral aspect of the ovary within the *suspensory ligament of the ovary,* which actually constitutes the lateral part of the mesovarium of the broad ligament. The ovary also attaches to the uterus by the *ligament of the ovary*, which runs within the mesovarium. This ligament is a remnant of the superior part of the ovarian gubernaculum of the fetus (see Fig. 2.14). The ligament of the ovary connects the proximal (uterine) end of the ovary to the lateral angle of the uterus, just inferior to the entrance of the uterine tube. Because the ovary is suspended in the peritoneal cavity and its surface is not covered by peritoneum, the oocyte expelled at ovulation passes into the peritoneal cavity. However, its intraperitoneal life is short because it is usually trapped by the fimbriae of the infundibulum of the uterine tube and carried into the ampulla, where it may be fertilized.

Laparoscopic Examination of Pelvic Viscera

Visual examination of the pelvic viscera is especially useful in diagnosing many conditions affecting the pelvic viscera, such as *ovarian cysts* and tumors, *endometriosis* (the presence of functioning endometrial tissue outside the uterus), and ectopic pregnancies. **Laparoscopy** involves inserting a *laparoscope* into the peritoneal cavity through a small (approximately 2 cm) incision below the umbilicus (Fig. B3.22). Insufflation of inert gas creates a pneumoperitoneum to provide space to visualize, and the pelvis is elevated so that gravity will pull the intestines into the abdomen. The uterus can be externally manipulated to facilitate visualization, or additional openings (ports) can be made to introduce other instruments for manipulation or to enable therapeutic procedures (e.g., ligation of the tubes). ✚

Laparoscopic view of normal pelvis

Figure B3.22

THE BOTTOM LINE: The ovaries are suspended by two peritoneal folds (the mesovarium from the posterosuperior aspect of the broad ligament and the vascular suspensory ligament of the ovary from the lateral wall of the pelvis) and attached to the uterus by the ovarian ligament. The peritoneum ends at the ovary itself. It is replaced on the surface of the ovary with a duller, cuboidal epithelium.

Neurovascular Structures Serving the Ovaries and Uterine Tubes

Arterial Supply of the Ovaries and Uterine Tubes. The *ovarian arteries* arise from the abdominal aorta (Table 3.5) and descend along the posterior abdominal wall. At the pelvic brim, they cross over the external iliac vessels and enter the suspensory ligaments (Fig. 3.31*A*), approaching the lateral aspects of the ovaries and uterine tubes. The ascending branches of the *uterine arteries* (branches of the internal iliac arteries), course along the lateral aspects of the uterus to approach the medial aspects of the ovaries and tubes (Figs. 3.12*B* and 3.29). Both the ovarian and ascending uterine arteries terminate by bifurcating into *ovarian* and *tubal branches*, which supply ovaries and tubes from opposite ends and anastomose with each other, providing a collateral circulation from abdominal and pelvic sources to both structures.

Venous and Lymphatic Drainage of the Ovaries and Uterine Tubes. Veins draining the ovary form a vine-like **pampiniform plexus of veins** in the broad ligament near the ovary and uterine tube (Fig. 3.29). The veins of the plexus usually merge to form a singular **ovarian vein**, which leaves the lesser pelvis with the ovarian artery. The right ovarian vein ascends to enter the *inferior vena cava;* the left ovarian vein drains into the *left renal vein* (Fig. 3.13). The *tubal veins* drain into the *ovarian veins* and *uterine (uterovaginal) venous plexus* (Fig. 3.29). The lymphatic vessels from the ovary join those from the uterine tubes and fundus and follow the ovarian blood vessels as they ascend to the *right* and *left lumbar (caval/aortic) lymph nodes* (Fig. 3.30).

Innervation of the Ovaries and Uterine Tubes. The nerve supply derives partly from the *ovarian plexus,* descending with the ovarian vessels, and partly from the *uterine (pelvic) plexus* (Fig. 3.32). The ovaries and uterine tubes are intraperitoneal and, therefore, are superior to the *pelvic pain line.* Thus visceral afferent pain fibers ascend retrogradely with the descending sympathetic fibers of the ovarian plexus and lumbar splanchnic nerves to cell bodies in the T11–L1 spinal sensory ganglia. Visceral afferent reflex fibers follow parasympathetic fibers retrogradely through the uterine (pelvic) and inferior hypogastric plexuses and the pelvic splanchnic nerves to cell bodies in the S2–S4 spinal sensory ganglia.

THE BOTTOM LINE: The ovaries and uterine tubes receive a double (collateral) blood supply from the abdominal aorta via the ovarian arteries and from the internal iliac artery via the uterine arteries. This collateral circulation allows the ovaries to be spared to supply estrogen when a hysterectomy necessitates ligation of the uterine arteries. Lymphatic drainage and sympathetic and visceral afferent pain fibers travel with the ovarian vessels. Parasympathetic and visceral afferent reflex fibers traverse pelvic plexuses and pelvic splanchnic nerves.

Rectum

The **rectum** (L. *rectus,* straight; a term coined during ancient studies on animals to describe the distal part of the gut) is the pelvic part of the alimentary tract and is continuous proximally with the sigmoid colon (Fig. 3.33) and distally with the

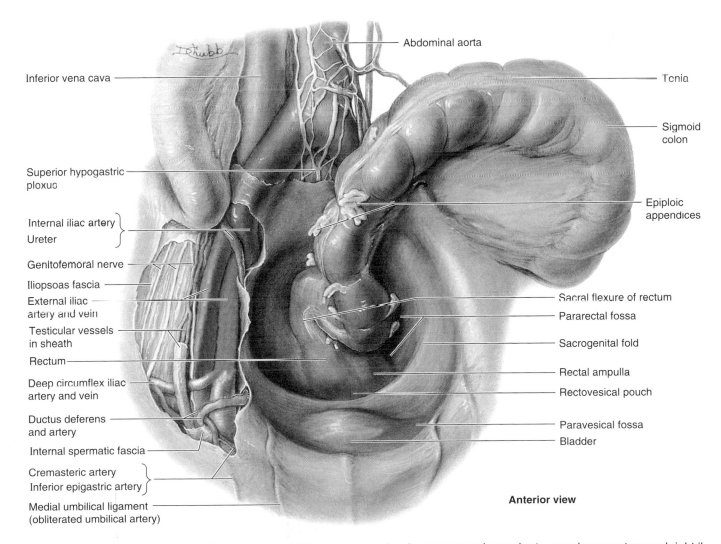

Inferior vena cava

Superior hypogastric plexus

Internal iliac artery
Ureter

Genitofemoral nerve

Iliopsoas fascia

External iliac artery and vein

Testicular vessels in sheath

Rectum

Deep circumflex iliac artery and vein

Ductus deferens and artery

Internal spermatic fascia

Cremasteric artery
Inferior epigastric artery

Medial umbilical ligament (obliterated umbilical artery)

Abdominal aorta

Tenia

Sigmoid colon

Epiploic appendices

Sacral flexure of rectum

Pararectal fossa

Sacrogenital fold

Rectal ampulla

Rectovesical pouch

Paravesical fossa

Bladder

Anterior view

Figure 3.33. Male greater and lesser pelves. The peritoneum has been removed superior to sacral promontory and right iliac fossa, revealing the superior hypogastric plexus lying in the bifurcation of the abdominal aorta and the common/external iliac vessels above the pelvic brim. The internal iliac artery, ureter, and ductus deferens cross the pelvic brim to enter the lesser pelvis, deep (external) to the peritoneum.

anal canal. The **rectosigmoid junction** lies anterior to the S3 vertebra. At this point, the teniae of the sigmoid colon spread out to form a continuous outer longitudinal layer of smooth muscle, and the fatty omental appendices are discontinued (see Fig. 2.41). The rectum follows the curve of the sacrum and coccyx, forming the **sacral flexure of the rectum.** The rectum ends anteroinferior to the tip of the coccyx, immediately before a sharp posteroinferior angle (the **anorectal flexure of the anal canal**) that occurs as the gut perforates the pelvic diaphragm (levator ani). The roughly 80° anorectal flexure is an important mechanism for fecal continence, being maintained during the resting state by the tonus of the puborectalis muscle and by its active contraction during peristaltic contractions if defecation is not to occur. With the flexures of the rectosigmoid junction superiorly and the anorectal junction inferiorly, the rectum has an S shape when viewed laterally.

Three sharp **lateral flexures of the rectum (superior, intermediate,** and **inferior)** are apparent when the rectum is viewed anteriorly. The flexures are formed in relation to three internal infoldings (**transverse rectal folds**): two on the left and one on the right side. The folds overlie thickened parts of the circular muscle layer of the rectal wall (Fig. 3.34B). The dilated terminal part of the rectum, lying directly superior to and supported by the pelvic diaphragm (levator ani) and anococcygeal ligament, is the **ampulla of the rectum** (Figs.

3.17B, 3.33, and 3.34). The ampulla receives and holds an accumulating fecal mass until it is expelled during defecation. The ability of the ampulla to relax to accommodate the initial and subsequent arrivals of fecal material is another essential element of maintaining fecal continence.

Peritoneum covers the anterior and lateral surfaces of the superior third of the rectum, only the anterior surface of the middle third, and no surface of the inferior third because it is subperitoneal (Table 3.3). In males, the peritoneum reflects from the rectum to the posterior wall of the bladder, where it forms the floor of the *rectovesical pouch.* In females, the peritoneum reflects from the rectum to the posterior part of the fornix of the vagina, where it forms the floor of the *rectouterine pouch.* In both sexes, lateral reflections of peritoneum from the superior third of the rectum form *pararectal fossae* (Fig. 3.33), which permit the rectum to distend as it fills with feces.

The rectum lies posteriorly against the inferior three sacral vertebrae and the coccyx, anococcygeal ligament, median sacral vessels, and inferior ends of the sympathetic trunks and sacral plexuses. In males, the rectum is related anteriorly to the fundus of the urinary bladder, terminal parts of the ureters, ductus deferentes, seminal glands, and prostate (Fig. 3.23). The *rectovesical septum* lies between the fundus of the bladder and the ampulla of the rectum and is closely associated with the seminal glands and prostate. In females, the rec-

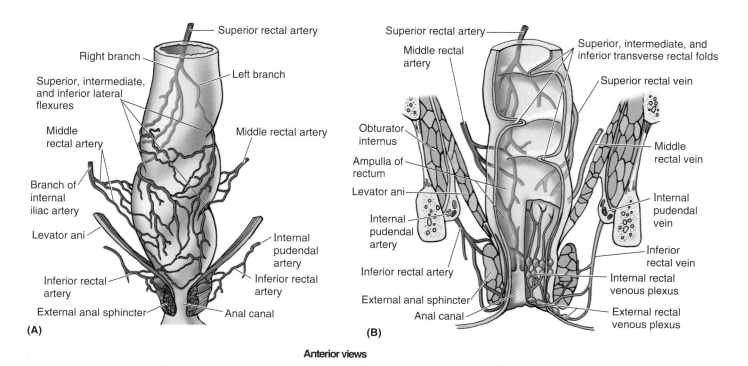

Anterior views

Figure 3.34. Arteries and veins of rectum and anal canal. A. In this anterior view of the arteries, there are two right middle rectal arteries. Despite their name, the inferior rectal arteries, which are branches of the internal pudendal arteries, mainly supply the anal canal. The three sharp lateral flexures of the rectum reflect the way in which the lumen navigates the transverse rectal folds (shown in part **B**) on the internal surface. **B.** This coronal section of the rectum and anal canal shows the arterial supply and venous drainage. The internal and external rectal venous plexuses are most directly related to the anal canal. The flexures and transverse rectal folds help support the weight of the feces.

tum is related anteriorly to the vagina and is separated from the posterior part of the fornix and the cervix by the *rectouterine pouch* (Fig. 3.27). Inferior to this pouch, the weak rectovaginal septum separates the superior half of the posterior wall of the vagina from the rectum.

Arterial Supply of the Rectum

The *superior rectal artery,* the continuation of the inferior mesenteric artery, supplies the proximal part of the rectum (Fig. 3.34). The right and left *middle rectal arteries,* usually arising from the inferior vesical arteries, supply the middle and inferior parts of the rectum. The **inferior rectal arteries,** arising from the internal pudendal arteries, supply the anorectal junction and anal canal. Anastomoses between these arteries provide potential collateral circulation.

Venous and Lymphatic Drainage of the Rectum

Blood from the rectum drains through the superior, middle, and inferior rectal veins (Fig. 3.34*B*). Anastomoses occur between the portal and systemic veins in the wall of the anal canal. Because the superior rectal vein drains into the portal venous system and the middle and inferior rectal veins drain into the systemic system, these anastomoses are clinically important areas of portacaval anastomosis (see Fig. 2.59). The submucosal rectal venous plexus surrounds the rectum and communicates with the vesical venous plexus in males and the uterovaginal venous plexus in females. The **rectal venous plexus** consists of two parts (Fig. 3.34*B*): the **internal rectal venous plexus** just deep to the mucosa of the anorectal junction and the subcutaneous **external rectal venous plexus**

external to the muscular wall of the rectum. Although these plexuses bear the term *rectal,* they are primarily "anal" in terms of location, function, and clinical significance (see "Venous and Lymphatic Drainage of the Anal Canal," later in this chapter).

Lymphatic vessels from the superior half of the rectum pass to the **pararectal lymph nodes** (located directly on the muscle layer of the rectum) and then ascend to the *inferior mesenteric lymph nodes,* either via *sacral lymph nodes* or more directly passing through nodes along the superior rectal vessels (Fig. 3.35; Table 3.6). The inferior mesenteric nodes drain into the *lumbar (caval/aortic) lymph nodes.* Lymphatic vessels from the inferior half of the rectum drain directly to *sacral lymph nodes* or, especially from the distal ampulla, follow the middle rectal vessels to drain into the *internal iliac lymph nodes.*

Innervation of the Rectum

The nerve supply to the rectum is from the sympathetic and parasympathetic systems (Fig. 3.36). The sympathetic supply is from the lumbar spinal cord, conveyed via lumbar splanchnic nerves and the hypogastric/pelvic plexuses and through the periarterial plexus of the inferior mesenteric and superior rectal arteries. The parasympathetic supply is from the S2–S4 spinal cord level, passing via the pelvic splanchnic nerves and the left and right inferior hypogastric plexuses to the rectal (pelvic) plexus. Because the rectum is inferior (distal) to the pelvic pain line, all visceral afferent fibers follow the parasympathetic fibers retrogradely to the S2–S4 spinal sensory ganglia.

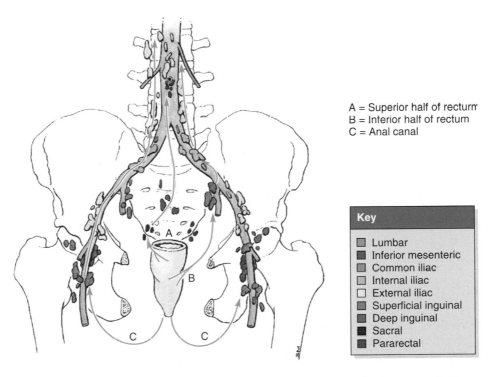

A = Superior half of rectum
B = Inferior half of rectum
C = Anal canal

Key
☐ Lumbar
◼ Inferior mesenteric
☐ Common iliac
☐ Internal iliac
☐ External iliac
◼ Superficial inguinal
◼ Deep inguinal
◼ Sacral
◼ Pararectal

Figure 3.35. Lymphatic drainage of rectum and anal canal. The *arrows* indicate the direction of lymph flow to the lymph nodes.

Upper lumbar
sympathetic trunk

Spinal ganglia

T12

L1

L2

L3

L4

L5

S1

S2

S3

S4

Lumbar
splanchnic
nerves

Spinal
ganglia

Pelvic splanchnic
nerves

Pelvic
plexus

Sacral
plexus

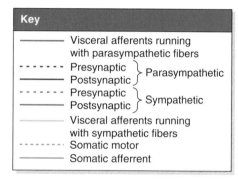

Key

————	Visceral afferents running with parasympathetic fibers
- - - - Presynaptic	Parasympathetic
———— Postsynaptic	
- - - - Presynaptic	Sympathetic
———— Postsynaptic	
————	Visceral afferents running with sympathetic fibers
- - - -	Somatic motor
————	Somatic afferent

Prevertebral
ganglia

Para-aortic
plexus

Superior
rectal nerves

Superior
hypogastric
plexus

Inferior
hypogastric
plexuses

Pelvic
plexus

Pudendal
nerve

Internal anal
sphincter

External anal sphincter

Inferior anal
(rectal) nerve

Figure 3.36 Innervation of rectum and anal canal. The lumbar and pelvic splanchnic nerves and hypogastric plexuses have been retracted laterally for clarity.

Rectal Examination

Many structures related to the anteroinferior part of the rectum may be palpated through its walls (e.g., the prostate and seminal glands in males and the cervix in females). In both sexes, the pelvic surfaces of the sacrum and coccyx may be palpated. The ischial spines and tuberosities may also be palpated. Enlarged internal iliac lymph nodes, pathological thickening of the ureters, swellings in the ischioanal fossae (e.g., ischioanal abscesses and abnormal contents in the rectovesical pouch in the male or the rectouterine pouch in the female) may also be palpated. Tenderness of an inflamed appendix may also be detected rectally if it descends into the lesser pelvis (pararectal fossa).

The internal aspect of the rectum can be examined with a *proctoscope,* and biopsies of lesions may be taken through this instrument. During insertion of a *sigmoidoscope,* the curvatures of the rectum and its acute flexion at the rectosigmoid junction have to be kept in mind so that the patient does not undergo unnecessary discomfort. The operator must also know that the *transverse rectal folds,* which provide useful landmarks for the procedure, may temporarily impede passage of these instruments.

Resection of the Rectum

When resecting the rectum in males (e.g., during cancer treatment), the plane of the rectovesical septum (a fascial septum extending superiorly from the perineal body) is located so that the prostate and urethra can be separated from the rectum. In this way, these organs are not damaged during the surgery. ○

THE BOTTOM LINE: The rectum accumulates and temporarily stores feces. It begins at the rectosigmoid junction as the teniae of the sigmoid colon spread and unite into a continuous longitudinal layer of smooth muscle and the omental appendices cease. It ends with the anorectal flexure as the gut penetrates the pelvic diaphragm, becoming the anal canal. Despite the Latin meaning of the term (straight), the rectum is concave anteriorly as the sacral flexure and has three lateral flexures formed in relation to the internal transverse rectal folds. The rectum enlarges into the rectal ampulla directly above the pelvic floor. Its superior, middle, and inferior parts are, respectively, intraperitoneal, retroperitoneal, and subperitoneal. Collateral arterial circulation and a portocaval venous anastomosis result from anastomoses of the superior and middle rectal vessels. Lymphatic vessels from the superior rectum pass to inferior mesenteric lymph nodes, many passing through pararectal nodes en route; those from the inferior rectum drain to sacral and internal iliac nodes. Sympathetic nerve fibers pass to the rectum (especially blood vessels and internal anal sphincter) from lumbar spinal cord segments via the hypogastric/pelvic plexuses and the periarterial plexus of the superior rectal artery. Parasympathetic and visceral afferent fibers involve the middle sacral spinal cord segments and spinal ganglia.

Perineum

The **perineum** refers to both an external surface area and a shallow "compartment" of the body. The perineum (*perineal compartment*) is bounded by the pelvic outlet and is separated from the pelvic cavity by the pelvic diaphragm, which is formed by the levator ani and coccygeus muscles. In the anatomical position, the surface of the perineum (*perineal area*) is the narrow region between the proximal parts of the thighs; however, when the lower limbs are abducted, it is a diamond-shaped area extending from the mons pubis anteriorly, the medial surfaces (insides) of the thighs laterally, and the gluteal folds and superior end of the intergluteal (natal) cleft posteriorly (Fig. 3.37).

The osseofibrous structures marking the boundaries of the perineum (perineal compartment) (Fig. 3.38) are the:

- *Pubic symphysis,* anteriorly.
- *Inferior pubic rami* and *ischial rami,* anterolaterally.
- *Ischial tuberosities,* laterally.
- *Sacrotuberous ligaments,* posterolaterally.
- Inferiormost *sacrum* and *coccyx,* posteriorly.

A transverse line joining the anterior ends of the ischial tuberosities divides the diamond-shaped perineum into two triangles, the oblique planes of which intersect at the transverse line (Fig. 3.38*A* & *B*). The **anal triangle** lies posterior to this line. The anal canal and its orifice, the anus, constitute the major deep and superficial features of the triangle, lying centrally surrounded by ischioanal fat. The **urogenital (UG) triangle** is anterior to this line. In contrast to the open anal triangle, the UG triangle is "closed" by a thin sheet of tough, deep fascia, the **perineal membrane,** which stretches between the two sides of the pubic arch, covering the anterior part of the pelvic outlet (Fig. 3.39*C*). The perineal membrane thus fills the anterior gap in the pelvic diaphragm (the urogenital hiatus, Fig. 3.39*A*) but is perforated by the urethra in both sexes and by the vagina of the female. The membrane and the ischiopubic rami to which it attaches provide a foundation for the erectile bodies of the external genitalia—the penis and scrotum of males and the vulva of females—which are the superficial features of the triangle (Fig. 3.37).

(A)

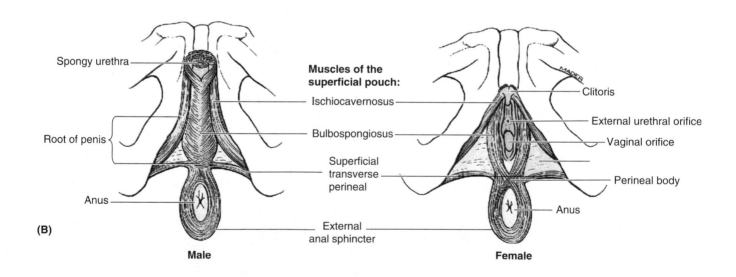

(B)

Figure 3.37. Male and female perineum. A. Surface features and projections of the osseous boundaries and structures in the perineal compartment. The penis and some of the scrotum (part of the perineum) are retracted anteriorly and thus not shown. **B.** The muscles of the superficial perineal pouch (space) are shown, corresponding to the projected structures in part **A.**

(A)

(B) Female

(C) Male

Figure 3.38. Disposition and boundaries of perineum.
A. The diamond-shaped perineum overlies the pelvic outlet; the perineum and outlet are bounded by the same osseofibrous structures. The two triangles (urogenital and anal) that together make up the perineum do not occupy the same plane. **B.** This view of the female pelvis is the one that the obstetrician visualizes in his or her mind's eye when the patient is on the examining table. **C.** The features bounding the pelvic outlet and perineum are identified on this male pelvis.

The midpoint of the line joining the ischial tuberosities is the **central point of the perineum** (Figs. 3.37A and 3.38A). This is the location of the **perineal body**, which is an irregular mass, variable in size and consistency and containing collagenous and elastic fibers and both skeletal and smooth muscle (Fig. 3.37B). The perineal body lies deep to the skin, with relatively little overlying subcutaneous tissue, posterior to the vestibule or bulb of the penis and anterior to the anus and anal canal. The perineal body is the site of convergence and interlacing of fibers of several muscles, including the:

- Bulbospongiosus.
- External anal sphincter.
- Superficial and deep transverse perineal muscles.
- Smooth and voluntary slips of muscle from the external urethral sphincter, levator ani, and muscular coats of the rectum.

Anteriorly, the perineal body blends with the posterior border of the perineal membrane (Fig. 3.39D & E) and superiorly with the rectovesical or rectovaginal septum.

Disruption of the Perineal Body

The perineal body is an especially important structure in women because it is the final support of the pelvic viscera, linking muscles that extend across the pelvic outlet, like crossing beams supporting the overlying pelvic diaphragm. Stretching or tearing the attachments of perineal muscles from the perineal body can occur during childbirth, removing support from the pelvic floor. As a result, *prolapse of pelvic viscera,* including prolapse of the bladder (through the urethra) and prolapse of the uterus and/or vagina (through the vaginal orifice) may occur. (Various degrees of prolapse are illustrated in clinical correlation [blue] box "Disposition of the Uterus and Uterine Prolapse," in this chapter). The perineal body can also be disrupted by trauma, inflammatory disease, and infection, which can result in the formation of a *fistula* (abnormal canal) connected to the vestibule (see clinical correlation [blue] box "Vaginal Fistulae," in this chapter). Attenuation of the perineal body, associated with diastasis (separation) of the puborectalis and pubococcygeus parts of the levator ani, may also result in the formation of a *cystocele, rectocele,* and/or *enterocele,* hernial protrusions of part of the bladder, rectum, or rectovaginal pouch, respectively, into the vaginal wall (Fig. B3.23).▶

Figure B3.23

Inferior view (lithotomy position)

Figure B3.24

Episiotomy

During vaginal surgery and labor, an **episiotomy** (surgical incision of the perineum and inferoposterior vaginal wall) is often made to enlarge the vaginal orifice. It was long held that episiotomy decreases the prevalence of excessive perineal body attenuation and decreases trauma to the pelvic diaphragm, preventing jagged tears of the perineal muscles. Episiotomies are still performed in > 50% of vaginal deliveries in the United States (Gabbe et al., 2002). It is generally agreed that episiotomy is indicated when descent of the fetus is arrested or protracted, when instrumentation is necessary (e.g., use of obstetrical forceps), or to expedite delivery when there are signs of fetal distress. However, routine prophylactic episiotomy is widely debated.

The perineal body is the major structure incised during a **median episiotomy** (Fig. B3.24*A*). The rationale of the median incision is that the scar produced as the wound heals will not be greatly different from the fibrous tissue surrounding it. Also, because the incision extends only partially into this fibrous tissue, some physicians believe that the incision is more likely to be self-limiting, resisting further tearing. However, when further tearing does occur, it is directed toward the anus, and sphincter damage or anovaginal fistulae are potential sequelae. Recent studies indicate median episiotomies are associated with an increased incidence of severe lacerations, associated in turn with an increased incidence of long-term incontinence and pelvic prolapse.

Mediolateral episiotomies are also performed (Fig. B3.24*A*). These episiotomies do not appear to increase the incidence of severe laceration and are less likely to be associated with damage to the anal sphincters and canal. (*Note:* the clinical use of the term *mediolateral* is technically inappropriate here; it actually refers to an incision that is initially a median incision that then turns laterally as it proceeds posteriorly, circumventing the perineal body and directing further tearing away from the anus.) ⊙

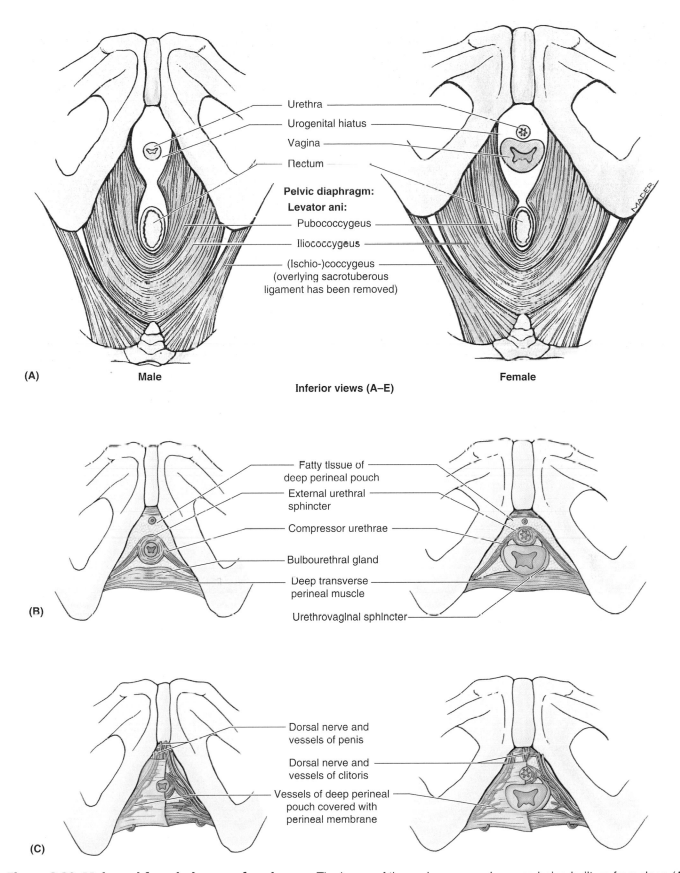

Urethra

Urogenital hiatus

Vagina

Rectum

Pelvic diaphragm:
Levator ani:

Pubococcygeus

Iliococcygeus

(Ischio-)coccygeus
(overlying sacrotuberous
ligament has been removed)

(A)

Male

Female

Inferior views (A–E)

Fatty tissue of
deep perineal pouch

External urethral
sphincter

Compressor urethrae

Bulbourethral gland

Deep transverse
perineal muscle

Urethrovaginal sphincter

(B)

Dorsal nerve and
vessels of penis

Dorsal nerve and
vessels of clitoris

Vessels of deep perineal
pouch covered with
perineal membrane

(C)

Figure 3.39. Male and female layers of perineum. The layers of the perineum are shown as being built up from deep (**A**) to superficial (**E**) layers. **A.** The pelvic outlet is almost closed by the pelvic diaphragm (levator ani and coccygeus muscles), forming the floor of the pelvic cavity and, as viewed here, the roof of the perineum. The urethra (and vagina in females) and rectum pass through the urogenital hiatus of the pelvic diaphragm. **B and C.** The external urethral sphincter and deep transverse perineal muscle span the region of the urogenital hiatus, which is closed inferiorly by the perineal membrane extending between the ischiopubic rami.

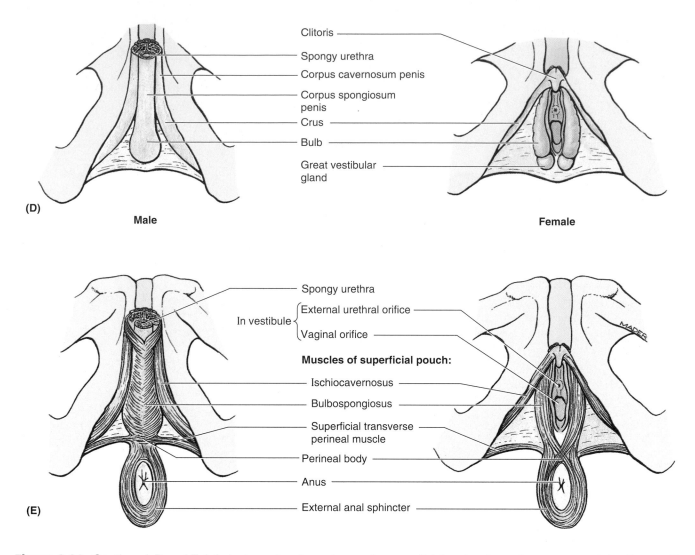

Male   Female

(D)

In vestibule

Clitoris
Spongy urethra
Corpus cavernosum penis
Corpus spongiosum penis
Crus
Bulb
Great vestibular gland

Spongy urethra
External urethral orifice
Vaginal orifice

Muscles of superficial pouch:

Ischiocavernosus
Bulbospongiosus
Superficial transverse perineal muscle
Perineal body
Anus
External anal sphincter

(E)

Figure 3.39 *Continued.* **D and E.** Inferior to perineal membrane, the superficial perineal pouch or space contains the erectile bodies and the muscles associated with them.

THE BOTTOM LINE: The perineum is the diamond-shaped compartment bounded peripherally by the osseofibrous pelvic outlet and deeply (superiorly) by the pelvic diaphragm. The term is also applied to the surface area overlying this compartment. The urogenital triangle (anteriorly) and anal triangle (posteriorly) that together compose this diamond-shaped area lie at angles to each other. Their intersecting planes define the transverse line (extending between ischial tuberosities) that is the base of each triangle. Centrally, the UG triangle is perforated by the urethra and, in females, by the vagina; the anal triangle is perforated by the anal canal. The perineal body is a musculofibrous mass between the UG and the anal perforating structures at the center point of the perineum.

Fasciae and Pouches of the Urogenital Triangle

Perineal Fasciae[2]

The perineal fascia consists of superficial and deep layers. The **subcutaneous tissue of the perineum,** or *superficial perineal fascia,* like that of the inferior anterior abdominal wall (see

[2]The terminology used in this section (in boldface) was recommended by the *Federative International Committee on Anatomical Terminology* (FICAT) in 1998; however, because many clinicians concerned with the perineum use eponyms, the authors have placed commonly used terms in parentheses so that the FICAT terminology will be understood by all readers.

Chapter 2) consists of a superficial *fatty layer* and a deep *membranous layer* (Colles fascia) (Fig. 3.40A & B). In females, the fatty layer makes up the substance of the labia majora and mons pubis and is continuous anteriorly and superiorly with the fatty layer of subcutaneous tissue of the abdomen (Camper fascia) (Fig. 3.40A & C). In males, the fatty layer is greatly diminished in the urogenital triangle, being replaced altogether in the penis and scrotum with smooth (dartos) muscle. It is continuous between the penis or scrotum and thighs with the fatty layer of subcutaneous tissue of the abdomen (Fig. 3.40B & E). In both sexes, the fatty layer of subcutaneous tissue of the perineum is continuous posteriorly with the ischioanal fat pad in the anal region (Fig. 3.40D).

The **membranous layer of subcutaneous tissue of the perineum** does not extend into the anal triangle, being attached posteriorly to the posterior margin of the perineal membrane and the perineal body (Fig. 3.40A & B). Laterally it is attached to the fascia lata (deep fascia) of the superiormost medial aspect of the thigh (Fig. 3.40C & E). Anteriorly in the male, the membranous layer of subcutaneous tissue is continuous with the **dartos fascia** of the penis and scrotum; however, on each side of and anterior to the scrotum, the membranous layer becomes continuous with the membranous layer of subcutaneous tissue of the abdomen (Scarpa fascia) (Fig. 3.40B). In females, the membranous layer passes superior to the fatty layer forming the labia majora and becomes continuous with the membranous layer of subcutaneous tissue of the abdomen (Fig. 3.40A & C).

The (**deep**) **perineal fascia** (investing or Gallaudet fascia) intimately invests the ischiocavernosus, bulbospongiosus, and superficial transverse perineal muscles (Fig. 3.40A & E). It is also attached laterally to the ischiopubic rami. Anteriorly it is fused to the suspensory ligament of the penis (Fig. 3.50) and is continuous with the deep fascia covering the external oblique muscle of the abdomen and the rectus sheath. In females, the perineal fascia is fused with the suspensory ligament of the clitoris and, as in males, with the deep fascia of the abdomen.

THE BOTTOM LINE: The subcutaneous tissue of the perineum includes a superficial fatty layer and a deeper membranous layer (Colles fascia), which are continuous with corresponding layers of the inferior anterior abdominal wall. In females, the fatty layer is thick within the mons pubis and labia majora, but in males, it is replaced by smooth dartos muscle in the penis and scrotum. The membranous layer is limited to the UG triangle, fusing with the deep fascia at the posterior border (base) of the triangle. In males, this layer extends into the penis and scrotum, where it is closely associated with the loose, mobile skin of those structures.

Superficial Perineal Pouch

The **superficial perineal pouch** (compartment) is a potential space between the membranous layer of subcutaneous tissue and the perineal membrane, bounded laterally by the ischiopubic rami (Figs. 3.39D & E and 3.40).

In males, the superficial perineal pouch contains the:

- *Root* (bulb and crura) *of the penis* and associated muscles (*ischiocavernosus* and *bulbospongiosus*).
- Proximal (bulbous) part of the *spongy urethra.*
- *Superficial transverse perineal muscles.*
- *Deep perineal branches* of the internal pudendal vessels and pudendal nerves.

In females, the superficial perineal pouch contains the:

- *Clitoris* and associated muscles (ischiocavernosus).
- *Bulbs of the vestibule* and surrounding muscle (bulbospongiosus).
- *Greater vestibular glands.*
- *Superficial transverse perineal muscles.*
- Related vessels and nerves (*deep perineal branches* of the internal pudendal vessels and pudendal nerves).

The structures of the superficial perineal pouch will be discussed in greater detail, specific to each sex, under "Male Perineum" and "Female Perineum," later in this chapter.

Deep Perineal Pouch

The **deep perineal pouch** (space) is bounded inferiorly by the perineal membrane, superiorly by the inferior fascia of the pelvic diaphragm, and laterally by the inferior portion of the obturator fascia (covering the obturator internus muscle) (Fig. 3.40C & E). It includes the fat-filled anterior recesses of the ischioanal fossa. The superior boundary in the region of the urogenital hiatus is indistinct.

In both sexes, the deep perineal pouch contains

- Part of the urethra, centrally.
- The inferior part of the external urethral sphincter muscle, above the center of the perineal membrane, surrounding the urethra.
- Anterior extensions of the ischioanal fat pads.

In males, the deep perineal pouch contains the:

- *Intermediate part of the urethra,* the narrowest part of the male urethra.
- *Deep transverse perineal muscles,* immediately superior to the perineal membrane (on its superior surface), running transversely along its posterior aspect.
- *Bulbourethral glands,* embedded within the deep perineal musculature.
- Dorsal neurovascular structures of the penis.

In females, the deep perineal pouch contains the:

- *Proximal part of the urethra.*

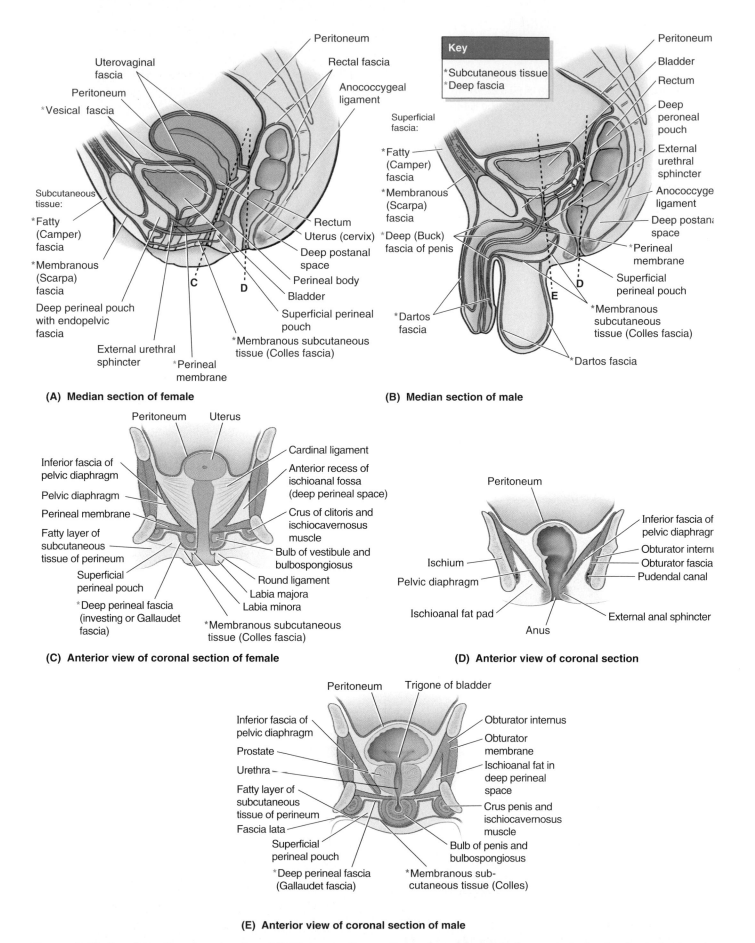

(A) Median section of female

Peritoneum
Uterovaginal fascia
Peritoneum
*Vesical fascia
Subcutaneous tissue:
*Fatty (Camper) fascia
*Membranous (Scarpa) fascia
Deep perineal pouch with endopelvic fascia
External urethral sphincter
*Perineal membrane

Peritoneum
Rectal fascia
Anococcygeal ligament
Rectum
Uterus (cervix)
Deep postanal space
Perineal body
Bladder
Superficial perineal pouch
*Membranous subcutaneous tissue (Colles fascia)

C   D

(B) Median section of male

Key
*Subcutaneous tissue
*Deep fascia

Superficial fascia:
*Fatty (Camper) fascia
*Membranous (Scarpa) fascia
*Deep (Buck) fascia of penis
*Dartos fascia

Peritoneum
Bladder
Rectum
Deep peroneal pouch
External urethral sphincter
Anococcygeal ligament
Deep postanal space
*Perineal membrane
Superficial perineal pouch
*Membranous subcutaneous tissue (Colles fascia)
*Dartos fascia

E   D

(C) Anterior view of coronal section of female

Peritoneum   Uterus
Inferior fascia of pelvic diaphragm
Pelvic diaphragm
Perineal membrane
Fatty layer of subcutaneous tissue of perineum
Superficial perineal pouch
*Deep perineal fascia (investing or Gallaudet fascia)

Cardinal ligament
Anterior recess of ischioanal fossa (deep perineal space)
Crus of clitoris and ischiocavernosus muscle
Bulb of vestibule and bulbospongiosus
Round ligament
Labia majora
Labia minora
*Membranous subcutaneous tissue (Colles fascia)

(D) Anterior view of coronal section

Peritoneum
Ischium
Pelvic diaphragm
Ischioanal fat pad
Anus
Inferior fascia of pelvic diaphragm
Obturator internus
Obturator fascia
Pudendal canal
External anal sphincter

(E) Anterior view of coronal section of male

Peritoneum   Trigone of bladder
Inferior fascia of pelvic diaphragm
Prostate
Urethra
Fatty layer of subcutaneous tissue of perineum
Fascia lata
Superficial perineal pouch
*Deep perineal fascia (Gallaudet fascia)

Obturator internus
Obturator membrane
Ischioanal fat in deep perineal space
Crus penis and ischiocavernosus muscle
Bulb of penis and bulbospongiosus
*Membranous subcutaneous tissue (Colles)

Figure 3.40. Fasciae of perineum. A and B. These median sections, viewed from left, demonstrate the fasciae in the female and male. The planes of the sections shown in parts **C–E** are indicated. **C.** This coronal section of the female UG triangle is in the plane of the vagina. **D.** This coronal section of the anal triangle is in the plane of the lower rectal and anal canals. **E.** This coronal section of the male UG triangle is in the plane of the prostatic urethra.

- A mass of smooth muscle in the place of deep transverse perineal muscles on the posterior edge of the perineal membrane, associated with the perineal body.

- Dorsal neurovasculature of the clitoris.

Past and Current Concepts of Deep Perineal Pouch and External Urethral Sphincter. Traditionally, a trilaminar, triangular *UG diaphragm* has been described as making up the deep perineal pouch. Although the classical descriptions appear justified when viewing only the superficial aspect of the structures occupying the deep pouch (Fig. 3.41*A*), the long-held concept of a flat, essentially two-dimensional diaphragm is erroneous. According to this concept, the UG diaphragm consisted of the perineal membrane (inferior fascia of the UG diaphragm) inferiorly and a superior fascia of the UG diaphragm superiorly. The deep pouch was the space between the two fascial membranes, occupied by a flat muscular sheet consisting of a disc-like sphincter urethra anterior to or within an equally two-dimensional, transversely oriented deep transverse perineal muscle. In males, the bulbourethral glands were also considered occupants of the pouch. Only the descriptions of the perineal membrane and deep transverse perineal muscles of the male (with embedded glands) appear to be supported by evidence, which includes medical imaging of live subjects (Myers et al., 1998a, 1998b).

In the female, the posterior edge of the perineal membrane is typically occupied by a mass of smooth muscle in the place of the deep transverse perineal muscles (Wendell-Smith, 1995). Immediately superior to the posterior half of the perineal membrane, the flat, sheet-like, deep transverse perineal muscle, when developed (typically only males), offers dynamic support for the pelvic viscera. As described by Oelrich (1980), however, the urethral sphincter muscle is not a flat, planar structure, and the only "superior fascia" is the intrinsic fascia of the external urethral sphincter muscle. Contemporary views consider the *inferior fascia of the pelvic diaphragm* to be the superior boundary of the deep pouch

(Fig. 3.40*C–E*). In both views, the strong *perineal membrane* is the inferior boundary (floor) of the deep pouch, separating it from the superficial pouch. The perineal membrane is indeed, with the perineal body, the final passive support of the pelvic viscera.

The *external urethral sphincter* is more like a tube or trough than like a disc. In the male only the inferior part of the muscle forms a circular investment (a true sphincter) for the intermediate part of the urethra inferior to the prostate (Fig. 3.41*B*). Its larger, trough-like part extends vertically to the neck of the bladder as part of the isthmus of the prostate, displacing glandular tissue and investing the prostatic urethra anteriorly and anterolaterally only. Apparently, the muscular primordium is established around the whole length of the urethra before development of the prostate. As the prostate develops from urethral glands, the posterior and posterolateral muscle atrophies or is displaced by the prostate. Whether this part of the muscle compresses or dilates the prostatic urethra is a matter of some controversy.

In the female, the external urethral sphincter is more properly a "urogenital sphincter," according to Oelrich (1983). Here, too, he describes a part forming a true anular sphincter around the urethra (Fig. 3.41*C*), with several additional parts extending from it: a superior part, extending to the neck of the bladder; a subdivision described as extending inferolaterally to the ischial ramus on each side (the compressor urethrae muscle); and yet another band-like part, which encircles both the vagina and the urethra (urethrovaginal sphincter). In both the male and female, the musculature described is oriented perpendicular to the perineal membrane, rather than lying in a plane parallel to it. Other authors substantiate most of Oelrich's description but dispute the encircling of the urethra in the female, claiming that the muscle is not capable of sphincteric action. Furthermore, they assert that sectioning the perineal nerve supplying the "sphincter" does not result in incontinence, but this may be a consequence of innervation from multiple sources.

Rupture of the Urethra in Males and Extravasation of Urine

Fractures of the pelvic girdle, especially those resulting from separation of the pubic symphysis and puboprostatic ligaments, often cause a *rupture of the intermediate part of the urethra*. Rupture of this part of the urethra results in the extravasation of urine and blood into the deep perineal pouch (Fig. B3.25*A*); the fluid may pass superiorly through the urogenital hiatus and distribute extraperitoneally around the prostate and bladder.

The common site of *rupture of the spongy urethra* and *extravasation* (escape) *of urine* is in the bulb of the penis (Fig.

B3.25*B*). This injury usually results from a forceful blow to the perineum (*straddle injury*), such as falling on a metal beam or, less commonly, from the incorrect passage (*false passage*) of a transurethral catheter or device that fails to negotiate the angle of the urethra in the bulb of the penis. Rupture of the corpus spongiosum and spongy urethra results in urine passing from it (extravasating) into the superficial perineal space. The attachments of the perineal fascia determine the direction of flow of the extravasated urine. Urine may pass into the loose connective tissue in the scrotum, around the penis, and superiorly, deep to the membranous layer of subcutaneous connective tissue of the inferior anterior abdominal wall. ▶

The urine cannot pass far into the thighs because the membranous layer of superficial perineal fascia blends with the fascia lata, enveloping the thigh muscles, just distal to the inguinal ligament. In addition, urine cannot pass posteriorly into the anal triangle because the superficial and deep layers of perineal fascia are continuous with each other around the superficial perineal muscles and with the posterior edge of the perineal membrane between them. Rupture of a blood vessel into the superficial perineal pouch resulting from trauma would result in a similar containment of blood in the superficial perineal pouch. ⊙

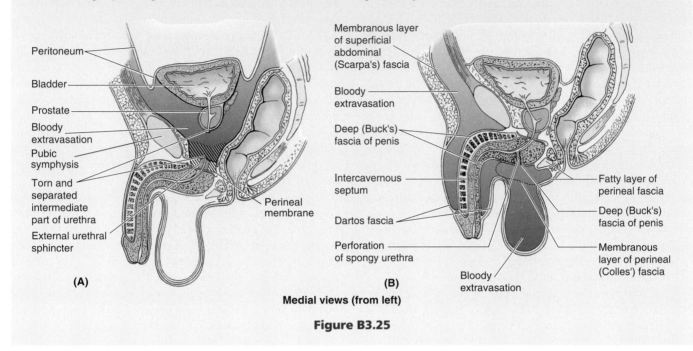

(A)

Peritoneum
Bladder
Prostate
Bloody extravasation
Pubic symphysis
Torn and separated intermediate part of urethra
External urethral sphincter
Perineal membrane

(B)

Membranous layer of superficial abdominal (Scarpa's) fascia
Bloody extravasation
Deep (Buck's) fascia of penis
Intercavernous septum
Dartos fascia
Perforation of spongy urethra
Bloody extravasation
Fatty layer of perineal fascia
Deep (Buck's) fascia of penis
Membranous layer of perineal (Colles') fascia

Medial views (from left)

Figure B3.25

THE BOTTOM LINE: The planar perineal membrane divides the urogenital triangle of the perineum into superficial and deep perineal pouches. The superficial perineal pouch is between the membranous layer of subcutaneous tissue of the perineum and the perineal membrane and is bounded laterally by the ischiopubic rami. The deep perineal pouch is between the perineal membrane and the inferior fascia of the pelvic diaphragm and is bounded laterally by the obturator fascia. The superficial pouch contains the erectile bodies of the external genitalia and associated muscles, the superficial transverse perineal muscle, deep perineal nerves and vessels, and in females the greater vestibular glands. The deep pouch includes the fat-filled anterior recesses of the ischioanal fossae (laterally), the deep perineal muscle and inferiormost part of the external urethral sphincter, the part of the urethra traversing the perineal membrane and inferiormost external urethral sphincter (the intermediate urethra of males), the dorsal nerves of the penis/clitoris, and in males the bulbourethral glands.

Features of the Anal Triangle

Ischioanal Fossae

The **ischioanal fossae** (formerly called ischiorectal fossae) on each side of the anal canal are large fascia-lined, wedge-shaped spaces between the skin of the anal region and the pelvic diaphragm (Figs. 3.40D, 3.42A, and 3.43). The apex of each fossa lies superiorly where the levator ani muscle arises from the obturator fascia. The ischioanal fossae, wide inferiorly and narrow superiorly, are filled with fat and loose connective tissue. The two ischioanal fossae communicate by means of the *deep postanal space* over the *anococcygeal ligament* (body), a fibrous mass located between the anal canal and the tip of the coccyx (Figs. 3.40A & B and 3.42B).

Each ischioanal fossa is bounded

- Laterally by the ischium and overlapping inferior part of the obturator internus, covered with obturator fascia.

- Medially by the external anal sphincter, with a sloping superior medial wall or roof formed by the levator ani as it descends to blend with the sphincter; both structures surround the anal canal.

- Posteriorly by the sacrotuberous ligament and gluteus maximus.

- Anteriorly by the bodies of the pubic bones, inferior to the origin of the puborectalis. These parts of the fossae, extending into the UG triangle superior to the perineal membrane (and musculature on its superior surface), are known as the **anterior recesses of the ischioanal fossae.**

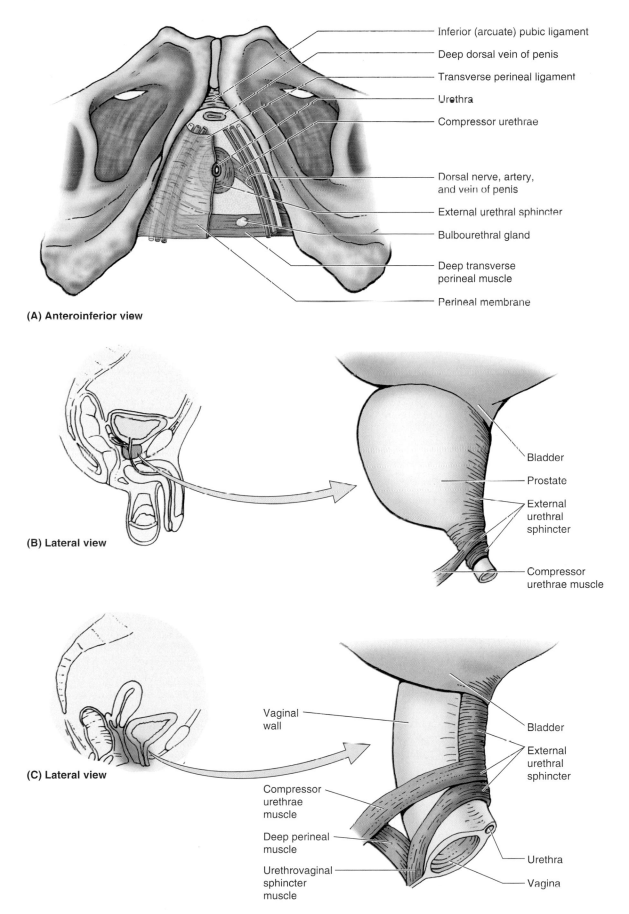

(A) Anteroinferior view

- Inferior (arcuate) pubic ligament
- Deep dorsal vein of penis
- Transverse perineal ligament
- Urethra
- Compressor urethrae
- Dorsal nerve, artery, and vein of penis
- External urethral sphincter
- Bulbourethral gland
- Deep transverse perineal muscle
- Perineal membrane

(B) Lateral view

- Bladder
- Prostate
- External urethral sphincter
- Compressor urethrae muscle

(C) Lateral view

- Vaginal wall
- Compressor urethrae muscle
- Deep perineal muscle
- Urethrovaginal sphincter muscle
- Bladder
- External urethral sphincter
- Urethra
- Vagina

Figure 3.41. Deep perineal pouch and male and female external urethral sphincters. A. The deep perineal pouch is seen through (left side) and after removal of the perineal membrane (right side). **B.** The trough-like fibers of the male external urethral sphincter ascend to neck of bladder as part of isthmus of prostate. **C.** The female urethral sphincter is shown.

(A) Anterior view of schematic coronal section

(B) Inferior view of perineum (lithotomy position)

Figure 3.42. Pelvic diaphragm and ischioanal fossae. A. Coronal section of the pelvis in the plane of the rectum, anal canal, and ischioanal fossae. **B.** Inferior view of pelvic diaphragm in situ. Left sacrospinous ligament has been removed.

Each ischioanal fossa is filled with a **fat body of the ischioanal fossa.** These fat bodies support the anal canal but they are readily displaced to permit descent and expansion of the anal canal during the passage of feces. The fat bodies are traversed by tough, fibrous bands, as well as by several neurovascular structures, including the inferior anal/rectal vessels and nerves and two other cutaneous nerves, the perforating branch of S2 and S3 and the perineal branch of S4 nerve.

Pudendal Canal and Its Neurovascular Bundle

The **pudendal canal** (Alcock canal) is an essentially horizontal passageway within the obturator fascia that covers the medial aspect of the obturator internus and lines the lateral wall of the ischioanal fossa (Figs. 3.42A and 3.43). The internal pudendal artery and vein, the pudendal nerve, and the nerve to the obturator internus enter this canal at the lesser sciatic notch, inferior to the ischial spine. The internal pudendal vessels and the pudendal nerve supply and drain blood from and innervate, respectively, most of the perineum. As the artery and nerve enter the canal, they give rise to the **inferior rectal** artery and **nerve,** which pass medially to supply the external anal sphincter and the perianal skin (Figs. 3.43 and 3.44; Table 3.8). Toward the distal (anterior) end of the pudendal canal, the artery and nerve both bifurcate, giving rise to the *perineal nerve* and *artery,* which are distributed mostly to the superficial pouch (inferior to the perineal membrane), and to the *dorsal artery* and *nerve of the penis or clitoris,* which run in the deep pouch (superior to the membrane). When the latter structures reach the dorsum of the penis or clitoris, the nerves run distally on the lateral side of the continuation of the internal pudendal artery as they both proceed to the glans.

The perineal nerve has two branches: the **superficial perineal nerves** give rise to posterior scrotal or labial (cutaneous) branches, and the **deep perineal nerve** supplies the muscles of the deep and superficial perineal pouches, the skin of the vestibule, and the mucosa of the inferiormost part of the vagina. The inferior rectal nerve communicates with the posterior scrotal or labial and perineal nerves. The **dorsal nerve of the penis or clitoris** is the primary sensory nerve serving the male or female organ, especially the sensitive glans at the distal end.

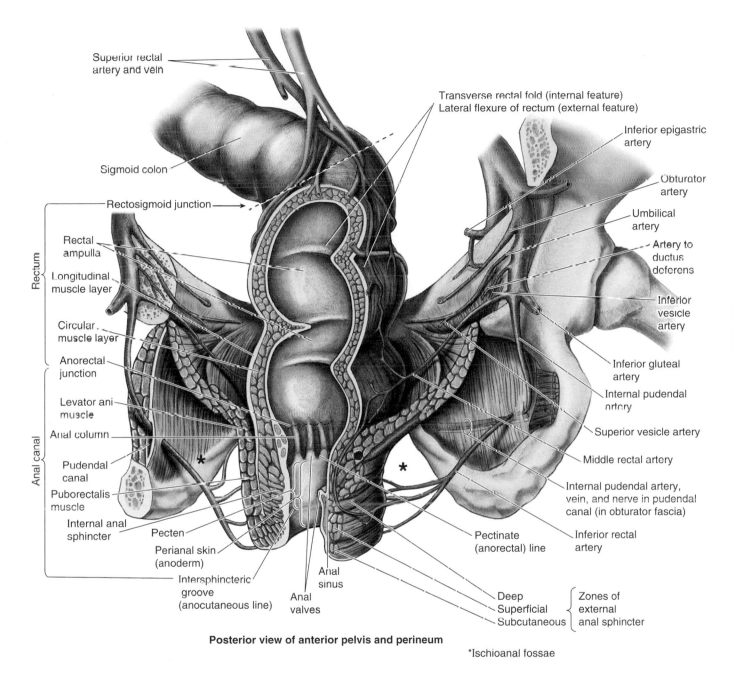

Superior rectal artery and vein

Transverse rectal fold (internal feature)
Lateral flexure of rectum (external feature)

Inferior epigastric artery

Sigmoid colon

Obturator artery

Rectosigmoid junction

Umbilical artery

Rectum

Rectal ampulla

Artery to ductus deferens

Longitudinal muscle layer

Inferior vesicle artery

Circular muscle layer

Anorectal junction

Inferior gluteal artery

Levator ani muscle

Internal pudendal artery

Anal column

Superior vesicle artery

Anal canal

Pudendal canal

Middle rectal artery

Puborectalis muscle

Internal pudendal artery, vein, and nerve in pudendal canal (in obturator fascia)

Internal anal sphincter

Pecten

Pectinate (anorectal) line

Inferior rectal artery

Perianal skin (anoderm)

Anal sinus

Intersphincteric groove (anocutaneous line)

Anal valves

Deep
Superficial
Subcutaneous

Zones of external anal sphincter

Posterior view of anterior pelvis and perineum

*Ischioanal fossae

Figure 3.43. Rectum and anal canal, levator ani, and ischioanal fossa. The left posterolateral third of the rectum and anal canal have been removed to demonstrate the luminal features. The pudendal canal, the space within the obturator fascia covering the medial surface of the obturator internus and lining the lateral wall of the ischioanal fossa, transmits the pudendal vessels and nerves.

Starvation and Rectal Prolapse

The fat bodies of the ischioanal fossae, along with the buccal fat pads (see Chapter 7), are among the last reserves of fatty tissue to disappear with starvation. In the absence of the support provided by the ischioanal fat, rectal prolapse is relatively common. ⊕

THE BOTTOM LINE: The ischioanal fossae are fascia-lined, wedge-shaped spaces occupied by ischioanal fat bodies. The fat bodies provide supportive packing that can be compressed or pushed aside to permit the temporary descent and expansion of the anal canal or vagina for passage of feces or a fetus. The fat bodies are traversed by inferior anal/rectal neurovasculature. The pudendal canal is an important passageway in the lateral wall of the fossa,

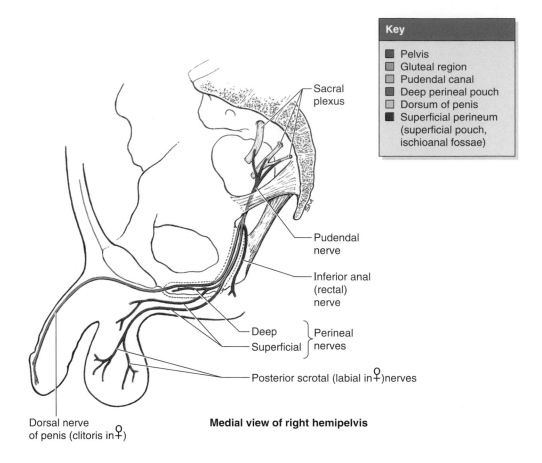

Sacral
plexus

Pudendal
nerve

Inferior anal
(rectal)
nerve

Deep
Superficial } Perineal
nerves

Posterior scrotal (labial in ♀)nerves

Dorsal nerve
of penis (clitoris in ♀)

Medial view of right hemipelvis

Key
- ■ Pelvis
- ■ Gluteal region
- □ Pudendal canal
- ■ Deep perineal pouch
- □ Dorsum of penis
- ■ Superficial perineum
  (superficial pouch,
  ischioanal fossae)

Figure 3.44. Distribution of pudendal nerve. The five regions traversed by the nerve are shown. The pudendal nerve supplies the skin, organs, and muscles of the perineum; therefore, it is concerned with micturition, defecation, erection, ejaculation, and, in the female, parturition. Although the pudendal nerve is shown here in the male, its distribution is similar in the female because the parts of the female perineum are homologs of those in the male.

between layers of the obturator fascia, for neurovasculature passing to and from the UG triangle.

Anal Canal

The **anal canal** is the terminal part of the large intestine, and of the entire alimentary canal. It extends from the superior aspect of the pelvic diaphragm to the **anus** (Figs. 3.42*B* and 3.43). The canal (2.5–3.5 cm long) begins where the rectal ampulla narrows at the level of the U-shaped sling formed by the puborectalis muscle (Fig. 3.7). The canal ends at the anus, the external outlet of the alimentary tract. The anal canal, surrounded by internal and external anal sphincters, descends posteroinferiorly between the anococcygeal ligament and the perineal body. The canal is collapsed, except during passage of feces. Both sphincters must relax before defecation can occur.

The **internal anal sphincter** (Figs. 3.42*A* and 3.43) is an involuntary sphincter surrounding the superior two thirds of the anal canal. It is a thickening of the circular muscle layer. Its contraction (tonus) is stimulated and maintained by sympathetic fibers from the superior rectal (periarterial) and hypogastric plexuses; its contraction is inhibited by parasym-

pathetic fiber stimulation, both intrinsically in relation to peristalsis and extrinsically by fibers passing through the pelvic splanchnic nerves. This sphincter is tonically contracted most of the time to prevent leakage of fluid or flatus; however, it relaxes (is inhibited) temporarily in response to distension of the rectal ampulla by feces or gas, requiring voluntary contraction of the puborectalis and external anal sphincter if defecation or flatulence is not to occur. The ampulla relaxes after initial distension (when peristalsis subsides) and tonus returns until the next peristalsis or until a threshold level of distension occurs, at which point inhibition of the sphincter is continuous until distension is relieved.

The **external anal sphincter** is a large voluntary sphincter that forms a broad band on each side of the inferior two thirds of the anal canal (Figs. 3.39*E*, 3.42, and 3.43). This sphincter is attached anteriorly to the perineal body and posteriorly to the coccyx via the anococcygeal ligament (body); it blends superiorly with the puborectalis muscle. For descriptive purposes, it is described as having subcutaneous, superficial, and deep parts; these are zones rather than muscle bellies and are often indistinct. The external anal sphincter is supplied mainly by S4 through the inferior rectal nerve (Fig. 3.44),

Table 3.8. Arteries of the Perineum

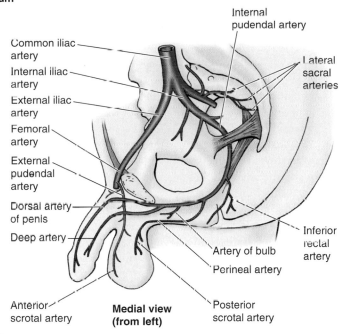

Internal
pudendal artery

Common iliac
artery

Internal iliac
artery

External iliac
artery

Femoral
artery

External
pudendal
artery

Dorsal artery
of penis

Deep artery

Anterior
scrotal artery

**Medial view
(from left)**

Lateral
sacral
arteries

Inferior
rectal
artery

Artery of bulb

Perineal artery

Posterior
scrotal artery

Artery	Origin	Course	Distribution in Perineum
Internal pudendal	Anterior division of internal iliac artery	Leaves pelvis through greater sciatic foramen; hooks around ischial spine to enter perineum via lesser sciatic foramen; immediately enters pudendal canal	Primary artery of perineum and external genital organs
Inferior rectal	Internal pudendal artery	Arises at entrance to pudendal canal; traverses ischioanal fossa to anal canal	Anal canal inferior to pectinate line; anal sphincters; perianal skin
Perineal	Terminal branch of perineal artery	Arises within pudendal canal; passes to superficial pouch (space) on exit	Supplies superficial perineal muscles and scrotum of male/vestibule of female
Posterior scrotal or labial	Terminal branch of perineal artery	Runs in superficial fascia of posterior scrotum or labia majora	Skin of scrotum or labia majora and minora
Artery of bulb of penis or vestibule	Terminal branch	Pierces perineal membrane to reach bulb of penis or vestibule	Supplies bulb of penis (including bulbar urethra) and bulbourethral gland (male) or bulb of vestibule and greater vestibular gland (female)
Deep artery of penis or clitoris	Terminal branch	Pierces perineal membrane to enter crura of corpora cavernosa of penis or clitoris; branches run proximally and distally	Supplies most erectile tissue of corpora cavernosa of penis or clitoris via helicine arteries
Dorsal artery of penis or clitoris		Passes to deep pouch; pierces perineal membrane and traverses suspensory ligament of penis or clitoris to run along dorsum of penis or clitoris to glans	Deep perineal pouch; skin of penis; fascia of penis or clitoris; distal corpus spongiosum of penis, including spongy urethra; glans of penis or clitoris
External pudendal, superficial, and deep branches	Femoral artery	Pass medially from thigh to reach anterior aspect of the urogenital triangle of perineum	Anterior aspect of scrotum and skin at root of penis of male; mons pubis and anterior aspect of labia of female

although its deep part also receives fibers from the nerve to the levator ani, in common with the puborectalis, with which it contracts in unison to maintain continence when the internal sphincter is relaxed (except during defecation).

Internally, the superior half of the mucous membrane of the anal canal is characterized by a series of longitudinal ridges called **anal columns** (Fig. 3.43). These columns contain the terminal branches of the superior rectal artery and vein. The **anorectal junction,** indicated by the superior ends of the anal columns, is where the rectum joins the anal canal. At this point, the wide rectal ampulla abruptly narrows as it traverses the pelvic diaphragm. The inferior ends of the anal columns are joined by **anal valves.** Superior to the valves are small recesses called **anal sinuses.** When compressed by feces, the anal sinuses exude mucus, which aids in evacuation of feces from the anal canal. The inferior comb-shaped limit of the anal valves forms an irregular line (the **pectinate line**),which indicates the junction of the superior part of the anal canal (visceral; derived from the embryonic hindgut) and the inferior part (somatic; derived from the embryonic proctodeum).

The anal canal superior to the pectinate line differs from the part inferior to the pectinate line in its arterial supply, innervation, and venous and lymphatic drainage (Fig. 3.45). These differences result from the different embryological origins of the superior and inferior parts of the anal canal (Moore and Persaud, 2003).

Arterial Supply of the Anal Canal. The *superior rectal artery* supplies the anal canal superior to the pectinate line (Figs. 3.34A and 3.45). The two *inferior rectal arteries* supply the inferior part of the anal canal as well as the surrounding muscles and perianal skin. The *middle rectal arteries* assist with the blood supply to the anal canal by forming anastomoses with the superior and inferior rectal arteries.

Venous and Lymphatic Drainage of the Anal Canal. The *internal rectal venous plexus* drains in both directions from the level of the pectinate line. Superior to the pectinate line, the internal rectal plexus drains chiefly into the *superior rectal vein* (a tributary of the inferior mesenteric vein) and the portal system (Figs. 3.34B and 3.45). Inferior to the pectinate line, the internal rectal plexus drains into the *inferior rectal veins* (tributaries of the caval venous system) around the margin of the external anal sphincter. The *middle rectal veins* (tributaries of the internal iliac veins) mainly drain the muscularis externa of the ampulla and form anastomoses with the superior and inferior rectal veins. In addition to the abundant venous anastomoses, the rectal plexuses receive multiple arteriovenous anastomoses (AVAs) from the superior and middle rectal arteries.

The normal submucosa of the anorectal junction is markedly thickened and in section has the appearance of cavernous (erectile) tissue owing to the presence of the sacculated veins of the internal rectal venous plexus. The vascular submucosa is especially thickened in the left lateral, right anterolateral, and right posterolateral positions, forming "anal cushions" (also referred to as threshold pads, corpora cavernosa recti, and anorectal cavernous bodies) at the point of closure of the anal canal. Because these cushions contain plexuses of saccular veins capable of directly receiving arterial blood via multiple AVAs, they are variably pliable and turgid and form a sort of flutter valve that contributes to the normally water- and gas-tight closure of the anal canal.

Superior to the pectinate line, the lymphatic vessels drain deeply into the *internal iliac lymph nodes* and through them into the common iliac and lumbar lymph nodes (Figs. 3.35 and 3.47). Inferior to the pectinate line, the lymphatic vessels drain superficially into the **superficial inguinal lymph nodes,** as does most of the perineum (Table 3.6).

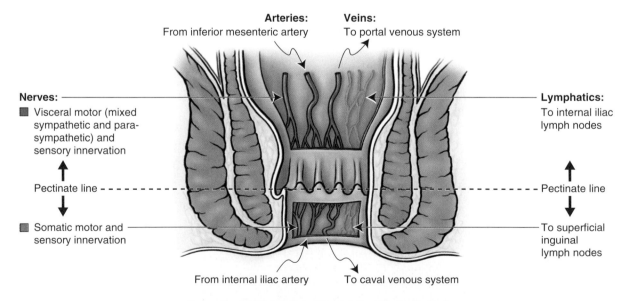

Separation of "visceral" and "parietal" at the pectinate line

Figure 3.45. Changes occurring at pectinate line. Vessels and nerves superior to the pectinate line are visceral; those inferior to the pectinate line are parietal or somatic. This orientation reflects the embryological development of the anorectum.

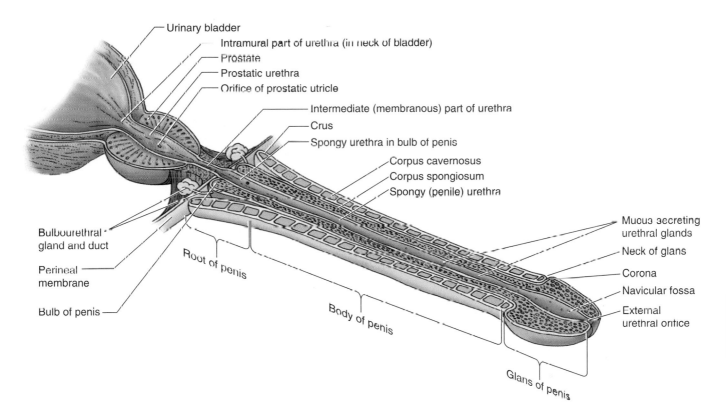

Figure 3.46 Male urethra and associated structures. The urethra has four parts: the vesicular part (in the bladder neck), the prostatic urethra, the intermediate part (membranous urethra), and the spongy (cavernous) urethra. The ducts of the bulbourethral glands open into the proximal part of the spongy urethra. The urethra is not uniform in its caliber: the external urethral orifice and intermediate part are narrowest. Attempting to approach this "straight-line" position as much as possible facilitates passage of a catheter or other transurethral device.

Innervation of the Anal Canal. The nerve supply to the anal canal superior to the pectinate line is visceral innervation from the *inferior hypogastric plexus,* involving sympathetic, parasympathetic, and visceral afferent fibers (Figs. 3.36 and 3.45). Sympathetic fibers maintain the tonus of the internal anal sphincter. Parasympathetic fibers inhibit the tonus of the internal sphincter and evoke peristaltic contraction for defecation. The superior part of the anal canal, like the rectum superior to it, is inferior to the pelvic pain line; all visceral afferents travel with the parasympathetic fibers to spinal sensory ganglia S2–S4. Superior to the pectinate line, the anal canal is sensitive only to stretching, which evokes sensations at both the conscious and the unconscious (reflex) levels. For example, distension of the rectal ampulla inhibits (relaxes) the tonus of the internal sphincter. The nerve supply of the anal canal inferior to the pectinate line is somatic innervation derived from the *inferior anal* (*rectal*) *nerves,* branches of the pudendal nerve. Therefore, this part of the anal canal is sensitive to pain, touch, and temperature. Somatic efferent fibers stimulate contraction of the voluntary external anal sphincter.

The Pectinate Line—A Clinically Important Landmark

The *pectinate line* (also called the dentate or mucocutaneous line by some clinicians) is a particularly important landmark because it is visible and approximates the level of important anatomical changes related to the transition from visceral to parietal (Fig. 3.45), affecting such things as the types of tumors that occur, and the direction in which they metastasize.

Anal Fissures and Perianal Abscesses

The ischioanal fossae are occasionally the sites of infection, which may result in the formation of **ischioanal abscesses** (Fig. B3.26A). These collections of pus are ▶

quite painful. Infections may reach the ischioanal fossae in several ways:

- After *cryptitis* (inflammation of the anal sinuses).

- Extension from a pelvirectal abscess.

- After a tear in the anal mucous membrane.

- From a penetrating wound in the anal region.

Diagnostic signs of an ischioanal abscess are fullness and tenderness between the anus and the ischial tuberosity. A perianal abscess may rupture spontaneously, opening into the anal canal, rectum, or perianal skin.

Because the ischioanal fossae communicate posteriorly through the *deep postnatal space,* an abscess in one fossa may spread to the other one and form a semicircular "horseshoe-shaped" abscess around the posterior aspect of the anal canal. In chronically constipated persons, the anal valves and mucosa may be torn by hard feces. An **anal fissure** (slit-like lesion) is usually located in the posterior midline, inferior to the anal valves. It is painful because this region is supplied by sensory fibers of the inferior rectal nerves. **Perianal abscesses** may follow infection of anal fissures, and the infection may spread to the ischioanal fossae and form ischioanal abscesses or spread into the pelvis and form **pelvirectal abscesses**. An *anal fistula* may result from the spread of an anal infection and cryptitis. One end of this abnormal canal (fistula) opens into the anal canal and the other end opens into an abscess in the ischioanal fossa or into the perianal skin.

Hemorrhoids

Internal hemorrhoids (piles) are prolapses of rectal mucosa (more specifically, of the so-called rectal cushions) containing the normally dilated veins of the *internal rectal venous plexus* (Fig. B3.26*B*). Internal hemorrhoids are thought to result from a breakdown of the muscularis mucosae, a smooth muscle layer deep to the mucosa. They occur quite predictably in the left lateral, right anterolateral, and right posterolateral positions (positions of anal cushions). Internal hemorrhoids that prolapse through the anal canal are often compressed by the contracted sphincters, impeding blood flow. As a result, they tend to strangulate and ulcerate. Because of the presence of abundant arteriovenous anastomoses, bleeding from internal hemorrhoids is characteristically bright red. Although all forms of internal hemorrhoids (including normal anal cushions misinterpreted as abnormalities) were once treated aggressively, current practice is to treat only prolapsed, ulcerated internal hemorrhoids. **External hemorrhoids** are thromboses (blood clots) in the veins of the *external rectal venous plexus* and are covered by skin. Predisposing factors for hemorrhoids include pregnancy, chronic constipation and

prolonged toilet sitting and straining, and any disorder that impedes venous return, including increased intra-abdominal pressure.

The anastomoses between the superior, middle, and inferior rectal veins form clinically important communications between the portal and systemic venous systems ▶

Pelvirectal space

Levator ani

Obturator internus

Pudendal canal

Perianal abscess in ischioanal fossa

Fistula

Pectinate line

Inferior transverse rectal fold

Rectum

External anal sphincter

(A)

Internal iliac vein

Middle rectal vein

Internal pudendal vein

Internal rectal plexus

Inferior rectal vein

External rectal plexus

Rectum

Internal hemorrhoid

External anal sphincter

External hemorrhoid

(B)

Anterior views of coronal sections

Figure B3.26

Plane of coronal sections

(see Fig. 2.59). The superior rectal vein drains into the inferior mesenteric vein, whereas the middle and inferior rectal veins drain through the systemic system into the inferior vena cava. Any abnormal increase in pressure in the valveless portal system or veins of the trunk may cause enlargement of the superior rectal veins, resulting in an increase in blood flow or stasis in the internal rectal venous plexus. In the *portal hypertension* that occurs in relation to *hepatic cirrhosis*, the portocaval anastomosis between the superior and the middle and inferior rectal veins, along with portocaval anastomoses elsewhere, may become varicose. Those in the esophagus are especially prone to rupture. It is important to note that the veins of the rectal plexuses *normally* appear varicose (dilated and tortuous), even in newborns, and that internal hemorrhoids occur most commonly in the *absence* of portal hypertension.

Regarding pain from and the treatment of hemorrhoids, it is important to note that the anal canal superior to the pectinate line is visceral; thus it is innervated by visceral afferent pain fibers, so that an incision or needle insertion in this region is painless. Internal hemorrhoids are not painful and can be treated without anesthesia. However, inferior to the pectinate line, the anal canal is somatic, supplied by the inferior anal (rectal) nerves containing somatic sensory fibers. Therefore, it is sensitive to painful stimuli (e.g., to the prick of a hypodermic needle). External hemorrhoids can be painful but often resolve in a few days.

Anorectal Incontinence

Stretching of the pudendal nerve(s) during a traumatic childbirth can result in *pudendal nerve damage* and anorectal incontinence. ☉

THE BOTTOM LINE: The anal canal is the terminal part of both the large intestine and the alimentary tract, the anus being the external outlet. Closure (and thus fecal continence) is maintained by the coordinated action of the involuntary internal and voluntary external anal sphincters. The sympathetically stimulated tonus of the internal sphincter maintains closure, except during filling of the rectal ampulla and when inhibited during a parasympathetically stimulated peristaltic contraction of the rectum. During these moments, closure is maintained (unless defecation is permitted) by voluntary contraction of the puborectalis and external anal sphincter. Internally, the pectinate line demarcates the transition from visceral to somatic neurovascular supply and drainage. The canal is surrounded by superficial and deep venous plexuses, the veins of which normally have a varicose appearance. Thromboses in the superficial plexus, and mucosal prolapse, including portions of the deep plexus, constitute painful external and insensitive internal hemorrhoids, respectively.

Male Perineum

The **male perineum** includes the external genitalia, perineal muscles, and anal canal. The **male external genitalia** include the urethra, scrotum, and penis.

Distal Male Urethra

The male urethra is subdivided into four parts: intramural (preprostatic), prostatic, intermediate, and spongy. The intramural and prostatic parts are described with the pelvis (earlier in this chapter). Details concerning all four parts of the male urethra are provided and compared in Table 3.7.

The intermediate (membranous) part of the urethra begins at the apex of the prostate and traverses the deep perineal pouch, surrounded by the external urethral sphincter. It then penetrates the perineal membrane, ending as the urethra enters the bulb of the penis (Fig. 3.46). Posterolateral to this part of the urethra are the small *bulbourethral glands* and their slender ducts, which open into the proximal part of the spongy urethra.

The **spongy urethra** begins at the distal end of the intermediate part of the urethra and ends at the *external urethral orifice,* which is slightly narrower than any of the parts of the urethra. The lumen of the spongy urethra is approximately 5 mm in diameter; however, it is expanded in the bulb of the penis to form the **intrabulbar fossa** and in the glans of the penis to form the **navicular fossa.** On each side, the slender *ducts of the bulbourethral glands* open into the proximal part of the spongy urethra; the orifices of these ducts are extremely small. There are also many minute openings of the ducts of mucus-secreting **urethral glands** (Littré glands) into the spongy urethra.

Arterial Supply of the Distal Male Urethra. The arterial supply of the intermediate and spongy parts of the urethra is from branches of the *dorsal artery of the penis* (Fig. 3.39C; Table 3.8).

Venous and Lymphatic Drainage of the Distal Male Urethra. Veins accompany the arteries and have similar names. Lymphatic vessels from the intermediate part of the urethra drain mainly into the *internal iliac lymph nodes* (Fig. 3.47; Table 3.6); whereas most vessels from the spongy urethra pass to the *deep inguinal lymph nodes,* but some lymph passes to the external iliac nodes.

Innervation of the Distal Male Urethra. The innervation of the intermediate part of the urethra is the same as that

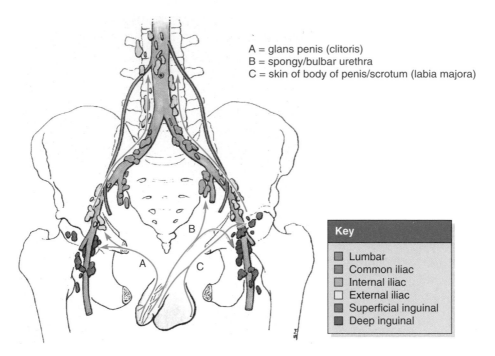

A = glans penis (clitoris)
B = spongy/bulbar urethra
C = skin of body of penis/scrotum (labia majora)

Key

■ Lumbar
■ Common iliac
■ Internal iliac
□ External iliac
■ Superficial inguinal
■ Deep inguinal

Figure 3.47. Lymphatic drainage of penis, spongy urethra, and scrotum.
The *arrows* indicate the direction of lymph flow to the lymph nodes.

of the prostatic part: autonomic (efferent) innervation via the *prostatic nerve plexus,* arising from the *inferior hypogastric plexus.* The sympathetic innervation is from the lumbar spinal cord levels via the lumbar splanchnic nerves, and the parasympathetic innervation is from the sacral levels via the *pelvic splanchnic nerves.* The visceral afferent fibers follow the parasympathetic fibers retrogradely to sacral spinal sensory ganglia. The dorsal nerve of the penis, a branch of the *pudendal nerve,* provides somatic innervation of the spongy part of the urethra (Fig. 3.44).

Urethral Catheterization

Urethral catheterization is done to remove urine from a person who is unable to micturate. It is also performed to irrigate the bladder and to obtain an uncontaminated sample of urine. When inserting catheters and *urethral sounds* (slightly conical instruments for exploring and dilating a constricted urethra) the curves of the male urethra must be considered. Just distal to the perineal membrane, the spongy urethra is well covered inferiorly and posteriorly by erectile tissue of the bulb of the penis; however, a short segment of the intermediate part of the urethra is unprotected (Fig. B3.27). Because the urethral wall is thin and because of the angle that must be negotiated to enter the intermediate part of the spongy urethra, it is vulnerable to rupture during the insertion of urethral catheters and sounds. The intermediate part, the least distensible part, runs inferoanteriorly as it passes through the external urethral sphincter. Proximally, the prostatic part takes a slight curve that is concave anteriorly as it traverses the prostate. ▶

Bladder

Medial view (from left)

Figure B3.27

THE BOTTOM LINE: The intermediate urethra is the shortest and narrowest part of the male urethra, the limit of its distension normally being the same as that of the external urethral orifice. It is encircled by voluntary muscle of the inferior part of the external urethral sphincter before perforating the perineal membrane. Immediately inferior to the membrane, the urethra enters the corpus spongiosum and becomes the spongy urethra, the longest part of the male urethra. The spongy urethra has expansions at each end, the intrabulbar and navicular fossae. The intermediate and spongy parts are supplied and drained by the same dorsal (blood) vessels of the penis but differ in terms of innervation and lymphatic drainage, that for the intermediate part following visceral paths and that for the spongy part follows somatic paths.

Scrotum

The **scrotum** is a cutaneous fibromuscular sac for the testes and associated structures. It is situated posteroinferior to the penis and inferior to the pubic symphysis. The bilateral embryonic formation of the scrotum is indicated by the midline **scrotal raphe** (Fig. 3.48), which is continuous on the ventral surface of the penis with the **penile raphe** and posteriorly along the median line of the perineum with the **perineal raphe**. Internally, deep to the scrotal raphe, the scrotum is divided into two compartments, one for each testis, by a prolongation of the dartos fascia, the **septum of the scrotum**. The testes and epididymides and their coverings are described with the abdomen (see Chapter 2).

Arterial Supply of the Scrotum. Anterior scrotal arteries, terminal branches of the **external pudendal arteries** (from the femoral artery), supply the anterior aspect of the scrotum; **posterior scrotal arteries**, terminal branches of the superficial perineal branches of the *internal pudendal arteries,* supply the posterior aspect (Table 3.8). The scrotum also receives branches from the cremasteric arteries (branches of the inferior epigastric arteries).

Venous and Lymphatic Drainage of the Scrotum. The scrotal veins accompany the arteries, sharing the same names but draining primarily to the *external pudendal veins.* Lymphatic vessels from the scrotum carry lymph to the *superficial inguinal lymph nodes* (Fig. 3.47; Table 3.6).

Innervation of the Scrotum. The anterior aspect of the scrotum is supplied by derivatives of the *lumbar plexus:* **anterior scrotal nerves,** derived from the *ilioinguinal nerve,* and the *genital branch of the genitofemoral nerve.* The posterior aspect of the scrotum is supplied by derivatives of the sacral plexus: **posterior scrotal nerves,** branches of the *superficial perineal branches* of the *pudendal nerve,* and the *perineal branch of the posterior femoral cutaneous nerve* (Figs. 3.44 and 3.49A). Sympathetic fibers conveyed by these nerves assist in the thermoregulation of the testes (see Chapter 2), stimulating contraction of the smooth dartos muscle in response to cold or stimulating the scrotal sweat glands while inhibiting contraction of the dartos muscle in response to excessive warmth.

Distension of the Scrotum

The scrotum is easily distended. In persons with large indirect inguinal hernias, for example (see Chapter 2), the intestine may enter the scrotum, making it as large as a soccer ball. Similarly, inflammation of the testes (**orchitis**), associated with mumps, bleeding in the subcutaneous tissue, or chronic lymphatic obstruction (as occurs in the parasitic disease *elephantiasis*), may produce an enlarged scrotum.

Palpation of the Testes

The soft, pliable skin of the scrotum makes it easy to palpate the testes and the structures related to them (e.g., the epididymis and ductus deferens). The left testis commonly lies at a more inferior level than does the right one. ⊙

THE BOTTOM LINE: The scrotum is a dynamic, fibromuscular cutaneous sac for the testes and epididymides. Its internal subdivision by a septum of dartos fascia is demarcated externally by a median scrotal raphe. The anterior aspect of the scrotum is served by anterior scrotal blood vessels and nerves, continuations of external pudendal blood vessels and branches of the lumbar nerve plexus; the posterior aspect of the scrotum is served by posterior scrotal blood vessels and nerves, continuations of internal pudendal blood vessels and branches of the sacral nerve plexus. Sympathetic innervation of smooth dartos muscle and sweat glands assists thermoregulation of the testes.

Penis

The **penis** is the male copulatory organ and, by conveying the urethra, provides the common outlet for urine and semen (Figs. 3.46, 3.48, and 3.49). The penis consists of a *root, body,* and *glans.* It is composed of three cylindrical bodies of erectile cavernous tissue: the paired **corpora cavernosa** dorsally and

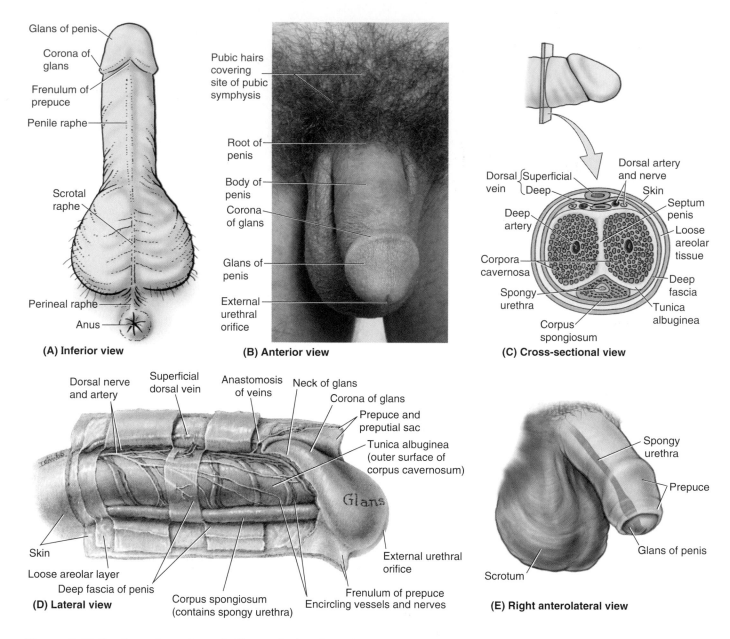

Figure 3.48. Penis and scrotum. A. The urethral surface of the circumcised penis is shown. The spongy urethra is deep to the cutaneous penile raphe. The scrotum is divided into right and left halves by the cutaneous scrotal raphe, which is continuous with the penile and perineal raphes. **B.** The dorsum of the circumcised penis and the anterior surface of the scrotum are shown. The penis comprises a root, body, and glans. **C.** The penis contains three erectile masses: two corpora cavernosa and a corpus spongiosum (containing the spongy urethra). **D.** The skin of the penis extends distally as the prepuce, overlapping the neck and corona of the glans. **E.** An uncircumcised penis.

single **corpus spongiosum** ventrally. (Note that in the anatomical position, the penis is erect; when the penis is flaccid, its dorsum is directed anteriorly.) Each *cavernous body* has an outer fibrous covering or capsule, the **tunica albuginea** (Fig. 3.48C). Superficial to the outer covering is the **deep fascia of the penis** (Buck fascia), the continuation of the deep perineal fascia that forms a strong membranous covering for the corpora cavernosa and corpus spongiosum, binding them together (Fig. 3.48C & D). The corpus spongiosum contains the spongy urethra. The corpora cavernosa are fused with

each other in the median plane, except posteriorly where they separate to form the **crura of the penis** (Figs. 3.47 and 3.50). Internally, the cavernous tissue of the corpora is separated (usually incompletely) by the **septum penis** (Fig. 3.48C).

The **root of the penis** (L. *radix penis*), the attached part, consists of the crura, bulb, and ischiocavernosus and bulbospongiosus muscles (Fig. 3.46). The root is located in the superficial perineal pouch, between the perineal membrane superiorly and the deep perineal fascia inferiorly. The **crura** and **bulb of the penis** contain masses of erectile tissue. Each

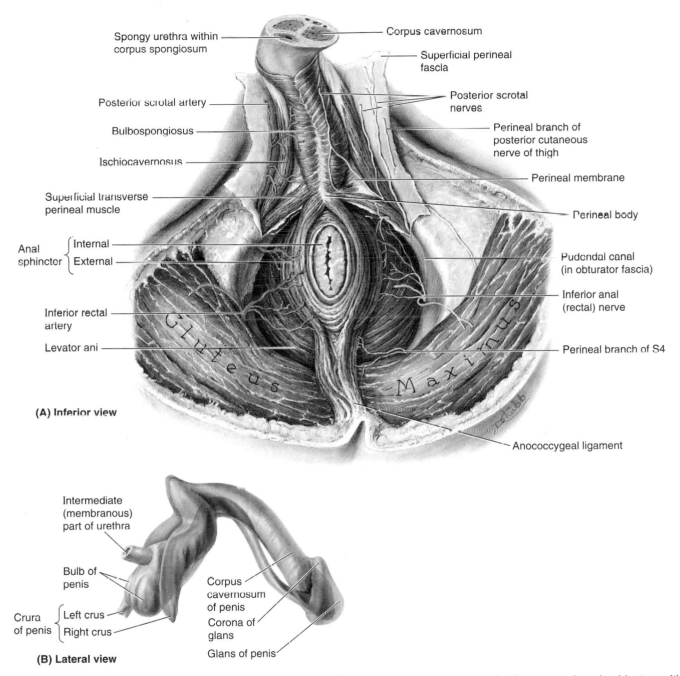

Spongy urethra within corpus spongiosum

Corpus cavernosum

Superficial perineal fascia

Posterior scrotal artery

Posterior scrotal nerves

Bulbospongiosus

Perineal branch of posterior cutaneous nerve of thigh

Ischiocavernosus

Perineal membrane

Superficial transverse perineal muscle

Perineal body

Anal sphincter { Internal / External }

Pudendal canal (in obturator fascia)

Inferior anal (rectal) nerve

Inferior rectal artery

Levator ani

Perineal branch of S4

Gluteus

Maximus

(A) Inferior view

Anococcygeal ligament

Intermediate (membranous) part of urethra

Bulb of penis

Corpus cavernosum of penis

Crura of penis { Left crus / Right crus }

Corona of glans

Glans of penis

(B) Lateral view

Figure 3.49. Male perineum and structure of penis. A. The anal canal is surrounded by the external anal sphincter, with an ischioanal fossa on each side. The inferior anal (rectal) nerve branches from the pudendal nerve at the entrance to the pudendal canal and, with the perineal branch of S4, supplies the external anal sphincter. **B.** The corpus spongiosum has been separated from the corpora cavernosa. The natural flexures of the penis are preserved. The glans penis fits like a cap over the blunt ends of the corpora cavernosa.

crus is attached to the inferior part of the internal surface of the corresponding ischial ramus (Fig. 3.39D), anterior to the ischial tuberosity. The enlarged posterior part of the bulb of the penis is penetrated superiorly by the urethra, continuing from its intermediate part (Fig. 3.49B).

The **body of the penis** is the free pendulous part that is suspended from the pubic symphysis (Figs. 3.46 and 3.48B). Except for a few fibers of the bulbospongiosus near the root

of the penis and the ischiocavernosus that embrace the crura, the body of the penis has no muscles. The penis consists of thin skin, connective tissue, blood and lymphatic vessels, fascia, the corpora cavernosa, and the corpus spongiosum containing the spongy urethra (Fig. 3.48C). Distally, the corpus spongiosum expands to form the conical **glans of the penis,** or head of the penis (Figs. 3.48A, B, & D and 3.49B). The margin of the glans projects beyond the ends of the corpora

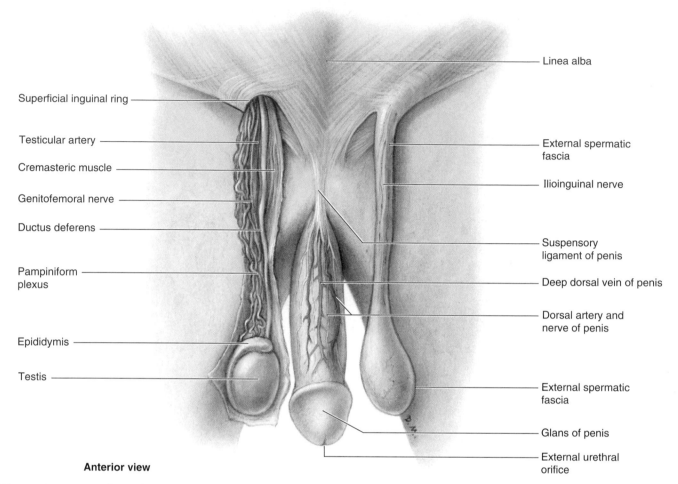

Superficial inguinal ring

Testicular artery

Cremasteric muscle

Genitofemoral nerve

Ductus deferens

Pampiniform plexus

Epididymis

Testis

Linea alba

External spermatic fascia

Ilioinguinal nerve

Suspensory ligament of penis

Deep dorsal vein of penis

Dorsal artery and nerve of penis

External spermatic fascia

Glans of penis

External urethral orifice

Anterior view

Figure 3.50. Vessels and nerves on dorsum of penis and contents of spermatic cord. This dissection of the penis and spermatic cord shows their vessels and nerves. The skin, including the scrotum, has been removed. The superficial (dartos) fascia covering the penis has also been removed to expose the midline deep dorsal vein and the bilateral dorsal arteries and nerves of the penis. The triangular suspensory ligament of the penis attaches to the pubic symphysis and blends with the deep fascia of the penis.

cavernosa to form the **corona of the glans.** The corona overhangs an obliquely grooved constriction, the **neck of the glans,** which separates the glans from the body of the penis. The slit-like opening of the spongy urethra, the *external urethral orifice* (meatus), is near the tip of the glans.

The skin of the penis is thin, darkly pigmented relative to adjacent skin, and connected to the tunica albuginea by loose connective tissue. At the neck of the glans, the skin and fascia of the penis are prolonged as a double layer of skin, the **prepuce** (foreskin), which in uncircumcised males covers the glans to a variable extent (Fig 3.48E). The **frenulum of the prepuce** is a median fold that passes from the deep layer of the prepuce to the urethral surface of the glans (Fig. 3.48A & D).

The **suspensory ligament of the penis** is a condensation of deep fascia that arises from the anterior surface of the pubic symphysis (Fig. 3.50). The ligament passes inferiorly and splits to form a sling that is attached to the deep fascia of the penis at the junction of its root and body. The fibers of the suspensory ligament are short and taut, anchoring the erectile bodies of the penis to the pubic symphysis. The **fundiform**

ligament of the penis is an irregular mass or condensation of collagen and elastic fibers of the subcutaneous tissue that descends in the midline from the linea alba superior to the pubic symphysis. The ligament splits to surround the penis and then unites and blends inferiorly with the dartos fascia forming the scrotal septum. The fibers of the fundiform ligament are relatively long and loose and lie superficial (anterior) to the suspensory ligament.

Arterial Supply of the Penis. The penis is supplied mainly by *branches of the internal pudendal arteries* (Figs. 3.48C & D and 3.50; Table 3.8).

- **Dorsal arteries of the penis:** run on each side of the deep dorsal vein in the dorsal groove between the corpora cavernosa, supplying the fibrous tissue around the corpora cavernosa, the corpus spongiosum and spongy urethra, and the penile skin.

- **Deep arteries of the penis:** pierce the crura proximally and run distally near the center of the corpora cavernosa, supplying the erectile tissue in these structures.

- **Arteries of the bulb of the penis:** supply the posterior (bulbous) part of the corpus spongiosum and the urethra within it as well as the bulbourethral gland.

In addition, **superficial** and **deep branches of the external pudendal arteries** supply the penile skin, anastomosing with branches of the internal pudendal arteries.

The deep arteries of the penis are the main vessels supplying the cavernous spaces in the erectile tissue of the corpora cavernosa and are, therefore, involved in the erection of the penis. They give off numerous branches that open directly into the cavernous spaces. When the penis is flaccid, these arteries are coiled, restricting blood flow; they are called **helicine arteries of the penis** (G. *helix,* a coil).

Venous and Lymphatic Drainage of the Penis. Blood from the cavernous spaces is drained by a venous plexus that joins the **deep dorsal vein of the penis** in the deep fascia (Figs. 3.48*C* and 3.50). This vein passes between the laminae of the suspensory ligament of the penis, inferior to the arcuate pubic ligament and anterior to the perineal membrane, to enter the pelvis, where it drains into the prostatic venous plexus. Blood from the superficial coverings of the penis drain into the **superficial dorsal vein**(s), which drain(s) into the *superficial external pudendal vein.* Some blood also passes to the

internal pudendal vein. Lymph from the skin of the penis drains initially to the *superficial inguinal lymph nodes,* that from the glans and distal spongy urethra drain to the *deep inguinal* and *external iliac nodes,* and that from the cavernous bodies and proximal spongy urethra drain to the *internal iliac nodes* (Fig. 3.47; Table 3.6).

Innervation of the Penis The nerves derive from the S2–S4 spinal cord segments and spinal ganglia, passing through the pelvic splanchnic and pudendal nerves, respectively (Fig. 3.51). Sensory and sympathetic innervation is provided primarily by the *dorsal nerve of the penis,* a terminal branch of the *pudendal nerve,* which arises in the pudendal canal and passes anteriorly into the deep perineal pouch. It then runs to the dorsum of the penis, where it runs lateral to the dorsal artery (Figs. 3.48*C* and 3.50). It supplies both the skin and glans of the penis. The penis is richly provided with a variety of sensory nerve endings, especially the glans penis. Branches of the *ilioinguinal nerve* supply the skin at the root of the penis. Cavernous nerves, conveying parasympathetic fibers independently from the prostatic nerve plexus, innervate the helicine arteries of the erectile tissue. The sexual functions of the penis are explained under "Erection, Emission, and Ejaculation," later in this chapter.

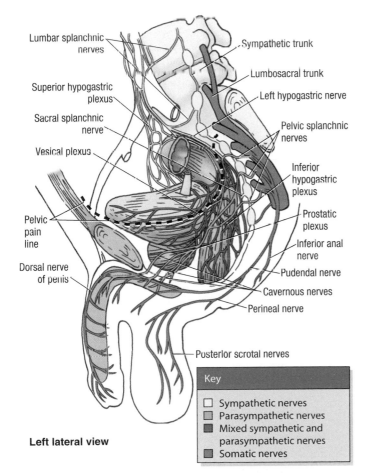

Left lateral view

Key
- ☐ Sympathetic nerves
- ☐ Parasympathetic nerves
- ■ Mixed sympathetic and parasympathetic nerves
- ■ Somatic nerves

Labels: Lumbar splanchnic nerves; Superior hypogastric plexus; Sacral splanchnic nerve; Vesical plexus; Pelvic pain line; Dorsal nerve of penis; Posterior scrotal nerves; Sympathetic trunk; Lumbosacral trunk; Left hypogastric nerve; Pelvic splanchnic nerves; Inferior hypogastric plexus; Prostatic plexus; Inferior anal nerve; Pudendal nerve; Cavernous nerves; Perineal nerve

Figure 3.51. Nerves of perineum. The pudendal nerve conveys the majority of sensory, sympathetic, and somatic motor fibers to the perineum. Although originating from the same spinal cord segments from which the pudendal nerve is derived, the parasympathetic fibers of the cavernous nerves course independently of the pudendal nerve. With the exception of the cavernous nerves, parasympathetic fibers do not occur outside of the head, neck, or cavities of the trunk. The cavernous nerves arise from the prostatic plexus of males and from the vesical plexus of females. They terminate on the arteriovenous anastomoses and helicine arteries of the erectile bodies, which, when stimulated, produce erection of the penis or engorgement of the clitoris and vestibular bulb in females.

Hypospadias

Hypospadias is a common congenital anomaly of the penis, occurring in 1 in 300 newborns. In the simplest and most common form, *glanular hypospadias,* the external urethral orifice is on the ventral aspect of the glans. In other infants, the defect is in the body of the penis (*penile hypospadias*) (Fig. B3.28), or in the perineum (*penoscrotal* or *scrotal hypospadias*). Hence, the external urethral orifice is on the urethral surface of the penis. The embryological basis of glanular and penile hypospadias is failure of the *urogenital folds* to fuse on the ventral surface of the developing penis and form the spongy urethra. The embryological basis of scrotal hypospadias is failure of the *labioscrotal folds* to fuse and form the scrotum. The cause of hypospadias is not clearly understood, but it appears to have a multifactorial origin (i.e., genetic and environmental factors are involved). Close relatives of patients with hypospadias are more likely than the general population to have the anomaly. It is generally believed that hypospadias is associated with an inadequate production of androgens by the fetal testes. Differences in the timing and degree of hormonal insufficiency probably account for the different types of hypospadias (Moore and Persaud, 2003). The less common but more severe forms of hypospadias, in which the external urethral orifice is located on the penile body or in the perineum, may interfere with normal urination in the usual male standing position. (Walsh, 1998)

Phimosis, Paraphimosis, and Circumcision

The prepuce of the penis is usually sufficiently elastic for it to be retracted over the glans penis. In some males, it fits tightly over the glans and cannot be retracted easily (*phimosis*) if at all. As there are modified sebaceous glands in the prepuce, the oily secretions of cheesy consistency (*smegma*) from them accumulate in the **preputial sac**, located between the glans and prepuce, causing irritation. In some males, retraction of the prepuce over the glans constricts the neck of the glans so much that there is interference with the drainage of blood and tissue fluid. In patients with this condition (*paraphimosis*) the glans may enlarge so much that the prepuce cannot be drawn over it. Circumcision is commonly performed in such cases. **Circumcision**, surgical excision of the prepuce, is the most commonly performed minor surgical operation on male infants. Although it is a religious practice in Islam and Judaism, it is often done routinely for non-religious reasons (a preference usually explained in terms of tradition or hygiene) in North America. In adults, circumcision is usually performed when phimosis or paraphimosis is present. ✛

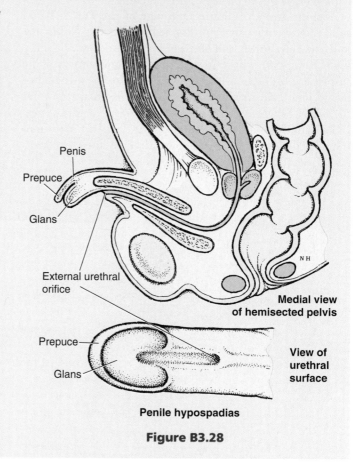

Penis

Prepuce

Glans

External urethral orifice

Medial view of hemisected pelvis

Prepuce

Glans

View of urethral surface

Penile hypospadias

Figure B3.28

THE BOTTOM LINE: The penis is the male copulatory organ and common final conveyor of urine and semen. It is formed mainly of thin, mobile skin overlying three cylindrical bodies of erectile cavernous tissue, the paired corpora cavernosa, and a single corpus spongiosum containing the spongy urethra. The erectile bodies are bound together by deep fascia of the penis, except posteriorly (at the root) where they separate into the crura and bulb of the penis. The crura attach to the ischiopubic rami, but all parts of the root are attached to the perineal membrane. At the junction of root and body, the penis is attached to the pubic syphysis by the suspensory ligament of the penis.

The ischiocavernosus muscles ensheath the crura, and the bulbospongiosus ensheaths the bulb, its most anterior fibers encircling the most proximal part of the body (which otherwise has no muscles) and deep dorsal vessels. The glans of the penis is a distal expansion of the corpus spongiosum, which has the external urethral orifice at its tip and a projecting corona that overhangs the neck of the glans. Unless removed by circumcision, the neck is covered by the prepuce or foreskin.

Except for skin near its root, the penis is supplied mainly by branches of the internal pudendal arteries. The dorsal arteries supply most of the body and glans, whereas the deep arteries supply the cavernous tissue, their terminal helicine arteries opening to engorge the sinuses with blood at arterial pressure, causing erection. Superficial structures drain via the superficial dorsal vein to external pudendal veins, whereas the erectile bodies drain via the deep dorsal vein to the prostatic venous plexus. Sensory and sympathetic innervation is provided mainly by the dorsal nerve of the penis, but the helicine arteries that directly produce erection are innervated by cavernous nerves, extensions of the prostatic nerve plexus.

Perineal Muscles of the Male

The **superficial perineal muscles**, located in the superficial perineal pouch, include the superficial transverse perineal, bulbospongiosus, and ischiocavernosus muscles (Fig. 3.49A). Details about the attachments, innervation, and actions of these muscles are provided in Table 3.9. The **superficial transverse perineal muscles** and bulbospongiosus muscles join the external anal sphincter in attaching centrally to the perineal body, crossing the pelvic outlet like intersecting beams, supporting the perineal body to aid the pelvic diaphragm in supporting the pelvic viscera. Simultaneous contraction of the superficial perineal muscles (plus the deep transverse perineal muscle) during penile erection provides a firmer base for the penis.

The *bulbospongiosus muscles* form a constrictor that compresses the bulb of the penis and the corpus spongiosum, thereby aiding in emptying the spongy urethra of residual urine and/or semen. The anterior fibers of the bulbospongiosus, encircling the most proximal part of the body of the penis, also assist erection by increasing the pressure on the erectile tissue in the root of the penis. At the same time, they also compress the deep dorsal vein of the penis, impeding venous drainage of the cavernous spaces and helping promote enlargement and turgidity of the penis.

The **ischiocavernosus muscles** surround the crura in the root of the penis. They force blood from the cavernous spaces in the crura into the distal parts of the corpora cavernosa, which increases the turgidity (firm distension) of the penis during erection. Contraction of the ischiocavernosus muscles also compresses the tributaries of deep dorsal vein of the penis leaving the crus of the penis, thereby restricting venous outflow from the penis and helping maintain the erection.

Because of their function during erection and the activity of the bulbospongiosus subsequent to urination and ejaculation to expel the last drops of urine and semen, the perineal muscles are generally more developed in males than in females.

THE BOTTOM LINE: In addition to their bony origins, the voluntary superficial and deep muscles of the perineum are also attached to the perineal membrane (by which they are separated) and the perineal body. In addition to the sphincteric functions of the external anal and urethral sphincters for maintaining fecal and urinary continence, the male perineal muscles function as a group to provide a base for the penis and support for the perineal body (which in turn sup-

ports the pelvic diaphragm). The ischiocavernosus and bulbospongiosus muscles both constrict venous outflow from the erectile bodies to assist erection, simultaneously pushing blood from the penile root into the body. In addition, the bulbospongiosus muscle constricts around the bulb of the penis to express the final drops of urine or semen. Because of these multiple functions, the perineal muscles are generally relatively well developed in males. The perineal muscles are innervated by muscular branches of the pudendal nerve.

Erection, Emission, and Ejaculation

When a male is stimulated erotically, arteriovenous anastomoses, by which blood is normally able to bypass the "empty" potential spaces or sinuses of the corpora cavernosa, are closed. The smooth muscle in the fibrous trabeculae and coiled helicine arteries relaxes (is inhibited) as a result of parasympathetic stimulation (S2–S4 through the cavernous nerves from the **prostatic nerve plexus**). Consequently, the helicine arteries straighten, enlarging their lumina and allowing blood to flow into and dilate the cavernous spaces in the corpora of the penis. The bulbospongiosus and ischiocavernosus muscles compress veins egressing from the corpora cavernosa, impeding the return of venous blood. As a result, the corpora cavernosa and corpus spongiosum become engorged with blood at venous pressure, causing the erectile bodies to become turgid (enlarged and rigid), and an **erection** occurs.

During **emission**, semen (sperms and secretions) is delivered to the prostatic urethra through the ejaculatory ducts after peristalsis of the ductus deferentes and seminal glands. Prostatic fluid is added to the seminal fluid as the smooth muscle in the prostate contracts. Emission is a sympathetic response (L1–L2 nerves). During **ejaculation**, semen is expelled from the urethra through the external urethral orifice. Ejaculation results from:

- Closure of the internal urethral sphincter at the neck of the urinary bladder, a sympathetic response (L1–L2 nerves).

- Contraction of the urethral muscle, a parasympathetic response (S2–S4 nerves).

- Contraction of the bulbospongiosus muscles, from the pudendal nerves (S2–S4).

After ejaculation, the penis gradually returns to a flaccid state (**remission**), resulting from sympathetic stimulation, which causes constriction of the smooth muscle in the coiled arteries. The bulbospongiosus and ischiocavernosus muscles relax, allowing more blood to be drained from the cavernous spaces in the penile corpora into the deep dorsal vein.

When a lesion of the prostatic plexus or cavernous nerves results in an inability to achieve an erection (**impotence**), a surgically implanted, semirigid or inflatable penile prosthesis may assume the role of the erectile bodies, providing the rigidity necessary to insert and move the penis within the vagina during intercourse.

Table 3.9. Muscles of the Perineum

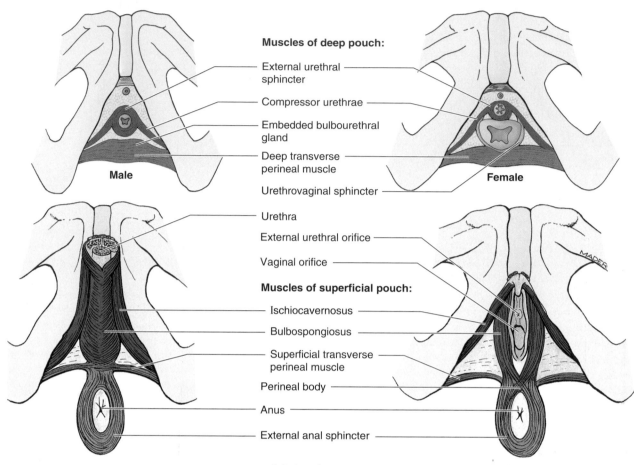

Muscles of deep pouch:

External urethral sphincter

Compressor urethrae

Embedded bulbourethral gland

Deep transverse perineal muscle

Urethrovaginal sphincter

Male

Female

Urethra

External urethral orifice

Vaginal orifice

Muscles of superficial pouch:

Ischiocavernosus

Bulbospongiosus

Superficial transverse perineal muscle

Perineal body

Anus

External anal sphincter

Inferior views

Muscle	Origin	Course and distribution	Innervation	Main Action
External and sphincter	Skin and fascia surrounding anus; coccyx via anococcygeal ligament	Passes around lateral aspects of anal canal, insertion into perineal body	Inferior anal (rectal) nerve, a branch of pudendal nerve (S2–S4)	Constricts anal canal during peristalsis, resisting defecation; supports and fixes perineal body and pelvic floor
Bulbospongiosus	*Male:* median raphe on ventral surface of bulb of penis; perineal body	*Male:* surrounds lateral aspects of bulb of penis and most proximal part of of body of penis, inserting into perineal membrane, dorsal aspect of corpora spongiosum and cavernosa, and fascia of bulb of penis		*Male:* supports and fixes perineal body/pelvic floor; compresses bulb of penis to expel last drops of urine/semen; assists erection by compressing outflow via deep perineal vein and by pushing blood from bulb into body of penis
	Female: perineal body	*Female:* passes on each side of lower vagina, enclosing bulb and greater vestibular gland; inserts into pubic arch and fascia of corpora cavernosa of clitoris	Muscular (deep) branch of perineal nerve, a branch of pudendal nerve (S2–S4)	*Female:* supports and fixes perineal body/pelvic floor; "sphincter" of vagina; assists in erection of clitoris (and perhaps bulb of vestibule); compresses greater vestibular gland
Ischiocavernosus	Internal surface of ischiopubic ramus and ischial tuberosity	Embraces crus of penis or clitoris, inserting onto the inferior and medial aspects of crus and to perineal membrane medial to crus		Maintains erection of penis or clitoris by compressing outflow veins and pushing blood from the root of penis or clitoris into the body of penis or clitoris

(continues)

Table 3.9. Muscles of the Perineum *(Continued)*

Muscle	Origin	Course and distribution	Innervation	Main action
Superficial transverse perineal	Internal surface of ischiopubic ramus and ischial tuberosity	Passes along inferior aspect of posterior border of perineal membrane to perineal body	Muscular (deep) branch of perineal nerve, a branch of pudendal nerve (S2–S4)	Supports and fixes perineal body/pelvic floor to support abdominopelvic viscera and resist increased intra-abdominal pressure
Deep transverse perineal		Passes along superior aspect of posterior border of perineal membrane to perineal body and external anal sphincter		
External urethra sphincter	(Compressor urethra portion only)	Surrounds urethra superior to perineal membrane; in males, it also ascends anterior aspect of prostate; in females, some fibers also enclose vagina (urethrovaginal sphincter)	Dorsal nerve of penis or clitoris, the terminal branch of the pudendal nerve (S2–S4)	Compresses urethra to maintain urinary continence; in females, urethrovaginal sphincter portion also compresses vagina

Female Perineum

The **female perineum** includes the female external genitalia, perineal muscles, and anal canal.

Female External Genitalia

The **female external genitalia** (Figs. 3.52–3.55) include the mons pubis and labia majora (enclosing the pudendal cleft), labia minora (enclosing the vestibule), clitoris, bulbs of the vestibule, and greater and lesser vestibular glands. The synonymous terms **vulva** and **pudendum** include all these parts;

the term *pudendum* is commonly used clinically. The vulva serves:

- As sensory and erectile tissue for sexual arousal and intercourse.

- To direct the flow of urine.

- To prevent entry of foreign material into the urogenital tract.

Mons Pubis. The **mons pubis** is the rounded, fatty eminence anterior to the pubic symphysis, pubic tubercles, and

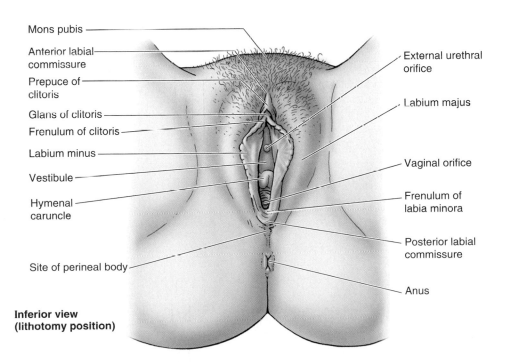

Mons pubis

Anterior labial commissure

Prepuce of clitoris

Glans of clitoris

Frenulum of clitoris

Labium minus

Vestibule

Hymenal caruncle

Site of perineal body

External urethral orifice

Labium majus

Vaginal orifice

Frenulum of labia minora

Posterior labial commissure

Anus

Inferior view (lithotomy position)

Figure 3.52. Female external genitalia. The labia majora and minora are separated to show the vestibule, into which the external urethral orifice and the vaginal orifice open.

Figure 3.53. Female perineum. A. A superficial dissection of the superficial pouch is shown. Encapsulated digital processes of fat pass deep to the thick superficial fatty tissue of the mons pubis, largely filling the labia majora. The prepuce of the clitoris forms a hood over the clitoris. Notice the ischioanal fossae lateral to the anal canal. **B.** This deeper dissection of the superficial pouch reveals the bulbs of the vestibule and the greater vestibular glands and ducts. The internal pudendal vessels and pudendal nerve are shown emerging from the pudendal canal.

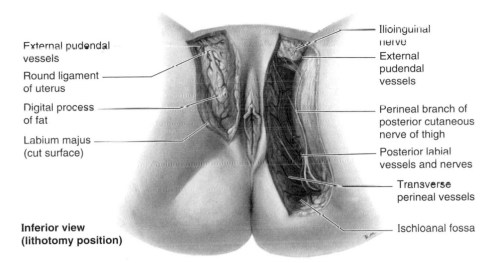

External pudendal
vessels

Round ligament
of uterus

Digital process
of fat

Labium majus
(cut surface)

Ilioinguinal
nerve

External
pudendal
vessels

Perineal branch of
posterior cutaneous
nerve of thigh

Posterior labial
vessels and nerves

Transverse
perineal vessels

Ischioanal fossa

**Inferior view
(lithotomy position)**

Figure 3.54. Female perineum. This subcutaneous dissection demonstrates the posterior labial vessels and nerves (S2–S3), joined by the perineal branch of the posterior cutaneous nerve of the thigh (S1–S3) running anteriorly almost to the mons pubis. The vessels anastomose here with the external pudendal vessels and the terminal branches of the nerves overlapping with those of the ilioinguinal nerve (L1). On the right side, the round ligament of the uterus terminates in the fat of the labium majus.

superior pubic rami (Fig. 3.52). The eminence is formed by a mass of fatty subcutaneous tissue (Fig. 3.53A). The amount of fat increases at puberty and decreases after menopause. The surface of the mons is continuous with the anterior abdominal wall. After puberty, the mons pubis is covered with coarse pubic hairs.

Labia Majora. The labia majora are prominent folds of skin that indirectly provide protection for the urethral and vaginal orifices. Each labium majus—largely filled with a finger-like "digital process" of loose subcutaneous tissue containing smooth muscle and the termination of the round ligament of the uterus (Figs. 3.53B and 3.54)—passes inferoposteriorly from the mons pubis toward the anus. The labia majora lie on the sides of a central depression (a narrow slit

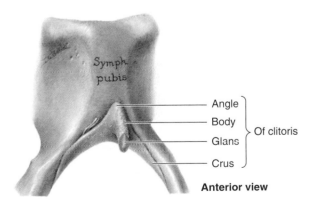

Anterior view

Figure 3.55. Clitoris. The surrounding soft tissues have been removed to reveal the parts of the clitoris. In many details, the clitoris resembles the structure of the penis, of which it is a homolog, although it is of reduced scale and has no association with the urethra.

when the thighs are adducted), the **pudendal cleft,** within which are the labia minora and vestibule (Fig. 3.52). The external aspects of the labia majora in the adult are covered with pigmented skin containing many sebaceous glands and are covered with crisp pubic hair. The internal aspects of the labia are smooth, pink, and hairless. The labia are thicker anteriorly where they join to form the **anterior commissure.** Posteriorly, in nulliparous women (never having borne children) they merge to form a ridge, the **posterior commissure,** which overlies the perineal body and is the posterior limit of the vulva. This commissure usually disappears after the first vaginal birth.

Labia Minora. The **labia minora** are rounded folds of fat-free, hairless skin. They are enclosed in the pudendal cleft and immediately surround the *vestibule* into which both the external urethral and the vaginal orifices open. They have a core of spongy connective tissue containing erectile tissue at their base and many small blood vessels. Anteriorly, the labia minora form two laminae. The medial laminae of each side unite as the **frenulum of the clitoris.** The lateral laminae unite anterior to (or often anterior and inferior to, thus overlapping and obscuring) the glans of the clitoris, forming the **prepuce** (foreskin) **of the clitoris.** In young women, especially virgins, the labia minora are connected posteriorly by a small transverse fold, the **frenulum of the labia minora** (fourchette). Although the internal surface of each labium minus consists of thin moist skin, it has the pink color typical of mucous membrane and contains many sebaceous glands and sensory nerve endings.

Clitoris. The **clitoris** is an erectile organ located where the labia minora meet anteriorly. The clitoris consists of a **root** and a **body,** which are composed of two crura; two corpora cavernosa; and the **glans of the clitoris,** which is covered by a prepuce (Figs. 3.53 and 3.55). Together, the body and glans of the clitoris are approximately 2 cm in length and < 1 cm in diameter. In contrast to the penis, the clitoris is not functionally related to the urethra or to urination. It functions solely as an organ of sexual arousal. The clitoris is highly sensitive and enlarges on tactile stimulation. The glans of the clitoris is the most highly innervated part of the clitoris and is densely supplied with sensory endings.

Vestibule. The **vestibule** is the space surrounded by the labia minora into which the orifices of the urethra and vagina and the ducts of the greater and lesser vestibular glands open (Figs. 3.52 and 3.53B). The *external urethral orifice* is located 2–3 cm posteroinferior to the glans of the clitoris and anterior to the vaginal orifice (Figs. 3.52 and 3.53A). On each side of the external urethral orifice are the openings of the ducts of the **paraurethral glands.** The size and appearance of the **vaginal orifice** vary with the condition of the **hymen,** a thin anular fold of mucous membrane immediately within the vaginal orifice surrounding the lumen. After its rupture, only remnants of the hymen, **hymenal caruncles** (tags), are visible. These remnants demarcate the vagina from the vestibule. The hymen has no established physiological function. It is considered primarily a developmental vestige, but its condition (and that of the frenulum of the labia minora) often provides critical evidence in cases of child abuse and rape.

Bulbs of the Vestibule. The **bulbs of the vestibule** are paired masses of elongated erectile tissue, approximately 3 cm in length (Fig. 3.53B). The bulbs lie along the sides of the vaginal orifice, superior or deep to (not within) the labia minora, immediately inferior to the perineal membrane (see Fig. 3.40C). They are covered inferiorly and laterally by the bulbospongiosus muscles extending along their length. The bulbs are homologous with the bulb of the penis of the corpus spongiosum.

Female Circumcision

Although illegal and now being actively discouraged in most countries, female circumcision is widely practiced in some cultures. The operation performed during childhood removes the prepuce of the clitoris and commonly also removes part or all of the clitoris and the labia minora. This disfiguring procedure is thought to inhibit sexual arousal and gratification.

Vulvar Trauma

The highly vascular bulbs of the vestibule are susceptible to disruption of vessels as the result of trauma (e.g., athletic injuries such as jumping hurdles, sexual assault, and obstetrical injury). These injuries often result in vulvar hematomas in the labia majora, for example. ⊙

Vestibular Glands. The **greater vestibular glands,** approximately 0.5 cm in diameter, are located on each side of the vestibule, posterolateral to the vaginal orifice and inferior to the perineal membrane; thus they are in the superficial perineal pouch (Fig. 3.53B). The greater vestibular glands (Bartholin glands) are round or oval and are partly overlapped posteriorly by the *bulbs of the vestibule,* and like the bulbs, are partially surrounded by the bulbospongiosus muscles. The slender ducts of these glands pass deep to the bulbs of the vestibule and open into the vestibule on each side of the vaginal orifice. These glands secrete mucus into the vestibule during sexual arousal. The **lesser vestibular glands** are small glands on each side of the vestibule that open into it between the urethral and the vaginal orifices. These glands secrete mucus into the vestibule, which moistens the labia and vestibule.

Infection of the Greater Vestibular Glands

The greater vestibular glands are usually not palpable, but are so when infected. Occlusion of the vestibular gland duct can predispose the individual to infection of the gland. The greater vestibular gland is the site or origin of most vulvar adenocarcinomas. **Bartholinitis,** inflammation of the greater vestibular glands, may result from a number of pathogenic organisms. Infected glands may enlarge to a diameter of 4–5 cm and impinge on the wall of the rectum. Occlusion of the vestibular gland duct without infection can result in the accumulation of mucin (**Bartholin cyst**). ⊙

Arterial Supply of the Vulva. The abundant arterial supply to the vulva is from the *external* and *internal pudendal arteries* (Figs. 3.53B and 3.54). The *internal pudendal artery* supplies most of the skin, external genitalia, and perineal muscles. The labial arteries are branches of the internal pudendal artery, as are those of the clitoris.

Venous and Lymphatic Drainage of the Vulva. The labial veins are tributaries of the *internal pudendal veins* and accompanying veins (L. *venae comitantes*) of the internal pudendal artery. Venous engorgement during the excitement phase of the sexual response causes an increase in the size and consistency of the clitoris and the bulbs of the vestibule. The clitoris becomes turgid, elongating in approximately 10% of women. The vulva contains a rich network of lymphatic vessels that pass laterally to the *superficial inguinal lymph nodes* (Fig. 3.56). The glans of the clitoris and anterior labia minora may also drain to the deep inguinal nodes or directly to the internal iliac nodes.

Innervation of the Vulva. The anterior aspect of the vulva (mons pubis, anterior labia) is supplied by derivatives of the lumbar plexus: the **anterior labial nerves,** derived from

A = vulva
B = glans clitoris, labia minora
C = urethra

Key

☐ Lumbar
☐ Common iliac
☐ Internal iliac
☐ External iliac
☐ Superficial inguinal
☐ Deep inguinal
☐ Sacral

Figure 3.56. Lymphatic drainage of vulva or pudendum. The *arrows* indicate the direction of lymph flow to the lymph nodes.

the *ilioinguinal nerve,* and the *genital branch of the genitofemoral nerve.* The posterior aspect of the vulva is supplied by derivatives of the sacral plexus: the *perineal branch of the posterior cutaneous nerve of the thigh* laterally and the *pudendal nerve* centrally (Figs. 3.54 and 3.57; Table 3.4). The latter is the primary nerve of the perineum. Its **posterior labial nerves** (terminal *superficial branches of the perineal nerve*) supply the labia; *deep* and *muscular branches of the perineal nerve* supply

the orifice of the vagina and superficial perineal muscles; and the *dorsal nerve of the clitoris* supplies deep perineal muscles and sensation to the clitoris. The bulb of the vestibule and erectile bodies of the clitoris receive parasympathetic fibers via *cavernous nerves* from the uterovaginal nerve plexus. Parasympathetic stimulation produces increased vaginal secretion, erection of the clitoris, and engorgement of erectile tissue in the bulbs of the vestibule.

Administration of Pudendal and Ilioinguinal Nerve Blocks

To relieve perineal pain during childbirth, **pudendal nerve block anesthesia** may be performed by injecting a local anesthetic agent into the tissues surrounding the pudendal nerve (Fig. B3.29). The injection is made where the pudendal nerve crosses the lateral aspect of the sacrospinous ligament, near its attachment to the ischial spine. The needle may be passed through the overlying skin (as illustrated) or, more commonly perhaps, through the vagina parallel to the palpating finger. Because the fetus's head is usually sta-

tioned within the lesser pelvis at this stage, it is important that the physician's finger is always positioned between the needle tip and the baby's head during the procedure. To abolish sensation from the anterior part of the perineum, an **ilioinguinal nerve block** is performed. When patients continue to complain of pain sensation after proper administration of a pudendal or pudendal and ilioinguinal nerve blocks, it is usually the result of overlapping innervation by the perineal branch at the posterior cutaneous nerve of the thigh. Other types of anesthesia for childbirth are explained and compared in the clinical correlation (blue) box "Anesthesia for Childbirth," in this chapter. ▶

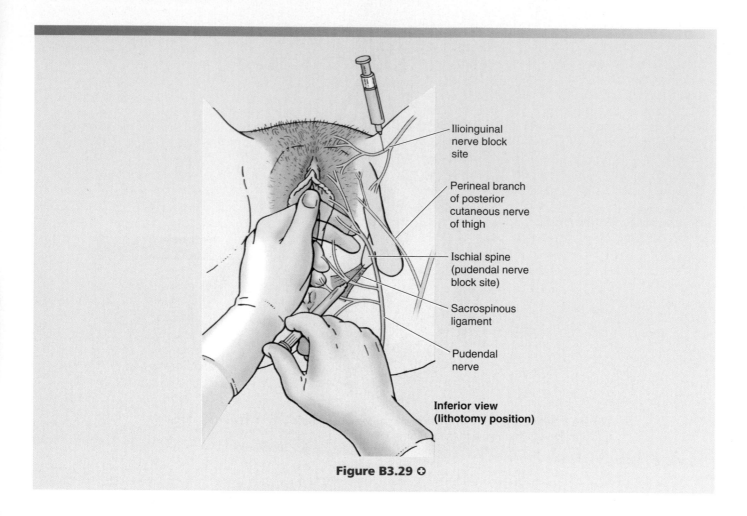

Ilioinguinal
nerve block
site

Perineal branch
of posterior
cutaneous nerve
of thigh

Ischial spine
(pudendal nerve
block site)

Sacrospinous
ligament

Pudendal
nerve

**Inferior view
(lithotomy position)**

Figure B3.29 ⊕

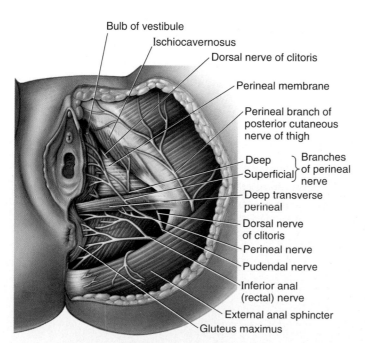

Bulb of vestibule

Ischiocavernosus

Dorsal nerve of clitoris

Perineal membrane

Perineal branch of
posterior cutaneous
nerve of thigh

Deep ⎤ Branches
Superficial ⎦ of perineal
nerve

Deep transverse
perineal

Dorsal nerve
of clitoris

Perineal nerve

Pudendal nerve

Inferior anal
(rectal) nerve

External anal sphincter

Gluteus maximus

Inferior view (lithotomy position)

Figure 3.57. Nerves of female perineum. In this view, the skin, subcutaneous tissue (fatty and membranous layers), and ischioanal fat bodies have been removed. Most of the area and most features of the perineum are innervated by branches of the pudendal nerve (S2–S4). The origin of the inferior anal nerve from the pudendal nerve is obscured from view by the inferior margin of the gluteus maximus muscle.

THE BOTTOM LINE: The female external genitalia consist of concentric folds (labia) surrounding an organ for sexual stimulation (clitoris) and the separate orifices of the urinary and reproductive systems. The fat-filled mons pubis and labia majora surround the pudendal cleft, covering and protecting its contents (e.g., bearing the body's weight when sitting on a bicycle). The fat-free labia minora attach to and cover the glans of the clitoris while surrounding the vestibule, into which the external urethral and vaginal orifices and vestibular glands open. The erectile clitoris, consisting of a highly sensitive glans, short body, and crura that attach to the pubic rami and perineal membrane, functions solely as a tactile sensory organ. A hymen or it remnants, hymenal caruncles, demarcate the vagina from the vestibule and the vaginal orifice. Immediately superior to the bases of the labia minora on each side of the vaginal orifice, the bulbs of the vestibule are paired masses of erectile tissue, homologous with the bulb of the penis. The internal pudendal vessels serve most of the vulva, with the external pudendal vessels serving a smaller anterior area. Except for the glans of the clitoris and associated structures (which drain to deep inguinal and external iliac nodes), lymph from the perineum drains to the superficial inguinal nodes.

Innervation is primarily from the pudendal nerve, with additional cutaneous innervation anteriorly from anterior labial nerves (ilioinguinal and genitofemoral nerves), and laterally from the posterior cutaneous nerve of the thigh. Parasympathetic fibers, passing independently from the pelvis to the perineum as cavernous nerves, innervate the erectile tissues.

Perineal Muscles of the Female

The *superficial perineal muscles* include the *superficial transverse perineal*, **ischiocavernosus**, and *bulbospongiosus muscles* (Fig. 3.53A & B). Details of their attachments, innervation and action are provided in Table 3.9.

Kegel Exercises for Increased Development of Female Perineal Muscles

In females, the superficial transverse perineal muscle, bulbospongiosus, and external anal sphincter, through their common attachment to the perineal body, form crossing beams over the pelvic outlet to support the perineal body, as in males. In the absence of the functional demands related to urination, penile erection, and ejaculation in males, the muscles are commonly relatively undeveloped in women. However, when developed, they contribute to the support of the pelvic viscera, and help prevent urinary stress incontinence and postpartum ▶

prolapse of pelvic viscera. Therefore, many gynecologists as well as prepartum classes for participatory childbirth recommend that women practice Kegel exercises (named for J. H. Kegel, a 20th-century U.S. gynecologist) using the perineal muscles, such as successive interruption of the urine flow during urination. Prepartum childbirth classes emphasize that in learning to voluntarily contract and relax the perineal muscles, women become prepared to resist the tendency to contract the musculature during uterine contractions, allowing a less obstructed passage for the fetus and decreasing the likelihood of tearing the perineal muscles.

Vaginismus

The initial distension of the bulbospongiosus and transverse perineal muscles are thought to trigger the involuntary spasms of the perivaginal and levator ani muscles of *vaginismus*, an emotional (psychosomatic) gynecological disorder. Vaginismus is encountered clinically when pelvic examination is attempted. In mild forms, it causes *dyspareunia* (painful intercourse); in severe forms, it prevents vaginal entry and is reportedly a cause of unconsummated marriages (Fromm, 2003). ☯

THE BOTTOM LINE: Although homologous to the male muscles, the perineal muscles of the female are generally less well developed. In addition to the sphincteric functions of the external anal and urethral sphincters for maintaining fecal and urinary continence, the female perineal muscles are also capable of supporting the perineal body (which in turn support the pelvic diaphragm). Learning to control perineal muscles through routine (Kegel) exercises may reduce the risk of obstetrical laceration of perineal muscles and of prolapse of the pelvic viscera. The perineal muscles are innervated by muscular branches of the pudendal nerve.

Medical Imaging of the Pelvis and Perineum

Various diagnostic imaging techniques are used to diagnose pelvic disease and fractures and to assess congenital anomalies of the pelvis and pelvic organs.

Radiography

Plain radiographs of the pelvis (Fig. 3.58) are often used as initial screening studies in patients with symptoms of pelvic disease (e.g., ureteric calculi, bowel obstruction). ▶

Figure 3.58. Radiograph of pelvis. A. This female pelvis demonstrates a wide subpubic angle and separation of the ischial spines. (Courtesy of Dr. E. L. Lansdown, Professor of Medical Imaging, University of Toronto, Toronto, ON, Canada.) **B.** The bony pelvis.

Contrast agents enhance the visualization of pelvic organs and vessels.

Hysterosalpingography, in which radiopaque dye is injected into the uterine cavity and tubes, is used for demonstrating tubal anatomy and patency (Fig. 3.59*A*) and for detecting uterine and tubal abnormalities (e.g., bicornuate uteri) (Fig. 3.59*B*).

Arteriography, visualization of arteries by X-ray imaging after injection of a radiopaque contrast medium, is used to demonstrate the pelvic arteries (Fig. 3.59*C*).

Ultrasonography

Ultrasonography (US; sonography) is used for obstetrical examination and for early evaluation of pelvic problems, such as screening examinations of high-risk patients for carcinoma and evaluation of congenital anomalies. Transabdominal US scanning requires a fully distended urinary bladder to displace the bowel loops from the pelvis and to provide an acoustical window through which to observe pelvic anatomy. The introduction of transrectal and ▶

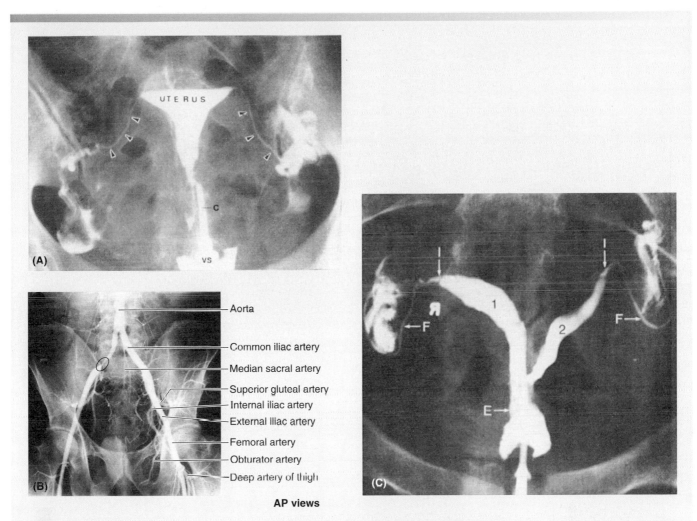

AP views

Figure 3.59. Radiograph of uterus and uterine tubes (hysterosalpingogram). A. Radiopaque material was injected into the uterus through the external os of the uterus. The contrast medium traveled through the triangular uterine cavity and uterine tubes (*arrowheads*) and passed into the pararectal fossae of the peritoneal cavity (lateral to the *arrowheads*). The female genital tract is in direct communication with the peritoneal cavity and is, therefore, a potential pathway for the spread of an infection from the vagina and uterus. *c,* catheter in the cervical canal, *vs,* vaginal speculum. **B.** For this iliac arteriogram, radiopaque dye has been injected into the aorta in the lumbar region. Features demonstrated include bifurcation of the aorta into right and left common iliac arteries (anterior to L4), bifurcation of the common iliacs into internal and external iliac arteries (opposite the sacroiliac joint at the level of the lumbosacral disc), and a site of narrowing (stenosis) of the right common iliac artery (*circled area* on the arteriogram). (Courtesy of Dr. D. Sniderman, Associate Professor of Medical Imaging, University of Toronto, Toronto, ON, Canada.) **C.** This hysterosalpingogram shows a bicornate uterus. *1* and *2,* uterine cavity; *E,* cervical canal; *F,* uterine tube; *I,* isthmus of tube. (Reprinted with permission from Stuart GCE, Reid DF: Diagnostic studies. *In* Copeland LJ (ed): *Textbook of Gynecology*. Philadelphia, Saunders, 1993.)

transvaginal ultrasonography has resulted in enhanced resolution of pelvic structures (Fig. 3.60). Transvaginal and transrectal ultrasonography enables the placing of the probe closer to the structures of interest, allowing increased resolution. For example, intrauterine blastocyst implantations can be distinguished 7–10 days earlier than with transabdominal scanning.

Computed Tomography

The anatomy of the pelvis is well demonstrated by CT. The presence of extraperitoneal fat and the relative absence of motion artifacts makes it possible to obtain excellent resolution (Fig. 3.61). An **axial scan**, a CT scan that is transverse to the axis of the body, is usually satisfactory; ▶

Figure 3.60. Ultrasound scans. A. In this transverse (transrectal) scan, the probe was inserted into the rectum to scan the anteriorly located prostate. The ducts of the glands in the peripheral zone open into the prostatic sinuses, whereas the ducts of the glands in the central (internal) zone open into the prostatic sinuses and the seminal colliculus. **B.** A transverse scan of a female's pelvis is shown. **C.** A sagittal scan is shown. (Courtesy of Dr. A. M. Arenson, Assistant Professor of Medical Imaging, University of Toronto, Toronto, ON, Canada.)

Spermatic cord
Rectus femoris
Vastus lateralis
Ischial tuberosity
Ischioanal fossa
(A)

Body of penis
Sartorius
Tensor of fascia lata
Left femur
Bulb of penis

Round ligament of uterus
Ligament of the ovary
Right ilium
Sigmoid colon
Sacral hiatus
(B)

Uterus
Gluteus medius
Gluteus maximus
Piriformis

Figure 3.61. Transverse CT images of pelvis. The male (**A**) and female (**B**) pelves are shown. (Courtesy of Dr. Donald R. Cahill, Department of Anatomy, Mayo Medical School, Rochester, MN.)

however, reformation of images into sagittal and coronal planes can provide additional information. CT is an important modality for assessing local tumor extent and in detecting metastases. It is also accurate in detecting postoperative and other abscesses.

Magnetic Resonance Imaging

MRI provides excellent evaluation of pelvic structures (Figs. 3.62 and 3.63) and permits outstanding delineation of the uterus and ovaries (Fig. 3.64). It also permits the identification of tumors (e.g., a myoma, or benign neoplasm) and congenital anomalies (e.g., bicornuate uterus). ○

(A) Median section from left

(B) Coronal section

(C) Coronal section

(D) Median section

Figure 3.62 MRI of male pelvis and perineum. A. A median section is shown. The plane for the section shown in **B** is indicated. **B.** This coronal section (of the same patient as in part **A**) is at the level of the femoral heads. **C.** A coronal section showing the normal penis and testes. **D.** In this median section of the female pelvis, the bladder is distended causing a retroversion of the uterus and making potential spaces of the vesicouterine and rectouterine pouches.

Key for A
BL	Urinary bladder
es	External anal sphincter
ms	Membranous urethra
PR	Prostate
R	Rectum
RA	Rectus abdominis
su	Prevesical (retropubic) space
sv	Seminal gland
sy	Pubic symphyses

Key for B
BL	Urinary bladder
oe	Obturator externus
oi	Obturator internus
PR	Prostate

Key for C
Large arrows	Spermatic cords
Arrow-heads	Tunica albuginea of testis and erectile bodies of penis
C	Corpus cavernosum
P	Pampiniform venous plexus
s	Corpus spongiosum
T	Testis

Key for D
a	Rectus abdominis muscle
b	Peritoneal cavity
c	Fundus of uterus
d	Body of uterus
e	Retrovesicular pouch
f	Cervical os of uterus
g	Bladder
h	Urethra
i	Mons pubis
j	Pubic symphyses
k	Labia majora
l	Central perineal tendon
m	Anus
n	Coccyx
o	Rectouterine pouch
p	Sacral promontory
q	Erector spinae muscle
L	Lumbar vertebrae (followed by the number of the specific vertebra)
S	Sacral vertebrae (followed by the number of the specific vertebra)

Planes of coronal scans in (A) and (B)

Figure 3.63. MRI studies of female pelvis. A and B. Coronal sections, along with an orientation drawing, are shown.

Key		IIV	Internal iliac vein	PM	Perineal membrane
BL	Broad ligament	IS	Internal urethral sphincter	S	Sigmoid colon
E	Endometrium	LS	Lumbosacral trunk	Sc	Sacrum
F	Follicle in ovary	M	Myometrium	SI	Sacroiliac joint
FU	Fundus of uterus	O	Ovary	U	Urethra
HdF	Head of femur	OE	Obturator externus	UB	Urinary bladder
I	Ilium	OI	Obturator internus	Ut	Uterus
IIA	Internal iliac artery	P	Pectineus	V	Vagina

(A) Median section ← Plane of coronal section (below)

Small intestine

Fluid in rectouterine pouch

Internal os

External os

Vaginal lumen

Wall of vagina

Myoma (benign muscle tumor)

Rectus abdominis

Endometrium

Body of uterus (myometrium)

Urinary bladder

Pubis

(B) Coronal section ← Plane of median section (above)

External iliac vessels

External iliac vessels

Bowel

Right ovary and follicles

Endometrium

Bladder

Left ovary and follicles

Body of uterus

Figure 3.64. MRI studies of female pelvis. A and B. The urinary bladder, body of the uterus, vagina, and intestine are demonstrated. Compare the coronal section (part **B**) with the dissected specimen shown in Figure 3.31*A*. (Courtesy of Dr. Shirley McCarthy, Department of Diagnostic Radiology, Yale University and Yale-New Haven Hospital, New Haven, CT.)

References and Suggested Readings

Beckmann CRB, Ling FW, Laube DW, Smith RP, Barzansky BM, Herbert WNP: *Obstetrics and Gynecology,* 4th ed., Baltimore, Lippincott Williams & Wilkins, 2002.

Behrman RE, Kliegman RM, Arvin AM (eds): *Nelson Textbook of Pediatrics*, 16th ed. Philadelphia, Saunders, 2000.

Berek JS: *Novak's Gynecology*, 12th ed., Baltimore, Lippincott, Williams & Wilkins, 1996.

Cahill DR, Orland MJ, Miller G: *Atlas of Human Cross-Sectional Anatomy*, 3rd ed. New York, Wiley-Liss, 1994.

Copeland LJ (ed): *Textbook of Gynecology*, 2nd ed. Philadelphia, Saunders, 2000.

Federative International Committee on Anatomical Terminology [FICAT]: *Terminologia Anatomica: International Anatomical Nomenclature.* Stuttgart, Thieme, 1998.

Fromm LM: Psychological aspects of gynecology. *In* Copeland LJ (ed): *Textbook of Gynecology*, 2nd ed. Philadelphia, Saunders, 2000.

Gabbe SG, Niebyl JR, Simpson JL: *Obstetrics—Normal and Problem Pregnancies*, 4th ed., New York, Churchill Livingstone, 2002.

Hatch K: Urinary tract injury and fistula. *In* Copeland LJ (ed): *Textbook of Gynecology*, 2nd ed. Philadelphia, Saunders, 2000.

Krebs H-B: Premalignant lesions of the cervix. *In* Copeland LJ (ed): *Textbook of Gynecology*, 2nd ed. Philadelphia, Saunders, 2000.

Moore KL, Persaud TVN: *The Developing Human. Clinically Oriented Embryology*, 7th ed. Philadelphia, Saunders, 2003.

Morris M, Burke TW: Cervical cancer. *In* Copeland LJ (ed): *Textbook of Gynecology*, 2nd ed. Philadelphia, Saunders, 2000.

Myers RP, Cahill DR, Devine RM, King BF: Anatomy of radical prostatectomy as defined by magnetic resonance imaging. *J Urol* 159:2148, 1998a.

Myers RP, King BF, Cahill DR: Deep perineal "space" as defined by magnetic resonance imaging. *Clin Anat* 11:132, 1998b.

Oelrich TM: The urethral sphincter muscle in the male. *Am J Anat* 158:229, 1980.

Oelrich TM: The striated urogenital sphincter muscle in the female. *Anat Rec* 205:223, 1983.

O'Rahilly R: *Gardner-Gray-O'Rahilly Anatomy. A Regional Study of Human Structure*, 5th ed. Philadelphia, Saunders, 1986.

Stormont TJ, Cahill DR, King BF, Myers RP: Fascias of the male external genitalia and perineum. *Clin Anat* 7:115, 1994.

Stuart GCE, Reid DF: Diagnostic studies. *In* Copeland LJ (ed): *Textbook of Gynecology*, 2nd ed Philadelphia, Saunders, 2000.

Walsh PC, Retnik AB, Vaughn ED, Wein AJ: *Campbell's Urology*, 7th ed. Philadelphia, Saunders, 1998.

Wendell-Smith CP, Wilson PM: The vulva, vagina, and urethra and the musculature of the pelvic floor. *In* Phillip E, Setchell M, Ginsburg J (eds): *Scientific Foundations of Obstetrics and Gynecology*. Oxford, Butterworth-Heinemann, 1991.

Wendell-Smith CP: Muscles and fasciae of the pelvis. *In* Williams PL, Bannister LH, Berry MM, Collins P, Dussek JE, Fergusson MWJ (eds): *Gray's Anatomy, The Anatomical Basis of Medicine and Surgery*, 38th ed. Edinburgh, Churchill-Livingstone, 1995.

Williams PL, Bannister LH, Berry MM, Collins P, Dussek JE, Fergusson MWJ (eds): *Gray's Anatomy, The Anatomical Basis of Medicine and Surgery*, 38th ed. Edinburgh, Churchill Livingstone, 1995.

4

Back

Overview of Back and Vertebral Column

The **back** comprises the posterior aspect of the trunk, inferior to the neck and superior to the buttocks (L. *nates*).

It is the region of the body to which the head, neck, and limbs are attached. The back includes the:

- Skin and subcutaneous tissue.

- Muscles: a superficial layer, primarily concerned with positioning and moving the limbs, and deeper layers ("true back muscles"), specifically concerned with moving or maintaining the position of the axial skeleton (posture).

- Vertebral column: the vertebrae, intervertebral (IV) discs, and associated ligaments (Fig. 4.1).

- Ribs (in the thoracic region): particularly their posterior portions, medial to the angles of the ribs.

- Spinal cord and meninges (membranes that cover the spinal cord).

- Various segmental nerves and vessels.

Because of their close association with the trunk, the back of the neck and the posterior and deep cervical muscles and vertebrae are also described in this chapter. The scapulae, although located in the back, are part of the appendicular skeleton and are considered with the upper limb (Chapter 6).

Study of the soft tissues of the back is best preceded by examination of the *vertebrae* and the fibrocartilaginous *intervertebral discs* that are interposed between the bodies of adjacent vertebrae. The vertebrae and IV discs collectively make up the *vertebral column* (spine), which extends from the cranium (skull) to the apex of the coccyx. The vertebral column forms the skeleton of the neck and back and is the main part of the **axial skeleton** (i.e., the articulated bones of the cranium, vertebral column, ribs, and sternum) (Fig. 4.1D). The adult vertebral column is 72–75 cm long, of which approximately one quarter is formed by the IV discs, which separate and bind the vertebrae together (Fig. 4.1D & E). The vertebral column:

- Protects the spinal cord and spinal nerves.

- Supports the weight of the body superior to the level of the pelvis.

- Provides a partly rigid and flexible axis for the body and an extended base on which the head is placed and pivots.

- Plays an important role in posture and **locomotion** (the movement from one place to another).

Backache and Back Pain

At least 10% of the population consults a physician, physiotherapist, or chiropractor each year about back pain. *Backache* is a nonspecific term used to describe back pain. More than 80% of people experience back complaints during their lifetime. *Low back pain,* the most common complaint, typically occurs between the ages of 30 and 70. *Back injuries* occur frequently in competitive sports and in industrial and automobile accidents. In severe injuries, the examiner must be careful not to cause further damage. For example, if an injured person complains of back pain and is unable to move the limbs, the vertebral column may be fractured. If the neck is flexed or the injured person sits up, the spinal cord may be (further) injured. Improper handling of an injured person can convert an unstable lesion without a neurological deficit into one with a deficit that produces permanent disability. ⊙

Vertebrae

The vertebral column in an adult typically consists of 33 vertebrae arranged in five regions: 7 cervical, 12 thoracic, 5 lumbar, 5 sacral, and 4 coccygeal (Fig. 4.1A–D). Significant motion occurs only between the 25 superior vertebrae. Of the 9 inferior vertebrae, the 5 sacral vertebrae are fused in adults to form the *sacrum* and, after approximately age 30, the 4 coccygeal vertebrae fuse to form the *coccyx*. The **lumbosacral angle** occurs at the junction of, and is formed by, the long axes of the lumbar region of the vertebral column and the sacrum (Fig.4.1D). The vertebrae gradually become larger as the vertebral column descends to the sacrum and then become progressively smaller toward the apex of the coccyx (Fig. 4.1A–D). The change in size is related to the fact that successive vertebrae bear increasing amounts of the body's weight as the column descends. The vertebrae reach maximum size immediately superior to the sacrum, which transfers the weight to the pelvic girdle at the sacroiliac joints.

The vertebral column is flexible because it consists of many relatively small bones, called **vertebrae** (singular = **vertebra**), that are separated by resilient IV discs (Fig. 4.2). The 25 cervical, thoracic, lumbar, and first sacral vertebrae also articulate at synovial *zygapophysial joints* (Fig. 4.2D), which facilitate and control the vertebral column's flexibility. Although the movement between two adjacent vertebrae is small, in aggregate the vertebrae and IV discs uniting them form a remarkably flexible yet rigid column that protects the spinal cord they surround.

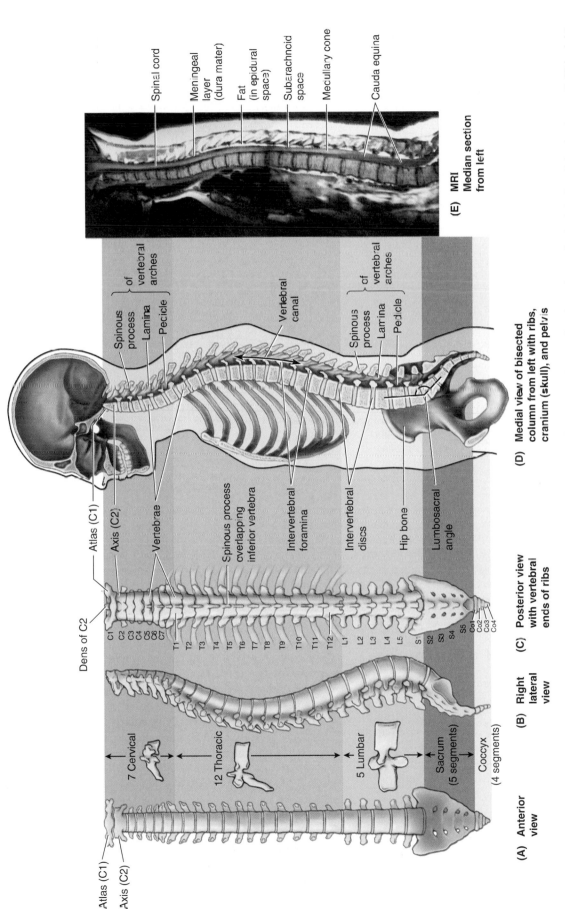

Figure 4.1. Vertebral column and vertebral canal, demonstrating its five regions. A. This anterior view shows the isolated vertebral column. **B.** This right lateral view shows the isolated vertebral column. Note the increase in size of the vertebrae as the column descends. **C.** This posterior view of the vertebral column includes the vertebral ends of ribs, representing the skeleton of the back. **D.** This medial view of the axial skeleton in situ demonstrates its regional curvatures and its relationship to the cranium (skull), thoracic cage, and hip bone. The continuous, weight-bearing column of vertebral bodies and IV discs forms the anterior wall of the vertebral canal. The lateral and posterior walls of the canal are formed by the series of vertebral arches. The IV foramina (seen also in part **B**) are openings in the lateral wall through which spinal nerves exit the vertebral canal. The posterior wall is formed by overlapping laminae and spinous processes, like shingles on a roof. **E.** This sagittal MRI study shows the primary contents of the vertebral canal. The medullary cone (L. *conus medullaris*) is the cone-shaped inferior end of the spinal cord, which typically ends at the L1–L2 level in adults. The dura mater, the external covering of the spinal cord (*gray*), is separated from the spinal cord by a fluid-filled space (*black*) and from the wall of the vertebral canal by fat (*white*) and thin-walled veins (not visible here).

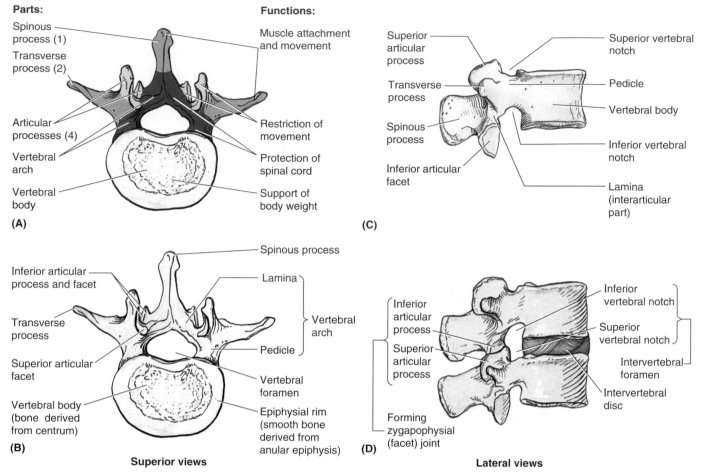

Parts:

Spinous process (1)

Transverse process (2)

Articular processes (4)

Vertebral arch

Vertebral body

(A)

Functions:

Muscle attachment and movement

Restriction of movement

Protection of spinal cord

Support of body weight

Inferior articular process and facet

Transverse process

Superior articular facet

Vertebral body (bone derived from centrum)

(B)

Spinous process

Lamina

Pedicle

Vertebral foramen

Epiphysial rim (smooth bone derived from anular epiphysis)

Vertebral arch

Superior views

Superior articular process

Transverse process

Spinous process

Inferior articular facet

(C)

Superior vertebral notch

Pedicle

Vertebral body

Inferior vertebral notch

Lamina (interarticular part)

Inferior articular process

Superior articular process

Forming zygapophysial (facet) joint

(D)

Inferior vertebral notch

Superior vertebral notch

Intervertebral foramen

Intervertebral disc

Lateral views

Figure 4.2. A "typical" vertebra, represented by L2. A. Functional components include the vertebral body (*bone color*), a vertebral arch (*red*), and seven processes: three for muscle attachment and leverage (*blue*) and four that participate in synovial joints with adjacent vertebrae (*yellow*). **B and C.** Bony formations of the vertebrae are demonstrated. The vertebral foramen is bounded by the vertebral arch and body. A small superior vertebral notch and a larger inferior vertebral notch flank the pedicle. **D.** The superior and inferior notches of adjacent vertebrae plus the IV disc that unites them form the IV foramen for the passage of a spinal nerve and its accompanying vessels. Note that each articular process has an articular facet where contact occurs with the articular facets of adjacent vertebrae (**B–D**).

Structure and Function of the Vertebrae

Vertebrae normally vary in size and other characteristics from one region of the vertebral column to another and to a lesser degree within each region; however, their basic structure is the same. A *typical vertebra* (Fig. 4.2) consists of a vertebral body, a vertebral arch, and seven processes.[1]

The **vertebral body** is the more massive, roughly cylindrical, anterior part of the bone that gives strength to the ver-

tebral column and supports body weight. The size of the vertebral bodies increases as the column descends, most markedly from T4 inferiorly, as each bears progressively greater body weight.

The vertebral body consists of vascular, trabecular (spongy, cancellous) bone enclosed by a thin external layer of compact bone (Fig. 4.3). The trabecular bone is a meshwork of mostly tall vertical trabeculae intersecting with short, horizontal trabeculae. The interstices of these trabeculae are occupied by red marrow that is among the most actively hematopoietic (blood-forming) tissues of the mature individual. One or more large foramina in the posterior surface of the body accommodate basivertebral veins that drain the marrow (Fig. 4.20).

In life, most of the superior and inferior surfaces of the vertebral body are covered with discs of hyaline cartilage (vertebral "end plates"), which are remnants of the cartilaginous model from which the bone develops (Bogduk, 1997). In dried

[1]In contemporary usage, the terms *vertebral body* and *centrum* and the terms *vertebral arch* and *neural arch* are often erroneously used as synonyms. Technically, however, in each case the former is a gross anatomy term applied to parts of the adult vertebrae, and the latter is an embryology term referring to parts of a developing vertebra ossifying from primary centers. The vertebral body includes the centrum and part of the neural arch; the vertebral arch is thus less extensive than the neural arch, and the centrum is less extensive than the vertebral body (O'Rahilly, 1986; Williams et al., 1995).

laboratory and museum skeletal specimens, this cartilage is absent, and the exposed bone appears spongy, except at the periphery where an **epiphysial rim** or ring of smooth bone, derived from an *anular epiphysis,* is fused to the body (Fig. 4.2*B*). In addition to serving as growth zones, the anular epiphyses and their cartilaginous remnants provide some protection to the vertebral bodies and permit some diffusion of fluid between the IV disc and the capillaries in the vertebral body. The superior and inferior epiphyses usually unite with the **centrum,** the primary ossification center for the central mass of the vertebral body (Fig. 4.2*B*), early in adult life (at approximately age 25) (see "Ossification of Vertebrae" in this chapter).

The **vertebral arch** is posterior to the vertebral body and consists of two (right and left) pedicles and laminae (Fig. 4.2*A*). The **pedicles** are short, stout cylindrical processes that project posteriorly from the vertebral body to meet two broad, flat plates of bone, called **laminae,** which unite in the midline. The vertebral arch and the posterior surface of the vertebral body form the walls of the **vertebral foramen** (Fig. 4.2*B* & *C*). The succession of vertebral foramina in the articulated vertebral column forms the **vertebral canal** (spinal canal), which contains the spinal cord and the roots of the spinal nerves that emerge from it, along with the membranes (meninges), fat, and vessels that surround and serve them (Fig. 4.1*E*). The **vertebral notches** are indentations observed in lateral views of the vertebrae superior and inferior to each pedicle between the superior and inferior articular processes posteriorly and the corresponding projections of the body an-

teriorly (Fig. 4.2*C* & *D*). The superior and inferior vertebral notches of adjacent vertebrae and the IV discs connecting them form the **intervertebral foramina** (Fig. 4.2*D*), in which the spinal (posterior root) ganglia are located and through which the spinal nerves emerge from the vertebral column with their accompanying vessels.

Seven processes arise from the vertebral arch of a typical vertebra (Fig. 4.2*A–C*):

- One median **spinous process** projects posteriorly (and usually inferiorly, typically overlapping the vertebra below) from the vertebral arch at the junction of the laminae.

- Two **transverse processes** project posterolaterally from the junctions of the pedicles and laminae.

- Four **articular processes** (G. *zygapophyses*)—two **superior** and two **inferior**—also arise from the junctions of the pedicles and laminae, each bearing an **articular surface** (**facet**).

The former three processes, one spinous and two transverse, afford attachments for deep back muscles and serve as levers, facilitating the muscles that fix or change the position of the vertebrae.

The latter four (articular) processes are in apposition with corresponding processes of vertebrae adjacent (superior and inferior) to them, forming *zygapophysial (facet) joints* (Fig. 4.2*D*). Through their participation in these joints, these processes determine the types of movements permitted and restricted between the adjacent vertebrae of each region. The articular

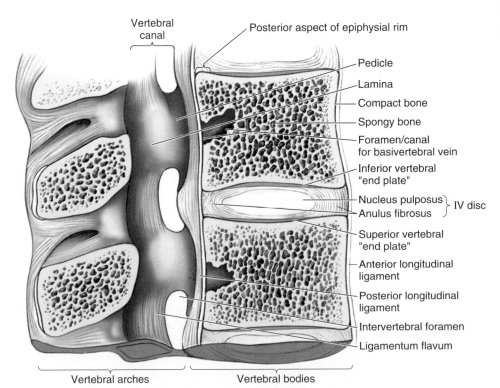

Vertebral canal

Posterior aspect of epiphysial rim

Pedicle

Lamina

Compact bone

Spongy bone

Foramen/canal for basivertebral vein

Inferior vertebral "end plate"

Nucleus pulposus

Anulus fibrosus

} IV disc

Superior vertebral "end plate"

Anterior longitudinal ligament

Posterior longitudinal ligament

Intervertebral foramen

Ligamentum flavum

Vertebral arches   Vertebral bodies

Medial view of left halves of two adjacent hemisected vertebrae

Figure 4.3. Internal aspects of vertebral body and vertebral canal. Vertebral bodies consist largely of spongy bone, with tall, vertical supporting trabeculae linked by short horizontal trabeculae, covered by a relatively thin layer of compact bone. Hyaline cartilage end plates cover the superior and inferior surfaces of the bodies, surrounded by smooth bony epiphysial rims. The posterior longitudinal ligament, covering the posterior aspect of the vertebral bodies and linking the IV discs, forms the anterior wall of the vertebral canal. Lateral and posterior walls of the vertebral canal are formed by vertebral arches (pedicles and laminae) alternating with IV foramina and ligamenta flava.

processes also assist in keeping adjacent vertebrae aligned, particularly preventing one vertebra from slipping anteriorly on the vertebra below. Generally, the articular processes bear weight only temporarily, as when one rises from the flexed position, and unilaterally when the cervical vertebrae are laterally flexed to their limit. However, the inferior articular processes of the L5 vertebra bear weight even in the erect posture.

THE BOTTOM LINE: Vertebrae consist of vertebral bodies, which bear weight and increase in size proportionately, and vertebral arches, which collectively house and protect the spinal cord. Processes extending from the arch provide attachment and leverage for muscles or direct movements between vertebrae.

Laminectomy

The surgical excision of one or more spinous processes and the adjacent supporting vertebral laminae in a particular region of the vertebral column is called a **laminectomy** (*1* in Fig. B4.1). The term is also commonly used to denote removal of most of the vertebral arch by transecting the pedicles (*2* in Fig. B4.1). Laminectomies are performed surgically (or anatomically in the dissection laboratory) to gain access to the vertebral canal, providing posterior exposure of the spinal cord (if performed above the L2 level) and/or the roots of specific spinal nerves. Surgical laminectomy is often performed to relieve pressure on the spinal cord or nerve roots caused by a tumor, herniated IV disc, or bony hypertrophy (excess growth). ✪

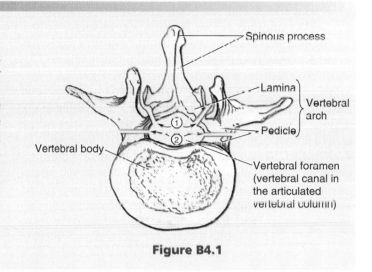

Figure B4.1

Regional Characteristics of the Vertebrae

Each of the 33 vertebrae is unique. However, most of the vertebrae demonstrate characteristic features identifying them as belonging to one of the five regions of the vertebral column (e.g., vertebrae having foramina in their transverse processes are cervical vertebrae). In addition, certain individual vertebrae have distinguishing features; the C7 vertebra, for example, has the longest spinous process. It forms a prominence under the skin at the back of the neck, especially when the neck is flexed.

In each region, the articular facets are oriented on the articular processes of the vertebrae in a characteristic direction that determines the type of movement permitted between the adjacent vertebrae and, in aggregate, for the region. For example, the articular facets of thoracic vertebrae are nearly vertical, and together define an arc centered in the IV disc; this arrangement permits rotation and lateral flexion of the vertebral column in this region (Table 4.2). Regional variations in the size and shape of the vertebral canal accommodate the varying thickness of the spinal cord (Fig 4.1*D* & *E*).

Cervical Vertebrae

Cervical vertebrae form the skeleton of the neck (Fig. 4.1). The smallest of the 24 movable vertebrae, the cervical vertebrae are located between the cranium and the thoracic vertebrae. Their smaller size reflects the fact that they bear less weight than do the larger inferior vertebrae. Although the cervical IV discs are thinner than those of inferior regions, they are relatively thick compared to the size of the vertebral bodies they connect. The relative thickness of the discs, the nearly horizontal orientation of the articular facets, and the small amount of surrounding body mass give the cervical region the greatest range and variety of movement of all the vertebral regions.

The distinctive features of cervical vertebrae are illustrated and listed in Table 4.1. The single-most distinctive feature of each cervical vertebra is the oval **transverse foramen** in the *transverse process* (L. *foramen transversarium*). The vertebral arteries and their accompanying veins pass through the transverse foramina, except those in C7, which transmit only small accessory veins. Thus the foramina are smaller in C7 than those in other cervical vertebrae, and occasionally they are absent. The transverse processes of cervical vertebrae end laterally in two projections: an **anterior tubercle** and a **posterior tubercle**. The tubercles provide attachment for a laterally placed group of cervical muscles (*levator scapulae* and *scalenes*). Grooves on the transverse processes between tubercles (the floor of the groove being formed by a **costotransverse bar**) accommodate the anterior rami of the cervical spinal nerves (Table 4.1*B*).

Table 4.1. Cervical Vertebrae[a]

Posterior arch
- Posterior tubercle
- Groove for vertebral artery

Anterior arch
- Facet for dens
- Anterior tubercle

Tubercle for transverse ligament
Superior articular surface (process)
Transverse foramen
Transverse process
} Lateral mass

Atlas (C1)

Inferior articular process
Transverse process
Superior articular facet
Dens

Axis (C2)

Transverse process
- Posterior tubercle
- Costotransverse bar
- Anterior tubercle

C3

Vertebral foramen
Transverse foramen
Spinous process

C4

Uncus of body (uncinate process)

C5

Articular process
- Inferior
- Superior
Carotid tubercle

C6

"Vestigial anterior tubercle"

C7

(A) Superior views, vertebrae C1–C7

Transverse process
Superior articular facet
Vertebral arch
Bifid spinous process
Uncus of body (uncinate process)
Vertebral foramen
Transverse foramen
Anterior tubercle
Pars articularis
Inferior articular facet
Posterior tubercle
Groove of spinal nerve

(B) Left anterior superior oblique view of "typical" cervical vertebra

Part	Characteristics
Body	Small and wider from side to side than anteroposteriorly; superior surface concave with uncus of body (uncinate process); inferior surface convex
Vertebral foramen	Large and triangular
Transverse processes	Transverse foramina small or absent in C7; vertebral arteries and accompanying venous and sympathetic plexuses pass through foramina, except C7, which transmits only small accessory vertebral veins; anterior and posterior tubercles
Articular processes	Superior facets directed superioposteriorly; inferior facets directed inferioanteriorly; obliquely placed facets are most nearly horizontal in this region
Spinous processes	Short (C3–C5) and bifid (C3–C6); process of C6 long, that of C7 is longer (thus C7 called "vertebra prominens")

[a] The C1 and C2 vertebrae are atypical

Typical intercostal nerves (3rd through 6th) run along the intercostal spaces posteriorly, between the parietal pleura (serous lining of the thoracic cavity)

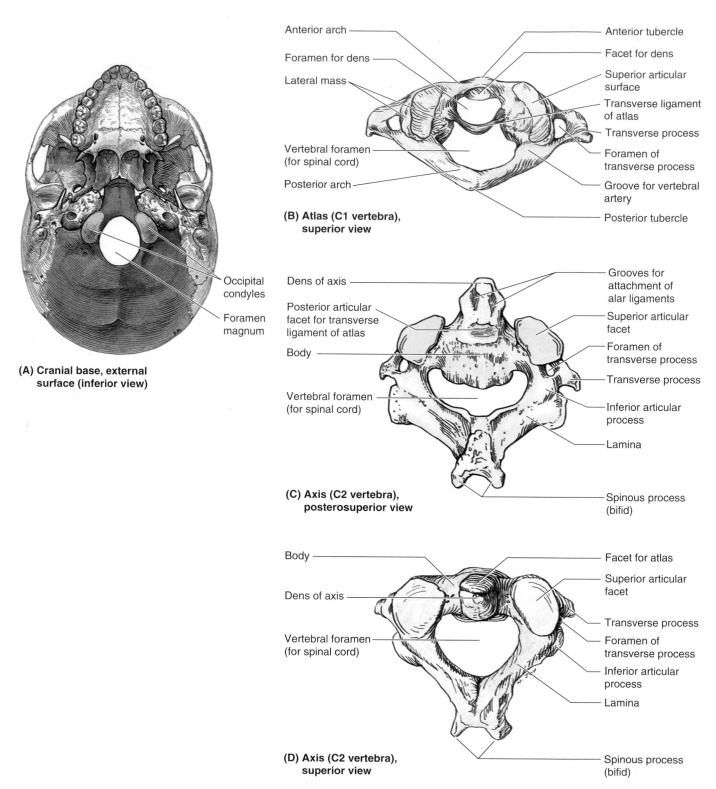

(A) Cranial base, external surface (inferior view)

Occipital condyles

Foramen magnum

Anterior arch

Foramen for dens

Lateral mass

Vertebral foramen (for spinal cord)

Posterior arch

Anterior tubercle

Facet for dens

Superior articular surface

Transverse ligament of atlas

Transverse process

Foramen of transverse process

Groove for vertebral artery

Posterior tubercle

(B) Atlas (C1 vertebra), superior view

Dens of axis

Posterior articular facet for transverse ligament of atlas

Body

Vertebral foramen (for spinal cord)

Grooves for attachment of alar ligaments

Superior articular facet

Foramen of transverse process

Transverse process

Inferior articular process

Lamina

Spinous process (bifid)

(C) Axis (C2 vertebra), posterosuperior view

Body

Dens of axis

Vertebral foramen (for spinal cord)

Facet for atlas

Superior articular facet

Transverse process

Foramen of transverse process

Inferior articular process

Lamina

Spinous process (bifid)

(D) Axis (C2 vertebra), superior view

Figure 4.4. Cranial base and C1 and C2 vertebrae. A. Observe the occipital condyles that articulate with the superior articular surfaces (facets) of the atlas (vertebra C1). **B.** The atlas, on which the cranium rests, has neither a spinous process nor a body. It consists of two lateral masses connected by anterior and posterior arches. **C and D.** The tooth-like dens characterizes the axis (vertebra C2) and provides a pivot around which the atlas turns and carries the cranium. It articulates anteriorly with the anterior arch of the atlas ("Facet for dens" in part **B**) and posteriorly with the transverse ligament of the atlas (see part **B**).

The **carotid tubercles** of vertebra C6 are so called **carotid tubercles** because the common carotid arteries may be compressed here, in the groove between the tubercle and body, to control bleeding from these vessels. Bleeding may continue because of the carotid's multiple anastomoses of distal branches with adjacent and contralateral branches, but at a slower rate.

Vertebrae C3–C7 demonstrate all the features typical of cervical vertebrae indicated in Table 4.1. They have large vertebral foramina to accommodate the enlargement of the spinal cord in this region in relation to the innervation of the upper limbs. The superior borders of the transversely elongated bodies of the cervical vertebrae are elevated posteriorly and especially laterally but are depressed anteriorly, resembling somewhat a sculpted seat (Table 4.1B). The inferior border of the body of the superiorly placed vertebra is reciprocally shaped. The adjacent cervical vertebrae articulate in a way that permits free flexion and extension and some lateral flexion but restricted rotation. The planar, nearly horizontal articular facets of the articular processes are also favorable for these movements. The elevated superolateral margin is the **uncus of the body (uncinate process)**. The spinous processes of the C3–C6 vertebrae are short and usually bifid in whites but usually not in people of African descent. C7 is a prominent vertebra that is characterized by a long spinous process; because of this prominent process, C7 is called the **vertebra prominens**. Run your finger along the midline of the posterior aspect of your neck until you feel the prominent C7 spinous process.

The two superior-most cervical vertebrae are atypical. Vertebra C1, also called the **atlas**, is unique in that it has neither a body nor a spinous process (Fig. 4.4B; Table 4.1A). This ring-shaped bone has paired **lateral masses** that serve the place of a body by bearing the weight of the globe-like cranium in a manner similar to the way that Atlas of Greek mythology bore the weight of the world on his shoulders. The

transverse processes of the atlas arise from the lateral masses, causing them to be more laterally placed than those of the inferior vertebrae. This feature makes the atlas the widest of the cervical vertebrae, thus providing increased leverage for attached muscles. The kidney-shaped, concave **superior articular surfaces** of the lateral masses receive two large cranial protuberances called the **occipital condyles** at the sides of the foramen magnum (Fig. 4.4A). **Anterior** and **posterior arches**, each of which bears a **tubercle** in the center of its external aspect, extend between the lateral masses, forming a complete ring (Fig 4.4B). The posterior arch, which corresponds to the lamina of a typical vertebra, has a wide **groove for the vertebral artery** on its superior surface. The C1 nerve also runs in this groove.

Vertebra C2, also called the **axis**, is the strongest of the cervical vertebrae. C1, carrying the cranium, rotates on C2, as when a person turns the head to indicate "no." The axis has two large, flat bearing surfaces, the **superior articular facets**, on which the atlas rotates (Fig. 4.4C). The distinguishing feature of the axis is the blunt tooth-like **dens** (odontoid process), which projects superiorly from its body. Both the dens (G. tooth) and the spinal cord inside its coverings are encircled by the atlas. The dens lies anterior to the spinal cord and serves as the pivot about which the rotation occurs. The dens is held in position against the posterior aspect of the anterior arch of the atlas by the **transverse ligament of the atlas** (Fig. 4.4B). This ligament extends from one lateral mass of the atlas to the other, passing between the dens and spinal cord, forming the posterior wall of the "socket" that receives the dens. Thus it prevents posterior (horizontal) displacement of the dens and anterior displacement of the atlas. Either displacement would compromise the portion of the vertebral foramen of C1 that gives passage to the spinal cord. C2 has a large bifid spinous process (Fig. 4.4C & D) that can be felt deep in the *nuchal groove,* the superficial vertical groove at the back of the neck.

Dislocation of the Cervical Vertebrae

Because of their more horizontally oriented articular facets, the cervical vertebrae are less tightly interlocked than other vertebrae. The cervical vertebrae, stacked like books, can be dislocated in neck injuries with less force than is required to fracture them (Fig. B4.2A–F). Because of the large vertebral canal in the cervical region, slight dislocation can occur here without damaging the spinal cord (Fig. B4.2B). Severe dislocations, or dislocations combined with fractures (fracture–dislocations) injure the spinal cord. If the dislocation does not result in "facet jumping" with locking of the displaced articular processes (Fig. B4.2F & G), the cervical vertebrae may self-reduce (slip back into place) so that a radiograph may not indicate

that the cord has been injured. MRI, however, may reveal the resulting soft tissue damage.

Fracture and Dislocation of the Atlas

Vertebra C1 is a bony ring, with two wedge-shaped lateral masses connected by relatively thin anterior and posterior arches and a transverse ligament (Fig. B4.3A). Because the thick side of the lateral mass wedges is directed laterally, vertical forces (as would result from a blow to the top of the head from a falling object, or striking the bottom of a pool in a diving accident) compressing the lateral masses between the occipital condyles and the axis drive them apart, fracturing one or both of the bony arches. If the force is sufficient, rupture of ▶

the transverse ligament that links them will occur (Fig. B4.3*B*). The resulting *Jefferson* or *burst fracture* (Fig. B4.3*C–E*) in itself does not necessarily result in spinal cord injury, because the dimensions of the bony ring actually increase. Spinal cord injury is more likely, however, if the transverse ligament has also been ruptured (see clinical correlation [blue] box "Rupture of the Transverse Ligament of the Atlas," in this chapter), indicated radiographically by widely spread lateral masses.

Fracture and Dislocation of the Axis

Fractures of the vertebral arch of the axis are one of the most common injuries of the cervical vertebrae (up to 40%) ▶

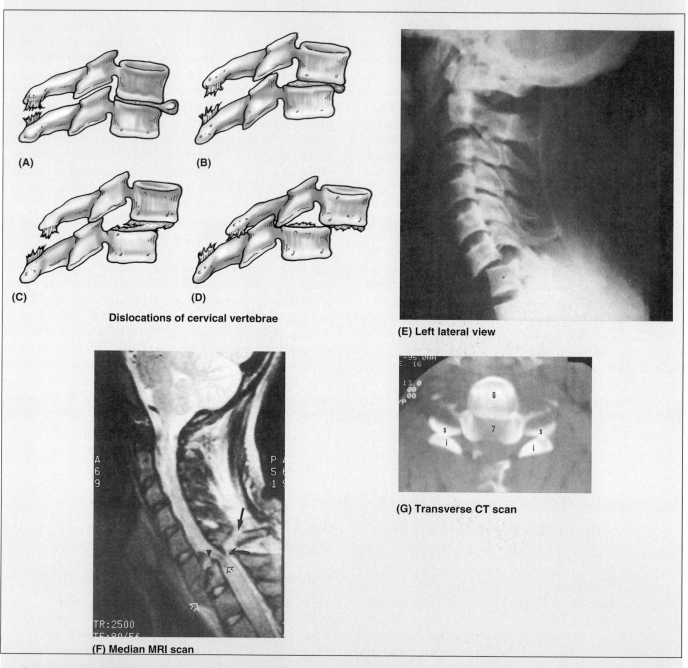

(A)

(B)

(C)

(D)

Dislocations of cervical vertebrae

(E) Left lateral view

(F) Median MRI scan

(G) Transverse CT scan

Figure B4.2. Dislocations of cervical vertebrae. Four stages of injury are shown: (**A**) stage I, flexion sprain; (**B**) stage II, anterior subluxation with 25% anterior translation; (**C**) stage III, 50% translation; and (**D**) stage IV, complete dislocation. **E.** This lateral view radiograph shows a stage III dislocation with 50% translation. **F.** This MRI study of a stage IV dislocation with cord injury reveals that the body of C7 is fractured (*open white arrowhead*). The ligamentum flavum is disrupted (*curved black arrow*), and the spinous process is avulsed (*straight black arrow*). **G.** This transverse CT scan (same as shown in part **F**) reveals the reversed position of the articular processes of the C6 and C7 vertebrae owing to "facet jumping." The flat articular surfaces should be in contact, forming C6–C7 zygapophysial joints.

(Yochum and Rowe, 2004). Usually the fracture occurs in the bony column formed by the superior and inferior articular processes of the axis, the pars interarticularis (Table 4.1*B*). A fracture in this location, called a **traumatic spondylolysis of C2** (Fig. B4.4*A*, *B*, & *D*), usually occurs as a result of *hyperextension of the head on the neck,* rather than the combined hyperextension of the head and neck, which results in *whiplash* injury. Such hyperextension of the head was used to execute criminals by hanging, in which the knot was placed under the chin before the body suddenly dropped its length through the gallows floor (Fig. B4.4*C*); thus this fracture is called a *hangman's fracture.* In more severe injuries, the body of the C2 vertebra is displaced anteriorly with respect to the body of the C3 vertebra. With or without such subluxation (incomplete dislocation) of the axis, injury of the spinal cord and/or of the brainstem is likely, sometimes resulting in **quadriplegia** (paralysis of all four limbs) or death. *Fractures of the dens* are also common axis injuries (40–50%), which may result from a horizontal blow to the head or as a complication of *osteopenia* (pathological loss of bone mass) (see clinical correlation [blue] box "Fracture of the Dens," in this chapter). ▶

(A) Anterior view of occipital condyles, atlas and axis

(B) Anterior view of coronal section of craniovertebral [atlanto-occipital (AO) and lateral atlantoaxial (AA)] joints

(C) Inferor view of Jefferson (burst) fracture of C1

(D) Inferior view of CT scan of Jefferson fracture

(E) Anterior view of reconstructed CT image of Jefferson fracture showing fragment of anterior arch and outward (lateral) shift of lateral masses of C1

Figure B4.3

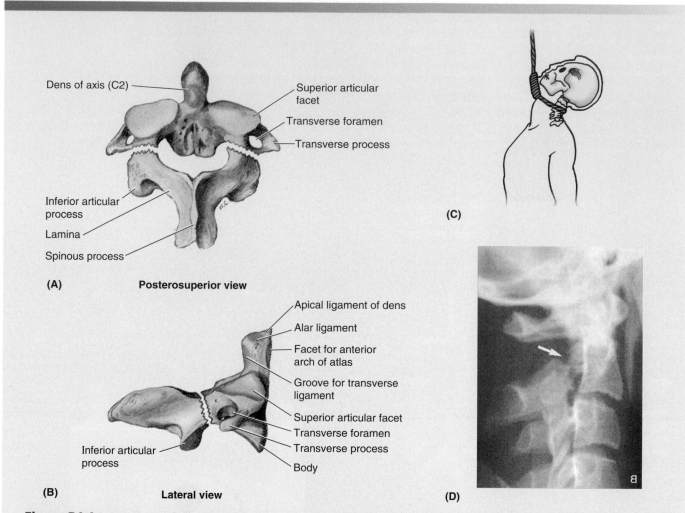

Figure B4.4 Fracture and dislocation of axis. Posterosuperior (**A**) and lateral (**B**) views of a hangman's fracture of the C2 vertebra are shown. **C.** This position of the knot produces hyperextension during hanging. **D.** This right lateral view radiograph reveals a hangman's fracture (*arrow*) of C2. ◉

Thoracic Vertebrae

The **thoracic vertebrae** lie in the upper back and provide attachment for the ribs (Fig. 4.1). Thus the primary characteristic features of thoracic vertebrae are the **costal facets** for articulation with ribs. The costal facets and other characteristic features of thoracic vertebrae are illustrated and listed in Table 4.2. The middle four thoracic vertebrae (T5–T8) demonstrate all the features typical of thoracic vertebrae. The articular processes of thoracic vertebrae extend vertically with paired, nearly coronally oriented articular facets that define an arc centered in the IV disc. This arc permits rotation and some lateral flexion of the vertebral column in this region, in fact, the greatest degree of rotation is permitted here (Table 4.2*A*). Attachment of the rib cage combined with the vertical orientation of articular facets and overlapping spinous processes limits flexion and extension as well as lateral flexion.

The T1–T4 vertebrae share some features of cervical vertebrae. T1 is atypical of thoracic vertebrae in that it has a long, almost horizontal spinous process that may be nearly as prominent as that of the vertebra prominens. T1 also has a complete costal facet on the superior edge of its body for the 1st rib and a demifacet on its inferior edge that contributes to the articular surface for the 2nd rib.

The T9–T12 vertebrae have some features of lumbar vertebrae, including tubercles similar to the accessory and mammillary processes of lumbar vertebrae. However, most of the transition in characteristics from thoracic to lumbar region occurs over the length of a single vertebra: vertebra T12. Generally, its superior half is thoracic in character, having costal facets and articular processes that permit primarily rotatory movement, whereas its inferior half is lumbar in character, devoid of costal facets and having articular processes that permit only flexion and extension. Consequently, vertebra T12 is

Table 4.2. Thoracic Vertebrae

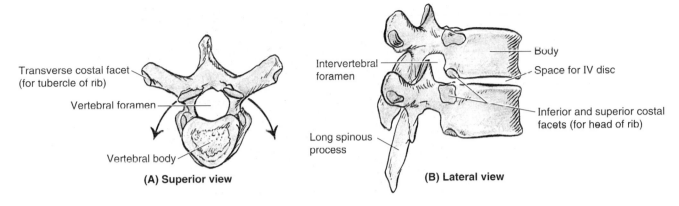

Transverse costal facet (for tubercle of rib)

Vertebral foramen

Vertebral body

(A) Superior view

Intervertebral foramen

Body

Space for IV disc

Inferior and superior costal facets (for head of rib)

Long spinous process

(B) Lateral view

Part	Characteristics
Body	Heart shaped; one or two costal facets for articulation with head of rib
Vertebral foramen	Circular and smaller than those of cervical and lumbar vertebrae
Transverse processes	Long and strong and extend posterolaterally; length diminishes from T1 to T12 (T1–T10 have facets for articulation with tubercle of rib)
Articular processes	Superior facets directed posteriorly and slightly laterally; inferior facets directed anteriorly and slightly medially; plane of facets lies on arc centered about vertebral body
Spinous processes	Long; slope posteroinferiorly; tips extend to level of vertebral body below

subject to transitional stresses that cause it to be the most commonly fractured vertebra.

Lumbar Vertebrae

Lumbar vertebrae are located in the lower back between the thorax and sacrum (Fig. 4.1). Characteristic features of the lumbar vertebrae are illustrated and listed in Table 4.3. Because the weight they support increases toward the inferior end of the vertebral column, lumbar vertebrae have massive bodies, accounting for much of the thickness of the lower trunk in the median plane. Their articular processes extend vertically, with articular facets sagittally oriented initially (beginning abruptly with the T12–L1 joints) but becoming more coronally oriented as the column descends. The L5–S1 facets are distinctly coronal in orientation. In the more sagittally oriented superior joints, the laterally facing facets of the inferior processes of the vertebra above are "gripped" by the medially facing facets of the superior processes of the vertebra below, in a manner that facilitates flexion and extension, allows lateral flexion, but prohibits rotation (Figs. 4.1 and 4.2). The transverse processes project somewhat posterosuperiorly as well as laterally. On the posterior surface of the base of each transverse process is a small **accessory process**, which provides an attachment for the medial intertransverse lumborum muscle. On the posterior surface of the superior articular processes are **mammillary processes**, which give attachment to the multifidus and medial intertransverse muscles (back muscles).

Vertebra L5 is the largest of all movable vertebrae; it carries the weight of the whole upper body. L5 is distinguished by its massive body and transverse processes. Its body is markedly deeper anteriorly; therefore, it is largely responsible for the lum-

bosacral angle between the long axis of the lumbar region of the vertebral column and that of the sacrum (Fig. 4.1D). Body weight is transmitted from L5 vertebra to the *base of the sacrum,* formed by the superior surface of S1 vertebra (Fig. 4.5A).

Lumbar Spinal Stenosis

Lumbar spinal stenosis describes a stenotic (narrow) vertebral foramen in one or more lumbar vertebrae (Fig. B4.5A). This condition may be a hereditary anomaly that can make a person more vulnerable to age-related degenerative changes such as IV disc bulging (Rowland and McCormick, 2000). The narrowing is usually maximal at the level of the IV discs. However, stenosis of a lumbar vertebral foramen alone may cause compression of one or more of the spinal nerve roots occupying the inferior vertebral canal (Fig. 4.1E). Electromyography can confirm that the denervation is restricted to muscles innervated by the lumbosacral nerve roots. Surgical treatment of lumbar stenosis may consist of decompressive laminectomy (see clinical correlation [blue] box "Laminectomy," in this chapter). When IV disc protrusion occurs in a patient with spinal stenosis (Fig. B4.5B), it further compromises a vertebral canal that is already limited, as does arthritic proliferation and ligamentous degeneration (McCormick, 2000). ▶

Normal vertebral foramen   Stenotic vertebral foramen

(A) Superior views

IV disc

Spinous
process

(B)

Lumbar myelogram   CT scan

Figure B4.5 Lumbar spinal stenosis. A. Normal and stenotic vertebral foramina are compared. **B.** The lumbar myelogram and CT scan demonstrate a high-grade stenosis caused by the IV disc bulging at the L4–L5 space.⊕

Sacrum

The large, triangular, wedged-shaped **sacrum** is usually composed of five fused sacral vertebrae in adults (Fig. 4.5). It is located between the hip bones and forms the roof and posterosuperior wall of the posterior pelvic cavity. The triangular shape of the sacrum results from the rapid decrease in the size of the lateral masses of the sacral vertebrae during development. The inferior half of the sacrum is not weight bearing; therefore, its bulk is diminished considerably. The sacrum (L. sacred or holy bone) provides strength and stability to the pelvis and transmits the weight of the body to the pelvic girdle, the bony ring formed by the hip bones and sacrum, to which the lower limbs are attached.

The **sacral canal** is the continuation of the vertebral canal in the sacrum (Fig. 4.5C). It contains the bundle of spinal nerve roots arising inferior to the L1 vertebra, known as the *cauda equina* (L. horse tail), that descend past the termination of the spinal cord. On the pelvic and posterior surfaces of the sacrum between its vertebral components are typically four pairs of **sacral foramina** for the exit of the posterior and anterior rami of the spinal nerves (Fig. 4.5A & B). The anterior (pelvic) sacral foramina are larger than the posterior (dorsal) ones.

The **base of the sacrum** is formed by the superior surface of the S1 vertebra. Its superior articular processes articulate with the inferior articular processes of the L5 vertebra. The anterior projecting edge of the body of the S1 vertebra is the **sacral promontory** (L. mountain ridge), an important obstetrical landmark (see Chapter 3). The **apex of the sacrum**, its

Table 4.3. Lumbar Vertebrae

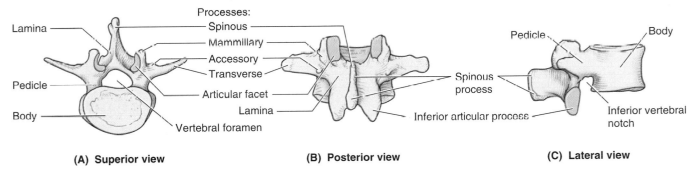

(A) Superior view   (B) Posterior view   (C) Lateral view

Superior articular process of vertebra below

Part	Characteristics
Body	Massive; kidney shaped when viewed superiorly
Vertebral foramen	Triangular; larger than in thoracic vertebrae and smaller than in cervical vertebrae
Transverse processes	Long and slender; accessory process on posterior surface of base of each process
Articular processes	Superior facets directed posteromedially (or medially); inferior facets directed anterolaterally (or laterally); mammillary process on posterior surface of each superior articular process
Spinous processes	Short and sturdy; thick, broad, and hatchet shaped

tapering inferior end, has an oval facet for articulation with the coccyx.

The sacrum supports the vertebral column and forms the posterior part of the bony pelvis. The sacrum is tilted so that it articulates with the L5 vertebra at the *lumbosacral angle* (Fig. 4.1*D*), which varies from 130° to 160°. The sacrum is often wider in proportion to length in the female than in the male, but the body of the S1 vertebra is usually larger in males.

The **pelvic surface of the sacrum** is smooth and concave (Fig. 4.5*A*). Four transverse lines on this surface of sacra from adults indicate where fusion of the sacral vertebrae occurred. During childhood, the individual sacral vertebrae are connected by hyaline cartilage and separated by IV discs. Fusion of the sacral vertebrae starts after age 20; however, most of the IV discs remain unossified up to or beyond middle life (Williams et al., 1995).

The **dorsal surface of the sacrum** is rough, convex, and marked by five prominent longitudinal ridges (Fig. 4.5*B*). The central ridge, the **median sacral crest**, represents the fused

rudimentary spinous processes of the superior three or four sacral vertebra; S5 has no spinous process. The **intermediate sacral crests** represent the fused articular processes, and the **lateral sacral crests** are the tips of the transverse processes of the fused sacral vertebrae. The clinically important features of the dorsal surface of the sacrum are the inverted U-shaped sacral hiatus and the sacral cornua (L. horns). The **sacral hiatus** results from the absence of the laminae and spinous process of S5 and sometimes S4. The sacral hiatus leads into the sacral canal. Its depth varies, depending on how much of the spinous process and laminae of S4 are present. The **sacral cornua**, representing the inferior articular processes of S5 vertebra, project inferiorly on each side of the sacral hiatus and are a helpful guide to its location.

The superior part of the **lateral surface of the sacrum** looks somewhat like an auricle (L. external ear, dim. of *auris*, ear); because of its shape, this area is called the **auricular surface** (Fig. 4.5*B* & *C*). It is the site of the synovial part of the sacroiliac joint between the sacrum and ilium. During life, the auricular surface is covered with hyaline cartilage.

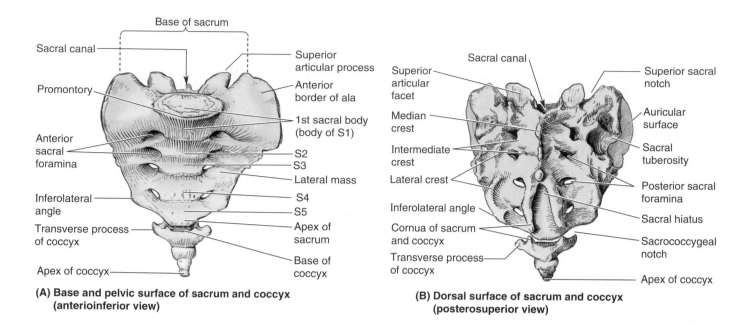

(A) Base and pelvic surface of sacrum and coccyx (anterioinferior view)

(B) Dorsal surface of sacrum and coccyx (posterosuperior view)

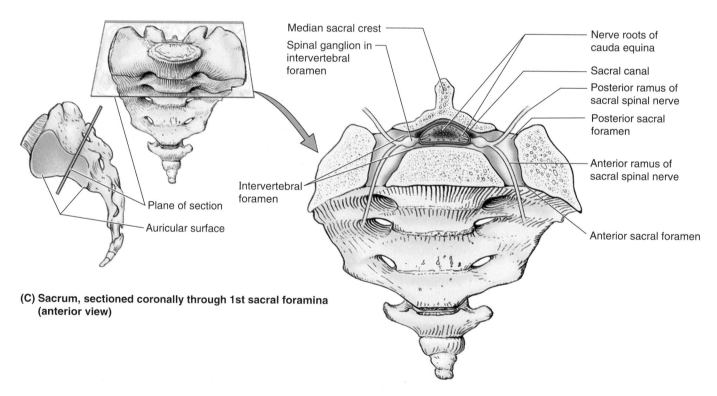

(C) Sacrum, sectioned coronally through 1st sacral foramina (anterior view)

Figure 4.5. Sacrum and coccyx. A. The base of the adult sacrum is the anterosuperior surface of the sacrum (i.e., the aspect of the sacrum opposite its apex). The base includes the articular surface of vertebra S1 (the anterior margin of which forms the sacral promontory), the sacral canal (the inferior part of the vertebral canal), and the right and left alae. Only the first of the four coccygeal vertebrae has transverse processes. **B.** The absence of the S4 and S5 spinous processes has resulted in the formation of a large sacral hiatus. The cornua, or horns, of the sacrum and coccyx are palpable clinical landmarks. **C.** Lateral and anterior orientation drawings of the sacrum in its anatomical position demonstrate the essentially frontal or coronal plane and level at which the sacrum has been sectioned to reveal the sacral canal containing the cauda equina. Spinal ganglia lie within the IV foramina, as they do at superior vertebral levels. However, the sacral posterior and anterior rami of the spinal nerves exit via posterior and anterior (pelvic) sacral foramina, respectively. The lateral orientation drawing demonstrates the auricular surface that joins the ilium to form the synovial part of the sacroiliac joint. In the anatomical position, the S1–S3 vertebrae lie in an essentially transverse plane, forming a roof for the pelvic cavity.

Caudal Epidural Anesthesia

In living persons, the sacral hiatus is closed by the membranous **sacrococcygeal ligament,** which is pierced by the *terminal filum* (a connective tissue strand extending from the tip of the spinal cord to the coccyx). Deep (superior) to the ligament, the epidural space of the sacral canal is filled with fatty connective tissue (Fig. B4.6*A*). In **caudal epidural anesthesia** or *caudal analgesia,* a local anesthetic agent is injected into the fat of the sacral canal that surrounds the proximal portions of the sacral nerves. This can be accomplished by several routes, including the sacral hiatus (Fig. B4.6*B* & *C*). Because the sacral hiatus is located between

the sacral cornua and inferior to the S4 spinous process or median sacral crest, these palpable bony landmarks are important for locating the hiatus (Fig. B4.6*A*). The anesthetic solution spreads superiorly and extradurally, where it acts on the S2–Co spinal nerves of the cauda equina. The height to which the anesthetic ascends is controlled by the amount injected and the position of the patient. Sensation is lost inferior to the epidural block. Anesthetic agents can also be injected through the posterior sacral foramina into the sacral canal around the spinal nerve roots (**transsacral epidural anesthesia**) (Fig. B4.6*B*). The role of epidural anesthesia during childbirth and the areas anesthetized are discussed in Chapter 3. ▶

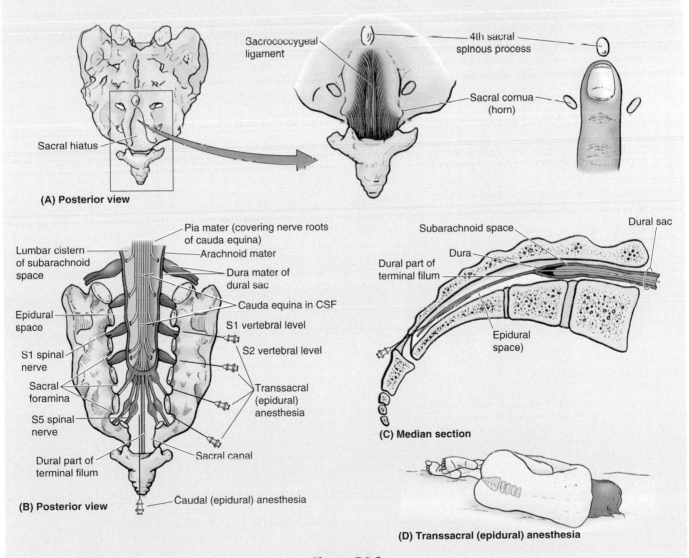

(A) Posterior view

Sacrococcygeal ligament

4th sacral spinous process

Sacral cornua (horn)

Sacral hiatus

Pia mater (covering nerve roots of cauda equina)

Lumbar cistern of subarachnoid space

Arachnoid mater

Dura mater of dural sac

Cauda equina in CSF

Epidural space

S1 vertebral level

S2 vertebral level

S1 spinal nerve

Sacral foramina

Transsacral (epidural) anesthesia

S5 spinal nerve

Dural part of terminal filum

Sacral canal

(B) Posterior view   Caudal (epidural) anesthesia

Subarachnoid space

Dural sac

Dura

Dural part of terminal filum

Epidural space)

(C) Median section

(D) Transsacral (epidural) anesthesia

Figure B4.6

Abnormal Fusion of Vertebrae

In approximately 5% of people, L5 is partly or completely incorporated into the sacrum—conditions known as **hemisacralization** and **sacralization of the L5 vertebra** (Fig. B4.7*A*), respectively. In others, S1 is more or less separated from the sacrum and is partly or completely fused with L5 vertebra, which is called **lumbarization of the S1 vertebra** (Fig. B4.7*B*). When L5 is sacralized, the L5–S1 level is strong and the L4–L5 level degenerates, often producing painful symptoms. ⊕

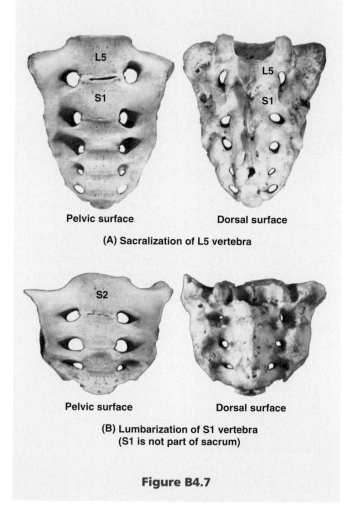

Pelvic surface   **Dorsal surface**

(A) Sacralization of L5 vertebra

Pelvic surface   **Dorsal surface**

**(B) Lumbarization of S1 vertebra
(S1 is not part of sacrum)**

Figure B4.7

Coccyx

The **coccyx** (tail bone) is a small triangular bone that is usually formed by fusion of the four rudimentary coccygeal vertebrae, although in some people, there may be one less or one more (Fig. 4.5). The coccygeal vertebra 1 (Co1) may be separate. The coccyx is the remnant of the skeleton of the embryonic tail-like caudal eminence, which is present in human embryos from the end of the 4th week until the beginning of the 8th week (Moore and Persaud, 2003). The pelvic surface of the coccyx is concave and relatively smooth, and the posterior surface has rudimentary articular processes. Co1 is the largest and broadest of all the coccygeal vertebrae. Its short transverse processes are connected to the sacrum, and its rudimentary articular processes form **coccygeal cornua**, which articulate with the sacral cornua. The last three coccygeal vertebrae often fuse during middle life, forming a beak-like coccyx; this accounts for its name (G. *coccyx,* cuckoo). With increasing age, Co1 often fuses with the sacrum, and the remaining coccygeal vertebrae usually fuse to form a single bone. The coccyx does not participate with the other vertebrae in support of the body weight when standing; however, when sitting it may flex anteriorly somewhat, indicating that it is receiving some weight. The coccyx provides attachments for parts of the gluteus maximus and coccygeus muscles and the *anococcygeal ligament,* the median fibrous intersection of the pubococcygeus muscles (see Chapter 3).

Injury of the Coccyx

An abrupt fall onto the lower back may cause a painful subperiosteal bruising or fracture of the coccyx, or a fracture–dislocation of the sacrococcygeal joint. Displacement is common, and surgical removal of the fractured bone may be required to relieve pain. An especially difficult childbirth occasionally injures the mother's coccyx. A troublesome syndrome, *coccygodynia,* often follows coccygeal trauma; pain relief is commonly difficult. ⊕

THE BOTTOM LINE: The chief regional characteristics of vertebrae are (1) transverse foramina for cervical vertebrae, (2) costal facets for thoracic vertebrae, (3) the absence of transverse foramina and costal facets for lumbar vertebrae, (4) the fusion of adjacent sacral vertebrae, and (5) the rudimentary nature of coccygeal vertebrae.

Ossification of the Vertebrae

Vertebrae begin to develop during the embryonic period as mesenchymal condensations around the notochord (Moore and Persaud, 2003). Later, these mesenchymal bone models chondrify and cartilaginous vertebrae form. Typically, vertebrae begin to ossify toward the end of the embryonic period (8th week), with three **primary ossification centers** developing in each cartilaginous vertebra: an endochondral *centrum,* which will eventually constitute most of the body of the vertebra, and two perichondral centers, one in each half of the **neural arch** (Fig. 4.6*A–I* & *M*). Ossification continues throughout the fetal period. At birth, each typical vertebra and the superiormost sacral vertebrae consists of three bony parts united by hyaline cartilage. The inferior sacral vertebrae and all the coccygeal vertebrae are still entirely cartilaginous; they ossify during infancy. The halves of the neural arches articulate at **neurocentral joints,** which are primary cartilaginous joints (Fig. 4.6*G*). The halves of the neural/vertebral arch begin to fuse with each other posterior to the vertebral canal during the 1st year, beginning in the lumbar region and then in the thoracic and cervical regions. The neural arches begin fusing with the centra in the upper cervical region around the end of the 3rd year, but usually the process is not completed in the lower lumbar region until after the 6th year.

Five **secondary ossification centers** develop during puberty in each typical vertebra: one at the tip of the spinous process; one at the tip of each transverse process; and two anular epiphyses (ring epiphyses), one on the superior and one on the inferior edges of each vertebral body (i.e., around the margins of the superior and inferior surfaces of the vertebral body) (Fig. 4.6*F* & *I–L*). The hyaline **anular epiphyses,** to which the IV discs attach, are sometimes referred to as *epiphysial growth plates* and form the zone from which the vertebral body grows in height (see "Cartilage and Bones" in the Introduction). When growth ceases early in the adult period, the epiphyses usually unite with the vertebral body. This union results in the characteristic smooth raised margin, the *epiphysial rim,* around the edges of the superior and inferior surfaces of the body of the adult vertebra (Figs. 4.2*B* and 4.3). All secondary ossification centers have usually united with the vertebrae by age 25; however, the ages at which specific unions are made vary.

Exceptions to the typical pattern of ossification occur in vertebrae C1, C2, and C7 (Fig. 4.6*A–C*) and in the sacrum (Fig. 4.6*M* & *N*) and coccyx. For example, 56–58 primary and secondary centers of ossification have been described in the sacrum.

In addition, at all levels, primordial "ribs" (**costal elements**) appear in association with the secondary ossification centers of the transverse processes (**transverse elements**). The costal elements normally develop into ribs only in the thoracic region; they become part of the transverse process or its equivalent at other levels.

In the cervical region, the costal element normally remains diminutive as part of the transverse process. *Transverse foramina* develop as gaps between the two lateral ossification centers, medial to a linking *costotransverse bar,* which forms the lateral boundary of the foramina (Fig. 4.6*A–F*). Also as a result of the cervical transverse processes being formed from the two developmental elements, the transverse processes of cervical vertebrae end laterally in an

anterior tubercle (from the costal element) and a *posterior tubercle* (from the transverse element). The atypical morphology of vertebrae C1 and C2 is also established during development. The centrum of C1 becomes fused to that of C2 and loses its peripheral connection to the remainder of C1, thus forming the *dens* (Fig. 4.6*C*). Since these first two centra are fused and are now part of C2, no IV disc is formed between C1 and C2 to connect them together. The part of the body that remains with C1 is represented by the *anterior arch* and *tubercle of C1.*

In the thoracic region, the costal elements separate from the developing vertebrae and elongate into ribs, and the transverse elements alone form the transverse processes (Fig. 4.6*I*).

All but the base of the transverse processes of the lumbar vertebrae develop from the costal element (Fig. 4.6*J*); this projecting bar of the mature bone is therefore called the **costal process.** The transverse elements of the lumbar vertebrae form the *mammillary processes.*

The ala and auricular surfaces of the sacrum are formed by the fusion of the transverse and costal elements. (For more information about the ossification of vertebrae, see Williams et al., 1995.)

Cervical Ribs

A relatively common anomaly is a *cervical rib.* In 1–2% of people, the developmental costal element of C7, which normally becomes a small part of the transverse process that lies anterior to the transverse foramen (Fig. 4.6*F*), becomes abnormally enlarged. This structure may vary in size from a small protuberance to a complete rib that occurs bilaterally about 60% of the time. The supernumerary (extra) rib or a fibrous connection extending from its tip to the first thoracic rib may elevate and place pressure on structures that emerge from the superior thoracic aperture: notably the subclavian artery or inferior trunk of the brachial plexus and may cause *thoracic outlet syndrome* (see clinical correlation [blue] box "Supernumerary Ribs," in Chapter 1).

Effect of Aging on Vertebrae

Between birth and age 5, the body of a typical lumbar vertebra increases in height threefold (from 5–6 mm to 15–18 mm), and between ages 5 and 13, it increases another 45–50%. Longitudinal growth continues throughout adolescence, but the rate decreases and is completed between ages 18 and 25. During middle and older age, there is an overall decrease in bone density and strength, particularly centrally within the vertebral body. Consequently, the articular surfaces gradually bow inward, so that both the superior and inferior ▶

surfaces of the vertebrae become increasingly concave (Fig. B4.8*A*) and the IV discs become increasingly convex. The bone loss and consequent change in shape of the vertebral bodies may account in part for the slight loss in height that occurs with aging.

The development of these concavities may cause an apparent narrowing of the intervertebral "space" on radiographs based on the distance between the margins of the vertebral bodies; however, this should not be interpreted as a loss of IV disc thickness. Aging of the IV discs combined with the changing shape of the vertebrae results in an increase in compressive forces at the periphery of the vertebral bodies, where the discs attach. In response, osteophytes (bony spurs) commonly develop around the margins of the vertebral body (along the attachments of the fibers outer part of the disc), especially anteriorly and posteriorly (Fig. B4.8*B*). Similarly, as altered mechanics place greater stresses on the zygapophysial joints, osteophytes develop along the attachments of the joint capsules and accessory ligaments, especially those of the superior articular process, whereas extensions of the articular cartilage ("wraparound bumpers") develop around the articular facets of the inferior processes. This bony or cartilaginous growth during advanced age has traditionally been viewed as a disease process (*spondylosis* in the case of the vertebral bodies, *osteoarthrosis* in the case of the zygapophysial joints), but it may be more realistic to view it as an expected morphological change with age, representing *normal anatomy* for a particular age range.

Correlation of these findings with pain is often difficult: Some patients with these manifestations present with pain,

others demonstrate the same age-related changes but have no pain, and still others exhibit little morphological change but complain of the same types of pain as those with evident change. In view of this and the typical occurrence of these findings, some have suggested that consideration of such age-related changes as pathological processes is not justified (Bogduk, 1997).

Anomalies of the Vertebrae

Sometimes the epiphysis of a transverse process fails to fuse. Caution must be exercised so that a persistent epiphysis is not mistaken for a vertebral fracture in a radiograph or CT scan.

A common congenital anomaly of the vertebral column is **spina bifida occulta,** in which the laminae (neural arches) of L5 and/or S1 fail to develop normally and fuse posterior to the vertebral canal. This bony defect, present in up to 24% of the population (Greer, 2000), usually occurs in the vertebral arch of L5 and/or S1. The defect is concealed by the overlying skin, but its location is often indicated by a tuft of hair (Moore and Persaud, 2003). Most people with spina bifida occulta have no back problems. When examining a newborn, adjacent vertebrae should be palpated in sequence to be certain the vertebral arches are intact and continuous from the cervical to the sacral regions.

In severe types of spina bifida, **spina bifida cystica,** one or more vertebral arches may fail to develop completely. Spina bifida cystica is associated with herniation of the meninges (*meningocele,* a spina bifida associated with ▶

(A) Medial view of right half of lumbar vertebra   **(B) Left anterior superior oblique view**   ✳ = osteophytes

Figure B4.8. Effects of aging on vertebrae.

a meningeal cyst) and/or the spinal cord (*meningomyelo-cele*) (Fig. B4.9). Neurological symptoms are usually present in severe cases of meningomyelocele (e.g., paralysis of the limbs and disturbances in bladder and bowel control). Severe forms of spina bifida result from **neural tube defects**, such as the defective closure of the neural tube during the 4th week of embryonic development (Moore and Persaud, 2003). ☻

Figure B4.9. Posterior view of spina bifida cystica.

Variations in the Vertebrae

Most people have 33 vertebrae, but developmental errors may result in 32 or 34 vertebrae. Estimates of the frequency of abnormal numbers of vertebrae superior to the sacrum (the normal number is 24) range between 5% and 12%. Variations in vertebrae are affected by race, sex, and developmental factors (genetic and environmental). An increased number of vertebrae occurs more often in males and a reduced number occurs more frequently in females. Some races show more variation in the number of vertebrae. Variations in the number of vertebrae may be clinically important: An increased length of the presacral region of the vertebral column increases the strain on the inferior part of the lumbar region of the column owing to the increased leverage. However, most numerical variations are detected incidentally during diagnostic medical imaging studies being performed for other reasons and during dissections and autopsies of persons with no history of back problems.

Caution is necessary, however, when describing an injury (e.g., when reporting the site of a vertebral fracture). When counting the vertebrae, begin at the base of the neck. *The number of cervical vertebrae (seven) is remarkably constant* (and not just in humans, but among mammals—even giraffes and snakes have seven cervical vertebrae!). When considering a numerical variation, the thoracic and lumbar regions must be considered together because some people have more than five lumbar vertebrae and a compensatory decrease in the number of thoracic vertebrae (O'Rahilly, 1986).

Variations in vertebrae also involve the relationship between the vertebrae and ribs, and the number of vertebrae that fuse to form the sacrum (Fig. 4.7). The relationship of presacral vertebrae to ribs and/or sacrum may occur higher (*cranial shift*) or lower (*caudal shift*) than normal. Note, however, that a C7 vertebra articulating with a rudimentary cervical rib(s) is still considered a cervical vertebra. The same is true for lumbar vertebrae and lumbar ribs. Likewise, an L5 vertebra fused to the sacrum is referred to as a "sacralized 5th lumbar vertebrae" (see clinical correlation [blue] box "Abnormal Fusion of Vertebrae," in this chapter).

THE BOTTOM LINE: Vertebrae typically ossify from three primary ossification centers within a cartilaginous model: a centrum that will form most of the body and a center in each half of the neural arch. Thus by the time of birth, most vertebrae consist of three bony parts united by hyaline cartilage. Fusion occurs during the first 6 years in a centrifugal pattern from the lumbar region. During puberty, five secondary ossification centers appear: three related to the spinous and transverse processes, and two anular epiphyses around the superior and inferior margins of the vertebral body. Costal elements formed in association with the ossification center of the transverse process usually form ribs only in the thoracic region. They form components of the transverse processes or their equivalents in other regions. Knowledge of the pattern of ossification of the vertebrae allows understanding of the normal structure of typical and atypical vertebrae, as well as variations and malformations.

Vertebral Column

The **vertebral column** is an aggregate structure, normally made up of all 33 vertebrae and the components that unite them into a single structural, functional entity—the "axis" of the axial skeleton. Because it provides the semirigid, central "core" about which movements of the trunk occur, "soft" or hollow structures that run a longitudinal course are subject to damage or kinking (e.g., the spinal cord, descending aorta, venae cavae, thoracic duct, and esophagus). Thus they lie in close proximity to the vertebral axis, where they receive its semirigid support and torsional stresses on them are minimized.

Joints of the Vertebral Column

The joints of the vertebral column include the:

- Joints of the vertebral bodies.
- Joints of the vertebral arches.
- Craniovertebral (atlantoaxial and atlanto-occipital) joints.
- Costovertebral joints (see Chapter 1).
- Sacroiliac joints (see Chapter 3).

(A) Atlas (inferior view)
Transverse element
Costal element
1° center of neural arch

(B) Axis (inferior view)
1° center of neural arch
Transverse element
Centrum of C2

(C) Anterior view of axis
Centrum of C1
Centrum of C2
Costal element

(D) Primary ossification centers of typical cervical vertebra
Centrum
1° center of neural arch
Cartilage

(E) Inferior view
SC

(F) Typical cervical vertebra (inferior view)
Transverse element
Costal element
1° center of neural arch
Costo-transverse bar

(G) Primary ossification centers of typical thoracic vertebra
Cartilage
Vertebral arch
Neurocentral joint
Centrum
Costovertebral synchondrosis (cartilaginous union between rib and vertebra)
Costal element
Primary ossification elements

(H) Bony parts of vertebra at birth (hyaline cartilage removed)
Halves of vertebral arch
Centrum
Site of hyaline cartilage

(I) Thoracic vertebra and ribs (inferior view)
Transverse process
1° center of neural arch
Rib

(J) Lumbar vertebra (inferior view)
Costal element (costal process of developed vertebra)
1° center of neural arch
Centrum

(K) Left superior view of lumbar vertebra
Superior anular epiphysis
Inferior anular epiphysis

(L) Anterior view of lumbar vertebra
Superior anular epiphysis
Centrum
Inferior anular epiphysis

(M) Sacrum (superior view)
Transverse element
Centrum

Key
- ■ Primary ossification center
- ■ Secondary ossification center
- ■ Costal element
- □ Hyaline cartilage

(N) Anterior view of sacrum

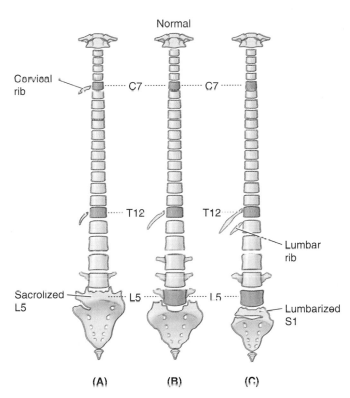

Figure 4.7. **Variations in vertebrae and their relationship to ribs. A.** A "cranial shift" is demonstrated, in which there are 13 ribs, including a cervical rib articulating with vertebra C7 and a diminished 12th rib articulating with vertebra T12. Vertebra L5 is shown partially incorporated into the sacrum, but such "sacralization" can also be complete. The lowest sacral segment (S5) is partially segmented. **B.** The common arrangement of the vertebrae and the position of 1st and 12th ribs are shown. **C.** A "caudal shift" is shown, in which the 12th rib is increased in size, and there is a small lumbar rib. The transverse process of vertebra L4 is increased in size, whereas those of vertebra L5 are greatly reduced. The first sacral segment is shown partially separated from the rest of the sacrum, but such "lumbarization" can also be complete. The 1st coccygeal segment is incorporated into the sacrum—that is, it is "sacralized."

Joints of the Vertebral Bodies

The joints of the vertebral bodies are *symphyses* (*secondary cartilaginous joints*) designed for weight bearing and strength. The articulating surfaces of adjacent vertebrae are connected by IV discs and ligaments (Fig. 4.8). The IV discs provide strong attachments between the vertebral bodies, uniting them into a continuous semirigid column and forming the inferior half of the anterior border of the IV foramen. In aggregate, the discs account for 20–25% of the length (height) of the vertebral column (Fig. 4.1). As well as permitting movement between adjacent vertebrae, their resilient deformability allows them to serve as shock absorbers. Each IV disc consists of an *anulus fibrosus*, an outer fibrous part, composed of

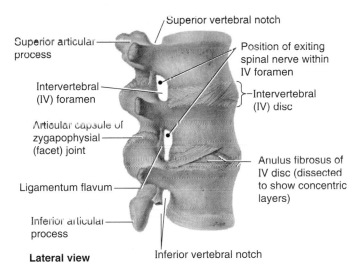

Lateral view

Figure 4.8 **Lumbar vertebrae and IV discs.** This view of the superior lumbar region shows the structure of the anuli fibrosi of the discs and the structures involved in formation of IV foramina. The disc forms the inferior half of the anterior boundary of an IV foramen (except in the cervical region). Thus herniation of the disc will not affect the spinal nerve exiting from the superior bony part of that foramen.

Figure 4.6. **Ossification of vertebrae.** Typical vertebrae develop from three primary ossification centers that are present at birth and five secondary ossifications centers that appear at puberty. Costal elements are usually incorporated into the transverse processes, except in the thoracic region where they become ribs. **A.** Vertebra C1 (atlas) lacks a centrum. **B and C.** Vertebra C2 (axis) has two centra, one of which forms most of the dens. **D–F.** The development of "typical" cervical vertebrae is shown, including (**D**) the primary ossification centers within the hyaline cartilage, (**E**) a CT scan of the vertebra shown in part **D** (*SC,* spinal cord), and (**F**) the primary and secondary ossification centers. **G–I.** The development of thoracic vertebrae is shown, including (**G**) the three primary ossification centers in a cartilaginous vertebra of a 7-week-old embryo (observe the joints present at this stage), (**H**) the bony parts of a thoracic vertebra after skeletonization (cartilage removed), and (**I**) the primary and secondary ossification centers (with ribs developed from costal elements). **J–L.** The development of the lumbar vertebrae is shown, including (**J**) the primary and secondary ossification centers, (**K**) the anular epiphyses separated from the body, and (**L**) the anular epiphyses in place. **M and N.** The development of the sacrum is shown. Note that the ossification and fusion of sacral vertebrae may not be completed until age 35.

concentric lamellae of fibrocartilage, and a gelatinous central mass, called the *nucleus pulposus.*

The **anulus fibrosus** is a fibrous ring consisting of concentric lamellae of fibrocartilage forming the circumference of the IV disc (Figs. 4.8 & 4.9*A*). The anuli insert into the smooth, rounded *epiphysial rims* on the articular surfaces of the vertebral bodies formed by the fused *anular epiphyses* (Fig. 4.2*B*). The fibers forming each lamella run obliquely from one vertebra to another; the fibers of one lamella typically run at right angles to those of the adjacent ones. This arrangement, allows some movement between adjacent vertebrae, while providing a strong bond between them.

The **nucleus pulposus** (L. *pulpa,* fleshy) is the central core of the IV disc (Fig. 4.9*A*). At birth, these pulpy nuclei are about 88% water and are initially more cartilaginous than fibrous. Their semifluid nature is responsible for much of the flexibility and resilience of the IV disc and of the vertebral column as a whole. Vertical forces deform the discs, which thus serve as shock absorbers. The pulpy nuclei become broader when compressed and thinner when tensed or stretched (as when hanging or suspended) (Fig. 4.9*C*). Compression and tension occur simultaneously in the same disc during anterior and lateral flexion and extension of the vertebral column (Fig. 4.9*D*). During these movements, as well as during rotation, the turgid nucleus acts as a semifluid fulcrum. Because the lamellae of the anulus fibrosus are thinner and less numerous posteriorly than they are anteriorly or laterally, the nucleus pulposus is not centered in the disc but is more posteriorly placed. The nucleus pulposus is avascular; it receives its nourishment by diffusion from blood vessels at the periphery of the anulus fibrosus and vertebral body.

There is no IV disc between C1 and C2 vertebrae; the most inferior functional disc is between L5 and S1 vertebrae. The discs vary in thickness in different regions; they are thickest relative to the size of the bodies they connect in the cervical and lumbar regions (and absolutely thickest in the latter) and thinnest in the superior thoracic region. Their relative thickness is clearly related to the range of movement, and their varying shapes produce the secondary curvatures of the vertebral column. The discs are thicker anteriorly in the cervical and lumbar regions, and their thickness is most uniform in the thoracic region.

Uncovertebral "joints" (of Luschka) are located between the unci of the bodies of C3–C6 vertebrae and the beveled inferolateral surfaces of the vertebral bodies superior to them (Fig. 4.10). The joints are at the lateral and posterolateral margins of the IV discs. The articulating surfaces of these joint-like structures are covered with cartilage moistened by fluid contained within an interposed potential space, or "capsule." They are considered synovial joints by some; others consider them to be degenerative spaces (fissures) in the discs occupied

| (A) Anterosuperior view, vertebral column transversely sectioned through IV disc | (B) Lateral view of disc when recumbent | (C) Lateral view of disc when erect (weight bearing) | (D) Anterior view during lateral flexion |

Figure 4.9. Structure and function of IV discs. A. The disc consists of a nucleus pulposus and an anulus fibrosus. The superficial layers of the anulus have been cut and spread apart to show the direction of the fibers. Note that the combined thickness of the rings of the anulus is diminished posteriorly—that is, the anulus is thinner posteriorly. **B.** The fibrogelatinous nucleus pulposus occupies the center of the disc and acts as a cushion and shock-absorbing mechanism. **C.** The pulpy nucleus flattens and the anulus bulges when weight is applied, as occurs during standing and more so during lifting. **D.** During flexion and extension movements, the nucleus pulposus serves as a fulcrum. The anulus is simultaneously placed under compression on one side and tension on the other.

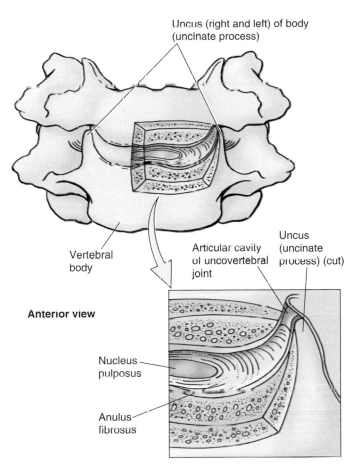

Figure 4.10. Uncovertebral joints. These small, synovial joint-like structures are between the unci of the bodies of the lower vertebrae and the beveled surfaces of the vertebral bodies superior to them. These joints are at the posterolateral margins of the IV discs.

vessels between the ligament and the bony surface. This ligament weakly resists hyperflexion of the vertebral column and helps prevent or redirect posterior herniation of the nucleus pulposus. It is well provided with nociceptive (pain) nerve endings.

Anterior view

Figure 4.11. Relationship of ligaments to vertebrae and IV discs. The lower thoracic (T9–T12) and upper lumbar (L1–L2) vertebrae, with associated discs and ligaments, are shown. The pedicles of the T9–T11 vertebrae have been sawn through and their bodies and intervening discs removed to provide an anterior view of the posterior wall of the vertebral canal formed by the laminae of the vertebral arches and the ligamenta flava extending between them. Between the adjacent left or right pedicles, the inferior and superior articular processes and the zygapophysial joints between them (from which joint capsules have been removed) and the lateralmost extent of the ligamenta flava form the posterior boundaries of IV foramina. The anterior longitudinal ligament is broad, whereas the posterior longitudinal ligament is narrow. Although thickest on the anterior aspect of the vertebral bodies (and often only this thickest part is illustrated), the anterior longitudinal ligament covers both the anterior and the lateral aspects of the bodies to the IV foramen.

by extracellular fluid. The uncovertebral joints are frequent sites of spur formation, which may cause neck pain.

The **anterior longitudinal ligament** is a strong, broad fibrous band that covers and connects the anterolateral aspects of the vertebral bodies and IV discs (Fig. 4.11). The ligament extends from the pelvic surface of the sacrum to the anterior tubercle of vertebra C1 and the occipital bone anterior to the foramen magnum. This ligament prevents hyperextension of the vertebral column, maintaining stability of the joints between the vertebral bodies. The anterior longitudinal ligament is the only ligament that limits extension, all other IV ligaments limit forms of flexion.

The **posterior longitudinal ligament** is a much narrower, somewhat weaker band than the anterior longitudinal ligament (Fig. 4.11). The posterior longitudinal ligament runs within the vertebral canal along the posterior aspect of the vertebral bodies. It is attached mainly to the IV discs and less so to the posterior aspects of the vertebral bodies from C2 to the sacrum, often bridging fat and

Aging of the Intervertebral Discs

With age, the nuclei pulposi dehydrate and lose elastin and proteoglycans while gaining collagen. As a result, the IV discs lose their turgor, becoming stiffer and more resistant to deformation. As the nucleus dehydrates and gains collagen, the two parts of the disc appear to merge as the distinction between them becomes increasingly diminished. With advancing age, the nucleus becomes dry and granular and may disappear altogether as a distinct formation. As this occurs, the anulus fibrosis assumes an increasingly greater share of the vertical load and the stresses and strains that come with it. The lamellae of the anulus thicken with age and often develop fissures and cavities.

Previously, a loss of disc thickness (height) was usually described as typical of the aging process and said to account for loss of trunk stature. Although the margins of adjacent vertebral bodies may approach more closely as the superior and inferior surfaces of the body become shallow concavities (the most probable reason for slight loss of height with aging), it has been shown that the intervertebral bodies *increase* in size with age. Not only do they become increasing convex but, between the ages of 20 and 70, their anteroposterior (AP) diameter increases about 10% in females and 2% in males, while thickness (height) increases centrally about 10% in both sexes. Thus disc height (as measured in the center of the disc) is normally maintained with aging; overt or marked cases of disc narrowing, especially when it is greater than that of more superiorly located discs, suggests pathology, not normal aging (Bogduk, 1997).

Herniation of the Nucleus Pulposus

Herniation or protrusion of the gelatinous nucleus pulposus into or through the anulus fibrosus is a well-recognized cause of low back and lower limb pain (Fig. B4.10*A* & *D*). The IV discs in young persons are strong—usually so strong that the vertebrae often fracture during a fall before the discs rupture. Furthermore, the water content of their nuclei pulposi is high (approaching 90%), giving them great turgor (fullness). However, violent hyperflexion of the vertebral column may rupture an IV disc and fracture the adjacent vertebral bodies. Flexion of the vertebral column produces compression anteriorly and stretching or tension posteriorly, squeezing the nucleus pulposus further posteriorly toward the thinnest part of the anulus fibrosus. If the anulus fibrosus has degenerated, the nucleus pulposus may herniate into the vertebral canal and compress the spinal cord (Fig. B4.10*B* & *C*) or the nerve roots of the cauda equina (Fig. B4.10*A* & *D*). A herniated IV disc is inappropriately called a "slipped disc" by some people. Sports writers often call the injury a "ruptured disc."

Herniations of the nucleus pulposus usually extend posterolaterally, where the anulus fibrosus is relatively thin and does not receive support from either the posterior or the anterior longitudinal ligaments. A posterolateral herniated IV disc is more likely to be symptomatic because of the proximity of the spinal nerve roots. The *localized back pain* of a herniated disc, which is usually acute, results from pressure on the longitudinal ligaments and periphery of the anulus fibrosus and from local inflammation caused by chemical irritation by substances from the ruptured nucleus pulposus. *Chronic pain* resulting from compression of the spinal nerve roots by the herniated disc is referred to the area (dermatome) supplied by that nerve. Because the IV discs are largest in the lumbar and lumbosacral regions, where movements are consequently greater, posterolateral herniations of the nucleus pulposus are most common here. Approximately 95% of lumbar disc protrusions occur at the L4–L5 or L5–S1 levels. The marked decrease in the radiographic intervertebral space (i.e., in disc height) that may occur as a result of acute herniation of a nucleus may also result in narrowing of the IV foramina, perhaps exacerbating the compression of the spinal nerve roots, especially if hypertrophy of the surrounding bone has also occurred. Because the nucleus pulposus becomes increasingly dehydrated and fibrous or even granular or solid with aging, a diagnosis of acute herniation in a patient of advanced years should be regarded with suspicion. Rather, it is likely that the nerve roots are being compressed by increased ossification of the IV foramen as they exit.

Lumbago, an acute middle and low back pain, may be caused by a mild posterolateral protrusion of a lumbar IV disc at the L5–S1 level that affects nociceptive (pain) endings in the region, such as those associated with the posterior longitudinal ligament. The clinical picture varies considerably, but pain of acute onset in the lower back is a common presenting symptom. Because muscle spasm is associated with low back pain, the lumbar region of the vertebral column becomes tense and increasingly cramped as a relative ischemia occurs, causing painful movement. With treatment, the lumbago type of back pain usually begins to fade after a few days; however, it may gradually be replaced by sciatica.

Sciatica, pain in the lower back and hip radiating down the back of the thigh into the leg, is often caused by a herniated lumbar IV disc that compresses and compromises the L5 or S1 component of the sciatic nerve. The IV foramina in the lumbar region decrease in size and the lumbar nerves increase in size, which may explain why sciatica is so common. New bone (osteophytes) deposited around the zygapophysial joints or the posterolateral margins during aging may narrow the foramina even more, causing shooting pains down the lower limbs. Any maneuver that stretches the sciatic nerve, such as flexing ▶

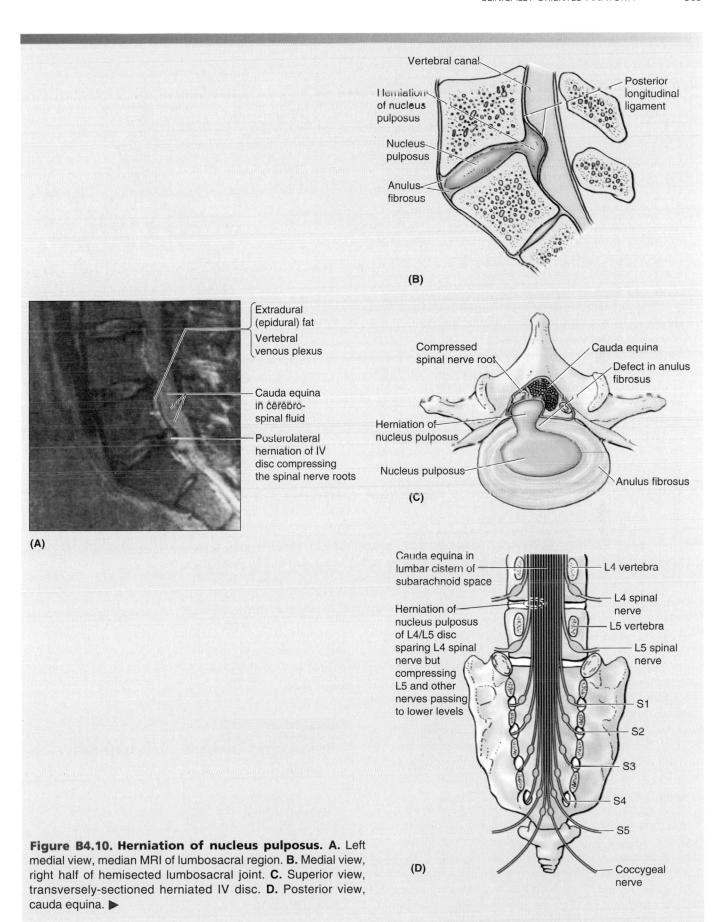

Figure B4.10. Herniation of nucleus pulposus. A. Left medial view, median MRI of lumbosacral region. **B.** Medial view, right half of hemisected lumbosacral joint. **C.** Superior view, transversely-sectioned herniated IV disc. **D.** Posterior view, cauda equina. ▶

Labels in the figure:

(B)
- Vertebral canal
- Herniation of nucleus pulposus
- Nucleus pulposus
- Anulus fibrosus
- Posterior longitudinal ligament

(A)
- Extradural (epidural) fat
- Vertebral venous plexus
- Cauda equina in cerebrospinal fluid
- Posterolateral herniation of IV disc compressing the spinal nerve roots

(C)
- Compressed spinal nerve root
- Herniation of nucleus pulposus
- Nucleus pulposus
- Cauda equina
- Defect in anulus fibrosus
- Anulus fibrosus

(D)
- Cauda equina in lumbar cistern of subarachnoid space
- Herniation of nucleus pulposus of L4/L5 disc sparing L4 spinal nerve but compressing L5 and other nerves passing to lower levels
- L4 vertebra
- L4 spinal nerve
- L5 vertebra
- L5 spinal nerve
- S1
- S2
- S3
- S4
- S5
- Coccygeal nerve

the thigh with the knee extended (Kernig maneuver), may produce or exacerbate (but in some individuals relieves) the pain caused by disc herniation.

IV discs may also be damaged by violent rotation or flexing of the vertebral column. The general rule is that when an IV disc protrudes, it usually compresses the nerve root numbered one inferior to the disc; for example, the L5 nerve is compressed by an L4–L5 IV disc herniation and the S1 nerve by a L5–S1 IV disc herniation. Recall that in the thoracic and lumbar regions the IV disc forms the inferior half of the anterior border of the IV foramen and that the superior half is formed by the bone of the body of the superior vertebra (Fig. 4.8). The spinal nerve roots descend to the IV foramen from which the spinal nerve formed by their merging will exit. The nerve that exits a given IV foramen passes through the superior bony half of the foramen and thus lies above and is not affected by a herniating disc at that level. However, the nerve roots passing to the IV foramen immediately and farther below pass directly across the area of herniation (i.e., herniation of the L4–L5 disc affects the L5 nerve root). Symptom-producing IV disc protrusions occur in the cervical region almost as often as in the lumbar region.

Chronic or sudden forcible *hyperflexion of the cervical region,* as might occur during a head-on collision or during illegal head blocking in football, for example, may rupture the IV disc posteriorly without fracturing the vertebral body (Fig. B4.11). In this region, the IV discs are centrally placed in the anterior border of the IV foramen, and a herniating disc compresses the nerve actually exiting at that level (rather than the level below as in the lumbar region). However, recall that cervical spinal nerves exit superior to

Ligament tear

Rupture of intervertebral disc C5/C6 with nucleus pulposus compressing C6 spinal nerve roots

Figure B4.11

the vertebra of the same number, so the numerical relationship of herniating disc to nerve affected is the same (e.g., the cervical IV discs most commonly ruptured are those between C5–C6 and C6–C7, compressing spinal nerve roots C6 and C7, respectively). IV disc protrusions result in pain in the neck, shoulder, arm, and hand. Any sport in which movement causes downward or twisting pressure on the neck or lower back may produce herniation of the nucleus pulposus. The most common sports involved are bowling, tennis, jogging, football, hockey, weight lifting, and gymnastics. ✛

Joints of the Vertebral Arches

The joints of the vertebral arches are the **zygapophysial joints** (often called *facet joints* for brevity). These articulations are plane synovial joints between the superior and the inferior articular processes (G. *zygapophyses*) of adjacent vertebrae (Figs. 4.9 and 4.11). Each joint is surrounded by a thin, loose **joint (articular) capsule.** Those in the cervical region are especially thin and loose, reflecting the wide range of movement (Fig. 4.12). The capsule is attached to the margins of the articular surfaces of the articular processes of adjacent vertebrae. Accessory ligaments unite the laminae, transverse processes, and spinous processes and help stabilize the joints.

The zygapophysial joints permit gliding movements between the articular processes; the shape and disposition of the articular surfaces determine the types of movement possible. The range (amount) of movement is determined by the size of the IV disc relative to that of the vertebral body. In the cervical and lumbar regions, these joints bear some weight, sharing this function with the IV discs particularly during lateral flexion. The zygapophysial joints are innervated by articular branches

that arise from the medial branches of the posterior rami of spinal nerves (Fig. 4.13). As these nerves pass posteroinferiorly, they lie in grooves on the posterior surfaces of the medial parts of the transverse processes. Each articular branch supplies two adjacent joints; therefore, each joint is supplied by two nerves.

Injury and Disease of Zygapophysial Joints

The zygapophysial joints are of clinical interest because they are close to the IV foramina through which the spinal nerves emerge from the vertebral canal. When these joints are injured or develop osteophytes during aging (*osteoarthritis*), the related spinal nerves are often affected. This causes pain along the distribution patterns of the *dermatomes* and spasm in the muscles derived from the associated *myotomes* (a myotome ▶

(A) Right lateral view

External occipital protuberance

Posterior atlanto-occipital membrane

Nuchal ligament

Ligamenta flava

Interspinous ligaments

Spinous process of C7 vertebra

Supraspinous ligament

Atlas

Axis

Articular capsule of zygapophysial joints

Anterior longitudinal ligament

(B) Right posterior oblique view

Intervertebral disc

Posterior longitudinal ligament

Pedicle (cut)

Inter-transverse ligament

Transverse process

Lateral costo-transverse ligament

Interspinous ligament

Supraspinous ligament

Figure 4.12. Joints and ligaments of vertebral column. A. The ligaments in the cervical region are shown. Superior to the prominent spinous process of C7 (vertebra prominens), the spinous processes are deeply placed and attached to an overlying nuchal ligament. **B.** The ligaments in the thoracic region are shown. The pedicles of the superior two vertebrae have been sawn through and the vertebral arches removed to reveal the posterior longitudinal ligament. Intertransverse, supraspinous, and interspinous ligaments are demonstrated in association with the vertebrae with intact vertebral arches.

consists all the muscles or parts of muscles receiving innervation from one spinal nerve).

Denervation of lumbar zygapophysial joints is a procedure historically used for treatment of back pain caused by disease of these joints. The nerves are sectioned near the joints or are destroyed by radiofrequency *percutaneous rhizolysis* (G. *rhiza*, root + G. *lysis*, dissolution). The denervation is directed at the articular branches of two adjacent posterior rami of the spinal nerves because each joint receives innervation from both the nerve exiting that level and the superjacent nerve. ○

Accessory Ligaments of the Intervertebral Joints

The laminae of adjacent vertebral arches are joined by broad, pale yellow elastic tissue called the **ligamenta flava** (L. *flavus*, yellow). These yellow ligaments extend almost vertically from the lamina above to the lamina below, those of opposite sides meeting and blending in the midline (Fig. 4.11). The ligaments bind the lamina of the adjoining vertebrae together, forming alternating sections of the posterior wall of the verte-

bral canal. The ligamenta flava are long, thin, and broad in the cervical region, thicker in the thoracic region, and thickest in the lumbar region. These ligaments resist separation of the vertebral lamina by arresting abrupt flexion of the vertebral column and thereby preventing injury to the IV discs. The strong elastic ligamenta flava help preserve the normal curvatures of the vertebral column and assist with straightening of the column after flexing.

Adjoining spinous processes are united by weak, almost membranous **interspinous ligaments** and strong fibrous supraspinous ligaments (Fig. 4.12A). The thin interspinous ligaments connect adjoining spinous processes, attaching from the root to the apex of each process. The cord-like **supraspinous ligament,** which connects the apices (tips) of the spinous processes from C7 to the sacrum, merges superiorly with the **nuchal ligament** (L. *ligamentum nuchae*), the strong, broad, median band at the back of the neck (Fr. *nuque*, back of neck) (Fig. 4.12A). Unlike the interspinous and supraspinous ligaments, the nuchal ligament is composed of thickened fibroelastic tissue, extending from the external occipital protuberance and posterior border of the foramen magnum to the spinous processes of the cervical vertebrae. Because of the shortness of the C3–C5 spinous processes, the nuchal ligament substitutes for bone in providing muscular

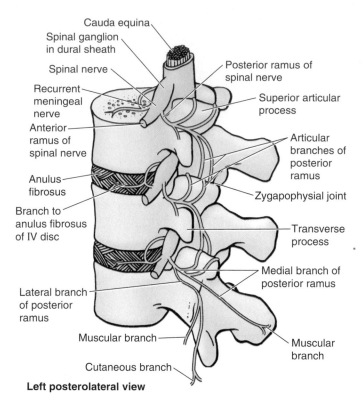

Cauda equina
Spinal ganglion in dural sheath
Spinal nerve
Recurrent meningeal nerve
Anterior ramus of spinal nerve
Anulus fibrosus
Branch to anulus fibrosus of IV disc
Lateral branch of posterior ramus
Muscular branch
Cutaneous branch
Left posterolateral view

Posterior ramus of spinal nerve
Superior articular process
Articular branches of posterior ramus
Zygapophysial joint
Transverse process
Medial branch of posterior ramus
Muscular branch

Figure 4.13. Innervation of zygapophysial joints. The posterior rami arise from the spinal nerves outside the IV foramen and divide into medial and lateral branches; the medial branch gives rise to articular branches distributed to the zygapophysial joint at that level and to the joint one level inferior to its exit. Thus, each zygapophysial joint receives articular rami from the medial branch of the posterior rami of two adjacent spinal nerves; the medial branches of both posterior rami would have to be ablated to denervate a zygapophysial joint.

attachments. The **intertransverse ligaments,** connecting adjacent transverse processes, consist of scattered fibers in the cervical region and fibrous cords in the thoracic region (Fig. 4.12B). The intertransverse ligaments in the lumbar region are thin and membranous.

THE BOTTOM LINE: Vertebrae are joined into a semirigid column by IV discs and zygapophysial joints. The relative thickness of the discs determines the degree of mobility. The disposition of the zygapophysial joints controls the type of movement between adjacent vertebrae. The anterior longitudinal ligament resists hyperextension; all other ligaments resist forms of flexion.

Craniovertebral Joints

There are two sets of craniovertebral joints, the atlanto-occipital joints. formed between the atlas (C1 vertebra) and the occipital bone of the cranium, and the atlantoaxial joints, formed between the atlas and axis (C2 vertebra) (Fig. 4.14). The Greek word *atlanto* refers to the atlas. The craniovertebral joints are synovial joints that have no IV discs. Their design gives a wider range of movement than in the rest of the vertebral column. The articulations involve the occipital condyles, atlas, and axis.

Atlanto-Occipital Joints. The articulations between the superior articular surfaces of the lateral masses of the atlas and the occipital condyles (Figs. 4.4A & B and 4.14A), the atlanto-occipital joints, permit nodding of the head, such as the neck flexion and extension occurring when indicating approval (the "yes" movement). These joints also permit side-

ways tilting of the head. The main movement is flexion, with a little lateral bending and rotation. They are synovial joints of the condyloid type and have thin, loose articular capsules. The cranium and C1 are also connected by **anterior** and **posterior atlanto-occipital membranes,** which extend from the anterior and posterior arches of C1 to the anterior and posterior margins of the foramen magnum (Figs. 4.14B and 4.15). The anterior membranes are composed of broad, densely woven fibers (especially centrally where they are continuous with the anterior longitudinal ligament); the posterior membranes are broad but relatively weak. The atlanto-occipital membranes help prevent excessive movement of these joints.

Atlantoaxial Joints. There are three atlantoaxial articulations (Fig. 4.14A–C): two (right and left) **lateral atlantoaxial joints** (between the inferior facets of the lateral masses of C1 and the superior facets of C2), and one **median atlantoaxial joint** (between the dens of C2 and the anterior arch of the atlas). The lateral atlantoaxial joints are gliding-type synovial joints, whereas the median atlantoaxial joint is a pivot joint. Movement at all three atlantoaxial joints permits the head to be turned from side to side (Fig. 4.14D), as occurs when rotating the head to indicate disapproval (the "no" movement). During this movement, the cranium and C1 rotate on C2 as a unit. During rotation of the head, the dens of C2 is the axis or pivot that is held in a socket or collar formed anteriorly by the anterior arch of the atlas and posteriorly by the *transverse ligament of the atlas* (Fig. 4.14A–C), a strong band extending between the tubercles on the medial aspects of the lateral masses of C1 vertebrae. Vertically oriented but much weaker superior and inferior **longitudinal bands** pass from the trans-

(A) Posterior view

Occipital bone

Left atlanto-occipital joint

Cruciate ligament (cut)
- Superior longitudinal band
- Transverse ligament of atlas
- Inferior longitudinal band

Tectorial membrane (cut)

Alar ligament

Articular facet of dens for transverse ligament of atlas (part of median atlanto axial joint)

Capsule of atlanto-occipital joint

Atlas (C1)

Tectorial membrane (accessory part)

Capsule of right lateral atlantoaxial joint

Posterior longitudinal ligament becoming tectorial membrane (cut)

Axis (C2)

Three atlantoaxial joints

Dens

Atlas (C1)

Median / Lateral } Atlanto-axial joints

Axis (C2)

(B) Medial view of right half of hemisected head and upper neck

Tectorial membrane

Anterior atlanto-occipital membrane

Anterior arch of atlas (C1)

Articular cavity between dens and anterior arch (median atlanto-axial joint)

Anterior atlanto-axial membrane

Becomes / Becomes

Anterior longitudinal ligament

Posterior longitudinal ligament

Dens of axis (C2)

Vertebral artery

Posterior atlanto-occipital membrane

Posterior arch of atlas (C1)

Posterior atlanto-axial membrane

Superior longitudinal band

Transverse ligament of atlas } Cruciate ligament

Inferior longitudinal band

Body of axis (C2)

Ligamentum flavum

Becomes

Figure 4.14. Craniovertebral joints and ligaments. A. Ligaments of the atlanto-occipital and atlantoaxial joints. The tectorial membrane and the right side of the cruciate ligament of the atlas have been removed to show the attachment of the right alar ligament to the dens of vertebra C2 (axis). **B.** The hemisected craniovertebral region shows the median joints and membranous continuities of the ligamenta flava and longitudinal ligaments in the craniovertebral region. **C.** The articulated atlas and axis showing that the median atlantoaxial joint is formed as the anterior arch and the transverse ligament of the atlas form a socket for the dens of the axis. **D.** During rotation of head, the cranium and atlas rotate as a unit around the pivot of the dens when the head is turned side to side (the "no" movement).

Anterior articular cavity of median atlantoaxial joint between dens and anterior arch of atlas

Anterior arch of atlas

Superior articular facet of atlas

Dens of axis

Posterior articular cavity of median atlantoaxial joint between dens and transverse ligament

Transverse ligament of atlas

Vertebral canal

Spinous process of axis

Posterior arch of atlas

(C) Superior view

Skull and atlas rotate left around pivot of dens

Head turned left

Skull and atlas rotate right around pivot of dens

Head turned right

(D) Superior views

Figure 4.14. *(Continued)*

Anterior atlanto-occipital membrane

Anterior atlantoaxial membrane

Anterior longitudinal ligament

Articular capsule

Axis

(A) Anterior view

Posterior atlanto-occipital membrane

Foramen for vertebral artery

Posterior atlantoaxial membrane

Occipital bone

Articular capsule

(B) Posterior view

Figure 4.15. Membranes of craniovertebral joints. A. Only the thicker, most anterior part of the anterior longitudinal ligament is included here to demonstrate its superior continuation as the anterior atlantoaxial membrane and anterior atlanto-occipital membrane. Laterally, the membranes blend with the articular capsules of the lateral atlantoaxial and atlanto-occipital joints. **B.** The posterior atlanto-occipital and atlantoaxial membranes span the gaps between the posterior arch of the atlas (C1) and the occipital bone (posterior margin of the foramen magnum) superiorly and the laminae of the axis (C2) inferiorly. The vertebral arteries penetrate the atlanto-occipital membrane before traversing the foramen magnum.

The **alar ligaments** extend from the sides of the dens to the lateral margins of the foramen magnum (Fig. 4.14*A*). These short, rounded cords, approximately 0.5 cm in diameter (just smaller than a pencil), attach the cranium to vertebra C1 and serve as check ligaments, preventing excessive rotation at the joints.

The **tectorial membrane** (Fig. 4.14*A* & *B*) is the strong superior continuation of the posterior longitudinal ligament across the median atlantoaxial joint through the foramen magnum to the central floor of the cranial cavity. It runs from the body of C2 to the internal surface of the occipital bone and covers the alar and transverse ligaments.

verse ligament to the occipital bone superiorly and to the body of C2 inferiorly. Together, the transverse ligament and the longitudinal bands form the **cruciate ligament** (formerly the cruciform ligament), so named because of its resemblance to a cross.

THE BOTTOM LINE: The atlanto-occipital joints enable the yes (nodding) movement of the head. The atlantoaxial joints enable the "no" (rotational) movement of the head. Alar ligaments limit rotation.

Fracture of the Dens

The transverse ligament of the atlas is stronger than the dens of the C2 vertebra. Fractures of the dens make up about 40% of axis fractures. The most common dens fracture occurs at its base—that is, at its junction with the body of the axis (Fig. B4.12*A*). Often these fractures are unstable (do not reunite) because the transverse ligament of the atlas becomes interposed between fragments (Crockard et al., 1993) and because the separated fragment (the dens) no longer has a blood supply, resulting in avascular necrosis. Almost as common are fractures of the vertebral body inferior to the base of the dens (Fig. B4.12*B–E*). This type of fracture heals more readily because the fragments retain their blood supply. Other dens fractures result from abnormal ossification patterns.

Rupture of the Transverse Ligament of the Atlas

When the transverse ligament of the atlas ruptures, the dens is set free, resulting in *atlantoaxial subluxation* or incomplete dislocation of the median atlantoaxial joint (Fig. B4.13*A*). Pathological softening of the transverse and adjacent ligaments, usually resulting from disorders of connective tissue, may also cause atlantoaxial subluxation (Bogduk and Macintosh, 1984); 20% of people with Down syndrome exhibit laxity or agenesis of this ligament. Dislocation owing to transverse ligament rupture or agenesis is more likely to cause spinal cord compression than that resulting from fracture of the dens (Fig. B4.13*B*). In fractures of the dens, the dens fragment is held in place against the anterior arch of the atlas by the transverse ligament, and the dens and atlas move as a unit. In the absence of a competent ligament, the upper cervical region of the spinal cord may be compressed between the approximated posterior arch of the atlas and the dens (Fig. B4.13*A*), causing paralysis of all four limbs (*quadriplegia*), or into the medulla of the brainstem, resulting in death. Approximately one third of the atlas ring is occupied by the dens, one third by the spinal cord, and the remaining third by the fluid-filled space and tissues surrounding the cord: *Steele Rule of Thirds* (Fig. B4.13*C* & *D*). This explains why some patients with anterior displacement of the atlas may be relatively asymptomatic until a large degree of movement (greater than one third of the diameter of the atlas ring) occurs. Sometimes inflammation in the craniovertebral area may produce softening of the ligaments ▶

(A)   (B)
Anterior views

(D) Transverse CT scan

(C) Median MRI scan

(E) Reconstructed median CT scan

Figure B4.12. Fractures of dens. *Black arrowheads* (in **C**, **D**, & **E**), fracture lines at root or base of dens; *white arrow* (in **C**), transverse ligament of atlas.

(A) Left lateral view

(B) Left lateral view

(C) Inferior view

(D) Superior view

¹/₃ Dens (*D*)
¹/₆ Space (*S*)
¹/₃ Spinal cord (*C*)
¹/₆ Space (*S*)

Figure B4.13. Rupture of transverse ligament of atlas. A. This left lateral view demonstrates that subluxation of the median atlantoaxial joint is allowed by rupture of the transverse ligament of the atlas. The atlas moves, but the dens is fixed. **B.** This left lateral view of a fracture of the dens shows that the dens and atlas move together as a unit because the transverse ligament holds the dens to the anterior arch of the atlas. **C and D.** Inferior view transverse CT scan and interpretive drawing showing a normal median atlantoaxial joint and demonstrating Steele's Rule of Thirds

of the craniovertebral joints and cause dislocation of the atlantoaxial joints. Sudden movement of a patient from a bed to a chair, for example, may produce posterior displacement of the dens and injury to the spinal cord.

Rupture of the Alar Ligaments

The alar ligaments are weaker than the transverse ligament of the atlas. Consequently, combined flexion and rotation of the head may tear one or both alar ligaments. Rupture of an alar ligament results in an increase of approximately 30% in the range

of movement to the contralateral side (Dvorak et al., 1988).

Compression of C2 Spinal Ganglion

Although uncommon, atlantoaxial rotation may compress the C2 spinal nerve. When the neck is severely hyperextended while the head is turned to the side, the spinal ganglion of the C2 nerve on the opposite side may be compressed between C1 and C2 vertebrae. This may be followed by prolonged severe headaches and excruciating cervico-occipital pain. ⊙

Movements of the Vertebral Column

The range of movement of the vertebral column varies according to the region and the individual. Some people are capable of extraordinary movements, such as acrobats who began their training during early childhood. The normal range of movement possible in healthy young adults is typically reduced by 50% or more as they age.

The mobility of the vertebral column results primarily from the compressibility and elasticity of the IV discs. The vertebral column is capable of flexion, extension, lateral flexion and extension, and rotation (torsion) (Fig. 4.16). Bending of the vertebral column to the right or left from the neutral (erect) position is *lateral flexion* (bending); returning to the erect posture from a position of lateral flexion is *lateral extension*.

The range of movement of the vertebral column is limited by the:

- Thickness, elasticity, and compressibility of the IV discs.
- Shape and orientation of the zygapophysial joints.
- Tension of the joint capsules of the zygapophysial joints.
- Resistance of the back muscles and ligaments (e.g., the ligamenta flava and the posterior longitudinal ligament).
- Attachment to the thoracic (rib) cage.
- Bulk of surrounding tissue.

The back muscles that produce movements of the vertebral column are discussed later in this chapter. Movements are not produced exclusively, however, by the back muscles. They are assisted by gravity and the action of the anterolateral abdominal muscles (see Chapter 2).

Movements between adjacent vertebrae occur at the resilient nuclei pulposi of the IV discs (serving as the axis of movement) and at the zygapophysial joints. The orientation of the latter joints permits some movements and restricts others. With the exception perhaps of C1–C2, movement never occurs at a single segment of the column. Although movements between adjacent vertebrae are relatively small, especially in the thoracic region, the summation of all the small movements produces a considerable range of movement of the vertebral column as a whole (e.g., when flexing to touch the toes). Movements of the vertebral column are freer in the cervical and lumbar regions than elsewhere. Flexion, extension, lateral flexion, and rotation of the neck are especially free because the:

- IV discs, although thin relative to most other discs, are thick relative to the size of the vertebral bodies at this level.
- Articular surfaces of the zygapophysial joints are relatively large and the joint planes are almost horizontal.
- Joint capsules of the zygapophysial joints are loose.
- Neck is relatively slender (with less surrounding soft tissue bulk compared with the trunk).

Flexion of the vertebral column is greatest in the cervical region (Fig. 4.16A). The sagittally oriented joint planes of the lumbar region are conducive to flexion and extension. Extension of the vertebral column is most marked in the lumbar region and is usually more extensive than flexion; however, the interlocking articular processes here prevent rotation (Table 4.3). The lumbar region, like the cervical region, has IV discs that are large (the largest discs occur here) relative to the size of the vertebral bodies. Lateral flexion of the vertebral column is greatest in the cervical and lumbar regions (Fig. 4.16B).

The thoracic region, in contrast, has IV discs that are thin relative to the size of the vertebral bodies. Relative stability is also conferred on this part of the vertebral column, through its connection to the sternum by the ribs and costal cartilages. The joint planes here lie on an arc that is centered on the vertebral body, permitting rotation in the thoracic region (Fig. 4.16C). This rotation of the upper trunk, in combination with the rotation permitted in the cervical region and that at the atlantoaxial joints, enables the torsion of the axial skeleton that occurs as one looks back over the shoulder. However, flexion is limited in the thoracic region, including lateral flexion.

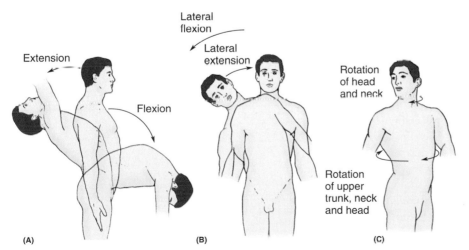

(A)   **(B)**   **(C)**

Figure 4.16. Movements of vertebral column. A. Flexion (forward bending) and extension (backward bending), both in the median plane, are shown. Flexion and extension are occurring primarily in the cervical and lumbar regions. **B.** Lateral flexion (to the right or left in a frontal plane) is shown, also occurring mostly in the cervical and lumbar regions. **C.** Rotation around a longitudinal axis, which occurs primarily at the craniovertebral joints (augmented by the cervical region) and the thoracic region, is shown.

Fractures and Dislocations of the Vertebrae

Although the construction of the vertebral column permits a considerable amount of movement as well as support and protection, excessive or sudden violent movement or movement of a type not permitted in a specific region, is likely to result in fractures, dislocations, and fracture–dislocations of the vertebral column. Sudden forceful flexion, as occurs in automobile accidents or from a violent blow to the back of the head, commonly produces a **crush or compression fracture** of the body of one or more vertebrae. If violent anterior movement of the vertebra occurs in combination with compression, a vertebra may be displaced anteriorly on the vertebra inferior to it (e.g., dislocation of C6 or C7 vertebrae) (see clinical correlation [blue] box "Dislocation of the Cervical Vertebrae," in this chapter). Usually this displacement dislocates and fractures the articular facets between the two vertebrae and ruptures the interspinous ligaments. Irreparable injuries to the spinal cord accompany most severe flexion injuries of the vertebral column.

Sudden, forceful extension of the neck can also injure the vertebral column and spinal cord. Head butting or illegal face blocking in football may lead to a **hyperextension injury of the neck** (Fig. B4.14A). Such severe hyperextension is most likely to injure posterior parts of the vertebrae, fracturing by crush or compression of the vertebral arches and their processes. Fractures of cervical vertebrae may radiate pain to the back of the neck and scapular region because the same spinal sensory ganglia and spinal cord segments receiving pain impulses from the vertebrae are also involved in supplying neck muscles. Hyperextension ("whiplash" injury) of the neck also occurs during rear-end motor vehicle collisions (Fig. B4.14B), an association especially well known to litigation lawyers. In these types of hyperextension injuries, the anterior longitudinal ligament is severely stretched and may be torn.

Hyperflexion injury of the vertebral column may also occur as the head "rebounds" after the hyperextension, snapping the head forward onto the thorax. "Facet jumping" or locking of the cervical vertebrae may occur because of dislocation of the vertebral arches (see clinical correlation (blue) box "Dislocation of the Cervical Vertebrae," in this chapter). Severe hyperextension of the head on the upper neck may, in addition to producing a cervical spondylolysis or hangman's fracture (see clinical correlation (blue) box "Fracture and Dislocation of the Axis," in this chapter), rupture the anterior longitudinal ligament and the adjacent anulus fibrosus of the C2–C3 IV disc. If this occurs, the cranium, C1, and the anterior portion (dens and body) of C2 are separated from the ▶

(A) Hyperextension of neck

(B) Hyperextension (whiplash) injury

(C) Hangman's fracture with disruption of C2/C3 disc and anterior longitudinal ligament

Figure B4.14

rest of the axial skeleton (Fig. B4.14C), and the spinal cord is usually severed. Persons with this severe injury seldom survive. Football, diving, falls from horses, and motor vehicle collisions cause most fractures of the cervical region of the vertebral column. Symptoms range from vague aches to progressive loss of motor and sensory functions.

Dislocation of vertebrae in the thoracic and lumbar regions is uncommon because of the interlocking of their articular processes. The transition from the relatively inflexible thoracic region to the much more mobile lumbar region occurs abruptly, unfortunately. Consequently, vertebrae T11 and especially T12 (which participates in rotatory movements superiorly but only flexion and extension movements inferiorly) are the most commonly fractured noncervical vertebrae (i.e., a "broken back" vs. a "broken neck").

Failure or fracture of the intercarticular parts of the vertebral laminae of L5 (*spondylolysis of L5*) may result in forward displacement of the L5 vertebral body relative to the sacrum (S1 vertebra)—*spondylolisthesis* (Fig. B4.15). Most agree that spondylolysis of L5, or susceptibility to it, probably results from a failure of the centrum of L5 to unite adequately with the neural arches at the neurocentral joint during development (see "Ossification of Vertebrae," earlier in this chapter). The anatomical basis of spondylolisthesis was discussed in Chapter 3 in relation to impinge-

Figure B4.15. Spondylolisthesis secondary to spondylolysis.

ment on the pelvic inlet. Spondylolisthesis at the L5–S1 articulation may (but does not necessarily) result in pressure on the spinal nerves of the cauda equina as they pass into the superior part of the sacrum, causing back and lower limb pain. ☉

THE BOTTOM LINE: The cervical and lumbar regions are most mobile (and consequently most vulnerable to injury). Flexion and extension occur primarily in the cervical and lumbar regions, whereas rotation occurs in the cervical and thoracic regions.

Curvatures of the Vertebral Column

The vertebral column in adults has four curvatures: cervical, thoracic, lumbar, and sacral (Fig. 4.17). The **thoracic** and **sacral** (pelvic) **curvatures** (kyphoses; singular = kyphosis) are concave anteriorly, whereas the **cervical** and **lumbar curvatures** (lordoses; singular − lordosis) are concave posteriorly. The thoracic and sacral curvatures are **primary curvatures** that develop during the fetal period in relationship to the (flexed) fetal position. Compare the curvatures in Figure 4.17, noting that the primary curvatures are in the same direction as the main curvatures of the fetal vertebral column. The primary curvatures are retained throughout life as a consequence of differences in height between the anterior and posterior parts of the vertebrae.

The cervical and lumbar curvatures are **secondary curvatures** that result from extension from the flexed fetal position.

They begin to appear during the fetal period but do not become obvious until infancy. Secondary curvatures are maintained primarily by differences in thickness between the anterior and the posterior parts of the IV discs. The *cervical curvature* becomes fully evident when an infant begins to raise (extend) its head while prone and to hold its head erect while sitting. The *lumbar curvature* becomes apparent when an infant begins to assume the upright posture, standing and walking. This curvature, generally more pronounced in females, ends at the *lumbosacral angle* formed at the junction of L5 vertebra with the sacrum (Fig. 4.1D). The *sacral curvature* also differs in males and females, that of the female reduced so that the coccyx protrudes less into the pelvic outlet (see Chapter 3).

The curvatures provide additional flexibility (shock-absorbing resilience) to the vertebral column, further augmenting that provided by the IV discs. When the load borne by the vertebral column is markedly increased (as by carrying a heavy backpack or another person on one's shoulders), both the IV discs and the flexible curvatures are compressed (i.e., the curvatures tend to increase). While the flexibility provided by the IV discs is passive and limited primarily by the zygapophysial joints and longitudinal ligaments, that provided by the curvatures is actively (dynamically) resisted by the contraction of

Curvatures:

Cervical (2°)

Thoracic (1°)

Lumbar (2°)

Sacral (1°)

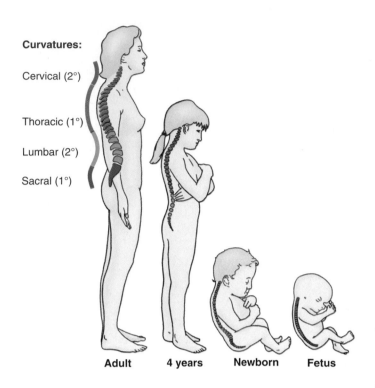

Adult   4 years   Newborn   Fetus

(A)   (B)

Figure 4.18. Flexion and extension while sitting. During prolonged sitting (especially when no back support is provided), flexion (**A**) and extension (**B**) occur alternately, transferring the load between muscles (active) and ligaments (passive).

Figure 4.17. Curvatures of vertebral column. The four curvatures of the adult vertebral column—cervical, thoracic, lumbar, and sacral—are contrasted with the C-shaped curvature of the vertebral column during fetal life, when only the primary (*1°*) curvatures exist. The secondary (*2°*) curvatures develop during infancy and childhood.

muscle groups antagonistic to the movement (e.g., the long extensors of the back resist increased thoracic kyphosis, whereas the abdominal flexors resist increased lumbar lordosis). Carrying additional weight anterior to the body's normal gravitational axis (e.g., abnormally large breasts, a pendulous abdomen, or carrying a young child) also tends to increase these curvatures. The muscles that provide resistance to the increase in curvature often ache when the weight is borne for extended periods.

When sitting, especially in the absence of back support for long periods of time, one usually "cycles" between back flexion (slumping) and extension (sitting up straight) to minimize stiffness and fatigue (Fig. 4.18). This allows alternation between the active support provided by the extensor muscles of the back and the passive resistance to flexion provided by ligaments.

THE BOTTOM LINE: Primary (thoracic and sacral) curvatures are developmental; secondary (cervical and lumbar) curvatures are acquired in relation to erect human posture. The curvatures provide shock-absorbing resilience and flexibility to the axial skeleton. Extensors of the back and abdominal flexors provide dynamic support to maintain the curvatures.

Abnormal Curvatures of the Vertebral Column

To detect an abnormal curvature of the vertebral column, have an individual stand in the anatomical position. Inspect the profile of the vertebral column from the person's side (Fig. B4.16*A–C*) and then from the posterior aspect (Fig. B4.16*D*). With the person bending over, observe the ability to flex directly forward and whether the back is level once the flexed position is assumed (Fig. B4.16*E*). Abnormal curvatures in some people result from developmental anomalies; in others, the curvatures result from pathological processes. The most prevalent metabolic disease of bone occurring in the elderly, especially in women, is *osteoporosis*. It is characterized by net demineralization of the bones caused by a disruption of the normal balance of calcium deposition and resorption. As a result, the quality of bone is reduced and atrophy of skeletal tissue occurs. Although osteoporosis affects the entire skeleton, the most affected areas are the neck of the femur (thigh bone), the vertebrae, the metacarpals (bones of the hand), and the radius (of the forearm). These bones become weakened and brittle, and are subject to fracture.

Excess thoracic kyphosis (clinically shortened to **kyphosis**, although this term actually applies to the normal curvature here, and colloquially known as *humpback* or *hunchback*) is characterized by an abnormal increase in the thoracic curvature; the vertebral column curves posteriorly (Fig. B4.16*B*). This abnormality can result from erosion of the anterior part of one ▶

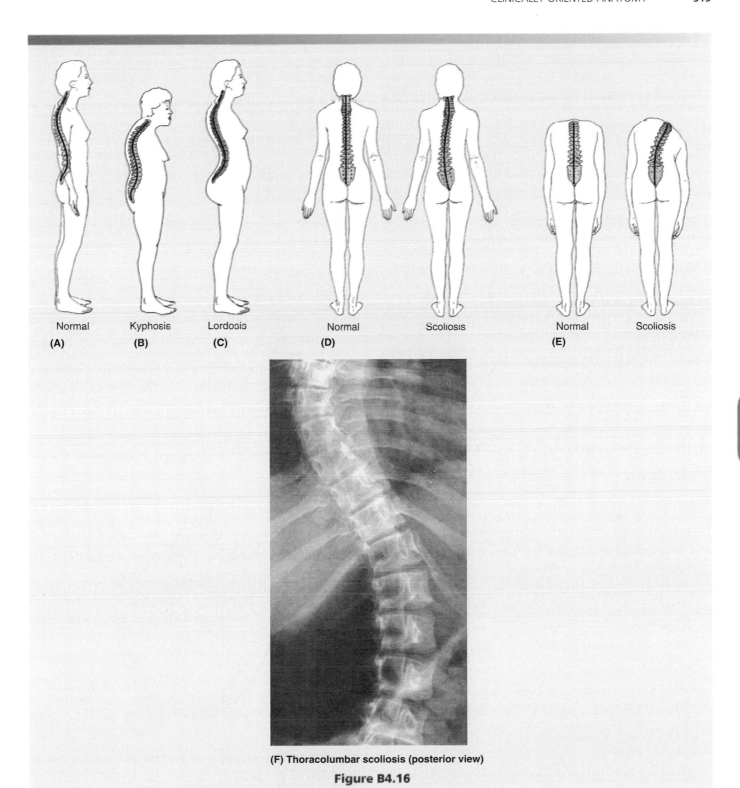

Normal
(A)

Kyphosis
(B)

Lordosis
(C)

Normal   Scoliosis
(D)

Normal   Scoliosis
(E)

(F) Thoracolumbar scoliosis (posterior view)

Figure B4.16

or more vertebrae (e.g., caused by osteoporosis). *Dowager's hump* is a colloquial name for excess thoracic kyphosis in older women resulting from osteoporosis. However, excess kyphosis also occurs in elderly men (Swartz, 2002). Osteoporosis especially affects the horizontal trabeculae of the trabecular (spongy) bone of the vertebral body (Fig. 4.3). The remaining, unsupported vertical trabeculae are less able to resist compression and sustain compression fractures, resulting in short and wedge-shaped thoracic vertebrae (Fig. B4.8A). Progressive erosion and collapse of vertebrae also result in an overall loss of height, and the excess kyphosis leads to an increase in the AP diameter of the thorax. ▶

Excess lumbar lordosis (clinically shortened to **lordosis,** although once again this term actually describes the normal curvature here. Colloquially, excess lumbar lordosis is known as *hollow back* or *sway back*) is characterized by an anterior rotation of the pelvis (the upper sacrum tilts anteroinferiorly) at the hip joints, producing an abnormal increase in the lumbar curvature; the vertebral column curves more anteriorly (Fig. B4.16C). This *abnormal extension deformity* is often associated with weakened trunk musculature, especially the anterolateral abdominal muscles. To compensate for alterations to their normal line of gravity, women develop a temporary excess lumbar lordosis during late pregnancy. This lordotic curvature may cause low back pain, but the discomfort normally disappears soon after childbirth. Obesity in both sexes can also cause excess lumbar lordosis and low back pain because of the increased weight of the abdominal contents (e.g., "pot-belly") anterior to the normal line of gravity. Loss of weight and exercise of the anterolateral abdominal muscles facilitate correction of this type of excess lordosis.

Scoliosis (crooked or curved back) is characterized by an abnormal lateral curvature that is accompanied by ro-tation of the vertebrae (Fig. B4.16*D* & *E*). The spinous processes turn toward the cavity of the abnormal curvature, and when the individual bends over, the ribs rotate posteriorly (protrude) on the side of the increased convexity. Scoliosis is the most common deformity of the vertebral column in pubertal girls (ages 12–15 years). Asymmetrical weakness of the intrinsic back muscles (*myopathic scoliosis*), failure of half of a vertebra to develop (*hemivertebra*), and a difference in the length of the lower limbs are causes of scoliosis. If the lengths of the lower limbs are not equal, a compensatory pelvic tilt may lead to a functional *static scoliosis.* When a person is standing, an obvious inclination or listing to one side may be a sign of scoliosis that is secondary to a herniated IV disc. *Habit scoliosis* is supposedly caused by habitual standing or sitting in an improper position. When the scoliosis is entirely postural, it disappears during maximum flexion of the vertebral column. Sometimes there is *kyphoscoliosis,* excess thoracic kyphosis combined with scoliosis, in which an abnormal AP diameter produces a severe restriction of the thorax and lung expansion (Swartz, 2002). ✹

Vasculature of the Vertebral Column

Vertebrae are supplied by *periosteal* and *equatorial branches* of the major cervical and segmental arteries and their **spinal branches** (Fig. 4.19). Parent arteries of periosteal, equatorial, and spinal branches occur at all levels of the vertebral column, in close association with it, and include the following arteries (described in detail in other chapters):

- *Vertebral* and *ascending cervical arteries* in the neck (Chapter 8).

- The major *segmental arteries* of the trunk:

- *Posterior intercostal arteries* in the thoracic region (Chapter 1).

- *Subcostal* and *lumbar arteries* in the abdomen (Chapter 2).

- *Iliolumbar* and *lateral and medial sacral arteries* in the pelvis (Chapter 3).

Periosteal and **equatorial branches** arise from these arteries as they cross the external (anterolateral) surfaces of the vertebrae. Spinal branches enter the IV foramina and divide. Smaller **anterior** and **posterior vertebral canal branches** pass to the vertebral body and vertebral arch, respectively, and give rise to ascending and descending branches that anastomose with the spinal canal branches of adjacent levels. Anterior vertebral canal branches send **nutrient arteries** anteriorly into the vertebral bodies that supply most of the red marrow of the central vertebral body (Bogduk, 1997). The

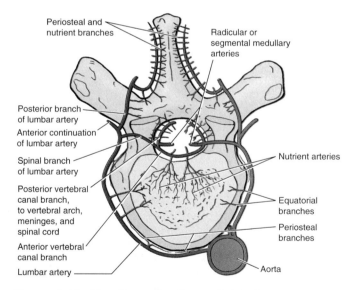

Figure 4.19. Blood supply of vertebrae. Typical vertebrae are supplied by segmental arteries—here lumbar arteries. In the thoracic and lumbar regions, each vertebra is encircled on three sides by paired intercostal or lumbar arteries that arise from the aorta. The segmental arteries supply equatorial branches to the vertebral body, and posterior branches supply the vertebral arch structures and the back muscles. Spinal branches enter the vertebral canal through the IV foramina to supply the bones, periosteum, ligaments, and meninges that bound the epidural space and radicular or segmental medullary arteries that supply nervous tissue (spinal nerve roots and spinal cord).

Basivertebral veins

Anterior external
vertebral
venous plexus

Intervertebral disc

Vertebral body

Internal
vertebral
(epidural)
plexus

Anterior internal
plexus

Posterior internal
plexus

Spinous
process

Posterior
external
vertebral
venous plexus

(A) Medial view of right half of hemisected vertebral column

Posterior external venous plexus

Anterior and posterior
longitudinal sinuses
(veins) of internal
vertebral (epidural) plexus

Lumbar vein

Ascending lumbar vein

Intervertebral vein

Basivertebral vein

Anterior external
vertebral venous plexus

(B) Superior view

Figure 4.20. Venous drainage of vertebral column. A. The venous drainage parallels the arterial supply and enters the external and internal vertebral venous plexuses. There is also anterolateral drainage from the external aspects of the vertebrae into segmental veins. **B.** The superior view of a lumbar vertebra is shown. The vertebral canal contains a dense plexus of thin-walled valveless veins, the internal vertebral venous plexuses, which surround the dura mater. Anterior and posterior longitudinal venous sinuses can be identified in the internal vertebral venous plexus. Basivertebral veins from the vertebral body drain primarily into the anterior internal vertebral venous plexus, but they may also drain to the anterior external plexus.

larger branches of the spinal branches continue as terminal *radicular* or *segmental medullary arteries* distributed to the posterior and anterior roots of the spinal nerves and their coverings and to the spinal cord, respectively (see "Vasculature of the Spinal Cord and Spinal Nerve Roots," later in this chapter).

Spinal veins form venous plexuses along the vertebral column both inside and outside the vertebral canal. These plexuses are the **internal vertebral venous plexus** (epidural venous plexuses) and **external vertebral venous plexuses**, re-

spectively (Fig. 4.20). These plexuses communicate through the intervertebral foramina. Both plexuses are densest anteriorly and posteriorly and relatively sparse laterally. The large, tortuous **basivertebral veins** form within the vertebral bodies. They emerge from foramina on the surfaces of the vertebral bodies (mostly the posterior aspect) and drain into the anterior external and especially the anterior internal vertebral venous plexuses, which may form large longitudinal sinuses. The **intervertebral veins** receive veins from the spinal cord and vertebral venous plexuses as they accompany the spinal nerves through the IV foramina to drain into the *vertebral veins* of the neck and *segmental* (intercostal, lumbar, and sacral) *veins* of the trunk.

from the vertebrae and drain, in turn, into the vertebral veins of the neck and the segmental veins of the trunk.

Nerves of the Vertebral Column

THE BOTTOM LINE: Spinal branches of the major cervical and segmental arteries supply the vertebral column. Internal and external vertebral venous plexuses collect blood

Other than the zygapophysial joints (innervated by *articular branches of the medial branches of the posterior rami,* as

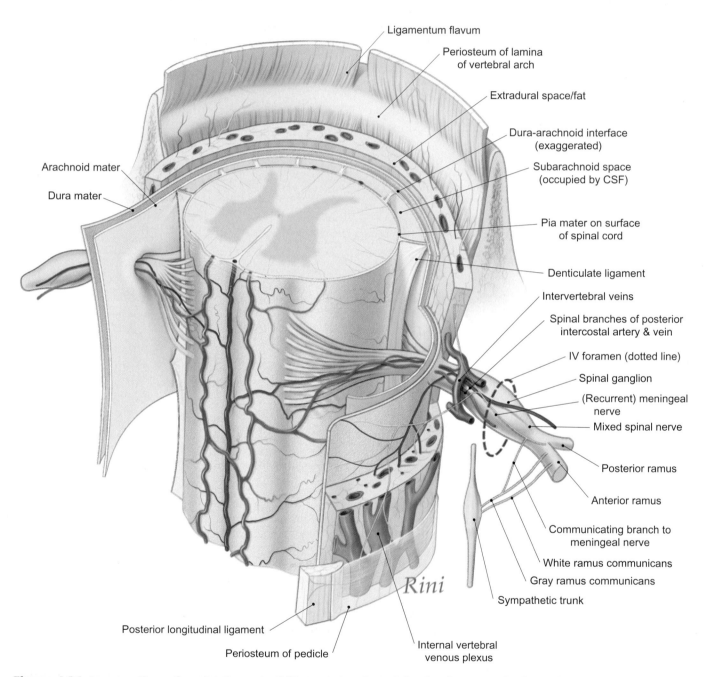

Ligamentum flavum
Periosteum of lamina of vertebral arch
Extradural space/fat
Dura-arachnoid interface (exaggerated)
Subarachnoid space (occupied by CSF)
Pia mater on surface of spinal cord
Denticulate ligament
Intervertebral veins
Spinal branches of posterior intercostal artery & vein
IV foramen (dotted line)
Spinal ganglion
(Recurrent) meningeal nerve
Mixed spinal nerve
Posterior ramus
Anterior ramus
Communicating branch to meningeal nerve
White ramus communicans
Gray ramus communicans
Sympathetic trunk

Arachnoid mater
Dura mater

Rini

Posterior longitudinal ligament
Periosteum of pedicle
Internal vertebral venous plexus

Figure 4.21. Innervation of periosteum and ligaments of vertebral column and of meninges. Except for the zygapophysial joints and external elements of the vertebral arch, the fibroskeletal structures of the vertebral column (and the meninges) are supplied by the (recurrent) meningeal nerves. Although usually omitted from diagrams and illustrations of spinal nerves, these fine nerves are the first branches to arise from all 31 pairs of spinal nerves and are the nerves that initially convey localized pain sensation from the back produced by acute herniation of an IV disc or from sprains, contusions, fractures, or tumors of the vertebral column itself. (Based on Frick H, Kummer B, Putz R: *Wolf-Heidegger's Atlas of Human Anatomy*, 4th ed. Basel, Karger AG, 1990:476.)

described with these joints), the vertebral column is innervated by (recurrent) **meningeal branches of the spinal nerves** (Fig. 4.21). These rarely described or depicted branches are the only branches to arise from the mixed spinal nerve, arising immediately after it is formed and before its division into anterior and posterior rami or from the anterior ramus immediately after its formation. Two to four of these fine branches arise on each side at all vertebral levels. Close to their origin, the meningeal branches receive communicating branches from the nearby gray rami communicantes. As the spinal nerves exit the IV foramina, most of the meningeal branches run back through the foramina into the vertebral canal (hence the alternate term *recurrent*). However, some branches remain outside the canal and are distributed to the anterolateral aspect of the vertebral bodies and IV discs. They supply the periosteum and especially the anuli fibrosi and anterior longitudinal ligament. Inside the vertebral canal, transverse, ascending, and descending branches distribute nerve fibers to the:

- Periosteum (covering the surface of the posterior vertebral bodies, pedicles, and laminae).

- Ligamenta flava.

- Anuli fibrosi of the posterior and posterolateral aspect of the IV discs.

- Posterior longitudinal ligament.

- Spinal dura mater.

- Blood vessels within the vertebral canal.

Nerve fibers to the periosteum, anuli fibrosi and ligaments supply pain receptors; those to the anuli fibrosi and ligaments also supply receptors for proprioception (the sense of one's position). Sympathetic fibers to the blood vessels stimulate vasoconstriction. Innervation of the dura mater is discussed later in this chapter.

THE BOTTOM LINE: Zygapophysial joints are innervated by medial branches of adjacent posterior rami. (Recurrent) meningeal branches of spinal nerves supply most bone (periosteum), IV discs, and ligaments as well as the coverings of the spinal cord. These two (groups of) nerves convey all localized pain from the vertebral column.

Back Pain

Back pain in general, and low back pain in particular, is an immense health problem, second only to the common cold as a reason people visit their doctors. In terms of health factors causing lost work days, backache is second only to headache. Annual costs for treatment of back pain are staggering. Yet the anatomical bases for the pain, especially the nerves initially involved in sensing and carrying pain from the vertebral column itself, are rarely described.

Five categories of structures receive innervation in the back and can be sources of pain:

- Fibroskeletal structures: periosteum, ligaments, and the anuli fibrosi of IV discs.

- Meninges: the coverings of the spinal cord.

- Synovial joints: the capsules of the zygapophysial joints.

- Muscles: the intrinsic muscles of the back.

- Nervous tissue: spinal nerves or nerve roots exiting the IV foramina.

Of these, the first two are innervated by (recurrent) meningeal branches of the spinal nerves and the next two are innervated by posterior rami (articular and muscular branches). Pain resulting from nervous tissue—that is, caused by compression or irritation of spinal nerves or nerve roots—is referred to the area (dermatome) supplied by that nerve (see clinical correlation [blue] box "Herniation of the Nucleus Pulposus," in this chapter) but may be accompanied by localized pain. Pain related to the meninges is relatively rare and is discussed later in this chapter; it is generally not considered to be a factor in back pain.

Localized back pain (pain perceived as coming from the back) is generally muscular, joint, or fibroskeletal pain. *Muscular pain* is usually related to reflexive cramping (spasms) producing *ischemia*, often secondarily as a result of *guarding* (contraction of muscles in anticipation of pain). *Zygapophysial joint pain* is generally associated with aging (osteoarthritis) or disease (rheumatoid arthritis) of the joints. Pain from vertebral fractures and dislocations is no different from that from other bones and joints. The sharp pain following a fracture is mostly periosteal in origin, whereas pain from dislocations is ligamentous. The acute localized pain associated with an IV disc herniation undoubtedly emanates from the disrupted posterolateral anulus fibrosis and impingement on the posterior longitudinal ligament. Pain in all of these latter instances is conveyed initially by the meningeal branches of the spinal nerves. ⊕

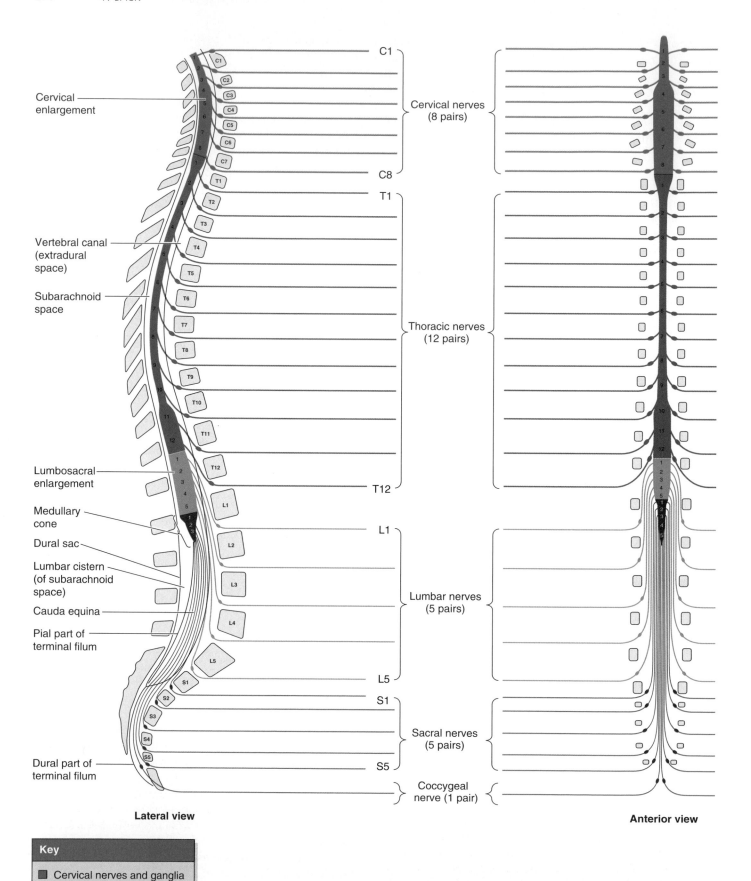

Cervical enlargement

Vertebral canal (extradural space)

Subarachnoid space

Lumbosacral enlargement

Medullary cone

Dural sac

Lumbar cistern (of subarachnoid space)

Cauda equina

Pial part of terminal filum

Dural part of terminal filum

C1

C8

T1

T12

L1

L5

S1

S5

Cervical nerves (8 pairs)

Thoracic nerves (12 pairs)

Lumbar nerves (5 pairs)

Sacral nerves (5 pairs)

Coccygeal nerve (1 pair)

Lateral view

Anterior view

Key

■ Cervical nerves and ganglia
■ Thoracic nerves and ganglia
□ Lumbar nerves and ganglia
■ Sacral and coccygeal nerves and ganglia

Figure 4.22. Vertebral column, spinal cord, spinal ganglia, and spinal nerves. Lateral and posterior views illustrating the relation of the spinal cord segments (the numbered segments) and spinal nerves to the adult vertebral column.

Contents of the Vertebral Canal

The spinal cord, spinal nerve roots, and spinal meninges and the neurovascular structures that supply them are located within the vertebral canal (Fig. 4.21).

Spinal Cord

The **spinal cord** is the major reflex center and conduction pathway between the body and the brain. This cylindrical structure, slightly flattened anteriorly and posteriorly, is protected by the vertebrae and their associated ligaments and muscles, the spinal meninges, and the cerebrospinal fluid (CSF). The spinal cord begins as a continuation of the **medulla oblongata** (commonly called the *medulla*), the caudal part of the brainstem. In adults, the spinal cord is 42–45 cm long and extends from the foramen magnum in the occipital bone to the level of the L1 or L2 vertebra (Fig. 4.22). However, its tapering inferior end, the **medullary cone,** may terminate as high as T12 vertebra or as low as L3 vertebra. Thus the spinal cord occupies only the superior two thirds of the vertebral canal.

The spinal cord is enlarged in two regions in relationship to innervation of the limbs. The **cervical enlargement** extends from the C4 through T1 segments of the spinal cord, and most of the anterior rami of the spinal nerves arising from it form the *brachial plexus of nerves* that innervates the upper limbs (see Chapter 6). The **lumbosacral (lumbar) enlargement** extends from T11 through S1 segments of the spinal cord, inferior to which the cord continues to diminish as the medullary cone. The anterior rami of the spinal nerves arising from this enlargement make up the *lumbar* and *sacral plexuses of nerves* that innervate the lower limbs (see Chapter 5).

Spinal Nerve Roots

The formation and composition of spinal nerves and nerve roots are discussed in the Introduction. Readers are urged to read this information now if they have not done so previously.

The portion of the spinal cord giving rise to the rootlets and roots that ultimately form one bilateral pair of spinal nerves is designated a **spinal cord segment,** the identity of which is the same as the spinal nerves arising from it. Cervical spinal nerves (except C8) bear the same alphanumeric designation as the vertebrae forming the inferior margin of the IV foramina through which the nerve exits the vertebral canal, whereas the more inferior spinal nerves bear the same alphanumeric designation as the vertebrae forming the superior margin of their exit. The first cervical nerves lack posterior roots in 50% of people, and the coccygeal nerve may be absent altogether.

In embryos, the spinal cord occupies the full length of the vertebral canal (Moore and Persaud, 2003); thus spinal cord segments lie approximately at the vertebral level of the same number, the spinal nerves passing laterally to exit the corresponding IV foramen. By the end of the embryonic period (8th week), the tail-like caudal eminence has disappeared, and the number of coccygeal vertebrae is reduced from six to four segments. The spinal cord in the vertebral canal of the coccyx atrophies. During the fetal period, the vertebral column grows faster than the spinal cord; as a result, the cord "ascends" relative to the vertebral canal. At birth, the tip of the medullary cone is at the L4–L5 level. Thus, in postnatal life, the spinal cord is shorter than the vertebral column; consequently, there is a progressive obliquity of the spinal nerve roots (Figs. 4.22 and 4.23). Because the distance between the origin of a nerve's roots from the spinal cord and the nerve's exit from the vertebral canal increases as the inferior end of the vertebral column is approached, the length of the nerve roots also increases progressively. The lumbar and sacral nerve roots are therefore the longest, extending far beyond the termination of the adult cord at approximately the L2 level to reach the remaining lumbar, sacral, and coccygeal IV foramina. This loose bundle of spinal nerve roots arising from the lumbosacral enlargement and the medullary cone and coursing within the *lumbar cistern* of CSF caudal to the termination of the spinal cord resembles a horse's tail, hence its name—the **cauda equina** (L. horse tail).

Arising from the tip of the medullary cone, the terminal filum descends among the spinal nerve roots in the cauda equina. The **terminal filum** (L. *filum terminale*) is the vestigial remnant of the caudal part of the spinal cord that was in the tail-like caudal eminence of the embryo. Its proximal end (the **pial part** or *internal terminal filum*) consists of vestiges of neural tissue, connective tissue, and neuroglial tissue covered by pia mater. The terminal filum perforates the inferior end of the dural sac, gaining a layer of dura and continuing through the sacral hiatus as the **dural part** or *external terminal filum* (also known as the *coccygeal ligament*) to attach to the dorsum of the coccyx. The terminal filum is an anchor for the inferior end of the spinal cord and the spinal meninges.

THE BOTTOM LINE: The spinal cord and spinal nerve roots and the CSF and membranes that surround them are the main contents of the vertebral canal. In adults, the spinal cord occupies only the superior two thirds of the canal and has two (cervical and lumbosacral) enlargements related to innervation of the limbs. The inferior, tapering end of the cord, the medullary cone, ends at the level of the L1 or L2 vertebrae. However, the terminal filament and the nerve roots from the lumbosacral part of the spinal cord that form the cauda equina continue inferiorly within the lumbar cistern containing CSF.

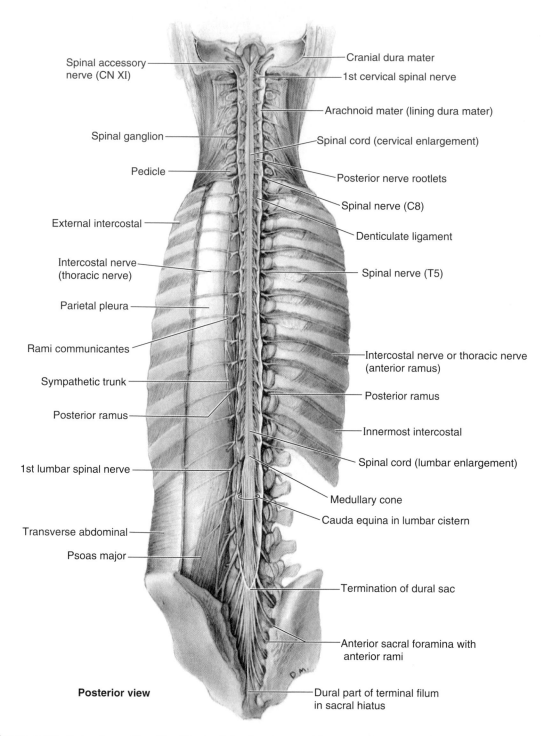

Spinal accessory nerve (CN XI)

Spinal ganglion

Pedicle

External intercostal

Intercostal nerve (thoracic nerve)

Parietal pleura

Rami communicantes

Sympathetic trunk

Posterior ramus

1st lumbar spinal nerve

Transverse abdominal

Psoas major

Posterior view

Cranial dura mater

1st cervical spinal nerve

Arachnoid mater (lining dura mater)

Spinal cord (cervical enlargement)

Posterior nerve rootlets

Spinal nerve (C8)

Denticulate ligament

Spinal nerve (T5)

Intercostal nerve or thoracic nerve (anterior ramus)

Posterior ramus

Innermost intercostal

Spinal cord (lumbar enlargement)

Medullary cone

Cauda equina in lumbar cistern

Termination of dural sac

Anterior sacral foramina with anterior rami

Dural part of terminal filum in sacral hiatus

Figure 4.23. Spinal cord in situ. The vertebral arches and the posterior aspect of the sacrum have been removed to expose the spinal cord in the vertebral canal. The spinal dural sac has also been opened to reveal the spinal cord and posterior nerve roots, the termination of the spinal cord between the L1 and the L2 vertebral level, and the termination of the spinal dural sac at the S2 segment.

Compression of the Lumbar Spinal Nerve Roots

The lumbar spinal nerves increase in size from superior to inferior, whereas the IV foramina decrease in diameter. Consequently, the L5 spinal nerve roots are the thickest and their foramina, the narrowest. This increases the chance that these nerve roots will be compressed if herniation of the nucleus pulposus occurs. ⊙

Spinal Meninges and Cerebrospinal Fluid

Collectively, the dura mater, arachnoid mater, and pia mater surrounding the spinal cord constitute the **spinal meninges** (Fig. 4.24; Table 4.4). These membranes surround, support, and protect the spinal cord and spinal nerve roots, including those of the cauda equina, and contain the cerebrospinal fluid (CSF) in which these structures are suspended.

Spinal Dura Mater

The **spinal dura mater**, composed mainly of tough fibrous with some elastic tissue, is the outermost covering membrane of the spinal cord. The spinal dura mater is separated from the periosteum-covered bone and the ligaments that form the walls of the vertebral canal by the **epidural space**. This space is occupied by the internal vertebral venous plexus embedded in a fatty matrix (**epidural fat**). The epidural space runs the length of the vertebral canal, terminating superiorly at the foramen magnum and laterally at the IV foramina, as the dura mater adheres to the periosteum surrounding each opening, and inferiorly, as the sacral hiatus is sealed by the sacrococcygeal ligament.

The dura mater forms the **spinal dural sac**, a long tubular sheath within the vertebral canal (Figs. 4.22 and 4.23). This sac adheres to the margin of the foramen magnum of the cranium, where it is continuous with the cranial dura mater. The spinal dural sac is anchored inferiorly to the coccyx by the *terminal filum*. The sac is evaginated by each pair of posterior and anterior roots as they extend laterally toward their exit from the vertebral canal (Fig. 4.25). Thus tapering lateral extensions of the spinal dura surround each pair of posterior and anterior nerve roots as **dural root sheaths**, or sleeves (Figs. 4.24, 4.26, and 4.27). Distal to the spinal ganglia, these sheaths blend with the *epineurium* (outer connective tissue covering of the spinal nerves) that adheres to the periosteum lining the IV foramina.

Innervation of the Dura Mater Nerve fibers are distributed to the dura mater by the (*recurrent*) *meningeal nerves* (Fig. 4.21). The function of these afferent and sympathetic fibers is unclear, although it is known that the afferent fibers supply pain receptors that are involved in the referred pain characteristic of spinal disorders and become irritated when there is inflammation of the meninges (*meningitis*).

Spinal Arachnoid Mater

The **spinal arachnoid mater** is a delicate, avascular membrane composed of fibrous and elastic tissue that lines the spinal dural sac and its dural root sheaths. It encloses the CSF-filled subarachnoid space containing the spinal cord, spinal nerve roots, and spinal ganglia (Figs. 4.24, 4.25, and 4.27). The arachnoid mater is not attached to the dura mater but is held against its inner surface by the pressure of the CSF. In a lumbar spinal puncture, the needle traverses the dura and arachnoid mater simultaneously. Their apposition is the **dura–arachnoid interface** (Table 4.4), often erroneously referred to as the "subdural space." No actual space occurs naturally at this site; it is, rather, a weak cell layer (Haines, 2002). Bleeding into this layer creates a pathological space at the dura–arachnoid junction in which a *subdural hematoma* is formed. In the cadaver, because of the absence of CSF, the arachnoid mater falls away from the inner surface of the dura mater and lies loosely on the spinal cord. The arachnoid

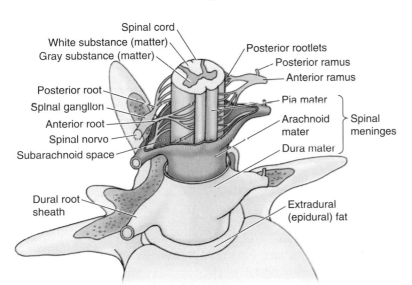

Figure 4.24. Spinal cord, spinal nerves, and spinal meninges. Three membranes (the spinal meninges) cover the spinal cord: dura mater, arachnoid mater, and pia mater. As the spinal nerve roots extend toward an IV foramen, they are surrounded by a dural root sheath (sleeve) that is continuous distally with the epineurium of the spinal nerve.

Table 4.4. Spaces Associated with the Spinal Meninges

Space	Location	Contents
Extradural (epidural)	Space between periosteum lining bony wall of vertebral canal and dura mater; position of extradural (epidural) herniation	Fat (loose connective tissue); internal vertebral venous plexuses; inferior to L2 vertebra, ensheathed roots of spinal nerves
Subarachnoid (leptomeningeal)	Naturally occurring space between arachnoid mater and pia mater	CSF; radicular, segmental, medullary, and spinal arteries; veins; arachnoid trabeculae

[a] Although it is common to refer to a "subdural space," there is no naturally occurring space at the arachnoid–dura junction (Haines, 2002).

mater is separated from the pia mater on the surface of the spinal cord by the *subarachnoid space* containing CSF. Delicate strands of connective tissue, the **arachnoid trabeculae,** span the subarachnoid space connecting the arachnoid mater and pia mater.

Spinal Pia Mater

The **spinal pia mater,** the innermost covering membrane of the spinal cord, consists of flattened cells with long, equally flattened processes that closely follow all the surface features of the spinal cord (Haines, 2002). The pia mater also directly covers the roots of the spinal nerves and the spinal blood vessels. Inferior to the medullary cone, the pia mater continues as the terminal filum (Fig. 4.22).

The spinal cord is suspended in the dural sac by the terminal filum and especially by the right and left sawtooth **denticulate ligaments** (L. *denticulus,* small tooth), which run longitudinally along each side of the spinal cord (Figs. 4.25

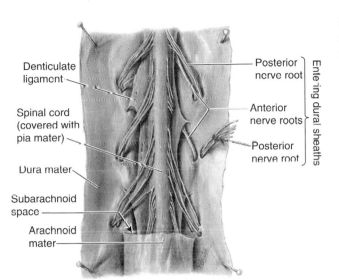

Denticulate ligament

Spinal cord (covered with pia mater)

Dura mater

Subarachnoid space

Arachnoid mater

Posterior nerve root

Anterior nerve roots

Posterior nerve root

Entering dural sheaths

Posterior view

Figure 4.25. Spinal cord within its meninges. The dura mater and arachnoid mater have been split and pinned flat to expose the spinal cord and spinal nerve roots.

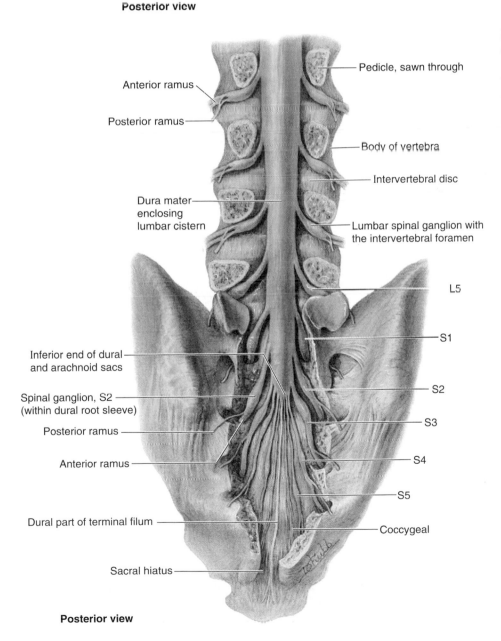

Anterior ramus

Posterior ramus

Dura mater enclosing lumbar cistern

Inferior end of dural and arachnoid sacs

Spinal ganglion, S2 (within dural root sleeve)

Posterior ramus

Anterior ramus

Dural part of terminal filum

Sacral hiatus

Pedicle, sawn through

Body of vertebra

Intervertebral disc

Lumbar spinal ganglion with the intervertebral foramen

L5

S1

S2

S3

S4

S5

Coccygeal

Posterior view

Figure 4.26. Inferior end of spinal dural sac. A laminectomy has been performed (i.e., most of the vertebral arches of the lumbar and sacral vertebrae have been removed) to show the inferior end of the dural sac, which encloses the lumbar cistern containing CSF and the cauda equina. The lumbar spinal ganglia lie within the IV foramina, but the sacral spinal ganglia (S1–S5) are in the sacral canal. In the lumbar region, the nerves exiting the IV foramina pass superior to the IV discs at that level; thus herniation of the nucleus pulposus tends to impinge on nerves passing to lower levels.

nerve roots in extensions of the subarachnoid space, protrude from the sides of the lumbar cistern (Fig. 4.26).

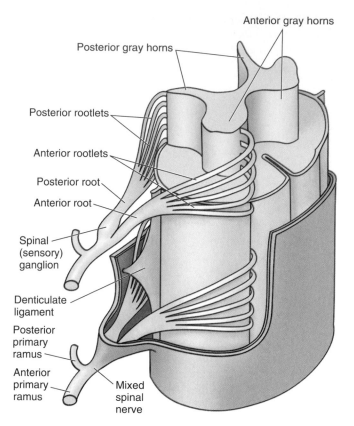

Figure 4.27. Spinal cord, anterior and posterior nerve rootlets and roots, spinal nerves, and spinal meninges. The structure of the spinal cord (gray and white substance) and the entrance and exit of nerve fibers via rootlets are demonstrated. The denticulate ligament is a serrated shelf-like extension of the spinal pia mater projecting between the posterior and the anterior nerve roots in a frontal plane from either side of the cervical and thoracic regions of the spinal cord. Its relatively strong, tooth-like processes anchor the spinal cord within the subarachnoid space.

and 4.27). The denticulate ligament consists of a fibrous sheet of pia mater extending midway between the posterior and the anterior nerve roots from the lateral surfaces of the spinal cord. The 20–22 processes, shaped much like shark's teeth, attach to the inner surface of the arachnoid-lined dural sac. The superior process of each denticulate ligament attaches to the cranial dura mater immediately superior to the foramen magnum, and the inferior process extends from the medullary cone, passing between the T12 and the L1 nerve roots.

Subarachnoid Space

The **subarachnoid space** is located between the arachnoid mater and the pia mater and is filled with CSF (Figs. 4.24 and 4.25; Table 4.4). The enlargement of the subarachnoid space in the dural sac, caudal to the medullary cone and containing CSF and the cauda equina, is the **lumbar cistern** (Figs. 4.22 and 4.23). It extends from the L2 vertebra to the second segment of the sacrum. Dural root sheaths, enclosing spinal

Development of the Meninges and Subarachnoid Space

Together, the pia mater and arachnoid mater form the **leptomeninges** (G. slender membranes). They develop as a single layer from the mesenchyme surrounding the embryonic spinal cord. Fluid-filled spaces form within this layer and coalesce to become the subarachnoid space (Moore and Persaud, 2003). The origin of the pia mater and arachnoid mater from a single membrane is reflected by the numerous arachnoid trabeculae passing between them (Table 4.4). The arachnoid mater in adults is thick enough to be manipulated with forceps. In contrast, the delicate pia mater is barely visible to the unaided eye, although it gives a shiny appearance to the surface of the spinal cord.

Lumbar Spinal Puncture

Lumbar spinal puncture (spinal tap), the extraction or sampling of CSF from the lumbar cistern, is an important diagnostic tool for evaluating a variety of central nervous system (CNS) disorders. *Meningitis* and diseases of the CNS may alter the cells in the CSF or change the concentration of its chemical constituents. Examination of CSF can also determine if blood is present. Lumbar spinal puncture is performed with the patient leaning forward or lying on the side with the back flexed (Fig. B4.17). Flexion of the vertebral column facilitates insertion of the needle by spreading the vertebral laminae and spinous processes apart, stretching the ligamenta flava.

Under aseptic conditions, the skin covering the lower lumbar vertebrae is anesthetized, and a *lumbar puncture needle,* fitted with a stylet, is inserted in the midline between the spinous processes of the L3 and L4 (or L4 and L5) vertebrae. Recall that a plane transecting the highest points of the iliac crests—the *supracristal plane*—usually passes through the L4 spinous process. At these levels, there is no danger of damaging the spinal cord. After passing 4–6 cm in adults (more in obese persons), the needle punctures the dura mater and arachnoid mater and enters the lumbar cistern. When the stylet is removed, CSF escapes at the rate of approximately one drop per second. If subarachnoid pressure is high, CSF flows out or escapes as a jet. Lumbar puncture is not performed in the presence of increased intracranial pressure. Intracranial pressure is now generally determined through CT scanning ▶

Figure B4.17

before lumbar puncture, but it may also be determined by examination of the fundus (back) of the interior of the eyeball with an ophthalmoscope (see clinical correlation [blue] box "Papilledema," in Chapter 7).

Spinal Block

An anesthetic agent can be injected into the CSF. Anesthesia usually occurs within 1 min. A headache may follow a *spinal block*, which likely results from the leakage of CSF

through the lumbar puncture. The clinical anatomy of spinal blocks for childbirth is discussed in Chapter 3.

Epidural Blocks

An anesthetic agent can be injected into the extradural (epidural) space using the position described in clinical correlation (blue) box "Lumbar Spinal Puncture," (lumbar epidural block), or through the sacral hiatus (caudal epidural block). Epidural block for anesthesia during childbirth is discussed in Chapter 3. ◗

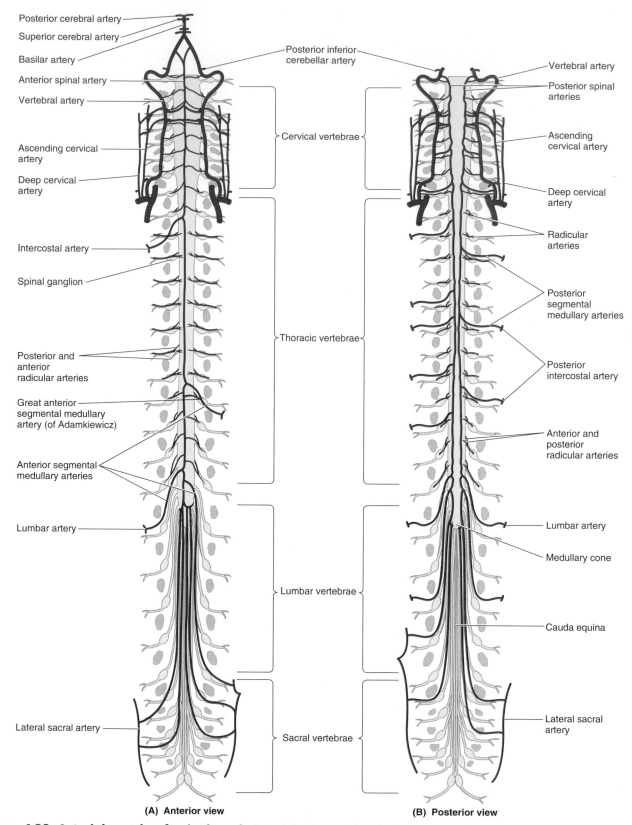

(A) Anterior view

(B) Posterior view

Figure 4.28. Arterial supply of spinal cord. A and B. The arteries derive from branches of the vertebral, ascending and deep cervical, intercostal, lumbar, and lateral sacral arteries. Three longitudinal arteries supply the spinal cord: an anterior spinal artery and two posterior spinal arteries. These vessels are reinforced by blood from the anterior and posterior segmental medullary arteries. Segmental medullary arteries supply the nerve roots that they course along and then contribute to the longitudinal arteries. The great anterior segmental medullary artery (of Adamkiewicz) is the largest segmental medullary artery, vital to the blood supply of the spinal cord between its cervical and lumbosacral enlargements. At levels where there are no segmental medullary arteries, radicular arteries supply the posterior and anterior roots of the spinal nerves. (Radicular arteries are shown at only the cervical and thoracic levels, but they also occur at the lumbar and sacral levels.)

THE BOTTOM LINE: Nerve tissues and neurovascular structures of the vertebral canal are suspended in CSF contained within the dural sac and sheaths. The fluid-filled subarachnoid space is lined with pia mater and arachnoid mater, which are continuous membranes. Because the spinal cord does not extend into the lumbar cistern (the inferior part of the subarachnoid space), it is an ideal site for sampling CSF or for injection of anesthetic agents.

Vasculature of the Spinal Cord and Spinal Nerve Roots

Arteries of the Spinal Cord and Nerve Roots

The arteries supplying the spinal cord are branches of the vertebral, ascending cervical, deep cervical, intercostal, lumbar, and lateral sacral arteries (Figs. 4.28 & 4.29). Three longitudinal arteries supply the spinal cord: an *anterior spinal artery* and paired *posterior spinal arteries*. These arteries run longitudinally from the medulla of the brainstem to the medullary cone of the spinal cord. The **anterior spinal artery**, formed by the union of branches of the vertebral arteries, runs inferiorly in the anterior median fissure. Sulcal arteries arise from the anterior spinal artery and enter the spinal cord through this fissure (Fig. 4.29B). The sulcal arteries supply approximately two thirds of the cross-sectional area of the spinal cord (Williams et al., 1995). Each **posterior spinal artery** is a branch of either the *vertebral artery* or the *posteroinferior cerebellar artery* (Figs. 4.28B and 4.29). The posterior spinal arteries commonly form anastomosing channels in the pia mater.

By themselves, the anterior and posterior spinal arteries can supply only the short superior part of the spinal cord. The circulation to much of the spinal cord depends on segmental medullary and radicular arteries running along the spinal nerve roots. The **anterior** and **posterior segmental**

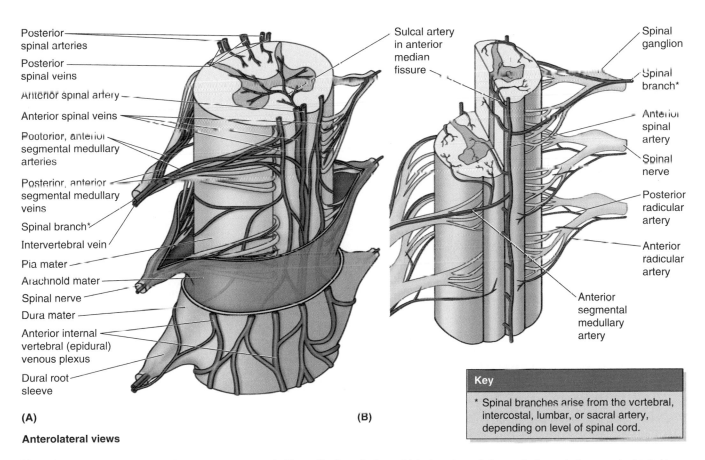

Posterior spinal arteries
Posterior spinal veins
Anterior spinal artery
Anterior spinal veins
Posterior, anterior segmental medullary arteries
Posterior, anterior segmental medullary veins
Spinal branch*
Intervertebral vein
Pia mater
Arachnoid mater
Spinal nerve
Dura mater
Anterior internal vertebral (epidural) venous plexus
Dural root sleeve

Sulcal artery in anterior median fissure

Spinal ganglion
Spinal branch*
Anterior spinal artery
Spinal nerve
Posterior radicular artery
Anterior radicular artery
Anterior segmental medullary artery

(A)

(B)

Anterolateral views

Key
* Spinal branches arise from the vertebral, intercostal, lumbar, or sacral artery, depending on level of spinal cord.

Most proximal spinal nerves and roots are accompanied by **radicular arteries**, which do not reach the posterior, anterior, or spinal arteries. **Segmental medullary arteries** occur irregularly *in the place of* radicular arteries—they are really just larger vessels that make it all the way to the spinal arteries.

Figure 4.29. Arterial supply and venous drainage of spinal cord and spinal nerve roots. A. The veins that drain the spinal cord, as well as the internal vertebral venous plexuses, drain into the intervertebral veins, which in turn drain into segmental veins. **B.** The pattern of the arterial supply of the spinal cord is from three longitudinal arteries: one anterior lying in the anteromedian position and the other two lying posterolaterally. These vessels are reinforced by medullary branches derived from the segmental arteries. The sulcal arteries are small branches of the anterior spinal artery coursing in the anterior median fissure.

medullary arteries are derived from spinal branches of the ascending cervical, deep cervical, vertebral, posterior intercostal, and lumbar arteries. The segmental medullary arteries are located chiefly where the need for a good blood supply to the spinal cord is greatest—the cervical and lumbosacral enlargements. They enter the vertebral canal through the IV foramina.

The **great anterior segmental medullary artery** (of Adamkiewicz), which is on the left side in about 65% of people, reinforces the circulation to two thirds of the spinal cord, including the lumbosacral enlargement (Fig. 4.28*A*). The great anterior segmental medullary artery, much larger than the other segmental medullary arteries, usually arises from an inferior intercostal or upper lumbar artery and enters the vertebral canal through the IV foramen at the lower thoracic or upper lumbar level.

The posterior and anterior roots of the spinal nerves and their coverings are supplied by **posterior** and **anterior radicular arteries** (L. *radix*, root), which run along the nerve roots (Figs. 4.28 and 4.29). Most spinal nerve roots and proximal spinal nerves and roots are accompanied by radicular arteries that do not reach the posterior, anterior, or spinal arteries. Segmental medullary arteries occur irregularly in the place of radicular arteries; they are really larger vessels that make it all the way to the spinal arteries. Most radicular arteries are small and supply only the nerve roots; however, some of them assist with the supply of superficial parts of the gray matter in the posterior and anterior horns of the spinal cord.

Veins of the Spinal Cord

In general, the veins draining the spinal cord have a distribution similar to that of the spinal arteries. There are usually three **anterior** and three **posterior spinal veins** (Fig. 4.29*A*). The spinal veins are arranged longitudinally, communicate freely with each other, and are drained by up to 12 **anterior** and **posterior medullary** and **radicular veins**. The veins draining the spinal cord join the internal vertebral (epidural) venous plexus in the epidural space (Fig. 4.20). The internal vertebral venous plexus passes superiorly through the foramen magnum to communicate with dural sinuses and vertebral veins in the cranium (see Chapter 7). The internal vertebral plexus also communicates with the external vertebral venous plexus on the external surface of the vertebrae.

The Bottom Line: Longitudinal spinal arteries supplying the spinal cord are reinforced by irregular and asymmetric segmental medullary arteries that also supply the spinal nerve roots they course along. Radicular arteries supply the remainder of the nerve roots. The veins draining the spinal cord have a distribution and drainage generally reflective of the spinal arteries, although there are normally three longitudinal spinal veins both anteriorly and posteriorly.

Ischemia of the Spinal Cord

The segmental reinforcements of the blood supply to the spinal cord from the segmental medullary arteries are important in supplying blood to the anterior and posterior spinal arteries. Fractures, dislocations, and fracture dislocations may interfere with the blood supply to the spinal cord from the spinal and medullary arteries.

Deficiency of the blood supply (ischemia) of the spinal cord affects its function and can lead to muscle weakness and paralysis. The spinal cord may also suffer circulatory impairment if the segmental medullary arteries, particularly the great anterior segmental medullary artery (of Adamkiewicz), are narrowed by *obstructive arterial disease.* Sometimes the aorta is purposely occluded (cross clamped) during surgery. Patients undergoing such surgeries, and those with ruptured aneurysms of the aorta or occlusion of the great anterior segmental medullary artery, may lose all sensation and voluntary movement inferior to the level of impaired blood supply to the spinal cord (*paraplegia*) secondary to death of neurons in the part of the spinal cord supplied by the anterior spinal artery (Figs. 4.28 and 4.29). Neurons with cell bodies distant from the site of ischemia will also be lost secondary to the degeneration of axons traversing the site. The likelihood of *iatrogenic paraplegia* depends on such factors as the age of the patient, the extent of the disease, and the length of time the aorta is cross clamped (Murray et al., 1992).

When systemic blood pressure drops severely for 3–6 min, blood flow from the segmental medullary arteries to the anterior spinal artery supplying the midthoracic region of the spinal cord may be reduced or stopped. These people may also lose sensation and voluntary movement in the areas supplied by the affected level of the spinal cord.

Spinal Cord Injuries

The vertebral canal varies considerably in size and shape from level to level, particularly in the cervical and lumbar regions. A narrow vertebral canal in the cervical region, into which the spinal cord fits tightly, is potentially dangerous because a minor fracture and/or dislocation of a cervical vertebra may damage the spinal cord. The protrusion of a cervical IV disc into the vertebral canal after a neck injury may cause *spinal cord shock* associated with paralysis inferior to the site of the lesion. In some people, no fracture or dislocation of cervical vertebrae can be found. If the individual dies and an autopsy is ▶

performed, a softening of the spinal cord may be detected at the site of the cervical disc protrusion. Encroachment of the vertebral canal by a protruding IV disc, by swollen ligamenta flava, or resulting from *osteoarthritis of the zygapophysial joints* may exert pressure on one or more of the spinal nerve roots of the cauda equina. Pressure may produce sensory and motor symptoms in the area of distribution of the involved spinal nerve. This group of bone and joint abnormalities, called **lumbar spondylosis** (degenerative joint disease), also causes localized pain and stiffness.

Transection of the spinal cord results in loss of all sensation and voluntary movement inferior to the lesion. Transection of the spinal cord between the following levels will result in the indicated effects:

- C1–C3: The patient has no function below head level; a ventilator is required to maintain respiration (otherwise fatal).

- C4–C5: Respiration occurs, but the patient is quadriplegic (no function of upper or lower limbs).

- C6–C8: The patient experiences a loss of hand and a variable amount of upper limb function; the individual may be able to self-feed or propel a wheelchair.

- T1–T9 (between cervical and lumbosacral enlargements): The individual is paraplegic (paralysis of both lower limbs); the amount of trunk control varies with the height of the lesion.

- T10–L1: The patient has some thigh muscle function, which may allow walking with long leg braces.

- L2–L3: The individual retains most leg muscle function; short leg braces may be required for walking. ⊕

Cervical lordosis
(2° curvature)

Thoracic kyphosis
(1° curvature)

Lumbar lordosis
(2° curvature)

Sacral kyphosis
(1° curvature)

Lateral view

Figure SA4.1. Normal curvatures of back.

Surface Anatomy of the Vertebral Column

When the posterior surface of the trunk is observed, especially in a lateral view, the normal **curvatures of the vertebral column** are especially apparent (Fig. SA4.1). Several of the **spinous processes** can usually be observed, especially when the back is flexed (Fig. SA4.2), most of them can be palpated—even in an obese patient—because fat does not normally accumulate in the midline.

Superiorly, the tip of the **C7 spinous process** is the most superior cervical spinous process that is usually evident superficially. Often, when the patient stands erect, this is the only spinous process visible; hence the name *vertebra prominens*. The *spinous process of C2* is the first bony point that can be felt deeply in the midline inferior to the *external occipital protuberance*, a median projection located a little inferior to the bulging part of the posterior aspect of the head at the junction of the head and neck. C1 has no spinous process, and its small posterior tubercle is neither visible nor palpable. The short bifid spinous processes of the C3–C5 vertebrae may be felt ▶

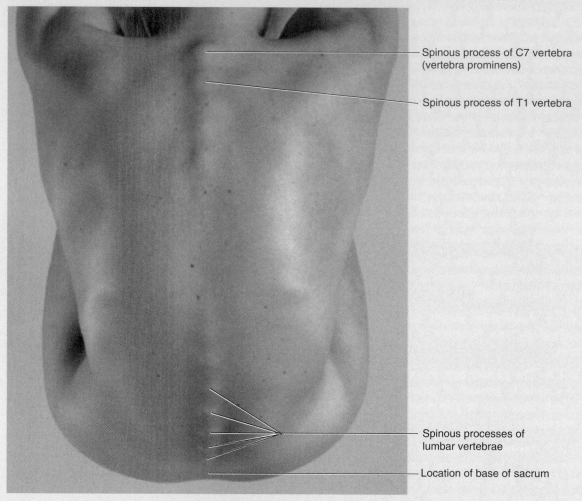

Spinous process of C7 vertebra (vertebra prominens)

Spinous process of T1 vertebra

Spinous processes of lumbar vertebrae

Location of base of sacrum

Posterior view during flexion of vertebral column

Figure SA4.2. Surface anatomy of back during flexion.

in the **nuchal groove** between the neck muscles, but they are not easy to palpate because the cervical curvature, which is concave posteriorly, places them deep to the surface from which they are separated by the nuchal ligament. The bifid *spinous process of C6 vertebra* is easily felt superior to the visible tip of the C7 process when the neck is flexed because of its long process. When the neck and back are flexed, the *spinous processes of the upper thoracic vertebra* may also be seen. If the individual is especially lean, a continuous ridge appears linking their tips—the *supraspinous ligament.*

Although C7 is the most superior process that is visible and readily palpable, the spinous process of T1 may actually be the most prominent. The spinous processes of the other thoracic vertebrae may be obvious in thin people and in others can be identified by superior to inferior palpation beginning at the C7 spinous process, immediately superior to the T1 spinous process. The tips of the *thoracic spinous processes* do not indicate the level of the corresponding vertebral bodies because they overlap (lie at the level of) the vertebra below (Fig. 4.1D). The tips of the spinous pro-

cesses are normally in line with each other, even if the collective line wanders slightly from the midline. A sudden shift in the alignment of adjacent spinous processes may be the result of a unilateral dislocation of a zygapophysial joint; however, slight irregular misalignments may also result from a fracture of the spinous process. The short 12th rib, the lateral end of which can be palpated in the posterior axillary line, can be used to confirm identity of the T12 spinous process.

The *transverse processes of C1* may be felt laterally by deep palpation between the **mastoid processes** (prominences of the temporal bones posterior to the ears) and the angles of the jaws. The *carotid tubercle,* the anterior tubercle of the transverse process of C6 vertebra, may be large enough to be palpable; the *carotid artery* lies anterior to it. In most people, the transverse processes of thoracic vertebrae can be palpated on each side of the spinous processes in the thoracic region; and in lean individuals, the ribs can be palpated from tubercle to angle, at least in the lower back (inferior to the scapula). ▶

The **spinous processes of lumbar vertebrae** are large and easy to observe when the trunk is flexed. They can also be palpated in the **posterior median furrow** (Fig. SA4.3A). The **L2 spinous process** provides an estimate of the position of the inferior end of the spinal cord. A horizontal line joining the highest points of the iliac crests passes through the tip of the L4 spinous process and the L4–L5 IV disc (Fig. SA4.3B). This is a useful landmark when performing a lumbar puncture to obtain a sample of CSF ▶

(A) Posterior view

Spinalis parts of erector spinae muscles

Posterior median furrow

Horizontal line indicating supracristal plane (high points of iliac crests) and crossing L4 spinous process, L4/L5 IV disc

Spinous process of S2

Dimples indicating location of posterior superior iliac spines

Superior part of intergluteal cleft

(B) Posterolateral view

Lumbar spinous processes

S2 spinous process

Median crest

Sacral hiatus

Coccyx

L4/L5 disc

Iliac crest

Iliac tubercle

Posterior superior iliac spine

Sacral triangle

Intergluteal cleft

Figure SA4.3. Surface anatomy of lower back.

(see clinical correlation [blue] box "Lumbar Spinal Puncture," in this chapter).

The **S2 spinous process** lies at the middle of a line drawn between the *posterior superior iliac spines*, indicated by the **skin dimples** formed by the attachment of skin and deep fascia to these spines (Fig. SA4.3*A*). This level indicates the inferior extent of the subarachnoid space (lumbar cistern). The *median crest of the sacrum*, formed by the fusion of the spinous processes of the superior three or four sacral vertebrae, can be felt inferior to the L5 spinous process (Fig. SA4.3*B*). The *sacral triangle* is formed by the lines joining the two posterior superior iliac spines and the **superior part**

of the **intergluteal** (**natal**) **cleft** between the buttocks. The sacral triangle outlining the sacrum is a common area of pain resulting from low back sprains. The *sacral hiatus* can be palpated at the inferior end of the sacrum located in the superior part of the intergluteal cleft (Fig. B4.6).

The transverse processes of thoracic and lumbar vertebrae are covered with thick muscles and may or may not be palpable. The *coccyx* can be palpated in the intergluteal cleft, inferior to the apex of the sacral triangle. The *apex* (*tip*) *of the coccyx* can be palpated approximately 2.5 cm posterosuperior to the anus. Clinically, the coccyx is examined with a gloved finger in the anal canal. ○

Muscles of the Back

Most body weight lies anterior to the vertebral column, especially in obese people; consequently, the many strong muscles attached to the spinous and transverse processes are necessary to support and move the vertebral column. There are two major groups of muscles in the back. The **extrinsic back muscles** include *superficial* and *intermediate muscles* that produce and control limb and respiratory movements, respectively. The *intrinsic (deep) back muscles* include muscles that specifically act on the vertebral column, producing its movements and maintaining posture.

Extrinsic Back Muscles

The **superficial extrinsic back muscles** (trapezius, latissimus dorsi, levator scapulae, and rhomboids) connect the upper limbs to the trunk and produce and control limb movements (Fig. 4.30*A*; see also Chapter 6). Although located in the back region, for the most part these muscles receive their nerve supply from the anterior rami of cervical nerves and act on the upper limb. The trapezius receives its motor fibers from a cranial nerve, the spinal accessory nerve (CN XI).

The **intermediate extrinsic back muscles** (serratus posterior) are thin muscles, commonly designated superficial respiratory muscles, but are more likely proprioceptive rather than motor in function (Vilensky et al., 2001). They are described with muscles of the thoracic wall (see Chapter 1). The **serratus posterior superior** lies deep to the rhomboids, and the **serratus posterior inferior** lies deep to the latissimus dorsi. Both serratus muscles are innervated by intercostal nerves, the superior by the first four intercostals and the inferior by the last four.

Intrinsic Back Muscles

The **intrinsic back muscles** (*muscles of back proper,* deep back muscles) are innervated by the posterior rami of spinal nerves and act to maintain posture and control movements of the vertebral column (Figs. 4.30*B* and 4.31). These muscles, which extend from the pelvis to the cranium, are enclosed by deep fascia that attaches medially to the nuchal ligament, the tips of the spinous processes of the vertebrae, the supraspinous ligament, and the median crest of the sacrum. The fascia attaches laterally to the cervical and lumbar transverse processes and to the angles of the ribs. The thoracic and lumbar parts of the deep fascia constitute the **thoracolumbar fascia**. It extends laterally from the spinous processes and forms a thin covering for the deep muscles in the thoracic region and a strong thick covering for muscles in the lumbar region. The deep back muscles are grouped into superficial, intermediate, and deep layers according to their relationship to the surface (Tables 4.5–4.7).

Superficial Layer of Intrinsic Back Muscles

The **splenius muscles** (L. *musculi splenii*) are thick and flat and lie on the lateral and posterior aspects of the neck, covering the vertical muscles somewhat like a bandage, which explains their name (L. *splenion,* bandage) (Fig. 4.31). The splenii arise from the midline and extend superolaterally to the cervical vertebrae (**splenius cervicis**) and cranium (**splenius capitis**). The splenii cover and hold the deep neck muscles in position. Information on the attachments, nerve supply, and actions of the superficial layer of intrinsic muscles is provided in Table 4.5.

Intermediate Layer of Intrinsic Back Muscles

The **erector spinae muscles** lie in a "groove" on each side of the vertebral column between the spinous processes centrally and the angles of the ribs laterally (Fig. 4.31). The massive erector spinae is the chief extensor of the vertebral column and is divided into three columns: The **iliocostalis** forms the lateral column, the **longissimus** forms the intermediate column, and the **spinalis** forms the medial column. Each column is divided regionally into three parts according to the superior attachments (e.g., iliocostalis lumborum, iliocostalis thoracis, and iliocostalis cervicis). The common origin of the three erector spinae columns is through a broad tendon that attaches inferiorly to the posterior part of the iliac crest, the posterior aspect of the sacrum, the sacroiliac ligaments, and

(cont'd on page 537)

Figure 4.30. Muscles of back. A. The superficial extrinsic muscles are shown. The trapezius is reflected on the left to show the spinal accessory nerve (CN XI), coursing on its deep surface, and the levator scapulae and rhomboid muscles. These muscles help attach the upper limb to the trunk. **B.** This transverse section of part of the back shows the location of the intrinsic back muscles and the layers of fascia associated with them. The combined posterior aponeuroses of the transverse abdominal and internal oblique muscles splits into two strong sheets, the middle and posterior layers of the thoracolumbar fascia, which enclose the intrinsic back muscles.

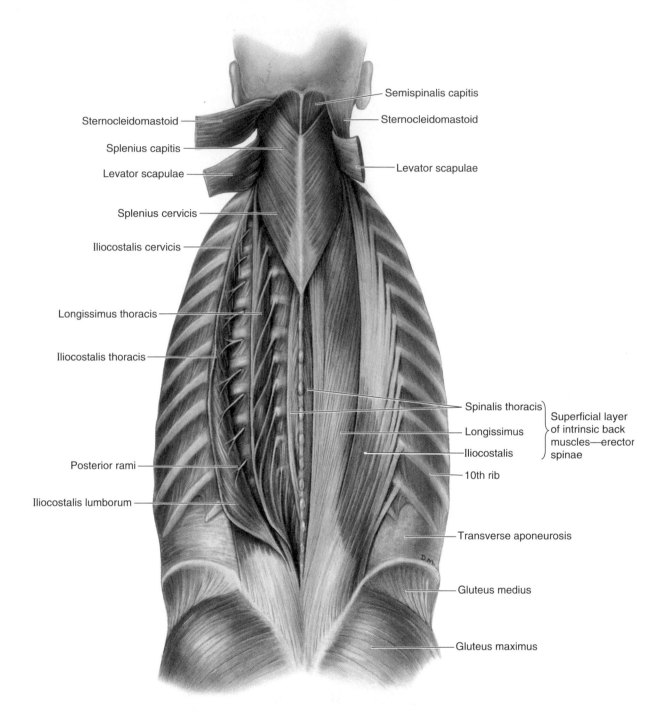

Figure 4.31. Superficial and intermediate layers of intrinsic back muscles: splenius and erector spinae. The sternocleidomastoid and levator scapulae muscles are reflected to reveal the splenius capitis and splenius cervicis muscles. On the right side, the erector spinae is undisturbed (in situ) and shows the three columns of this massive muscle. On the left side, the spinalis muscle, the thinnest and most medial of the erector spinae columns, is displayed as a separate muscle by reflecting the longissimus and iliocostalis columns of the erector spinae.

Table 4.5. Superficial Layer of Intrinsic Back Muscles

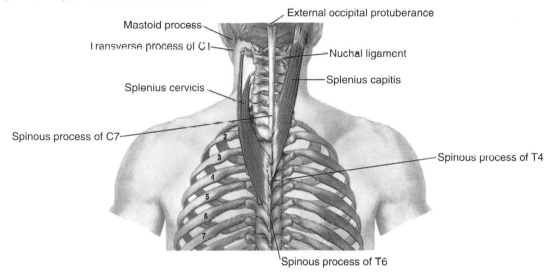

Muscle	Origin	Insertion	Nerve supply	Main action(s)
Splenius	Arises from nuchal ligament and spinous processes of C7–T3 or T4 vertebrae	*Splenius capitis:* fibers run superolaterally to mastoid process of temporal bone and lateral third of superior nuchal line of occipital bone *Splenius cervicis:* tubercles of transverse processes of C1–C3 or C4 vertebrae	Posterior rami of spinal nerves	*Acting alone:* laterally flex neck and rotate head to side of active muscles *Acting together:* extend head and neck

the sacral and inferior lumbar spinous processes. The erector spinae are often referred to as the "long muscles" of the back. In general, they are dynamic (motion-producing) muscles, acting bilaterally to extend (straighten) the flexed trunk. Information on the attachments, nerve supply, and actions of the intermediate layer of intrinsic muscles is provided in Table 4.6.

Deep Layer of Intrinsic Back Muscles

Deep to the erector spinae is an obliquely disposed group of much shorter muscles called the **transversospinal muscle group** (L. *transversospinalis*), consisting of the semispinalis, multifidus, and rotatores. These muscles originate from transverse processes of vertebrae and pass to spinous processes of more superior vertebrae. They occupy the "gutter" between the transverse and the spinous processes and are attached to these processes, the laminae between them, and the ligaments linking them together (Fig. 4.32).

The **semispinalis** is the superficial member of the group. As its name indicates, it arises from approximately half of the vertebral column (spine) (Fig. 4.31). It is divided into three parts according to the superior attachments: **semispinalis capitis, semispinalis thoracis,** and **semispinalis cervicis**. Semispinalis capitis is responsible for the longitudinal bulge in the back of the neck near the median plane. The **multifidus** is the middle layer of the group and consists of short, triangular muscular bundles that are thickest in the lumbar region (Fig. 4.32*A*). The **rotatores,** or rotator muscles, are the deepest of the three layers of transversospinal muscles and are best

developed in the thoracic region. Details concerning the attachments, innervation, and action of the transversospinalis group of the deep layer of intrinsic back muscles are provided in Table 4.7.

The **interspinal** (L. *interspinales*), **intertransverse** (L. *intertransversarii*), and **elevators of ribs** (L. *levatores costarum*) are minor deep back muscles that are poorly developed in the thoracic region. The interspinal and intertransverse muscles connect spinous and transverse processes, respectively. The elevators of the ribs represent the posterior intertransverse muscles of the neck. Details concerning the attachments, nerve supply, and actions of the minor muscles of the deep layer of intrinsic muscles are provided in Table 4.7.

Principal Muscles Producing Movements of the Intervertebral Joints

The principal muscles producing movements of the cervical, thoracic, and lumbar IV joints are summarized in Tables 4.8 and 4.9. Many of the muscles acting on the cervical vertebrae are specifically discussed in Chapter 8. The back muscles are relatively inactive in the stand-easy position, but they (especially the shorter deep layer of intrinsic muscles) act as static postural muscles (fixators, or steadiers) of the vertebral column, maintaining tension and stability as required for the erect posture. Note in Table 4.9 that all movements of the IV joints (i.e., all movements of the vertebral column) except pure extension involve or are solely produced by the *concentric contraction* of abdominal muscles. However, bear in mind that in these as in all move-

Table 4.6. Intermediate Layer of Intrinsic Back Muscles

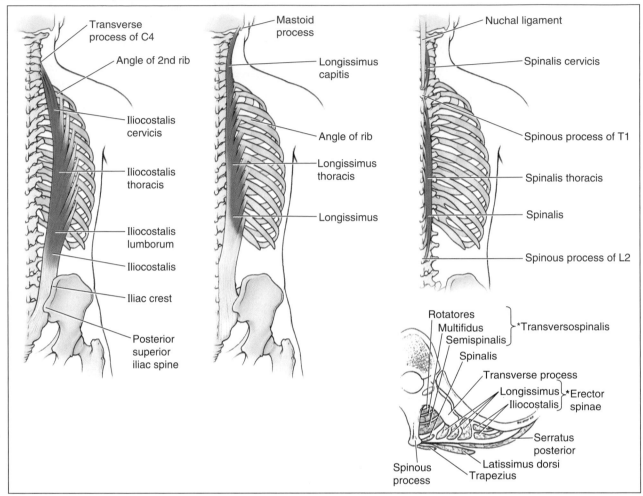

Muscle	Origin	Insertion	Nerve supply	Main action(s)
Erector spinae Iliocostalis Longissimus Spinalis	Arises by a broad tendon from posterior part of iliac crest, posterior surface of sacrum, sacroiliac ligaments, sacral and inferior lumbar spinous processes, and supraspinous ligament	*Iliocostalis:* lumborum, thoracis, cervicis; fibers run superiorly to angles of lower ribs and cervical transverse processes *Longissimus:* thoracis, cervicis, capitis; fibers run superiorly to ribs between tubercles and angles to transverse processes in thoracic and cervical regions, and to mastoid process of temporal bone *Spinalis:* thoracis, cervicis, capitis; fibers run superiorly to spinous processes in the upper thoracic region and to cranium	Posterior rami of spinal nerves	*Acting bilaterally:* extend vertebral column and head; as back is flexed, control movement by gradually lengthening their fibers *Acting unilaterally:* laterally flex vertebral column

ments, the *eccentric contraction* (controlled relaxation) of the antagonist muscles is vital to smooth, controlled movement (see "Muscle Tissue and the Muscular System" in the Introduction). Thus it is actually the interaction of anterior (abdominal) and posterior (back) muscles (as well as the contralateral pairs of each) that provides the stability and produces motion of the axial skeleton, much like guy (guide) wires support a pole. Often chronic back strain

(such as that caused by excessive lumbar lordosis) results from imbalance in this support (lack of tonus of abdominal muscles in the case of lordosis). To restore that balance, the patient may need to exercise or eliminate excessive, unevenly distributed weight.

Smaller muscles generally have higher densities of **muscle spindles** (sensors of proprioception that are interdigitated among the muscle's fibers) than do large muscles. It was as-

(*cont'd on page 543*)

Table 4.7. Deep Layers of Intrinsic Back Muscles

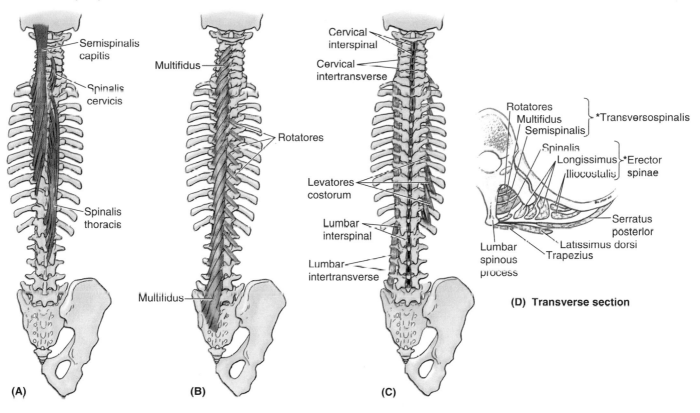

Posterior views

Muscle	Origin	Insertion	Nerve supply	Main action(s)
Deep layer				
Transversospinal Semispinalis Multifidus Rotatores (brevis and longus)	Transverse processes *Semispinalis:* arises from transverse processes of C4–T12 vertebrae *Multifidus:* arises from posterior sacrum, posterior superior iliac spine of ilium, aponeurosis of erector spinae, sacroiliac ligaments, mammillary processes of lumbar vertebrae, transverse processes of T1–T3, articular processes of C4–C7 *Rotatores:* arise from transverse processes of vertebrae; best developed in thoracic region	Spinous processes of more superior vertebrae *Semispinalis:* thoracis, cervicis, capitis; fibers run superomedially to occipital bone and spinous processes in thoracic and cervical regions, spanning 4–6 segments *Multifidus:* thickest in lumbar region; fibers pass obliquely superomedially to entire length of spinous processes of vertebrae, located 2–4 segments superior to origin *Rotatores:* fibers pass superomedially to attach to junction of lamina and transverse process or spinous process of vertebra immediately (brevis) or 2 segments (longus) superior to vertebra of origin	Posterior rami of spinal nerves	Extension *Semispinalis:* extends head and thoracic and cervical regions of vertebral column and rotates them contralaterally *Multifidus:* stabilizes vertebrae during local movements of vertebral column *Rotatores:* stabilize vertebrae and assist with local extension and rotatory movements of vertebral column; may function as organs of proprioception
Minor deep layer				
Interspinales	Superior surfaces of spinous processes of cervical and lumbar vertebrae	Inferior surfaces of spinous processes of vertebra superior to vertebra of origin	Posterior rami of spinal nerves	Aid in extension and rotation of vertebral column
Intertransversarii	Transverse processes of cervical and lumbar vertebrae	Transverse processes of adjacent vertebrae	Posterior and anterior rami of spinal nerves[a]	Aid in lateral flexion of vertebral column; acting bilaterally, stabilize vertebral column
Levatores costarum	Tips of transverse processes of C7 and T1–T11 vertebrae	Pass inferolaterally and insert on rib between tubercle and angle	Posterior rami of C8–T11 spinal nerves	Elevate ribs, assisting respiration; assist with lateral flexion of vertebral column

[a]Most back muscles are innervated by posterior rami of spinal nerves, but a few are innervated by anterior rami. Anterior intertransverse muscles of the cervical region are supplied by anterior rami.

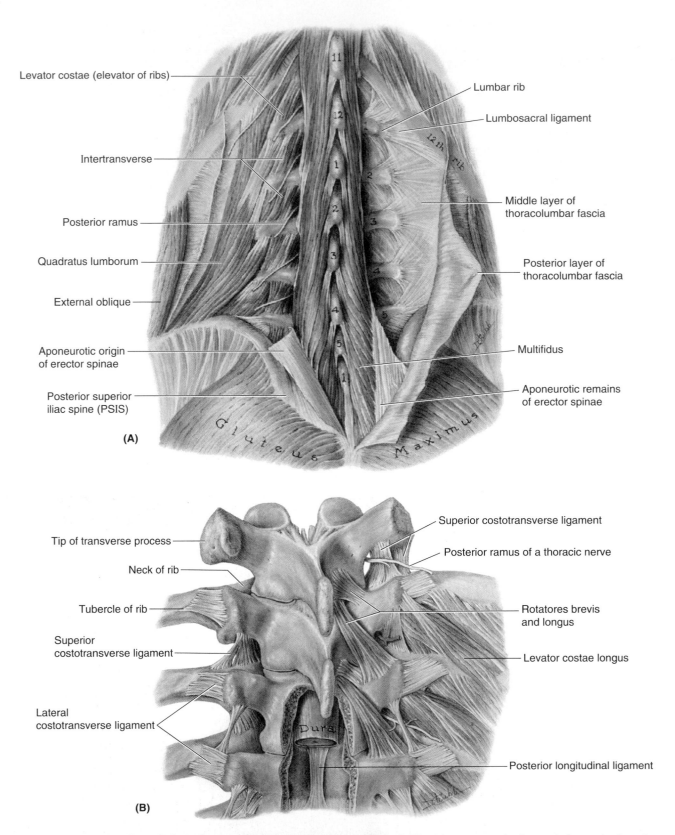

Figure 4.32. Muscles of deep layer of intrinsic back muscles. A. The transversospinal muscle group is deep to the erector spinae. It consists chiefly of a large number of small muscles that run obliquely upward and medially from transverse to spinous processes. The multifidus and quadratus lumborum muscles are shown as is the thoracolumbar fascia. The short lumbar rib is articulating with the transverse process of L1 vertebra. This common variation does not usually cause a problem; however, those unfamiliar with its possible presence may think it is a fractured transverse process. **B.** Deeper dissection showing the rotatores and costotransverse ligaments. Two of the three sets of costotransverse ligaments are seen: superior and lateral. The (medial) costotransverse ligaments extend between the neck of the rib and the transverse process of the vertebra of the same number (not shown). The levator muscles, which elevate the ribs, represent the posterior intertransverse muscles in the thoracic region.

Table 4.8. Principal Muscles Producing Movement of the Cervical Intervertebral Joints

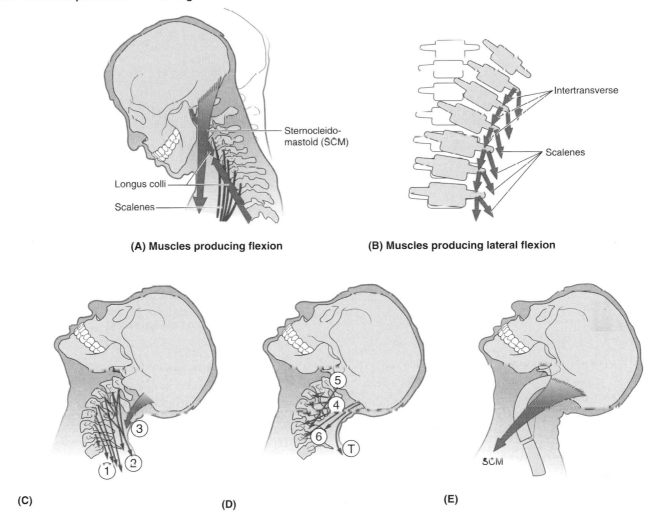

(A) Muscles producing flexion

(B) Muscles producing lateral flexion

B–D = Muscles Producing Extension

Flexion	Extension	Lateral bending	Rotation (not shown)

Bilateral action of
   Longus coli
   Scalene
   Sternocleidomastoid
	Deep neck muscles
	1, semispinalis cervicis and iliocostalis cervicis
	2, splenius cervicis and levator scapulae
	3, splenius capitis
	4, multifidus
	5, longissimus capitis
	6, semispinalis capitis
	T, trapezius
		Unilateral action of Iliocostalis cervicis
		   Longissimus capitis and cervics
		   Splenius capitis and cervicis
		   Intertransverse and scalenes
			Unilateral action of
			   Rotatores
			   Semispinalis capitis and cervicis
			   Multifidus
			   Splenius cervicis

Table 4.9. Principal Muscles Producing Movements of the Thoracic and Lumbar Intervertebral (IV) Joints

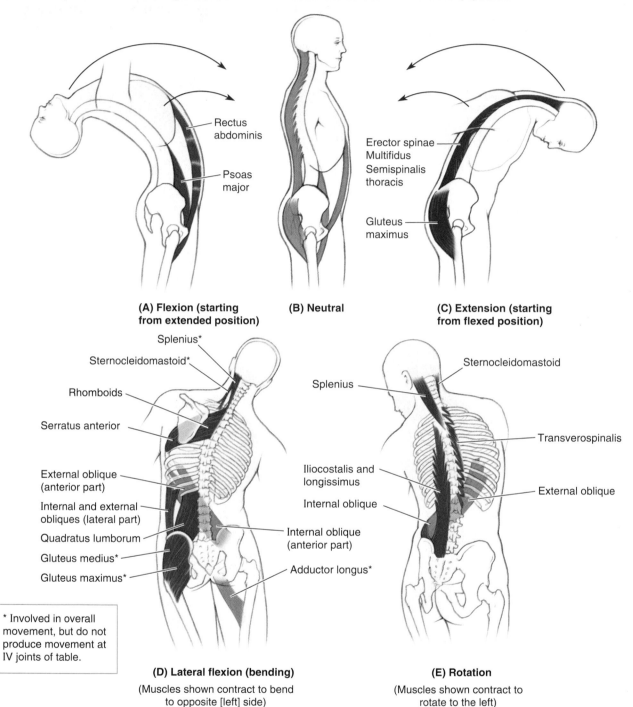

(A) Flexion (starting from extended position)

(B) Neutral

(C) Extension (starting from flexed position)

Rectus abdominis
Psoas major

Erector spinae
Multifidus
Semispinalis thoracis
Gluteus maximus

Splenius*
Sternocleidomastoid*
Rhomboids
Serratus anterior
External oblique (anterior part)
Internal and external obliques (lateral part)
Quadratus lumborum
Gluteus medius*
Gluteus maximus*

Internal oblique (anterior part)
Adductor longus*

Sternocleidomastoid
Splenius
Transverospinalis
Iliocostalis and longissimus
Internal oblique
External oblique

* Involved in overall movement, but do not produce movement at IV joints of table.

(D) Lateral flexion (bending)
(Muscles shown contract to bend to opposite [left] side)

(E) Rotation
(Muscles shown contract to rotate to the left)

Flexion	Extension	Lateral bending	Rotation (not shown)

Bilateral action of
  Rectus abdominis
  Psoas major
  Gravity
	Bilateral action of
	  Erector spinae
	  Multifidus
	  Semispinalis thoracis
		Unilateral action of
		  Iliocostalis thoracis and lumborum
		  Longissimus thoracis
		  Multifidus
		  External and internal oblique
		  Quadratus lumborum
		  Rhomboids
		  Serratus anterior
			Unilateral action of
			  Rotatores
			  Multifidus
			  Iliocostalis
			  Longissimus
			  External oblique acting synchronously
			    with opposite internal oblique
			  Splenius thoracis
			(See bracket to rotatores and multifidus:
			Transversospinalis)

sumed that the higher concentration of spindles occurred because small muscles produce the most precise movements, such as fine postural movements or manipulation and, therefore, require more proprioceptive feedback. The movements described for small muscles are deduced from the location of their attachments and the direction of the muscle fibers and from activity measured by electromyography as movements are performed. Muscles such as the rotatores, however, are so small and are placed in positions of such relatively poor mechanical advantage that their ability to produce the movements described is somewhat questionable. Furthermore, such small muscles are often redundant to other larger mus-

cles that have superior mechanical advantage. Hence it has been proposed (Buxton and Peck, 1989) that the smaller muscles of small–large muscle pairs function more as "kinesiological monitors," or organs of proprioception and that the larger muscles are the producers of motion.

THE BOTTOM LINE: Superficial (extrinsic) back muscles serve upper limbs. Deep (intrinsic) back muscles provide primarily extension and proprioception for posture and work synergistically with the muscles of the anterolateral abdominal wall to produce movements of the trunk.

Back Strains and Sprains

Adequate warmup and stretching may prevent many back strains and sprains. **Back sprain** is an injury in which only ligamentous tissue, or the attachment of ligament to bone, is involved, without dislocation or fracture. It results from excessively strong contractions related to movements of the vertebral column, such as excessive extension or rotation. **Back strain** is a common back problem in people who participate in sports; it results from overly strong muscular contraction. Back strain involves some degree of stretching or microscopic tearing of muscle fibers. The muscles usually involved are those producing movements of the lumbar IV joints, especially the erector spinae columns. If the weight is not

properly balanced on the vertebral column, strain is exerted on the muscles. This is undoubtedly a common cause of low back pain.

Using the back as a lever when lifting puts an enormous strain on the vertebral column and its ligaments and muscles. These strains can be minimized if the lifter crouches, holds the back as straight as possible, and uses the muscles of the buttocks and lower limbs to assist with the lifting. As a protective mechanism, the back muscles go into **spasm** after an injury or in response to inflammation of structures in the back, such as ligaments. A spasm is a sudden involuntary contraction of one or more muscle groups. Spasms are attended by cramps, pain, and interference with function, producing involuntary movement and distortion. ✪

Surface Anatomy of the Back Muscles

In the midline of the back there is a **posterior median furrow** that overlies the tips of the spinous processes of the vertebrae (Fig. SA4.4). The furrow is continuous superiorly with the **nuchal groove** in the neck. The posterior median furrow is deepest in the lower thoracic and upper lumbar regions. The **erector spinae** produce prominent vertical bulges on each side of the furrow. In the lumbar region, the erector spinae are readily palpable, and their lateral borders are indicated by shallow grooves in the skin. When the individual is standing, the lumbar

spinous processes may be indicated by depressions in the skin. These processes usually become visible when the vertebral column is flexed (Fig. SA4.2). The posterior median furrow ends in the flattened triangular area covering the sacrum and is replaced inferiorly by the **intergluteal cleft.**

When the upper limbs are elevated, the scapulae move laterally on the thoracic wall, making the **rhomboid** and *teres major* muscles visible. These muscles are described in Chapter 6. The superficially located **trapezius** and **latissimus dorsi** muscles connecting the upper limbs to the vertebral column are also clearly visible. ▶

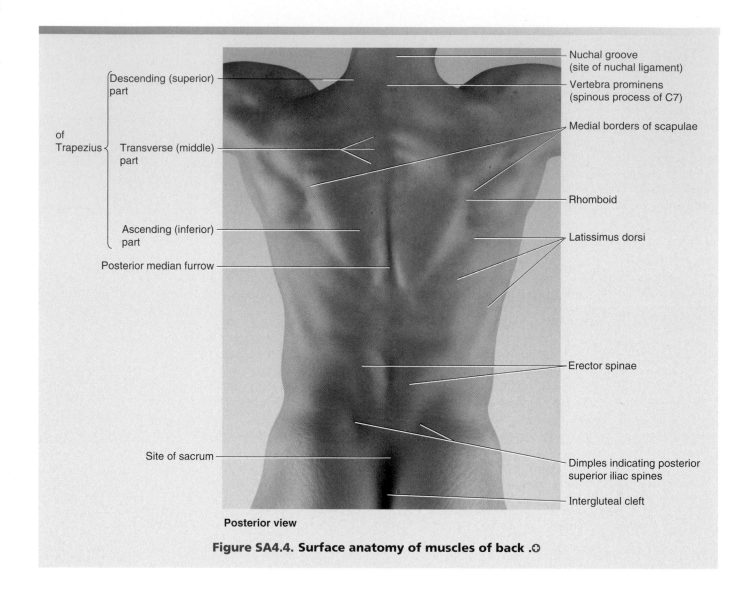

Posterior view

Figure SA4.4. Surface anatomy of muscles of back .☉

Suboccipital and Deep Neck Muscles

The **suboccipital region**, the superior part of the posterior cervical region, is the triangular area inferior to the occipital region of the head, including the posterior aspects of vertebrae C1 and C2. The four small muscles of the suboccipital region lie deep to the trapezius and semispinalis capitis muscles and consist of two rectus capitis posterior (major and minor) and two obliquus muscles. All four muscles are innervated by the *posterior ramus of C1,* the **suboccipital nerve.** The nerve emerges as the vertebra artery courses deeply between the occipital bone and the atlas (vertebra C1) within the **suboccipital triangle.** Details concerning the boundaries and contents of this triangle and the attachments of the suboccipital muscles are provided and illustrated in Table 4.10.

Note that the **inferior oblique of the head** (L. *obliquus capitis inferior*) is the only "capitis" muscle that has no attachment to the cranium. These muscles are mainly postural muscles, but actions are typically described for each muscle in terms of producing movement of the head. The muscles are considered to act on the head directly or indirectly (explaining the inclusion of *capitis* in their names) by extending it on vertebra C1 and rotating it on vertebrae C1 and C2. However, recall the discussion of the small member of the small–large muscle pair functioning as a kinesiological monitor for the sense of proprioception. The principal muscles producing movements of the craniovertebral joints are summarized in Tables 4.11 and 4.12, and the nerves of the suboccipital region and posterior neck are summarized in Table 4.13.

Table 4.10. Suboccipital Muscles and Suboccipital Triangle

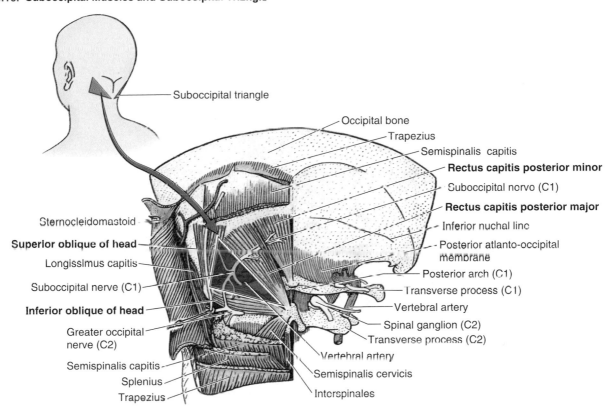

Suboccipital muscles		
Muscle	**Origin**	**Insertion**
Rectus capitis posterior major	Spinous process of vertebra C2	Lateral part of inferior nuchal line of occipital bone
Rectus capitis posterior minor	Posterior tubercle of posterior arch of vertebra C1	Medial part of inferior nuchal line of occipital bone
Inferior oblique of head (L. *m. obliquus capitis inferior*)	Spinous process of vertebra C2	Transverse process of vertebra C1
Superior oblique of head (L. *m. obliquus capitis superior*)	Transverse process of vertebra C1	Occipital bone between superior and inferior nuchal lines

Suboccipital triangle	
Aspect of Triangle	**Structures**
Superomedial boundary	Rectus capitis posterior major
Superolateral boundary	Superior oblique of head
Inferolateral boundary	Inferior oblique of head
Floor	Posterior atlanto-occipital membrane and posterior arch of vertebra C1
Roof	Semispinalis capitis
Contents	Vertebral artery and suboccipital nerve

Table 4.11. Principal Muscles Producing Movement of the Atlanto-Occipital Joints

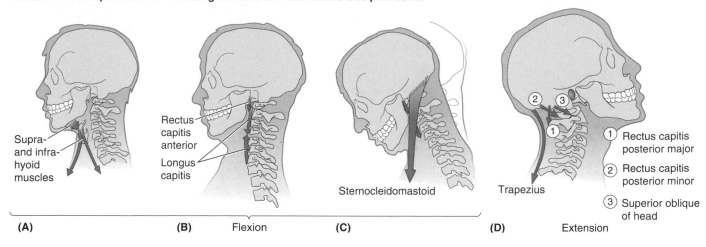

Flexion	Extension	Lateral bending (not shown)
Longus capitis Rectus capitis anterior Anterior fibers of sternocleidomastoid Suprahyoid and infrahyoid muscles	Rectus capitis posterior major and minor Superior oblique of head Splenius capitis Longissimus capitis Trapezius	Sternocleidomastoid Superior oblique of head Rectus capitis lateralis Longissimus capitis Splenius capitis

Table 4.12. Principal Muscles Producing Movement of the Atlanto-Axial Joints[a]

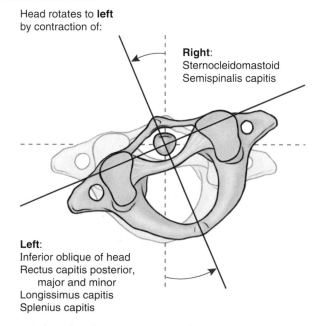

Head rotates to **left** by contraction of:

Right:
Sternocleidomastoid
Semispinalis capitis

Left:
Inferior oblique of head
Rectus capitis posterior, major and minor
Longissimus capitis
Splenius capitis

Ipsilateral[b]	Contralateral
Inferior oblique of head Rectus capitis posterior, major and minor Longissimus capitis Splenius capitis	Sternocleidomastoid Semispinalis capitis

[a] Rotation is the specialized movement at these joints. Movement of one joint involves the other.
[b] Same side to which head is rotated.

Table 4.13. Nerves of the Suboccipital Region/Posterior Neck

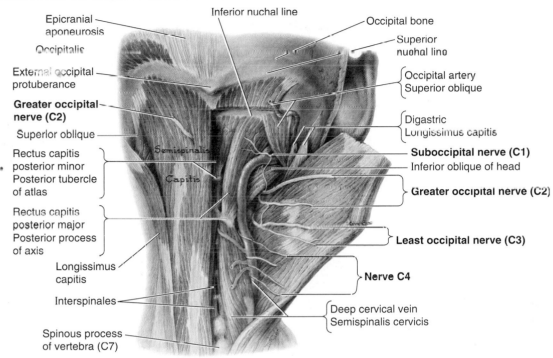

Nerve	Origin	Course	Distribution
Suboccipital	Posterior ramus of spinal nerve C1	Runs between cranium and C1 vertebra to reach suboccipital triangle	Muscles of suboccipital triangle
Greater occipital	Posterior ramus of spinal nerve C2	Emerges inferior to inferior oblique and ascends to posterior scalp	Skin over neck and occipital bone
Lesser occipital	Anterior rami of spinal nerves C2–C3	Passes directly to skin	Skin of superior posterolateral neck and scalp posterior to ear
Posterior rami, nerves C3–C7	Posterior rami of spinal nerves C3–C7	Pass segmentally to muscles and skin	Intrinsic muscles of back and overlying skin (adjacent to vertebral column)

Reduced Blood Supply to the Brainstem

The winding course of the vertebral arteries through the transverse foramina of the transverse processes of the cervical vertebrae and through the suboccipital triangles becomes clinically significant when blood flow through these arteries is reduced, as occurs with *arteriosclerosis*. Under these conditions, prolonged turning of the head, as occurs when backing up a motor vehicle, may cause light-headedness, dizziness, and other symptoms from the interference with the blood supply to the brainstem. ✪

Medical Imaging of the Back
Radiography

Radiographical examination of the vertebral column usually requires both AP and lateral views. The anatomical features visible in the regions of the vertebral column are illustrated and described in Figures 4.33–4.36. Conventional radiographs are excellent for high contrast structures such as bone. The advent of *digital radiography* allows improved contrast resolution.

Vertebral body osteoporosis is a common metabolic bone disease that is often detected during routine radiographical studies. Vertical striping may become apparent, reflecting the loss of the horizontal supporting trabeculae and thickening of the vertical struts (Fig. 4.37*A*). Radiographs taken during early to moderate ▶

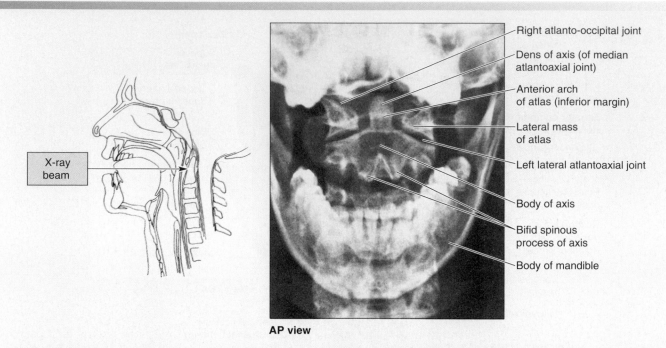

Right atlanto-occipital joint

Dens of axis (of median atlantoaxial joint)

Anterior arch of atlas (inferior margin)

Lateral mass of atlas

Left lateral atlantoaxial joint

Body of axis

Bifid spinous process of axis

Body of mandible

X-ray beam

AP view

Figure 4.33. Radiograph of superior part of cervical region of vertebral column. As shown in the orientation drawing, the radiograph was taken through the open mouth. The lateral atlantoaxial joint and the body of the axis (C2 vertebra), with its dens projecting superiorly between the lateral masses of the atlas (C1 vertebra), are seen.

osteoporosis demonstrate demineralization, which is evident as diminished radiodensity of the trabecular (spongy) bone of the vertebral bodies, causing the thinned cortical bone to appear relatively prominent (Fig. 4.37*B*). Radiographs in later stages may reveal vertebral collapse (compression fractures) and increased thoracic kyphosis (Fig. 4.37*C*). Vertebral body osteoporosis occurs in all vertebrae but is most common in thoracic vertebrae and is an especially common finding in postmenopausal females.

Myelography

Myelography is a radiopaque contrast study that allows visualization of the spinal cord and spinal nerve roots (Fig. 4.38). In this procedure, CSF is withdrawn by lumbar puncture and replaced with a contrast material injected into the spinal subarachnoid space. This technique shows the extent of the subarachnoid space and its extensions around the spinal nerve roots within the dural root sheaths. High-resolution MRI has largely supplanted myelography (McCormick et al., 2000).

Computed Tomography

CT differentiates between the white and gray matter of the brain and spinal cord. It has also improved the radiological assessment of fractures of the vertebral column, particularly in determining the degree of compression of the spinal cord (McCormick, 2000). CT images of the vertebral column are used to detect fractures, lesions, and congenital anomalies. The dense vertebrae attenuate much of the X-ray beam and, therefore, appear white on the scans (Fig. 4.39). The IV discs have a higher density than the surrounding adipose tissue in the epidural space and the CSF in the subarachnoid space. Herniations of the IV discs are thus recognizable in CT images, as are displaced fragments of the IV discs.

Magnetic Resonance Imaging

MRI, like CT, is a computer-assisted imaging procedure, but X-rays are not used, as with CT. MRI produces extremely good images of the vertebral column, spinal cord, and CSF (Fig.4.40). Until relatively recently, a ▶

Uncovertebral joint

Superior lip of
vertebral body C5

Pedicle

1st rib

Transverse process
of T2

Clavicle

Spinous process
of T2

C3

C7

(A) AP view

Dens (odontoid
process)

Posterior arch
of atlas (C1)

Angles of
mandible

Transverse
process

Hyoid bone

Inferior articular
process

Superior articular
process

Zygapophysial
(facet) joint

Spinous process
of C7

A

2

3

4

5

6

7

(B) Right lateral view

Figure 4.34. Radiographs of cervical region of vertebral column. A. The bifid spinous processes of C2–C6 vertebrae are overlapped by the radiotranslucency (*black shadow*) of the trachea. *Arrowheads,* margins of the column of air in the trachea; *boxed area,* the column of articular processes and the overlapping transverse processes. **B.** The anterior arch of the atlas (*A*) lies in a plane that is anterior to the curved line joining the anterior borders of the vertebral bodies. The bodies of the C2–C7 vertebrae are numbered. Observe also the long spinous process of the vertebra prominens (C7). (Courtesy of Dr. J. Heslin, Toronto, Ontario, Canada.)

Scapulae

Vertebra T5

Radiologic "disc space"
(intervertebral disc)

Intervertebral foramen

Pedicle

Head of 10th rib
(note position
of attachment
on vertebral body)

Spinous process

Articular facets { inferior
                  { superior

11th rib head

Body of vertebra T12

12th ribs

Right lateral view

Figure 4.35. Radiograph of thoracic region of vertebral column. In the lateral view of the thoracic vertebrae, the uniform vertebral bodies and radiographic disc "spaces" (caused by the radiolucency of the IV discs) are evident, except for the superior two or three, which are obscured by shoulder structures. The vertebral arch components, such as the transverse and spinous processes, are obscured by the posterior aspects of the overlapping ribs.

disadvantage of MRI was that the patient had to remain motionless in the scanner for long periods; however, new technologies have markedly decreased this time. MRI clearly demonstrates the components of the IV discs and shows their relationship to the vertebral bodies and longitudinal ligaments. Herniations of the nucleus pulposus and its relationship to the spinal nerve roots are also well defined (Fig. 4.41). MRI is the imaging procedure of choice for evaluating IV disc disorders and is gradually replacing myelography and CT for the study of these disorders (McCormick, 2000). MRI can demonstrate spinal cord or nerve root compression and indicate the degree of degenerative change within the IV disc (Fig. 4.37). MRI is also an ideal screening procedure for the differential diagnosis of structural disorders affecting the spinal cord and spinal nerve roots. ⊙

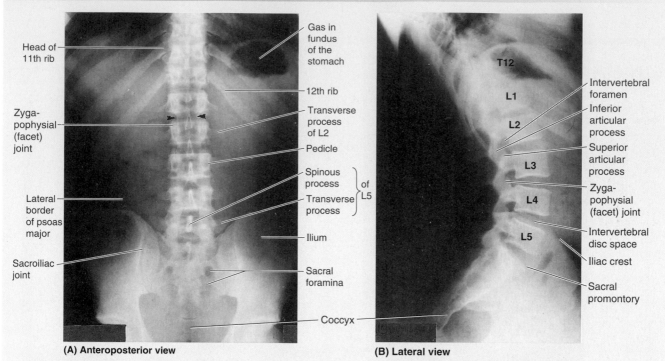

(A) Anteroposterior view

(B) Lateral view

Figure 4.36. Radiographs of inferior thoracic and lumbosacral regions of vertebral column. A. Spinous processes in the midline overlap the vertebral canal (columnar shadow between *arrowheads*), containing the spinal cord and spinal meninges (not visible). The coccyx is not well shown because of its oblique position relative to the film/detector. In addition, gas and feces in the rectum and sigmoid colon tend to obscure the coccyx. (Courtesy of Dr. J. Heslin, Toronto, Ontario, Canada.) **B.** The larger bodies of the lumbar vertebrae and the IV disc spaces, the IV foramina, and the angulation at the lumbosacral junction producing the sacral promontory are evident. The lumbar IV discs are wedge shaped, especially the L5–S1 disc. The zygapophysial (facet) joint between the superior articular process of vertebra L4 and the inferior articular process of vertebra L3 is clearly seen.

(A) Right lateral view

(B) Left lateral view

(C) Left lateral view

Figure 4.37. Effects of osteoporosis on vertebral column. A. A loss of the horizontal trabeculae with thickening of the vertical trabeculae produces a pattern of vertical striation in the vertebral bodies, indicating early to moderate osteoporosis. **B.** Later, the striated pattern is lost as the continued loss of spongy bone produces uniform radiolucency (less white, more "transparent"). In contrast, the cortical bone of the vertebral endplates, while thinned, appears relatively prominent. **C.** Osteoporotic thoracic region of the vertebral column demonstrates excessive thoracic kyphosis, a result of the evident collapse of the vertebral bodies, which have become wedge-shaped (*W*), planar (*P*), and biconcave (*B*).

Pedicle

L3 vertebral body

Dye in dural root sheaths
(extensions of subarachnoid
space around spinal
nerve roots)

Cauda equina

Lumbar cistern
within dural sac

AP view

Figure 4.38. Myelogram of lumbar region of vertebral column. Contrast medium was injected into the lumbar cistern. The lateral projections indicate the extensions of the subarachnoid space in the dural root sheaths around the spinal nerve roots.

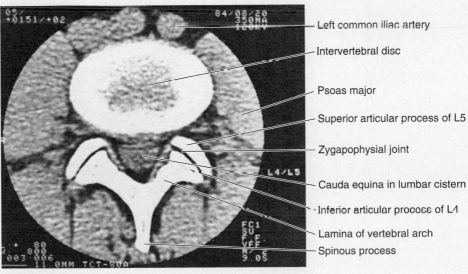

Left common iliac artery

Intervertebral disc

Psoas major

Superior articular process of L5

Zygapophysial joint

Cauda equina in lumbar cistern

Inferior articular process of L4

Lamina of vertebral arch

Spinous process

Inferior view

Figure 4.39. Transverse CT image of L4–L5 IV disc and vertebral arch. The two parts of the IV disc (anulus fibrosis and nucleus pulposus) are apparent. The superior articular processes of the inferior vertebra (L5) "grip" the inferior articular processes of the superior vertebra (L4), disallowing rotatory movements but permitting flexion and extension. The cauda equina is seen running through the lumbar cistern within the vertebral canal; it is composed of all the spinal nerves inferior to the conus medullaris.

- Cerebellum
- Medulla
- Foramen magnum
- Posterior arch of atlas
- Dens of axis
- Subarachnoid space
- Spinal cord
- Esophagus
- Trachea
- Nucleus pulposus of intervertebral disc

Median section (viewed from left)

Figure 4.40. Midsagittal MRI of lower head and neck. The cerebellum, medulla, spinal cord, and cervical region of the vertebral column are shown. The nuclei pulposi are evident in the IV discs of this young adult, interspersed between the spongy bone of the vertebral bodies. The anuli fibrosi and compact bone of the bodies produce little signal, and appear black.

(A) Left lateral view

(B) Inferior view

Figure 4.41. MRI studies of vertebral column. A. T1-weighted sagittal MRI showing a C5–C6 IV disc herniation (*arrow*). The bright signal surrounding the spinal cord indicates the CSF. **B.** This axial (transverse) MRI demonstrates an IV disc herniation (*arrow*) in a patient with radiculopathy, a disorder of the spinal nerve roots (McCormick, 2000).

References and Suggested Readings

Bergman RA, Thompson SA, Afifi AK, Saadeh FA: *Compendium of Human Anatomic Variation. Text, Atlas, and World Literature.* Baltimore, Urban & Schwarzenberg, 1988.

This useful source has been updated and is available from the Virtual Hospital's Web site *Illustrated Encyclopedia of Human Anatomic Variation* at www.vh.org/Providers/Textbooks/AnatomicVariants/AnatomyHP.html (accessed May 2004).

Bogduk N: *Clinical Anatomy of the Lumbar Spine and Sacrum,* 3rd ed. London: Churchill Livingstone, 1997.

Bogduk N, Macintosh JE: Applied anatomy of the thoracolumbar fascia. *Spine* 9:164, 1984.

Buxton DF, Peck D: Neuromuscular spindles relative to joint movement complexities. *Clin Anat* 2:211, 1989.

Clark CR: *The Cervical Spine,* 3rd ed., Philadelphia: Lippincott-Raven, 1997.

Crockard HA, Heilman AE, Stevens JM: Progressive myelopathy secondary to odontoid fractures: Clinical, radiological, and surgical features. *J Neurosurg* 78: 579, 1993.

Dvorak J, Schneider E, Saldinger P, Rahn B: Biomechanics of the craniovertebral region: The alar and transverse ligaments. *J Orthop Res* 6: 452, 1988.

Greer M: Structural malformations. *In* Rowland LP (ed): *Merritt's Textbook of Neurology*, 10th ed. Baltimore, Lippincott Williams & Wilkins, 2000.

Haines DE (ed): *Fundamental Neuroscience*, 2nd ed. New York, Churchill Livingstone, 2002.

McCormick PC: Intervertebral discs and radiculopathy. *In* Rowland LP (ed): *Merritt's Textbook of Neurology*, 10th ed. Baltimore, Lippincott Williams & Wilkins, 2000.

McCormick PC, Fetell MR, Roland LP: Spinal tumors. *In* Rowland LP (ed): *Merritt's Textbook of Neurology*, 10th ed. Baltimore, Lippincott Williams & Wilkins, 2000.

Moore KL, Persaud TVN: *The Developing Human: Clinically Oriented Embryology*, 7th ed. Philadelphia, Saunders, 2003.

Murray MJ, Bower TC, Carmichael SW: Anatomy of the anterior spinal artery in pigs. *Clin Anat* 5:452, 1992.

O'Rahilly R: *Gardner-Gray-O'Rahilly Anatomy. A Regional Study of Human Structures*, 5th ed. Philadelphia, Saunders, 1986.

Rickenbacher J, Landolt AM, Theiler K: *Applied Anatomy of the Back*. New York: Springer Verlag, 1985.

Rowland LP, McCormick PC: Lumbar spondylosis. *In* Rowland LP (ed): *Merritt's Textbook of Neurology*, 10th ed. Baltimore, Lippincott Williams & Wilkins, 2000.

Swartz MH: *Textbook of Physical Diagnosis. History and Examination*, 4th ed. Philadelphia, Saunders, 2002.

Vilensky JA, Baltes M, Weikel L, Fortin JD, Fourie LJ: Serratus posterior muscles: Anatomy, clinical relevance, and function. *Clin Anat* 14:237, 2001.

Williams PL, Bannister LH, Berry MM, Collins P, Dyson M, Dussek JE, Ferguson MWJ (eds.): *Gray's Anatomy*, 38th British ed. New York, Churchill Livingstone, 1995.

Yochum TR, Rowe LJ: *Essentials of Skeletal Radiology*, 3rd ed. Baltimore, Lippincott Williams & Wilkins, 2004.

5 Lower Limb

Overview of the Lower Limb

The lower limbs (extremities) are extensions from the trunk specialized to support body weight, for *locomotion,* the ability to move from one place to another and maintain balance.

It is customary when describing the lower limbs to include regions that are transitional between the trunk and the **free lower limbs** (the mobile part of the limbs extending from the trunk), such as the gluteal region (G. *gloutos,* buttocks). The lower limb has six major parts or regions (Fig. 5.1):

1. **Gluteal region** (L. *regio glutealis*). This transitional region between the trunk and free lower limb includes two parts of the lower limb: the rounded, prominent posterior region, the **buttocks** (L. *nates, clunes*), and the lateral, usually less prominent **hip** (L. *coxa*) or **hip region** (L. *regio coxae*), which overlies the hip joint and greater trochanter of the femur. Note that the "width of the hips" in common terminology is a reference to one's transverse dimensions at the level of the greater trochanter. The gluteal region is bounded superiorly by the iliac crest, medially by the **intergluteal (natal) cleft** (L. *natus,* to be born), and inferiorly by the skin fold (groove) underlying the buttock, the **gluteal fold** (L. *sulcus glutealis*). The gluteal muscles constitute the bulk of this region.

2. **Thigh** or **femoral region** (L. *regio femoris*). This part/ region of the free lower limb lies between the gluteal, abdominal, and perineal regions proximally and the knee region distally. It contains most of the *femur* (thigh bone), which connects the hip and knee. The

Anterior view

Figure 5.1. Regions and bones of lower limb. The pelvic girdle, consisting of the sacrum and right and left hip bones united by the pubic symphysis, attaches the appendicular skeleton of the free lower limb to the axial skeleton and transfers weight from the axial skeleton to the lower limbs.

transition between the trunk and free lower limb is abrupt anteriorly and medially. The boundary between the thigh and abdominal regions is demarcated by the *inguinal ligament* anteriorly and the ischiopubic ramus of the *hip bone* (part of the *pelvic girdle* or skeleton of the pelvis) medially. The junction of these regions is the *inguinal region* or groin.

3. **Knee** (L. *genu*) or **knee region** (L. *regio genus*). This part/region includes the prominences (condyles) of the distal femur and proximal tibia, the head of the fibula, and the *patella* (knee cap, which lies anterior to the distal end of the femur) as well as the joints between these bony structures. The **posterior part of the knee** (L. *poples*) includes a well-defined, fat-filled hollow, transmitting neurovascular structures, called the *popliteal fossa.*

4. **Leg** (L. *crus*) or **leg region** (L. *regio cruris*). Although laypersons refer incorrectly to the entire lower limb as "the leg," the leg is the part that lies between the knee and the rounded medial and lateral prominences (*malleoli*) that flank the ankle joint. The leg contains the *tibia* (shin bone) and *fibula* (L. *buckle*) and connects the knee and foot. The **calf** (L. *sura*) of the leg is the posterior prominence caused by the *triceps surae muscle,* from which the *calcaneal* (Achilles) *tendon* extends to reach the heel.

5. **Ankle** (L. *tarsus*) or **talocrural region** (L. *regio talocruralis*). This includes the narrow, distal part of the leg and the malleoli; the ankle (talocrural) joint is located between the malleoli.

6. **Foot** (L. *pes*) or **foot region** (L. *regio pedis*). The foot is the distal part of the lower limb containing the *tarsus, metatarsus,* and *phalanges* (toe bones). The superior surface is the **dorsum of the foot** and the inferior, ground-contacting surface is the **sole** or **plantar region.** The **toes** are the **digits of the foot.** The **great toe** (L. *hallux*), like the thumb, has only two *phalanges* (digital bones); the other digits have three.

Development of the Lower Limb

Development of the lower limb is illustrated, explained, and contrasted with that of the upper limb in Figure 5.2. Initially, the development of the lower limb is similar to that of the upper limb, although occurring about a week later. During the 5th week, *lower limb buds* bulge from the lateral aspect of the L2–S2 segments of the trunk (a broader base than for the upper limbs) (Fig. 5.2*A*). Both limbs initially extend from the trunk with their developing thumbs and great toes directed superiorly and the palms and soles directed anteriorly. Both limbs then undergo torsion around their long axes, but in opposite directions (Fig. 5.2*B–D*). The medial rotation and permanent pronation of the lower limb explain (1) how the knee, unlike the joints superior to it, extends anteriorly and

flexes posteriorly, as do the joints inferior to the knee (e.g., interphalangeal joints of the toes); (2) how the foot becomes oriented with the great toe on the medial side (Fig. 5.2*D*), whereas the hand (in the anatomical position) becomes oriented with the thumb on the lateral side; and (3) the "barber-pole" pattern of the segmental innervation of the skin (dermatomes) of the lower limb (see "Cutaneous Innervation of the Lower Limb," in this chapter). The torsion and twisting of the lower limb is still in progress at birth (note the way babies' feet tend to meet sole to sole when they are brought together, like clapping). Completion of the process coincides with the mastering of walking skills.

Lower Limb Injuries

Knee, leg, and foot injuries are the most common lower limb injuries. Injuries to the hips make up <3% of lower limb injuries. In general, most injuries result from acute trauma during contact sports such as hockey and football and from overuse during endurance sports such as marathon races. Adolescents are most vulnerable to these injuries because of the demands of sports on their slowly maturing musculoskeletal systems. The cartilaginous models of the bones in the developing lower limbs are transformed into bone by endochondral ossification (see "Bone Development" in the Introduction) (Fig. 5.2*E* & *F*). Because the process is not completed until early adulthood, cartilaginous epiphysial plates still exist during the teenage years when physical activity often peaks and involvement in competitive sports is most common. During growth spurts, bones actually grow faster than the attached muscle. The combined stress on the epiphysial plates resulting from physical activity and rapid growth may result in irritation and injury of the plates and developing bone (osteochondrosis). ✪

Bones of the Lower Limb

The skeleton of the lower limb (inferior appendicular skeleton) may be divided into two functional components: the pelvic girdle and the bones of the free lower limb (Fig. 5.1). The **pelvic girdle** (bony pelvis) is a bony ring composed of the sacrum and right and left hip bones joined anteriorly at the pubic symphysis. It attaches the free lower limb to the axial skeleton, the sacrum being common to the axial skeleton and the pelvic girdle. The pelvic girdle also makes up the skeleton of the lower part of the trunk. Its protective and supportive functions serve the abdomen, pelvis, and perineum as well as the lower limb. The bones of the free lower limb are contained within and specifically serve that part of the limb.

(A)

During early development, the trunk is divided into segments (metameres) that correspond to and receive innervation from the corresponding spinal cord segments. During the 4th week of development, the upper limb buds appear as elevations of the C5–T1 segments of the anterolateral body wall. Following the cranial to caudal pattern of development common to other systems, the lower limb buds appear about a week later (5th week). The lower limb buds grow laterally from broader bases formed by the L2–S2 segments.

(B)

The distal ends of the limb buds flatten into paddle-like hand and foot plates that are elongated in the craniocaudal axis. Initially, both the thumb and the great toe are on the cranial sides of the developing hand and foot, directed superiorly, with the palms and soles directed anteriorly. Flexures occur where gaps develop between the precursors of the long bones [see(E)]. At first, the limbs bend anteriorly, so that the elbow and knee are directed laterally, causing the palm and sole to be directed medially (toward the trunk).

(C)

By the end of the 7th week, the proximal parts of the upper and lower limbs undergo a 90° torsion around their long axes, but in opposite directions, so that the elbow becomes directed caudally and the knee cranially.

(D) In the lower limb, the torsion of the proximal limb is accompanied by a permanent pronation (twisting) of the leg, so that the foot becomes oriented with the great toe on the medial side.

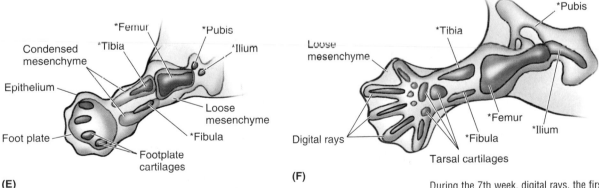

(E)

As the limb buds elongate, the loose mesenchyme within them condenses centrally, and cartilaginous models of the limb bones appear. The distal ends of the limb buds flatten into paddle-like plates (hand plates and foot plates) elongated in the craniocaudal axis. Gaps develop between precursors of the long bones where flexures (future elbow and knee joints) will occur.

*Cartilage models of indicated bones

(F)

During the 7th week, digital rays, the first indication of future digits, appear. The thinner tissue between the digital rays undergoes apoptosis (programmed cell death), causing notches to develop, so that the rays soon appear as webbed fingers and toes.

Figure 5.2. Development of lower limb. A–D. The upper and lower limbs develop from limb buds that arise from the lateral body wall during the 4th and 5th weeks, respectively. They then elongate, develop flexures, and rotate in opposite directions. Segmental innervation is maintained, the dermatomal pattern reflecting the elongation and spiraling of the limb. **E and F.** Future bones develop from cartilage models, demonstrated at the end of the 6th week (**E**) and beginning of the 7th week (**F**).

Arrangement of Lower Limb Bones

Body weight is transferred from the vertebral column through the *sacroiliac joints* (see Chapter 4) to the pelvic girdle and from the pelvic girdle through the hip joints to the femurs (L. *femora*) (Fig. 5.3*A*). To support the erect bipedal posture better, the femurs are oblique (directed inferomedially) within the thighs so that when standing the knees are adjacent and are placed directly inferior to the trunk, returning the center of gravity to the vertical lines of the supporting legs and feet

(Figs. 5.1, 5.3, and 5.4). Compare this oblique position of the femurs with that of quadrupeds, in whom the femurs are vertical and the knees are apart, with the trunk mass suspended between the limbs (Fig. 5.3*B*). The femurs of females are slightly more oblique than those of males, reflecting the greater width of their pelves. At the knees, the distal end of each femur articulates with the patella and tibia of the corresponding leg. Weight is transferred from the knee joint to the ankle joint by the tibia. The fibula does not articulate with the femur and

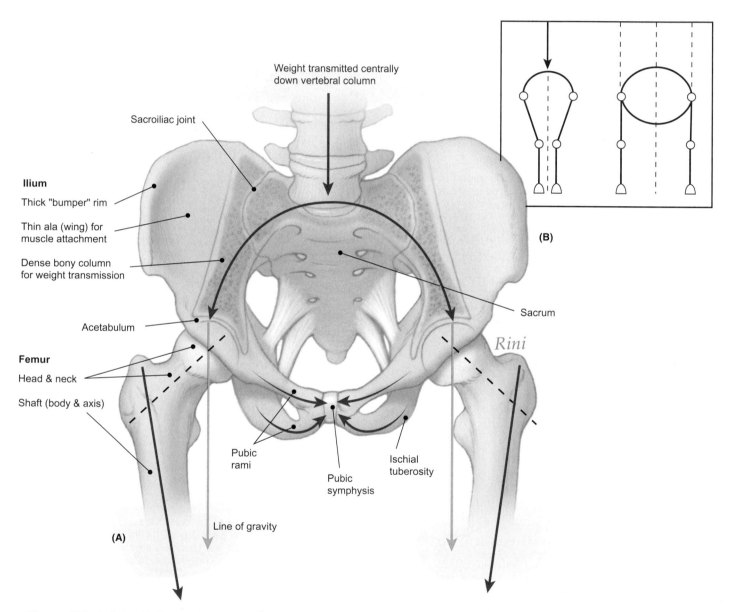

Figure 5.3. Pelvic Girdle and Related Joints, Demonstrating Transfer of Weight. A. The weight of the upper body, transmitted centrally through the vertebral column, is divided and directed laterally by means of the bony arch formed by the sacrum and ilia. Thick portions of the ilia transfer the weight to the femurs. The pubic rami form "struts" or braces that help maintain the integrity of the arch. **B.** The arrangement of the lower limb bones of bipeds is compared to that of quadrupeds. The diagonal disposition of the femur recenters support directly inferior to the trunk (body mass) to make bipedal standing more efficient and to enable bipedal walking, in which the full weight is borne alternately by each limb. In quadrupeds, the trunk is suspended between essentially vertical limbs, requiring simultaneous support from each side.

Iliac crest
Hip bone
Iliac fossa
Tubercle of iliac crest
Iliopubic eminence
Anterior superior iliac spine (ASIS)
Superior ramus of pubis
Anterior inferior iliac spine
Pubic crest
Greater trochanter
Pubic tubercle
Intertrochanteric line
Pubic symphysis
Lesser trochanter
Body of pubis
Femur
Obturator foramen
Head of femur
Patella
Adductor tubercle
Lateral epicondyle
Medial epicondyle
Lateral femoral condyle
Medial femoral condyle
Apex of head
Medial tibial condyle
Head
Intercondylar eminence
Neck
Tuberosity
Fibula
Anterior border
Lateral surface
Medial surface
Tibia
Medial malleolus
Lateral malleolus
Talus
Calcaneus
Cuboid
Navicular
Cuneiforms
First metatarsal
Proximal phalanx
Distal phalanx

(A) Anterior view

Hip bone
Iliac crest
Posterior gluteal line
Anterior gluteal line
Posterior superior iliac spine (PSIS)
Tubercle of iliac crest
Posterior inferior iliac spine
Inferior gluteal line
Greater sciatic notch
Ischium
Ischial spine
Head of femur
Lesser sciatic notch
Greater trochanter
Ischial tuberosity
Neck of femur
Acetabulum
Intertrochanteric crest
Gluteal tuberosity
Spiral line
Lesser trochanter
Lateral supracondylar line
Linea aspera
Medial supracondylar line
Femur
Adductor tubercle
Popliteal surface
Medial femoral condyle
Lateral femoral condyle
Intercondylar fossa
Medial tibial condyle
Lateral tibial condyle
Soleal line
Head
Vertical line
Neck
Tibia
Fibula
Medial malleolus
Talus
Talus
Lateral malleolus
Navicular
Calcaneus
Medial cuneiform
Cuboid
5th metatarsal
Proximal phalanx

(B) Posterior view

Figure 5.4. Bones of lower limb. A and B. Individual bones and bony formations are identified. The foot is in full plantarflexion. The hip joint is disarticulated (**B**) to demonstrate the acetabulum of the hip bone, which receives the head of the femur.

does not bear or transfer weight, but it provides for muscle attachment and contributes to the formation of the ankle joint.

At the ankle, the weight borne by the tibia is transferred to the *talus*. The talus is the keystone of a longitudinal arch formed by the tarsal and metatarsal bones of each foot that distributes the weight evenly between the heel and the forefoot when standing, creating a flexible but stable platform to support the body.

Hip Bone

The mature **hip bone** (L. *os coxae*), once called the innominate (unnamed) bone, is the large, flat pelvic bone formed by the fusion of three primary bones—*ilium, ischium,* and *pubis*—at the end of the teenage years. Each of the three bones is formed from its own primary center of ossification; five secondary centers of ossification appear later. At birth, the three primary bones are joined by hyaline cartilage; in children, they are incompletely ossified (Fig. 5.5). At puberty, the three bones are still separated by a Y-shaped **triradiate cartilage** centered in the acetabulum, although the two parts of the ischiopubic rami fuse by the 9th year (Fig. 5.5*B*). The bones begin to fuse between 15 and 17 years of age; fusion is complete between 20 and 25 years of age. Little or no trace of the lines of fusion of the primary bones is visible in older adults (Fig. 5.6). Although the bony components are rigidly fused, their names are still used in adults to describe the three parts of the hip bone.

Because much of the medial aspect of the hip bones/bony pelvis is primarily concerned with pelvic and perineal structures and functions (Chapter 3) or their union with the vertebral column (Chapter 4), it is described more thoroughly in those chapters. Aspects of the hip bones concerned with lower limb structures and functions, mainly involving their lateral aspects, are described in this chapter.

Ilium

The **ilium** composes the largest part of the hip bone and contributes the superior part of the acetabulum (Fig. 5.5*B*). The ilium has thick medial portions (columns) for weight bearing and thin, wing-like, posterolateral portions, the **alae** (L. wings), that provide broad surfaces for the fleshy attachment of muscles (Fig. 5.3). The **body of the ilium** joins the pubis and ischium to form the acetabulum. Anteriorly, the ilium has stout **anterior superior** and **anterior inferior iliac spines** that provide attachment for ligaments and tendons of lower limb muscles (Fig. 5.6). Beginning at the anterior superior iliac spine (ASIS), the long curved and thickened superior border of the ala of the ilium, the **iliac crest,** extends posteriorly, terminating at the **posterior superior iliac spine** (PSIS). The crest serves as a protective "bumper" and is an important site of aponeurotic attachment for thin, sheet-like muscles and deep fascia. A prominence on the external lip of the crest, the **tubercle of the iliac crest** (iliac tubercle), lies 5–6 cm posterior to the ASIS. The **posterior inferior iliac spine** marks the superior end of the *greater sciatic notch.*

(A) Anterior view

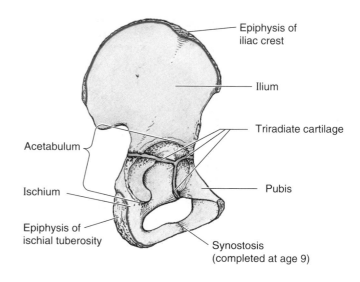

(B) Lateral view

Figure 5.5. Parts of hip bones. A. An anteroposterior radiograph of an infant's hips shows the three parts of the incompletely ossified hip bones (ilium, ischium, and pubis). **B.** The right hip bone of a 13-year-old demonstrating the Y-shaped triradiate cartilage extending through the acetabulum, uniting the three primary parts of the bone, and the ossified epiphyses along the iliac crest and ischial tuberosity. These bony parts fuse to form the one-part mature hip bone of the adult between the 16th and 18th years.

The lateral surface of the ala of the ilium has three rough curved lines—the posterior, anterior, and inferior **gluteal lines**—that demarcate the proximal attachments of the three large gluteal muscles (glutei). Medially, each ala has a large, smooth depression, the **iliac fossa** (Fig. 5.6*B*), that provides proximal attachment for the iliac muscle (L. *iliacus*). The bone forming the superior part of this fossa may become thin and translucent, especially in older women with osteoporosis. Posteriorly, the medial aspect of the ilium has a rough, ear-shaped articular area called the **auricular surface** (L. *auricula,* a little ear) and an even rougher **iliac**

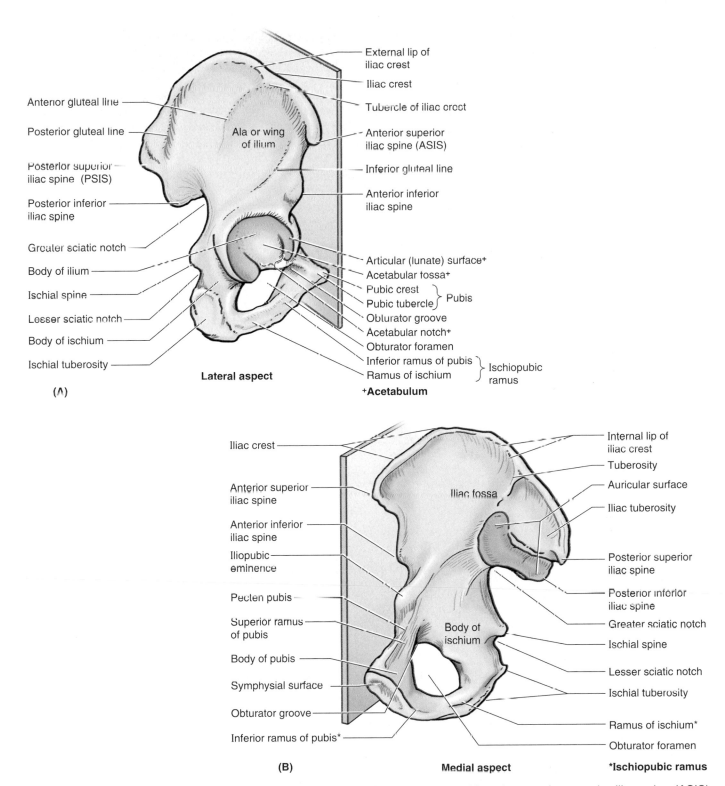

Figure 5.6. Right hip bone of adult in anatomical position. In this position, the anterior superior iliac spine (ASIS) and the anterior aspect of the pubis lie in the same coronal plane. **A.** The large hip bone is constricted in the middle and expanded at its superior and inferior ends. **B.** The symphysial surface of the pubis articulates with the corresponding surface of the contralateral hip bone. The auricular surface of the ilium articulates with a corresponding surface of the sacrum to form the sacroiliac joint.

tuberosity superior to it for synovial and syndesmotic articulation with the reciprocal surfaces of the sacrum at the sacroiliac joint (see Chapter 4).

Ischium

The **ischium** forms the posteroinferior part of the hip bone. The superior part of the **body of the ischium** fuses with the pubis and ilium, forming the posteroinferior aspect of the acetabulum. The **ramus of the ischium** joins the *inferior ramus of the pubis* to form a bar of bone, the **ischiopubic ramus** (Fig. 5.6A), which constitutes the inferomedial boundary of the *obturator foramen.* The posterior border of the ischium forms the inferior margin of a deep indentation called the **greater sciatic notch.** The large, triangular **ischial spine** at the inferior margin of this notch provides ligamentous attachment. This sharp demarcation separates the greater sciatic notch from a more inferior, smaller, rounded, and smooth-surfaced indentation, the **lesser sciatic notch.** The lesser sciatic notch serves as a trochlea or pulley for a muscle that emerges from the bony pelvis here. The rough bony projection at the junction of the inferior end of the body of the ischium and its ramus is the large **ischial tuberosity.** The body's weight rests on this tuberosity when sitting, and it provides the proximal, tendinous attachment of posterior thigh muscles.

Pubis

The **pubis** forms the anteromedial part of the hip bone, contributing the anterior part of the acetabulum, and provides proximal attachment for muscles of the medial thigh. The pubis is divided into a flattened body and two rami, superior and inferior (Fig. 5.6). The rami are strong yet relatively light skeletal "struts" (braces) that maintain the arch composed of the sacrum and the two ilia, by which axial weight is divided and transferred laterally to the limbs when standing and to the ischial tuberosities when sitting (Fig. 5.3). Medially, the symphysial surface of the **body of the pubis** articulates with the corresponding surface of the body of the contralateral pubis by means of the **pubic symphysis.** The anterosuperior border of the united bodies and symphysis forms the **pubic crest,** which provides attachment for abdominal muscles. Small projections at the lateral ends of this crest, the **pubic tubercles,** are important landmarks of the inguinal regions. The tubercles provide attachment for the main part of the inguinal ligament and thereby indirect muscle attachment. The posterior margin of the **superior ramus** of the pubis has a sharp raised edge, the **pecten pubis,** which forms part of the pelvic brim (see Chapter 3).

Obturator Foramen

The **obturator foramen** is a large oval or irregularly triangular aperture in the hip bone. It is bounded by the pubis and ischium and their rami. Except for a small passageway for the obturator nerve and vessels (the *obturator canal*), the obturator foramen is closed by the thin, strong *obturator membrane*

(see Chapter 3). The presence of the foramen minimizes bony mass (weight) while its closure by the obturator membrane still provides extensive surface area on both sides for fleshy muscle attachment.

Acetabulum

The acetabulum (L. shallow vinegar cup) is the large cup-shaped cavity or socket on the lateral aspect of the hip bone that articulates with the head of the femur to form the hip joint (Fig. 5.6A). All three primary bones forming the hip bone contribute to the formation of the acetabulum. The margin of the acetabulum is incomplete inferiorly at the *acetabular notch,* which makes the fossa resemble a cup with a piece of its lip missing. The rough depression in the floor of the acetabulum extending superiorly from the acetabular notch is the *acetabular fossa.* The acetabular notch and fossa also create a deficit in the smooth *lunate surface of the acetabulum,* which articulates with the head of the femur. The acetabulum is discussed further in relation to the hip joint.

THE BOTTOM LINE: Formed by the union of three primary bones (ilium, ischium, and pubis), the hip bones are joined to the sacrum posteriorly and to each other anteriorly (at the pubic symphysis) to form the pelvic girdle. Each hip bone is specialized to receive half the weight of the upper body when standing and all of it periodically during walking. Thick parts of the bone transfer weight to the femur. Thin parts of the bone provide a broad surface for attachment of powerful muscles that move the femur. The pelvic girdle encircles and protects pelvic viscera, particularly the reproductive organs.

Anatomical Position of the Hip Bone

Surfaces, borders, and relationships of the hip bone are described assuming that the body is in the *anatomical position* (see Introduction). To place an isolated hip bone or bony pelvis in this position, situate it so that the:

- ASIS and the anterosuperior aspect of the pubis lie in the same vertical plane.
- Symphysial surface of the pubis is vertical, parallel to the median plane (Fig. 5.6).

In the anatomical position, the:

- Acetabulum faces inferolaterally, with the acetabular notch directed inferiorly.
- Obturator foramen lies inferomedial to the acetabulum.
- Internal aspect of the body of the pubis faces almost directly superiorly (it essentially forms a floor on which the urinary bladder rests).
- The superior pelvic aperture (pelvic inlet) is more vertical than horizontal; in the anteroposterior (AP) view, the tip of the coccyx appears near its center (Fig. 5.3).

Injuries of the Hip Bone (Pelvic Injuries)

Fractures of the hip bone are commonly referred to as *pelvic fractures* (see clinical correlation [blue] box "Pelvic Fractures," in Chapter 3). The term *hip fracture* is most commonly applied (unfortunately) to fractures of the femoral head, neck, or trochanters.

Avulsion fractures of the hip bone may occur during sports that require sudden acceleration or deceleration forces, such as sprinting or kicking in football, soccer, hurdle jumping, basketball, and martial arts (Fig. B5.1). A small part of bone with a piece of a tendon or ligament attached is "avulsed" (torn away). These fractures occur at **apophyses** (bony projections that lack secondary ossification centers). Avulsion fractures occur where muscles are attached: anterior superior and inferior iliac spines, ischial tuberosities, and ischiopubic rami. ⊙

Ischial tuberosity

Hamstrings tendon (torn and avulsed from tuberosity)

Figure B5.1

Femur

The **femur** is the longest and heaviest bone in the body. It transmits body weight from the hip bone to the tibia when a person is standing (Fig. 5.4). Its length is approximately a quarter of the person's height. The femur consists of a **shaft (body)** and two ends, superior or proximal and inferior or distal (Fig. 5.7). The superior (proximal) end of the femur consists of a head, neck, and two trochanters (greater and lesser). The round **head of the femur** makes up two thirds of a sphere that is covered with articular cartilage, except for a medially placed depression or pit, the **fovea for the ligament of the head.** In early life, the ligament gives passage to an artery supplying the epiphysis of the head. The **neck of the femur** is trapezoidal, with its narrow end supporting the head and its broader base being continuous with the shaft. Its average diameter is three quarters that of the femoral head.

The proximal femur is "bent" (L-shaped) so that the long axis of the head and neck projects supromedially at an angle to that of the obliquely oriented shaft (Fig. 5.7A & B). This obtuse **angle of inclination** is greatest (most nearly straight) at birth and gradually diminishes (becomes more acute) until the adult angle is reached (115–140°, averaging 126°) (Fig. 5.7C D). The angle is less in females because of the increased width between the acetabula (a consequence of a wider lesser pelvis) and the greater obliquity of the shaft. The angle of inclination allows greater mobility of the femur at the hip joint because it places the head and neck more perpendicular to the acetabulum in the neutral position. The abductors and rotators of the thigh attach mainly to the apex of the angle (the *greater trochanter*) so they are pulling on a lever (the short limb of the *L*) that is more laterally than vertically directed. This provides increased leverage for the abductors and rotators of the thigh and allows the considerable mass of the abductors of the thigh to be placed superior to the femur (in the gluteal region) instead of lateral to it, freeing the lateral aspect of the femoral shaft to provide increased area for fleshy attachment of the extensors of the knee. The angle also allows the obliquity of the femur within the thigh, which permits the knees to be adjacent and inferior to the trunk, as explained previously. All of this is advantageous for bipedal walking; however, it imposes considerable strain on the neck of the femur. Consequently, fractures of the femoral neck can occur in older people as a result of a slight stumble if the neck has been weakened by osteoporosis.

The torsion of the proximal lower limb (femur) that occurred during development does not conclude with the long axis of the superior end of the femur (head and neck) parallel to the transverse axis of the inferior end (femoral condyles). When the femur is viewed superiorly (so that one is looking along the long axis of the shaft), it is apparent that the two axes lie at an angle (the **torsion angle**, or **angle of declination**), the mean of which is 7° in males and 12° in females. The torsion angle, combined with the angle of inclination, allows rotatory movements of the femoral head within the obliquely placed acetabulum to convert into flexion and

(A) Anterior view of right femur

- Long axis of shaft (body)
- Greater trochanter
- Intertrochanteric line
- Long axis of head and neck
- Head
- Fovea (pit) for ligament of head
- Neck
- Angle of inclination
- Lesser trochanter
- Anterior surface of shaft
- Weight-bearing line (line of gravity)
- Superior or proximal end
- Shaft (body)
- Inferior or distal end
- Lateral epicondyle
- Lateral condyle
- Horizontal plane
- Adductor tubercle
- Medial epicondyle
- Medial condyle
- Patellar surface

(B) Posterior view of right femur

- Trochanteric fossa
- Head
- Fovea (pit) for ligament of head
- Neck
- Intertrochanteric crest
- Lesser trochanter
- Pectineal line
- Medial lip of linea aspera
- Nutrient foramen
- Medial surface of body
- Medial supracondylar line
- Adductor tubercle
- Medial epicondyle
- Medial condyle
- Greater trochanter
- Quadrate tubercle
- Gluteal tuberosity
- Lateral lip of linea aspera
- Lateral surface of body
- Posterior surface of shaft
- Lateral supracondylar line
- Popliteal surface
- Intercondylar line
- Lateral epicondyle
- Lateral condyle
- Intercondylar fossa

(C) 45° — Angle of inclination in 3-year-old child

(D) 126° — Angle of inclination in adult

(E) 120° — Angle of inclination in old age

(F) Superior view demonstrating torsion angle of femur
- Axis of femoral head and neck
- Long axis of body of femur
- Inferior (distal) end of femur
- Transverse axis of femoral condyles
- Torsion angle of femur — 12°
- Trochanteric fossa
- Greater trochanter

Figure 5.7. Right femur. A and B. The bony features of an adult femur are shown. Functionally and morphologically, the bone consists of highly modified superior and inferior ends and an intervening cylindrical shaft. The nutrient foramen (**B**) is demonstrated entering the femoral shaft near the linea aspera. **A–E.** The femur is "bent" so that the long axis of the head and neck lies at an angle (angle of inclination) to that of the shaft. When the massive femoral condyles rest on a horizontal surface, the femur assumes its oblique anatomical position in which the center of the round femoral head lies directly superior to the intercondylar fossa. **C–E.** The angle of inclination decreases (becomes more acute) with age, resulting in greater stress at a time when bone mass is reduced. When the femur is viewed along the long axis of the femoral shaft, so that the proximal end is superimposed over the distal end (**F**), it can be seen that the axis of the head and neck of the femur forms a 12° angle with the transverse axis of the femoral condyles (angle of torsion).

extension, abduction and adduction, and rotational movements of the thigh.

Where the neck joins the femoral shaft are two large, blunt elevations called trochanters (Fig. 5.7*A*, *B*, & *F*). The abrupt, conical and rounded **lesser trochanter** (G. a runner) extends medially from the posteromedial part of the junction of the neck and shaft to give tendinous attachment to the primary flexor of the thigh (the iliopsoas). The **greater trochanter** is a large, laterally placed bony mass that projects superiorly and posteriorly where the neck joins the femoral shaft, providing attachment and leverage for abductors and rotators of the thigh. The site where the neck and shaft join is indicated by the **intertrochanteric line**, a roughened ridge formed by the attachment of a powerful ligament (iliofemoral ligament), that runs from the greater trochanter and winds around the lesser trochanter to continue posteriorly and inferiorly as a less distinct ridge, the **spiral line**. A similar but smoother and more prominent ridge, the **intertrochanteric crest**, joins the trochanters posteriorly. The rounded elevation on the crest is the **quadrate tubercle**. In anterior and posterior views (Fig. 5.7*A* & *B*), the greater trochanter is in line with the femoral shaft. In posterior and superior views (Fig. 5.7*B* & *F*), it overhangs a deep depression medially, the **trochanteric fossa**.

The **shaft of the femur** is slightly bowed (convex) anteriorly. This convexity may increase markedly, proceeding laterally as well as anteriorly, if the shaft is weakened by a loss of calcium, as occurs in rickets. Most of the shaft is smoothly rounded, providing fleshy origin to extensors of the knee, except posteriorly where a broad, rough line, the **linea aspera**, provides aponeurotic attachment for adductors of the thigh. This vertical ridge is especially prominent in the middle third of the femoral shaft, where it has **medial** and **lateral lips** (margins). Superiorly, the lateral lip blends with the broad, rough **gluteal tuberosity**, and the medial lip continues as a narrow, rough spiral line. The *spiral line* extends toward the lesser trochanter but then passes to the anterior surface of the femur, where it is continuous with the intertrochanteric line. A prominent intermediate ridge, the **pectineal line**, extends from the central part of the linea aspera to the base of the lesser trochanter. Inferiorly, the linea aspera divides into medial and lateral **supracondylar lines**, which lead to the spirally curved medial and lateral condyles (Fig. 5.7*B*).

The **medial** and **lateral femoral condyles** make up nearly the entire inferior (distal) end of the femur. The two condyles are on the same horizontal level when the bone is in its anatomical position, so that if an isolated femur is placed upright with both condyles contacting the floor or tabletop, the femoral shaft will assume the same oblique position it occupies in the living body (about 9° from vertical in males and slightly greater in females). The femoral condyles articulate with menisci (crescentic plates of cartilage) and tibial condyles to form the knee joint (Fig. 5.4). The menisci and tibial condyles glide as a unit across the inferior and posterior aspects of the femoral condyles during flexion and extension. The convexity of the articular surface of the condyles increases as it descends the anterior surface, covering the infe-

rior end, and then ascends posteriorly. The condyles are separated posteriorly and inferiorly by an **intercondylar fossa** (intercondylar notch) but merge anteriorly, forming a shallow longitudinal depression, the **patellar surface** (Fig. 5.7), which articulates with the patella. The lateral surface of the lateral condyle has a central projection called the *lateral epicondyle.* The medial surface of the medial condyle has a larger and more prominent *medial epicondyle,* superior to which another elevation, the **adductor tubercle**, forms in relation to a tendon attachment. The epicondyles provide proximal attachment for the collateral ligaments of the knee joint.

THE BOTTOM LINE: Through evolution and development, our largest bone, the femur, has developed a bend (angle of inclination) and has twisted (medial rotation and torsion so that the knee and all joints inferior to it flex posteriorly) to accommodate our erect posture and to enable bipedal walking and running. The angle of inclination and attachment of the abductors and rotators to the greater trochanter allow increased leverage, superior placement of the abductors, and oblique orientation of the femur in the thigh. Combined with the torsion angle, oblique rotatory movements at the hip joint are converted into movements of flexion–extension and abduction–adduction (in the sagittal and coronal planes, respectively) as well as of rotation.

Coxa Vara and Coxa Valga

The angle of inclination between the long axis of the femoral neck and the femoral shaft (Fig. 5.7*C–E*) varies with age, sex, and development of the femur (e.g., a congenital defect in the ossification of the femoral neck). It may also change with any pathological process that weakens the neck of the femur (e.g., rickets). When the angle of inclination is decreased, the condition is **coxa vara** (Fig. B5.2*A*); when it is increased, it is **coxa valga** (Fig. B5.2*B*). Coxa vara causes a mild shortening of the lower limb and limits passive abduction of the hip.

Dislocated ("Slipped") Epiphysis of the Femoral Head

In older children and adolescents (10–17 years of age), the epiphysis of the femoral head may slip away from the femoral neck because of a weakened epiphysial plate. This injury may be caused by acute trauma or repetitive microtraumas that place increased shearing stress on the epiphysis, especially with abduction and lateral rotation of the thigh. The epiphysis often dislocates (slips) slowly and results in a progressive *coxa vara.* The common initial symptom of the injury is hip discomfort that may be referred to the knee. Radiographic examination of ▶

Posterior views

Figure B5.2.

the superior end of the femur is usually required to confirm a diagnosis of a dislocated epiphysis of the head of the femur.

Femoral Fractures

Despite its large size and strength, the femur is commonly fractured. The type of fracture sustained is frequently age- and even sex-related. The neck of the femur is most frequently fractured because it is the narrowest and weakest part of the bone and it lies at a marked angle to the line of weight bearing (pull of gravity). It becomes increasingly vulnerable with age, especially in females, secondary to *osteoporosis*. Fractures of the proximal femur occur at several locations; two examples are transcervical (middle of neck) and intertrochanteric (Fig. B5.3). These fractures usually occur as a result of indirect trauma (stumbling or stepping down hard, as off a curb or step). Because of the angle of inclination, these fractures are inherently unstable and **impaction** (overriding of fragments resulting in foreshortening of the limb) occurs. Muscle spasm also contributes to the shortening of the limb. Intracapsular fractures (occurring within the hip joint capsule), are complicated by degeneration of the femoral head owing to vascular trauma (see clinical correlation [blue] boxes "Fractures of the Femoral Neck

('Hip Fractures')" and "Surgical Hip Replacement," both later in this chapter).

Fracture of the greater trochanter and femoral shaft usually result from direct trauma (direct blows sustained by the bone resulting from falls or being hit) and are most common during the more active years. They frequently occur during motor vehicle accidents and sports such as skiing and climbing. In some cases, a *spiral fracture* of the femoral shaft occurs, resulting in foreshortening as the fragments override, or the fracture may be comminuted (broken into several pieces), with the fragments displaced in various directions as a result of muscle pull and depending on the level of the fracture. Union of this serious type of fracture may take up to a year.

Fractures of the distal femur may be complicated by separation of the condyles, resulting in misalignment of the articular surfaces of the knee joint, or by hemorrhage from the large popliteal artery that runs directly on the surface of the bone, which compromises the blood supply to the leg (an occurrence that should always be considered in knee fractures–dislocations). ✱

Transcervical fracture of femoral neck   Intertrochanteric fracture   Spiral fracture

Anterior views

Figure B5.3

Tibia and Fibula

The tibia and fibula are the bones of the leg (Figs. 5.4 and 5.8). The *tibia* articulates with the condyles of the femur superiorly and the talus inferiorly and in so doing transmits the body's weight. The *fibula* mainly functions as an attachment for muscles, but it is also important for the stability of the ankle joint. The shafts (bodies) of the tibia and fibula are con-

nected by a dense interosseous membrane composed of strong oblique fibers.

Tibia

Located on the anteromedial side of the leg, nearly parallel to the fibula, the **tibia** (shin bone) is the second largest bone in the body. It flares outward at both ends to provide an increased area for articulation and weight transfer. The superior

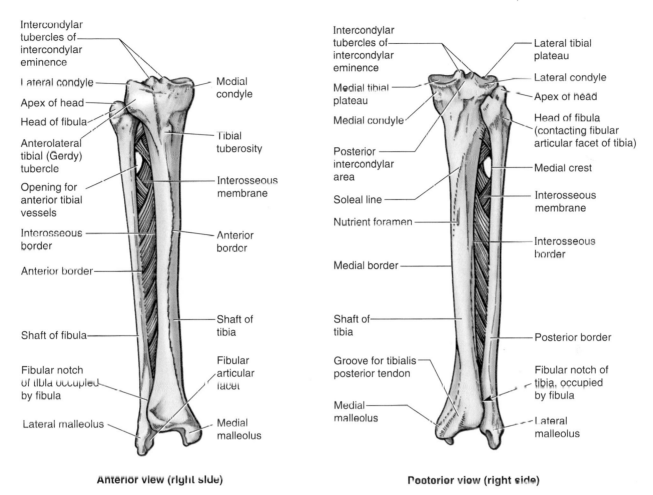

Figure 5.8. Right tibia and fibula. Tibiofibular syndesmoses, including the dense interosseous membrane, tightly connect the tibia and fibula. The interosseous membrane provides additional surface area for muscular attachment. The anterior tibial vessels traverse the opening in the membrane to enter the anterior compartment of the leg (Fig. 5.10).

(proximal) end widens to form **medial and lateral condyles** that overhang the shaft medially, laterally, and posteriorly, forming a relatively flat **superior articular surface**, or **tibial plateau.** This plateau consists of two smooth articular surfaces (the medial one slightly concave and the lateral one slightly convex) that articulate with the large condyles of the femur. The articular surfaces are separated by an **intercondylar eminence** formed by two **intercondylar tubercles** (medial and lateral) flanked by relatively rough **anterior** and **posterior intercondylar areas.** The tubercles fit into the intercondylar fossa between the femoral condyles (Fig. 5.7B). The intercondylar tubercles and areas provide attachment for the menisci and principal ligaments of the knee, which hold the femur and tibia together, maintaining contact between their articular surfaces. The anterolateral aspect of the lateral tibial condyle bears an **anterolateral tibial tubercle** (Gerdy tubercle) inferior to the articular surface (Fig. 5.8), which provides the distal attachment for a dense thickening of the fascia covering the lateral thigh, adding stability to the knee joint. The lateral condyle also bears a **fibular articular facet** posterolaterally on its inferior aspect for the head of the fibula.

Unlike that of the femur, the **shaft of the tibia** is truly vertical within the leg and somewhat triangular in cross section, having three surfaces and borders: medial, lateral/interosseous, and posterior. The **anterior border** of the tibia is the most prominent border; it and the adjacent anterior surface are subcutaneous throughout their lengths and are commonly known as the "shin" or "shin bone"; their periosteal covering and overlying skin is vulnerable to bruising. At the superior end of the anterior border, a broad, oblong **tibial tuberosity** provides distal attachment for the patellar ligament, which stretches between the inferior margin of the patella and the tibial tuberosity. The tibial shaft is thinnest at the junction of its middle and distal thirds. The distal end of the tibia is smaller than the proximal end, flaring only medially; the medial expansion extends inferior to the rest of the shaft as the **medial malleolus.** The inferior surface of the shaft and the lateral surface of the medial malleolus articulate with the talus and are covered with articular cartilage (Fig. 5.4). The **interosseous border** of the tibia is sharp where it gives attachment to the *interosseous membrane* that unites the two leg bones. Inferiorly, the sharp border is replaced by a groove, the **fibular notch,** that accommodates and provides fibrous attachment to the distal end of the fibula.

On the posterior surface of the proximal part of the tibial shaft is a rough diagonal ridge, called the **soleal line,** which runs inferomedially to the medial border; it is formed in relationship to the aponeurotic origin of the soleus muscle approximately one third of the way down the shaft. Immediately distal to the soleal line is an obliquely directed vascular groove, which leads to a large **nutrient foramen.** From it, the nutrient canal runs inferiorly in the tibia before it opens into the medullary (marrow) cavity.

Fibula

The slender **fibula** lies posterolateral to the tibia and is firmly attached to it by the *tibiofibular syndesmosis,* which includes the *interosseous membrane* (Fig. 5.8). Unlike the comparable bones of the forearm (radius and ulna), which are joined to enable mobility (pronation and supination), the leg is fixed in a permanently pronated position that places the great toe medially and directs the sole of the foot inferiorly, toward the ground. The fibula has no function in weight bearing; it serves mainly for muscle attachment, providing distal attachment (insertion) for one muscle and proximal attachment (origin) for eight muscles. The fibers of the tibiofibular syndesmosis are arranged to resist the resulting net downward pull on the fibula.

The distal end enlarges and is prolonged laterally and inferiorly as the **lateral malleolus.** The malleoli form the outer walls of a rectangular socket (mortise), which is the superior component of the ankle joint (Fig. 5.4A), and provide attachment for the ligaments that stabilize the joint. The lateral malleolus is more prominent and posterior than the medial malleolus and extends approximately 1 cm more distally. The proximal end of the fibula consists of an enlarged **head** and smaller **neck;** the head has a pointed **apex** formed in relationship to a tendinous attachment. The head articulates with the fibular facet on the posterolateral, inferior aspect of the lateral tibial condyle. The **shaft** of the fibula is twisted and marked by the sites of muscular attachments. Like the shaft of the tibia, it is triangular in cross section, having three borders (anterior, interosseous, and posterior) and three surfaces (medial, posterior, and lateral).

THE BOTTOM LINE: Our second largest bone, the tibia, is a vertical column bearing the weight of all superior to it. The slender fibula does not bear weight but, along with the interosseous membrane that binds it to the tibia, is accessory to the tibia in providing an additional surface area for fleshy muscle attachment and in forming the socket of the ankle joint. Through evolution and development, the two bones have become permanently pronated to accommodate bipedalism.

Tibial Fractures

The tibial shaft is narrowest at the junction of its middle and inferior thirds, which is the most frequent site of fracture. Unfortunately, this area of the bone also has the poorest blood supply. Because its anterior surface is subcutaneous, the tibial shaft is the most common site for a *compound fracture* (Fig. B5.4A). Compound tibial fractures may also result from direct trauma (e.g., a "bumper fracture" caused when a car bumper strikes the leg). Fracture of the tibia through the nutrient canal predisposes the patient to non-union of the bone fragments resulting from damage to the nutrient artery.

Transverse stress (march) fractures of the inferior third of the tibia (Fig. B5.4B) are common in people who take long hikes before they are conditioned for this activity. The strain may fracture the anterior cortex of the tibia. Indirect violence applied to the tibial shaft when the bone turns with the foot fixed during a fall may produce a fracture (e.g., when a person is tackled in football). In addition, severe torsion during skiing may produce a *diagonal fracture* (Fig. B5.4C) of the tibial shaft at the junction of the middle and inferior thirds as well as a *fracture of the fibula.* Diagonal fractures are often associated with limb shortening caused by overriding of the fractured ends. Frequently

during skiing, a fracture results from a high-speed forward fall, which angles the leg over the rigid ski boot, producing a "boot-top fracture" (Fig. B5.4D).

Because of its extensive subcutaneous location, the anterior tibia is accessible for obtaining pieces of bone for grafting in children; it is also used as a site for intramedullary infusion in dehydrated/shocked children.

Fractures Involving the Epiphysial Plates

The primary ossification center for the superior end of the tibia appears shortly after birth and joins the shaft of the tibia during adolescence (usually at 16–18 years of age). Tibial fractures in children are more serious if they involve the epiphysial plates because continued normal growth of the bone may be jeopardized. The tibial tuberosity usually forms by inferior bone growth from the superior epiphysial center at approximately 10 years of age, but a separate center for the tibial tuberosity may appear at approximately 12 years of age. Disruption of the epiphysial plate at the tibial tuberosity may cause inflammation of the tuberosity and chronic recurring pain during adolescence (**Osgood-Schlatter disease**), especially in young athletes. ▶

Fibular Fractures

Fibular fractures commonly occur 2–6 cm proximal to the distal end of the lateral malleolus and are often associated with *fracture–dislocations of the ankle joint,* which are combined with tibial fractures (Fig. B5.4F). When a person slips and the foot is forced into an excessively inverted position, the ankle ligaments tear, forcibly tilting the talus against the lateral malleolus and shearing it off (Fig. B5.4G). *Fractures of the lateral and medial malleoli* are relatively common in soccer and basketball players. Fibular fractures can be painful owing to disrupted muscle attachments; walking is compromised because of the bone's role in ankle stability. ▶

Lateral view   Anterior view

(A) Compound (open) fracture with external bleeding

(B) March (stress) fracture of tibia (*arrows*), most apparent in the MRI study at the right

(C) Diagonal fracture with shortening

(D) Transverse fractures with fibula intact

(E) Normal

(F) Tibial and fibular fractures

Eversion

Inversion

(G) Fibular fracture with excessive inversion of foot

Posterior views

Figure B5.4

Bone Grafts

If a part of a major bone is destroyed by injury or disease, the limb becomes useless. Replacement of the affected segment by a bone transplant may avoid amputation. The fibula is a common source of bone for grafting. Even after a segment of shaft has been removed, walking, running, and jumping can be normal. Free vascularized fibulas have been used to restore skeletal integrity to upper and lower limbs in which congenital bone defects exist and to replace segments of bone after trauma or excision of a malignant tumor (Fig. B5.5). The remaining parts of the fibula usually do not regenerate because the periosteum and nutrient artery are generally removed with the piece of bone so that the graft will remain alive and grow when transplanted to another site. Secured in its new site, the fibular segment restores the blood supply of the bone to which it is now attached. Healing proceeds as if a fracture had occurred at each of its ends.

Awareness of the location of the nutrient foramen in the fibula is important when performing free vascularized fibular transfers. Because the nutrient foramen is located in the middle third of the fibula in most cases, this segment of the bone is used for transplanting when the graft must include a blood supply to the marrow cavity as well as to the compact bone of the surface (via the periosteum). ✪

Posterior view

Section of left fibula grafted into right tibia

Figure B5.5

Bones of the Foot

The bones of the foot include the *tarsus, metatarsus,* and *phalanges.* There are 7 tarsal bones, 5 metatarsal bones, and 14 phalanges (Figs. 5.1, 5.4, and 5.9). Although knowledge of the characteristics of individual bones is necessary for an understanding of the structure of the foot, it is important to study the skeleton of the foot as a whole and to identify its principal bony landmarks in the living foot (see "Surface Anatomy of the Bones of the Foot," later in this chapter).

Tarsus

The **tarsus** (posterior or proximal foot; hindfoot) consists of seven bones (Fig. 5.9*A* & *B*): talus, calcaneus, cuboid, navicular, and three cuneiforms. Only one bone, the talus, articulates with the leg bones.

The **talus** (L. ankle, ankle bone) has a body, neck, and head (Fig. 5.9*C*). The superior surface, or **trochlea of the talus,** is gripped by the two malleoli (Fig. 5.4) and receives the weight of the body from the tibia. It transmits that weight in turn, dividing it between the calcaneus, on which the **talar body** rests, and the forefoot, via an osseoligamentous "hammock' that receives the rounded and anteromedially directed **talar head.** The hammock (spring ligament) is suspended across a gap between the *talar shelf* (a bracket-like lateral projection of the calcaneus) and the navicular bone, which lies anteriorly (Fig. 5.9*B* & *D*). The talus is the only tarsal bone that has no muscular or tendinous attachments. Most of its surface is covered with articular cartilage. The talar body bears the trochlea superiorly and narrows into a **posterior process** that features a **groove for the tendon of the flexor hallucis longus** (Fig. 5.9*D*), flanked by a prominent **lateral tubercle** and a less prominent **medial tubercle** (Fig. 5.9*A*).

The **calcaneus** (heel bone) is the largest and strongest bone in the foot (Fig. 5.9). When standing, the calcaneus transmits the majority of the body's weight from the talus to the ground. The anterior two thirds of the calcaneus's superior surface articulates with the talus and its anterior surface articulates with the cuboid. The lateral surface of the calcaneus has an oblique ridge (Fig. 5.9*C*), the **fibular trochlea,** that anchors a tendon pulley for the evertors of the foot (muscles that move the sole of the foot away from the median plane). On the medial side, the **talar shelf** (L. *sustentaculum tali*), the shelf-like support of the talus, projects from the superior border of the medial surface of the calcaneus and participates in supporting the talar head (Fig. 5.9*B* & *D*). The posterior part of the calcaneus has a massive, weight-bearing prominence, the **calcaneal tuberosity** (L. *tuber calcanei*), which has **medial, lateral,** and **anterior tubercles.** Only the medial tubercle contacts the ground during standing.

The **navicular** (L. little ship) is a flattened, boat-shaped bone located between the talar head posteriorly and the three cuneiforms anteriorly (Fig. 5.9). The medial surface of the navicular projects inferiorly to form the **navicular tuberosity,**

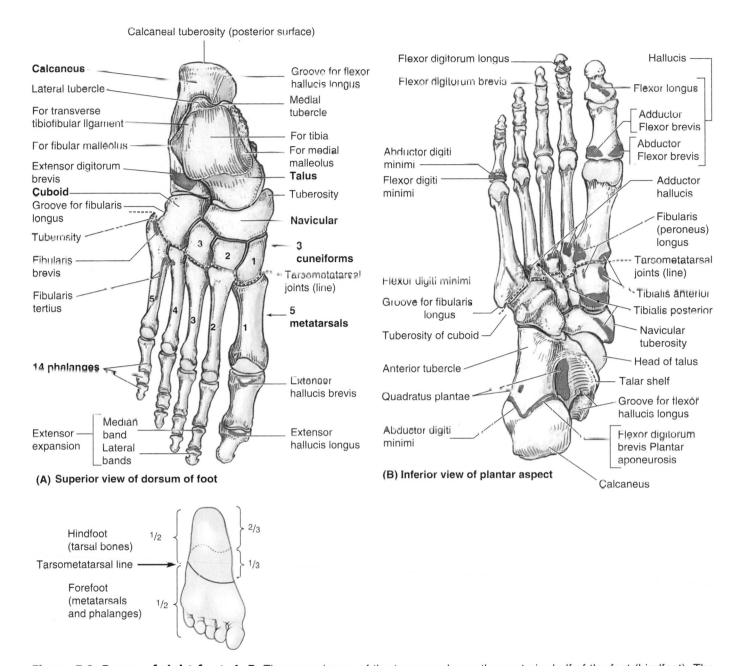

(A) Superior view of dorsum of foot

Calcaneal tuberosity (posterior surface)

Calcaneus
Lateral tubercle
For transverse tibiofibular ligament
For fibular malleolus
Extensor digitorum brevis
Cuboid
Groove for fibularis longus
Tuberosity
Fibularis brevis
Fibularis tertius
14 phalanges
Extensor expansion
Median band
Lateral bands

Groove for flexor hallucis longus
Medial tubercle
For tibia
For medial malleolus
Talus
Tuberosity
Navicular
3 cuneiforms
Tarsometatarsal joints (line)
5 metatarsals
Extensor hallucis brevis
Extensor hallucis longus

(B) Inferior view of plantar aspect

Flexor digitorum longus
Flexor digitorum brevis
Abductor digiti minimi
Flexor digiti minimi
Flexor digiti minimi
Groove for fibularis longus
Tuberosity of cuboid
Anterior tubercle
Quadratus plantae
Abductor digiti minimi

Hallucis
Flexor longus
Adductor Flexor brevis
Abductor Flexor brevis
Adductor hallucis
Fibularis (peroneus) longus
Tarsometatarsal joints (line)
Tibialis anterior
Tibialis posterior
Navicular tuberosity
Head of talus
Talar shelf
Groove for flexor hallucis longus
Flexor digitorum brevis Plantar aponeurosis
Calcaneus

Hindfoot (tarsal bones)
Tarsometatarsal line
Forefoot (metatarsals and phalanges)
1/2   2/3
1/3
1/2

Figure 5.9. Bones of right foot. A–D. The seven bones of the tarsus make up the posterior half of the foot (hindfoot). The talus and calcaneus occupy the posterior two thirds of the hindfoot, and the cuboid; navicular; and medial, lateral, and intermediate cuneiforms occupy the anterior third. Only the talus articulates with the leg bones. The metatarsus connects the tarsus posteriorly with the phalanges anteriorly. Together, the metatarsus and phalanges make up the anterior half of the foot (forefoot). Sites of muscle attachment are shown in parts **A, B,** and **D.** Proximal attachments are shown in *salmon* color and distal attachments in *blue.*

an important site for tendon attachment because the medial border of the foot does not rest on the ground, as does the lateral border. Instead, it forms a *longitudinal arch of the foot,* which must be supported centrally. If this tuberosity is too prominent, it may press against the medial part of the shoe and cause foot pain.

The **cuboid,** approximately cubical in shape, is the most lateral bone in the distal row of the tarsus (Fig. 5.9A & C). Anterior to the **tuberosity of the cuboid** on the lateral and in-

ferior surfaces of the bone is a **groove for the tendon of the fibularis longus** muscle.

The three cuneiforms (Fig. 5.9A, C, & D) are the medial (1st), intermediate (2nd), and lateral (3rd). The **medial cuneiform** is the largest bone, and the **intermediate cuneiform** is the smallest. Each cuneiform (L. *cuneus,* wedge shaped) articulates with the navicular posteriorly and the base of its appropriate metatarsal anteriorly. The **lateral cuneiform** also articulates with the cuboid.

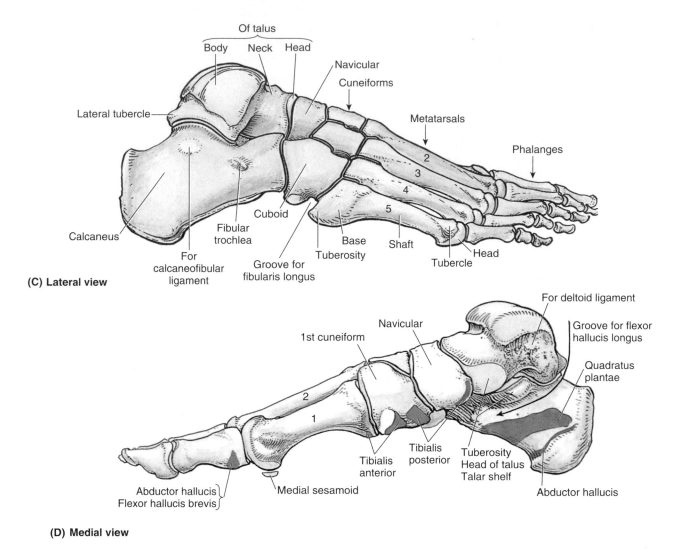

Figure 5.9. *(Continued)*

Metatarsus

The **metatarsus** (anterior or distal foot, forefoot) consists of five metatarsals that are numbered from the medial side of the foot (Fig. 5.9*A*). In the articulated skeleton of the foot (Figs. 5.1, 5.4, and 5.9), the tarsometatarsal joints form an oblique **tarsometatarsal line** joining the midpoints of the medial and shorter lateral borders of the foot; thus the metatarsals and phalanges are located in the anterior half (forefoot) and the tarsals are in the posterior half (hindfoot) (Fig. 5.9*A inset* & *B*).

The **1st metatarsal** is shorter and stouter than the others. The **2nd metatarsal** is the longest. Each metatarsal has a base proximally, a shaft, and a head distally (Fig. 5.9*C*). The base of each metatarsal is the larger, proximal end. The bases of the metatarsals articulate with the cuneiform and cuboid bones, and the heads articulate with the proximal phalanges. The bases of the 1st and 5th metatarsals have large tuberosities that provide for tendon attachment; the **tuberosity of the 5th metatarsal** projects laterally over the cuboid. On the plantar surface of the head of the 1st metatarsal are prominent medial

and lateral *sesamoid bones* (not shown); they are embedded in the tendons passing along the plantar surface (see "Bones of the Foot" in the following section on Surface Anatomy).

Phalanges

The 14 **phalanges** are as follows: the 1st digit (great toe) has 2 phalanges (proximal and distal); the other four digits have 3 phalanges each: proximal, middle, and distal (Fig. 5.9*A* & *C*). Each **phalanx** has a **base** (proximally), a **shaft**, and a **head** (distally). The phalanges of the 1st digit are short, broad, and strong. The middle and distal phalanges of the 5th digit may be fused in elderly people.

THE BOTTOM LINE: The many bones of the foot form a functional unit that allows weight to be distributed to a wide platform to maintain balance when standing, enable conformation and adjustment to terrain variations, and perform shock absorption. They also transfer weight from the heel to the forefoot as required in walking and running.

Surface Anatomy of the Lower Limb Bones

Bony landmarks are helpful during physical examinations and surgery because they can be used to evaluate normal development, detect and assess fractures and dislocations, and locate structures such as nerves and blood vessels.

Pelvic Girdle and Femur

When your hands are on your hips, they rest on your **iliac crests,** the curved superior borders of the alae or wings of the ilia (singular = ilium) (Fig. SA5.1A). The anterior third of the crests is easily palpated because the crests are subcutaneous (Fig. SA5.1C & D). The posterior two thirds of the crests are more difficult to palpate because they are usually covered with fat. The iliac crest ends anteriorly at the rounded **anterior superior iliac spine,** which is easy to palpate by tracing the iliac crest anteroinferiorly. The ASIS is often visible in thin individuals. In obese people these spines are covered with fat and may be difficult to locate; however, they are easier to palpate when the person is sitting and the muscles attached to them are relaxed. The **iliac tubercle,** 5–6 cm posterior to the ASIS, marks the widest point of the iliac crest. To palpate the iliac tubercle, place your thumb on the ASIS and move your fingers posteriorly along the external lip of the iliac crest (Fig. SA5.1B). The iliac tubercle lies at the level of the spinous process of L5 vertebra.

Approximately a hand's width inferior to the umbilicus, the **bodies** and **superior rami of the pubic bones** may be palpated (Fig. SA5.1C). Palpation of the *pubic tubercles* was discussed in Chapter 2. The iliac crest ends posteriorly at the sharp **posterior superior iliac spine** (Fig. SA5.1D), which may be difficult to palpate; however, its position is easy to locate because it lies at the bottom of a skin dimple, approximately 4 cm lateral to the midline (see Chapter 4). The dimple exists because the skin and underlying fascia attach to the PSIS. The **skin dimples** are useful landmarks when palpating the area of the sacroiliac joints in search of edema (swelling) or local tenderness. These dimples also indicate the termination of the iliac crests from which bone marrow and pieces of bone for grafts can be obtained (e.g., to repair a fractured tibia).

The **ischial tuberosity** is easily palpated in the inferior part of the buttock when the thigh is flexed (Fig. SA5.1E). The buttock covers and obscures the tuberosity when the thigh is extended (Fig. SA5.1D). The **gluteal fold (sulcus)** coincides with the inferior border of the gluteus maximus and indicates the separation of the buttock from the thigh.

The center of the **femoral head** can be palpated deep to a point approximately a thumb's breadth inferior to the midpoint of the inguinal ligament (Fig. SA5.1C). The *shaft of the femur* is covered with muscles and is not usually palpable. Only the superior and inferior ends of the femur are palpable. The laterally placed **greater trochanter** projects superior to the junction of the shaft with the femoral neck and can be palpated on the lateral side of the thigh approximately 10 cm inferior to the iliac crest (Fig. SA5.1B). The greater trochanter forms a prominence anterior to the hollow on the lateral side of the buttock. The prominences of the greater trochanters are normally responsible for the width of the adult pelvis. The posterior edge of the greater trochanter is relatively uncovered and most easily palpated when the limb is not weight bearing. The anterior and lateral parts of the trochanter are not easy to palpate because they are covered by fascia and muscle. Because it lies close to the skin, the greater trochanter causes discomfort when you lie on your side on a hard surface. In the anatomical position, a line joining the tips of the greater trochanters normally passes through the pubic tubercles and the center of the femoral heads. The **lesser trochanter** is indistinctly palpable superior to the lateral end of the gluteal fold. ▶

(A)

(B)

Figure SA5.1

Green = palpable features
of lower limb bones

(C) Anterior view

(D) Posterior view

Figure SA5.1. *(Continued)*

The **femoral condyles** are subcutaneous and easily palpated when the knee is flexed or extended (Fig. SA5.1*F*). At the center of the lateral aspect of each condyle is a prominent **epicondyle** that is easily palpable. The patellar surface of the femur is where the **patella** slides during flexion and extension of the leg at the knee joint. The lateral and medial margins of the patellar surface can be palpated when the leg is flexed. The **adductor tubercle,** a small prominence of bone, may be felt at the superior part of the medial femoral condyle by pushing your thumb inferiorly along the medial side of the thigh until it encounters the tubercle.

Tibia and Fibula

The **tibial tuberosity,** an oval elevation on the anterior surface of the tibia, is easily palpated approximately 5 cm distal to the apex of the patella. The subcutaneous, flat **anteromedial surface of the tibia** is also easy to palpate. The skin covering this surface is freely movable. The **tibial condyles** can be palpated anteriorly at the sides of the patellar ligament, especially when the knee is flexed. The **head of the fibula** is prominent at the level of the superior part of the tibial tuberosity because the knob-like head is subcutaneous at the posterolateral aspect of the knee. The **neck of the fibula** can be palpated just distal to the lateral ▶

Figure SA5.1. *(Continued)*

side of the head. Doing so may evoke a mildly unpleasant sensation because of the presence of a nerve passing there.

The **medial malleolus,** the prominence on the medial side of the ankle, is also subcutaneous and prominent (Fig. SA5.1*G* & *H*). Note that its inferior end is blunt and does not extend as far distally as the lateral malleolus. The medial malleolus lies approximately 1.25 cm proximal to the level of the tip of the lateral malleolus. Only the distal quarter of the shaft of the fibula is palpable. Feel your **lateral malleolus,** noting that it is subcutaneous and that its inferior end is sharp (Fig. SA5.1*G* & *I*). Note that the tip of the lateral malleolus extends farther distally and more posteriorly than does the tip of the medial malleolus.

Bones of the Foot

The **talar head** is palpable anteromedial to the proximal part of the lateral malleolus when the foot is inverted and anterior to the medial malleolus when the foot is everted (Fig. SA5.1*G*). Eversion of the foot makes the talar head more prominent as it moves away from the navicular. The head occupies the space between the talar shelf and the navicular tuberosity. If the talar head is difficult to palpate, draw a line from the tip of the medial malleolus to the navicular tuberosity; the talar head lies deep to the center of this line. When the foot is plantarflexed, the superior surface of the body of the talus can be palpated on the anterior aspect of the ankle, anterior to the inferior end of the tibia.

The weight-bearing **medial tubercle of the calcaneus** on the plantar surface of the foot is broad and large (Fig. SA5.1*J*), but often it is not palpable because of the overlying skin and subcutaneous tissue. The **talar shelf** is the only part of the medial aspect of the calcaneus that may be palpated as a small prominence approximately a finger's breadth distal to the tip of the medial malleolus. The entire lateral surface of the calcaneus is subcutaneous. The **fibular trochlea,** a small lateral extension of the calcaneus, may be detectable as a small tubercle on the lateral aspect of the calcaneus, anteroinferior to the tip of the lateral malleolus.

Usually, palpation of bony prominences on the plantar surface of the foot is difficult because of the thick skin, fascia, and pads of fat. The medial and lateral **sesamoid bones** inferior to the head of the 1st metatarsal can be felt to slide when the great toe is moved passively. The **heads of the metatarsals** can be palpated by placing the thumb on their plantar surfaces and the index finger on their dorsal surfaces. If **callosities** (calluses), thickenings of the keratin layer of the epidermis, are present, the metatarsal heads are difficult to palpate.

The **tuberosity of the 5th metatarsal** forms a prominent landmark on the lateral aspect of the foot (Fig. SA5.1*I* & *J*), which can easily be palpated at the midpoint of the lateral border of the foot. The **shafts of the metatarsals and phalanges** can be felt on the dorsum of the foot between the extensor tendons. The **cuboid** can be felt on the lateral aspect of the foot, posterior to the base of the 5th metatarsal. The **medial cuneiform** can be palpated between the tuberosity of the navicular and the base of the 1st metatarsal (Fig. SA5.1*H*). The **head of the 1st metatarsal** forms a prominence on the medial aspect of the foot. The **tuberosity of the navicular** is easily seen and palpated on the medial aspect of the foot (Fig. SA5.1*H*), inferoanterior to the tip of the medial malleolus. The cuboid and cuneiforms are difficult to identify individually by palpation. ◉

Calcaneal Fractures

A hard fall onto the heel, from a ladder for example, may fracture the calcaneus into several pieces, producing a *comminuted fracture* (Fig. B5.6*A*). A calcaneal fracture is usually disabling because it disrupts the subtalar (talocalcaneal) joint, where the talus articulates with the calcaneus.

Fractures of the Talar Neck

Fractures of the talar neck (Fig. B5.6*B*) may occur during severe dorsiflexion of the ankle (e.g., when a person is pressing extremely hard on the brake pedal of a vehicle during a head-on collision). In some cases, the body of the talus dislocates posteriorly.

Fractures of the Metatarsals

Metatarsal fractures occur when a heavy object falls on the foot, for example or when it is run over by a heavy object such as a metal wheel (Fig. B5.6*C*). Metatarsal fractures are also common in dancers, especially female ballet dancers who use the demi-pointe technique. The *dancer's fracture* usually occurs when the dancer loses balance, putting the full body weight on the metatarsal and fracturing the bone. *Fatigue fractures of the metatarsals* may result from prolonged walking. These fractures, usually transverse, result from repeated stress on the metatarsals.

When the foot is suddenly and violently inverted, the tuberosity of the 5th metatarsal may be avulsed by the ▶

(A) Lateral views

Comminuted fractures of calcaneus

Subtalar joint

Talus

Calcaneus

Medial tubercle

(B) Medial views

Tibia

Talar neck

Talus

Calcaneus

Fracture of talar neck

4th metatarsal

5th metatarsal

5th metatarsal tuberosity

Cuboid

(C) Dorsal view

Fractures of metatarsals

Figure B5.6

tendon of the fibularis brevis muscle. *Avulsion fractures of the 5th metatarsal tuberosity* (Fig. B5.6C) are common in basketball and tennis players. Part of the tuberosity is pulled off, producing pain and edema at the base of the 5th metatarsal.

Os Trigonum

During ossification of the talus, the secondary ossification center, which becomes the lateral tubercle of the talus, occasionally fails to unite with the body of the talus. This failure may be caused by applied stress (forceful plan-

tarflexion) during the early teens. Occasionally, a partly or even fully ossified center may fracture and progress to nonunion. Either event may result in a bone (accessory ossicle) known as an **os trigonum,** which occurs in 14–25% of adults, more commonly bilaterally (Fig. B5.7). It has an increased prevalence among soccer players and ballet dancers. Patients with an os trigonum may be symptomatic or pain free. Radionuclide bone scanning, which provides physiological as well as anatomical evidence, is useful in distinguishing symptomatic and asymptomatic ossicles. (Lawson, 1994) ▶

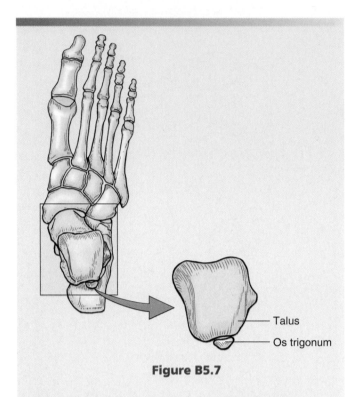

Talus

Os trigonum

Figure B5.7

Fracture of the Sesamoid Bones

The sesamoid bones of the great toe in the tendon of the flexor hallucis longus bear the weight of the body, especially during the latter part of the stance phase of walking (see "Posture and Gait," in this chapter). The sesamoids develop before birth and begin to ossify during late childhood. *Fracture of the sesamoids* may result from a crushing injury (e.g., when a heavy object falls on the great toe). ⊕

Fascia, Vessels, and Cutaneous Nerves of the Lower Limb

Subcutaneous Tissue and Fascia

The **subcutaneous tissue (superficial fascia)** lies deep to the skin (Fig. 5.10) and consists of loose connective tissue that contains a variable amount of fat, cutaneous nerves, superficial veins (great and small saphenous veins and their tributaries), lymphatic vessels, and lymph nodes. The subcutaneous tissue of the hip and thigh is continuous with that of the inferior part of the anterolateral abdominal wall and buttock. At the knee, the subcutaneous tissue loses its fat and blends with the deep fascia, but fat is again present distal to the knee in the subcutaneous tissue of the leg.

The **deep fascia** of the lower limb is especially strong, investing the limb like an elastic stocking (Fig. 5.10*A* & *B*). The deep fascia limits outward expansion of contracting muscles, making muscular contraction more efficient in compressing veins to push blood toward the heart. The *deep fascia of the thigh* is called **fascia lata** (L. *lata,* broad). It is continues inferior to the knee as the *deep fascia of the leg.*

The fascia lata attaches to/is continuous with:

- The inguinal ligament, pubic arch, body of pubis, and pubic tubercle superiorly; the membranous layer of subcutaneous tissue (Scarpa fascia) of the inferior abdominal wall also attaches to the fascia lata approximately a finger's breadth inferior to the inguinal ligament.

- The iliac crest laterally and posteriorly.

- The sacrum, coccyx, sacrotuberous ligament, and ischial tuberosity posteriorly.

- Exposed parts of bones around the knee and the deep fascia of the leg distally.

The fascia lata is substantial because it encloses the large thigh muscles, especially laterally where it is thickened and strengthened by additional reinforcing longitudinal fibers to form the **iliotibial tract** (Fig. 5.10*B*). This broad band of fibers is the conjoint aponeurosis of the *tensor of fascia lata* and *gluteus maximus* muscles. The iliotibial tract extends from the iliac tubercle to the anterolateral tibial tubercle.

The thigh muscles are separated into three compartments—anterior, medial, and posterior. The walls of these compartments are formed by the fascia lata and three fascial intermuscular septa that arise from its deep aspect and attach to the linea aspera of the femur (Fig. 5.10*D*). The **lateral intermuscular septum** is especially strong; the other two septa are relatively weak. The lateral intermuscular septum extends deeply from the iliotibial tract to the lateral lip of the linea aspera and lateral supracondylar line of the femur. This septum offers a welcome internervous plane to surgeons needing wide exposure of the femur.

The **saphenous opening** in the fascia lata (Fig. 5.10*A*) is a gap or hiatus in the fascia lata inferior to the medial part of the inguinal ligament, approximately 4 cm inferolateral to the pubic tubercle. The saphenous opening is usually approximately 3.75 cm in length and 2.5 cm in breadth, and its long axis is vertical. Its medial margin is smooth but its superior, lateral, and inferior margins form a sharp crescentic edge, the **falciform margin.** This margin is joined at its medial margin by fibrofatty tissue, the **cribriform fascia** (L. *cribrum,* a sieve). This sieve-like fascia is a localized membranous layer of subcutaneous tissue that spreads over the saphenous opening, closing it. This layer of spongy connective tissue is pierced by numerous openings (thus its name) for the passage of efferent lymphatic vessels from the superficial inguinal lymph nodes and by the great saphenous vein and its tributaries. After passing through the saphenous opening and cribriform fascia, the great saphenous

Figure 5.10. Fascia, intermuscular septa, and fascial compartments of lower limb. A. The anterior skin and subcutaneous tissue have been removed to reveal the deep fascia of the thigh (fascia lata) and leg (crural fascia). **B.** The fascia lata is reinforced laterally with longitudinal fibers to form the iliotibial tract, which also serves as an aponeurosis for the gluteus maximus and tensor of fascia lata muscles. **C and D.** The fascial compartments of the thigh and leg, containing muscles sharing common functions and innervation, are demonstrated in transverse sections.

vein enters the femoral vein (Figs. 5.10*A* and 5.11*A*). The lymphatic vessels enter the deep inguinal lymph nodes.

The **deep fascia of the leg,** the **crural fascia** (L. *crus,* leg), attaches to the anterior and medial borders of the tibia, where it is continuous with its periosteum. The deep fascia of the leg is thick in the proximal part of the anterior aspect of the leg, where it forms part of the proximal attachments of the underlying muscles. Although thinner distally, the deep fascia of the leg forms thickened bands both superior and anterior to the ankle joint, the **extensor retinacula** (Fig. 5.10*A*). **Anterior** and **posterior intermuscular septa** pass from the deep surface of the lateral deep fascia of the leg and attach to the corresponding margins of the fibula. The *interosseous membrane* and the intermuscular septa divide the leg into three compartments: anterior (dorsiflexor), lateral (fibular), and posterior (plantarflexor) (Fig. 5.10*C*). The muscles in the posterior compartment are subdivided into superficial and deep parts by the **transverse intermuscular septum.**

THE BOTTOM LINE: The lower limb is invested by subcutaneous tissue and deep fascia. The former insulates, stores fat, and provides passage for cutaneous nerves and superficial vessels (lymphatics and veins). The deep fascia of the thigh (fascia lata) and leg (crural fascia) (1) surround the thigh and leg, respectively, limiting outward bulging of muscles and facilitating venous return in deep veins; (2) separate muscles with similar functions and innervation into compartments, and (3) surround individual muscles, allowing them to act independently. Modifications of the deep fascia include openings that allow the passage of neurovascular structures (e.g., the saphenous opening) and thickenings that retain tendons close to the joints they act on (retinacula).

Venous Drainage of the Lower Limb

The lower limb has superficial and deep veins; the superficial veins are in the subcutaneous tissue, and the deep veins are deep to (beneath) the deep fascia and accompany all major arteries. Superficial and deep veins have valves, which are more numerous in deep veins.

Superficial Veins of the Lower Limb

The two major superficial veins in the lower limb are the great and small *saphenous veins* (Fig. 5.11*A* & *B*). Most of their tributaries are unnamed.

The **great saphenous vein** is formed by the union of the **dorsal vein of the great toe** and the **dorsal venous arch** of the foot. The great saphenous vein:

- Ascends anterior to the medial malleolus.

- Passes posterior to the medial condyle of the femur (about a hand's breadth posterior to the medial border of the patella) (Fig. 5.12 inset).

- Anastomoses freely with the small saphenous vein.

- Traverses the saphenous opening in the fascia lata.

- Empties into the femoral vein.

The *great saphenous vein* has 10–12 valves, which are more numerous in the leg than in the thigh. These valves are usually located just inferior to the perforating veins (Fig. 5.11*A*). The perforating veins also have valves. **Venous valves** are cusps (flaps) of endothelium with cup-like *valvular sinuses* that fill from above. When they are full, the valve cusps occlude the lumen of the vein, thereby preventing reflux of blood distally, making flow unidirectional. The valvular mechanism also breaks the column of blood in the saphenous vein into shorter segments, reducing back pressure. Both effects make it easier for the musculovenous pump to overcome the force of gravity to return the blood to the heart.

As it ascends in the leg and thigh, the great saphenous vein receives numerous tributaries and communicates in several locations with the small saphenous vein. Tributaries from the medial and posterior aspects of the thigh frequently unite to form an **accessory saphenous vein** (Fig. 5.11*B*). When present, this vein becomes the main communication between the great and the small saphenous veins. Also, fairly large vessels, the **lateral** and **anterior cutaneous veins,** arise from networks of veins in the inferior part of the thigh and enter the great saphenous vein superiorly, just before it enters the femoral vein. Near its termination, the great saphenous vein also receives the superficial circumflex iliac, superficial epigastric, and external pudendal veins (Fig. 5.11*A*).

The **small saphenous vein** arises on the lateral side of the foot from the union of the **dorsal vein of the little toe** with the *dorsal venous arch* (Fig. 5.11*B*). The small saphenous vein:

- Ascends posterior to the lateral malleolus as a continuation of the lateral marginal vein.

- Passes along the lateral border of the calcaneal tendon.

- Inclines to the midline of the fibula and penetrates the deep fascia.

- Ascends between the heads of the gastrocnemius muscle.

- Empties into the popliteal vein in the popliteal fossa.

Although many tributaries are received by the saphenous veins, their diameters remain remarkably uniform as they ascend the limb. This is possible because the blood received by the saphenous veins is continuously shunted from these superficial veins in the subcutaneous tissue to the deep veins by means of many perforating veins.

The **perforating veins** penetrate the deep fascia close to their origin from the superficial veins and contain valves that allow blood to flow only from the superficial veins to the deep veins. The perforating veins pass through the deep fascia at an oblique angle so that when muscles contract and the pressure

(*cont'd on page 583*)

Figure 5.11. Veins of lower limb. The veins are subdivided into superficial (**A and B**) and deep (**C and E**) groups. The superficial veins, usually unaccompanied, course within the subcutaneous tissue; the deep veins are internal to the deep fascia and usually accompany arteries. **A, inset.** The proximal ends of the femoral and great saphenous veins are opened and spread apart to show the valves. Although depicted as single veins in parts **C** and **E,** the deep veins usually occur as duplicate or multiple accompanying veins. **D.** Multiple perforating veins pierce the deep fascia to shunt blood from the superficial veins (e.g., the great saphenous vein) to the deep veins (e.g., the posterior tibial and fibular veins).

Superficial inguinal lymph nodes (superior or horizontal group)

Deep inguinal lymph nodes

Femoral vein

Superficial inguinal lymph nodes (inferior or vertical group)

Great saphenous vein

Superficial lymphatic vessels

Great saphenous vein

Great saphenous vein

Medial border of patella

Popliteal vein

Popliteal lymph nodes

Small saphenous vein

Lumbar lymphatic trunk

Lateral aortic nodes

Common iliac vein and nodes

External iliac vein and nodes

Superficial inguinal nodes

(A) Anteromedial view of left limb

(B) Posterior view of left limb

(C) Medial view: *Arrows* represent the continuation of lymph drainage from the lower limb via the superficial inguinal and iliac nodes

Figure 5.12. Superficial veins and lymphatics of lower limb. A. The great saphenous vein ascends the medial aspect of the limb, passing anterior to the medial malleolus and approximately a hand's breadth posterior to the patella (knee cap) (**inset**). The superficial lymphatic vessels from the medial foot, anteromedial leg, and thigh converge toward and accompany the great saphenous vein, draining into the inferior (vertical) group of superficial inguinal lymph nodes. **B.** Superficial lymphatic vessels of the lateral foot and posterolateral leg accompany the lesser saphenous vein and drain initially into the popliteal lymph nodes, which lie deep to the popliteal fascia. The efferent vessels from these nodes join other deep lymphatics, which accompany the femoral vessels to drain into the deep inguinal lymph nodes. **C.** Lymph from the superficial and deep inguinal lymph nodes traverses the external and common iliac nodes before entering the lateral aortic lymph nodes and the lumbar lymphatic trunk.

increases inside the deep fascia, the perforating veins are compressed. Compression of the perforating veins also prevents blood from flowing from the deep to the superficial veins. This pattern of venous blood flow—from superficial to deep—is important for proper venous return from the lower limb because it enables muscular contractions to propel blood toward the heart against the pull of gravity (*musculovenous pump;* see the Introduction).

Deep Veins of the Lower Limb

The deep veins accompany all the major arteries (L. *venae comitantes*) and their branches. Instead of occurring as a single vein in the limbs (although they are frequently illustrated as one and are often referred to as a single vein), the deep veins usually occur as paired, frequently interconnecting veins that flank the artery they accompany (Fig. 5.11C & F). They are contained within the vascular sheath with the artery, whose pulsations also help compress and move blood in the veins.

Although the *dorsal venous arch* drains primarily via the superficial saphenous veins, perforating veins penetrate the deep fascia, forming and continually supplying an anterior tibial vein in the anterior leg. **Medial** and **lateral plantar veins** from the plantar aspect of the foot form the **posterior tibial** and **fibular veins** posterior to the medial and lateral malleoli (Fig. 5.11C–E). All three deep veins from the leg flow into the **popliteal vein** posterior to the knee, which becomes the **femoral vein** in the thigh. Veins accompanying the perforating arteries of the deep artery of the thigh drain blood from the thigh muscles and terminate in the **deep vein of the thigh** (L. *vena profunda femoris*), which joins the terminal portion of the femoral vein. The femoral vein passes deep to the inguinal ligament to become the external iliac vein of the trunk.

Because of the effect of gravity, blood flow is slower when a person stands quietly. During exercise, blood received from the superficial veins by the deep veins is propelled by muscular contraction to the femoral and then the external iliac veins. Flow in the reverse direction—away from the heart or from the deep to the superficial veins—is prevented if the venous valves are competent (capable of performing their function). The deep veins are more variable and anastomose much more frequently than the arteries they accompany. Both superficial and deep veins can be ligated with impunity if necessary.

THE BOTTOM LINE: The veins of the lower limb include both superficial (in the subcutaneous tissue) and deep (internal to the deep fascia) veins. The superficial great and lesser saphenous veins mainly drain the integument or skin and, via many perforating veins, continuously shunting blood to the deep veins accompanying the arteries. Deep veins are subject to muscle compression (musculovenous pump) to aid venous return. All lower limb veins have valves to overcome the effects of gravity.

Varicose Veins, Thrombosis, and Thrombophlebitis

Frequently, the great saphenous vein and its tributaries become **varicose** (dilated so that the cusps of their valves do not close). *Varicose veins* are common in the posteromedial parts of the lower limb and may cause considerable discomfort (Fig. B5.8). Varicose veins form when the valves that usually prevent blood flow from the deep veins through the perforating veins to the superficial veins are incompetent. When the valves within the great saphenous vein itself are incompetent, the pull of gravity on the uninterrupted column of blood results in a higher intraluminal pressure, which also exacerbates varicosities. As a result, the superficial veins become tortuous and dilated.

The veins of the lower limb are subject to **venous thrombosis** (blood clotting) after a bone fracture. **Venous stasis** (stagnation) is an important cause of thrombus formation. Venous stasis can be caused by:

- Incompetent, loose fascia that fails to resist muscle expansion, diminishing the effectiveness of the musculovenous pump. ▶

Varicose veins

Figure B5.8

- External pressure on the veins from bedding during a prolonged hospital stay or from a tight cast or bandage.

- Muscular inactivity (e.g., during an overseas flight).

Venous inflammation with thrombus formation (**thrombophlebitis**) may develop around the vein. A thrombus that breaks free from a lower limb vein and travels to the lungs constitutes a **pulmonary thromboembolism** (obstruction of a pulmonary artery). A large embolus may obstruct a main pulmonary artery and cause death (see Chapter 1).

Saphenous Vein Grafts

The great saphenous vein is commonly used for coronary arterial bypasses because (1) it is readily accessible, (2) sufficient distance occurs between the tributaries and the perforating veins so that usable lengths can be harvested, and (3) its wall contains a higher percentage of muscular and elastic fibers than do other superficial veins. Saphenous vein grafts are used to bypass obstructions in blood vessels (e.g., in an intracoronary thrombus; see Chapter 1). When part of the great saphenous vein is removed for a bypass, the vein is reversed so that the valves do not obstruct blood flow in the graft. Because there are so many other leg veins, removal of the great saphenous vein rarely produces a significant problem in the lower limb or seriously affects circulation, provided the deep veins are intact. In fact, removal of this vein may facilitate the superficial to deep drainage pattern to take advantage of the musculovenous pump.

Saphenous Cutdown and Saphenous Nerve Injury

Even when it is not visible in infants, in obese people, or in patients in shock whose veins are collapsed, the great saphenous vein can always be located by making a skin incision anterior to the medial malleolus (Fig. 5.11A). This procedure, called a **saphenous cutdown**, is used to insert a cannula for prolonged administration of blood, plasma expanders, electrolytes, or drugs. The saphenous nerve accompanies the great saphenous vein anterior to the medial malleolus. Should this nerve be cut during a saphenous cutdown or caught by a ligature during closure of a surgical wound, the patient may complain of pain or numbness along the medial border of the foot. ⊙

Lymphatic Drainage of the Lower Limb

The lower limb has superficial and deep lymphatic vessels. The **superficial lymphatic vessels** converge on and accompany the saphenous veins and their tributaries (Fig. 5.12A). The lymphatic vessels accompanying the great saphenous vein end in the vertical group of **superficial inguinal lymph nodes.** Most lymph from these nodes passes directly to the **external iliac lymph nodes,** located along the external iliac vein; but lymph may also pass to the **deep inguinal lymph nodes.** These nodes lie under the deep fascia on the medial aspect of the femoral vein. The lymphatic vessels accompanying the small saphenous vein enter the **popliteal lymph nodes,** which surround the popliteal vein in the fat of the popliteal fossa (Fig. 5.12B). The **deep lymphatic vessels** from the leg accompany deep veins and enter the popliteal lymph nodes. Most lymph from these nodes ascends through deep lymphatic vessels to the deep inguinal lymph nodes. Lymph from the deep nodes passes to the external and common iliac lymph nodes and is then received by the **lumbar lymphatic trunks** (Fig. 5.12C).

veins to deep inguinal nodes. Lymph drainage from the lower limb then passes deep to the external and common iliac nodes of the trunk.

Enlarged Inguinal Lymph Nodes

Lymph nodes enlarge when diseased. **Abrasions** and **minor sepsis,** caused by pathogenic microorganisms or their toxins in the blood or other tissues, may produce slight enlargement of the superficial inguinal lymph nodes (**lymphadenopathy**) in otherwise healthy people. Because these enlarged nodes are located in the subcutaneous tissue, they are easy to palpate in healthy people. Those who are unaware of this may be concerned when they feel these nodes because they assume they have a serious genital disease, for example. When inguinal lymph nodes are enlarged, their entire field of drainage—the trunk inferior to the umbilicus, including the perineum, as well as the entire lower limb—should be examined to determine the cause of their enlargement. In ▶

THE BOTTOM LINE: Most lymph from the lower limb drains via lymphatics that follow the superficial veins to the superficial inguinal nodes. Some lymphatics follow deep

Cutaneous Innervation of the Lower Limb

Cutaneous nerves in the subcutaneous tissue supply the skin of the lower limb (Table 5.1). These nerves, except for some proximal unisegmental nerves arising from the T12 or L1 spinal nerves, are branches of the lumbar and sacral plexuses (see Chapters 3 and 4). The areas of skin supplied by the individual spinal nerves, including those contributing to the plexuses, are called **dermatomes**. The dermatomal (segmental) pattern of skin innervation is retained throughout life but is distorted by limb lengthening and the torsion of the limb that occurs during development (Fig. 5.13). Although simplified into distinct zones in dermatome maps, adjacent dermatomes overlap, except at the **axial line**, the line of junction of dermatomes supplied from discontinuous spinal levels. Dermatomes L1–L5 extend as a series of bands from the posterior midline of the trunk into the limbs, passing laterally and inferiorly around the limb to its anterior and medial aspects, reflecting the medial rotation that occurs developmentally. Dermatomes S1 and S2 pass inferiorly down the posterior aspect of the limb, separating near the ankle to pass to the lateral and medial margins of the foot. The cutaneous nerves of the lower limb are illustrated and their origin (including contributing spinal nerves), course, and distribution are listed in Table 5.1.

(A) Anterior view   **(B) Posterior view**   **(C) Anterior view**   **(D) Posterior view**

Figure 5.13. Dermatomes of lower limb. The dermatomal or segmental pattern of distribution of sensory nerve fibers persists despite the merging of spinal nerves in plexus formation during development. Two different dermatome maps are commonly used. **A and B.** The dermatome pattern of the lower limb according to Foerster (1933) is preferred by many because of its correlation with clinical findings. **C and D.** The dermatome pattern of the lower limb according to Keegan and Garrett (1948) is preferred by others for its aesthetic uniformity and obvious correlation with development. Although depicted as distinct zones, adjacent dermatomes overlap considerably, except along the axial line.

Table 5.1. Cutaneous Nerves of the Lower Limb

(A) Anterior view

(B) Posterior View

Nerve	Origin (contributing spinal nerves)	Course	Distribution in Lower Limb
Subcostal	T12 anterior ramus	Courses along inferior border of 12th rib; lateral cutaneous branch descends over iliac crest	Lateral cutaneous branch supplies skin of hip region interior to anterior iliac crest and anterior to greater trochanter
Iliohypogastric	Lumbar plexus (L1; occasionally T12)	Parallels iliac crest; divides into lateral and anterior cutaneous branches	Lateral cutaneous branch supplies superolateral quadrant of buttock
Ilioinguinal	Lumbar plexus (L1; occasionally T12)	Passes through inguinal canal; divides into femoral and scrotal or labial branches	Femoral branch supplies skin over medial femoral triangle
Genitofemoral	Lumbar plexus (L1–L2)	Descends anterior surface of psoas major; divides into genital and femoral branches	Femoral branch supplies skin over lateral femoral triangle; genital branch supplies anterior scrotum or labia majora
Lateral cutaneous nerve of thigh	Lumbar plexus (L2–L3)	Passes deep to inguinal ligament, 2–3 cm medial to anterior superior iliac spine	Supplies skin on anterior and lateral aspects of thigh
Anterior cutaneous branches	Lumbar plexus via femoral nerve (L2–L4)	Arise in femoral triangle; pierce fascia lata along path of sartorius muscle	Supply skin of anterior and medial aspects of thigh
Cutaneous branch of obturator nerve	Lumbar plexus via obturator nerve, ant. branch (L2–L4)	Following its descent between adductors longus and brevis, anterior division of obturator nerve pierces fascia lata to reach skin of thigh	Skin of middle part of medial thigh

Table 5.1. Cutaneous Nerves of the Lower Limb *(continued)*

Nerve	Origin (contributing spinal nerves)	Course	Distribution in Lower Limb
Posterior cutaneous nerve of thigh	Sacral plexus (S1–S3)	Enters gluteal region via infrapiriform portion of greater sciatic foramen deep to gluteus maximus; then descends deep to fascia lata	Terminal branches pierce fascia lata to supply skin of posterior thigh and popliteal fossa
Saphenous nerve	Lumbar plexus via femoral nerve (L3–L4)	Traverses adductor canal but does not pass through adductor hiatus; crossing medial side of knee deep to sartorius tendon	Skin on medial side of leg and foot
Superficial fibular nerve	Common fibular nerve (L4–S1)	Courses through lateral compartment of leg; after supplying fibular muscles, perforates crural fascia	Skin of anterolateral leg and dorsum of foot, excluding web between great and 2nd toes
Deep fibular nerve	Common fibular nerve (L5)	After supplying muscles on dorsum of foot, pierces deep fascia superior to heads of 1st and 2nd metatarsals	Skin of web between great and 2nd toes
Sural nerve	Tibial and common fibular nerves (S1–S2)	Medial sural cutaneous branch of tibial nerve and lateral sural cutaneous branch of fibular nerve merge at varying levels on posterior leg	Skin of posterolateral leg and lateral margin of foot
Medial plantar nerve	Tibial nerve (L4–L5)	Passes between first and second layers of plantar muscles; then between medial and middle muscles of first layer	Skin on medial side of sole and sides, plantar aspect, and nail beds of medial 3½ toes
Lateral plantar nerve	Tibial nerve (S1–S2)	Passes between first and second layers of plantar muscles; then between middle and lateral muscles of first layer	Skin on lateral side of sole and sides, plantar aspect, and nail beds of lateral 1½ toes
Calcaneal nerves	Tibial and sural nerves (S1–S2)	Lateral and medial branches of tibial and sural nerves, respectively, over calcaneal tuberosity	Skin of heel
Superior clunial nerves	L1–L3 posterior rami	Penetrate thoracodorsal fascia; course laterally and inferiorly in subcutaneous tissue	Skin overlying superior and central parts of buttock
Medial clunial nerves	S1–S3 posterior rami	Emerge from dorsal sacral foramina; directly enter overlying subcutaneous tissue	Skin of medial buttock and intergluteal cleft
Inferior clunial nerves	Posterior cutaneous nerve of thigh (S2–S3)	Arise deep to gluteus maximus; emerge from beneath inferior border of muscle	Skin of inferior buttock (overlying gluteal fold)

THE BOTTOM LINE: The cutaneous innervation of the lower limb reflects both the original segmental innervation of the skin via separate spinal nerves in its dermatomal pattern and the result of plexus formation in the distribution of multi-segmental peripheral nerves. Most innervation of the thigh is supplied by lateral and posterior cutaneous nerves of the thigh and anterior cutaneous branches of the femoral nerve, the names of which describe their distribution. The latter branches also supply most of the medial aspect of the thigh. The innervation of the leg and dorsum of the foot is supplied by saphenous (anteromedial leg), sural (posterolateral leg), and fibular nerves (anterolateral leg and dorsum of foot). The plantar aspect (sole) of the foot is supplied by calcaneal branches of the tibial and sural nerves (heel region) and the medial and lateral plantar nerves; the areas of distribution of the latter are demarcated by a line bisecting the 4th toe.

Regional Anesthetic Nerve Blocks of the Lower Limbs

The iliohypogastric and ilioinguinal nerves can be blocked by injecting an anesthetic agent 4–6 cm posterior to the ASIS, along the lateral aspect of the external lip of the iliac crest (see Chapter 2). This is where these nerves perforate the transverse abdominal (L. *transversus abdominis*) muscle. The femoral nerve (L2–L4) can be blocked 2 cm inferior to the inguinal ligament, approximately a finger's breadth lateral to the femoral artery. **Paresthesia** (tingling, burning, tickling) radiates to the knee and over the medial side of the leg if the saphenous nerve (terminal branch of femoral) is affected. ▶

Variations of the Cutaneous Nerves

Variations of the cutaneous nerves are common. For example, the iliohypogastric and ilioinguinal nerves may arise from a common trunk of variable length, or the ilioinguinal nerve may join the iliohypogastric nerve at the iliac crest. In the latter case, the iliohypogastric nerve supplies the cutaneous branches for both nerves. When the obturator nerve has a large cutaneous branch, the medial anterior cutaneous branches of the femoral nerve are correspondingly small.

Abnormalities of Sensory Function

In most instances, a peripheral nerve sensitizing an area of skin represents more than one segment of the spinal cord. Therefore, to interpret abnormalities of peripheral sensory function, peripheral nerve distribution of the major cutaneous nerves must be interpreted as anatomically different from dermatome distribution of the spinal cord segments (Fig. 5.13). Neighboring dermatomes may overlap. Pain sensation is tested by using a sharp object and asking the patient if pain is felt. If there is no sensation, the spinal cord segment(s) involved can be determined. ✪

Posture and Gait

The lower limbs function primarily in standing and walking. Typically the actions of the lower limb muscles are described as if the muscle were acting in isolation, which rarely occurs. In this book, including the comments in the tables, the role of each muscle (or of the functional group of which it is a member) is described in typical activities, especially standing and walking. It is important to be familiar with lower limb movements and concentric and eccentric contractions of muscles, as described in the Introduction, and to have a basic understanding of the processes of standing and walking.

Standing at Ease

When a person is standing at ease with the feet slightly apart and rotated laterally so the toes point outward, only a few of the back and lower limb muscles are active (Fig. 5.14). The mechanical arrangement of the joints and muscles are such that a minimum of muscular activity is required to keep from falling. In the stand-easy position, the hip and knee joints are extended and are in their most stable positions (maximal contact of articular surfaces for weight transfer, with supporting ligaments taut). The ankle joint is less stable than the hip and knee joints, and the line of gravity falls between the two limbs just anterior to the axis of rotation of the ankle joints. Consequently, a tendency to fall forward

(*forward sway*) must be countered periodically by bilateral contraction of calf muscles (plantarflexion). The spread and splay of the feet increase lateral stability. However, when *lateral sway* occurs, it is countered by the hip abductors (acting through the iliotibial tract); fibular collateral ligament of the knee joint; and the evertor muscles of one side acting with the thigh adductors, tibial collateral ligament, and invertor muscles of the contralateral side.

(A) Lateral view   **(B) Inferior view**

Figure 5.14. Relaxed standing. A. The relationship of the line of gravity to the transverse rotational axes of the pelvis and lower limb in the relaxed standing (stand-easy) position is demonstrated. Only minor postural adjustments, mainly by the extensors of the back and the plantarflexors of ankle, are necessary to maintain this position because the ligaments of the hip and knee are being tightly stretched to provide passive support. **B.** A bipedal platform is formed by the feet during relaxed standing. The weight of the body is symmetrically distributed around the center of gravity, which falls in the posterior third of a median plane between the slightly parted and laterally rotated feet, anterior to the rotational axes of the ankle joints.

Walking: The Gait Cycle

Locomotion is a complex function. The movements of the lower limbs during walking on a level surface may be divided into alternating swing and stance phases (Table 5.2). The **gait cycle** consists of one cycle of swing and stance by one limb. The **stance phase** begins with **heel strike**, when the heel strikes the ground and begins to assume the body's full weight (loading response), and ends with **push off** from the forefoot—a result of plantarflexion. The **swing phase** begins after push off when the toes leave the ground and ends when the heel strikes the ground. The swing phase occupies approximately 40% of the walking cycle and the stance phase, 60%. The stance phase of walking is longer than the swing phase because it begins and ends with relatively short periods (each 10% of the cycle) of double support (both feet are contacting the ground) as the weight is transferred from one side to the other, with a more extended period of single support (only one foot on the ground bearing all body weight) in between as the contralateral limb swings forward. In *running*, there is no period of double support; consequently, the time and percentage of the gait cycle represented by the stance phase are reduced.

Walking is a remarkably efficient activity taking advantage of gravity and momentum so that a minimum of physical exertion is required. Most energy is used (1) in the eccentric contraction of the dorsiflexors during the beginning (loading) phase of stance as the heel is lowered to the ground following heel strike and (2) especially at the end of stance as the plantarflexors concentrically contract, pushing the forefoot (metatarsals and phalanges) down to produce push off, thus providing most of the propulsive force. During the last part of the stance phase (push off), the toes flex to grip the ground and augment the push off initiated from the ball of the foot (sole underlying the heads of the medial two metatarsals). The long flexors and intrinsic muscles of the foot stabilize the forefoot and toes so that the effect of plantarflexion at the ankle and flexion of the toes is maximized.

The swing phase also involves flexion of the hip so that the limb accelerates faster than the forward movement of the body. Initially, the knee flexes almost simultaneously, owing to momentum (without expenditure of energy), followed by dorsiflexion (lifting the forefoot up) at the ankle joint. The latter two movements have the effect of shortening the free limb so that it will clear the ground as it swings forward; by midswing, knee extension is added to the flexion and momentum of the thigh to realize anterior swing fully. The extensors of the hip and flexors of the knee contract eccentrically at the end of swing to decelerate the forward movement, while extensors of the knee (quadriceps) contract as necessary to extend the leg for the desired length of stride and to position the foot (present the heel) for heel strike. Contraction of the knee extensors is maintained through heel strike into the loading phase to absorb shock and keep the knee from buckling until it reaches full extension. Because the unsupported side of the hip tends to drop during the swing phase (which would negate the effect of limb shortening), abductor muscles on the supported side contract strongly during the single support part of the stance phase, pulling on the fixed femur to resist the tilting and keep the pelvis level. These same muscles also rotate (advance) the contralateral side of the pelvis forward, concurrent with the swing of its free limb.

Of course, all these actions alternate from side to side with each step. The extensors of the hip normally make only minor contributions to level walking. Primarily, the hip is passively extended by momentum during stance, except when accelerating or walking fast, and becomes increasingly active with increase in slope (steepness) during walking uphill or up stairs. Concentric hip flexion and knee extension are used during the swing phase of level walking and so are not weight-bearing actions; however, they are effected by body weight when their eccentric contraction is necessary for deceleration or walking downhill or down stairs.

Stabilization and resilience are important during locomotion. The invertors and evertors of the foot are principal stabilizers of the foot during the stance phase. Their long tendons, plus those of the flexors of the digits, also help support the arches of the foot during the stance phase, assisting the intrinsic muscles of the sole.

Absence of Plantarflexion in Walking

If the muscles of the calf are paralyzed or the calcaneal tendon is ruptured, a much less effective and efficient push off (from the midfoot) can still be accomplished by the actions of the gluteus maximus and hamstrings in extending the thigh at the hip joint and the quadriceps in extending the knee. Because push off from the forefoot is not possible (in fact, the ankle will be passively dorsiflexed as the body's weight moves anterior to the foot), those attempting to walk in the absence of plantarflexion often rotate the foot as far laterally (externally) as possible during the stance phase to disable passive dorsiflexion and allow a more effective push off through hip and knee extension exerted at the midfoot. ✛

Thigh and Gluteal Region

In evolution, the development of a prominent gluteal region is closely associated with the assumption of bipedalism and an erect posture. The prominent gluteal region is unique to humans. Modification of the shape of the femur necessary for bipedal walking and running (specifically the "bending" of the bone, creating the angle of inclination and the trochanters, as discussed earlier in this chapter) allows the superior placement of the abductors of the thigh into the gluteal region. The remaining thigh muscles are organized into three compartments by intermuscular septa that pass deeply between the muscle groups from the inner surface of the fascia lata to the linea aspera of the femur (Fig. 5.10D). The

Table 5.2. Muscle Action during the Gait Cycle

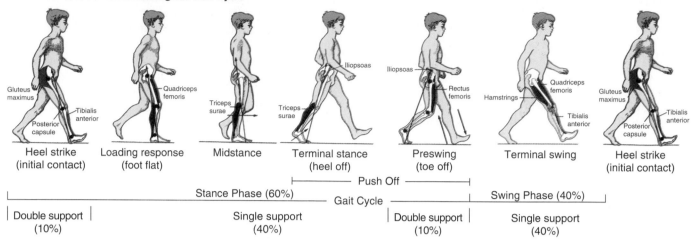

	Phase of Gait	Mechanical Goals	Active Muscle Groups	Examples
S T A N C E P H A S E	**Heel strike** (initial contact)	**Lower forefoot to ground**	Ankle dorsiflexors (eccentric contraction)	**Tibialis anterior**
		Continue deceleration (reverse forward swing)	Hip extensors	Gluteus maximus
		Preserve longitudinal arch of foot	Intrinsic muscles of foot	Flexor digitorum brevis
			Long tendons of foot	Tibialis anterior
	Loading response (flat foot)	**Accept weight**	Knee extensors	**Quadriceps**
		Decelerate mass (slow dorsiflexion)	Ankle plantarflexors	Triceps surae (soleus and gastrocnemius)
		Stabilize pelvis	Hip abductors	**Gluteus medius and minimus; tensor of fascia lata**
		Preserve longitudinal arch of foot	Intrinsic muscles of foot	Flexor digitorum brevis
			Long tendons of foot	Tibialis posterior; long flexors of digits
	Midstance	Stabilize knee	Knee extensors	Quadriceps
		Control dorsiflexion (preserve momentum)	Ankle plantarflexors (eccentric and gastrocnemius)	Triceps surae (soleus contraction)
		Stabilize pelvis	Hip abductors	**Gluteus medius and minimus, tensor of fascia lata**
		Preserve longitudinal arch of foot	Intrinsic muscles of foot	Flexor digitorum brevis
			Long tendons of foot	Tibialis posterior; long flexors of digits
	Terminal stance (heel off)	**Accelerate mass**	Ankle plantarflexors (concentric contraction)	**Triceps surae (soleus and gastrocnemius)**
		Stabilize pelvis	Hip abductors	**Gluteus medius and minimus, tensor of fascia lata**
		Preserve arches of foot; fix forefoot	Intrinsic muscles of foot	Adductor hallucis
			Long tendons of foot	Tibialis posterior; long flexors of digits

Table 5.2. Muscle Action during the Gait Cycle *(continued)*

<table>
<tr><th colspan="2">Phase of Gait</th><th>Mechanical Goals</th><th>Active Muscle Groups</th><th>Examples</th></tr>
<tr><td rowspan="15" style="writing-mode: vertical">S W I N G   P H A S E</td><td rowspan="4">Preswing
(toe off)</td><td>Accelerate mass</td><td>Long flexors of digits</td><td rowspan="2">Flexor hallucis longus; flexor digitorum longus Adductor hallucis</td></tr>
<tr><td>Preserve arches of foot; fix forefoot</td><td>Intrinsic muscles of foot</td></tr>
<tr><td></td><td>Long tendons of foot</td><td>Tibialis posterior; long flexors of digits</td></tr>
<tr><td>Decelerate thigh; prepare for swing</td><td>Flexor of hip (eccentric contraction)</td><td>Iliopsoas; rectus femoris</td></tr>
<tr><td rowspan="2">Initial swing</td><td>Accelerate thigh, vary cadence</td><td>Flexor of hip (concentric contraction)</td><td>Iliopsoas; rectus femoris</td></tr>
<tr><td>Clear foot</td><td>Ankle dorsiflexors</td><td>Tibialis anterior</td></tr>
<tr><td>Midswing</td><td>Clear foot</td><td>Ankle dorsiflexors</td><td>Tibialis anterior</td></tr>
<tr><td rowspan="4">Terminal swing</td><td>Decelerate thigh</td><td>Hip extensors (eccentric contraction)</td><td>Gluteus maximus; hamstrings</td></tr>
<tr><td>Decelerate leg</td><td>Knee flexors (eccentric contraction)</td><td>Hamstrings</td></tr>
<tr><td>Position foot</td><td>Ankle dorsiflexors</td><td>Tibialis anterior</td></tr>
<tr><td>Extend knee to place foot (control stride); prepare for contact</td><td>Knee extensors</td><td>Quadriceps</td></tr>
</table>

compartments are *anterior* or *extensor, medial* or *adductor,* and *posterior* or *flexor,* so named on the basis of their location or action at the knee joint. Generally, the anterior group is innervated by the femoral nerve, the medial group by the obturator nerve, and the posterior group by the tibial portion of the sciatic nerve. Although the compartments vary in absolute and relative size depending on level, the anterior compartment is largest overall and includes the femur.

To facilitate continuity and follow an approach commonly used in dissection courses, the anterior and medial thigh is addressed initially, followed by continuous examination of the posterior aspect of the proximal limb: gluteal region, posterior thigh, and popliteal fossa

Anterior Thigh Muscles

The large **anterior compartment of the thigh** contains the **anterior thigh muscles,** the *flexors of the hip* and *extensors of the knee* (Fig. 5.15). For attachments, nerve supply, and main actions of these muscles, see Table 5.3. The anterior thigh muscles include the pectineus, iliopsoas, sartorius, and quadriceps femoris.[1] The major muscles of the anterior compartment tend to atrophy (diminish) rapidly with disease, and physical therapy is often necessary to restore strength, tone, and symmetry with the opposite limb after immobilization of the thigh or leg.

[1] Because of its anterior position, the tensor of the fascia lata is often studied with the anterior thigh muscles for convenience (i.e., when the cadaver is supine); however, it is actually part of the gluteal group, and will be included with that group in this book.

Pectineus

The **pectineus** is a flat quadrangular muscle located in the anterior part of the superomedial aspect of the thigh. It often appears to be composed of two layers, superficial and deep, and these are generally innervated by two different nerves. Because of the dual nerve supply and the muscle's actions (the pectineus adducts and flexes the thigh and assists in medial rotation of the thigh), it is actually a transitional muscle between the anterior and the medial compartments.

Iliopsoas

The **iliopsoas** is the chief flexor of the thigh, the most powerful of the hip flexors with the longest range. Although it is one of the body's most powerful muscles, it is relatively hidden, with most of its mass located in the posterior wall of the abdomen and greater pelvis. Its broad lateral part, the **iliacus,** and its long medial part, the **psoas major,** arise from the iliac fossa and lumbar vertebrae, respectively (Table 5.3C). Thus it is the only muscle attached to the vertebral column, pelvis, and femur. It is in a unique position not only to produce movement but to stabilize (fixate). However, it can also perpetuate and even contribute to deformity and disability when it is malformed (especially if it is shortened for various reasons), dysfunctional, or diseased.

Concentric contraction of the iliopsoas typically moves the free limb, producing flexion at the hip to lift the limb and initiate its forward swing during walking (i.e., during the preswing and initial swing phases, as the opposite limb accepts weight; Table 5.2) or to elevate the limb during

Anterior views

Figure 5.15. Muscles of anterior thigh. A. The surface anatomy of the anterior thigh muscles is shown. In **B–C**, skin, subcutaneous tissue, and deep fascia have been removed to expose the anterior thigh muscles, the layers of which are demonstrated by removing the muscles sequentially, from superficial (**B**-right side) to deep (**C**-left side).

climbing. However, it is also capable of moving the trunk. Bilateral contraction initiates flexion of the trunk at the hip on the fixed thigh—as when (incorrectly) doing sit-ups—and increases the lumbar curvature of the vertebral column. It is active during walking downhill, its eccentric contraction resisting acceleration. The iliopsoas is also a postural muscle, active during standing in maintaining normal lumbar lordosis (and indirectly the compensatory thoracic kyphosis; see Chapter 4) and resisting hyperextension of the hip joint (Fig. 5.14). Unilateral weakness or spasticity may be a factor in the development of scoliosis.

Sartorius

The **sartorius,** the "tailor's muscle" (L. *sartus,* patched or repaired), is long and ribbon-like. It passes obliquely (lateral to medial) across the superoanterior part of the thigh (Fig. 5.15; Table 5.3D). The sartorius lies superficially inside the anterior compartment, within its own relatively distinct fascial sheath. This muscle descends inferiorly as far as the side of the knee. The sartorius, the longest muscle in the body, acts across two joints. It flexes the hip joint and participates in flexion of the knee joint. It also weakly abducts the thigh and laterally rotates it. The actions of both sartorius muscles bring

the lower limbs into the cross-legged sitting position. None of the actions of the sartorius is strong; therefore, it is mainly a synergist, acting with other thigh muscles that produce these movements.

Quadriceps Femoris

The **quadriceps femoris** (L. four-headed femoral muscle) forms the main bulk of the anterior thigh muscles and collectively constitutes the largest and one of the most powerful muscles in the body. It may be three times stronger than its antagonistic muscle group, the hamstrings. It covers almost all the anterior aspect and sides of the femur. The quadriceps femoris (quadriceps) consists of four parts: (1) rectus femoris, (2) vastus lateralis, (3) vastus intermedius, and (4) vastus medialis. Collectively, the quadriceps is a two-joint muscle capable of producing action at both the hip and the knee. The two major components of the quadriceps (rectus femoris and vasti) are discussed separately later in this chapter.

The quadriceps is the great extensor of the leg. Concentric contraction of the quadriceps to extend the knee against gravity is important during rising from sitting or squatting, during climbing and walking up stairs, and for acceleration and

Table 5.3-I. Muscles of the Anterior Thigh: Flexors of the Hip Joint

Anterior views

Muscle	Proximal Attachment	Distal Attachment	Innervation[a]	Main Action
Pectineus (A & B)	Superior ramus of pubis	Pectineal line of femur, just inferior to lesser trochanter	Femoral nerve (**L2**, L3); may receive a branch from obturator nerve	Adducts and flexes thigh; assists with medial rotation of thigh
Iliopsoas (A & C) Psoas major	Sides of T12–L5 vertebrae and discs between them; transverse processes of all lumbar vertebrae	Lesser trochanter of femur	Anterior rami of lumbar nerves (**L1, L2**, L3)	Act conjointly in flexing thigh at hip joint and in stabilizing this joint[b]
Psoas minor	Sides of T12–L1 vertebrae and intervertebral disc	Pectineal line, iliopectineal eminence via iliopectineal arch	Anterior rami of lumbar nerves (L1, L2)	
Iliacus	Iliac crest, iliac fossa, ala of sacrum, and anterior sacroiliac ligaments	Tendon of psoas major, lesser trochanter, and femur distal to it	Femoral nerve (**L2**, L3)	
Sartorius (A & D)	Anterior superior iliac spine and superior part of notch inferior to it	Superior part of medial surface of tibia	Femoral nerve (L2, L3)	Flexes, abducts, and laterally rotates thigh at hip joint; flexes leg at knee joint[c]

[a]The spinal cord segmental innervation is indicated (e.g., "L1, L2, L3" means that the nerves supplying the psoas major are derived from the first three lumbar segments of the spinal cord). Numbers in boldface (**L1, L2**) indicate the main segmental innervation. Damage to one or more of the listed spinal cord segments or to the motor nerve roots arising from them results in paralysis of the muscles concerned.

[b]The psoas major is also a postural muscle that helps control the deviation of the trunk and is active during standing.

[c]The four actions of the sartorius (L. *sartor*, tailor) produce the once common cross-legged sitting position used by tailors, hence the name.

projection (running and jumping). In level walking, it becomes active during the termination of the swing phase, preparing the knee to accept weight (Table 5.2). It is primarily responsible for absorbing the jarring shock of heel strike, and its activity continues as the weight is assumed during the early stance phase (loading response). It also functions much of the time as a fixator during bent-knee sports, such as skiing and tennis, and contracts eccentrically during downhill walking and descending stairs.

The tendons of the four parts of the quadriceps unite in the distal portion of the thigh to form a single, strong, broad quadriceps tendon (Table 5.3E). The patellar ligament (L.

ligamentum patellae), attached to the tibial tuberosity (Fig. 5.15B), is the continuation of the quadriceps tendon in which the patella is embedded. The patella is thus the largest sesamoid bone in the body. The medial and lateral vasti muscles also attach independently to the patella and form aponeuroses, the **medial** and **lateral patellar retinacula**, which reinforce the joint capsule of the knee on each side of the patella en route to attachment to the anterior border of the tibial plateau. The retinacula also play a role in keeping the patella aligned over the patellar articular surface of the femur.

The **patella** provides a bony surface that is able to withstand the compression placed on the quadriceps tendon

Table 5.3-II. Muscles of the Anterior Thigh: Extensors of the Knee

Anterior views   **Posterior views**

Muscle	Proximal Attachment	Distal Attachment	Innervation[a]	Main Action
Quadriceps femoris (fig. *E–H*)				
Rectus femoris	Anterior inferior iliac spine and ilium superior to acetabulum	Via common tendinous (quadriceps tendon) and independent attachments to base of patella; indirectly via patellar ligament to tibial tuberosity; medial and lateral vasti also attach to tibia and patella via aponeuroses (medial and lateral patellar retinacula)	Femoral nerve (L2, **L3, L4**)	Extend leg at knee joint; rectus femoris also steadies hip joint and helps iliopsoas flex thigh
Vastus lateralis	Greater trochanter and lateral lip of linea aspera of femur			
Vastus medialis	Intertrochanteric line and medial lip of linea aspera of femur			
Vastus intermedius	Anterior and lateral surfaces of shaft of femur			

[a]The spinal cord segmental innervation is indicated (e.g., "L1, L2, L3" means that the nerves supplying the quadriceps femoris are derived from the first three lumbar segments of the spinal cord). Numbers in boldface (**L3, L4**) indicate the main segmental innervation. Damage to one or more of the listed spinal cord segments or to the motor nerve roots arising from them results in paralysis of the muscles concerned.

during kneeling and the friction occurring when the knee is flexed and extended during running. The patella also provides additional leverage for the quadriceps in placing the tendon more anteriorly, farther from the joint's axis, causing it to approach the tibia from a position of greater mechanical advantage. The inferiorly directed apex of the patella indicates the level of the joint plane of the knee when the leg is extended and the patellar ligament is taut.

Testing the quadriceps is performed with the person in the supine position with the knee partly flexed. The person extends the knee against resistance. During the test, contraction of the rectus femoris should be observable and palpable if the muscle is acting normally, indicating that its nerve supply is intact.

Rectus Femoris. The **rectus femoris** received its name because it runs straight down the thigh (L. *rectus*, straight). Because of its attachments to the hip bone and tibia, the rec-

tus femoris crosses two joints; hence it is capable of flexing the thigh at the hip joint and extending the leg at the knee joint. The rectus femoris is the only part of the quadriceps that crosses the hip joint, and as a hip flexor it acts with and like the iliopsoas during the preswing and initial swing phases of walking (Table 5.2). The ability of the rectus femoris to extend the knee is compromised during hip flexion, but it does contribute to the extension force during the toe off phase, when the thigh is extended. It is particularly efficient in movements combining knee extension and hip flexion from a position of hip hyperextension and knee flexion, as in the preparatory position for kicking a soccer ball. The rectus femoris, the "kicking muscle," is susceptible to injury and avulsion from the anterior inferior iliac spine during kicking. A loss of function of the rectus femoris may reduce thigh flexion strength by as much as 17% (Markhede and Stener, 1981).

Vastus Muscles. The names of the three large **vastus muscles** (vasti) indicate their position around the femoral shaft (Fig. 5.15; Table 5.3-II):

- **Vastus lateralis,** the largest component of the quadriceps, lies on the lateral side of the thigh.

- **Vastus medialis** covers the medial side of the thigh.

- **Vastus intermedius** lies deep to the rectus femoris, between the vastus medialis and the vastus lateralis.

It is difficult to isolate the function of the three vastus muscles.

The small, flat **articular muscle of the knee** (L. *articularis genus*), a derivative of the vastus intermedius (Fig. 5.16), usually consists of a variable number of muscular slips that at-

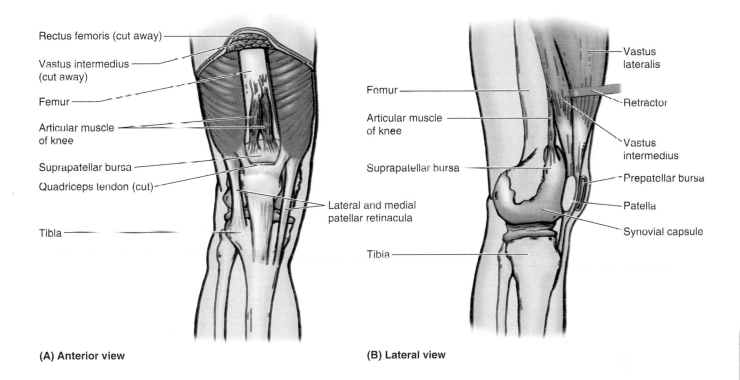

(A) Anterior view

(B) Lateral view

(C) Medial view

Figure 5.16. Suprapatellar bursa and articular muscle of knee. A and B. The large suprapatellar bursa, normally a potential space extending between the quadriceps and the femur, is depicted as if injected with latex. **C.** In this deep dissection of the knee region, the projected outline of the femur is indicated by a *red broken line* and the extent of the suprapatellar bursa is indicated by a *blue broken line.* **A–C.** The articular muscle of the knee is shown as extending from the distal femur to attach to the bursa. This muscle blends with the deep aspect of the vastus intermedius.

tach superiorly to the inferior part of the anterior aspect of the femur and inferiorly to the synovial membrane of the knee joint and the wall of the *suprapatellar bursa* (Table 5.3*A*). This muscle pulls the synovial membrane superiorly during extension of the leg, thereby preventing folds of the membrane from being compressed between the femur and the patella within the knee joint.

THE BOTTOM LINE: The large anterior compartment of the thigh includes the flexors of the hip and extensors of the knee, with most muscles innervated by the femoral nerve. The quadriceps femoris accounts for most of the mass of this compartment. It surrounds the femur on three sides and has a common tendon of attachment to the tibia, which includes the patella as a sesamoid bone. Major muscles of this compartment atrophy rapidly with disease or disuse, requiring physical therapy to retain or restore function.

Hip and Thigh Contusions

Sports broadcasters and trainers refer to a "hip pointer," which is a *contusion of the iliac crest* that usually occurs at its anterior part (e.g., where the sartorius attaches to the ASIS). This is one of the most common injuries to the hip region, usually occurring in association with collision sports, such as the various forms of football, ice hockey, and volleyball. **Contusions** cause bleeding from ruptured capillaries and infiltration of blood into the muscles, tendons, and other soft tissues. The term *hip pointer* may also refer to avulsion of bony muscle attachments, for example, of the sartorius or rectus femoris to the anterior iliac spines, of the hamstrings from the ischium (see clinical correlation [blue] box "Hamstring Injuries," in this chapter), or of the iliopsoas from the lesser trochanter of the femur). However, these injuries should be called *avulsion fractures*.

Another term commonly used is "charley horse," which may refer either to the cramping of an individual thigh muscle because of ischemia or to contusion and rupture of blood vessels sufficient enough to form a *hematoma*. The injury is usually the consequence of tearing of fibers of the rectus femoris; sometimes the quadriceps tendon is also partially torn. The most common site of a thigh hematoma is in the quadriceps. A charley horse is associated with localized pain and/or muscle stiffness and commonly follows direct trauma (e.g., a stick slash in hockey or a tackle in football).

Psoas Abscess

The psoas major arises in the abdomen from the intervertebral discs, the sides of the T12–L5 vertebrae, and their transverse processes. The medial arcuate ligament of the diaphragm arches obliquely over the proximal part of the psoas major (see Chapter 2). The transversalis fascia on the internal abdominal wall is continuous with the psoas fascia, where it forms a fascial covering for the psoas major that accompanies the muscle into the anterior region of the thigh.

There is a resurgence of tuberculosis (TB) in Africa, Asia, and elsewhere. A retroperitoneal **pyogenic** (pus-forming) infection in the abdomen or greater pelvis, characteristically occurring in association with TB of the vertebral column, or secondary to regional enteritis of the ileum (Crohn disease), may result in the formation of a *psoas abscess*. When the abscess passes between the psoas and its fascia to the inguinal and proximal thigh regions, severe pain may be referred to the hip, thigh, or knee joint. Consequently, a psoas abscess should always be considered when edema occurs in the proximal part of the thigh. Such an abscess may be palpated or observed in the inguinal region, just inferior or superior to the inguinal ligament, and may be mistaken for an indirect inguinal hernia or a femoral hernia, an enlargement of the inguinal lymph nodes, or a saphenous varix (see clinical correlation [blue] box "Saphenous Varix," in this chapter). The lateral border of the psoas is commonly visible in radiographs of the abdomen; an obscured psoas shadow may be an indication of abdominal pathology.

Paralysis of the Quadriceps

A person with a paralyzed quadriceps cannot extend the leg against resistance and usually presses on the distal end of the thigh during walking to prevent inadvertent flexion of the knee joint. Weakness of the vastus medialis or vastus lateralis, resulting from arthritis or trauma to the knee joint, for example, can result in abnormal patellar movement and loss of joint stability.

Chondromalacia Patellae

Chondromalacia patellae (runner's knee) is a common knee problem for marathon runners. Such overstressing of the knee can also occur in running sports such as basketball. The soreness and aching around or deep to the patella results from *quadriceps imbalance*. Chondromalacia patellae may result from a blow to the patella or extreme flexion of the knee (e.g., during squatting when power lifting).

Patellar Fractures

A direct blow to the patella may fracture it in two or more fragments. *Transverse patellar fractures* may result from a blow to the knee or sudden contraction of the ▶

quadriceps (e.g., when one slips and attempts to prevent a backward fall). The proximal fragment is pulled superiorly with the quadriceps tendon, and the distal fragment remains with the patellar ligament.

Abnormal Ossification of the Patella

The patella is cartilaginous at birth. It becomes ossified during the 3rd–6th years, frequently from more than one ossification center. Although these centers usually coalesce and form a single bone, they may remain separate on one or both sides, giving rise to a **bipartite** or **tripartite patella** (Fig. B5.9). An unwary observer might interpret this con-

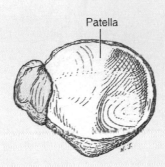

Patella

Figure B5.9

dition on a radiograph or CT as a patellar fracture. Ossification abnormalities are nearly always bilateral; therefore, diagnostic images should be examined from both sides. If the defects are bilateral, the abnormalities are likely ossification abnormalities.

Patellar Tendon Reflex

Tapping the patellar ligament with a reflex hammer normally elicits the **patellar reflex** (knee jerk). This myotatic (deep tendon) reflex is routinely tested during a physical examination by having the person sit with legs dangling. A firm strike on the ligament with a reflex hammer usually causes the leg to extend. If the reflex is normal, a hand on the person's quadriceps should feel the muscle contract. This tendon reflex tests the integrity of the femoral nerve and the L2–L4 spinal cord segments. Tapping the ligament activates muscle spindles in the quadriceps; afferent impulses from the spindles travel in the femoral nerve to the L2–L4 segments of the spinal cord. From here, efferent impulses are transmitted via motor fibers in the femoral nerve to the quadriceps, resulting in a jerk-like contraction of the muscle and extension of the leg at the knee joint. *Diminution or absence of the patellar tendon reflex* may result from any lesion that interrupts the innervation of the quadriceps (e.g., peripheral nerve disease). ○

Medial Thigh Muscles

The medial thigh muscles, collectively called the **adductor group**, are in the medial compartment of the thigh, innervated primarily by the obturator nerve (Figs. 5.15 and 5.17). The adductor group of thigh muscles consists of the adductor longus, adductor brevis, adductor magnus, gracilis, and obturator externus. In general, they attach proximally to the anteroinferior exterior of the bony pelvis (pubic bone, ischiopubic ramus, and ischial tuberosity) and adjacent obturator membrane and distally to the linea aspera of the femur (Table 5.4A). All adductor muscles, except the "hamstring part" of the adductor magnus—plus part of the pectineus—are supplied by the *obturator nerve* (L2–L4). The pectineus is supplied by the femoral nerve (L2–L4), and the hamstring part of the adductor magnus is supplied by the tibial part of the sciatic nerve (L4). The details of their attachments, nerve supply, and actions of the muscles are provided in Table 5.4. While collectively these muscles are the adductors of the thigh, the actions of some of these muscles are more complex.

Adductor Longus

The **adductor longus** is a large, fan-shaped muscle and is the most anteriorly placed of the adductor group. This triangular *long adductor* arises by a strong tendon from the anterior aspect of the body of the pubis just inferior to the pubic tubercle (apex of triangle) and expands to attach to the linea aspera

of the femur (base of triangle); in so doing it covers the anterior aspects of the adductor brevis and middle of the adductor magnus.

Adductor Brevis

The **adductor brevis**, or *short adductor,* lies deep to the pectineus and adductor longus where it arises from the body and inferior ramus of the pubis. It widens as it passes distally to attach to the uppermost part of the linea aspera. As the obturator nerve emerges from the obturator canal to enter the medial compartment of the thigh, it splits into an anterior and a posterior division, the two divisions passing anterior and posterior to the adductor brevis. This unique relationship is useful in identifying the muscle in dissection and in anatomical cross sections.

Adductor Magnus

The **adductor magnus** is the largest (most powerful) and most posterior muscle in the adductor group. This *large adductor* is a composite, triangular muscle with a thick, medial margin that has an *adductor part* and a *hamstring part*. The two parts differ in their attachments, nerve supply, and main actions (Table 5.4). The adductor part fans out widely for aponeurotic distal attachment along the entire length of the linea aspera of the femur, extending inferiorly onto the medial supracondylar ridge. The hamstring part has a tendinous distal attachment to the adductor tubercle.

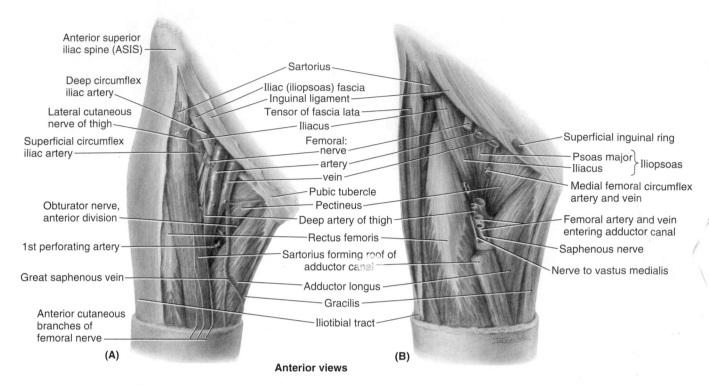

Figure 5.17. Femoral triangle. A. The boundaries and contents of the femoral triangle are shown. Observe the structures that bound the triangle: the inguinal ligament superiorly, the adductor longus medially, and the sartorius laterally. Superiorly, the femoral nerve and vessels enter the base of the triangle; inferiorly, they exit from its apex. **B.** In this deeper dissection, sections have been removed from the sartorius and the femoral vessels and nerve. Observe the muscles forming the floor of the femoral triangle: the iliopsoas laterally and the pectineus medially. Of the neurovascular structures at the apex of the femoral triangle, the two anterior vessels (femoral artery and vein) and the two nerves enter the adductor canal (anterior to adductor longus), and the two posterior vessels (deep artery and vein of thigh) pass deep (posterior) to the adductor longus.

Gracilis

The **gracilis** (L. slender) is a long, strap-like muscle and is the most medial muscle of the thigh. It is the most superficial of the adductor group and the weakest member. It is the only one of the group to cross the knee joint as well as the hip joint, joining with two other two-joint muscles from the other two compartments (the sartorius and semitendinosus muscles. Thus the three muscles are innervated by three different nerves). They have a common tendinous insertion, the **pes anserinus** (L. goose's foot), into the upper part of the medial surface of the tibia. The gracilis is a synergist in adducting the thigh, flexing the knee, and rotating the leg medially when the knee is flexed. It acts with the other "pes anserinus" muscles to add stability to the medial aspect of the extended knee, much as the gluteus maximus and tensor of the fascia lata do via the iliotibial tract on the lateral side.

Obturator Externus

The **obturator externus** is a flat, relatively small, fan-shaped muscle that is deeply placed in the superomedial part of the thigh. It extends from the external surface of the obturator membrane and surrounding bone of the pelvis to the posterior aspect of the greater trochanter, passing directly under the acetabulum and neck of the femur.

Actions of the Adductor Muscle Group

From the anatomical position, the main action of the adductor muscle group is to pull the thigh medially, toward or past the median plane. Three adductors (longus, brevis, and magnus) are used in all movements in which the thighs are adducted (e.g., pressed together when riding a horse). They are used to stabilize the stance when standing on both feet, to correct lateral sway of the trunk, or when there is a side-to-side shift of the surface on which one is standing (rocking a boat, standing on a balance board). They are also used in kicking with the medial side of the foot in soccer and in swimming. Finally, they contribute to flexion of the extended thigh and extension of the flexed thigh when running or against resistance.

The adductors as a group constitute a large muscle mass. Although they are important in many activities, it has been shown that a reduction of as much as 70% in their function will result in only a slight to moderate impairment of hip function (Markhede and Stener, 1981).

Testing of the medial thigh muscles is performed while the person is lying supine with the knee straight. The person adducts the thigh against resistance, and if the adductors are normal, the proximal ends of the gracilis and adductor longus can easily be palpated.

Table 5.4. Muscles of the Medial Thigh: Adductors of the Thigh

(A) Anterior view

- ▨ Adductor longus
- ▨ Adductor brevis
- ▨ Adductor magnus
- ▢ Gracilis
- ▨ Obturator extremus

(B) Anterior view   **(C) Anterior view**   **(D) Posterior view**

(E) Anterior view   **(F) Posterior view**   **(G) Anterior view**   **(H) Anterior view**

Muscle[a]	Proximal Attachment	Distal Attachment	Innervation[b]	Main Action
Adductor longus (E & G)	Body of pubis inferior to pubic crest	Middle third of linea aspera of femur	Obturator nerve, branch of anterior division (L2, **L3**, L4)	Adducts thigh
Adductor brevis (F & G)	Body and inferior ramus of pubis	Pectineal line and proximal part of linea aspera of femur	Obturator nerve (L2, **L3**, L4), branch of anterior division	Adducts thigh; to some extent flexes it
Adductor magnus (C, D, & G)	Adductor part: inferior ramus of pubis, ramus of ischium Hamstrings part: ischial tuberosity	Adductor part: gluteal tuberosity, linea aspera, medial supracondylar line Hamstrings part: adductor tubercle of femur	Adductor part: obturator nerve (L2, **L3**, L4), branches of posterior division Hamstrings part: tibial part of sciatic nerve (**L4**)	Adducts thigh Adductor part: flexes thigh Hamstrings part: extends thigh
Gracilis (H)	Body and inferior ramus of pubis	Superior part of medial surface of tibia	Obturator nerve (**L2**, L3)	Adducts thigh; flexes leg; helps rotate it medially
Obturator externus	Margins of obturator foramen and obturator membrane	Trochanteric fossa of femur	Obturator nerve (L3, **L4**)	Laterally rotates thigh; steadies head of femur in acetabulum

[a]Collectively, the five muscles listed are the adductors of the thigh, but their actions are more complex (e.g., they act as flexors of the hip joint during flexion of the knee joint and are active during walking).
[b]The spinal cord segmental innervation is indicated (e.g., "L2, L3, L4" means that the nerves supplying the adductor longus are derived from the second to fourth lumbar segments of the spinal cord). Numbers in boldface (**L3**) indicate the main segmental innervation. Damage to one or more of the listed spinal cord segments or to the motor nerve roots arising from them results in paralysis of the muscles concerned.

THE BOTTOM LINE: The muscles of the medial compartment of the thigh attach proximally to the anteroinferior bony pelvis and distally to the linea aspera of the femur. They are adductors of the thigh, innervated primarily by the obturator nerve. Use of these muscles as prime movers is relatively limited.

Adductor Hiatus

The **adductor hiatus** is an opening or gap between the aponeurotic distal attachment of the adductor part of the adductor magnus and the tendinous distal attachment of the hamstring part. The adductor hiatus transmits the femoral artery and vein from the adductor canal in the thigh to the popliteal fossa posterior to the knee (Table 5.4). The opening is located just lateral and superior to the adductor tubercle of the femur.

Transplantation of the Gracilis

Because the gracilis is a relatively weak member of the adductor group of muscles, it can be removed without noticeable loss of its actions on the leg. Hence, surgeons often transplant the gracilis, or part of it, with its nerve and blood vessels to replace a damaged muscle in the hand, for example. Once the muscle is transplanted, it soon produces good digital flexion and extension. Freed from its distal attachment, the muscle has also been relocated and repositioned to create a replacement for a non-functional external anal sphincter.

Groin Pull

Sports broadcasters refer to a "pulled groin" or "groin injury." These terms mean that a strain, stretching, and probably some tearing of the proximal attachments of the anteromedial thigh muscles has occurred. The injury usually involves the flexor and adductor thigh muscles. The proximal attachments of these muscles are in the inguinal region (groin), the junction of the thigh and trunk. Groin pulls usually occur in sports that require quick starts such as short-distance racing (e.g., a 60-m sprint), base stealing in baseball, and quick starts in basketball.

Injury to the Adductor Longus

Muscle strains of the adductor longus may occur in horseback riders and produce pain (rider's strain). Ossification sometimes occurs in the tendons of these muscles because the horseback riders actively adduct their thighs to keep from falling from their animals. The areas of the ossified tendons are sometimes called "riders' bones." ⊕

Neurovascular Structures and Relationships in the Anteromedial Thigh

Femoral Triangle

The femoral triangle, a subfascial space, is a triangular landmark useful in dissection and in understanding relationships in the groin. (Figs. 5.15*A* & *B*, and 5.17–5.19). In living people it appears as a triangular depression inferior to the inguinal ligament when the thigh is flexed, abducted, and laterally rotated. (Fig. 5.15*A*) The femoral triangle is bounded:

- Superiorly by the inguinal ligament (the thickened inferior margin of the external oblique aponeurosis) that forms the *base of the femoral triangle.*

- Medially by the adductor longus.

- Laterally by the sartorius; the *apex* is where the lateral border of the sartorius crosses the medial border of the adductor longus.

The muscular *floor of the femoral triangle* is formed by the iliopsoas laterally and the pectineus medially. The *roof of the femoral triangle* is formed by the fascia lata and cribriform fascia, subcutaneous tissue, and skin.

Deep to the inguinal ligament, the **subinguinal space** (created as the inguinal ligament spans the gap between the two bony prominences to which it is attached, the ASIS and public tubercle) is an important passageway connecting the trunk/abdominopelvic cavity to the lower limb. The inguinal ligament actually serves as a flexor retinaculum, retaining structures that pass anterior to the hip joint against the joint during flexion of the thigh. The passageway posterior to the ligament is divided into two compartments, or lacunae, by a thickening of the iliopsoas fascia, the **iliopectineal arch** (Fig. 5.19), which passes between the deep surface of the inguinal ligament and the *iliopubic eminence* (Fig. 5.6*B*). Lateral to the arch is the *muscular lacuna,* through which the iliopsoas muscle and femoral nerve pass from the greater pelvis into the anterior thigh; medial to the arch, the *vascular lacuna* allows passage of the major vascular structures (veins, artery, and lymphatics) between the greater pelvis and the femoral triangle of the anterior thigh. As they enter the femoral triangle, the names of the vessels change from *external iliac* to *femoral.*

The contents of the femoral triangle, from lateral to medial, are the:

- Femoral nerve and its (terminal) branches.

- Femoral sheath and its contents:

  - Femoral artery and several of its branches.

  - Femoral vein and its proximal tributaries (e.g., the great saphenous and deep femoral veins).

  - Deep inguinal lymph nodes and associated lymphatic vessels.

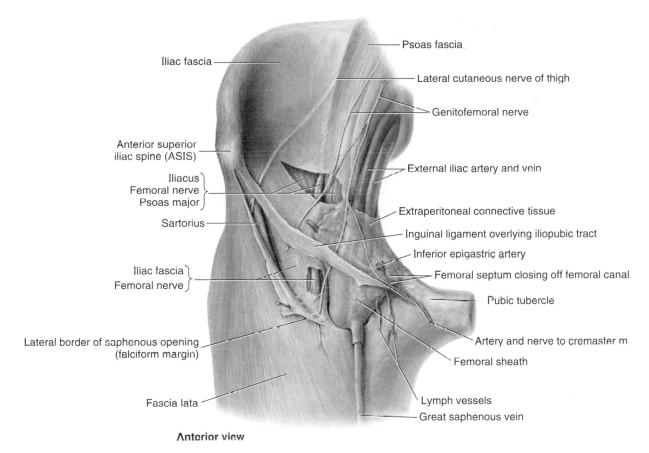

Iliac fascia

Psoas fascia

Lateral cutaneous nerve of thigh

Genitofemoral nerve

Anterior superior iliac spine (ASIS)

Iliacus
Femoral nerve
Psoas major

Sartorius

External iliac artery and vein

Extraperitoneal connective tissue

Inguinal ligament overlying iliopubic tract

Inferior epigastric artery

Iliac fascia
Femoral nerve

Femoral septum closing off femoral canal

Pubic tubercle

Lateral border of saphenous opening (falciform margin)

Artery and nerve to cremaster m

Femoral sheath

Fascia lata

Lymph vessels

Great saphenous vein

Anterior view

Figure 5.18. Dissection of femoral sheath in femoral triangle. The falciform margin of the saphenous opening in the fascia lata is cut and reflected. Note that the femoral nerve is external and lateral to the femoral sheath, whereas the femoral artery and vein occupy the sheath.

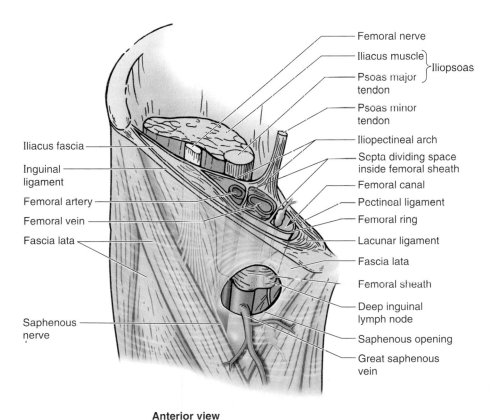

Femoral nerve

Iliacus muscle
Psoas major tendon

Iliopsoas

Psoas minor tendon

Iliopectineal arch

Septa dividing space inside femoral sheath

Femoral canal

Pectineal ligament

Femoral ring

Lacunar ligament

Fascia lata

Femoral sheath

Deep inguinal lymph node

Saphenous opening

Great saphenous vein

Iliacus fascia

Inguinal ligament

Femoral artery

Femoral vein

Fascia lata

Saphenous nerve

Anterior view

Figure 5.19. Structure and contents of femoral sheath. This dissection is of the superior end of the anterior aspect of the right thigh. Note the compartments within the femoral sheath. The proximal end (abdominal opening) of the femoral canal is the femoral ring.

The femoral triangle is bisected by the femoral artery and vein, which pass to and from the adductor canal inferiorly at its apex (Fig. 5.17A). The *adductor canal* is an intramuscular passageway by which the major neurovascular bundle of the thigh traverses its middle third (Figs. 5.17B and 5.20).

Femoral Nerve

The **femoral nerve** (L2–L4) is the largest branch of the lumbar plexus. The nerve originates in the abdomen within the psoas major and descends posterolaterally through the pelvis to approximately the midpoint of the inguinal ligament (Figs. 5.17A–5.19). It then passes deep to this ligament and enters the femoral triangle, lateral to the femoral vessels. After entering the triangle, the femoral nerve divides into several branches to the anterior thigh muscles. It also sends articular branches to the hip and knee joints and provides several cutaneous branches to the anteromedial side of the thigh (Table 5.1). The terminal cutaneous branch of the femoral nerve, the **saphenous nerve,** descends through the femoral triangle, lateral to the femoral sheath containing the femoral vessels (Fig. 5.17B and 5.19). The saphenous nerve accompanies the femoral artery and vein through the adductor canal and becomes superficial by passing between the sartorius and the gracilis when the femoral vessels traverse the adductor hiatus at the distal end of the canal. It runs anteroinferiorly to supply the skin and fascia on the anteromedial aspects of the knee, leg, and foot.

Femoral Sheath

The **femoral sheath** is a funnel-shaped fascial tube of varying length (usually 3–4 cm) that passes deep to the inguinal ligament, lining the *vascular lacuna* of the *subinguinal space*. It terminates inferiorly by blending with the adventitia of the femoral vessels. The sheath encloses proximal parts of the femoral vessels and creates the femoral canal medial to them (Figs. 5.18 and 5.19). The sheath is formed by an inferior prolongation of transversalis and iliopsoas fascia from the abdomen/greater pelvis (see Chapter 2). The femoral sheath does not enclose the femoral nerve because it passes through the muscular lacuna. When a long femoral sheath occurs (when it extends farther distally), its medial wall is pierced by the great saphenous vein and lymphatic vessels (Fig. 5.18). The femoral sheath allows the femoral artery and vein to glide deep to the inguinal ligament during movements of the hip joint.

The femoral sheath is subdivided internally into three compartments by vertical septa of extraperitoneal connective tissue that extend from the abdomen along the femoral vessels (Fig. 5.19). The compartments of the femoral sheath are the:

- *Lateral compartment* for the femoral artery.

- *Intermediate compartment* for the femoral vein.

- *Medial compartment,* which constitutes the femoral canal.

The **femoral canal** is the smallest of the three compartments. It is short (approximately 1.25 cm) and conical and lies between the medial edge of the femoral sheath and the femoral vein. The femoral canal (Fig. 5.19):

- Extends distally to the level of the proximal edge of the saphenous opening.

- Allows the femoral vein to expand when venous return from the lower limb is increased or when increased intraabdominal pressure causes a temporary stasis in the vein (as

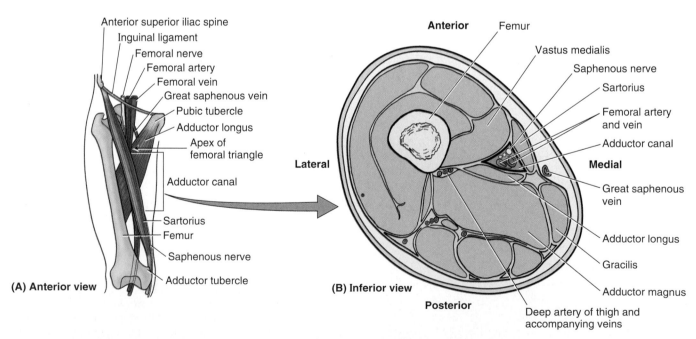

Figure 5.20. Adductor canal in medial part of middle third of thigh. A. Orientation drawing showing the canal formed between the three thigh muscles and the level of the section shown in part **B. B.** This transverse section of the thigh shows the muscles bounding the adductor canal and its neurovascular contents.

during a Valsalva maneuver, i.e., taking a breath and holding it, often while bearing down).

- Contains loose connective tissue, fat, a few lymphatic vessels, and sometimes a deep inguinal lymph node (Cloquet node).

The base of the femoral canal, formed by the small (approximately 1 cm wide) proximal opening at its abdominal end, is the oval **femoral ring**. This opening is closed by extraperitoneal fatty tissue that forms the transversely oriented **femoral septum** (Fig. 5.18). The abdominal surface of the septum is covered by parietal peritoneum (see Chapter 2). The femoral septum is pierced by lymphatic vessels connecting the inguinal and external iliac lymph nodes.

The boundaries of the femoral ring are

- *Laterally,* the vertical septum between the femoral canal and the femoral vein.

- *Posteriorly,* the superior ramus of the pubis covered by the pectineus and its fascia.

- *Medially,* the lacunar ligament.

- *Anteriorly,* the medial part of the inguinal ligament.

Femoral Artery

Details concerning the origin, course, and distribution of the arteries of the thigh are described in Table 5.5.

The **femoral artery,** the continuation of the external iliac artery distal to the inguinal ligament, is the chief artery to the lower limb (Figs. 5.17–20). It enters the femoral triangle deep to the midpoint of the inguinal ligament (midway between the ASIS and the pubic tubercle), lateral to the femoral vein (Fig. 5.20A). Its pulsations are palpable within the triangle because of its relatively superficial position deep (posterior) to the fascia lata, where it lies and descends on the adjacent borders of the iliopsoas and pectineus that make up the floor of the triangle. The superficial epigastric artery, superficial (and sometimes the deep) circumflex iliac arteries, and the superficial and deep external pudendal arteries arise from the anterior aspect of the proximal part of the femoral artery.

The **deep artery of the thigh** (L. *arteria profunda femoris*) is the largest branch of the femoral artery and the chief artery to the thigh. It arises from the lateral or posterior side of the femoral artery in the femoral triangle. In the middle third of the thigh, where it is separated from the femoral artery and vein by the adductor longus (Figs. 5.17B and 5.20B), it gives off perforating arteries that wrap around the posterior aspect of the femur. The perforating arteries supply muscles of all three fascial compartments (adductor magnus, hamstrings, and vastus lateralis).

The *circumflex femoral arteries* encircle the uppermost shaft of the femur and anastomose with each other and other arteries, supplying the thigh muscles and the superior (proximal) end of the femur. The **medial circumflex femoral artery** is especially important because it supplies most of the blood to the head and the neck of the femur via its branches, the **posterior retinacular arteries**. The retinacular arteries are often torn when the femoral neck is fractured or the hip joint is dislocated. The **lateral circumflex femoral artery,** less able to supply the femoral head and neck as it passes laterally across the thickest part of the joint capsule of the hip joint, mainly supplies muscles on the lateral side of the thigh.

Obturator Artery. The obturator artery helps the deep artery of the thigh supply the adductor muscles via anterior and posterior branches, which anastomose (Table 5.5). The posterior branch gives off an acetabular branch that supplies the head of the femur.

Palpation, Compression, and Cannulation of the Femoral Artery

The initial part of the femoral artery, proximal to the branching of the deep artery of the thigh, is superficial in position, making it especially accessible and useful for a number of clinical procedures. Some vascular surgeons refer to this part of the femoral artery as the *common femoral artery* and to its continuation distally as the *superficial femoral artery.* This terminology is not recommended by the Federative International Committee on Anatomical Terminology and is not used in this book because these terms may cause misunderstanding. Anterior to the initial part of the femoral artery are the skin, subcutaneous tissue, superficial inguinal lymph nodes, superficial circumflex iliac artery, cribriform fascia, and the anterior part of the femoral sheath (Figs. 5.10, 5.12, and 5.18).

With the person lying in the supine position, the *femoral pulse* is palpated midway between the ASIS and the pubic symphysis (Fig. B5.10A & B). By placing the tip of the little finger (of the right hand when dealing with the right side) on the ASIS and the tip of the thumb on the pubic tubercle, the femoral pulse can be palpated with the midpalm just inferior to the midpoint of the inguinal ligament by pressing firmly. Normally the pulse is strong; however, if the common or external iliac arteries are partially occluded, the pulse may be diminished.

Compression of the femoral artery may also be accomplished at this site by pressing directly posteriorly against the superior pubic ramus, psoas major, and femoral head (Fig. B5.10C). Compression at this point will reduce blood flow through the femoral artery and its branches, such as the deep artery of the thigh.

The femoral artery may be cannulated just inferior to the midpoint of the inguinal ligament. In *left cardial (cardiac) angiography,* a long, slender catheter is inserted into the artery and passed up the external iliac artery, common iliac artery, and aorta to the left ventricle of the heart (see Chapter 1). ▶

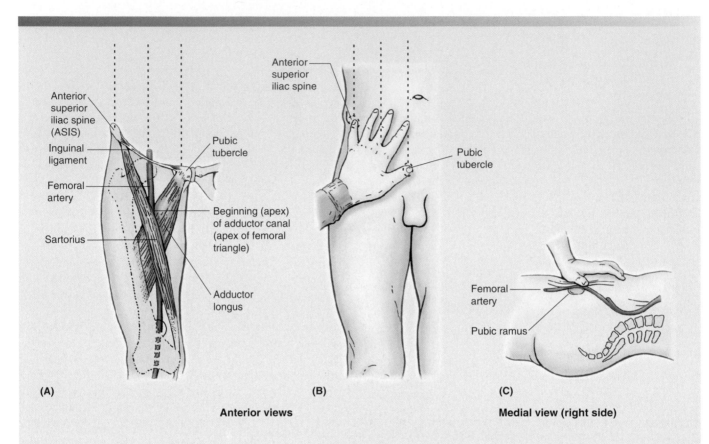

(A)

(B)

Anterior views

(C)

Medial view (right side)

Figure B5.10

This same approach via the femoral artery may be used to visualize the coronary arteries in *coronary arteriography*.

Laceration of the Femoral Artery

The superficial position of the femoral artery in the femoral triangle also makes it vulnerable to traumatic injury, especially laceration. Commonly, both the femoral artery and vein are lacerated in anterior thigh wounds because they lie close together. In some cases, an arteriovenous shunt occurs as a result of communication between the injured vessels. When it is necessary to ligate the femoral artery, anastomosis of branches of the femoral artery with other arteries that cross the hip joint, may supply blood to the lower limb. However, the *cruciate anastomosis,* consisting of a four-way common meeting of the medial and lateral circumflex femoral arteries with the inferior gluteal artery superiorly and the first perforating artery inferiorly posterior to the femur, occurs less commonly than its frequent description in textbooks and depiction in atlases implies.

Replaced or Accessory Obturator Artery

An enlarged pubic branch of the inferior epigastric artery either takes the place of the obturator artery (*replaced obturator artery*) or joins it as an *accessory obturator artery* in approximately 20% of people. This artery runs close to or across the femoral ring to reach the obturator foramen and would be closely related to the neck of a femoral hernia. Consequently, this artery could be involved in a *strangulated femoral hernia.* Surgeons placing staples during endoscopic repair of both inguinal and femoral hernias must also be vigilant concerning the possible presence of this common arterial variant. ⊙

Femoral Vein

The *femoral vein* is the continuation of the popliteal vein proximal to the adductor hiatus. As it ascends through the adductor canal, the femoral vein lies posterolateral and then posterior to the femoral artery (Figs. 5.17*A* & *B* and 5.19). The femoral vein enters the femoral sheath lateral to the femoral canal and ends posterior to the inguinal ligament, where it becomes the external iliac vein. In the inferior part of the femoral triangle, the femoral vein receives the deep vein of the thigh, the great saphenous vein, and other tributaries. The *deep vein of the thigh,* formed by the union of three or four perforating veins, enters the femoral vein approximately 8 cm inferior to the inguinal ligament and approximately 5 cm inferior to the termination of the great saphenous vein.

Table 5.5. Arteries of the Anterior and Medial Thigh

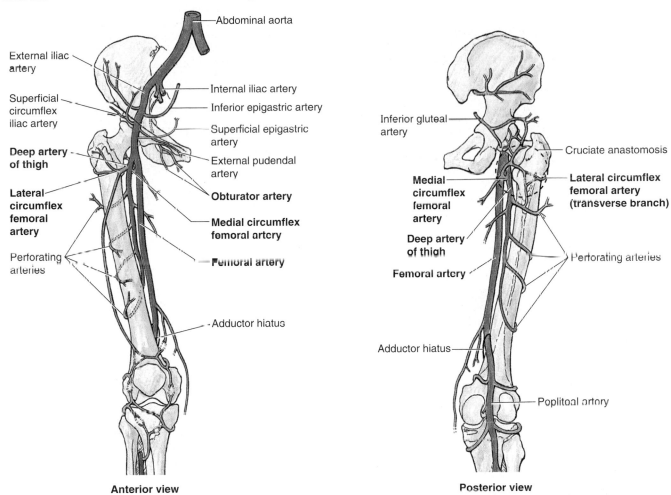

Anterior view

Posterior view

Artery	Origin	Course	Distribution
Femoral	Continuation of external iliac artery distal to inguinal ligament	Descends through femoral triangle bisecting it; then courses through adductor canal; terminates as it traverses adductor hiatus, where its name becomes popliteal artery	Branches supply anterior and anteromedial aspects of thigh
Deep artery of thigh	Femoral artery 1–5 cm inferior to inguinal ligament	Passes deeply between pectineus and adductor longus; descending posterior to latter on medial side of femur	Three to four perforating branches pass through adductor magnus muscle, winding around femur to supply muscles in medial, posterior, and lateral part of anterior compartments
Medial circumflex femoral	Deep artery of thigh; may arise from femoral artery	Passes medially and posteriorly between pectineus and iliopsoas; enters gluteal region and gives rise to posterior retinacular arteries; then terminates by dividing into transverse and ascending branches	Supplies most of blood to head and neck of femur; transverse branch takes part in cruciate anastomosis of thigh; ascending branch joins inferior gluteal artery
Lateral circumflex femoral	Deep artery of thigh; may arise from femoral artery	Passes laterally deep to sartorius and rectus femoris, dividing into ascending, transverse, and descending arteries	Ascending branch supplies anterior part of gluteal region; transverse branch winds around femur; descendingbranch joins genicular periarticular anastomosis
Obturator	Internal iliac artery or (in ~ 20%) as an accessory or replaced obturator artery from the inferior epigastric artery	Passes through obturator foramen; enters medial compartment of thigh and divides into anterior and posterior branches, which pass on respective sides of adductor brevis	Anterior branch supplies obturator externus, pectineus, adductors of thigh, and gracilis; posterior branch supplies muscles attached to ischial tuberosity

Potentially Lethal Misnomer

Clinical staff, some vascular laboratories, and even some text and reference books use the term "superficial femoral vein" when referring to the femoral vein before it is joined by the accompanying veins of the deep artery of the thigh (deep femoral veins). Some primary care physicians may not have been taught and/or may not realize that the so-called superficial femoral vein is actually a deep vein and that acute thrombosis of this vessel is potentially life threatening. The adjective *superficial* should not be used because it implies that this vein is a superficial vein. Most *pulmonary emboli* originate in deep veins, not in superficial veins. The risk of embolism can be greatly reduced by anticoagulant treatment. The use of imprecise language here creates the possibility that an acute thrombosis of this truly deep vessel could be overlooked as an acute clinical issue, and a life-threatening situation created. Anatomical terminology used in clinical reports must be accurate to avoid possible life-threatening situations.

Saphenous Varix

A localized dilation of the terminal part of the great saphenous vein, called a **saphenous varix** (L. dilated vein), may cause edema in the femoral triangle. A saphenous varix may be confused with other groin swellings such as a psoas abscess (see clinical correlation [blue] box "Psoas Abscess," in this chapter); however, a varix should be considered when varicose veins are present in other parts of the lower limb.

Location of the Femoral Vein

The femoral vein is not usually palpable but its position can be located inferior to the inguinal ligament by feeling the pulsations of the femoral artery, which is immediately lateral to the vein. In thin people, the femoral vein may be close to the surface and may be mistaken for the great saphenous vein. It is important therefore to know that the femoral vein has no tributaries at this level, except for the great saphenous vein that joins it approximately 3 cm inferior to the inguinal ligament. In *varicose vein operations,* it is obviously important to identify the great saphenous vein correctly and not tie off the femoral vein by mistake.

Cannulation of the Femoral Vein

To secure blood samples and take pressure recordings from the chambers of the right side of the heart and/or from the pulmonary artery and to perform *right cardiac angiography,* a long, slender catheter is inserted into the femoral vein as it passes through the femoral triangle. Under fluoroscopic control, the catheter is passed superiorly through the external and common iliac veins into the inferior vena cava and right atrium of the heart. Femoral venous puncture may also be used for the administration of fluids. ▶

Transversalis fascia

Fascia lata

Femoral hernia

Inguinal ligament

Femoral artery and vein

Iliopsoas muscle and fascia

Femoral nerve

External iliac artery and vein (cut)

Inferior epigastric artery

Intestine

Aberrant obturator artery

Femoral ring

Pubic tubercle

Pubic symphysis

Lacunar ligament

Saphenous opening

Femoral hernia

Great saphenous vein

Early stage

Anterior view

Late stage

Figure B5.11

Femoral Hernia

The femoral ring is a weak area in the anterior abdominal wall that normally is of a size sufficient to admit the tip of the little finger. The femoral ring is the usual originating site of a *femoral hernia,* a protrusion of abdominal viscera (often a loop of small intestine) through the femoral ring into the femoral canal. A femoral hernia appears as a mass, often tender, in the femoral triangle, *inferolateral to the pubic tubercle* (Fig. B5.11). The hernia is bounded by the femoral vein laterally and the lacunar ligament medially. The hernial sac compresses the contents of the femoral canal (loose connective tissue, fat, and lymphatics) and distends the wall of the canal. Initially, the hernia is small because it is contained within the canal; but it can enlarge by passing inferiorly through the saphenous opening into the subcutaneous tissue of the thigh. Femoral hernias are more common in females. *Strangulation of a femoral hernia* may occur because of the sharp, rigid boundaries of the femoral ring, particularly the concave margin of the lacunar ligament. Strangulation of a femoral hernia interferes with the blood supply to the herniated intestine. This vascular impairment may result in death of the tissues. ○

Adductor Canal

The **adductor canal** (subsartorial canal; Hunter canal) is a long (approximately 15 cm), narrow passageway in the middle third of the thigh. It extends from the apex of the femoral triangle, where the sartorius crosses over the adductor longus, to the *adductor hiatus* in the tendon of the adductor magnus (Fig. 5.20). The adductor canal provides an intermuscular passage for the femoral artery and vein, the saphenous nerve, and the nerve to vastus medialis, delivering the femoral vessels to the popliteal fossa where they become the popliteal vessels.

The adductor canal is bounded:

- Anteriorly and laterally by the vastus medialis.

- Posteriorly by the adductors longus and magnus.

- Medially by the sartorius, which overlies the groove between the above muscles, forming the roof of the canal.

In the inferior third to half of the canal, a tough subsartorial or vastoadductor fascia spans between the adductor longus and the vastus medialis muscles, forming the anterior wall of the canal deep to the sartorius. Because this fascia has a distinct superior margin, novices dissecting in this area commonly assume when they see the femoral vessels pass deep to this fascia that they are traversing the adductor hiatus. The adductor hiatus, however, is located at a more inferior level, just proximal to the medial supracondylar ridge. This hiatus is a gap between the aponeurotic adductor and the tendinous hamstrings attachments of the adductor magnus.

THE BOTTOM LINE: The primary neurovascular bundle of the thigh, like that of the arm, is placed on the medial side of the limb for protection. In the upper third of the thigh, the bundle is most superficial as it enters deep to the inguinal ligament. This relatively superficial position is important for clinical procedures. Although they are essentially adjacent, the femoral nerve traverses the muscular lacunae of the subinguinal space, whereas the femoral vessels traverse the vascular lacunae within the femoral sheath. The femoral vessels bisect the femoral triangle, where the primary vessels of the thigh, the deep artery and vein of the thigh, arise and terminate, respectively. The femoral nerve per se terminates within the triangle. However, two of its branches, a motor branch (nerve to vastus medialis) and sensory branch (saphenous nerve), are part of the neurovascular bundle that traverses the adductor canal in the middle third of the thigh. The vascular structures then pass through the adductor hiatus, becoming popliteal in name and location in the distal thigh/posterior knee region.

Hip and Buttocks: The Gluteal Region

Although the demarcation of trunk and limb is abrupt anteriorly at the inguinal ligament, posteriorly the gluteal region is a large transitional zone between trunk and limb. Physically part of the trunk, functionally the gluteal region is definitely part of the limb. The gluteal region is the prominent area posterior to the pelvis and inferior to the level of the iliac crests (the buttocks) and extending laterally and anteriorly to the greater trochanter according to some definitions and to the ASIS according to others (Fig. 5.21). The *intergluteal cleft* separates the buttocks from each other. The *gluteal muscles*

Level of iliac crests
Intergluteal cleft
Buttock
Thigh
Gluteal fold

Figure 5.21. Gluteal region—buttocks area. The intergluteal cleft separates the buttocks (right and left gluteal regions or prominences). The gluteal fold (sulcus) marks the lower limit of the buttock and the upper limit of the thigh.

(gluteus maximus, medius, and minimus and tensor of the fascia lata) form the bulk of the region. The *gluteal fold* demarcates the inferior boundary of the buttock and the superior boundary of the thigh.

Gluteal Ligaments

The parts of the bony pelvis—hip bones, sacrum, and coccyx—are bound together by dense ligaments (Fig. 5.22). The **sacrotuberous** and **sacrospinous ligaments** convert the sciatic notches in the hip bones into the greater and lesser sciatic foramina. The **greater sciatic foramen** is the passageway for structures entering or leaving the pelvis (e.g., sciatic nerve), whereas the **lesser sciatic foramen** is the passageway for structures entering or leaving the perineum (e.g., pudendal nerve). It is helpful to think of the greater sciatic foramen as the "door" through which all lower limb arteries and nerves leave the pelvis and enter the gluteal region. The *piriformis* (Table 5.6) also enters the gluteal region through the greater sciatic foramen and almost fills it.

Gluteal Muscles

The gluteal muscles (Fig. 5.23*A, C, & D*) share a common compartment but are organized into two layers, superficial and deep:

- The *superficial layer* consists of the three large glutei (maximus, medius, and minimus) and the tensor of the fascia lata. These muscles all have proximal attachments to the posterolateral (external) surface and margins of the ala of the ilium and are mainly extensors, abductors, and medial rotators of the thigh.

- The *deep layer* consists of smaller muscles (piriformis, obturator internus, externus gemelli, and quadratus femoris) covered by the inferior half of the gluteus maximus. They all have distal attachments on or adjacent to the intertrochanteric crest of the femur. These muscles are lateral rotators of the thigh but they also stabilize the hip joint, working with the strong ligaments of the hip joint to steady the femoral head in the acetabulum.

For the attachments, innervation, and main actions of these muscles, see Table 5.6.

Gluteus Maximus

The **gluteus maximus** is the most superficial gluteal muscle. It is the largest, heaviest, and most coarsely fibered muscle of the body. The gluteus maximus covers all of the other gluteal muscles (Figs. 5.23*A* & *C* and 5.24*A*) except for the anterosuperior third of the gluteus medius. The *ischial tuberosity* can be felt on deep palpation through the inferior part of the muscle, just superior to the medial part of the gluteal fold. When the thigh is flexed, the inferior border of the gluteus maximus moves superiorly, leaving the ischial tuberosity subcutaneous. You do not sit on your gluteus maximus; you sit on the fatty fibrous tissue and the ischial bursa that lie between the ischial tuberosity and the skin.

Posterior view

Figure 5.22. Ligaments of pelvic girdle. The sacrotuberous and sacrospinous ligaments pass from the ischial tuberosity and ischial spine, respectively, to the side of the sacrum and coccyx. These ligaments convert the greater and lesser sciatic notches into foramina. The greater sciatic foramen is the doorway of the true pelvis; the lesser sciatic foramen, the entrance to the perineum.

Table 5.6. Muscles of Gluteal Region: Abductors and Rotators of the Thigh

(A) Posterior view — Gluteus maximus, Gluteus medius, Gluteus minimus, Tensor of fascia lata, Gluteus medius and minimus, Quadratus femoris, Gemelli, Gluteus maximus

(B) Anterior view — Obturator internus and gemelli, Piriformis, Gluteus minimus

(C) Posterior view — Gluteus medius (cut), Attachment to anterior gluteal line, Gluteus minimus, Gluteus maximus (cut and reflected), Gluteus maximus, Attachment to greater trochanter

(D) Lateral views — Piriformis

(E) Lateral views — Posterior gluteal line, Gluteus medius, Anterior superior iliac spine, Gluteus minimus, Piriformis, Attachment to greater trochanter of femur

(F) Posterior view — Piriformis

(G) Anterior view — Piriformis

(H) Posterior views — Obturator internus inside pelvis, Inferior gemellus, Attachment to tendon of obturator internus, Superior gemellus, Obturator internus

(I) Posterior views — Ischial tuberosity, Lateral condyle of tibia, Quadratus femoris

(J) Anterior view — Tensor of fascia lata, Iliotibial tract, Anterior superior iliac spine

Muscle	Proximal Attachment	Distal Attachment	Innervation[a]	Main Action
Gluteus maximus (A & C)	Ilium posterior to posterior gluteal line; dorsal surface of sacrum and coccyx; sacrotuberous ligament	Most fibers end in iliotibial tract, which inserts into lateral condyle of tibia; some fibers insert on gluteal tuberosity	Inferior gluteal nerve (L5, **S1, S2**)	Extends thigh (especially from flexed position) and assists in its lateral rotation; steadies thigh and assists in rising from sitting position
Gluteus medius (A,C, & E)	External surface of ilium between anterior and posterior gluteal lines	Lateral surface of greater trochanter of femur	Superior gluteal nerve (**L5,** S1)	Abduct and medially rotate thigh; keep pelvis level when ipsilateral limb is weight bearing and advance opposite (unsupported) side during its swing phase
Gluteus minimus (A–D)	External surface of ilium between anterior and inferior gluteal lines	Anterior surface of greater trochanter of femur		
Tensor of fascia lata (J)	Anterior superior iliac spine; anterior part of iliac crest	Iliotibial tract, which attaches to lateral condyle of tibia		
Piriformis (F & G)	Anterior surface of sacrum; sacrotuberous ligament	Superior border of greater trochanter of femur	Branches of anterior rami of **S1**, S2	Laterally rotate extended thigh and abduct flexed thigh; steady femoral head in acetabulum
Obturator internus (H)	Pelvic surface of obturator membrane and surrounding bones	Medial surface of greater trochanter (trochanteric fossa) of femur[b]	Nerve to obturator internus (L5, **S1**)	
Superior and inferior gemelli (H)	Superior: ischial spine Inferior: ischial tuberosity	Medial surface of greater trochanter (trochanteric fossa) of femur[b]	Superior gemellus: same nerve supply as obturator internus Inferior gemellus: same nerve supply as quadratus femoris	
Quadratus femoris (I)	Lateral border of ischial tuberosity	Quadrate tubercle on intertrochanteric crest of femur and area inferior to it	Nerve to quadratus femoris (L5, S1)	Laterally rotates thigh;[c] steadies femoral head in acetabulum

[a]The spinal cord segmental innervation is indicated (e.g., "S1, S2" means that the nerves supplying the piriformis are derived from the first two sacral segments of the spinal cord). Numbers in boldface (**S1**) indicate the main segmental innervation. Damage to one or more of the listed spinal cord segments or to the motor nerve roots arising from them results in paralysis of the muscles concerned.
[b]The gemelli muscles blend with the tendon of the obturator internus as it attaches to the greater trochanter of the femur.
[c]There are six lateral rotators of the thigh: piriformis, obturator internus, superior and inferior gemelli, quadratus femoris, and obturator externus. These muscles also stabilize the hip joint.

The gluteus maximus slopes inferolaterally at a 45° angle from the pelvis to the buttock. The fibers of the superior and larger part of the gluteus maximus and superficial fibers of the inferior part insert into the *iliotibial tract* (Fig. 5.23*A, C, & D*). Some deep fibers of the inferior part of the muscle (roughly the deep anterior and inferior quarter) attach to the *gluteal tuberosity of the femur.* The inferior gluteal nerve and vessels enter the deep surface of the gluteus maximus at its center. It is supplied by both the inferior and superior gluteal arteries. In the superior part of its course, the *sciatic nerve* passes deep to the gluteus maximus (Fig. 5.24*A*).

The main actions of the gluteus maximus are extension and lateral rotation of the thigh. When the gluteus maximus is fixed proximally, the muscle extends the trunk on the lower limb. Although it is the strongest extensor of the hip, it acts mostly when force is necessary (rapid movement or move-ment against resistance) and functions primarily between the flexed and standing (straight) positions of the thigh, as when rising from the sitting position, straightening from the bend-ing position, walking uphill and up stairs, and running. It is used only briefly during casual walking and usually not at all when standing motionless. Paralysis of the gluteus maximus does not seriously affect walking on level ground. Verify this by placing your hand on your buttock when walking slowly. The gluteus maximus contracts only briefly during the earli-est part of the stance phase (from heel strike to when the foot is flat on the ground, to resist further flexion as weight is as-sumed by the partially flexed limb) (Table 5.2). If you climb stairs and put your hand on your buttock, you will feel the gluteus maximus contract strongly.

Because the iliotibial tract crosses the knee and attaches to the anterolateral tibial tubercle (Fig. 5.23*C & D;* Table 5.6),

(A)

Posterior views   †Attachment of inferior half of deep part of gluteus maximus to gluteal tuberosity

(B)

*Triceps coxae:
Tendon of obturator internus
Superior gemellus
Inferior gemellus

Figure 5.23. Muscles of gluteal region and posterior compartment of thigh. Superficial and deep dissections of the gluteal region (**A**) and the posterior compartment of the thigh (**B**) are demonstrated.

Figure 5.23. *(Continued)* Also shown are superficial (**C**) and deep (**D**) views of the lateral musculofibrous complex formed by the tensor of the fascia lata and gluteus maximus muscles and their shared aponeurotic tendon, the iliotibial tract. The iliotibial tract is continuous (posteriorly and deeply) with the dense lateral intermuscular septum, by which the tract is attached to the linea aspera of the femur.

the gluteus maximus and tensor of the fascia lata together are also able to assist in making the extended knee stable, but they are not usually called on to do so during normal standing. Because the iliotibial tract attaches to the femur via the lateral intermuscular septum, it does not have the freedom necessary to produce motion at the knee.

Testing the gluteus maximus is performed when the person is prone with the lower limb straight. The person tightens the buttock and extends the hip joint as the examiner observes and palpates the gluteus maximus.

Gluteal Bursae. Gluteal bursae (L. purses) separate the gluteus maximus from adjacent structures (Fig. 5.25). Bursae are membranous sacs lined by a synovial membrane containing a capillary layer of slippery fluid resembling egg white. Bursae are located in areas subject to friction (e.g., where the iliotibial tract crosses the greater trochanter); their purpose is to reduce friction and permit free movement. Usually three bursae are associated with the gluteus maximus:

1. The **trochanteric bursa** separates superior fibers of the gluteus maximus from the greater trochanter. The trochanteric bursa is commonly the largest of the bursae formed in relation to bony prominences and is present at birth. Other such bursae appear to form as a result of postnatal movement.

2. The **ischial bursa** separates the inferior part of the gluteus maximus from the ischial tuberosity; it is often absent.

3. The **gluteofemoral bursa** separates the iliotibial tract from the superior part of the proximal attachment of the vastus lateralis, a thigh muscle.

Gluteus Medius and Gluteus Minimus

The smaller gluteal muscles, **gluteus medius** and **gluteus minimus,** are fan shaped, and their fibers converge in the same manner toward essentially the same target (Figs. 5.23*A,* 5.24*A,* 5.25, and 5.26*D*). They share the same actions and nerve supply (Table 5.6) and are supplied by the same blood vessel, the superior gluteal artery. The gluteus minimus and most of the gluteus medius lie deep to the gluteus maximus on the external surface of the ilium. The gluteus medius and minimus abduct the thigh and rotate it medially (Fig. 5.26; Table 5.2).

Testing the gluteus medius and minimus is performed while the person is prone with the leg flexed to a right angle. The

person abducts the thigh against resistance. The gluteus medius can be palpated inferior to the iliac crest, posterior to the tensor of the fascia lata, which is also contracting during abduction of the thigh.

Tensor of the Fascia Lata

The **tensor of the fascia lata** (L. *tensor fasciae latae*) is a fusiform muscle approximately 15 cm long that is enclosed between two layers of fascia lata (Fig. 5.17*B*). Its attachments, innervation and action are provided in Table 5.6. The tensor and the superficial and anterior part of the gluteus maximus share a common distal attachment to the anterolateral tibial condyle via the *iliotibial tract,* which acts as

(*cont'd on page 615*)

(A) Posterior view

Figure 5.24. Dissection of gluteal region and abductors and rotators of thigh. A. In this deep dissection, the neurovascular structures of the gluteal region and proximal posterior thigh are revealed. Most of the gluteus maximus and medius are removed, and segments of the hamstrings are excised. Except for the superior gluteal artery and nerve, the neurovascular structures supplying or traversing the gluteal region and posterior thigh emerge from the pelvis via the greater sciatic foramen inferior to the piriformis; however, exceptions occur (Fig. 5.28). The sciatic nerve runs deep (anterior) to and is protected by the overlying gluteus maximus initially and then the biceps femoris.

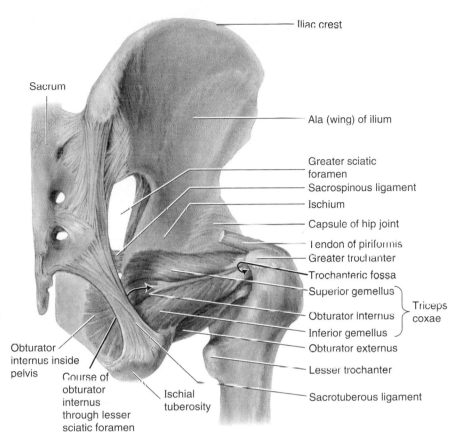

Iliac crest

Sacrum

Ala (wing) of ilium

Greater sciatic foramen

Sacrospinous ligament

Ischium

Capsule of hip joint

Tendon of piriformis

Greater trochanter

Trochanteric fossa

Superior gemellus

Obturator internus ⎤ Triceps coxae

Inferior gemellus ⎦

Obturator externus

Lesser trochanter

Sacrotuberous ligament

Obturator internus inside pelvis

Course of obturator internus through lesser sciatic foramen

Ischial tuberosity

(B) Posterior view

Figure 5.24. *(Continued)* **B.** This dissection shows some of the lateral rotators of the thigh: the piriformis (distal tendinous attachment only), the external and internal obturators (arising from opposite sides of the obturator membrane), and the gemelli muscles. Note that the components of the triceps coxae share a common attachment—adjacent to that of the obturator externus—into the trochanteric fossa.

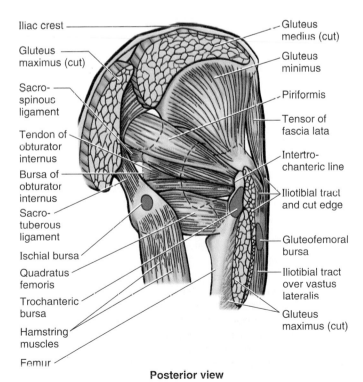

Iliac crest

Gluteus maximus (cut)

Sacrospinous ligament

Tendon of obturator internus

Bursa of obturator internus

Sacrotuberous ligament

Ischial bursa

Quadratus femoris

Trochanteric bursa

Hamstring muscles

Femur

Gluteus medius (cut)

Gluteus minimus

Piriformis

Tensor of fascia lata

Intertrochanteric line

Iliotibial tract and cut edge

Gluteofemoral bursa

Iliotibial tract over vastus lateralis

Gluteus maximus (cut)

Posterior view

Figure 5.25. Gluteal muscles and bursae. Three bursae (trochanteric, gluteofemoral, and ischial) usually separate the gluteus maximus from underlying bony prominences, allowing free muscular contraction or tendon movement. The bursa of the obturator internus allows the tendon of the obturator internus to glide freely over the lesser sciatic notch of the hip bone, which the muscle uses as a trochlea (pulley), changing its direction of pull by more than 90° before the gemelli muscles become attached to it.

Posterior views

(A) (B) (C)

Iliotibial tract

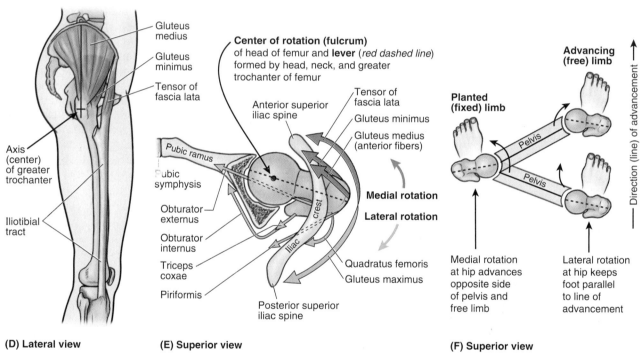

(D) Lateral view

- Gluteus medius
- Gluteus minimus
- Tensor of fascia lata
- Axis (center) of greater trochanter
- Iliotibial tract

(E) Superior view

Center of rotation (fulcrum) of head of femur and **lever** (*red dashed line*) formed by head, neck, and greater trochanter of femur

- Anterior superior iliac spine
- Pubic ramus
- Pubic symphysis
- Obturator externus
- Obturator internus
- Triceps coxae
- Piriformis
- Posterior superior iliac spine
- Tensor of fascia lata
- Gluteus minimus
- Gluteus medius (anterior fibers)
- Iliac crest

Medial rotation

Lateral rotation

- Quadratus femoris
- Gluteus maximus

(F) Superior view

- Advancing (free) limb
- Planted (fixed) limb
- Pelvis
- Pelvis
- Direction (line) of advancement

Medial rotation at hip advances opposite side of pelvis and free limb

Lateral rotation at hip keeps foot parallel to line of advancement

Figure 5.26. Action of abductors/medial rotators of thigh when walking. A–C. The role of the abductors (gluteus medius and minimus, tensor of fascia lata) is demonstrated. When the weight is on both feet (**A**), the pelvis is evenly supported and does not sag. When the weight is borne by one limb (**B**), the muscles on the supported side fix the pelvis so that it does not sag to the unsupported side. Keeping the pelvis level enables the non-weight-bearing limb to clear the ground as it is brought forward during the swing phase. When the right abductors are paralyzed (**C**), owing to a lesion of the right superior gluteal nerve, fixation by these muscles is lost and the pelvis tilts to the unsupported left side (positive Trendelenburg sign). The net effect is that the limb becomes "too long" for the hip height, requiring a compensatory limp to prevent the foot from hitting the ground during swing phase. **D–F.** The role of the rotators of the thigh is demonstrated. In the lateral (**D**) and superior (**E**) views, note that most abductors—the tensor of the fascia lata, gluteus minimus, and most (the anterior fibers) of the gluteus medius—lie anterior to the lever provided by the axis of the head, neck, and greater trochanter of the femur to rotate the thigh around the vertical axis traversing the femoral head. The superior view of the right hip joint (**E**) includes the superior pubic ramus, acetabulum, and iliac crest; the inferior part of the ilium has been removed to reveal the head and neck of the femur. The lines of pull of the rotators of the hip are indicated by arrows, demonstrating the antagonistic relationship resulting from their positions relative to the lever and the center of rotation (fulcrum). The medial rotators pull the greater trochanter anteriorly and the lateral rotators pull the trochanter posteriorly, resulting in rotation of the thigh around the vertical axis. Note that all of these muscles also pull the head and neck of the femur medially into the acetabulum, strengthening the joint. In walking (**F**), the same muscles that act unilaterally during the stance phase (planted limb) to keep the pelvis level via abduction can simultaneously produce medial rotation at the hip joint, advancing the opposite unsupported side of the pelvis (augmenting advancement of the free limb). The lateral rotators of the advancing (free) limb act during the swing phase to keep the foot parallel to the direction (line) of advancement.

a long aponeurosis for the muscles. However, unlike the gluteus maximus, the tensor is served by the superior gluteal neurovascular bundle. Despite its gluteal innervation and shared attachment, the tensor of the fascia lata is primarily a flexor of the thigh because of its anterior location; however, it generally does not act independently. To produce flexion, the tensor of the fascia lata acts in concert with the iliopsoas and rectus femoris. When the iliopsoas is paralyzed, the tensor of the fascia lata undergoes hypertrophy in an attempt to compensate. It also works in conjunction with other abductor/medial rotator muscles (gluteus medius and minimus) (Fig. 5.26). It lies too far anteriorly to be a strong abductor and thus probably contributes primarily as a synergist or fixator.

The tensor of the fascia lata also tenses the fascia lata and iliotibial tract, thereby helping support the femur on the tibia when standing. Because the iliotibial tract is attached to the femur via the lateral intermuscular septum, the tensor produces little if any movement of the leg (Fig. 5.23D). However, when the knee is fully extended, it contributes to (increases) the extending force, adding stability. When the knee is flexed by other muscles, the tensor can synergistically augment flexion and lateral rotation of the leg.

The abductors/medial rotators of the hip joint play an essential role during locomotion, advancing and preventing the sagging of the unsupported side of the pelvis during walking, as illustrated and explained in Figure 5.26. The supportive and action-producing functions of the abductors/medial rotators depends on normal:

- Muscular activity and innervation from the superior gluteal nerve.

- Articulation of the hip joint components.

- Strength and angulation of the femoral neck.

Piriformis

The narrow, pear-shaped **piriformis** (L. *pirum*, a pear) is located partly on the posterior wall of the lesser pelvis and partly posterior to the hip joint (Figs. 5.23A, 5.24A, and 5.25; Table 5.6). The piriformis leaves the pelvis through the *greater sciatic foramen*, almost filling it, to reach its attachment to the superior border of the greater trochanter. Because of its key position in the buttock, the piriformis is the landmark of the gluteal region. The piriformis provides the key to understanding relationships in the gluteal region because it determines the names of the blood vessels and nerves:

- The superior gluteal vessels and nerve emerge superior to it.

- The inferior gluteal vessels and nerve emerge inferior to it.

- The surface marking of the superior border of the piriformis is indicated by a line joining the skin dimple formed by the posterior superior iliac spine to the superior border of the greater trochanter of the femur (Fig. SA5.2G).

Obturator Internus and Gemelli

The **obturator internus** and the **superior** and **inferior gemelli** (L. *geminus*, small twin) form a tricipital (three-headed) muscle, the *triceps coxae* (triceps of the hip), which occupies the gap between the piriformis and the quadratus femoris (Figs. 5.23A and 5.24A & B; Table 5.6). The common tendon of these muscles lies horizontally in the buttock as it passes to the greater trochanter of the femur.

The obturator internus is located partly in the pelvis, where it covers most of the lateral wall of the lesser pelvis (Fig. 5.24B; Table 5.6). It leaves the pelvis through the *lesser sciatic foramen*, makes a right-angle turn (Fig. 5.26E), becomes tendinous, and receives the distal attachments of the gemelli before attaching to the medial surface of the greater trochanter (trochanteric fossa). The small gemelli are narrow, triangular extrapelvic reinforcements of the obturator internus. Although the inferior gemellus receives separate innervation from the nerve to the quadratus femoris, it is more realistic to consider these three muscles as a unit (i.e., as the triceps coxae) because they are incapable of independent action. The **bursa of the obturator internus** allows free movement of the muscle over the posterior border of the ischium, where the border forms the lesser sciatic notch and the trochlea over which the tendon glides as it turns (Fig. 5.25).

Quadratus Femoris

The **quadratus femoris** is a short, flat quadrangular muscle located inferior to the obturator internus and gemelli (Figs. 5.23A and 5.25). True to its name, the quadratus femoris is a rectangular muscle; it is a strong lateral rotator of the thigh.

Obturator Externus

Based on its location (posterior to the pectineus and the superior ends of the adductor muscles) and its innervation (obturator nerve), the obturator externus was described earlier in this chapter with the medial thigh muscles (Table 5.4). However, it functions as a lateral rotator of the thigh, and its distal attachment is visible only during dissection of the gluteal region (Fig. 5.24B) or hip joint. Thus it is mentioned again in this context. It lies deep in the proximal thigh, with its tendon passing deep to the quadratus femoris on the way to its attachment to the trochanteric fossa of the femur (Fig. 5.24A). The obturator externus, with other short muscles around the hip joint, stabilizes the head of the femur in the acetabulum (Fig. 5.26E). It is most effective as a lateral rotator of the thigh when the hip joint is flexed.

THE BOTTOM LINE: Because the femur is bent at the angle of inclination, the relatively transverse lever formed by the proximal femur allows superior placement of the abductors of the thigh and provides mechanical advantage for the deeper medial and lateral rotators of the thigh. This is critical for bipedal locomotion. Thus, despite their designations, the abductors/medial rotators (the superficial gluteal muscles) are most active during the stance phase when they simultaneously elevate and advance the contralateral unsupported side of the pelvis during ambulation. The lateral rotators (deep gluteal muscles) of the unsupported side rotate the free limb during the swing phase so that the foot remains parallel to the line of advancement.

Ischial Bursitis

Recurrent microtrauma resulting from repeated stress (e.g., as from cycling, rowing, or other activities involving repetitive hip extension while seated) may overwhelm the ischial bursa's ability to dissipate applied stress. The recurrent trauma results in inflammation of the bursa (**ischial bursitis**). Ischial bursitis is a **friction bursitis** resulting from excessive friction between the ischial bursae and the ischial tuberosities. Localized pain occurs over the bursa, and the pain increases with movement of the gluteus maximus. Calcification may occur in the bursa with chronic bursitis. Because the ischial tuberosities bear the body weight during sitting, these pressure points may lead to *pressure sores* in debilitated people, particularly paraplegic persons with poor nursing care.

Trochanteric Bursitis

Inflammation of the trochanteric bursae, or **trochanteric bursitis,** may result from repetitive actions such as climbing stairs while carrying heavy objects or running on a steeply elevated treadmill. These movements involve the gluteus maximus and move the superior tendinous fibers repeatedly back and forth over the bursae of the greater trochanter. Trochanteric bursitis causes deep diffuse pain in the lateral thigh region. This type of *friction bursitis* is characterized by point tenderness over the great trochanter; however, the pain radiates along the iliotibial tract that extends from the iliac tubercle to the tibia (Figs. 5.23*C* and 5.26*D*). This thickening of the fascia lata receives tendinous reinforcements from the tensor of the fascia lata and the gluteus maximus. The pain from an inflamed trochanteric bursa, usually localized just posterior to the greater trochanter, is generally elicited by manually resisting abduction and lateral rotation of the thigh while the person is lying on the unaffected side. ✛

Posterior Thigh Muscles

The attachments, innervation, and actions of the posterior thigh muscles are provided in Table 5.7. Three of the four muscles in the posterior aspect of the thigh are **hamstrings** (Fig. 5.27*A* & *B*): (1) semitendinosus, (2) semimembranosus,

and (3) biceps femoris (long head). The hamstrings share common features:

- Proximal attachment to the ischial tuberosity deep to the gluteus maximus.
- Spanning and acting on two joints: extension at the hip joint and flexion at the knee.
- Innervation by the tibial division of the sciatic nerve.

The long head of the biceps meets all these conditions, but the short head of the biceps, the fourth muscle of the posterior compartment, fails to meet any of them. The hamstrings received their name because it is common to tie hams (pork thighs) up for curing and/or smoking with a hook around these muscle tendons. This also explains the expression "hamstringing the enemy" by slashing these tendons lateral and medial to the knees.

The two actions of the hamstrings cannot be performed maximally at the same time: full flexion of the knee requires so much shortening of the hamstrings that they cannot provide the additional contraction that would be necessary for simultaneous full extension of the thigh; similarly, full extension of the hip shortens the hamstrings so they cannot further contract to act fully on the knee. When the thighs and legs are fixed, the hamstrings can help extend the trunk at the hip joint. They are active in thigh extension under all situations except full flexion of the knee, including maintenance of the relaxed standing posture (standing at ease). A person with paralyzed hamstrings tends to fall forward because the gluteus maximus muscles cannot maintain the necessary muscle tone to stand straight.

The hamstrings are the hip extensors involved in walking on flat ground, when the gluteus maximus demonstrates minimal activity. However, rather than producing either hip extension or knee flexion per se during normal walking, the hamstrings demonstrate most activity when they are eccentrically contracting, resisting (decelerating) hip flexion and knee extension during terminal swing (between midswing and heel strike) (Table 5.2).

The length of the hamstrings varies, but this is usually a matter of conditioning. In some people, they are not long enough to allow them to touch their toes when the knees are extended. Routine stretch exercise can lengthen these muscles and tendons.

To test the hamstrings the person flexes the leg against resistance. Normally, these muscles—especially their tendons on each side of the popliteal fossa—should be prominent as they bend the knee.

Semitendinosus

As its name indicates, the **semitendinosus** muscle is semitendinous. This muscle has a fusiform belly that is usually interrupted by a tendinous intersection and a long, cord-like tendon that begins approximately two thirds of the way down the thigh. Distally, the tendon attaches to the medial surface of the superior part of the tibia as part of the *pes anserinus*

Table 5.7. Muscles of the Posterior Thigh: Extensors of the Hip, Flexors of the Knee

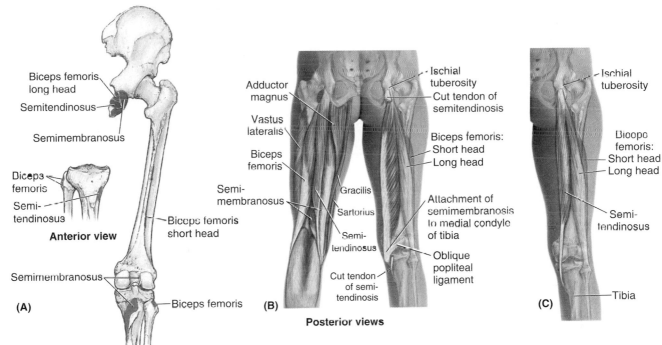

Muscle[a]	Proximal Attachment	Distal Attachment	Innervation[b]	Main Action
Semitendinosus	Ishchial tuberosity	Medial surface of superior part of tibia	Tibial division of sciatic nerve part of tibia (L5, **S1**, **S2**)	Extend thigh; flex leg and rotate it medially when knee is flexed; when thigh and leg are flexed, these muscles can extend trunk
Semimembranosus		Posterior part of medial condyle of tibia; reflected attachment forms oblique popliteal ligament (to lateral femoral condyle)		
Biceps femoris	Long head: ischial tuberosity Short head: linea aspera and lateral supracondylar line of femur	Lateral side of head of fibula; tendon is split at this site by fibular collateral ligament of knee	Long head: tibial division of sciatic nerve (L5, **S1**, S2) Short head: common fibular division of sciatic nerve (L5, **S1**, S2)	Flexes leg and rotates it laterally when knee is flexed; extends thigh (e.g., when starting to walk)

[a]Collectively these three muscles are known as hamstrings.
[b]The spinal cord segmental innervation is indicated (e.g., "L5, S1, S2" means that the nerves supplying the semitendinosus are derived from the fifth lumbar segment and first two sacral segments of the spinal cord). Numbers in boldface (**L5**, **S1**) indicate the main segmental innervation. Damage to one or more of the listed spinal cord segments or to the motor nerve roots arising from them results in paralysis of the muscles concerned.

formation in conjunction with the tendinous insertions of the sartorius and gracilis (discussed earlier in this chapter).

Semimembranosus

The **semimembranosus** is a broad muscle that is also aptly named because of the flattened membranous form of its proximal attachment to the ischial tuberosity (Fig. 5.27A). The tendon of the semimembranosus forms around the middle of the thigh and descends to the posterior part of the medial tibial condyle. Its tendon divides distally into three parts: (1) a direct attachment to the posterior aspect of the medial tibial condyle, (2) a part that blends with the popliteal fascia, and

(3) a reflected part that reinforces the intercondylar part of the joint capsule of the knee as the **oblique popliteal ligament** (Figs. 5.23B and 5.60).

When the knee is flexed to 90°, the tendons of the medial hamstrings or "semi-" muscles (semitendinosus and semimembranosus) pass to the medial side of the tibia; in this position, contraction of the medial hamstrings (and of synergists including the gracilis, sartorius, and popliteus) produces a limited amount (about 10°) of medial rotation of the tibia at the knee. The two medial hamstrings are not as active as the lateral hamstring, the biceps femoris, which is the "workhorse" of extension at the hip (Hamill and Knutzen, 1995).

(A) Posterior view

- Gluteus medius
- Piriformis
- Obturator internus and gemelli
- Sciatic nerve
- Ischial tuberosity
- Quadratus femoris
- Adductor magnus
- Gluteus maximus
- Iliotibial tract
- Level of section
- Biceps femoris
- Semitendinosus — Hamstrings
- Semimembranosus

(B) Inferior view

- Vastus medialis
- Rectus femoris
- Vastus intermedius
- Vastus lateralis
- Iliotibial tract
- Femoral vein and saphenous nerve
- Femoral artery and nerve to vastus medialis
- **Anterior**
- Sartorius
- **Lateral**
- **Medial**
- Femur
- Biceps femoris (short head)
- Deep femoral artery and veins
- Sciatic nerve
- Gracilis
- Adductor longus
- Adductor brevis
- Adductor magnus
- Hamstrings { Biceps femoris (long head), Semitendinosus, Semimembranosus }
- **Posterior**

(C) Inferior view

- Anterior compartment (femoral nerve territory): Flexors of hip, Extensors of knee
- Posterior compartment (sciatic nerve territory): Extensors of hip, Flexors of knee
- Medial compartment (obturator nerve territory): adductors of thigh

(D) Inferior view

- Rectus femoris
- Vastus intermedius
- Vastus lateralis
- Vastus medialis
- Sartorius
- Biceps femoris
- Sciatic nerve
- Semitendinosus and semimembranosus
- Femoral vessels
- Gracilis and adductor longus
- Adductor magnus

Figure 5.27. Muscles and fascial compartments of thigh. A. The gluteus maximus has been reflected to reveal the sciatic nerve entering the proximal thigh and the attachments of the hamstrings. The level of the sections shown in parts **B** and **C** is indicated. **B.** An anatomical transverse section through the middle thigh, 10–15 cm inferior to the inguinal ligament. **C.** The three compartments of the thigh are shown. Note that each has its own nerve supply and functional group(s) of muscles. **D.** This transverse MRI of the right thigh indicates the muscles of each compartment. (Courtesy of Dr. W. Kucharczyk, Chair of Medical Imaging, Faculty of Medicine, University of Toronto and Clinical Director of the Tri-Hospital Resonance Centre, Toronto, Ontario, Canada.)

Biceps Femoris

As its name indicates, the fusiform **biceps femoris** has two heads: a *long head* and a *short head* (Fig. 5.23*A* & *B*). In the inferior part of the thigh, the long head becomes tendinous and is joined by the short head. The rounded common tendon attaches to the head of the fibula and can easily be seen and felt as it passes the knee, especially when the knee is flexed against resistance (see "Surface Anatomy of the Gluteal Region and Thigh," in this chapter). The **long head of the biceps femoris** crosses and provides protection for the sciatic nerve after it descends from the gluteal region into the posterior aspect of the thigh (Fig. 5.27). When the sciatic nerve divides into its terminal branches, the lateral branch (common fibular nerve) continues this relationship, running with the biceps tendon.

The **short head of the biceps femoris** arises from the lateral lip of the inferior third of the linea aspera and supracondylar ridge of the femur. Whereas the hamstrings have a common nerve supply from the tibial division of the sciatic nerve, the short head of the biceps is innervated by the fibular division (Table 5.7). Because each of the two heads of the biceps femoris has a different nerve supply, a wound in the posterior thigh with nerve injury may paralyze one head and not the other.

When the knee is flexed to 90°, the tendons of the lateral hamstring (biceps) as well as the iliotibial tract pass to the lateral side of the tibia. In this position, contraction of the biceps and tensor of the fascia lata produces about 40° lateral rotation of the tibia at the knee. Rotation of the flexed knee is especially important in snow skiing.

THE BOTTOM LINE: Although they have only about two thirds the strength of the gluteus maximus, the hamstrings are the main extensors of the hip used in normal walking. They are two-joint muscles, and their concentric contraction produces either extension of the hip or flexion of the knee. However, in walking they are most active in eccentrically contracting to decelerate hip flexion and knee extension during terminal swing. The hamstrings also rotate the flexed knee. If resistance to hip extension is increased, or more vigorous extension is required, the gluteus maximus is called into action.

Hamstring Injuries

Hamstring strains (pulled and/or torn hamstrings) are common in individuals who run and/or kick hard (e.g., in running, jumping, and quick-start sports such as baseball, basketball, football, and soccer). The violent muscular exertion required to excel in these sports may tear part of the proximal tendinous attachments of the hamstrings to the ischial tuberosity. Hamstring strains are twice as common as quadriceps strains (Levandowski and Difiori, 1994).

Usually thigh strains are accompanied by contusion and tearing of muscle fibers, resulting in rupture of the blood vessels supplying the muscles. The resultant *hematoma* is contained by the dense stocking-like fascia lata. Tearing of hamstring fibers is often so painful when the athlete moves or stretches the leg that he or she falls and writhes in pain. These injuries often result from inadequate warming up before practice or competition. *Avulsion of the ischial tuberosity* (see clinical correlation [blue] box "Injuries of the Hip Bone (Pelvic Injuries)," in this chapter) at the proximal attachment of the biceps femoris and semitendinosus ("hurdler's injury") may result from forcible flexion of the hip with the knee extended (e.g., kicking a football). ○

Neurovascular Structures of the Gluteal Region and Posterior Thigh

Several important nerves arise from the sacral plexus and either supply the gluteal region (e.g., superior and inferior gluteal nerves) or pass through it to supply the perineum and thigh (e.g., the pudendal and sciatic nerves, respectively). Table 5.8 describes the origin, course, and distribution of the nerves of the gluteal region and posterior thigh.

Clunial (Superficial Gluteal) Nerves

The skin of the gluteal region is richly innervated by **superior**, **middle**, and **inferior clunial nerves** (L. *clunes*, buttocks). These superficial nerves supply the skin over the iliac crest, between the posterior superior iliac spines and over the iliac tubercles. Consequently, these nerves are vulnerable to injury when bone is taken from the ilium for grafting.

Deep Gluteal Nerves

The deep gluteal nerves are the superior and inferior gluteal nerves, sciatic nerve, nerve to quadratus femoris, posterior cutaneous nerve of the thigh, nerve to obturator internus, and pudendal nerve (Fig. 5.24*A*; Table 5.8, figure). All of these nerves are branches of the sacral plexus and leave the pelvis through the greater sciatic foramen. Except for the superior gluteal nerve, they all emerge inferior to the piriformis.

Superior Gluteal Nerve. The **superior gluteal nerve** runs laterally between the gluteus medius and minimus with the deep branch of the superior gluteal artery. It divides into a superior branch that supplies the gluteus medius and an inferior branch that continues to pass between the gluteus medius and the gluteus minimus to supply both muscles and the tensor of the fascia lata.

Inferior Gluteal Nerve. This **inferior gluteal nerve** leaves the pelvis through the greater sciatic foramen, inferior to the piriformis and superficial to the sciatic nerve, accompanied by multiple branches of the inferior gluteal artery and vein. It

Table 5.8. Nerves of Gluteal Region and Posterior Thigh

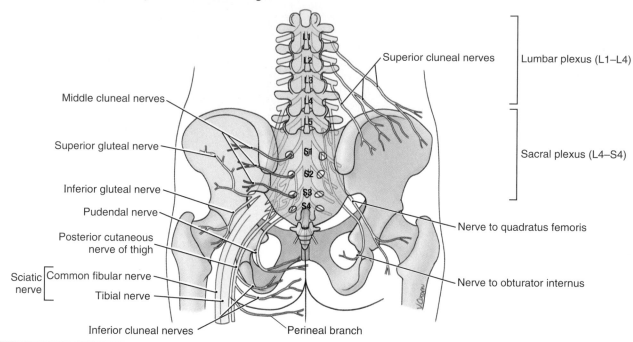

Nerve	Origin	Course	Distribution
Clunial Superior	As lateral cutaneous branches of posterior rami of L1–L3 spinal nerves	Pass inferolaterally across iliac crest	Supply skin of superior buttock as far as tubercle of iliac crest
Middle	As lateral cutaneous branches of posterior rami of S1–S3 spinal nerves	Exit through posterior sacral foramina and pass laterally to gluteal region	Supply skin over sacrum and adjacent area of buttock
Inferior	Posterior cutaneous nerve of thigh (anterior rami of S2–S3 spinal nerves)	Emerges from inferior border of gluteus maximus and ascends superficial to it	Supplies skin of inferior half of buttock as far as greater trochanter
Sciatic	Sacral plexus (anterior and posterior divisions of anterior rami of L4–S3 spinal nerves)	Enters gluteal region via greater sciatic foramen inferior to piriformis and deep to gluteus maximus; descends in posterior thigh deep to biceps femoris; bifurcates into tibial and common fibular nerves at apex of popliteal fossa.	Supplies no muscles in gluteal region; supplies all muscles of posterior compartment of thigh (tibial division supplies all but short head of biceps, which is supplied by common fibular division)
Posterior cutaneous nerve of thigh	Sacral plexus (anterior and posterior divisions of anterior rami of S1–S3 spinal nerves)	Enters gluteal region via greater sciatic foramen inferior to piriformis and deep to gluteus maximus, emerging from inferior border of latter; descends in posterior thigh deep to fascia lata	Supplies skin of inferior half of buttock (through inferior clunial nerves), skin over posterior thigh and popliteal fossa, and skin of lateral perineum and upper media thigh (via its perineal branch).
Superior gluteal	Sacral plexus (posterior divisions of anterior rami of L4–S1 spinal nerves)	Enters gluteal region via greater sciatic foramen superior to piriformis; courses laterally between gluteus medius and minimus as far as tensor of fascia lata	Innervates gluteus medius, gluteus minimus, and tensor of fascia lata muscles
Inferior gluteal	Sacral plexus (posterior divisions of anterior rami of L5–S2 spinal nerves)	Enters gluteal region via greater sciatic foramen inferior to piriformis and deep to inferior part of gluteus maximus, dividing into several branches	Supplies gluteus maximus
Nerve to quadratus femoris	Sacral plexus (anterior divisions of anterior rami of L4–S1 spinal nerves)	Enters gluteal region via greater sciatic foramen inferior to piriformis, deep (anterior) to sciatic nerve	Innervates hip joint, inferior gemellus, and quadratus femoris

Table 5.8. Nerves of Gluteal Region and Posterior Thigh *(continued)*

Nerve	Origin	Course	Distribution
Pudendal	Sacral plexus (anterior divisions of anterior rami of S2–S4 spinal nerves)	Exits pelvis via greater sciatic foramen inferior to piriformis; descends posterior to sacrospinous ligament; enters perineum through lesser sciatic foramen	Supplies no structures in gluteal region or posterior thigh (principal nerve to perineum)
Nerve to obturator internus	Sacral plexus (posterior divisions of anterior rami of L5–S2 spinal nerves)	Exits pelvis via greater sciatic foramen inferior to piriformis; descends posterior to sacrospinous ligament; enters perineum through lesser sciatic foramen	Supplies superior gemellus and obturator internus

also divides into several branches, which provide motor innervation to the overlying gluteus maximus.

Sciatic Nerve. The **sciatic nerve** is the largest nerve in the body and is the continuation of the main part of the sacral plexus. The rami converge at the inferior border of the piriformis to form the sciatic nerve, a thick, flattened band approximately 2 cm wide. The sciatic nerve is the most lateral structure emerging through the greater sciatic foramen inferior to the piriformis. Medial to it are the inferior gluteal nerve and vessels, the internal pudendal vessels, and the pudendal nerve. The sciatic nerve runs inferolaterally under cover of the gluteus maximus, midway between the greater trochanter and ischial tuberosity. The nerve rests on the ischium and then passes posterior to the obturator internus, quadratus femoris, and adductor magnus muscles. The sciatic nerve is so large that it receives a named branch of the inferior gluteal artery, the **artery to the sciatic nerve** (L. *arteria comitans nervi ischiadici*).

The sciatic nerve supplies no structures in the gluteal region. It supplies the posterior thigh muscles, all leg and foot muscles, and the skin of most of the leg and the foot. It also supplies the articular branches to all joints of the lower limb.

The sciatic nerve is really two nerves, the *tibial nerve*, derived from anterior (preaxial) divisions of the anterior rami, and the *common fibular nerve*, derived from posterior (postaxial) divisions of the anterior rami, which are loosely bound together in the same connective tissue sheath (Fig. 5.28A). *Perone* is Greek for the *fibula;* because of the close relationship of the nerve to the fibular neck, its name has been changed internationally from common peroneal to common fibular. The tibial and common fibular nerves usually separate approximately halfway or more down the thigh (Fig. 5.33); however, in approximately 12% of people, the nerves separate as they leave the pelvis (Fig. 5.28B). In these cases, the tibial nerve passes inferior to the piriformis, and the common fibular nerve pierces this muscle or passes superior to it (Fig. 5.28C).

Nerve to Quadratus Femoris. The **nerve to the quadratus femoris** leaves the pelvis anterior to the sciatic nerve and obturator internus and passes over the posterior surface of the hip joint. It supplies an articular branch to this joint and innervates the inferior gemellus and quadratus femoris.

Posterior Cutaneous Nerve of the Thigh. The **posterior cutaneous nerve of the thigh** supplies more skin than any other cutaneous nerve. Its fibers from the anterior divisions of S2 and S3 supply the skin of the perineum. Some of the fibers from the posterior divisions of the anterior rami of S1 and S2 supply the skin of the inferior part of the buttock (via the inferior clunial nerves); others continue inferiorly in branches that supply the skin of the posterior thigh and proximal part of the leg. Unlike most nerves bearing the name *cutaneous,* the main part of this nerve lies deep to the deep fascia (fascia lata), with only its terminal branches penetrating the subcutaneous tissue for distribution to the skin.

Pudendal Nerve. The **pudendal nerve** is the most medial structure to exit the pelvis through the greater sciatic foramen inferior to the piriformis muscle. It descends posterolateral to the sacrospinous ligament and enters the perineum through the lesser sciatic foramen to supply structures in the perineum (see Chapter 3); it supplies no structures in the gluteal region or posterior thigh.

Nerve to Obturator Internus. The **nerve to the obturator internus** arises from the anterior divisions of the anterior rami of the L5–S2 nerves and parallels the course of the pudendal nerve. As it passes around the base of the ischial spine, it supplies the superior gemellus. After entering the perineum via the lesser sciatic foramen, it supplies the obturator internus muscle.

Injury to the Superior Gluteal Nerve

Injury to the superior gluteal nerve results in a characteristic motor loss, resulting in a disabling *gluteus medius limp,* to compensate for weakened abduction of the thigh by the gluteus medius and minimus, and/or a *gluteal gait,* a compensatory list of the body to the weakened gluteal side. This compensation places the center of gravity over the supporting lower limb. Medial rotation of the thigh is also severely impaired. When a person is asked to stand on one leg, the gluteus medius and ▶

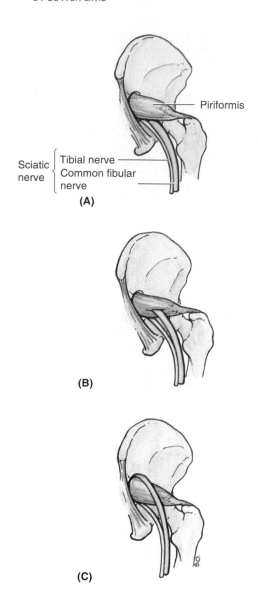

Posterior views

Figure 5.28. Relationship of sciatic nerve to piriformis. A. The sciatic nerve usually emerges from the greater sciatic foramen inferior to the piriformis. **B.** In 12.2% of 640 limbs studied, the sciatic nerve divided before exiting the greater sciatic foramen, the common fibular division (*yellow*) passed through the piriformis. **C.** In 0.5% of cases, the common fibular division passed superior to the muscle, where it is especially vulnerable to injury during intragluteal injections.

minimus normally contract as soon as the contralateral foot leaves the floor, preventing tipping of the pelvis to the unsupported side (Fig. B5.12*A*). When a person who has suffered a lesion of the superior gluteal nerve is asked to stand on one leg, the pelvis on the unsupported side descends (Fig. B5.12*B*), indicating that the gluteus

medius and minimus on the supported side are weak or non-functional. This observation is referred to clinically as a **positive Trendelenburg test.** Other causes of this sign include *fracture of the greater trochanter* (the distal attachment of gluteus medius) and *dislocation of the hip joint.*

When the pelvis descends on the unsupported side, the lower limb becomes, in effect, too long and does not clear the ground when the foot is brought forward in the swing phase of walking. To compensate, the individual leans away from the unsupported side, raising the pelvis to allow adequate room for the foot to clear the ground as it swings forward. This results in a characteristic "waddling" or gluteal gait. Other ways to compensate is to lift the foot higher as it is brought forward, resulting in the so-called steppage gait, or to swing the foot outward (laterally), the so-called swing-out gait. These same gaits are adopted to compensate for the *footdrop* that results from common fibular nerve paralysis (see clinical correlation [blue] box "Injury to the Common Fibular Nerve and Footdrop," in this chapter), which also makes the limb too long.

Anesthetic Block of the Sciatic Nerve

Sensation conveyed by the sciatic nerve can be blocked by the injection of an anesthetic agent a few centimeters ▶

Figure B5.12

inferior to the midpoint of the line joining the PSIS and the superior border of the greater trochanter. Paresthesia radiates to the foot because of anesthesia of the plantar nerves, which are terminal branches of the tibial nerve derived from the sciatic nerve.

Injury to the Sciatic Nerve

A pain in the buttock may result from compression of the sciatic nerve by the piriformis muscle (**piriformis syndrome**). Individuals involved in sports that require excessive use of the gluteal muscles (e.g., ice skaters, cyclists, and rock climbers) and women are more likely to develop this syndrome. In approximately 50% of cases, the case histories indicate trauma to the buttock associated with hypertrophy and *spasm of the piriformis*. In the approximately 12% of people in whom the common fibular division of the sciatic nerve passes through the piriformis (Fig. 5.28*B*), this muscle may compress the nerve.

Complete section of the sciatic nerve is uncommon. When this occurs, the leg is useless because extension of the hip is impaired, as is flexion of the leg. All ankle and foot movements are also lost. *Incomplete section of the sciatic nerve* (e.g., from stab wounds) may also involve the inferior gluteal and/or the posterior femoral cutaneous nerves. Recovery from a sciatic lesion is slow and usually incomplete.

With respect to the sciatic nerve, the buttock has a side of safety (its lateral side) and a side of danger (its medial side). Wounds or surgery on the medial side of the buttock are liable to injure the sciatic nerve and its branches to the hamstrings (semitendinosus, semimembranosus, and biceps femoris) on the posterior aspect of the thigh. Paralysis of these muscles results in impairment of thigh extension and leg flexion.

Intragluteal Injections

The gluteal region is a common site for intramuscular injection of drugs. *Gluteal intramuscular injections* penetrate the skin, fascia, and muscles. The gluteal region is a favorable injection site because the muscles are thick and large; consequently, they provide a substantial volume for absorption of injected substances by intramuscular veins. It is important to be aware of the extent of the gluteal region and the safe region for giving injections. Some people restrict the area of the buttock to the most prominent part, which may be dangerous because the sciatic nerve lies deep to this area (Fig. B5.13*A*).

Injections into the buttock are safe only in the superolateral quadrant of the buttock or superior to a line ▶

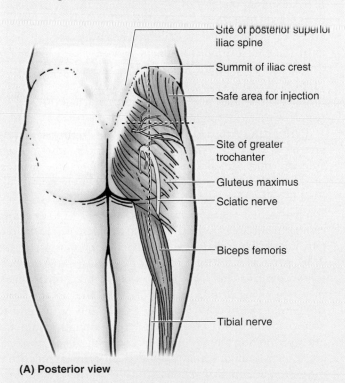

Site of posterior superior iliac spine
Summit of iliac crest
Safe area for injection
Site of greater trochanter
Gluteus maximus
Sciatic nerve
Biceps femoris
Tibial nerve

(A) Posterior view

Tubercle of iliac crest
Site of safe area for injection
Anterior superior iliac spine
Location of sciatic nerve

(B) Lateral view

Figure B5.13.

extending from the PSIS to the superior border of the greater trochanter (approximating the superior border of the gluteus maximus). Intramuscular injections can also be given safely into the anterolateral part of the thigh, where the needle enters the tensor of the fascia lata (Fig. 5.23*C*) as it extends distally from the iliac crest and ASIS. The index finger is placed on the ASIS, and the fingers are spread posteriorly along the iliac crest until the tubercle of the crest is felt by the middle finger (Fig. B5.13*B*). An intragluteal injection can be made safely in the triangular area between the fingers (just anterior to the proximal joint of the middle finger) because it is superior to the sciatic nerve. Complications of improper technique include nerve injury, hematoma, and abscess formation. ⊙

THE BOTTOM LINE: Because it overlies the major doorway (the greater sciatic foramen) by which derivatives of the sacral plexus exit the bony pelvis, the gluteal region includes a disproportionate number of nerves of all sizes, both motor and sensory. Fortunately, most are placed in the inferomedial quadrant; thus properly administered intramuscular injections avoid these structures. Because the sciatic nerve includes fibers from the L4–S3 spinal nerves, it is affected by the most common nerve compression syndromes (e.g., radiculopathies of the L4 and L5 spinal nerve roots; see Chapter 4). Even though occurring outside the lower limb per se, these syndromes result in sciatica—pain that radiates down the lower limb along the course of the nerve and its terminal branches. Pain experienced in the lower limb may not necessarily arise from a problem in the limb!

Arteries of the Gluteal Region and Posterior Thigh

The arteries of the gluteal region arise, directly or indirectly, from the *internal iliac arteries,* but the patterns of origin of the arteries are variable (Fig. 5.24*A;* Table 5.9). The major branches of the internal iliac artery that supply or traverse the gluteal region are the (1) superior gluteal artery, (2) inferior gluteal artery, and (3) internal pudendal artery. After birth, the posterior compartment of the thigh has no major artery exclusive to the compartment; it receives blood from multiple sources: inferior gluteal, medial circumflex femoral, perforating, and popliteal arteries.

Superior Gluteal Artery. The **superior gluteal artery** is the largest branch of the internal iliac artery and passes posteriorly between the lumbosacral trunk and the S1 nerve. The superior gluteal artery leaves the pelvis through the greater sciatic foramen, superior to the piriformis, and divides immediately into superficial and deep branches. The *superficial branch* supplies the gluteus maximus and skin over the proximal attachment of this muscle; the *deep branch* supplies the

gluteus medius, gluteus minimus, and tensor of the fascia lata. The superior gluteal artery anastomoses with the inferior gluteal and medial circumflex femoral arteries.

Inferior Gluteal Artery. The **inferior gluteal artery** arises from the internal iliac artery and passes posteriorly through the parietal pelvic fascia, between the S1 and the S2 (or S2 and S3) nerves. The inferior gluteal artery leaves the pelvis through the greater sciatic foramen, inferior to the piriformis. It enters the gluteal region deep to the gluteus maximus and descends medial to the sciatic nerve.

The inferior gluteal artery supplies the gluteus maximus, obturator internus, quadratus femoris, and superior parts of the hamstrings. It anastomoses with the superior gluteal artery and frequently participates in the *cruciate anastomosis of the thigh,* involving the first perforating arteries of the deep artery of the thigh and the medial and lateral circumflex femoral arteries (Table 5.5). Whether the cruciate anastomosis is formed or not, these vessels all participate in supplying the structures of the proximal posterior thigh.

Developmentally, the inferior gluteal artery is the major artery of the posterior compartment, traversing its length and becoming continuous with the popliteal artery. This part of the artery diminishes, however, persisting postnatally as the *artery to the sciatic nerve.*

Internal Pudendal Artery. The **internal pudendal artery** arises from the internal iliac artery and lies anterior to the inferior gluteal artery. Its course parallels that of the pudendal nerve, entering the gluteal region through the greater sciatic foramen inferior to the piriformis. The internal pudendal artery leaves the gluteal region immediately by crossing the ischial spine/sacrospinous ligament and enters the perineum through the lesser sciatic foramen. Like the pudendal nerve, it supplies the skin, external genitalia, and muscles in the perineal region. It does not supply any structures in the gluteal region or posterior thigh.

Perforating Arteries. There are usually **four perforating arteries of the deep artery of the thigh,** three arising in the anterior compartment and the fourth being the terminal branch of the deep artery itself. The perforating arteries are large vessels, unusual in the limbs for their transverse, intercompartmental course. Surgeons operating in the posterior compartment are careful to identify them to avoid inadvertent injury. They perforate the aponeurotic portion of the distal attachment of the adductor magnus to enter the posterior compartment. Within the posterior compartment, they typically give rise to muscular branches to the hamstrings and anastomotic branches that ascend or descend to unite with those arising superiorly or inferiorly from the other perforating arteries or the inferior gluteal and popliteal artery. A continuous anastomotic chain thus extends from the gluteal to popliteal regions, which gives rise to additional branches to muscles and to the sciatic nerve. After giving off their posterior compartment branches, the perforating arteries pierce the lateral intermuscular septum to enter the anterior compartment, where they supply the vastus lateralis muscle.

Table 5.9. Arteries of the Gluteal Region and Posterior Thigh

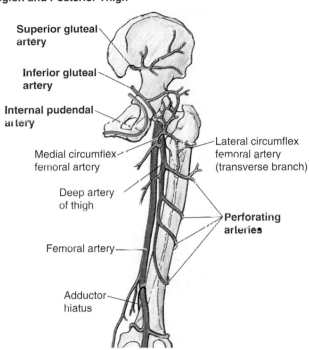

Superior gluteal artery

Inferior gluteal artery

Internal pudendal artery

Medial circumflex femoral artery

Deep artery of thigh

Femoral artery

Adductor hiatus

Lateral circumflex femoral artery (transverse branch)

Perforating arteries

Artery[a]	Course	Distribution
Superior gluteal	Enters gluteal region through greater sciatic foramen superior to piriformis; divides into superficial and deep branches; anastomoses with inferior gluteal and medial circumflex arteries (not shown in figure)	Superficial branch: supplies gluteus maximus Deep branch: runs between gluteus medius and minimus and supplies them and tensor of fascia lata
Inferior gluteal	Enters gluteal region through greater sciatic foramen inferior to piriformis; descends on medial side of sciatic nerve; anastomoses with superior gluteal artery and participates in cruciate anastomosis of thigh, involving first perforating artery of deep femoral and medial and lateral circumflex arteries (not shown in figure)	Supplies gluteus maximus, obturator internus, quadratus femoris, and superior parts of hamstrings
Internal pudendal	Enters gluteal region through greater sciatic foramen; descends posterior to ischial spine; enters perineum through lesser sciatic foramen	Supplies external genitalia and muscles in perineal region; does not supply gluteal region
Perforating	Enters posterior compartment by perforating aponeurotic portion of adductor magnus attachment and medial intermuscular septum; after providing muscular branches to hamstrings, continues on to anterior compartment by piercing lateral intermuscular septum	Supplies majority (central portions) of hamstring muscles, then continues to supply vastus lateralis in anterior compartment

[a]All of these arteries arise from the internal iliac artery (see Table 5.5 for an anterior view).

Veins of the Gluteal Region and Posterior Thigh

The *gluteal veins* are tributaries of the internal iliac veins that drain blood from the gluteal region. The **superior and inferior gluteal veins** accompany the corresponding arteries through the greater sciatic foramen, superior and inferior to the piriformis, respectively (Fig. 5.29A). They communicate with tributaries of the femoral vein, thereby providing alternate routes for the return of blood from the lower limb if the femoral vein is occluded or has to be ligated. The **internal pudendal veins** accompany the internal pudendal arteries and join to form a single vein that enters the internal iliac vein. These veins drain blood from the external genitalia or pudendum (L. *pudere*, to be ashamed). *Perforating veins* accompany the arteries of the same name to drain blood from the posterior compartment of the thigh into the *deep vein of the thigh*. The perforating veins, like the arteries, usually also communicate inferiorly with the popliteal vein and superiorly with the inferior gluteal vein.

Lymphatic Drainage of the Gluteal Region and Thigh

Lymph from the deep tissues of the buttocks follows the gluteal vessels to the superior and inferior **gluteal lymph nodes** and from them to the internal, external, and common **iliac lymph nodes** (Fig. 5.29A) and from them to the **lateral**

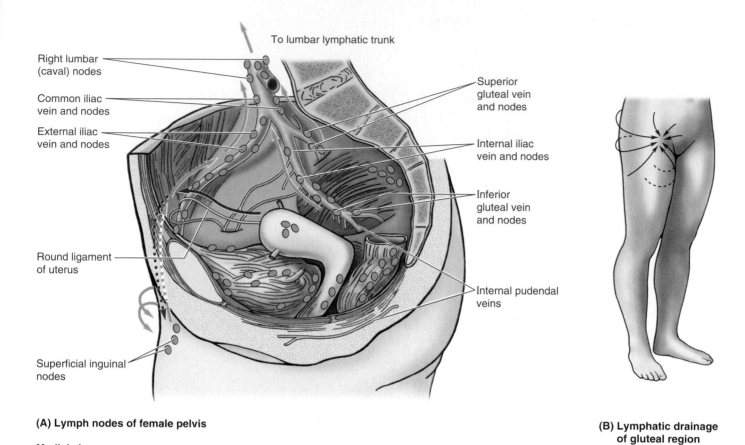

(A) Lymph nodes of female pelvis

Medial view

**(B) Lymphatic drainage
of gluteal region
and thigh**

Figure 5.29. Lymphatic drainage of gluteal region and thigh. A. Lymph from the deep tissues of the gluteal region enters the pelvis along the gluteal veins, draining to the superior and inferior gluteal lymph nodes; from them, it passes to the iliac and lateral lumbar (caval/aortic) lymph nodes. **B.** Lymph from superficial tissues of the gluteal region passes initially to the superficial inguinal nodes, which also receive lymph from the thigh. Lymph from all the superficial inguinal nodes passes via efferent lymph vessels to the external and common iliac and right and left lumbar (caval/aortic) lymph nodes, draining via lumbar lymphatic trunks to the chyle cistern.

aortic lumbar **(caval/lymph) nodes.** Lymph from the superficial tissues of the gluteal region enters the *superficial inguinal lymph nodes,* which also receive lymph from the thigh. All the superficial inguinal nodes send efferent lymphatic vessels to the external iliac lymph nodes.

THE BOTTOM LINE: Arteries and veins serving the gluteal region and the proximal part of the posterior compartment of the thigh are branches and tributaries of the internal iliac artery and vein that pass to and from the region via the greater sciatic foramen. All but the superior gluteal vessels exit the foramen inferior to the piriformis muscle. Although the pudendal vessels follow the same route, they traverse the gluteal region only briefly en route to and from the perineum via the lesser sciatic foramen. The posterior compartment of the thigh does not have a major artery coursing through it with primary responsibility for the compartment. Rather, branches are sent from several arteries in other compartments to supply it.

In terms of the vascular supply to the lower limb as a whole, the majority of the arterial blood coming to the limb and most of the venous blood and lymph exiting from it pass along the more protected anteromedial aspect of the limb. Flexor aspects are generally better protected than are extensor aspects, the latter being exposed and therefore vulnerable in the flexed, defensive position.

Surface Anatomy of the Gluteal Region and Thigh

The skin of the gluteal region is usually thick and course, especially in men, whereas the skin of the thigh is relatively thin and loosely attached to the underlying subcutaneous tissue. A line joining the highest points of the **iliac crests** (Fig. SA5.2A) crosses the L4–L5 intervertebral (IV) disc and is a useful landmark when a ▶

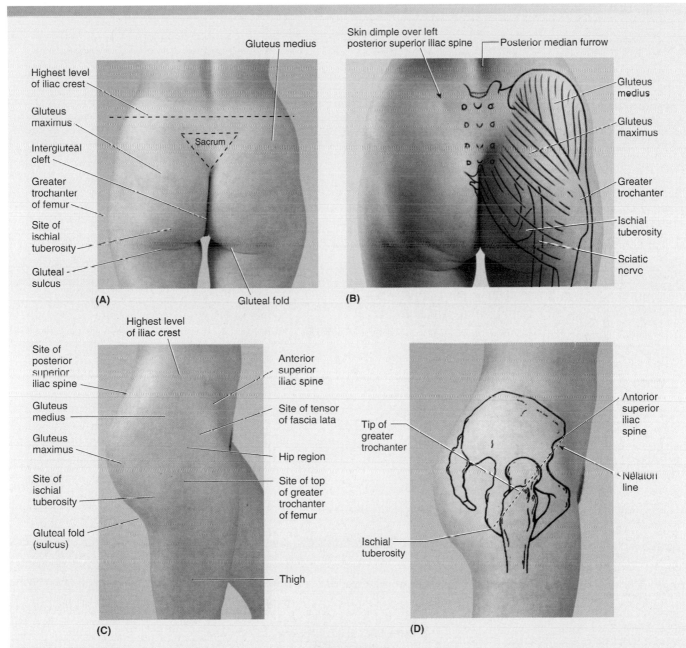

Figure SA5.2

lumbar puncture is performed (see Chapter 4), indicating the middle of the lumbar cistern (Fig. SA5.2A–D). The **intergluteal cleft**, beginning inferior to the apex of the sacrum, is the deep groove between the buttocks. It extends as far superiorly as the S3 or S4 segment. The coccyx is palpable in the superior part of the intergluteal cleft. The **posterior superior iliac spines** are located at the posterior extremities of the iliac crests and may be difficult to palpate; however, their position can always be located at the bottom of the permanent skin dimples approximately 3.75 cm from midline (Fig. SA5.2B). A line joining these dimples, often more visible in women than in men, passes

through the S2 spinous process, indicating the level of the lowest limit of the dural sac or lumbar cistern, the middle of the sacroiliac joints, and the bifurcation of the common iliac arteries.

The location of only two of the gluteal muscles can be observed. The *gluteus maximus* covering most structures in the gluteal region can be felt to contract when straightening up from bending over. The inferior edge of this large muscle is located just superior to the **gluteal fold**, which contains a variable amount of subcutaneous fat (Fig. SA5.2A & C). The gluteal fold disappears when the hip joint is flexed. The degree of prominence of the ▶

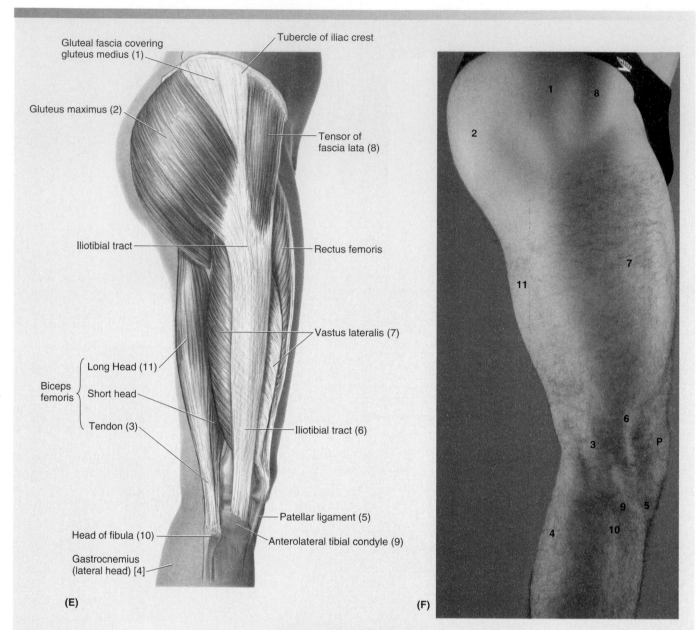

Gluteal fascia covering
gluteus medius (1)

Tubercle of iliac crest

Gluteus maximus (2)

Tensor of
fascia lata (8)

Iliotibial tract

Rectus femoris

Vastus lateralis (7)

Long Head (11)

Biceps
femoris

Short head

Tendon (3)

Iliotibial tract (6)

Patellar ligament (5)

Head of fibula (10)

Anterolateral tibial condyle (9)

Gastrocnemius
(lateral head) [4]

(E)

(F)

Figure SA5.2. *(Continued)*

gluteal fold changes in certain abnormal conditions, such as atrophy of the gluteus maximus. An imaginary line drawn from the coccyx to the ischial tuberosity indicates the inferior edge of the gluteus maximus (Fig. SA5.2*B*). Another line drawn from the PSIS to a point slightly superior to the greater trochanter indicates the superior edge of this muscle.

The **gluteal sulcus**, the skin crease inferior to the gluteal fold, delineates the buttock from the posterior aspect of the thigh (Fig. SA5.2*A* & *C*). When the thigh is extended as in the figures, the **ischial tuberosity** is covered by the inferior part of the gluteus maximus; however, the tuberosity is easy to palpate when the thigh is flexed because the

gluteus maximus slips superiorly off the tuberosity, which is then subcutaneous. Feel the ischial tuberosity as you bend to sit. The superior part of the *gluteus medius* can be palpated between the superior part of the gluteus maximus and the iliac crest (Fig. SA5.2*E* & *F*). The gluteus medius of one buttock can be felt when all the body weight shifts onto the ipsilateral limb (the one on the same side).

The **greater trochanter**, the most lateral bony point in the gluteal region, may be felt on the lateral aspect of the hip, especially its inferior part (Fig. SA5.2*A–C*). It is easier to palpate when you passively abduct your lower limb to relax the gluteus medius and minimus. The top of the trochanter lies approximately a hand's breadth inferior to ▶

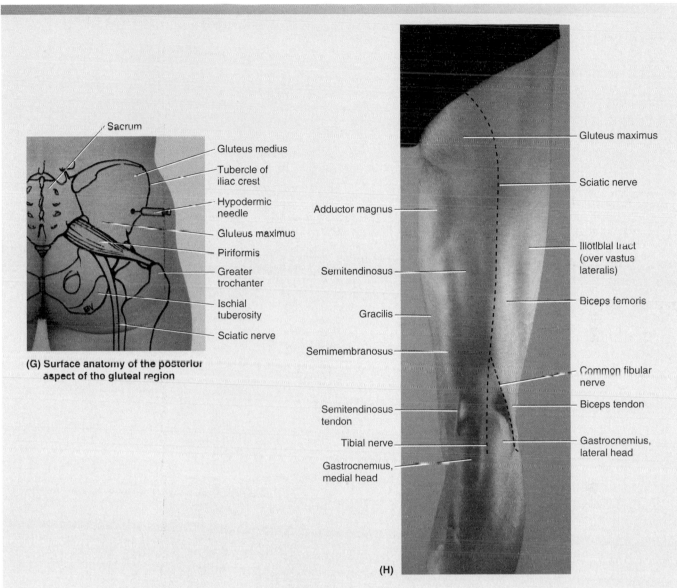

(G) Surface anatomy of the posterior aspect of the gluteal region

Figure SA5.2. *(Continued)*

the tubercle of the iliac crest. The prominence of the trochanter increases when a dislocated hip causes atrophy of the gluteal muscles and displacement of the trochanter. A line drawn from the ASIS to the ischial tuberosity (*Nélaton line*), passing over the lateral aspect of the hip region, normally passes over or near the top of the greater trochanter (Fig. SA5.2*D*). The trochanter can be felt superior to this line in a person with a dislocated hip or a fractured femoral neck. The **lesser trochanter** is palpable with difficulty from the posterior aspect when the thigh is extended and rotated medially.

The *sciatic nerve,* the most important structure inferior to the piriformis, is represented by a line that extends from a point midway between the greater trochanter and the ischial tuberosity (Fig. SA5.2*G*) down the middle of the

posterior aspect of the thigh (Fig. SA5.2*H*). The level of the bifurcation of the sciatic nerve into the tibial and common fibular nerves varies. The separation usually occurs in the inferior third of the thigh, but the division of the sciatic nerve may occur as it passes through the sciatic foramen. The *tibial nerve* bisects the popliteal fossa, and the *common fibular nerve* follows the biceps femoris, which covers it. The sciatic nerve stretches when the thigh is flexed and the knee is extended, and it relaxes when the thigh is extended and the knee is flexed.

The **hamstrings** can be felt as a group as they arise from the ischial tuberosity and extend along the lateral and posterior aspects of the thigh (Fig. SA5.2*E*). The **iliotibial tract,** the fibrous band that reinforces the fascia lata laterally, can be observed on the lateral aspect of the thigh as it ▶

Semimem-
branosus

Semitendinosus

Gastrocnemius,
medial head

Fibularis brevis

Calcaneal
tendon

Vastus lateralis

Biceps femoris

Head of fibula

Gastrocnemius
lateral head

Fibularis longus

Soleus

Fibularis longus
tendon

Lateral malleolus

(I)

Vastus lateralis

Vastus medialis

Iliotibial tract

Patella

Head of fibula

Patellar ligament

Tibial tuberosity

(J)

Figure SA5.2. *(Continued)*

passes to the *lateral tibial condyle*. While sitting down with your lower limb extended, raise your heel off the floor and feel the anterior border of the iliotibial tract passing a finger's breadth posterior to the lateral border of the patella (Fig. SA5.2*E* & *F*). Note that the iliotibial tract is prominent and taut when the heel is raised and indistinct when the heel is lowered. The *tendons of the hamstrings* can be observed and palpated at the borders of the popliteal fossa (Fig. SA5.2*I* & *J*). The **biceps femoris tendon** is on the lateral side of the fossa. The most lateral tendon on the medial side when the knee is flexed against resistance is the **semimembranosus tendon.** While sitting on a chair with your knee flexed, press your heel against the leg of the chair and feel your biceps femoris tendon laterally and trace it to the head of the fibula. Also feel the narrow and more prominent **semitendinosus tendon** medially, which pulls away from the semimembranosus tendon that attaches to the superomedial part of the tibia.

In fairly muscular individuals, some of the bulky anterior thigh muscles can be observed. The prominent muscles are the **quadriceps** and **sartorius,** whereas laterally the tensor of the fascia lata is palpable as is the iliotibial tract to

which this muscle attaches (Fig. SA5.2*F*). Three of the four parts of the *quadriceps* are visible or can be approximated (Fig. SA5.2*J* & *K*); the fourth part (vastus intermedius) is deep and almost hidden by the other muscles and cannot be palpated. (Fig. SA5.2*K* & *L*). The **rectus femoris** may be easily observed as a ridge passing down the thigh when the lower limb is raised from the floor while sitting. Observe the large bulges formed by the vastus lateralis and medialis at the knee (Fig. SA5.2*J*). The **patellar ligament** is easily observed, especially in thin people, as a thick band running from the patella to the tibial tuberosity. You can also palpate the **infrapatellar fat pads,** the masses of loose fatty tissue on each side of the patellar ligament.

On the medial aspect of the inferior part of the thigh, the **gracilis** and *sartorius* muscles form a well-marked prominence, which is separated by a depression from the large bulge formed by the **vastus medialis** (Fig. SA5.2*K*). Deep in this depressed area, the **large tendon of the adductor magnus** can be palpated as it passes to its attachment to the adductor tubercle of the femur.

Measurements of the lower limb are taken to detect shortening (e.g., resulting from a femoral fracture). To ▶

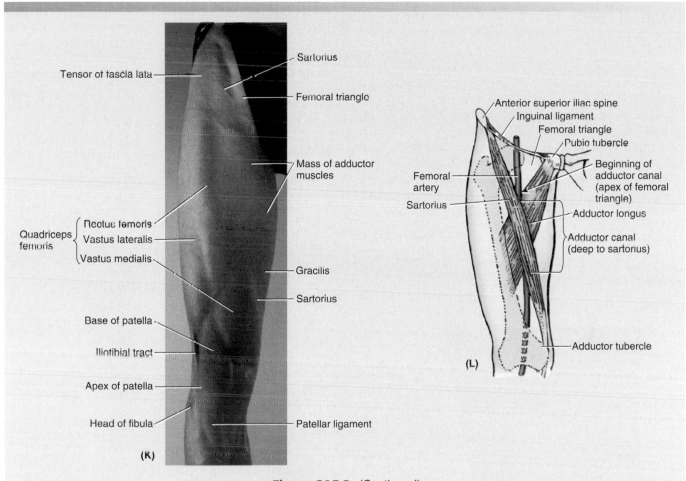

Figure SA5.2. (Continued)

make such measurements, compare the affected limb with the corresponding limb. Real limb shortening is detected by comparing the measurements from the ASIS to the distal tip of the medial malleolus on both sides. To determine if the shortening is in the thigh, the measurement is taken from the top of the ASIS to the distal edge of the lateral femoral condyle on both sides. Keep in mind that small differences between the two sides—such as a difference of 1.25 cm in total length of the limb—may be normal.

The proximal two thirds of a line drawn from the midpoint of the inguinal ligament to the **adductor tubercle** when the thigh is flexed, abducted, and rotated laterally represents the course of the *femoral artery* (Fig. SA5.2*L*). The proximal third of the line represents this artery as it passes through the *femoral triangle,* whereas the middle third represents the artery while it is in the *adductor canal.* Approximately 3.75 cm along this line distal to the inguinal ligament, the deep artery of the thigh arises from the femoral artery. The *femoral vein* is

- Medial to the femoral artery at the base of the femoral triangle (indicated by inguinal ligament)

- Posterior to the femoral artery at the apex of the femoral triangle.

- Posterolateral to the artery in the adductor canal.

The **femoral triangle,** in the superoanterior aspect of the thigh, is not a prominent surface feature in most people. When some people sit cross-legged, the sartorius and adductor longus stand out, delineating the femoral triangle. The surface anatomy of the femoral triangle is clinically important because of its contents. The *femoral artery* can be felt pulsating just inferior at the midinguinal point. When you palpate the femoral pulse, the *femoral vein* is just medial, the femoral nerve is a finger's breadth lateral, and the *femoral head* is just posterior. The femoral artery runs a 5-cm superficial course through the femoral triangle before it is covered by the sartorius in the adductor canal.

The *great saphenous vein* enters the thigh posterior to the medial femoral condyle and passes superiorly along a line from the adductor tubercle to the **saphenous opening.** The central point of this opening, where the great saphenous vein enters the femoral vein, is located 3.75 cm inferior and 3.75 cm lateral to the pubic tubercle. ✚

Popliteal Fossa

The **popliteal fossa** is a mostly fat-filled compartment of the lower limb. Superficially, when the knee is flexed, the popliteal fossa is evident as a diamond-shaped depression posterior to the knee joint, bound superiorly by the diverging hamstrings and inferiorly by the converging heads of the gastrocnemius and plantaris (Fig. 5.30). The size of this gap between muscles is misleading, however, in terms of the actual size and extent of the popliteal fossa. Deeply, it is much larger than the superficial depression indicates because the heads of the gastrocnemius forming the inferior boundary superficially

form a roof over the inferior half of the deep part. When the knee is extended, the fat within the fossa protrudes through the gap between muscles, producing a rounded elevation flanked by shallow longitudinal grooves overlying the hamstring tendons. In dissection, if the heads of the gastrocnemius are separated and retracted (Fig. 5.31), a much larger space is revealed.

Superficially, the popliteal fossa is bound:

- Superolaterally by the biceps femoris (superolateral border).

- Superomedially by the semimembranosus, lateral to which is the semitendinosus (superomedial border).

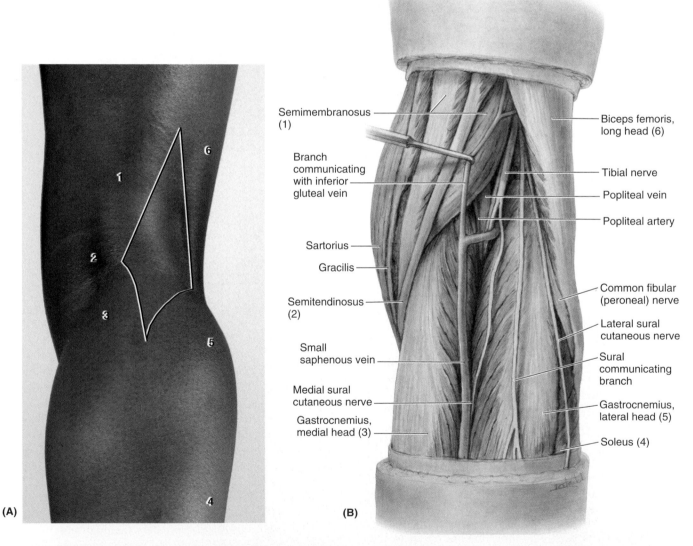

Figure 5.30. Superficial popliteal region. A. *Numbers* on the surface anatomy refer to structures identified in part **B.** The diamond-shaped gap in the roof of the popliteal fossa, formed by the overlying muscles, is outlined. **B.** Superficial dissection of the popliteal region showing the muscles that cover most of the popliteal fossa. The medial sural cutaneous nerve and the sural communicating branch of the common fibular nerve unite at various levels to form the sural nerve. In this specimen, the union occurs inferior to the level of this dissection. Compare this with the high union within the popliteal fossa in the specimen shown in Figure 5.31.

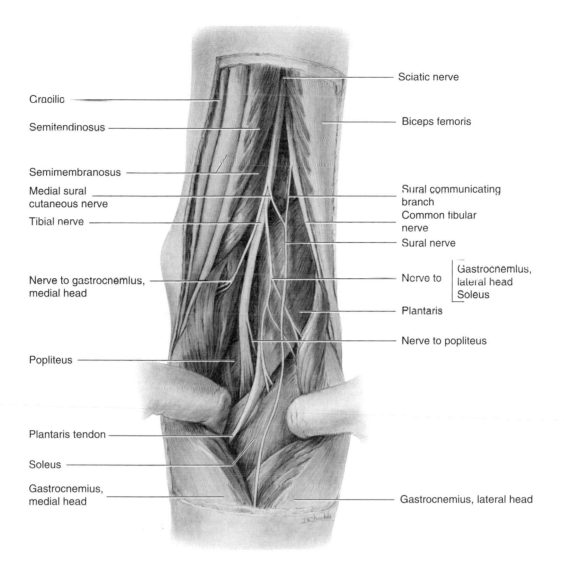

Gracilis

Semitendinosus

Semimembranosus

Medial sural
cutaneous nerve

Tibial nerve

Nerve to gastrocnemius,
medial head

Popliteus

Plantaris tendon

Soleus

Gastrocnemius,
medial head

Sciatic nerve

Biceps femoris

Sural communicating
branch

Common fibular
nerve

Sural nerve

Nerve to { Gastrocnemius, lateral head / Soleus }

Plantaris

Nerve to popliteus

Gastrocnemius, lateral head

Posterior view

Figure 5.31. Exposure of popliteal fossa and nerves of fossa. The two heads of the gastrocnemius muscle have been separated and are being retracted. The sciatic nerve separates into its components at the apex of the popliteal fossa (or higher; Fig. 5.28*B*). The common fibular nerve courses along the medial border of the biceps femoris. All the motor branches arising from the tibial nerve, except one, arise from the lateral side; consequently, in surgery it is safer to dissect on the medial side. The level at which the medial and lateral sural nerves merge to form the sural nerve—occurring high here—is quite variable; it may even occur at the level of the ankle.

- Inferolaterally and inferomedially by the lateral and medial heads of the gastrocnemius, respectively (inferolateral and inferomedial borders).

- Posteriorly by skin and popliteal fascia (roof).

Deeply, the superior boundaries are formed by the diverging medial and lateral supracondylar lines of the femur. The inferior boundary is formed by the soleal line of the tibia (Fig. 5.1*B*). These boundaries surround a relatively large diamond-shaped floor (anterior wall), formed by the **popliteal surface**

of the femur superiorly, the posterior capsule of the knee joint centrally, and the popliteus fascia covering the popliteus muscle inferiorly (Fig. 5.60).

The contents of the popliteal fossa (Figs. 5.30*B*, 5.31, and 5.32) include the:

- Termination of the small saphenous vein.

- Popliteal arteries and veins and their branches and tributaries.

- Tibial and common fibular nerves.

Gracilis

Semitendinosus

Semimembranosus

Popliteal artery
Popliteal vein
Tibial nerve

Medial superior
genicular artery

Semitendinosus (2)

Semimembranosus (1)

Bursa

Gastrocnemius

Fibrous (articular)
capsule of knee joint

Medial inferior
genicular artery

Deep popliteus fascia

Gastrocnemius,
medial head (3)

Biceps femoris,
long head (6)

Biceps femoris,
short head

Lateral intermuscular
septum

Common fibular
nerve

Biceps femoris

Lateral superior
genicular artery

Popliteal face
of femur

Gastrocnemius

Plantaris
Lateral inferior
genicular artery

Popliteus

Nerve to popliteus

Soleus (4)

Plantaris

Gastrocnemius,
lateral head (5)

Posterior view

Figure 5.32. Deep dissection of popliteal fossa. The popliteal artery runs on the floor of the fossa, formed by the popliteal surface of the femur, the joint capsule of the knee, and the popliteus fascia. The floor of the fossa, which extends superiorly to the diverging supracondylar lines of the femur and inferiorly to the soleal line of (superior attachment of the soleus to) the tibia, is much larger than the gap between the overlying muscles (outlined in Figure 5.30A), often mistaken as representing the extent of the fossa. *Numbers* refer to the surface anatomy shown in Figure 5.30A.

- Posterior cutaneous nerve of thigh (Table 5.1B).

- Popliteal lymph nodes and lymphatic vessels (Fig. 5.13B).

Fascia of the Popliteal Fossa

The *subcutaneous tissue* overlying the popliteal fossa (Fig. 5.10B) contains the small saphenous vein (unless it has penetrated the deep fascia at a more inferior level), and three cutaneous nerves: the terminal branch(es) of the *posterior cutaneous nerve of the thigh* and the *medial* and *lateral sural cutaneous nerves*. The deep **popliteal fascia** is a strong sheet of deep fascia, continuous superiorly with the *fascia lata* and inferiorly with the *deep fascia of the leg*. The popliteal fascia forms a protective covering for neurovascular structures passing from the thigh through the popliteal fossa to the leg and a relatively loose but functional retaining "retinaculum"

for the hamstring tendons. Often it is pierced by the small saphenous vein. When the leg extends, the fat within the fossa is relatively compressed as the popliteal fascia becomes taut, and the semimembranosus moves laterally, providing further protection to the contents of the popliteal fossa. The contents, most important the popliteal artery and lymph nodes, are most easily palpated with the knee in semiflexion. Because of the deep fascial roof and osseofibrous floor, the popliteal fossa is a relatively confined space. Many disorders produce swelling of the fossa, making knee extension painful.

Neurovascular Structures and Relationships in the Popliteal Fossa

All important neurovascular structures that pass from the thigh to the leg do so by traversing the popliteal fossa.

Progressing from superficial to deep (posterior to anterior) within the fossa, as in dissection, the nerves are encountered first, then the veins. The arteries lie deepest, directly on the surface of the femur, joint capsule, and popliteal fascia forming the floor of the fossa.

Nerves in the Popliteal Fossa

The *sciatic nerve* usually ends at the superior angle of the popliteal fossa by dividing into the tibial and common fibular nerves (Figs. 5.30B–5.32). The **tibial nerve** is the medial, larger terminal branch of the sciatic nerve derived from anterior (preaxial) divisions of the anterior rami of the L4–S3 spinal nerves. The tibial nerve is the most superficial of the three main central components of the popliteal fossa (i.e., nerve, vein, and artery); however, it is still in a deep and protected position. The tibial nerve bisects the fossa as it passes from its superior to its inferior angle. While in the fossa, the tibial nerve gives branches to the soleus, gastrocnemius, plantaris, and popliteus muscles. The **medial sural cutaneous nerve** is also derived from the tibial nerve in the popliteal fossa and is joined by the **sural communicating branch** of the common fibular nerve at a highly variable level to form the *sural nerve*. This nerve supplies the lateral side of the leg and ankle.

The **common fibular nerve** is the lateral, smaller terminal branch of the sciatic nerve derived from posterior (postaxial) divisions of the anterior rami of the L4–S2 spinal nerves. It begins at the superior angle of the popliteal fossa and follows closely the medial border of the biceps femoris and its tendon along the superolateral boundary of the popliteal fossa. The common fibular nerve leaves the fossa by passing superficial to the lateral head of the gastrocnemius and then passes over the posterior aspect of the head of the fibula. The common fibular nerve winds around the fibular neck and divides into its terminal branches.

The most inferior branches of the *posterior cutaneous nerve of the thigh* supply the skin that overlies the popliteal fossa. The nerve traverses most of the length of the posterior compartment of the thigh deep to the fascia lata; only its terminal branches enter the subcutaneous tissue as cutaneous nerves per se.

Blood Vessels in the Popliteal Fossa

The **popliteal artery,** the continuation of the femoral artery (Fig. 5.32), begins when the latter passes through the adductor hiatus. The popliteal artery passes inferolaterally through the fossa and ends at the inferior border of the popliteus by dividing into the anterior and posterior tibial arteries. The deepest (most anterior) structure in the fossa, the popliteal artery, runs in close proximity to the joint capsule of the knee as it spans the intercondylar fossa. Five genicular branches of the popliteal artery supply the capsule and ligaments of the knee joint. The genicular arteries are the **superior lateral, superior medial, middle, inferior lateral,** and **inferior medial genicular arteries** (Fig. 5.33). They participate in the formation of the periarticular **genicular anastomosis,** a network of vessels surrounding the knee that provides collateral circulation capable of maintaining blood supply to the leg during

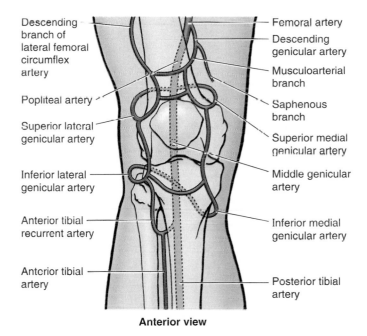

Anterior view

Figure 5.33. Genicular anastomosis. The many arteries making up the periarticular anastomosis around the knee provide an important collateral circulation for bypassing the popliteal artery when the knee has been maintained too long in a fully flexed position or when the vessels are narrowed or occluded.

full knee flexion, which may kink the popliteal artery. Other contributors to this important anastomosis are the:

- Descending genicular branch of the femoral artery, superomedially.

- Descending branch of the lateral femoral circumflex artery, superolaterally.

- Anterior tibial recurrent branch of the anterior tibial artery, inferolaterally.

Muscular branches of the popliteal artery supply the hamstring, gastrocnemius, soleus, and plantaris muscles. The superior muscular branches of the popliteal artery have clinically important anastomoses with the terminal part of the deep femoral and gluteal arteries.

The **popliteal vein** begins at the distal border of the popliteus as a continuation of the *posterior tibial vein* (Fig. 5.32). Throughout its course, the vein lies close to the popliteal artery, lying superficial to it and in the same fibrous sheath. The popliteal vein is initially posteromedial to the artery and lateral to the tibial nerve. More superiorly, the popliteal vein lies posterior to the artery, between this vessel and the overlying tibial nerve. Superiorly, the popliteal vein, which has several valves, becomes the *femoral vein* as it traverses the adductor hiatus. The small saphenous vein passes from the posterior aspect of the lateral malleolus to the popliteal fossa, where it pierces the deep popliteal fascia and enters the popliteal vein.

Popliteal Abscesses and Tumors

Because the deep popliteal fascia is strong and limits expansion, pain from an abscess or tumor in the popliteal fossa is usually severe. *Popliteal abscesses* tend to spread superiorly and inferiorly because of the toughness of the popliteal fascia. A *popliteal cyst* (Baker cyst), a *saphenous varix*, and an *aneurysm of the popliteal artery* should be considered in the differential diagnosis of masses within this space (see clinical correlation [blue] boxes "Popliteal Cysts," "Saphenous Varix," and "Popliteal Aneurysm and Hemorrhage," in this chapter).

Popliteal Pulse

Because the popliteal artery is deep, it may be difficult to feel the *popliteal pulse.* Palpation of this pulse is commonly performed with the person in the prone position with the knee flexed to relax the popliteal fascia and hamstrings. The pulsations are best felt in the inferior part of the fossa where the popliteal artery is related to the tibia. Weakening or loss of the popliteal pulse is a sign of a femoral artery obstruction.

Popliteal Aneurysm and Hemorrhage

A **popliteal aneurysm** (abnormal dilation of all or part of the popliteal artery) usually causes edema and pain in the popliteal fossa. A popliteal aneurysm may be distinguished from other masses by palpable pulsations (*thrills*)

and abnormal arterial sounds (*bruits*) detectable with a stethoscope. Because the artery lies deep to the tibial nerve, an aneurysm may stretch the nerve or compress its blood supply (vasa vasorum). Pain from such nerve compression is usually referred, in this case to the skin overlying the medial aspect of the calf, ankle or foot. Because the artery is closely applied to the popliteal surface of the femur and the joint capsule, fractures of the distal femur or dislocations of the knee may rupture the artery, resulting in hemorrhage. Furthermore, because of their proximity and confinement within the fossa, an injury of the artery and vein may result in an **arteriovenous fistula** (communication between an artery and a vein). Failure to recognize these occurrences and to act promptly may result in the loss of the leg and foot. If the femoral artery must be ligated, blood can bypass the occlusion through the genicular anastomosis and reach the popliteal artery distal to the ligation.

Injury to the Tibial Nerve

Injury to the tibial nerve is uncommon because of its deep and protected position in the popliteal fossa; however, the nerve may be injured by deep lacerations in the popliteal fossa. *Posterior dislocation of the knee joint* may also damage the tibial nerve. *Severance of the tibial nerve* produces paralysis of the flexor muscles in the leg and the intrinsic muscles in the sole of the foot. People with a tibial nerve injury are unable to plantarflex their ankle or flex their toes. Loss of sensation also occurs on the sole of the foot. ☉

Lymph Nodes in the Popliteal Fossa

The **superficial popliteal lymph nodes** are usually small and lie in the subcutaneous tissue. A lymph node lies at the termination of the small saphenous vein and receives lymph from the lymphatic vessels that accompany this vein (Fig. 5.12*B*). The **deep popliteal lymph nodes** surround the vessels and receive lymph from the joint capsule of the knee and the lymphatic vessels that accompany the deep veins of the leg. The lymphatic vessels from the popliteal lymph nodes follow the femoral vessels to the *deep inguinal lymph nodes.*

THE BOTTOM LINE: The popliteal fossa is a fat-filled and relatively confined compartment posterior to the knee that is traversed by all neurovascular structures passing between the thigh and the leg. The sciatic nerve bifurcates at the apex of the fossa, with the common fibular nerve passing laterally along the biceps tendon. The tibial nerve, popliteal vein, and popliteal artery bisect the fossa—in that order, from superficial (posterior) to deep (anterior). Genicular branches of the popliteal artery form a periarticular genicular anastomosis around the knee, providing collateral circulation to maintain blood flow in all positions of the knee.

Leg

The bones of the leg (*tibia* and *fibula*) that connect the knee and ankle, and the three fascial compartments (*anterior, lateral,* and *posterior compartments of the leg*), formed by the *anterior* and *posterior intermuscular septa,* the *interosseous membrane,* and the two leg bones to which they attach, were discussed at the beginning of this chapter and are illustrated in cross-section in Figure 5.34. It was pointed out that the muscles of each compartment share common functions and innervations.

Compartment Infections and Syndromes in the Leg

The fascial compartments of the limbs are generally closed spaces, ending proximally and distally at the joints. Inflammations within the anterior and posterior compartments spread chiefly in a distal direction. Suppuration (formation of pus) from purulent ▶

(cont'd on page 638)

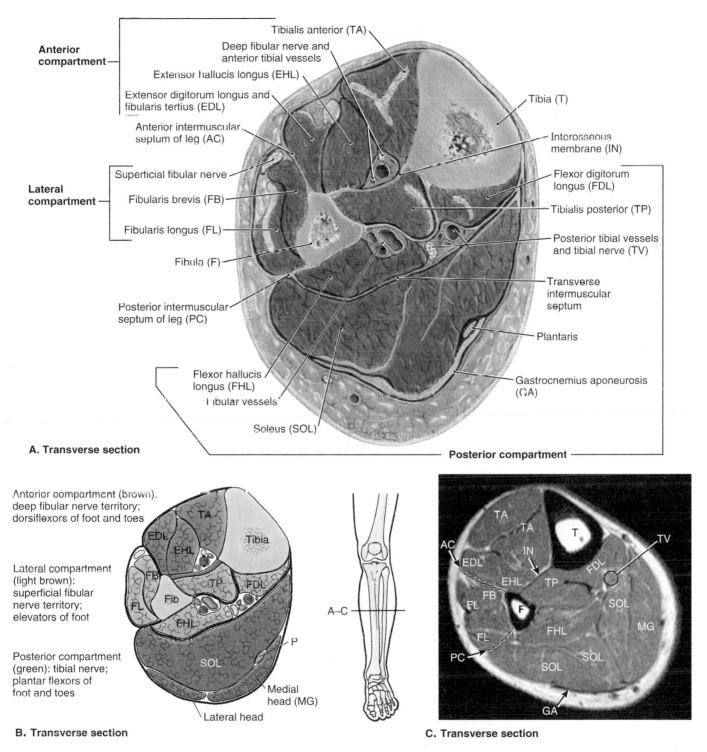

A. Transverse section

Anterior compartment —
Tibialis anterior (TA)
Deep fibular nerve and anterior tibial vessels
Extensor hallucis longus (EHL)
Extensor digitorum longus and fibularis tertius (EDL)
Anterior intermuscular septum of leg (AC)

Lateral compartment —
Superficial fibular nerve
Fibularis brevis (FB)
Fibularis longus (FL)
Fibula (F)
Posterior intermuscular septum of leg (PC)
Flexor hallucis longus (FHL)
Fibular vessels
Soleus (SOL)

Tibia (T)
Interosseous membrane (IN)
Flexor digitorum longus (FDL)
Tibialis posterior (TP)
Posterior tibial vessels and tibial nerve (TV)
Transverse intermuscular septum
Plantaris
Gastrocnemius aponeurosis (GA)

Posterior compartment —

Anterior compartment (brown): deep fibular nerve territory; dorsiflexors of foot and toes

Lateral compartment (light brown): superficial fibular nerve territory; elevators of foot

Posterior compartment (green): tibial nerve; plantar flexors of foot and toes

B. Transverse section

C. Transverse section

Figure 5.34. Compartments of leg at midcalf level in transverse anatomical section. **A.** The anterior (dorsiflexor or extensor) compartment contains four muscles (the fibularis tertius lies inferior to the level of this section). The lateral (fibular) compartment contains two evertor muscles. The posterior (plantarflexor or flexor) compartment, containing seven muscles, is subdivided by an intracompartmental transverse intermuscular septum into a superficial group of three (two of which are commonly tendinous/aponeurotic at this level) and a deep group of four. The popliteus (part of the deep group) lies superior to the level of this section. **B.** Overview of compartments of leg. **C.** MRI of the leg. Abbreviations are defined in the labels for parts **A** and **B.**

(pus-forming) infections in the lateral compartment of the leg, however, can ascend proximally into the popliteal fossa.

Trauma to muscles and/or vessels in the compartments may produce hemorrhage, edema, and inflammation of the muscles. Because the septa and deep fascia of the leg forming the boundaries of the leg compartments are strong, the increased volume consequent to any of these processes increases intracompartmental pressure. With arterial bleeding, the pressure may reach levels high enough to compress structures significantly in the compartment(s) concerned. Structures distal to the compressed area may become ischemic and permanently injured (e.g., loss of motor function in muscles whose blood supply and/or innervation is affected). These conditions, in which increased pressure in a confined anatomical space adversely affects the circulation and threatens the function and viability of tissue within or distally, constitute **compartment syndromes.** Loss of distal pulses is an obvious sign of arterial compression, as is a lowering of the temperature of tissues distal to the compression. A **fasciotomy** (incision of the overlying fascia or a septum) may be performed to relieve the pressure in the compartment(s) concerned. ⊘

Anterior Compartment of the Leg

The **anterior compartment,** or *dorsiflexor (extensor) compartment,* is located anterior to the *interosseous membrane,* between the lateral surface of the tibial shaft and the medial surface of the fibular shaft, and anterior to the intermuscular septum that connects them. The anterior compartment is bounded anteriorly by the deep fascia of the leg and skin. The deep fascia of the leg overlying the anterior compartment is dense superiorly, providing part of the proximal attachment of the muscle immediately deep to it. With unyielding structures on three sides (the two bones and the interosseous membrane) and a dense fascia on the remaining side, the relatively small anterior compartment is especially confined and therefore most susceptible to compartment syndromes. Inferiorly, two band-like thickenings of the fascia form retinacula that bind the tendons of the anterior compartment muscles before and after they cross the ankle joint, preventing them from bowstringing anteriorly during dorsiflexion of the joint (Fig. 5.35):

1. The **superior extensor retinaculum** is a strong, broad band of deep fascia, passing from the fibula to the tibia, proximal to the malleoli.

2. The **inferior extensor retinaculum,** a Y-shaped band of deep fascia, attaches laterally to the anterosuperior surface of the calcaneus. It forms a strong loop around the tendons of the fibularis tertius and the extensor digitorum longus muscles.

Muscles of the Anterior Compartment

The four muscles in the anterior compartment are the tibialis anterior, extensor digitorum longus, extensor hallucis longus, and fibularis tertius (Fig. 5.34A & B; Table 5.10). These muscles pass and insert anterior to the transversely oriented axis of the ankle (talocrural) joint and, therefore, are dorsiflexors of the ankle joint, elevating the forefoot and depressing the heel. The long extensors also pass along and attach to the dorsal aspect of the digits and are thus extensors (elevators) of the toes.

Although it is a relatively weak and short movement—only about a quarter the strength of plantarflexion (Soderberg, 1986), with a range of about 20° from neutral—dorsiflexion is actively used in the swing phase of walking, when concentric contraction keeps the forefoot elevated to clear the ground as the free limb swings forward, and immediately after in the stance phase, as eccentric contraction controls the lowering of the forefoot to the floor following heel strike (Table 5.2). The latter is important to a smooth gait and is important to deceleration (braking) relative to running and walking downhill. During standing, the dorsiflexors reflexively pull the leg (and thus the center of gravity) anteriorly on the fixed foot when the body starts to lean (the center of gravity begins to shift too far) posteriorly. When descending a slope, especially if the surface is loose (sand, gravel or snow), dorsiflexion is used to "dig in" one's heels.

Tibialis Anterior. The **tibialis anterior** (TA), the most medial and superficial dorsiflexor, is a slender muscle that lies against the lateral surface of the tibia (Figs. 5.34 and 5.36). The long tendon of the TA begins halfway down the leg and descends along the anterior surface of the tibia. The tendon passes within its own synovial sheath deep to the superior and inferior extensor retinacula (Fig. 5.35) to its attachment on the medial side of the foot. In so doing, its tendon is located farthest from the axis of the ankle joint, giving it the most mechanical advantage and making it the strongest dorsiflexor. Although antagonists at the ankle joint, the TA and the tibialis posterior (from the posterior compartment) both cross the subtalar and transverse tarsal joints to attach to the medial border of the foot and thus act synergistically to invert the foot.

To test the TA, the individual is asked to stand on the heels or dorsiflex the foot against resistance; if normal, its tendon can be seen and palpated.

Extensor Digitorum Longus. The **extensor digitorum longus** (EDL) is the most lateral of the anterior leg muscles (Figs. 5.34–5.36). A small part of the proximal attachment of the muscle is to the lateral tibial condyle; however, most of it attaches to the medial surface of the fibula and the superior part of the anterior surface of the interosseous membrane (Table 5.10A). The muscle becomes tendinous superior to the ankle, forming four tendons that attach to the phalanges of the lateral four toes. A common synovial sheath surrounds the four tendons of the EDL (plus that of the fibularis tertius) as they diverge on the dorsum of the foot and pass to their distal attachments (Fig. 5.35B).

(cont'd on page 642)

Superior extensor retinaculum

Extensor digitorum longus (EDL)
Lateral malleolus
Fibularis tertius (FT)
Inferior fibular retinaculum

Inferior extensor retinaculum

Extensor hallucis brevis (EHB)

Fibularis tertius (FT)

Extensor digitorum longus (EDL)

Extensor digitorum brevis (EDB)

Extensor expansion

Anterior tibial artery

Extensor hallucis longus (EHL)

Medial malleolus

Tibialis anterior (TA)

Deep fibular nerve

Dorsal artery of foot
(L. *arteria dorsalis pedis*)

Extensor hallucis longus (EHL)

1st dorsal interosseous

Extensor expansion

Central band

Lateral bands

(A) Anterosuperior view of dorsum of foot

Tibialis anterior (TA)

Anterior tibial artery

Inferior extensor retinaculum

Common synovial sheath covering extensor digitorum longus (EDL) and fibularis tertius (FT)

Medial terminal branch of deep fibular nerve
Extensor hallucis longus (EHL)
Dorsal artery of foot
Extensor hallucis brevis (EHB)

Superior extensor retinaculum

Fibularis longus (FL) **Fibularis brevis (FB)** **Extensor digitorum brevis (EDB)** **Fibularis tertius (FT)**

(B) Anterolateral view

Figure 5.35. Dissections of foot. These dissections demonstrate the continuation of the anterior and lateral leg muscles into the foot. The thinner portions of the deep fascia of the leg have been removed, leaving the thicker portions that make up the extensor and fibular retinacula, which retain the tendons as they cross the ankle. **A.** The vessels and nerves are cut short. At the ankle, the vessels and the deep fibular nerve lie midway between the malleoli and between the tendons of the long dorsiflexors of the toes. **B.** Synovial sheaths surround the tendons as they pass beneath the retinacula of the ankle.

Table 5.10. Muscles of the Anterior and Lateral Compartments of the Leg

(A) Anterior muscle attachments

(B) Anterior and lateral compartments

(C)

(D)

(E)

(F)

Muscle[a]	Proximal Attachment	Distal Attachment	Innervation[b]	Main Action[a]
Anterior compartment Tibialis anterior (1)	Lateral condyle and superior half of lateral surface of tibia and interosseous membrane	Medial and inferior surfaces of medial cuneiform and base of 1st metatarsal	Deep fibular nerve (**L4**, L5)	Dorsiflexes ankle and inverts foot
Extensor digitorum longus (2)	Lateral condyle of tibia and superior three quarters of medial surface of fibula and interosseous membrane	Middle and distal phalanges of lateral four digits	Deep fibular nerve (L5, S1)	Extends lateral four digits and dorsiflexes ankle
Extensor hallucis longus (3)	Middle part of anterior surface of fibula and interosseous membrane	Dorsal aspect of base of distal phalanx of great toe (hallux)	Deep fibular nerve (L5, S1	Extends great toe and dorsiflexes ankle
Fibularis tertius (4)	Inferior third of anterior surface of fibula and interosseous membrane	Dorsum of base of 5th metatarsal	Deep fibular nerve (L5, S1	Dorsiflexes ankle and aids in inversion of foot
Lateral compartment Fibularis longus (5)	Head and superior two thirds of lateral surface of fibula	Base of 1st metatarsal and medial cuneiform	Superficial fibular nerve (**L5, S1**, S2)	Everts foot and weakly plantarflexes ankle
Fibularis brevis (6)	Inferior two thirds of lateral surface of fibula	Dorsal surface of tuberosity on lateral side of base of 5th metatarsal	Superficial fibular nerve (**L5, S1**, S2)	Everts foot and weakly plantarflexes ankle

[a]Numbers refer to the figure, parts A and B.
[b]The spinal cord segmental innervation is indicated (e.g., "L4, L5" means that the nerves supplying the tibialis anterior are derived from the fourth and fifth lumbar segments of the spinal cord). Numbers in boldface (**L4**) indicate the main segmental innervation. Damage to one or more of the listed spinal cord segments or to the motor nerve roots arising from them results in paralysis of the muscles concerned.

Iliotibial tract

Biceps femoris tendon

Patellar retinaculum

Plantaris

Common fibular nerve

Gastrocnemius

Fibularis longus (FL)

Soleus

Superficial fibular nerve

Fibularis brevis (FB)

Superior fibular retinaculum

Calcaneal tendon

Inferior fibular retinaculum

Fibularis brevis (FB)

Fibularis tertius (FT)

Patella

Fibular collateral ligament, uncovered by retracting fascia

Head of fibula

Patellar ligament

Deep fibular nerve

Deep fascia of leg

Tibialis anterior (TA)

Extensor digitorum longus (EDL)

Extensor hallucis longus (EHL)

Superior extensor retinaculum

Fibularis tertius (FT)

Perforating branch of fibular artery

Inferior extensor retinaculum

Extensor hallucis brevis (EHB)

Extensor digitorum brevis (EDB)

Extensor digitorum longus (EDL)

Lateral branch to articulations and extensor digitorum brevis

Anterior tibial artery

Vascular twig of nerve

Vascular twig of nerve

Inferior extensor retinaculum (medial portion, retracted)

Medial branch to articulations and skin between 1st and 2nd digits

(A) Anterolateral view

(B) Anterior oblique view

Figure 5.36. Dissections of anterior and lateral compartments of leg. A. This dissection shows the muscles of the anterolateral leg and dorsum of the foot. The common fibular nerve, coursing subcutaneously across the lateral aspect of the head and neck of the fibula, is the most commonly injured peripheral nerve. **B.** In this deeper dissection of the anterior compartment, the muscles and inferior extensor retinaculum are retracted to display the arteries and nerves.

Each tendon forms a membranous *extensor expansion* (dorsal aponeurosis) over the dorsum of the proximal phalanx of the toe, which divides into two lateral bands and one central band (Fig. 5.35*A*). The central band inserts into the base of the middle phalanx, and the lateral slips converge to insert into the base of the distal phalanx.

To test the EDL, the lateral four toes are dorsiflexed against resistance; if acting normally, the tendons can be seen and palpated.

Fibularis Tertius. The **fibularis tertius** (FT) is a separated part of the EDL, which shares its synovial sheath (Figs. 5.35 and 5.36). Proximally, the attachments and fleshy parts of the EDL and FT are continuous; however, distally, the FT tendon is separate and attaches to the 5th metatarsal, not to a phalanx (Table 5.10*F*). Although the FT does contribute (weakly) to dorsiflexion, it also acts at the subtalar and transverse tarsal joints, contributing to pronation (eversion) of the foot. It may play a special proprioceptive role in sensing sudden inversion and then contracting reflexively to protect the anterior tibiofibular ligament, the most commonly sprained ligament of the body. The FT is not always present.

Extensor Hallucis Longus. The **extensor hallucis longus** (EHL) is a thin muscle that lies deeply between the TA and the EDL at its superior attachment to the middle half of the fibula and interosseous membrane. The EHL rises to the surface in the distal third of the leg, passing deep to the extensor retinacula (Figs. 5.35 and 5.36). It courses distally along the crest of the dorsum of the foot to the great toe.

To test the EHL, the great toe is dorsiflexed against resistance; if normal, its entire tendon can be seen and palpated.

Nerve of the Anterior Compartment

The **deep fibular nerve** is the nerve of the anterior compartment (Figs. 5.34*A* and 5.36*B;* Table 5.11). It is one of the two terminal branches of the common fibular nerve, arising between the fibularis longus muscle and the neck of the fibula. After its entry into the anterior compartment, the deep fibular nerve accompanies the anterior tibial artery, first between the TA and the EDL and then between the TA and the EHL. It then exits the compartment, continuing across the ankle joint to supply intrinsic muscles and a small area of the skin of the foot. A lesion of this nerve results in an inability to dorsiflex (footdrop).

Artery in the Anterior Compartment

The **anterior tibial artery** supplies structures in the anterior compartment (Figs. 5.34*A* and 5.38*B;* Table 5.12). The smaller terminal branch of the popliteal artery, the anterior tibial artery, begins at the inferior border of the popliteus muscle (i.e., as the popliteal artery passes deep to the tendinous arch of the soleus) and immediately passes anteriorly through a gap in the superior part of the interosseous membrane to descend on the anterior surface of this membrane between the TA and the EDL muscles. At the ankle joint, midway between the malleoli, the anterior tibial artery changes names, becoming the dorsal artery of the foot (L. *arteria dorsalis pedis*).

Tibialis Anterior Strain (Shin Splints)

Shin splints—edema and pain in the area of the distal two-thirds of the tibia—result from repetitive microtrauma of the TA, which causes small tears in the periosteum covering the shaft of the tibia and/or of fleshy attachments to the overlying deep fascia of the leg. Shin splints are a mild form of the anterior compartment syndrome. Shin splints commonly occur during traumatic injury or athletic overexertion of muscles in the anterior compartment, especially the TA, by untrained persons. Often persons who lead sedentary lives develop shin splints when they participate in walk-a-thons (long-distance walks). Shin splints also occur in trained runners who do not warm up and cool down sufficiently. Muscles in the anterior compartment swell from sudden overuse, and the edema and muscle–tendon inflammation reduce the blood flow to the muscles. The swollen muscles are painful and tender to pressure.

Deep Fibular Nerve Entrapment

Excessive use of muscles supplied by the deep fibular nerve (e.g., during skiing, running, and dancing) may result in muscle injury and edema in the anterior compartment. This entrapment may cause compression of the deep fibular nerve and pain in the anterior compartment. Compression of the nerve by tight-fitting ski boots, for example, may occur where the nerve passes deep to the inferior extensor retinaculum and the extensor hallucis brevis. Pain occurs in the dorsum of the foot and usually radiates to the web space between the 1st and 2nd toes. Because ski boots are a common cause of this type of nerve entrapment, this condition has been called the "ski boot syndrome"; however, the syndrome also occurs in soccer players and runners and can result from tight shoes. ○

THE BOTTOM LINE: The anterior compartment, confined by mostly unyielding bones and membranes, is susceptible to compartment syndromes. The contained muscles are ankle dorsiflexors/toe extensors that are active in walking as they (1) concentrically contract to raise the forefoot to clear the ground during the swing phase of the gait cycle and (2) eccentrically contract to lower the forefoot to the ground after the heel strike of the stance phase. The deep fibular nerve and anterior tibial artery course within and supply the compartment. Injury of the common or deep fibular nerve results in footdrop (see clinical correlation [blue] box, "Injury to the Common Fibular Nerve and Footdrop," in this chapter).

Table 5.11. Nerves of the Leg

Anterior view

Common fibular nerve
Superficial fibular nerve
Fibularis longus
Fibularis brevis
Extensor digitorum brevis
Deep fibular nerve
Tibialis anterior
Extensor hallucis longus
Extensor digitorum longus
Fibularis tertius
Saphenous nerve

Posterior view

Sciatic nerve
Tibial nerve
Gastrocnemius
Medial sural cutaneous nerve
Flexor digitorum longus
Flexor hallucis longus
Medial plantar nerve
Abductor hallucis
Flexor digitorum brevis
Flexor hallucis brevis
Lumbrical to 2nd digit
Common fibular nerve
Plantaris
Gastrocnemius
Popliteus
Soleus
Tibialis posterior
Lateral sural cutaneous nerve
Sural nerve
Lateral plantar nerve
All other muscles in sole of foot

Nerve	Origin	Course	Distribution in Leg
Saphenous	Femoral nerve	Descends with femoral vessels through femoral triangle and adductor canal and then descends with great saphenous vein	Supplies skin on medial side of ankle and foot
Sural	Usually arises from both tibial and common fibular nerves	Descends between heads of gastrocnemius and becomes superficial at middle of leg; descends with small saphenous vein and passes inferior to lateral malleolus to lateral side of foot	Supplies skin on posterior and lateral aspects of leg and lateral side of foot
Tibial	Sciatic nerve	Forms as sciatic bifurcates at apex of popliteal fossa; descends through popliteal fossa and lies on popliteus; runs inferiorly on tibialis posterior with posterior tibial vessels; terminates beneath flexor retinaculum by dividing into medial and lateral plantar nerves	Supplies posterior muscles of leg and knee joint
Common fibular	Sciatic nerve	Forms as sciatic bifurcates at apex of popliteal fossa and follows medial border of biceps femoris and its tendon; passes over posterior aspect of head of fibula and then winds around neck of fibula deep to fibularis longus, where it divides into deep and superficial fibular nerves	Supplies skin on lateral part of posterior aspect of leg via its branch (lateral sural cutaneous nerve); also supplies knee joint via its articular branch
Superficial fibular	Common fibular nerve	Arises between fibularis longus and neck of fibula and descends in lateral compartment of leg; pierces deep fascia at distal third of leg to become subcutaneous	Supplies fibularis longus and brevis and skin on distal third of anterior surface of leg and dorsum of foot
Deep fibular	Common fibular nerve	Arises between fibularis longus and neck of fibula; passes through extensor digitorum longus and descends on interosseous membrane; crosses distal end of tibia and enters dorsum of foot	Supplies anterior muscles of leg, dorsum of foot, and skin of first interdigital cleft; sends articular branches to joints it crosses

Table 5.12. Arteries of the Leg

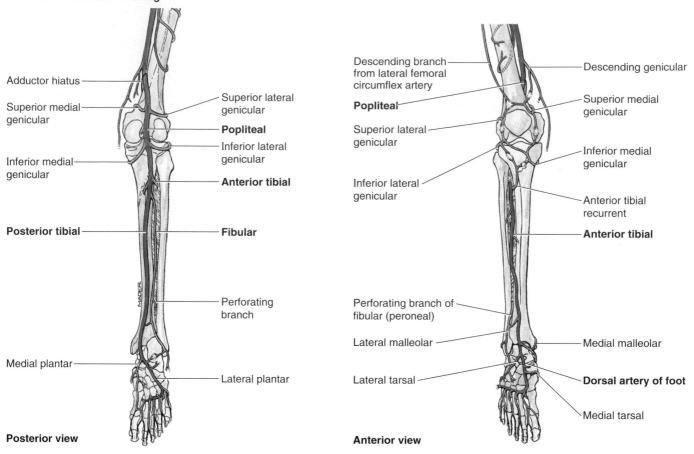

Posterior view   **Anterior view**

Artery	Origin	Course	Distribution in Leg
Popliteal	Continuation of femoral artery at adductor hiatus in adductor magnus	Passes through popliteal fossa to leg; ends at lower border of popliteus muscle by dividing into anterior and posterior tibial arteries	Superior, middle, and inferior genicular arteries to both lateral and medial aspects of knee
Anterior tibial	Popliteal	Passes between tibia and fibula into anterior compartment through gap in superior part of interosseous membrane and descends this membrane between tibialis anterior and extensor digitorum longus	Anterior compartment of leg
Doral artery of foot (L. *dorsalis pedis*)	Continuation of anterior tibial artery distal to inferior extensor retinaculum	Descends anteromedially to first interosseous space and divides into plantar and arcuate arteries	Muscles on dorsum of foot; pierces first dorsal interosseous muscles as deep plantar artery to contribute to formation of plantar arch
Posterior tibial	Popliteal	Passes through posterior compartment of leg and terminates distal to flexor retinaculum by dividing into medial and lateral plantar arteries	Posterior and lateral compartments of leg; circumflex fibular branch joins anastomoses around knee; nutrient artery passes to tibia
Fibular	Posterior tibial	Descends in posterior compartment adjacent to posterior intermuscular septum	Posterior compartment of leg: perforating branches supply lateral compartment of leg

Lateral Compartment of the Leg

The **lateral compartment** or *evertor compartment,* is the smallest (narrowest) of the leg compartments, bounded by the lateral surface of the fibula, the anterior and posterior intermuscular septa, and the deep fascia of the leg (Fig. 5.34A

& *B;* Table 5.10). The compartment ends inferiorly at the **superior fibular retinaculum,** which spans between the distal tip of the fibula and the calcaneus (Fig. 5.36A). Here the tendons of the two muscles of the lateral compartment enter a common synovial sheath to accommodate their passage between the superior fibular retinaculum and the lateral malleolus, using the latter as a trochlea as they cross the ankle joint.

Muscles in the Lateral Compartment

The lateral compartment contains the fibularis longus and brevis muscles. These muscles have their fleshy bellies in the lateral compartment but are tendinous as they exit the compartment within the common synovial sheath deep to the superior fibular retinaculum. Both muscles are evertors of the foot, elevating the lateral margin of the foot. Developmentally, the fibularis muscles are postaxial muscles, receiving innervation from the posterior divisions of the spinal nerves, which contribute to the sciatic nerve. However, because the fibularis longus and brevis pass posterior to the transverse axis of the ankle (talocrural) joint, they contribute to plantarflexion at the ankle—unlike the postaxial muscles of the anterior compartment (including the fibularis tertius), which are dorsiflexors.

As evertors, the fibularis muscles act at the subtalar and transverse tarsal joints. From the neutral position, only a few degrees of eversion are possible. In practice, the primary function of the evertors of the foot is not to elevate the lateral margin of the foot (the common description of eversion) but to depress or fix the medial margin of the foot in support of the toe off phase of walking and, especially, running and to resist inadvertent or excessive inversion of the foot (the position in which the ankle is most vulnerable to injury). When standing (and particularly when balancing on one foot), the fibularis muscles contract to resist medial sway (to recenter a line of gravity, which has shifted medially) by pulling laterally on the leg while depressing the medial margin of the foot.

To test the fibularis longus and brevis, the foot is everted strongly against resistance; if acting normally, the muscle tendons can be seen and palpated inferior to the lateral malleolus.

Fibularis Longus. The **fibularis longus** (FL) is the longer and more superficial of the two fibularis muscles, arising much more superiorly on the shaft of the fibula (Figs. 5.34 and 5.36A; Table 5.10). The narrow FL extends from the head of the fibula to the sole of the foot. Its tendon can be palpated and observed proximal and posterior to the lateral malleolus. Distal to the superior fibular retinaculum, the common sheath shared by the fibular muscles splits to extend through separate compartments deep to the **inferior fibular retinaculum** (Figs. 5.35A and 5.36). The FL passes through the inferior compartment—inferior to the *fibular trochlea* on the calcaneus—and enters a groove on the anteroinferior aspect of the cuboid bone (Fig. 5.9C). It then crosses the sole of the foot, running obliquely and distally to reach its attachment to the 1st metatarsal and medial cuneiform bones (see Fig. 5.9B). When a person stands on one foot, the FL helps steady the leg on the foot.

Fibularis Brevis. The **fibularis brevis** (FB) is a fusiform muscle that lies deep to the FL and, true to its name, the FB is shorter than its partner in the lateral compartment (Figs. 5.34 and 5.36A; Table 5.10). Its broad tendon grooves the

posterior aspect of the lateral malleolus and can be palpated inferior to it. The narrower tendon of the FL lies on that of the FB and does not contact the lateral malleolus. The tendon of the FB traverses the superior compartment of the inferior fibular retinaculum, passing superior to the fibular trochlea of the calcaneus; it can be easily traced to its distal attachment to the base of the 5th metatarsal (Fig. 5.9C). The tendon of the *fibularis tertius,* a slip of muscle from the extensor digitorum longus, often merges with the tendon of the FB (Fig. 5.36A). Occasionally, however, the fibularis tertius passes anteriorly to attach directly to the proximal phalanx of the 5th digit.

Nerves in the Lateral Compartment

The **superficial fibular nerve,** a terminal branch of the common fibular nerve, is the nerve of the lateral compartment (Figs. 5.34A and 5.36A; Table 5.11). After supplying the FL and FB, the superficial fibular nerve continues as a cutaneous nerve, supplying the skin on the distal part of the anterior surface of the leg and nearly all the dorsum of the foot.

Blood Vessels of the Lateral Compartment

The lateral compartment does not have an artery coursing through it. Instead, perforating branches and accompanying veins supply blood to and drain blood from the compartment. Proximally, perforating branches of the anterior tibial artery penetrate the anterior intermuscular septum. Inferiorly, perforating branches of the *fibular artery* penetrate the posterior intermuscular septum, along with their accompanying veins (L. *venae comitantes*) (Table 5.12).

THE BOTTOM LINE: The small lateral compartment contains the primary evertors of the foot and the superficial fibular nerve that supplies them. Because no artery courses within the compartment, perforating branches from the anterior tibial and fibular arteries (and their accompanying veins) penetrate the intermuscular septa to supply (and drain) blood. Eversion is used to support/depress the medial foot during the toe off of the stance phase and to resist inadvertent inversion, preventing injury.

The Fibularis Muscles and Evolution of the Human Foot

Whereas the feet of anthropoids (higher primates) are inverted so that they walk on the outer border of the foot, feet of humans are relatively everted (pronated) so that the soles lie more fully on the ground. This pronation is the result, at least in part, to the medial migration of the distal attachment of the fibularis longus across the sole of the foot and the development of a fibularis tertius that is attached to the base of the 5th metatarsal. These features are unique to the human foot. ▶

Injury to the Common Fibular Nerve and Footdrop

Because of its superficial position, the common fibular is the nerve most often injured in the lower limb, mainly because it winds subcutaneously around the fibular neck, leaving it vulnerable to direct trauma. This nerve may also be severed during fracture of the fibular neck or severely stretched when the knee joint is injured or dislocated. *Severance of the common fibular nerve* results in flaccid paralysis of all muscles in the anterior and lateral compartments of the leg (dorsiflexors of the ankle and evertors of the foot). The loss of dorsiflexion of the ankle causes *footdrop,* which is further exacerbated by unopposed inversion of the foot. This has the effect of making the limb "too long": The toes do not clear the ground during the swing phase of walking (Fig. B5.14A).

There are several other conditions that may result in a lower limb that is "too long" functionally, for example, pelvic tilt (Fig. 5.26C) and spastic paralysis or contraction of the soleus. There are at least three means of compensating for this problem:

1. A *waddling gait,* in which the individual leans to the side opposite the long limb, "hiking" the hip (Fig. B5.14B).

2. A *swing-out gait,* in which the long limb is swung out laterally (abducted) to allow the toes to clear the ground (Fig. B5.14C).

3. A high-stepping *steppage gait,* in which extra flexion is employed at the hip and knee to raise the foot as high as necessary to keep the toes from hitting the ground (Fig. B5.14D).

Because the dropped foot makes it difficult to make the heel strike the ground first as in a normal gait, a steppage gait is commonly employed in the case of flaccid paralysis. Sometimes an extra "kick" is added as the free limb swings forward in an attempt to flip the forefoot upward just before setting the foot down. In addition, the braking action normally produced by eccentric contraction of the dorsiflexors is also lost in flaccid paralysis footdrop. Therefore, the foot is not lowered to the ground in a controlled manner after heel strike but instead slaps the ground suddenly, producing a distinctive *clop* and greatly increasing the shock both received by the forefoot and transmitted up the tibia to the knee. Individuals with a fibular nerve injury may also experience a variable loss of sensation on the anterolateral aspect of the leg and the dorsum of the foot.

Superficial Fibular Nerve Entrapment

Chronic ankle sprains may produce recurrent stretching of the superficial fibular nerve, which may cause pain along the lateral side of the leg and the dorsum of the ankle and foot. Numbness and *paresthesia* (tickling or tingling) may be present and increase with activity.

Avulsion of the Tuberosity of the 5th Metatarsal

Violent inversion of the foot may cause *avulsion of the tuberosity of the 5th metatarsal,* the distal attachment of fibularis brevis. This avulsion fracture is associated with a severely sprained ankle. Injury to the associated superficial fibular nerve causes inversion of the foot because of paralysis of the fibular muscles in the lateral compartment. ⊕

(A)   (B)   (C)   (D)

Figure B5.14

Posterior Compartment of the Leg

The **posterior compartment** (*plantarflexor compartment*, is the largest of the three leg compartments (Fig. 5.34A). The posterior compartment and the *calf muscles* within it are divided into superficial and deep subcompartments/muscle groups by the **transverse intermuscular septum**. The tibial nerve and posterior tibial and fibular vessels supply both parts of the posterior compartment but run in the deep subcompartment deep (anterior) to the transverse intermuscular septum. The larger superficial subcompartment is the least confined compartmental area. The smaller deep subcompartment, like the anterior compartment, is bounded by the two leg bones and the *interosseous membrane* that binds them together plus the transverse intermuscular septum; therefore, the deep subcompartment is quite tightly confined. Because the nerve and blood vessels supplying the entire posterior compartment and the sole of the foot pass through the deep subcompartment, when swelling occurs it leads to a compartment syndrome that has serious consequences.

Inferiorly, the deep subcompartment tapers as the muscles it contains become tendinous. The transverse intermuscular septum ends as reinforcing transverse fibers that extend between the tip of the medial malleolus and the calcaneus to form the flexor retinaculum. The retinaculum is subdivided deeply, forming separate compartments for each tendon of the deep muscle group, as well as for the tibial nerve and posterior tibial artery as they bend around the medial malleolus.

Muscles of the posterior compartment produce plantarflexion at the ankle, inversion at the subtalar and transverse tarsal joints, and flexion of the toes. Plantarflexion is a powerful movement (four times stronger than dorsiflexion) produced over a relatively long range (approximately 50° from neutral) by muscles that pass posterior to the transverse axis of the ankle joint. The movement develops thrust, applied primarily at the ball of the foot, that is used to propel the body forward and upward and is the major component of the forces generated during the push-off (heel off and toe off) parts of the stance phase of walking and running (Table 5.2).

Superficial Muscle Group in the Posterior Compartment

The superficial group of calf muscles includes the gastrocnemius, soleus, and plantaris. Details concerning their attachments, innervation and actions are provided in Table 5.13. The two-headed gastrocnemius and soleus share a common tendon, the calcaneal tendon, which attaches to the calcaneus. Collectively these two muscles make up the three-headed **triceps surae** (L. *sura*, calf) (Fig. 5.37). This powerful muscular mass tugs on the lever provided by the calcaneal tuberosity, elevating the heel and thus depressing the forefoot, generating as much as 93% of the plantarflexion force. The large size of the gastrocnemius and soleus muscles is a human characteristic that is directly related to our upright stance. These muscles are strong and heavy because they lift, propel, and accelerate the weight of the body when walking, running, jumping, or standing on the toes.

The **calcaneal tendon** (L. *tendo calcaneus*, Achilles tendon) is the most powerful (thickest and strongest) tendon in the body. Approximately 15 cm in length, it is a continuation of the flat aponeurosis, formed halfway down the calf where the bellies of the gastrocnemius terminate. The aponeurosis receives fleshy fibers of the soleus directly on its deep surface proximally but thickens as the soleus fibers become tendinous inferiorly. The tendon thus becomes thicker (deeper) but narrower as it descends until it becomes essentially round in cross-section superior to the calcaneus. It then expands as it inserts centrally on the posterior surface of the *calcaneal tuberosity*. It typically spirals a quarter turn (90°) during its descent, so that the gastrocnemius fibers attach laterally and the soleal fibers attach medially. This arrangement is thought to be significant to the tendon's elastic ability to absorb energy (shock) and recoil, releasing the energy as part of the propulsive force it exerts. Although they share a common tendon, the two muscles of the triceps surae are capable of acting alone, and often do so: "You stroll with the soleus but win the long jump with the gastrocnemius."

A *subcutaneous calcaneal bursa,* located between the skin and the calcaneal tendon, allows the skin to move over the taut tendon, and a deep *bursa of the calcaneal tendon* (retrocalcaneal bursa), located between the tendon and the calcaneus, allows the tendon to glide over the bone.

To test the triceps surae, the foot is plantarflexed against resistance (e.g., by "standing on the toes," in which case body weight [gravity] provides resistance). If normal, the calcaneal tendon and triceps surae can be seen and palpated.

Gastrocnemius. The **gastrocnemius** is the most superficial muscle in the posterior compartment and forms the proximal, most prominent part of the calf (Fig. 5.37; Table 5.13). It is a fusiform, two-headed, two-joint muscle with the medial head slightly larger and extending more distally than its lateral partner. The heads come together at the inferior margin of the popliteal fossa, where they form the inferolateral and inferomedial boundaries of this fossa. Because its fibers are mainly vertical, and largely of the white, fast-twitch (type 2) variety, contractions of the gastrocnemius produce rapid movements during running and jumping (Table 5.13). It is recruited into action only intermittently during symmetrical standing. The gastrocnemius crosses and is capable of acting on both the knee and the ankle joints; however, it cannot exert its full power on both joints at the same time. It functions most effectively when the knee is extended (and is maximally activated when knee extension is combined with dorsiflexion, as in the sprint start). It is incapable of producing plantarflexion when the knee is fully flexed.

Soleus. The **soleus** is located deep to the gastrocnemius and is considered to be the "workhorse" of plantarflexion. It is a large muscle, flatter than the gastrocnemius, that is named for its resemblance to a sole—the flat fish that reclines on its side on the sea floor. The soleus has a continuous proximal attachment in the shape of an inverted U to the posterior aspects of the fibula and tibia and a tendinous arch between them, the **tendinous arch of the soleus** (L. *arcus tendineus*

Table 5.13-I. Superficial Muscles of the Posterior Compartment of the Leg

Posterior muscle attachments

(A)

Muscle[a]	Proximal Attachment	Distal Attachment	Innervation[b]	Main Action
Gastrocnemius (1)	Lateral head: lateral aspect of lateral condyle of femur Medial head: popliteal surface of femur, superior to medial condyle	Posterior surface of calcaneus via calcaneal tendon	Tibial nerve (S1, S2)	Plantarflexes ankle when knee is extended; raises heel during walking; flexes leg at knee joint
Soleus (2)	Posterior aspect of head of fibula; superior quarter of posterior surface of fibula soleal line, medial border, and of tibia			Plantarflexes ankle independent of position of knee; steadies leg on foot
Plantaris (3)	Inferior end of lateral supracondylar line of femur; oblique popliteal ligament			Weakly assists gastrocnemius in plantarflexing ankle

[a] Numbers refer to the figure, part A.
[b] The spinal cord segmental innervation is indicated (e.g., "S1, S2" means that the nerves supplying these muscles are derived from the first and second sacral segments of the spinal cord). Damage to one or more of the listed spinal cord segments or to the motor nerve roots arising from them results in paralysis of the muscles concerned.

soleus) (Fig. 5.38A). The popliteal artery and tibial nerve exit the popliteal fossa by passing through this arch, the popliteal artery simultaneously bifurcating into its terminal branches, the anterior and posterior tibial arteries. The soleus can be palpated on each side of the gastrocnemius when the individual is standing on the tiptoes.

The soleus may act with the gastrocnemius in plantarflexing the ankle joint; it cannot act on the knee joint and acts alone when the knee is flexed. The fibers of the soleus slope posteriorly and inferomedially. When the foot is planted, it pulls posteriorly on the bones of the leg. This is important to standing because the line of gravity passes anterior to the leg's

bony axis. The soleus is thus an antigravity muscle (the predominant plantarflexor for standing and strolling), which contracts antagonistically but cooperatively (alternately) with the dorsiflexor muscles of the leg to maintain balance. Composed largely of red, fatigue-resistant, slow-twitch (type 1) muscle fibers, it is a strong but relatively slow plantarflexor of the ankle joint, capable of sustained contraction. Electromyography (EMG) studies show that during symmetrical standing, the soleus is continuously active.

Plantaris. The **plantaris** is a small muscle with a short belly and a long tendon (Figs. 5.31 and 5.34A; Table 5.13). This vestigial muscle is absent in 5–10% of people and is

Table 5.13-II. Deep Muscles of the Posterior Compartment of the Leg

(B)

Muscle[a]	Proximal Attachment	Distal Attachment	Innervation[b]	Main Action
Popliteus	Lateral surface of lateral condyle of femur and lateral meniscus	Posterior surface of tibia, superior to soleal line	Tibial nerve (L4, L5, S1)	Weakly flexes knee and unlocks it by rotating femur 5° on fixed tibia; medially rotates tibia of unplanted limb
Flexor hallucis longus (4)	Inferior two thirds of posterior surface of fibula; inferior part of interosseous membrane	Base of distal phalanx of great toe (hallux)	Tibial nerve (S2, S3)	Flexes great toe at all joints; weakly plantarflexes ankle; supports medial longitudinal arches of foot
Flexor digitorum longus (5)	Medial part of posterior surface of tibia inferior to soleal line; by a broad tendon to fibula	Bases of distal phalanges of lateral four digits		Flexes lateral four digits; plantarflexes ankle; supports longitudinal arches of foot
Tibialis posterior (6)	Interosseous membrane; posterior surface of tibia inferior to soleal line; posterior surface of fibula	Tuberosity of navicular, cuneiform, and cuboid; bases of 2nd, 3rd, and 4th metatarsals	Tibial nerve (L4, L5)	Plantarflexes ankle; inverts foot

[a] Numbers refer to the figure, part A.
[b] The spinal cord segmental innervation is indicated (e.g., "S2, S3" means that the nerves supplying the flexor hallucis longus are derived from the second and third sacral segments of the spinal cord). Damage to one or more of the listed spinal cord segments or to the motor nerve roots arising from them results in paralysis of the muscles concerned.

highly variable in size and form when present (most commonly a tapering slip about the size of the small finger). It acts with the gastrocnemius but is insignificant as either a flexor of the knee or a plantarflexor of the ankle. It has been considered to be an organ of proprioception for the larger plantarflexors, as it has a high density of muscle spindles (receptors for proprioception). Its long, slender tendon is easily mistaken for a nerve (and hence dubbed by some the "freshman's nerve"). It runs distally between the gastrocnemius and the soleus (Fig. 5.34A) and occasionally suddenly ruptures with a painful *pop* during activities such as racquet sports. Because of its minor role, the plantaris tendon can be removed for grafting (e.g., during reconstructive surgery of the tendons of the hand) without causing disability.

Fabella in the Gastrocnemius

Close to its proximal attachment, the lateral head of the gastrocnemius contains a sesamoid bone, the *fabella* (L. bean), which articulates with the lateral femoral condyle and is visible in lateral radiographs of the knee in 3–5% of people (Fig. B5.15).

Calcaneal Tendinitis

Inflammation of the calcaneal tendon constitutes 9–18% of running injuries. Microscopic tears of ▶

(cont'd on page 652)

Semitendinosus

Semimembranosus

Medial sural
cutaneous nerve

Gracilis

Vastus
medialis

Sartorius

Biceps femoris

Tibial nerve

Sural communicating
branch

Common fibular
nerve

Lateral sural
cutaneous nerve

Sural nerve

Gastrocnemius,
lateral head

Triceps
surae

Gastrocnemius,
medial head

Soleus

Fibularis
longus (FL)

Fibularis
brevis (FB)

Flexor
digitorum
longus (EDL)

Tibialis
posterior (TP)

Flexor
retinaculum

Calcaneal
tendon

Superior fibular
retinaculum

Posterior view

Figure 5.37. Superficial dissection of posterior aspect of leg. Except for the retinacula in the ankle region, the deep fascia has been removed to reveal the nerves and muscles. Visible nerves include the
tibial and common fibular nerves and their contributions to the formation of the sural nerve. The three heads
of the triceps surae muscle attach distally to the calcaneus via the spiraling fibers of the calcaneal tendon.

Tendinous arch of soleus

Popliteus

Soleus

Flexor digitorum longus (FDL)

Posterior tibial artery

Tibial nerve

Fibula

Tibialis posterior (TP)

Fibular artery

Flexor hallucis longus

Transverse intermuscular septum

Flexor retinaculum

Tibialis posterior (TP) tendon

Flexor digitorum longus (FDL) tendon

Medial plantar nerve and artery

Calcaneal tendon

Lateral plantar nerve and artery

(A) Posteromedial view

Femur

Gastrocnemius, lateral head

Lateral meniscus (with attachment of popliteus muscle)

Fibular collateral ligament

Popliteus tendon

Biceps femoris

Popliteus bursa

Popliteus

Posterior menisco-femoral ligament

Posterior cruciate ligament

(B) Posterior aspect of the knee joint

Figure 5.38. Deep dissection of posterior aspect of right leg and knee joint. A. The gastrocnemius and most of the soleus are removed, leaving only a horseshoe-shaped section of the soleus close to its proximal attachments and the distal part of the calcaneal tendon in the superficial part of the posterior compartment The transverse intermuscular septum has been split to reveal the deep muscles, vessels, and nerves. **B.** The popliteus tendon attaches in part to the lateral meniscus and is separated from the proximal end of the tibia by the popliteus bursa.

Femur

Fabella

Fibula

Tibia

Patella

Lateral view

Figure B5.15

collagen fibers in the tendon, particularly just superior to its attachment to the calcaneus, result in *tendinitis,* which causes pain during walking, especially when wearing rigid-soled shoes. Calcaneal tendinitis often occurs during repetitive activities, especially in individuals who take up running after prolonged inactivity or suddenly increase the intensity of their training, but it may also result from poor footwear or training surfaces.

Ruptured Calcaneal Tendon

Rupture of the calcaneal tendon is often sustained by poorly conditioned people with a history of *calcaneal tendinitis.* The injury is typically experienced as an audible snap during a forceful push off (plantarflexion with the knee extended) followed immediately by sudden calf pain and sudden dorsiflexion of the plantarflexed foot. In a completely ruptured tendon, a gap is palpable, usually 1–5 cm proximal to the calcaneal attachment.

    Calcaneal tendon rupture is probably the most severe acute muscular problem of the leg. Individuals with this injury cannot plantarflex against resistance (cannot raise the heel from the ground or balance on the affected side), and passive dorsiflexion (usually limited to 20° from neutral) is excessive. Ambulation is possible only when the limb is externally rotated, rolling over the transversely placed foot during the stance phase without push off. Bruising appears in the malleolar region, and a lump usually appears in the calf owing to shortening of the triceps surae. In older or non-athletic people, non-surgical repairs are often adequate, but surgical intervention is usually advised for those with active lifestyles.

Calcaneal Tendon Reflex

The ankle (jerk) reflex, the calcaneal tendon reflex, is a myotatic reflex elicited while the person's legs are dangling over the side of the examining table. The calcaneal tendon is struck briskly with a reflex hammer just proximal to the calcaneus. The normal result is plantarflexion of the ankle joint. The calcaneal tendon reflex tests the S1 and S2 nerve roots. If the S1 nerve root is injured or compressed, the ankle reflex is virtually absent.

Gastrocnemius Strain

Gastrocnemius strain (tennis leg) is a painful acute injury resulting from the partial tearing of the medial belly of the gastrocnemius at or near its musculotendinous junction, often seen in individuals older than 40 years of age. It is caused by overstretching the muscle by concomitant full extension of the knee and dorsiflexion of the ankle joint. Usually, an abrupt onset of stabbing pain is followed by edema and spasm of the gastrocnemius.

Calcaneal Bursitis

Calcaneal bursitis (retroachilles bursitis) results from *inflammation of the bursa of the calcaneal tendon* located between the calcaneal tendon and the superior part of the posterior surface of the calcaneus (Fig. B5.16). Calcaneal bursitis causes pain posterior to the heel and occurs quite commonly during long-distance running, basketball, and tennis. It is caused by excessive friction on the bursa as the tendon continuously slides over it. *Inflammation of the subcutaneous calcaneal bursa* also results from repetitive microtrauma from the backs of shoes, usually new ones.

Venous Return from the Leg

A venous plexus deep to the triceps surae is involved in the return of blood from the leg. When a person is standing, the venous return from the leg depends largely on the ▶

Calcaneal tendon

Deep calcaneal bursa

Figure B5.16

muscular activity of the triceps surae (see "Venous Drainage of the Lower Limb," earlier in this chapter). Contraction of the calf muscles pumps blood superiorly in the deep veins. The efficiency of the calf pump is improved by the deep fascia that invests the muscles like an elastic stocking. Normally, blood is prevented from flowing into the superficial veins by the valves in the perforating veins. If these valves are incompetent, blood is forced into the superficial veins during contraction of the triceps surae and by hydrostatic pressure when straining or standing. As a consequence, the vessels become dilated and tortuous *varicose veins*.

Accessory Soleus

An accessory soleus is present in approximately 3% of people (Fig. B5.17). The accessory muscle usually appears as a distal belly medial to the calcaneal tendon. Clinically, an accessory soleus may be associated with pain and edema during prolonged exercise. ○

Posterior view

Figure B5.17

Deep Muscle Group in the Posterior Compartment

Four muscles make up the deep group in the posterior compartment of the leg (Figs. 5.34, 5.38–5.40): popliteus, flexor digitorum longus, flexor hallucis longus, and tibialis posterior. Details concerning the attachments, innervation, and actions of these muscles are provided in Table 5.13. The popliteus acts on the knee joint, whereas the other muscles

Medial view

Figure 5.39. Dissection demonstrating continuation of plantarflexor tendons across ankle joint. The foot is raised as in the push-off phase of walking. Observe the sesamoid bone acting as a "foot stool" for the 1st metatarsal, giving it extra height and protecting the flexor hallucis longus tendon.

plantarflex the ankle and flex the toes. However, because of their smaller size and the close proximity of their tendons to the axis of the ankle joint, the "non-triceps" plantarflexors collectively produce only about 7% of the total force of plantarflexion, and in this the fibularis longus and brevis are most significant. When the calcaneal tendon is ruptured, these muscles cannot generate the power necessary to lift the body's weight (i.e., to stand on the toes).

The two muscles of the posterior compartment that pass to the toes are criss-crossed—that is, the muscle attaching to the medial (great) toe (flexor hallucis longus) arises laterally (from the fibula) in the deep subcompartment, and the muscle attaching to the lateral four toes (flexor digitorum longus) arises medially (from the tibia) (Fig. 5.40). Their tendons cross in the sole of the foot.

Popliteus. The **popliteus** is a thin, triangular muscle that forms the inferior part of the floor of the popliteal fossa (Figs. 5.31, 5.32, and 5.38B). Proximally, its tendinous attachment to the lateral aspect of the lateral femoral condyle and its broader attachment to the lateral meniscus occur between the fibrous layer and the synovial membrane of the joint capsule of the knee. The apex of its fleshy belly emerges from the joint capsule of the knee joint. It has a fleshy distal attachment to the tibia that is covered by popliteal fascia reinforced by a fibrous expansion from the semimembranosus muscle.

Soleus

Gastrocnemius
tendon

Calcaneal
tendon

Flexor hallucis
longus (FHL)

Flexor
digitorum longus
(FDL)

Tibialis
posterior (TP)
tendon

Tibialis
anterior (TA)
tendon

Tuberosity of
navicular

Sesamoid
bones

Calcaneus

Quadratus plantae

Fibularis longus (FL)

Fibularis brevis (FB)

Flexor digitorum
longus (FDL) tendon

Slip from flexor
hallucis longus (FHL)

Flexor hallucis
longus (FHL) tendon

Lumbricals

Posteroinferior view

Figure 5.40. Dissection demonstrating continuation of plantarflexor tendons in second layer of sole of foot. This layer of foot muscles includes the tendons of the flexor hallucis longus and flexor digitorum longus, the four lumbrical (L. *lumbricus,* earthworm) muscles, and the quadratus plantae.

The popliteus is insignificant as a flexor of the knee joint per se; but during flexion at the knee, it assists in pulling the lateral meniscus posteriorly, a movement otherwise produced passively by compression (as it is for the medial meniscus; some have claimed this is part of the reason the lateral meniscus is injured less often). When a person is standing with the knee partly flexed, the popliteus contracts to assist the posterior cruciate ligament (PCL) in preventing anterior displacement of the femur on the inclined tibial plateau.

The **popliteus bursa** lies deep to the popliteus tendon (Fig. 5.38*B*). When standing with the knees locked in the fully extended position, the popliteus acts to rotate the femur laterally 5° on the tibial plateaus (see "Tibia," earlier in this chapter), releasing the knee from its close-packed or locked position so that flexion can occur. When the foot is off the ground and the knee is flexed, the popliteus can aid the medial hamstrings (the "semimuscles") in rotating the tibia medially beneath the femoral condyles.

Flexor Hallucis Longus. The **flexor hallucis longus** (FHL) is a powerful flexor of all of the joints of the great

toe. Immediately after the triceps surae has delivered the thrust of plantarflexion to the *ball of the foot* (the prominence of the sole underlying the heads of the 1st and 2nd metatarsals), the FHL delivers a final thrust via flexion of the great toe for the preswing phase (toe off) of the gait cycle (Table 5.2). When barefoot, this thrust is delivered by the great toe; but with soled shoes on, it becomes part of the thrust of plantarflexion delivered by the forefoot. The tendon of the FHL passes posterior to the distal end of the tibia and occupies a shallow groove on the posterior surface of the talus, which is continuous with the groove on the plantar surface of the talar shelf (Figs. 5.39 and 5.40). The tendon then crosses deep to the tendon of the flexor digitorum longus in the sole of the foot. As it passes to the distal phalanx of the great toe, the FHL tendon runs between two **sesamoid bones** in the tendons of the flexor hallucis brevis (Fig. 5.40). These bones protect the tendon from the pressure of the head of the 1st metatarsal bone.

To test the FHL, the distal phalanx of the great toe is flexed against resistance; if normal, the tendon can be seen and palpated on the plantar aspect of the great toe as it crosses the joints of the toe.

Flexor Digitorum Longus. The **flexor digitorum longus** (FDL) is smaller than the FHL, even though it moves four digits (Figs. 5.38*A*, 5.39, and 5.40). It passes diagonally into the sole of the foot, superficial to the tendon of the FHL. However, its direction of pull is realigned by the *quadratus plantae muscle,* which is attached to the posterolateral aspect of the FDL tendon as it divides into four tendons (Fig. 5.40), which in turn pass to the distal phalanges of the lateral four digits.

To test the FDL, the distal phalanges of the lateral four toes are flexed against resistance; if they are acting normally, the tendons of the toes can be seen and palpated.

Tibialis Posterior. The **tibialis posterior** (TP), the deepest (most anterior) muscle in the posterior compartment, lies between the FDL and the FHL in the same plane as the tibia and fibula within the deep subcompartment (Figs. 5.38*A*, 5.39, and 5.40). Distally, the TP attaches primarily to the navicular bone (in close proximity to the high point of the medial longitudinal arch of the foot) but has attachments to other tarsal and metatarsal bones (Figs. 5.44*D* and 5.68*A*; Table 5.13).

The TP is traditionally described as an invertor of the foot. Indeed, when the foot is off the ground, it can act synergistically with the TA to invert the foot, their otherwise antagonistic functions canceling each other out. However, the primary role of the TP is to support or maintain (fix) the medial longitudinal arch during weight bearing; consequently, the muscle contracts statically throughout the stance phase of gait (Fig. 5.69*C* & *E;* Table 5.2). In so doing, it acts independently of the TA because, once the foot is flat on the ground after heel strike, that muscle is relaxed during the stance phase (the dorsiflexion that occurs as the body passes over the planted foot is passive), unless braking requires its eccentric contraction. While standing (especially on one foot), however, the two muscles may cooperate to depress the lateral side of the foot and pull medially on the leg as needed to counteract lateral leaning for balance.

To test the tibialis posterior, the foot is inverted against resistance with the foot in slight plantarflexion; if normal, the tendon can be seen and palpated posterior to the medial malleolus.

Nerves in the Posterior Compartment

The *tibial nerve* (L4, L5, and S1–S3) is the larger of the two terminal branches of the *sciatic nerve.* It runs vertically through the popliteal fossa with the popliteal artery, passing between the heads of the gastrocnemius, the two structures exiting the fossa by passing deep to the tendinous arch of the soleus. The tibial nerve supplies all muscles in the posterior compartment of the leg (Figs. 5.34*A* and 5.38*A*; Table 5.11). At the ankle, the nerve lies between the tendons of the FHL and the FDL. Posteroinferior to the medial malleolus, the tibial nerve divides into the medial and lateral plantar nerves. A branch of the tibial nerve, the *medial sural cutaneous nerve,* is usually joined by the *sural communicating branch of the common fibular nerve* to form the **sural nerve.** This nerve supplies the skin of the lateral and posterior part of the inferior third of the leg and the lateral side of the foot. Articular branches of the tibial nerve supply the knee joint, and medial calcaneal branches supply the skin of the heel.

Arteries in the Posterior Compartment

The **posterior tibial artery,** the larger and more direct terminal branch of the popliteal artery, provides the blood supply to the posterior compartment of the leg and to the foot (Figs. 5.34*A*, 5.38*A*, and 5.41; Table 5.12). It begins at the distal border of the popliteus as the popliteal artery passes deep to the tendinous arch of the soleus and simultaneously bifurcates into its terminal branches. Close to its origin, the posterior tibial artery gives rise to its largest branch, the fibular artery (see below), which runs lateral and parallel to it, also within the deep subcompartment. During its descent, the posterior tibial artery is accompanied by the tibial nerve and veins. The artery runs posterior to the medial malleolus, from which it is separated by the tendons of the tibialis posterior and flexor digitorum longus. Inferior to the medial malleolus, it runs between the tendons of the flexor hallucis longus and flexor digitorum longus. Deep to the flexor retinaculum and the origin of the abductor hallucis, the posterior tibial artery divides into *medial and lateral plantar arteries,* the arteries of the sole of the foot.

The **fibular artery,** the largest and most important branch of the tibial artery, arises inferior to the distal border of the popliteus and the tendinous arch of the soleus (Figs. 5.38*A* and 5.41; Table 5.12). It descends obliquely toward the fibula and passes along its medial side, usually within the FHL. The fibular artery gives muscular branches to the popliteus and other muscles in both the posterior and the lateral compartments of the leg. It also gives rise to the *nutrient artery of the*

Posterior view with foot plantar flexed

Figure 5.41. Arteries of knee, posterior leg, and sole of foot. The popliteal artery bifurcates into the anterior and posterior tibial arteries; the latter gives rise to the fibular artery and terminates as it enters the foot, bifurcating into the medial and lateral plantar arteries.

fibula (Fig. 5.41). Distally, the fibular artery gives rise to a perforating branch and terminal lateral malleolar and calcaneal branches. The perforating branch pierces the *interosseous membrane* and passes to the dorsum of the foot, where it anastomoses with the arcuate artery. The *lateral calcaneal branches* supply the heel, and the *lateral malleolar branch* joins other malleolar branches to form a periarticular *arterial anastomosis of the ankle.*

The **circumflex fibular artery** arises from the origin of the anterior or posterior tibial artery at the knee and passes laterally over the neck of the fibula to the anastomoses around the knee.

The **nutrient artery of the tibia,** the largest nutrient artery in the body, arises from the origin of the anterior or posterior tibial artery. It pierces the tibialis posterior, to which it supplies branches, and enters the nutrient foramen in the proximal third of the posterior surface of the tibia.

Posterior Tibial Pulse

The posterior tibial pulse can usually be palpated between the posterior surface of the medial malleolus and the medial border of the calcaneal tendon (Fig. B5.18). Because the posterior tibial artery passes deep to the flexor retinaculum, it is important when palpating this pulse to have the person invert the foot to relax the retinaculum. Failure to do so may lead to the erroneous conclusion that the pulse is absent. Both arteries are examined simultaneously for equality of force. Palpation of the posterior tibial pulses is essential for examining patients with occlusive *peripheral arterial disease.* Although posterior tibial pulses are absent in approximately 15% of normal young people, absence of posterior tibial pulses is considered to be a sign of occlusive peripheral arterial disease in people older than 60 years. For example, *intermittent claudication,* characterized by leg pain and cramps, develops during walking and disappears after rest. These conditions result from ischemia of the leg muscles caused by narrowing or occlusion of the leg arteries. ☉

Medial malleolus
Posterior tibial artery
Calcaneal tendon

Figure B5.18

THE BOTTOM LINE: The posterior or plantarflexor compartment is subdivided by the transverse intermuscular septum into superficial and deep subcompartments. In the superficial subcompartment, the gastrocnemius and soleus muscles (the triceps surae) share a common tendon (the calcaneal tendon, the body's strongest tendon). The triceps surae provides the power of plantarflexion that propels the body in walking and plays a major role in running and jumping via push off. The deep muscles augment the action through flexion of the digits and support of the longitudinal arch of the foot. The contents of the compartment are supplied by the tibial nerve and two arteries, the (medial)

posterior tibial and fibular arteries. All three structures course within the confined deep subcompartment, where swelling may have profound consequences for the entire posterior compartment, the distal lateral compartment, and the foot.

Surface Anatomy of the Leg

The **tibial tuberosity** is an easily palpable elevation on the anterior aspect of the proximal part of the tibia, approximately 5 cm distal to the apex of the patella (Fig. SA5.3A). The tibial tuberosity indicates the level of the head of the fibula and the bifurcation of the popliteal artery into the anterior and posterior tibial arteries. The **patellar ligament** may be felt as it extends from the inferior border of the apex of the patella. It is most easily felt when the knee is extended. When the knee flexes to a right angle, a depression may be felt on each side of the patellar ligament. The joint cavity is superficial in these depressions. The **head of the fibula** is subcutaneous and may be palpated at the posterolateral aspect of the knee, at the level of the tibial tuberosity. The **neck of the fibula** can be palpated just distal to the head. The **tendon of the biceps femoris** may be traced by palpating its distal attachment to the lateral side of the head of the fibula. This tendon and the neck of the fibula guide the examining finger to the **common fibular nerve** (Fig. 5.37). The nerve is indicated by a line along the biceps femoris tendon, posterior to the head of the fibula, and around the lateral aspect of the fibular neck to its anterior aspect, just distal to the fibular head. The common fibular nerve can usually be palpated just posterior to the fibular head and rolled against the fibular neck with the fingertips.

The **anterior border of the tibia** is sharp, subcutaneous, and easily followed distally by palpation from the tibial tuberosity to the medial malleolus (Fig. SA5.3A–C). It is not usually perfectly straight. The medial surface of the **shaft of the tibia** is also subcutaneous, except at its proximal end. Its inferior third is crossed obliquely by the great saphenous vein as it passes proximally to the medial aspect of the knee.

The **tibialis anterior** lies superficially and is easily palpable just lateral to the anterior border of the tibia. As the foot is inverted and dorsiflexed, the large **tendon of the TA** can be seen and palpated as it runs distally and slightly medially over the anterior surface of the ankle joint to the medial side of the foot (Fig SA5.3C). If the 1st digit is dorsiflexed, the **tendon of the EHL** can be palpated just lateral to the tendon of the tibialis anterior. The **tendon of the extensor hallucis brevis** may also be visible. ▶

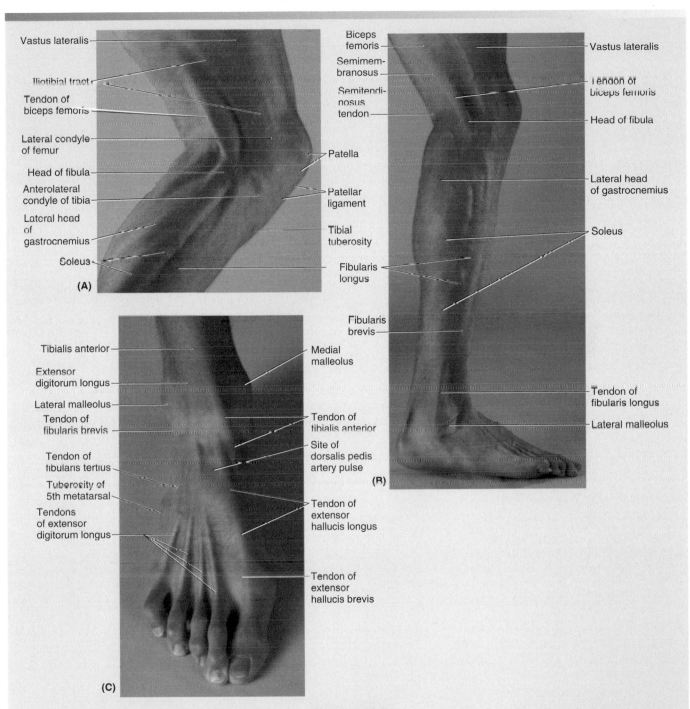

Figure SA5.3

As the toes are dorsiflexed, the **tendons of the EDL** can be palpated lateral to the extensor hallucis longus and followed to the four lateral digits. The **tendon of the FT** may be palpable lateral to the tendons of the EDL, especially when the foot is dorsiflexed and everted.

The **shaft of the fibula** is subcutaneous only in its distal part, proximal to the lateral malleolus; this part is the common site of fractures. The **medial** and **lateral malleoli** are subcutaneous and prominent. Palpate them, noting

that the tip of the lateral malleolus extends farther distally and posteriorly than the medial malleolus.

The **fibularis longus** is subcutaneous throughout its course (Fig. SA5.3B). The tendons of this muscle and the **fibularis brevis** are palpable when the foot is everted as they pass around the posterior aspect of the lateral malleolus. These tendons may be followed anteriorly along the lateral side of the foot. The tendon of the fibularis longus runs as far anteriorly as the cuboid and then disappears ▶

by turning into the sole of the foot. The **tendon of the FB** may be traced to its attachment to the base of the 5th metatarsal.

The **calcaneal tendon** can be easily followed to its attachment to the posterior part of the calcaneus. The ankle joint is fairly superficial in the depression on each side of the calcaneal tendon. The **heads of the gastrocnemius** are easily recognizable in the superior part of the calf of the leg (Fig. SA5.3*A* & *B*). The **soleus** can be palpated deep to and at the sides of the superior part of the calcaneal tendon. The **triceps surae** (soleus and gastrocnemius together) is easy to palpate when the individual is standing on the toes. The soleus can be distinguished from the gastrocnemius during squatting (flexing the knees while standing on toes) because flexion of the knee to approximately 90° makes the gastrocnemius flaccid; plantarflexion in this position is maintained by the soleus. The deep muscles of the posterior compartment are not easily palpated, but their tendons can be observed just posterior to the medial malleolus, especially when the foot is inverted and the toes are flexed. ☉

Foot

The clinical importance of the foot is indicated by the considerable amount of time primary care physicians devote to foot problems. *Podiatry* is the specialized field that deals with the study and care of the feet.

The *ankle* refers to the narrowest and malleolar parts of the distal leg, proximal to the dorsum and heel of the foot, including the ankle joint. The *foot,* distal to the ankle, provides a platform for supporting the body when standing and has an important role in locomotion. The skeleton of the foot consists of 7 tarsals, 5 metatarsals, and 14 phalanges (Fig. 5.42; Table 5.14). The foot and its bones

Figure 5.42. Retinacula of ankle and parts of foot. The disposition of the bones of the foot and the superior and inferior extensor and fibular retinacula relative to surface features are demonstrated.

Table 5.14-I. Muscles of the Foot: 1st and 2nd Layers of the Sole

Plantar view

(A)

Muscle	Proximal Attachment	Distal Attachment	Innervation[a]	Main Action[b]
1st layer				
Abductor hallucis	Medial tubercle of tuberosity of calcaneus; flexor retinaculum; plantar aponeurosis	Medial side of base of proximal phalanx of 1st digit	Medial plantar nerve (S2, S3)	Abducts and flexes 1st digit (great toe, hallux)
Flexor digitorum brevis	Medial tubercle of tuberosity of calcaneus; plantar aponeurosis; intermuscular septa	Both sides of middle phalanges of lateral four digits	Medial plantar nerve (S2, S3)	Flexes lateral four digits
Abductor digiti minimi	Medial and lateral tubercles of tuberosity of calcaneus; plantar aponeurosis; intermuscular septa	Lateral side of base of proximal phalanx of 5th digit	Lateral plantar nerve (S2, S3)	Abducts and flexes little toe (5th digit)
2nd layer				
Quadratus plantae	Medial surface and lateral margin of plantar surface of calcaneus	Posterolateral margin of tendon of flexor digitorum longus	Lateral plantar nerve (S2, S3)	Assists flexor digitorum longus in flexing lateral four digits (toes)
Lumbricals	Tendons of flexor digitorum longus	Medial aspect of expansion over lateral four digits	Medial one: medial plantar nerve (S2, S3) Lateral three: lateral plantar nerve (S2, S3)	Flex proximal phalanges, extend middle and distal phalanges of lateral four digits (toes)

[a] The spinal cord segmental innervation is indicated (e.g., "S2, S3" means that the nerves supplying the abductor hallucis are derived from the second and third sacral segments of the spinal cord). Damage to one or more of the listed spinal cord segments or to the motor nerve roots arising from them results in paralysis of the muscles concerned.
[b] Despite individual actions, the primary function of the intrinsic muscles of the sole of the foot is to resist flattening or maintain the arch of the foot.

may be considered in terms of three anatomical and functional parts:

- The **hindfoot:** talus and calcaneus.
- The **midfoot:** navicular, cuboid, and cuneiforms.
- The **forefoot:** metatarsals and phalanges.

The part/region of the foot contacting the floor or ground is the *sole* (L. *planta*) or *plantar region* (L. *regio plantaris*), and the part directed superiorly is the *dorsum of the foot* (L. *dorsum pedis*) or **dorsal region of the foot** (L. *regio dorsalis pedis*). The sole of the foot underlying the calcaneus is the *heel* or **heel region** (L. *regio calcanea*) and the sole underlying the heads of the medial two metatarsals is the *ball of the foot*. The *great toe*

Table 5.14-II. Muscles of the Foot: 3rd and 4th layers of the Sole

Plantar view

(B)

Layer 3   Layer 4

Plantar view   Dorsal view

Muscle	Proximal Attachment	Distal Attachment	Innervation[a]	Main Action[b]
3rd layer				
Flexor hallucis brevis	Plantar surfaces of cuboid and lateral cuneiforms	Both sides of base of proximal phalanx of 1st digit	Medial plantar nerve (S2, S3)	Flexes proximal phalanx of 1st digit
Adductor hallucis	Oblique head: bases of metatarsals 2–4 Transverse head: plantar ligaments of metatarsophalangeal joints	Tendons of both heads attach to lateral side of base of proximal phalanx of 1st digit	Deep branch of lateral plantar nerve (S2, S3)	Traditionally said to adduct 1st digit; assists in transverse arch of foot by metatarsals medially
Flexor digit minimi brevis	Base of 5th metatarsal	Base of proximal phalanx of 5th digit	Superficial branch of lateral plantar nerve (S2, S3)	Flexes proximal phalanx of 5th digit, thereby assisting with its flexion
4th layer				
Plantar interossei (three muscles)	Bases and medial sides of metatarsals 3–5	Medial sides of bases of phalanges of 3rd–5th digits	Lateral plantar nerve (S2, S3)	Adduct digits (2–4) and flex metatarsophalangeal joints
Dorsal interossei (four muscles)	Adjacent sides of metatarsals 1–5	1st: medial side of proximal phalanx of 2nd digit; 2nd–4th: lateral sides of 2nd–4th digits	Lateral plantar nerve (S2, S3)	Abduct digits (2–4) and flex metatarsophalangeal joints

[a] The spinal cord segmental innervation is indicated (e.g., "S2, S3" means that the nerves supplying the flexor hallucis brevis are derived from the second and third sacral segments of the spinal cord). Damage to one or more of the listed spinal cord segments or to the motor nerve roots arising from them results in paralysis of the muscles concerned.

[b] Despite individual actions, the primary function of the intrinsic muscles of the sole of the foot is to resist flattening or maintain the arch of the foot.

(L. *hallux*) is also the **1st toe** (L. *digitus primus*); the *little toe* (L. *digitus minimus*) is also the **5th toe** (L. *digitus quintus*).

Skin and Fascia of the Foot

Marked variations occur in the thickness (strength) and texture of skin, subcutaneous tissue (superficial fascia), and deep fascia in relationship to weight bearing and distribution, ground contact (grip, abrasion), and the need for containment or compartmentalization.

Skin and Subcutaneous Tissue

The skin of the dorsum of the foot is much thinner and less sensitive than skin on most of the sole. The subcutaneous

Table 5.14-III. **Muscles of the Foot: Dorsum of the Foot**

Calcaneus

Extensor hallucis brevis

Extensor digitorum brevis

Dorsal interossei

Extensor hallucis brevis

Extensor digitorum longus tendons (cut)

(C) Anterosuperior views

Adductor hallucis (transverse head)

Flexor hallucis brevis

Adductor hallucis (oblique head)

Flexor digiti minimi brevis

Layer 3

(D)

Plantar interossei

Dorsal interossei

Layer 4

Muscle	Proximal Attachment	Distal Attachment	Innervation[a]	Main Action
Extensor digitorum brevis	Calcaneus (floor of tarsal sinus); Interosseous talocalcaneal ligament; stem of inferior extensor retinaculum	Long flexor tendons of four medial toes (digits 2–5)	Deep fibular nerve (L5 or S1, or both)	Aids the extensor digitorum longus in extending the four medial toes at the metatarsophalangeal and interphalangeal joints
Extensor hallucis brevis	In common with extensor digitorum brevis (above)	Dorsal aspect of base of proximal phalanx of great toe (digit 1)		Aids the extensor hallucis longus in extending the great toe at the metatarsophalangeal joint

[a] The spinal cord segmental innervation is indicated (e.g., "L5 or S1" means that the nerve supplying the extensor digitorum brevis is derived from either the fifth lumbar segment or first sacral segment of the spinal cord). Damage to one or more of the listed spinal cord segments or to the motor nerve roots arising from them results in paralysis of the muscles concerned.

tissue is loose deep to the dorsal skin; therefore, *edema* (G. *oide ̄ma,* a swelling) is most marked over this surface, especially anterior to and around the medial malleolus. The skin over the major weight-bearing areas of the sole—the heel, lateral margin, and ball of the foot—is thick. The subcutaneous tissue in the sole is more fibrous than in other areas of the foot. **Fibrous septa** (highly developed skin ligaments, retinac-

ula cutis; see Introduction) divide this tissue into fat-filled areas, making it a shock-absorbing pad, especially over the heel. The skin ligaments also anchor the skin to the underlying deep fascia (plantar aponeurosis), improving the "grip" of the sole. The skin of the sole is hairless and sweat glands are numerous; the entire sole is sensitive (ticklish), especially the thinner-skinned area underlying the arch.

Deep Fascia of the Foot

The deep fascia is thin on the dorsum of the foot, where it is continuous proximally with the *inferior extensor retinaculum* (Fig. 5.43*A*). Over the lateral and posterior aspects of the foot, the deep fascia is continuous with the **plantar fascia**, the deep fascia of the sole (Fig. 5.43*B & C*). The plantar fascia has a thick central part and weaker medial and lateral parts. The thick, central part forms the strong **plantar aponeurosis**, longitudinally arranged bundles of dense fibrous connective tissue investing the central plantar muscles. It resembles the palmar aponeurosis of the palm of the hand (Chapter 6) but is tougher, denser, and elongated. The plantar fascia holds the parts of the foot together, helps protect the sole from injury, and helps support the longitudinal arches of the foot.

The plantar aponeurosis arises posteriorly from the calcaneus and functions like a superficial ligament. Distally, the longitudinal bundles of collagen fibers of the aponeurosis divide into five bands that become continuous with the *fibrous digital sheaths* that enclose the flexor tendons that pass to the toes. At the anterior end of the sole, inferior to the heads of the metatarsals, the aponeurosis is reinforced by transverse fibers forming the **superficial transverse metatarsal ligament.**

In the midfoot and forefoot, vertical *intermuscular septa* extend deeply (superiorly) from the margins of the plantar aponeurosis toward the 1st and 5th metatarsals, forming the three *compartments of the sole* (Fig. 5.43*C*):

1. The **medial compartment of the sole** is covered superficially by thinner *medial plantar fascia*. It contains the

(A) **Fascia of dorsum of foot (anterolateral view)**

Inferior extensor retinaculum

Dorsal fascia of foot

Key

- ■ Medial compartment of sole
- □ Central compartment of sole
- □ Lateral compartment of sole
- □ Interosseous compartment of foot
- ■ Dorsal compartment of foot

Dorsal fascia

Plantar fascia

(C) **Transverse section of foot compartments (anterior view)**

Flexor digitorum longus

Fibrous digital sheaths

Superficial transverse metatarsal ligament

Lateral plantar fascia

Cutaneous branches of lateral plantar vessels and nerves

Fat pad

Flexor hallucis longus

Site of sesamoid bones of great toe

Plantar digital nerves and arteries

Medial plantar fascia

Cutaneous branches of medial plantar nerve and artery

Medial calcaneal nerve and artery

(B) **Plantar aspect or sole of foot (inferior view)**

Figure 5.43. Fascia and compartments of foot. A. The skin and subcutaneous tissue have been removed to demonstrate the deep fascia of the leg and dorsum of the foot. **B.** The deep plantar fascia consists of the thick plantar aponeurosis and the thinner medial and lateral plantar fascia. The aponeurosis consists of longitudinal bands of dense fibrous connective tissue. Thinner parts of the plantar fascia have been removed, revealing the plantar digital vessels and nerves. **C.** The bones and muscles of the foot are surrounded by the deep dorsal and plantar fascia. A large central and smaller medial and lateral compartments of the sole are created by intermuscular septa that extend deeply from the plantar aponeurosis.

abductor hallucis, flexor hallucis brevis, the tendon of the flexor hallucis longus, and the medial plantar nerve and vessels.

2. The **central compartment of the sole** is covered superficially by the dense *plantar aponeurosis*. It contains the flexor digitorum brevis, the tendons of the flexor hallucis longus and flexor digitorum longus plus the muscles associated with the latter, the quadratus plantae and lumbricals, and the adductor hallucis. The lateral plantar nerve and vessels are also located here.

3. The **lateral compartment of the sole** is covered superficially by the thinner *lateral plantar fascia* and contains the abductor and flexor digiti minimi brevis.

In the forefoot only, a fourth compartment, the **interosseous compartment of the foot**, is surrounded by the plantar and dorsal interosseous fascias. It contains the metatarsals, the dorsal and plantar interosseous muscles, and the deep plantar and metatarsal vessels. Whereas the plantar interossei and plantar metatarsal vessels are distinctly plantar in position, the remaining structures of the compartment are located intermediate between the plantar and the dorsal aspects of the foot.

A fifth compartment, the **dorsal compartment of the foot**, lies between the dorsal fascia of the foot and the tarsal bones and the dorsal interosseous fascia of the midfoot and forefoot. It contains the muscles (extensors hallucis brevis and extensor digitorum brevis) and neurovascular structures of the dorsum of the foot.

Muscles of the Foot

Of the 20 individual muscles of the foot, 14 are located on the plantar aspect, 2 are on the dorsal aspect, and 4 are intermediate in position. From the plantar aspect, muscles of the sole are arranged in four layers within four compartments. The muscles of the foot are illustrated and their attachments, innervation, and actions are described by compartment and by layer in Figures 5.43C, 5.44, and 5.45B and Table 5.14.

Despite their compartmental and layered arrangement, the plantar muscles function primarily as a group during the support phase of stance, maintaining the arches of the foot (Table 5.2). They basically resist forces that tend to reduce the longitudinal arch as weight is received at the heel (posterior end of the arch) and is then transferred to the ball of the foot and great toe (anterior end of the arch). The muscles become most active in the later portion of the movement to stabilize the foot for propulsion (push off), a time when forces also tend to flatten the foot's transverse arch. Concurrently, they are also able to refine further the efforts of the long muscles, producing supination and pronation in enabling the platform of the foot to adjust to uneven ground. The muscles of the foot are of little importance individually because fine control of the individual toes is not important to most people. Rather than producing actual movement, they are most active in fixing the foot or in increasing the pressure applied against the ground by various aspects of the sole or toes to maintain balance.

Although the adductor hallucis resembles a similar muscle of the palm that adducts the thumb and despite its name, the

(cont'd on page 666)

Plantar Fasciitis

Straining and inflammation of the plantar aponeurosis, a condition called *plantar fasciitis,* may result from running and high-impact aerobics, especially when inappropriate footwear is worn. Plantar fasciitis is the most common hindfoot problem in runners (Middleton and Kolodon, 1992). It causes pain on the plantar surface of the heel and on the medial aspect of the foot. The pain is often most severe after sitting and when beginning to walk in the morning, but dissipates after 5–10 minutes of activity, often recurring again following rest. Point tenderness is located at the proximal attachment of the aponeurosis to the medial tubercle of the calcaneus and on the medial surface of this bone. The pain increases with passive extension of the great toe and may be further exacerbated by dorsiflexion of the ankle and/or weight bearing. If a *calcaneal spur* (abnormal bony process) protrudes from the medial tubercle, plantar fasciitis is likely to cause pain on the medial side of the foot when walking (Fig. B5.19). Usually a bursa develops at the end of the spur that may also become inflamed and tender. ✺

Calcaneus

Calcaneal spur

Bursa

Figure B5.19

Plantar digital nerves and arteries

Plantar digital nerves

Branch connecting lateral and medial plantar nerves

Flexor digiti minimi

Abductor digiti minimi*

Flexor digitorum brevis* (FDB)

Tendon of flexor hallucis longus (FHL)

1st lumbrical

Flexor hallucis brevis (FHB)

Abductor hallucis* (AH)

Plantar aponeurosis, reflected

*First layer muscles

(A) 1st layer

Flexor digitorum brevis (FDB) (cut tendons)

Lumbrical muscles*

Interosseous muscles

Quadratus plantae*

Abductor digiti minimi

Abductor digiti minimi (deep head)

Sesamoid bones

Tendon of flexor hallucis longus* (FHL)

Flexor hallucis brevis (FHB)

Tendons of flexor digitorum longus* (FDL)

Abductor hallucis

Flexor digitorum brevis (FDB)

Calcaneal tuberosity

*Second layer tendons and muscles

(B) 2nd layer

Plantar ligament (plate)

Deep transverse metatarsal ligament

Adductor hallucis (transverse head)*

Flexor digiti minimi*

Deep branch of lateral plantar artery and nerve

Lateral plantar artery and nerve

Abductor digiti minimi

Flexor digitorum brevis (FDB) Plantar aponeurosis

Fibrous digital sheath

Adductor hallucis (oblique head)*

Lateral head of flexor hallucis brevis* (FHB)

Medial head of flexor hallucis brevis*(FHB)

Flexor hallucis longus (FHL)

Flexor digitorum longus (FDL)

Medial plantar nerve

Abductor hallucis (AH)

Quadratus plantae

*Third layer muscles

(C) 3rd layer

Flexor digitorum longus (FDL)

Flexor digitorum brevis (FDB)

Dorsal (D) and plantar (P) interosseous muscles*

Flexor digiti minimi brevis

Lateral "cord" of plantar aponeurosis

Fibularis longus (FL)

Abductor digiti minimi

Flexor digitorum brevis (FDB) Plantar aponeurosis

Flexor hallucis longus (FHL)

Sesamoids

Plantar ligament (plate)

Flexor hallucis brevis (FHB) (medial head)

Flexor hallucis brevis (FHB) (lateral head)

Tibialis posterior (TP) (insertion)

Plantar calcaneonavicular ligament (spring ligament)

Long plantar ligament

Abductor hallucis

*Fourth layer muscles

(D) 4th layer

Inferior views (plantar aspect of foot)

Figure 5.44. Layers of plantar muscles. A. The 1st layer consists of the abductors of the large and small toes, and the short flexor of the toes. **B.** The 2nd layer consists of the long flexor tendons and associated muscles: four lumbricals and the quadratus plantae. **C.** The 3rd layer consists of the flexor of the little toe and the flexor and adductor of the great toe. Also demonstrated are the neurovascular structures that course in a plane between the 1st and 2nd layers. **D.** The 4th layer consists of the dorsal and plantar interosseous muscles.

(A)

Plantar digital arteries proper

Perforating artery (deep plantar artery-from dorsal artery of foot)

Plantar metatarsal arteries

Deep plantar arch

Perforating branches

Superficial arch

Medial plantar artery

Lateral plantar artery

Posterior tibial artery

Calcaneal branch

Posterolateral views

Key for layers

■	1st
■ □	2nd
■	3rd
□ ■	4th*

* The 4th layer (interosseous muscles) is indirectly represented by the bones, representing the layer in which the interosseous muscles occur.

Schema

Interosseous muscles

Dorsal artery of foot

Transverse head of adductor hallucis

Flexor hallucis brevis

Abductor hallucis

Oblique head of adductor hallucis

Flexor digitorum brevis

Medial plantar artery

Flexor hallucis longus (FHL) tendon

Posterior tibial artery

Deep plantar artery

Perforating branches

Deep branch of lateral plantar nerve

Deep plantar arch

Lumbrical muscles

Lateral plantar artery and nerve

Flexor digiti minimi

Flexor digitorum longus (FDL) tendon

Quadratus plantae muscles

Abductor digiti minimi

(B)

Figure 5.45. Arteries and muscle layers of foot. A and B. The posterior tibial artery terminates as it enters the foot by dividing into the medial and lateral plantar arteries. Observe the distal anastomoses of these vessels with the deep plantar artery from the dorsal artery of the foot and the perforating branches to the arcuate artery on the dorsum of the foot (Fig. 5.47). Note that the plantar arteries enter and run in the plane between the 1st and the 2nd layers, with the lateral plantar artery passing from medial to lateral. The deep branches of the artery then pass from lateral to medial between the 3rd and the 4th layers adductor hallucis is probably most active during the push-off phase of stance in pulling the lateral four metatarsals toward the great toe, fixing the transverse arch of the foot, and resisting forces that would spread the metatarsal heads as weight and force are applied to the forefoot (Table 5.2).

In Table 5.14, note that the:

• **P**lantar interossei **AD**duct (**PAD**) and arise from a single metatarsal as unipennate muscles.

• **D**orsal interossei **AB**duct (**DAB**) and arise from two metatarsals as bipennate muscles.

There are two neurovascular planes between the muscle layers of the sole of the foot (Figs. 5.44 and 5.45*B*): (1) a superficial one between the 1st and the 2nd muscular layers, and (2) a deep one between the 3rd and the 4th muscular layers. The *tibial nerve* divides posterior to the medial malleolus into the *medial* and *lateral plantar nerves* (Figs. 5.38*A* and 5.46; Table 5.15). These nerves supply the intrinsic muscles of the plantar aspect of the foot. The medial plantar nerve courses within the medial compartment of the sole between the 1st and the 2nd muscle layers. Initially, the lateral plantar artery and nerve run laterally between the muscles of the 1st and 2nd layers of plantar muscles (Figs. 5.44*C* and 5.45*B*). Their deep branches then pass medially between the muscles of the 3rd and 4th layers (Fig. 5.45*B*).

Two closely connected muscles on the dorsum of the foot are the **extensor digitorum brevis** (EDB) and **extensor hallucis brevis** (EHB) (Figs. 5.35*A* & *B* and 5.36*A*). These thin, broad muscles form a fleshy mass on the lateral part of the dorsum of the foot, anterior to the lateral malleolus. The EHB is actually part of the EDB. Its small fleshy belly may be felt when the toes are extended.

THE BOTTOM LINE: The intrinsic muscles of the plantar surface of the foot are arranged in four layers and divided into four fascial compartments. A tough plantar aponeurosis overlies the central compartment, passively contributing to arch maintenance and, along with firmly bound fat, protecting the vessels and nerves from compression. There is similarity to the arrangement of muscles in the palm of the hand, but the muscles of the foot generally respond as a group rather than individually, acting to fix the foot or push a portion of it harder against the ground to maintain balance. The movements of abduction and adduction produced by the interossei are toward or away from the 2nd digit. The foot has two intrinsic muscles on its dorsum that augment the long extensor muscles. The plantar intrinsic muscles function throughout the stance phase of gait, from heel strike to toe off, resisting forces that tend to spread the arches of the foot. They are especially active in fixing the medial forefoot for the propulsive push off. The plantar intrinsic muscles are innervated by the medial and lateral plantar nerves, whereas the dorsal muscles are innervated by the deep fibular nerve.

(A)

(B)

Figure 5.46. Arteries of foot: branching and communicating. A. The arteries of the midfoot and forefoot resemble those of the hand in that (1) arches on the two aspects give rise to metatarsal (metacarpal) arteries, which in turn give rise to digital arteries; (2) the dorsal arteries are exhausted before reaching the distal ends of the digits, so the plantar (palmar) digital arteries send branches dorsally to supply the distal dorsal aspects of the digits, including the nail beds; and (3) perforating branches extend between the metatarsals (metacarpals) forming anastomoses between the arches of each side. **B.** The parent neurovascular structures giving rise to plantar vessels and nerves pass posterior to the medial malleolus and then divide, their terminal plantar branches entering the sole by passing deep to the abductor hallucis and coursing between the 1st and the 2nd muscle layers of the sole.

Infections of the Foot

Foot infections are common, especially in seasons, climates, and cultures where shoes are less commonly worn. A neglected puncture wound may lead to an extensive deep infection, resulting in swelling, pain, and fever. Deep infections of the foot often localize ▶

(*cont'd on page 668*)

Table 5.15. Nerves of the Foot

Dorsal view   Plantar view

Nerve[a]	Origin	Course	Distribution in Foot
Saphenous (1)	Femoral nerve	Arises in femoral triangle and descends through thigh and leg; accompanies great saphenous vein anterior to medial malleolus; ends on medial side of foot	Supplies skin on medial side of foot as far anteriorly as head of 1st metatarsal
Superficial fibular (2)	Common fibular nerve	Pierces deep fascia in distal third of leg to become cutaneous; then sends branches to foot and digits	Supplies skin on dorsum of foot and all digits, except lateral side of 5th and adjoining sides of the 1st and 2nd digits
Deep fibular (3)		Passes deep to extensor retinaculum to enter dorsum of foot	Supplies extensor digitorum brevis and skin on contiguous sides of 1st and 2nd digits
Medial plantar (4)	Larger terminal branch of tibial nerve	Passes distally in foot between abductor hallucis and flexor digitorum brevis; divides into muscular and cutaneous branches	Supplies skin of medial side of sole of foot and sides of first three digits; also supplies abductor hallucis, flexor digitorum brevis, flexor hallucis brevis, and first lumbrical
Lateral plantar (5)	Smaller terminal branch of tibial nerve	Passes laterally in foot between quadratus plantae and flexor digitorum brevis muscles; divides into superficial and deep branches	Supplies quadratus plantae, abductor digiti minimi, digiti minimi brevis; deep branch supplies plantar and dorsal interossei, lateral three lumbricals, and adductor hallucis; supplies skin on sole lateral to a line splitting 4th digit
Sural (6)	Usually arises from both tibial and common fibular nerves	Passes inferior to the lateral malleolus to lateral side of foot	Lateral aspect of hindfoot and midfoot
Calcaneal branches (7)	Tibial and sural nerves	Pass from distal part of the posterior aspect of leg to skin on heel	Skin of heel

[a]Numbers refer to the figure.

within the compartments between the muscular layers. A well-established infection in one of the enclosed fascial or muscular spaces usually requires surgical incision and drainage. When possible, the incision is made on the medial side of the foot, passing superior to the abductor hallucis to allow visualization of critical neurovascular structures, while avoiding production of a painful scar in a weight-bearing area.

Contusion of the Extensor Digitorum Brevis

Functionally, the EDB and EHB muscles are relatively unimportant. Clinically, knowing the location of the belly of the EDB is important for distinguishing it from abnormal edema. Contusion and tearing of the muscle's fibers and associated blood vessels result in a *hematoma,* producing edema anteromedial to the lateral malleolus. Most people who have not seen this inflamed muscle assume they have a severely sprained ankle. ⊕

Neurovascular Structures and Relationships in the Foot

Nerves of the Foot

The cutaneous innervation of the foot is supplied (Table 5.15):

- Medially by the saphenous nerve, which extends distally to the head of 1st metatarsal.

- Superiorly (dorsum of foot) by the superficial (primarily) and deep fibular nerves.

- Inferiorly (sole of foot) by the medial and lateral plantar nerves; the common border of their distribution extends along the 4th metacarpal and digit. (This is similar to the pattern of innervation of the palm; see Chapter 6.)

- Laterally by the sural nerve, including part of the heel.

- Posteriorly (heel) by calcaneal branches of the tibial and sural nerves.

Saphenous Nerve. The *saphenous nerve* is the largest (longest and most widely distributed) cutaneous branch of the femoral nerve; it is the only branch to extend beyond the knee (Fig. 5.48*B;* Table 5.1). In addition to supplying the skin and fascia on the anteromedial aspect of the leg, the saphenous nerve passes anterior to the medial malleolus to the dorsum of the foot, where it supplies articular branches to the ankle joint and continues to supply skin along the medial side of the foot as far anteriorly as the head of the 1st metatarsal (Table 5.15).

Superficial and Deep Fibular Nerves. After coursing between and supplying the fibular muscles in the lateral compartment of the leg, the *superficial fibular nerve* emerges as a cutaneous nerve about two thirds of the way down the leg. It then supplies the skin on the anterolateral aspect of the leg and divides into the **medial** and **intermediate dorsal cutaneous nerves,** which continue across the ankle to supply most of the skin on the dorsum of the foot. Its terminal branches are the dorsal digital nerves (common and proper) that supply the skin of the proximal aspect of the medial half of the great toe and that of the lateral three and a half digits.

After supplying the muscles of the anterior compartment of the leg, the *deep fibular nerve* passes deep to the extensor retinaculum and supplies the intrinsic muscles on the dorsum of the foot (extensors digitorum and hallucis longus) and the tarsal and tarsometatarsal joints. When it finally emerges as a cutaneous nerve, it is so far distal in the foot that only a small area of skin remains available for innervation: the web of skin between and contiguous sides of the 1st and 2nd toes. It innervates this area as the **1st common dorsal** (and then **proper dorsal) digital nerve(s).**

Medial Plantar Nerve. The **medial plantar nerve,** the larger and more anterior of the two terminal branches of the tibial nerve, arises deep to the flexor retinaculum and enters the sole of the foot by passing deep to the abductor hallucis (Figs. 5.44*C* and 5.46*B*). It then runs anteriorly between this muscle and the flexor digitorum brevis, supplying both with motor branches on the lateral side of the medial plantar artery (Fig. 5.44*A* and *C*). After sending motor branches to the flexor hallucis brevis and 1st lumbrical muscle, the medial plantar nerve terminates near the bases of the metatarsals by dividing into three sensory branches (common plantar digital nerves). These branches supply the skin of the medial three and a half digits (including the dorsal skin and nail beds of their distal phalanges), and the skin of the sole proximal to them. Compared to the other terminal branch of the tibial nerve, the medial plantar nerve supplies more skin area but fewer muscles. Its distribution to both skin and muscles of the foot is comparable to that of the median nerve in the hand (Chapter 6).

Lateral Plantar Nerve. The **lateral plantar nerve,** the smaller and more posterior of the two terminal branches of the tibial nerve, also courses deep to the abductor hallucis (Fig. 5.46*B*) but runs anterolaterally between the 1st and 2nd layers of plantar muscles, on the medial side of the lateral plantar artery (Fig. 5.44*C*). The lateral plantar nerve terminates as it reaches the lateral compartment, dividing into superficial and deep branches (Table 5.15). The superficial branch divides, in turn, into two plantar digital nerves (one common and one proper) that supply the skin of the plantar aspects of the lateral one and a half digits, the dorsal skin and nail beds of their distal phalanges, and skin of the sole proximal to them. The deep branches of the lateral plantar nerve course with the plantar arterial arch between the 3rd and the 4th muscle layers. The superficial and deep branches supply all muscles of the sole not supplied by the medial plantar nerve. Compared to the latter, the lateral plantar nerve supplies less skin area but more individual muscles. Its distribution to both skin and muscles of the foot is comparable to that of the ulnar nerve in the hand (Chapter 6). The medial and lateral plantar nerves also provide innervation to the plantar aspects of all the joints of the foot.

Sural Nerve. The *sural nerve* is formed by union of the *medial sural cutaneous nerve* (from the tibial nerve) and *sural communicating branch of the common fibular nerve,* respectively (Fig. 5.48*B*; Table 5.11). The level of junction of these branches is variable; it may be high (in the popliteal fossa) or low (proximal to heel), and sometimes the branches do not join and, therefore, no sural nerve is formed. In these people, the skin normally innervated by the sural nerve is supplied by the medial and lateral sural cutaneous branches. The sural nerve accompanies the small saphenous vein and enters the foot posterior to the lateral malleolus to supply the ankle joint and skin along the lateral margin of the foot (Table 5.15).

Sural Nerve Grafts

Pieces of the sural nerve are often used for nerve grafts in procedures such as repairing nerve defects resulting from wounds. The surgeon is usually able to locate this nerve in relation to the small saphenous vein (Fig. 5.48*B*). Because of the variations in the level of formation of the sural nerve, the surgeon may have to make incisions in both legs, and then select the better specimen.

Anesthetic Block of the Superficial Fibular Nerve

After the superficial fibular nerve pierces the deep fascia to become a cutaneous nerve, it divides into medial and intermediate cutaneous nerves. In thin people, these branches can often be seen or felt as ridges under the skin when the foot is plantarflexed. Injections of an anesthetic agent around these branches in the ankle region, anterior to the palpable portion of the fibula, anesthetizes the skin on the dorsum of the foot (except the web between and adjacent surfaces of the 1st and 2nd toes) more broadly and effectively than more local injections on the dorsum of the foot for superficial surgery.

Plantar Reflex

The **plantar reflex** (L4, L5, S1, and S2 nerve roots) is a myotatic (deep tendon) reflex that is routinely tested during neurologic examinations. The lateral aspect of the sole of the foot is stroked with a blunt object, such as a tongue depressor, beginning at the heel and crossing to the base of the great toe. The motion is firm and continuous but neither painful nor ticklish. Flexion of the toes is a normal response. Slight fanning of the lateral four toes and dorsiflexion of the great toe is an abnormal response (*Babinski sign*), indicating brain injury or cerebral disease, except in infants. Because the corticospinal tracts are not fully developed in newborns, a Babinski sign is usually elicited and may be present until children are 4 years of age.

Medial Plantar Nerve Entrapment

Compressive irritation of the medial plantar nerve as it passes deep to the flexor retinaculum or curves deep to the abductor hallucis may cause aching, burning, numbness, and tingling (paresthesia) on the medial side of the sole and in the region of the navicular tuberosity. *Medial plantar nerve compression* may occur during repetitive eversion of the foot (e.g., during gymnastics and running). Because of its frequency in runners, these symptoms have been called "jogger's foot." ⊙

THE BOTTOM LINE: Most of the dorsum of the foot receives cutaneous innervation from the superficial fibular nerve, the exception being the skin of the web between and the adjacent sides of the 1st and 2nd toes. The latter receives innervation from the deep fibular nerve after it supplies the muscles on the dorsum of the foot. The skin of the medial and lateral sides of the foot is innervated by the saphenous and sural nerves, respectively. The plantar aspect of the foot receives innervation from the larger medial and smaller lateral plantar nerves, the former supplying more skin (the plantar aspect of the medial three and half toes and adjacent sole) but fewer muscles (the medial hallux and 1st lumbrical muscles only) than the latter, which supplies the remaining muscles and skin of the plantar aspect. The distribution of the medial and lateral plantar nerves is comparable to that of the median and ulnar nerves in the palm.

Arteries of the Foot

The arteries of the foot are terminal branches of the anterior and posterior tibial arteries (Figs. 5.46*B* and 5.47), respectively: the dorsal and plantar arteries.

Dorsal Artery of the Foot. The **dorsal artery of the foot** (L. *arteria dorsalis pedis*)—often a major source of blood supply to the forefoot (e.g., during extended periods of standing)—is the direct continuation of the anterior tibial artery (Fig. 5.47*A*). The dorsal artery begins midway between the malleoli and runs anteromedially, deep to the inferior extensor retinaculum between the extensor hallucis longus and the extensor digitorum longus tendons on the dorsum of the foot. The dorsal artery passes to the first interosseous space, where

(A) Dorsum of foot

(B) Plantar aspect of foot

Figure 5.47. Arteries of foot: overview. A. Observe the anterior tibial artery becoming the dorsal artery of the foot (L. *arteria dorsalis pedis*) and the arcuate artery. **B.** Observe the posterior tibial artery and its terminal branches, the medial and lateral plantar arteries. The deep plantar arch is formed by the lateral plantar artery. Note the anastomoses between the dorsal and the plantar arteries through the deep plantar artery and perforating branches of the deep plantar arch.

it divides into the 1st dorsal metatarsal artery and a **deep plantar artery.** The latter passes deeply between the heads of the first dorsal interosseous muscle to enter the sole of the foot, where it joins the lateral plantar artery to form the **deep plantar arch** (Fig. 5.47*B*). The course and destination of the dorsal artery and its major continuation, the deep plantar artery, are comparable to the radial artery of the hand, which completes a deep arterial arch in the palm (Chapter 6).

The **lateral tarsal artery,** a branch of the dorsal artery of the foot, runs laterally in an arched course beneath the extensor digitorum brevis to supply this muscle and the underlying tarsals and joints (Fig. 5.47*A*). It anastomoses with other branches, such as the arcuate artery.

The **1st dorsal metatarsal artery** divides into branches that supply both sides of the great toe and the medial side of the 2nd toe.

The **arcuate artery** runs laterally across the bases of the lateral four metatarsals, deep to the extensor tendons, to reach the lateral aspect of the forefoot where it may anastomose with the lateral tarsal artery to form an arterial loop. The arcuate artery gives rise to the **2nd, 3rd,** and **4th dorsal metatarsal arteries.** These vessels run distally to the clefts of

the toes and are connected to the plantar arch and to the plantar metatarsal arteries by *perforating branches* (Figs. 5.45*A* & *B*, 5.46*A*, and 5.47*B*). Distally, each dorsal metatarsal artery divides into two **dorsal digital arteries** for the dorsal aspect of the sides of adjoining toes (Fig. 5.47*A*); however, these arteries generally end proximal to the distal interphalangeal joint (Fig. 5.46*A*) and are replaced by or receive replenishment from dorsal branches of the plantar digital arteries.

Palpation of the Dorsalis Pedis Pulse

The pulse of the dorsal artery of the foot (referred to clinically as the **dorsalis pedis pulse**) is evaluated during a physical examination of the peripheral vascular system. Dorsalis pedis pulses may be palpated with the feet slightly dorsiflexed. The pulses are usually easy to palpate because the dorsal arteries of the foot are subcutaneous and pass along a line from the extensor retinaculum to a point just lateral to the ▶

EHL tendons (Swartz, 2002) (Fig. B5.20). A diminished or absent dorsalis pedis pulse usually suggests vascular insufficiency resulting from arterial disease. The five **P signs of acute arterial occlusion** are pain, pallor, paresthesia, paralysis, and pulselessness. Some healthy adults (and even children) have *congenitally non-palpable dorsalis pedis pulses;* the variation is usually bilateral. In these cases, the dorsal artery of the foot is replaced by an enlarged perforating fibular artery. ○

— Extensor hallucis longus

— Dorsalis pedis artery

— Tibialis anterior tendon

Figure B5.20

Arteries of the Sole of the Foot

The sole of the foot has a prolific blood supply that is derived from the posterior tibial artery, which divides deep to the flexor retinaculum (Figs. 5.44A, 5.46B, and 5.47B). The terminal branches pass deep to the abductor hallucis as the medial and lateral plantar arteries, which accompany the similarly named nerves.

Medial Plantar Artery. The **medial plantar artery** is the smaller terminal branch of the posterior tibial artery. It gives rise to a deep branch (or branches) that supplies mainly muscles of the great toe. The larger superficial branch of the medial plantar artery supplies the skin on the medial side of the sole and has digital branches that accompany digital branches of the medial plantar nerve, the more lateral of which anastomose with medial plantar metatarsal arteries. Occasionally, a **superficial plantar arch** is formed when the superficial branch anastomoses with the lateral plantar artery or the (deep) plantar arch.

Lateral Plantar Artery. The **lateral plantar artery,** much larger than the medial plantar artery, arises with and accompanies the nerve of the same name (Figs. 5.44C, 5.45B, 5.46B, and 5.47B). It runs laterally and anteriorly, at first deep to the adductor hallucis and then between the flexor digitorum brevis and quadratus plantae (Figs. 5.44C and 5.45B). The lateral plantar artery arches medially across the foot with the deep branch of the lateral plantar nerve to form the **deep plantar arch,** which is completed by union with the *deep plantar artery,* a branch of the dorsal artery of the foot (Figs. 5.44C, 5.45, and 5.47B). As it crosses the foot, the deep plantar arch gives rise to four **plantar metatarsal arteries;** three **perforating branches** (Figs. 5.45, 5.46A, and 5.47B); and many branches to the skin, fascia, and muscles in the sole. The plantar metatarsal arteries divide near the base of the proximal phalanges to form the **plantar digital arteries,** supplying the adjacent digits; the more medial metatarsal arteries are joined by superficial digital branches of the medial plantar artery. The plantar digital arteries typically provide most of the blood reaching the distal toes, including the nail bed, via perforating and dorsal branches (Fig. 5.46A)—an arrangement that also occurs in the fingers.

Hemorrhaging Wounds of the Sole of the Foot

Puncture wounds of the sole of the foot involving the deep plantar arch and its branches usually result in severe bleeding, typically from both ends of the cut artery because of the abundant anastomoses. Ligature of the arch is difficult because of its depth and the structures that surround it. ○

THE BOTTOM LINE: The dorsal and plantar arteries of the foot are terminal branches of the anterior and posterior tibial arteries, respectively. The dorsal artery of the foot supplies all of the dorsum of the foot and, via the arcuate artery, the proximal dorsal aspect of the toes. It also contributes to formation of the plantar (arterial) arch via its terminal deep plantar artery. The smaller medial and larger lateral plantar arteries supply the plantar aspect of the foot, the latter running in vascular planes between the 1st and 2nd and then, as the plantar arch, the 3rd and 4th layers of the intrinsic muscles. Anastomoses between the dorsal and the plantar arteries are abundant and important for the health of the foot. Except for the scarcity of a superficial arch, the arterial pattern of the foot is similar to that of the hand.

Venous Drainage of the Foot

As in the rest of the lower limb, there are both superficial and deep veins in the foot. The deep veins take the form of interanastomosing paired veins accompanying all arteries internal to the deep fascia (Fig. 5.48*A*). The superficial veins are subcutaneous and unaccompanied by arteries (Fig. 5.48*B*). Unlike the leg and thigh, however, the venous drainage in the foot is primarily to the major superficial veins, both from the deep accompanying veins and other smaller superficial veins. Perforating veins begin the one-way shunting of blood from superficial to deep veins, a pattern essential to operation of the musculovenous pump (see "Venous Drainage of the Lower Limb," in this chapter), proximal to the ankle joint. Most blood is drained from the foot through the superficial veins.

Dorsal digital veins continue proximally as **dorsal metatarsal veins,** which also receive branches from **plantar digital veins.** These veins drain to the **dorsal venous arch** of the foot, proximal to which a **dorsal venous network** covers the remainder of the dorsum of the foot. Both the arch and the network are located in the subcutaneous tissue. For the main part, superficial veins from a **plantar venous network** either drain around the medial border of the foot to converge with the medial part of the dorsal venous arch and network to form a **medial marginal vein,** which becomes the *great saphenous vein,* or drain around the lateral margin to converge with the lateral part of the dorsal venous arch and network to form the **lateral marginal vein,** which becomes the *small saphenous vein* (Fig. 5.48*B*). Perforating veins from the great and small saphenous veins then continuously shunt blood deeply as they ascend to take advantage of the musculovenous pump.

Lymphatic Drainage of the Foot

The lymphatics of the foot begin in subcutaneous plexuses. The collecting vessels consist of superficial and deep lymphatic vessels that follow the superficial veins and major vascular bundles, respectively. Superficial lymphatic vessels are most numerous in the sole. The *medial superficial lymphatic vessels,* larger and more numerous than the lateral ones, drain the medial side of the dorsum and sole of the foot (Fig. 5.49). These vessels converge on the *great saphenous vein* and ac-

company it to the vertical group of *superficial inguinal lymph nodes,* located along the vein's termination, and then to the *deep inguinal lymph nodes* along the proximal femoral vein. The *lateral superficial lymphatic vessels* drain the lateral side of the dorsum and sole of the foot. Most of these vessels pass posterior to the lateral malleolus and accompany the small saphenous vein to the popliteal fossa, where they enter the *popliteal lymph nodes* (Fig. 5.12). The *deep lymphatic vessels* from the foot follow the main blood vessels: fibular, anterior and posterior tibial; then popliteal and femoral. The deep vessels from the foot also drain into the popliteal lymph nodes. Lymphatic vessels from them follow the femoral vessels, carrying lymph to the deep inguinal lymph nodes. From the deep inguinal nodes, all lymph from the lower limb passes deep to the inguinal ligament to the iliac nodes.

Lymphadenopathy

Infections of the foot may spread proximally, causing enlargement of popliteal and inguinal lymph nodes (*lymphadenopathy*). Infections on the lateral side of the foot initially produce enlargement of popliteal lymph nodes (**popliteal lymphadenopathy**); later, the inguinal lymph nodes may enlarge. **Inguinal lymphadenopathy** without popliteal lymphadenopathy can result from infection of medial side of the foot, leg, or thigh; however, enlargement of these nodes can also result from an infection or tumor in the vulva, penis, scrotum, perineum, and gluteal region and from terminal parts of the urethra, anal canal, and vagina. ⊕

THE BOTTOM LINE: Venous drainage of the foot primarily follows a superficial route, draining to the dorsum of the foot and then medially via the greater or laterally via the lesser saphenous veins. From these veins, blood is shunted by perforating veins to the deep veins of the leg and thigh that participate in the musculovenous pump. The lymphatics carrying lymph from the foot drain toward and then along the superficial veins draining the foot. Lymph from the medial foot follows the greater saphenous vein and drains directly to superficial inguinal lymph nodes. Lymph from the lateral foot follows the lesser saphenous vein and drains initially to the popliteal lymph nodes and then by deep lymphatic channels to the deep inguinal nodes.

Joints of the Lower Limb

The joints of the lower limb include the articulations of the pelvic girdle—lumbosacral joints, sacroiliac joints, and pubic symphysis, which are discussed in Chapter 3. The remaining joints of the lower limb are the hip joint, knee joint, tibiofibular joints, ankle joint, and foot joints (Fig. 5.50).

Anterior tibial vein (accompanying veins of anterior tibial artery)

Deep veins on dorsum of foot, which communicate with superficial veins — Accompanying veins of arcuate and dorsal arteries — Accompanying veins of dorsal metatarsal arteries

(A) Deep veins of leg and foot   **Anterior view**

Posterior tibial vein (accompanying veins of posterior tibial artery)

Fibular vein (accompanying veins of fibular artery)

Plantar venous arch

Plantar digital veins

Plantar metatarsal veins

Posterior view of leg and plantarflexed foot

Saphenous nerve

Perforating veins

Great saphenous vein

Medial malleolus

Medial marginal vein of foot

Dorsal venous arch of foot

Dorsal venous network

Dorsal metatarsal veins

(B) Superficial veins of leg and foot   **Medial view**

Medial sural cutaneous branch (of tibial nerve)

Lateral sural cutaneous branch (of common fibular nerve)

Perforating veins

Small saphenous vein

Sural nerve

Lateral marginal vein of foot

Plantar venous network

Posterior view of leg and plantarflexed foot

Figure 5.48. Veins of leg and foot. A. The deep veins accompany the arteries and their branches (L. *venae comitantes*); they anastomose frequently and have numerous valves. **B.** The main superficial veins are the great and small saphenous veins, which drain into the deep veins as they ascend the limb by means of perforating veins so that muscular compression can propel blood toward the heart against the pull of gravity. Note that the distal great saphenous vein is accompanied by the saphenous nerve, and the small saphenous vein is accompanied by the sural nerve and its medial root (medial sural cutaneous nerve).

Superficial inguinal lymph nodes (superior or horizontal group)

Deep inguinal lymph nodes

Femoral vein

Superficial inguinal lymph nodes (inferior or vertical group)

Great saphenous vein

Superficial lymphatic vessels

Great saphenous vein

Great saphenous vein

Medial border of patella

Popliteal vein

Popliteal lymph nodes

Small saphenous vein

Lumbar lymphatic trunk

Lateral lumbar (caval/aortic) nodes

Common iliac vein and nodes

External iliac vein and nodes

Superficial inguinal nodes

(A) Anteromedial view of left limb

(B) Posterior view of left limb

(C) Medial view: *Arrows* represent the continuation of lymph drainage from the lower limb via the superficial inguinal and iliac nodes

Figure 5.49. Lymphatic drainage of foot. A. Superficial lymphatic vessels from the medial foot drain are joined by those from the anteromedial leg in draining to the superficial inguinal lymph nodes via lymphatics that accompany the greater saphenous vein. **B.** Superficial lymphatic vessels from the lateral foot join those from the posterolateral leg, converging to vessels accompanying the lesser saphenous vein and draining into the popliteal lymph nodes. The popliteal lymph nodes drain via lymphatics accompanying the femoral vein to the deep inguinal lymph nodes.

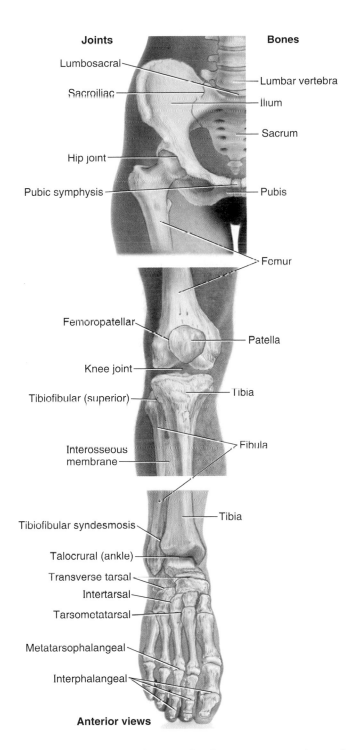

Joints | Bones

Lumbosacral — Lumbar vertebra
Sacroiliac — Ilium
— Sacrum
Hip joint —
Pubic symphysis — Pubis

— Femur

Femoropatellar — Patella
Knee joint —
Tibiofibular (superior) — Tibia
Interosseous membrane — Fibula

— Tibia
Tibiofibular syndesmosis —
Talocrural (ankle) —
Transverse tarsal —
Intertarsal —
Tarsometatarsal —
Metatarsophalangeal —
Interphalangeal —

Anterior views

Figure 5.50. Joints of lower limb. The joints are those of the pelvic girdle connecting the free lower limb to the vertebral column, the knee, the tibiofibular articulations, and the many joints of the foot.

Hip Joint

The **hip joint** forms the connection between the lower limb and the pelvic girdle. It is a strong and stable multiaxial ball and socket type of synovial joint. The femoral head is the ball, and the acetabulum is the socket (Fig. 5.51). The hip joint is designed for stability over a wide range of movement. Next to the glenohumeral (shoulder) joint, it is the most movable of all joints. During standing, the entire weight of the upper body is transmitted through the hip bones to the heads and necks of the femurs.

Articular Surfaces of the Hip Joint

The round head of the femur articulates with the cup-like acetabulum of the hip bone (Figs. 5.50 5.52). The *head of the femur* forms approximately two thirds of a sphere. Except for the pit or *fovea for the ligament of the femoral head,* all of the head is covered with articular cartilage, which is thickest over weight-bearing areas. The *acetabulum,* a hemispherical hollow on the lateral aspect of the hip bone, is formed by the fusion of three bony parts (Fig. 5.5). The heavy, prominent rim of the acetabulum consists of a semilunar articular part covered with articular cartilage, the **lunate surface of the acetabulum.** The acetabular rim and lunate surface form approximately three quarters of a circle; the missing inferior segment of the circle is the **acetabular notch.**

The fibrocartilaginous **acetabular labrum** (L. *labrum,* lip) attaches to the acetabular rim, increasing the acetabular articular area by nearly 10%. The **transverse acetabular ligament,** a continuation of the acetabular labrum, bridges the acetabular notch. As a result of the height of the rim and labrum, more than half of the femoral head fits within the acetabulum (Fig. 5.52C). In other words, the acetabular labrum enables the acetabulum to "grasp" the femoral head beyond its equator; thus during dissection, the femoral head must be cut from the acetabular rim to enable disarticulation of the joint. Centrally a deep non-articular part, called the **acetabular fossa,** is formed mainly by the ischium (Figs. 5.51 and 5.52C). This fossa is thin walled (often translucent) and continuous inferiorly with the acetabular notch.

(cont'd on page 678)

Bipedalism and Congruity of the Articular Surfaces of the Hip Joint

The acetabulum is directed inferiorly, laterally, and anteriorly in humans. The weight-bearing iliac portion of the acetabular rim overlies the femoral head, which is important for transfer of weight to the femur in the erect (standing/walking) position (Figs. 5.50A and 5.52C). Consequently, of the positions commonly assumed by humans, the hip joint is mechanically most stable when a person is bearing weight, as when lifting a heavy object, for example. Decreases in the degree to which the ilium overlies the femoral head (detectable radiographically as the *angle of Wiberg*) may indicate joint instability. Because of the anterior direction the axis of the acetabulum and the posterior direction of the axis of the femoral head and neck as it extends laterally (owing to the torsion angle—discussed earlier in this ▶

Figure 5.51. Hip joint. The hip joint was disarticulated by cutting the ligament of the head of the femur and retracting the head from the acetabulum. The transverse acetabular ligament is retracted superiorly to show the obturator canal, which transmits the obturator nerve and vessels passing from the pelvic cavity to the medial thigh.

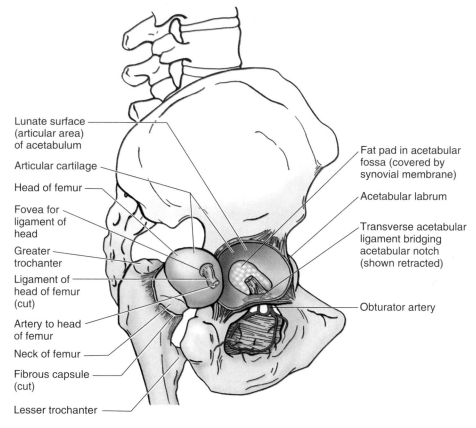

Lunate surface (articular area) of acetabulum

Articular cartilage

Head of femur

Fovea for ligament of head

Greater trochanter

Ligament of head of femur (cut)

Artery to head of femur

Neck of femur

Fibrous capsule (cut)

Lesser trochanter

Fat pad in acetabular fossa (covered by synovial membrane)

Acetabular labrum

Transverse acetabular ligament bridging acetabular notch (shown retracted)

Obturator artery

Lateral view

chapter), there is an angle of 30–40° between their axes (Fig. B5.21). Consequently, the articular surfaces of the head and acetabulum are not fully congruent in the erect (bipedal) posture. The anterior part of the femoral head is "exposed" and articulates mostly with the joint capsule (Figs. 5.52*B*, 5.53*A*,

and 5.56). Nonetheless, rarely is <40% of the available articular surface of the femoral head in contact with the surface of the acetabulum in any position. Relative to other joints and in view of the large size of the hip joint, this is extensive contact, contributing considerably to the joint's great stability. ✪

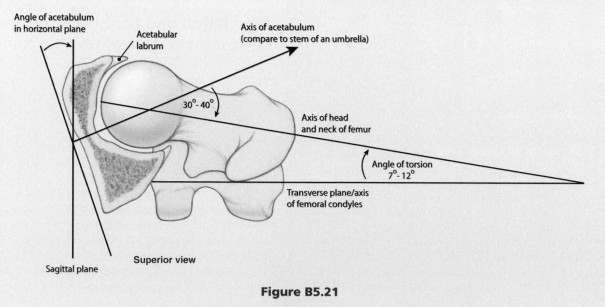

Angle of acetabulum in horizontal plane

Acetabular labrum

Axis of acetabulum (compare to stem of an umbrella)

30°- 40°

Axis of head and neck of femur

Angle of torsion 7°- 12°

Transverse plane/axis of femoral condyles

Sagittal plane

Superior view

Figure B5.21

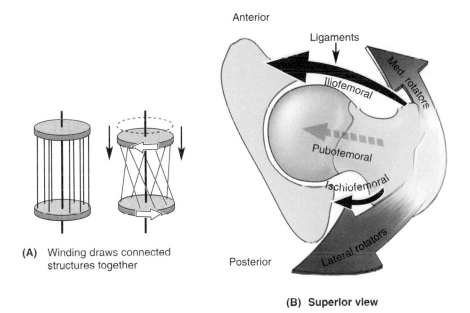

(A) Winding draws connected structures together

Anterior

Ligaments

Iliofemoral

Med. rotators

Pubofemoral

Ischiofemoral

Lateral rotators

Posterior

(B) Superior view

Angle of Wiberg

Fibrous layer of joint capsule

Acetabular labrum

Orbicular zone

Retinacula

Greater trochanter

Ilium

Articular cartilage

Acetabular fossa

Epiphysis of head

Ligament of head of femur

Epiphysial plate of head

Transverse acetabular ligament (region of acetabular notch)

Synovial membrane

Retinacula

Plane of acetabular rim

Vertical

(C) Anterior view of coronal section

Figure 5.52. Factors increasing stability of hip joint. A. Parallel fibers linking two discs resemble those making up the tube-like fibrous layer of the hip joint capsule. When one disc (the femur) rotates relative to the other (the acetabulum), the fibers become increasingly oblique and draw the two discs together. Similarly, extension of the hip joint winds (increases the obliquity of) the fibers of the fibrous layer, pulling the head and neck of the femur tightly into the acetabulum, increasing the stability of the joint. Flexion unwinds the fibers of the capsule. **B.** This transverse section through the hip joint demonstrates the medial and reciprocal pull of the periarticular muscles (medial and lateral rotators; *reddish brown arrows*) and intrinsic ligaments of the hip joint (*black arrows*) on the femur. Relative strengths are indicated by arrow width: Anteriorly, the muscles are less abundant but the ligaments are robust; posteriorly, the muscles predominate. **C.** In this coronal section of hip joint, the acetabular labrum and transverse acetabular ligament, spanning the acetabular notch (and included in the plane of section here), extend the acetabular rim so that a complete socket is formed. Thus the acetabular complex engulfs the head of the femur. The epiphysis of the femoral head is entirely within the joint capsule. The thick weight-bearing bone of the ilium normally lies directly superior to the head of the femur for efficient transfer of weight to the femur (Fig. 5.3). The angle of Wiberg (see text) is used radiographically to determine the degree to which the acetabulum overhangs the head of the femur.

The articular surfaces of the acetabulum and femoral head are most congruent when the hip is flexed 90°, abducted 5°, and rotated laterally 10° (the position in which the axis of the acetabulum and the axis of the femoral head and neck are aligned), which is the quadruped position! In other words, in assuming the upright position, a relatively small degree of joint stability was sacrificed to maximize weight bearing when erect. Even so, the hip joint is our most stable joint, owing also to its complete ball and socket construction (depth of the socket); the strength of its capsule; and the attachments of muscles crossing the joint, many of which are located at some distance from the center of movement (Palastanga et al., 2002).

Joint Capsule of the Hip Joint

The hip joints are enclosed within strong yet loose **joint capsules**, formed of an external *fibrous layer* (fibrous capsule) and an internal *synovial membrane* (Fig. 5.52C). Proximally, the fibrous layer attaches to the acetabulum, just peripheral to the rim to which the labrum is attached, and to the transverse acetabular ligament (Figs. 5.51, 5.52C, and 5.53). Distally, the fibrous layer attaches to the femoral neck only anteriorly at the *intertrochanteric line* and root of the greater trochanter (Fig. 5.55B). Posteriorly, the fibrous layer crosses the neck proximal to the *intertrochanteric crest* but is not attached to it (Fig. 5.55C).

Most fibers of the fibrous layer take a spiral course from the hip bone to the intertrochanteric line, but some deep fibers pass circularly around the neck, forming the **orbicular zone**. Thick parts of the fibrous layer of the capsule form the **ligaments of the hip joint**, which pass in a spiral fashion from the pelvis to the femur. Extension winds its spiraling ligaments and fibers more tightly, constricting the capsule and drawing the femoral head tightly into the acetabulum (Fig. 5.52A). The tightened fibrous layer increases the stability of the joint, but restricts extension of the joint to 10–20° beyond the vertical position. Flexion increasingly unwinds the spiraling ligaments and fibers. This permits considerable flexion of the hip joint with increasing mobility.

Of the three intrinsic ligaments of the joint capsule below it is the first one that reinforces and strengthens the joint:

- *Anteriorly and superiorly* is the strong, Y-shaped **iliofemoral ligament** (Bigelow ligament), which attaches to the anterior inferior iliac spine and the acetabular rim proximally and the intertrochanteric line distally (Fig. 5.53A & B). Said to be the body's strongest ligament, the iliofemoral ligament specifically prevents hyperextension of the hip joint during standing by screwing the femoral head into the acetabulum via the mechanism described above.

- *Anteriorly and inferiorly* is the **pubofemoral ligament**, which arises from the obturator crest of the pubic bone and passes laterally and inferiorly to merge with the fibrous layer of the joint capsule (Fig. 5.53A). This ligament blends with the medial part of the iliofemoral ligament and tightens during both extension and abduction of the hip joint. The pubofemoral ligament prevents overabduction of the hip joint.

- *Posteriorly* is the **ischiofemoral ligament**, which arises from the ischial part of the acetabular rim (Fig. 5.53C). The weakest of the three ligaments, it spirals superolaterally to the femoral neck, medial to the base of the greater trochanter.

The relative size, strengths, and positions of the three ligaments of the hip joint are shown in Figure 5.52B. The ligaments and periarticular muscles (the medial and lateral rotators of the thigh) play a vital role in maintaining the structural integrity of the joint, as demonstrated in the above figure. Both muscles and ligaments pull the femoral head medially into the acetabulum, and they are reciprocally balanced when doing so. The medial flexors, located anteriorly, are fewer, weaker, and less mechanically advantaged, whereas the anterior ligaments are strongest. Conversely, the ligaments are weaker posteriorly where the medial rotators are abundant, stronger, and more mechanically advantaged.

In all synovial joints, synovial membrane lines all internal surfaces of the fibrous layer as well as any intracapsular bony surfaces not lined with articular cartilage. Thus in the hip joint, where the fibrous layer attaches to the femur distant from the articular cartilage covering the femoral head, the **synovial membrane of the hip joint** reflects proximally along the femoral neck to the edge of the femoral head. Longitudinal **synovial folds** (retinacula) occur in the membrane covering the femoral neck (Fig. 5.52C). Subsynovial **retinacular arteries** (branches of the medial, and a few of the lateral, circumflex femoral artery) that supply the femoral head and neck course within the synovial folds (Fig. 5.54).

The **ligament of the head of the femur** (Figs. 5.51, 5.52C, and 5.54), primarily a synovial fold conducting a blood vessel, is weak and of little importance in strengthening the hip joint. Its wide end attaches to the margins of the acetabular notch and the *transverse acetabular ligament*; its narrow end attaches to the *fovea for the ligament of the head*. Usually, the ligament contains a small artery to the head of the femur. A fat pad in the *acetabular fossa* fills the part of the acetabular fossa that is not occupied by the ligament of the femoral head. Both the ligament and the fat-pad are covered with synovial membrane. The malleable nature of the fat-pad permits it to change shape to accommodate the variations in the congruity of the femoral head and acetabulum as well as changes in the position of the ligament of the head during joint movements. A **synovial protrusion** beyond the free margin of the joint capsule onto the posterior aspect of the femoral neck forms a bursa for the obturator externus tendon. (Fig. 5.53C)

Movements of the Hip Joint

Hip movements are flexion–extension, abduction–adduction, medial–lateral rotation, and circumduction (Fig. 5.55). Movements of the trunk at the hip joints are also important, such as those occurring when a person lifts the trunk from the supine position during sit-ups or keeps the pelvis level when one foot is off the ground.

(A) Anterior view

Transverse process of L5 vertebra
Anterior longitudinal ligament
Iliac crest
Iliolumbar ligament
Anterior superior iliac spine
Anterior sacroiliac ligament
Greater sciatic foramen
Anterior inferior iliac spine
Sacrotuberous and sacrospinous ligaments
Ventral sacrococcygeal ligament
Iliofemoral ligament
Head of femur (joint capsule removed)
Pubofemoral ligament
Intertrochanteric line
Obturator membrane
Pubic symphysis

*Thin area of joint capsule (floor of iliopectineal bursa) has been removed here

Anterior superior iliac spine
Acetabular labrum
* Head of femur
Anterior inferior iliac spine
Pectineus
Pectineal fascia
Rectus femoris
Pectineal ligament
Pubic tubercle
Obturator externus
Iliofemoral ligament
Greater trochanter
Inter-trochanteric line
Lesser trochanter
Obturator nerve, anterior and posterior divisions
Sacrospinous ligament and ischial spine
(B) Anterior view
Obturator internus tendon
Obturator internus bursa
Course of obturator externus

Ischiofemoral ligament
Rectus femoris, reflected head
Iliofemoral ligament
Orbicular zone
Neck of femur
Intertrochanteric crest
Synovial protrusion
Psoas major and lesser trochanter
(C) Posterior view

Figure 5.53. Ligaments of pelvis and hip joint. A. Weight transfer from the vertebral column to the pelvic girdle is a function of the sacroiliac ligaments. Weight transfer at the hip joint is accomplished primarily by the disposition of the bones, with the ligaments limiting the range of movement and adding stability. **B.** The strong, triangular iliofemoral ligament attaches at its apex to the rim of the acetabulum inferior to the anterior inferior iliac spine and at its base to the anterior intertrochanteric line of the femur. The pubofemoral ligament, a thickened part of the fibrous layer of the joint capsule, extends from the superior ramus of the pubis to the intertrochanteric line of the femur, passing deep to the iliofemoral ligament. **C.** The ischiofemoral ligament, also a thickened part of the fibrous layer, passes superolaterally from the ischium over the neck of the femur. The joint capsule does not attach to the posterior aspect of the femur. Thus the synovial membrane is able to protrude from the joint capsule, forming the obturator externus bursa to facilitate movement of the tendon of the obturator externus (shown in part **B**) over the bone.

Anterior view of coronally sectioned hip joint

Figure 5.54. Blood supply of head and neck of femur. Branches of the medial and lateral circumflex femoral arteries, branches of the deep artery of the thigh, and the artery to the femoral head (a branch of the obturator artery) supply the head and neck of the femur. In the adult, the medial circumflex femoral artery is the most important source of blood to the femoral head and adjacent (proximal) neck.

The degree of flexion and extension possible at the hip joint depends on the position of the knee. If the knee is flexed, relaxing the hamstrings, the thigh can be actively flexed until it almost reaches the anterior abdominal wall, and can reach it via further passive flexion. Not all this movement occurs at the hip joint; some results from flexion of the vertebral column. During extension of the hip joint, the fibrous layer of the joint capsule, especially the iliofemoral ligament, is taut; therefore, the hip can usually be extended only slightly beyond the vertical except by movement of the bony pelvis (flexion of lumbar vertebrae).

From the anatomical position, the range of abduction of the hip joint is usually somewhat greater than for adduction. About 60° of abduction is possible when the thigh is extended, and more when it is flexed. Lateral rotation is much more powerful than medial rotation. The main muscles producing movements of the hip joint are listed in Figure 5.55*B*. Note that:

1. The *iliopsoas* is the strongest flexor of the hip.

2. In addition to its function as an adductor, the *adductor magnus* also serves as a flexor (anterior or aponeurotic part) and an extensor (posterior or hamstrings part).

3. Several muscles participate in both flexion and adduction (*pectineus* and *gracilis* as well all three "adductor" muscles).

4. In addition to serving as abductors, the anterior portions of the *gluteus medius* and *minimus* are also medial rotators.

5. The *gluteus maximus* serves as the primary extensor from the flexed to the straight (standing) position; and

from this point posteriorly, extension is achieved primarily by the hamstrings. The gluteus maximus is also a lateral rotator.

Blood Supply of the Hip Joint

Arteries supplying the hip joint include (Fig. 5.54) the following:

- The *medial* and *lateral circumflex femoral arteries,* which are usually branches of the *deep artery of the thigh* but occasionally arise as branches of the *femoral artery.*

- The **artery to the head of the femur,** which is a branch of the obturator artery of variable size; it traverses the ligament of the head.

The main blood supply of the hip joint is from the *retinacular arteries* arising as branches of the circumflex femoral arteries. Retinacular arteries arising from the medial circumflex femoral artery are most abundant, bringing more blood to the head and neck of the femur because they are able to pass beneath the unattached posterior border of the joint capsule. Retinacular arteries arising from the lateral circumflex femoral must penetrate the thick iliofemoral ligament and are smaller and fewer.

Nerve Supply of the Hip Joint

Hilton's law states that the nerves supplying the muscles extending directly across and acting at a given joint also innervate the joint. Articular rami arise from the intramuscular rami of the muscular branches and directly from named nerves. A knowledge of the nerve supply of the muscles and their relationship to the joints can allow one to deduce the nerve supply

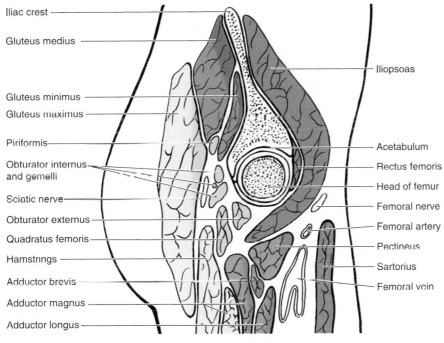

(A) Lateral view of sagittal section through femoral head

Labels (A), top to bottom left:
- Iliac crest
- Gluteus medius
- Gluteus minimus
- Gluteus maximus
- Piriformis
- Obturator internus and gemelli
- Sciatic nerve
- Obturator externus
- Quadratus femoris
- Hamstrings
- Adductor brevis
- Adductor magnus
- Adductor longus

Labels (A), right:
- Iliopsoas
- Acetabulum
- Rectus femoris
- Head of femur
- Femoral nerve
- Femoral artery
- Pectineus
- Sartorius
- Femoral vein

(B) Diagrammatic lateral view

Gluteal group (externally)
Iliopsoas group (internally)

MEDIAL ROTATORS
ABDUCTORS
Anterior
Posterior
EXTENSORS
FLEXORS
LATERAL ROTATORS
ADDUCTORS

Hamstrings and lateral rotator group

Adductor group

Circular Zones =
The zones represent the position of origin of functional groups relative to center of humeral head in acetabulum (point of rotation). Pull is applied on the femur (femoral trochanters or shaft) from these positions.

Colored Arrows =
The arrows show the direction of rotation of femoral head caused by activity of functional groups.

Functional groups of muscles acting at hip joint

Flexors

Iliopsoas
Sartorius
Tensor of fascia lata
Rectus femoris
Pectineus
Adductor longus
Adductor brevis
Adductor magnus—anterior part
Gracilis

Adductors

Adductor longus
Adductor brevis
Adductor magnus
Gracilis
Pectineus
Obturator externus

Lateral rotators

Obturator externus
Obturator internus
Gemelli
Piriformis
Quadratus femoris
Gluteus maximus

Extensors

Hamstrings:
Semitendinosus
Semimembranosus
Long head, biceps femoris
Adductor magnus—posterior part
Gluteus maximus

Abductors

Gluteus medius
Gluteus minimus
Tensor of fascia lata

Medial rotators

Gluteus medius ⎫ Anterior parts
Gluteus minimus ⎭
Tensor of fascia lata

Figure 5.55. Relations of hip joint and muscles producing movements of joint. A. Sagittal section of the hip joint showing the muscles, vessels, and nerves related to it. The muscles are color coded to indicate their function(s). Applying Hilton's law, it is possible to deduce the innervation of the hip joint by knowing which muscles directly cross and act on the joint and their nerve supply. **B.** The relative positions of the muscles producing movements of the hip joint and the direction of the movement are demonstrated.

of many joints. Possible deductions regarding the hip joint and its muscular relationships include (Fig. 5.55):

- Flexors innervated by the femoral nerve pass anterior to the hip joint; the anterior aspect of the hip joint is innervated by the femoral nerve (directly and via articular rami of the muscular branches to the pectineus and rectus femoris).

- Lateral rotators pass inferior and posterior to the hip joint; the inferior aspect of the joint is innervated by the obtura-

tor nerve (directly and via articular rami of the muscular branch to the obturator externus), and the posterior aspect is innervated by the nerve to the quadratus femoris.

- Adductors innervated by the superior gluteal nerve pass superior to the hip joint; the superior aspect of the joint is innervated by the superior gluteal nerve.

Pain perceived as coming from the hip joint may be misleading because pain can be referred from the vertebral column.

Fractures of the Femoral Neck ("Hip Fractures")

Fractures of the neck of the femur (unfortunately referred to as "fractured hips," implying that the hip bone is broken) are uncommon in most contact sports because the participants are usually young and the femoral neck is strong in people <40 years of age. When they do occur in this age group, these fractures usually result from high-energy impacts (e.g., during race-car accidents, skiing, trampoline, and equestrian events) when the lower limb is extended and the force of the impact is transmitted to the hip joint, even if applied at some distance from the joint. For example, if the foot is firmly braced against the car floor with the knee locked, or if the knee is braced against the dashboard during a head-on collision, the force of the impact may be transmitted superiorly and produce a femoral neck fracture. These fractures are especially common in individuals >60 years, especially in women because their femoral necks are more often weak and brittle as a result of *osteoporosis* (Fig. B5.22). Fractures of the femoral neck are often intracapsular, and realignment of the neck fragments requires internal skeletal fixation. Femoral neck fractures are among the most troublesome and problematic of all fractures (Salter, 1999).

Fractures of the femoral neck often disrupt the blood supply to the head of the femur. Most of the blood to the head and neck of the femur is supplied by the medial circumflex femoral artery (Fig. 5.54). The retinacular arteries arising from this artery are often torn when the femoral neck is fractured or the hip joint is dislocated. Following some femoral neck fractures, the artery to the ligament of the femoral head may be the only remaining source of blood to the proximal fragment. This artery is frequently inadequate for maintaining the femoral head; consequently, the fragment may undergo *aseptic vascular necrosis*.

Surgical Hip Replacement

Although the hip joint is strong and stable, it is subject to severe traumatic injury and degenerative disease. *Osteoarthritis of the hip joint*, characterized by pain, edema, limitation of motion, and erosion of articular cartilage, is a common cause of disability (Fig. B5.23). During hip replacement, a metal prosthesis anchored to the person's femur by bone cement replaces the femoral head and neck. A plastic socket cemented to the hip bone replaces the acetabulum.

Necrosis of the Femoral Head in Children

In children, traumatic dislocations of the hip joint disrupt the artery to the head of the femur. Fractures that result in separation of the superior femoral epiphysis (the growth plate between the femoral head and neck) are also likely ▶

Cartilage

Normal hip

Hip with moderate arthritis

Hip prothesis

Figure B5.22

Figure B5.23

to result in an inadequate blood supply to the femoral head and in *post-traumatic avascular necrosis of the head*. As a result, incongruity of the joint surfaces develops, and growth at the epiphysis is retarded. Such conditions, most common in children 3–9 years of age, produce hip pain that may radiate to the knee (Salter, 1999).

Dislocation of the Hip Joint

Congenital dislocation of the hip joint is common, occurring in approximately 1.5 per 1000 live births; it is bilateral in approximately half the cases. Girls are affected at least eight times more often than boys (Salter, 1999). Dislocation occurs when the femoral head is not properly located in the acetabulum. Inability to abduct the thigh is characteristic of congenital dislocation. In addition, the affected limb appears (and functions as if) shorter because the dislocated femoral head is more superior than on the normal side, resulting in a positive *Trendelenburg sign* (hip appears to drop on one side during walking). Approximately 25% of all cases of arthritis of the hip in adults are the direct result of residual defects from congenital dislocation of the hip.

Acquired dislocation of the hip joint is uncommon because this articulation is so strong and stable. Nevertheless, dislocation may occur during an automobile accident when the hip is flexed, adducted, and medially rotated, the usual position of the lower limb when a person is riding in a car. Posterior dislocations are most common. A head-on collision that causes the knee to strike the dashboard may dislocate the hip when the femoral head is forced out of the acetabulum (Fig. B5.24A). The joint capsule ruptures inferiorly and posteriorly, allowing the femoral head to pass through the tear in the capsule and over the posterior margin of the acetabulum onto the lateral surface of the ilium, shortening and medially rotating the affected limb (Fig. B5.24B). Because of the close relationship of the *sciatic nerve* to the hip joint (Fig. 5.56A), it may be injured (stretched and/or compressed) during posterior dislocations or fracture–dislocations of the hip joint. This kind of injury may result in paralysis of the hamstrings and muscles distal to the knee supplied by the sciatic nerve. Sensory changes may also occur in the skin over the posterolateral aspects of the leg and over much of the foot because of injury to sensory branches of the sciatic nerve.

Anterior dislocation of the hip joint results from a violent injury that forces the hip into extension, abduction, and lateral rotation (e.g., catching a ski tip when snow skiing). In these cases, the femoral head is inferior to the acetabulum. Often, the acetabular margin fractures, producing a *fracture–dislocation of the hip joint*. When the femoral head dislocates, it usually carries the acetabular bone fragment and acetabular labrum with it. ○

(A)

(B)

Posterior dislocation
of the right hip joint

Head of femur is driven
posteriorly, out of acetabulum

Figure B5.24

THE BOTTOM LINE: The hip joint is our strongest and most stable joint. Its stability results from (1) the mechanical strength of its ball and (deep) socket construction, allowing extensive articular surface contact; (2) its strong joint capsule; and (3) its many surrounding muscles. However, it remains vulnerable, especially in older age, because of the angle of the femoral neck (inclination) and close association of the blood supply of the femoral head to the neck. Thus fractures result in avascular necrosis of the femoral head. Major movements are flexion and extension, possible over a wide range; medial and lateral rotation with abduction are part of every step of normal, bipedal walking.

Knee Joint

The **knee joint** is our largest and most superficial joint. It is primarily a hinge type of synovial joint, allowing flexion and extension; however, the hinge movements are combined with gliding and rolling and with rotation about a vertical axis. Although the knee joint is well constructed, its function is commonly impaired when it is hyperextended (e.g., in body contact sports, such as ice hockey).

Articulations, Articular Surfaces, and Stability of the Knee Joint

Relevant anatomical details of the involved bones, including their articulating surfaces, were discussed in "Bones of the Lower Limb," earlier in this chapter. The articular surfaces of the knee joint are characterized by their large size and their complicated and incongruent shapes. The knee joint consists of three articulations (Fig. 5.56):

- Two **femorotibial articulations** (**lateral** and **medial**) between the lateral and the medial femoral and tibial condyles.

- One intermediate **femoropatellar articulation** between the patella and the femur.

The fibula is not involved in the knee joint.

The knee joint is relatively weak mechanically because of the incongruence of its articular surfaces, which has been compared to two balls sitting on a warped tabletop. The stability of the knee joint depends on (1) the strength and actions of the surrounding muscles and their tendons and (2) the ligaments that connect the femur and tibia. Of these supports, the muscles are most important; therefore, many sport injuries are preventable through appropriate conditioning and training. The most important muscle in stabilizing the knee joint is the large *quadriceps femoris,* particularly the inferior fibers of the vastus medialis and lateralis (Fig. 5.57*A*). The knee joint will function surprisingly well after a ligament strain if the quadriceps is well conditioned.

The erect, extended position is the most stable position of the knee. In this position the articular surfaces are most congruent (contact is minimized in all other positions), the primary ligaments of the joint (collateral and cruciate ligaments)

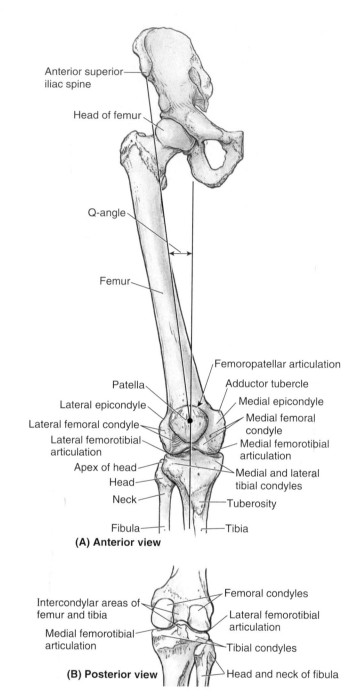

(A) Anterior view

(B) Posterior view

Figure 5.56. Bones of knee joint. A The bones articulating at the knee joint are shown. The hip bone and proximal femur are included to demonstrate the Q-angle, determined during physical examination to indicate alignment of the femur and tibia and to evaluate valgus or varus stress at the knee. **B.** The bones and bony features of the posterior aspect of the knee joint and knee are shown.

are taut, and the many tendons surrounding the joint provide a splinting effect.

Joint Capsule of the Knee Joint

The **joint capsule of the knee joint** is typical in consisting of an external *fibrous layer* (fibrous capsule) and an internal

(A) Anterior view

Rectus femoris (cut away)
Vastus intermedius (cut away)
Femur
Vastus lateralis
Articular muscle of knee
Vastus medialis
Suprapatellar bursa
Quadriceps femoris tendon
Iliotibial tract
Patellar retinacula
Tibial collateral ligament
Fibular collateral ligament
Tibia
Patellar ligament
Pes anserinus

(B) Posterior view

Adductor magnus
Adductor hiatus
Vastus medialis
Tendon of "hamstring" portion of adductor magnus
Medial head of gastrocnemius
Adductor tubercle
Tibial collateral ligament
Semimembranosus tendon
Fibrous layer extending across intercondylar fossa
Oblique popliteal ligament
Pes anserinus
Semimembranosus contribution to fascia of popliteus
Tendinous arch of soleus
Soleus

Linea aspera
Lateral intermuscular septum covering vastus lateralis
Popliteal surface of femur
Plantaris
Lateral head of gastrocnemius
Fibular collateral ligament
Biceps femoris tendon
Arcuate popliteal ligament and opening for popliteus tendon
Common fibular nerve
Popliteus

Figure 5.57. Joint capsule of knee. The external aspect (fibrous layer) of the joint capsule is relatively thin in some places and thickened in others to form reinforcing intrinsic (capsular) ligaments. **A.** Modifications of the anterior aspect and sides of the fibrous layer include the patellar retinacula, which attach to the sides of the quadriceps tendon, patella, and patellar ligament, and incorporation of the iliotibial tract (laterally) and the medial collateral ligament (medially). **B.** The hamstring and gastrocnemius muscles and the posterior intermuscular septum have been cut and removed to expose the adductor magnus, lateral intermuscular septum, and the floor of the popliteal fossa. Posterior modifications of the fibrous layer include the oblique and arcuate popliteal ligaments and a perforation inferior to the arcuate popliteal ligament to allow passage of the popliteus tendon.

synovial membrane that lines all internal surfaces of the articular cavity not covered with articular cartilage. The fibrous layer has a few thickened parts that make up intrinsic ligaments but, for the main part, it is thin and is actually incomplete in some areas. The fibrous layer attaches to the femur superiorly, just proximal to the articular margins of the condyles. Posteriorly, the fibrous layer encloses the condyles and the *intercondylar fossa* (Fig. 5.57B). The fibrous layer has an opening posterior to the lateral tibial condyle to allow the tendon of the popliteus to pass out of the joint capsule to attach to the tibia. Inferiorly, the fibrous layer attaches to the margin of the superior articular surface (tibial plateau) of the tibia, except where the tendon of the popliteus crosses the bone (Figs. 5.57A & B and 5.58A). The quadriceps tendon, patella, and patellar ligament replace the fibrous layer anteriorly—that is, the fibrous layer is continuous with the lateral and medial margins of these structures, and there is no separate fibrous layer in the region of these structures (Figs. 5.57A and 5.58A).

The extensive *synovial membrane* lines all surfaces bounding the articular cavity (the space containing synovial fluid) not covered by articular cartilage (Fig. 5.58A & B). Thus it attaches to the periphery of the articular cartilage covering the femoral and tibial condyles; the posterior surface of the patella; and the edges of the *menisci*, the fibrocartilaginous discs between the tibial and femoral articular surfaces. It lines the internal surface of the fibrous layer laterally and medially, but centrally it becomes separated from the fibrous layer. From the posterior aspect of the joint, the synovial membrane reflects anteriorly into the intercondylar region, covering the cruciate ligaments and the **infrapatellar fat-pad,** so that they are excluded from the articular cavity. This creates a median **infrapatellar synovial fold,** a vertical fold of synovial membrane that approaches the posterior aspect of the patella, occupying all but the most anterior part of the intercondylar region. Thus it almost subdivides the articular cavity into right and left femorotibial articular cavities; indeed, this is how arthroscopic surgeons consider the articular

Patellar ligament

Alar folds

Lateral patellar
retinaculum

Infrapatellar
synovial
fold

Articular
surface of
medial condyle

Posterior intercondylar area

Anterior intercondylar area

Lateral patellar retinaculum

Fibrous layer (blue)
Synovial membrane (red)
} Joint capsule

Site of attachment of
anterior cruciate ligament

Articular surface of lateral condyle

Site of attachment of
posterior cruciate ligament

Gap in fibrous capsule for popliteus tendon

**(A)   Superior view of superior articular
surface of tibia (tibial plateau)**

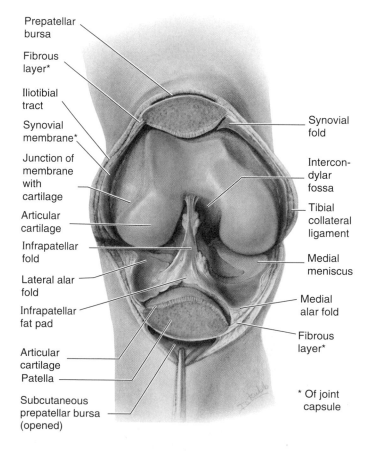

Prepatellar
bursa

Fibrous
layer*

Iliotibial
tract

Synovial
membrane*

Junction of
membrane
with
cartilage

Articular
cartilage

Infrapatellar
fold

Lateral alar
fold

Infrapatellar
fat pad

Articular
cartilage
Patella

Subcutaneous
prepatellar bursa
(opened)

Synovial
fold

Intercon-
dylar
fossa

Tibial
collateral
ligament

Medial
meniscus

Medial
alar fold

Fibrous
layer*

* Of joint
capsule

(B)   Anterior view of flexed knee

**Figure 5.58. Layers of joint
capsule, articular cavity,
and articular surfaces of
knee joint. A.** The attachments of the fibrous layer and
synovial membrane to the tibia
are shown. Note that, although
they are adjacent on each side,
they part company centrally to
accommodate intercondylar and
infrapatellar structures that are
intracapsular (inside the fibrous
layer) but extra-articular (excluded from the articular cavity
by synovial membrane). **B.** The
joint capsule was incised transversely, the patella was sawn
through, and then the knee was
flexed, opening the articular cavity. The infrapatellar fold of synovial membrane encloses the
cruciate ligaments, excluding
them from the joint cavity. All internal surfaces not covered with
or made of articular cartilage
(*blue,* or *gray* in the case of the
menisci) are lined with synovial
membrane (mostly *purple,* but
transparent and colorless where
it is covering non-articular surfaces of the femur).

cavity. Fat-filled **lateral** and **medial alar folds** cover the inner surface of fat-pads that occupy the space on each side of the patellar ligament internal to the fibrous layer.

Superior to the patella, the knee joint cavity extends deep to the vastus intermedius as the suprapatellar bursa (Figs. 5.57A and 5.59A). The synovial membrane of the joint capsule is continuous with the synovial lining of this bursa. This large bursa usually extends approximately 5 cm superior to the patella; however, it may extend halfway up the anterior aspect of the femur. Muscle slips deep to the vastus intermedius form the *articular muscle of the knee,* which attaches to the synovial membrane and retracts the bursa during extension of the knee (Figs. 5.16 and 5.57A).

Extracapsular Ligaments of the Knee Joint

The joint capsule is strengthened by five extracapsular or capsular (intrinsic) ligaments: patellar ligament, fibular collateral ligament, tibial collateral ligament, oblique popliteal ligament, and arcuate popliteal ligament (Fig. 5.57A & B). They are sometimes called *external ligaments* to differentiate them from internal ligaments, such as the cruciate ligaments.

The *patellar ligament,* the distal part of the quadriceps tendon, is a strong, thick fibrous band passing from the apex and adjoining margins of the patella to the tibial tuberosity (Fig. 5.57A). The patellar ligament is the anterior ligament of the knee joint. Laterally, it receives the *medial* and *lateral patellar retinacula,* aponeurotic expansions of the vastus medialis and lateralis and overlying deep fascia. The retinacula make up the joint capsule of the knee on each side of the patella (Figs. 5.57A and 5.58A) and play an important role in maintaining alignment of the patella relative to the patellar articular surface of the femur. The oblique placement of the femur and/or line of pull of the quadriceps femoris muscle relative to the axis of the patellar tendon and tibia, assessed clinically as the *Q-angle,* favors lateral displacement of the patella (Fig. 5.56).

The *collateral ligaments of the knee* are taut when the knee is fully extended, contributing to stability while standing (Fig. 5.59). As flexion proceeds, they become increasingly slack, permitting and limiting (serving as check ligaments for) rotation at the knee. The **fibular collateral ligament** (FCL; lateral collateral ligament), a cord-like extracapsular ligament, is strong. It extends inferiorly from the lateral epicondyle of the femur to the lateral surface of the fibular head (Fig. 5.59A & B). The tendon of the popliteus passes deep to the FCL, separating it from the lateral meniscus. The tendon of the biceps femoris is split into two parts by this ligament (Fig. 5.59A). The **tibial collateral ligament** (TCL; medial collateral ligament) is a strong, flat, intrinsic (capsular) band that extends from the medial epicondyle of the femur to the medial condyle and the superior part of the medial surface of the tibia (Fig. 5.59C & D). At its midpoint, the deep fibers of the TCL are firmly attached to the medial meniscus. The TCL, weaker than the FCL, is more often damaged. As a result, the TCL and medial meniscus are commonly torn during contact sports such as football and ice hockey.

The **oblique popliteal ligament** is a recurrent expansion of the tendon of the semimembranosus that reinforces the joint capsule posteriorly as it spans the intracondylar fossa (Fig. 5.57B). The ligament arises posterior to the medial tibial condyle and passes superolaterally toward the lateral femoral condyle, blending with the central part of the posterior aspect of the joint capsule.

The **arcuate popliteal ligament** also strengthens the joint capsule posterolaterally. It arises from the posterior aspect of the fibular head, passes superomedially over the tendon of the popliteus, and spreads over the posterior surface of the knee joint. Its development appears to be inversely related to the presence and size of a fabella in the proximal attachment of the lateral head of gastrocnemius (see clinical correlation [blue] box "Fabella in the Gastrocnemius," in this chapter). Both structures are thought to contribute to posterolateral stability of the knee.

Genu Valgum and Genu Varum

The femur is placed diagonally within the thigh, whereas the tibia is almost vertical within the leg, creating an angle at the knee between the long axes of the bones (Fig. B5.25A). The angle between the two bones, referred to clinically as the **Q-angle,** is assessed by drawing a line from the ASIS to the middle of the patella and extrapolating a second (vertical) line passing through the middle of the patella and tibial tuberosity (Fig. 5.56). The Q-angle is typically greater in adult females, owing to their wider pelves. When normal, the angle of the femur within the thigh places the middle of the knee joint directly inferior to the head of the femur when standing, centering the weight-bearing line in the intercondylar region of the knee (Fig. B5.25A).

A medial angulation of the leg in relation to the thigh, in which the femur is abnormally vertical and the Q-angle is small, is a deformity called **genu varum** (bowleg) that causes unequal weight bearing: The line of weight bearing falls medial to the center of the knee (Fig. B5.25B). Excess pressure is placed on the medial aspect of the knee joint, which results in **arthrosis** (destruction of knee cartilages), and the fibular collateral ligament is overstressed (Fig. B.25D). A lateral angulation of the leg (large Q-angle, >17°) in relation to the thigh (exaggeration of the knee angle) is called **genu valgum** (knock-knee) (Fig. B5.25C). Because of the exaggerated knee angle in genu valgum, the weight-bearing line falls lateral to the center of the knee. Consequently, the tibial collateral ligament is overstretched, and there is excess stress on the lateral meniscus and cartilages of the lateral femoral and tibial condyles. The patella, normally pulled laterally by the tendon of the vastus lateralis, is pulled even farther laterally when the leg is extended in the presence of genu valgum so that its articulation with the femur is abnormal. ▶

(cont'd on page 689)

(A)

Femur

Gastrocnemius lateral head, turned superiorly

Fibular collateral ligament (FCL)

Popliteus muscle and tendon

Biceps femoris (turned inferiorly)

Fib. Tibia

Quadriceps femoris muscle and tendon

Suprapatellar bursa

Subcutaneous prepatellar bursa

Patella

Lateral meniscus

Patellar ligament

Fibrous layer of capsule of proximal tibiofibular joint

Iliotibial tract (turned inferiorly)

(B)

Gastrocnemius

Fibular collateral ligament

Popliteus

Lateral part of tibial plateau

Biceps femoris

Fibular collateral ligament

Iliotibial tract

Patellar ligament

Lateral views

(C)

Vastus Medialis

Meniscus

Adductor magnus tendon

Medial superior genicular artery

Gastrocnemius tendon (of proximal attachment)

Semimembranosus tendon

Tibial collateral ligament (TCL)

Coronary ligament (in which a window has been cut)

Medial inferior genicular artery

Gracilis
Semitendinosus } Pes anserinus
Sartorius

Popliteus fascia overlying popliteus muscle

(D)

Adductor magnus

Gastrocnemius

Tibial collateral ligament

Tibial collateral ligament

Semimembranosus

Patellar ligament

Sartorius
Gracilis
Semi-tendinosus

Tibial collateral ligament

Medial views

Figure 5.59. Collateral ligaments of knee joint. A. The fibular collateral ligament is shown. Purple latex was injected into the articular cavity to demonstrate the extensive and complex synovial membrane surrounding it. The articular cavity/synovial membrane extends superiorly deep to the quadriceps, forming the suprapatellar bursa. **B.** The attachment sites of the FCL (*green*) and related muscles (*red,* proximal; *blue,* distal) on the lateral aspect of the bones of the knee region are indicated. The tendon of the biceps femoris bifurcates, its site of attachment embracing the inferior attachment of the FCL. **C.** The band-like part of the tibial collateral ligament (isolated here from the fibrous layer of the joint capsule, of which it is a part) attaches to the medial epicondyle (almost in line with the adductor magnus tendon); crosses the insertion of the semimembranosus muscle; and passes deep to the pes anserinus, the combined attachment sites of the tendinous distal attachment of the gracilis, semitendinosus, and sartorius muscles. **D.** The attachment sites of the TCL and related muscles on the medial aspect of the bones of the knee region are indicated.

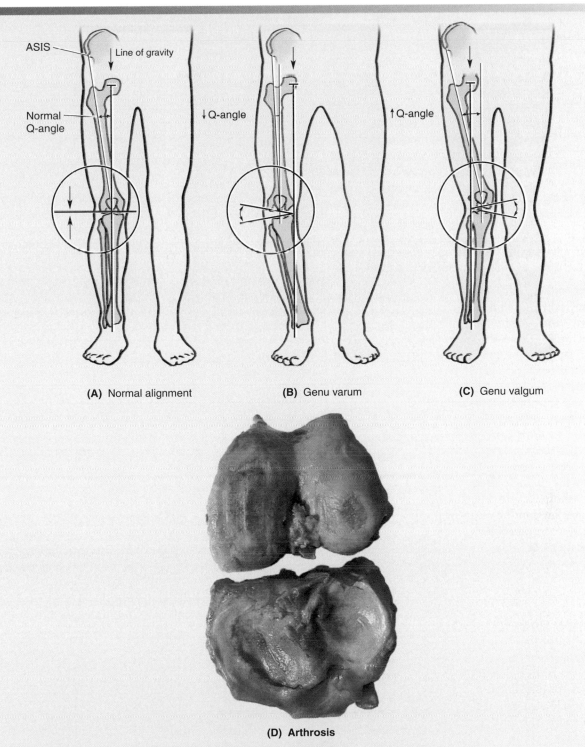

(A) Normal alignment   (B) Genu varum   (C) Genu valgum

(D) Arthrosis

Figure B5.25

Children commonly appear bowlegged for 1–2 years after starting to walk, and knock-knees are frequently observed in children 2–4 years of age. Persistence of these abnormal knee angles in late childhood usually means congenital deformities exist that may require correction. Any irregularity of a joint eventually leads to wear and tear (arthrosis) of the articular cartilages.

Patellar Dislocation

When the patella is dislocated, it nearly always dislocates laterally. Patellar dislocation is more common in women, presumably because of their greater Q-angle which, in addition to representing the oblique placement of the femur relative to the tibia, represents the angle of pull of ▶

the quadriceps relative to the axis of the patella and tibia (the term *Q-angle* was actually coined in reference to the angle of pull of the quadriceps). The tendency toward lateral dislocation is normally counterbalanced by the medial, more horizontal pull of the powerful vastus medialis. In addition, the more anterior projection of the lateral femoral condyle and deeper slope for the larger lateral patellar facet provide a mechanical deterrent to lateral dislocation. An imbalance of the lateral pull and the mechanisms resisting it result in abnormal tracking of the patella within the patellar groove and chronic patellar pain, even if actual dislocation does not occur.

Patellofemoral Syndrome

Pain deep to the patella often results from excessive running, especially downhill; hence, this type of pain is often called "runner's knee." The pain results from repetitive microtrauma caused by abnormal tracking of the patella relative to the patellar surface of the femur, a condition known as the **patellofemoral syndrome**. This syndrome may also result from a direct blow to the patella and from **osteoarthritis of the patellofemoral compartment** (degenerative wear and tear of articular cartilages). In some cases, strengthening of the vastus medialis corrects *patellofemoral dysfunction*. This muscle tends to prevent lateral dislocation of the patella resulting from the Q-angle because the vastus medialis attaches to and pulls on the medial border of the patella. Hence, weakness of the vastus medialis predisposes the individual to the patellofemoral dysfunction and patellar dislocation. ✚

Intra-Articular Ligaments of the Knee Joint

The intra-articular ligaments within the knee joint consist of the cruciate ligaments and menisci. The popliteal tendon is also intra-articular during part of its course.

The *cruciate ligaments* (L. *crux,* a cross) crisscross within the joint capsule of the joint but outside the synovial cavity (Figs. 5.60 and 5.61). The cruciate ligaments are located in the center of the joint and cross each other obliquely, like the letter *X*. During medial rotation of the tibia on the femur, the cruciate ligaments wind around each other; thus the amount of medial rotation possible is limited to about 10°. Because they become unwound during lateral rotation, nearly 60° of lateral rotation is possible when the knee is flexed >90°, the movement being ultimately limited by the TCL. The chiasm (point of crossing) of the cruciate ligaments serves as the pivot for rotatory movements at the knee. Because of their oblique orientation, in every position one cruciate ligament, or parts of one or both ligaments, is tense. It is the cruciate ligaments

that maintain contact with the femoral and tibial articular surfaces during flexion of the knee.

The **anterior cruciate ligament** (ACL), the weaker of the two cruciate ligaments, arises from the anterior intercondylar area of the tibia, just posterior to the attachment of the medial meniscus (Fig. 5.60*A*). The ACL has a relatively poor blood supply. It extends superiorly, posteriorly, and laterally to attach to the posterior part of the medial side of the lateral condyle of the femur (Fig. 5.60*C*). It limits posterior rolling (turning and traveling) of the femoral condyles on the tibial plateau during flexion, converting it to spin (turning in place). It also prevents posterior displacement of the femur on the tibia and hyperextension of the knee joint. When the joint is flexed at a right angle, the tibia cannot be pulled anteriorly (like pulling out a drawer) because it is held by the ACL.

The **posterior cruciate ligament** (PCL), the stronger of the two cruciate ligaments, arises from the posterior intercondylar area of the tibia (Fig. 5.60*A* & *D*). The PCL passes superiorly and anteriorly on the medial side of the ACL to attach to the anterior part of the lateral surface of the medial condyle of the femur (Fig. 5.60*B* & *C*). The PCL limits anterior rolling of the femur on the tibial plateau during extension, converting it to spin. It also prevents anterior displacement of the femur on the tibia or posterior displacement of the tibia on the femur and helps prevent hyperflexion of the knee joint. In the weight-bearing flexed knee, the PCL is the main stabilizing factor for the femur (e.g., when walking downhill).

The **menisci of the knee joint** are crescentic plates ("wafers") of fibrocartilage on the articular surface of the tibia that deepen the surface and play a role in shock absorption (Fig. 5.61). The menisci (G. *meniskos,* crescent) are thicker at their external margins and taper to thin, unattached edges in the interior of the joint. Wedge shaped in transverse section, the menisci are firmly attached at their ends to the *intercondylar area of the tibia* (Fig. 5.60*A*). Their external margins attach to the joint capsule of the knee. The **coronary ligaments** are portions of the joint capsule extending between the margins of the menisci and most of the periphery of the tibial condyles (Fig. 5.60*B*). A slender fibrous band, the **transverse ligament of the knee** joins the anterior edges of the menisci (Fig. 5.61*A*), tethering them to each other during knee movements.

The **medial meniscus** is C shaped, broader posteriorly than anteriorly. Its anterior end (horn) is attached to the anterior intercondylar area of the tibia, anterior to the attachment of the ACL (Fig. 5.60*A*). Its posterior end is attached to the posterior intercondylar area, anterior to the attachment of the PCL. The medial meniscus firmly adheres to the deep surface of the TCL (Figs. 5.59*C* and 5.61). Because of its widespread attachments laterally to the tibial intercondylar area and medially to the TCL, the medial meniscus is less mobile on the tibial plateau than is the lateral meniscus.

The **lateral meniscus** is nearly circular, smaller, and more freely movable than the medial meniscus. The tendon of the popliteus has two parts proximally. One part attaches to the lateral epicondyle of the femur and passes between the lateral meniscus and inferior part of the lateral epicondylar surface of

(*cont'd on page 694*)

Attachments of:

- ■ Medial meniscus
- ☐ Lateral meniscus
- ■ Cruciate ligaments

Medial intercondylar tubercle

Articular surface of medial condyle

Anterior intercondylar area

Lateral intercondylar tubercle

Articular surface of lateral condyle

Posterior intercondylar area

(A) Superior view of superior articular surface of tibia (tibial plateau)

Patellar surface

Groove for lateral meniscus

Popliteus tendon

Lateral meniscus

Coronary ligament (cut edge)

Fibular collateral ligament

Biceps femoris, extension to deep fascia of leg

Groove for medial meniscus

Notch for anterior cruciate ligament

Posterior cruciate ligament

Anterior cruciate ligament

Medial meniscus

Coronary ligament (cut edge)

Tibial collateral ligament

Sartorius tendon

Lig. patellae

Apex of patella

Nonarticular area

Inferior facets

Middle facets

Superior facets

Medial vertical facet

Base of patella

Quadriceps tendon

(B) Anterior view with knee flexed

Figure 5.60. Cruciate ligaments of knee joint. A. Superior aspect of the superior articular surface of the tibia (tibial plateau) showing the medial and lateral condyles (articular surfaces) and the intercondylar eminence between them. The sites of attachment of the cruciate ligaments are colored *green;* those of the medial meniscus, *purple;* and those of the lateral meniscus, *orange.* **B.** The quadriceps tendon has been severed and the patella (within the tendon and its continuation, the patellar ligament) has been reflected inferiorly. The knee is flexed to demonstrate the cruciate ligaments. (continued)

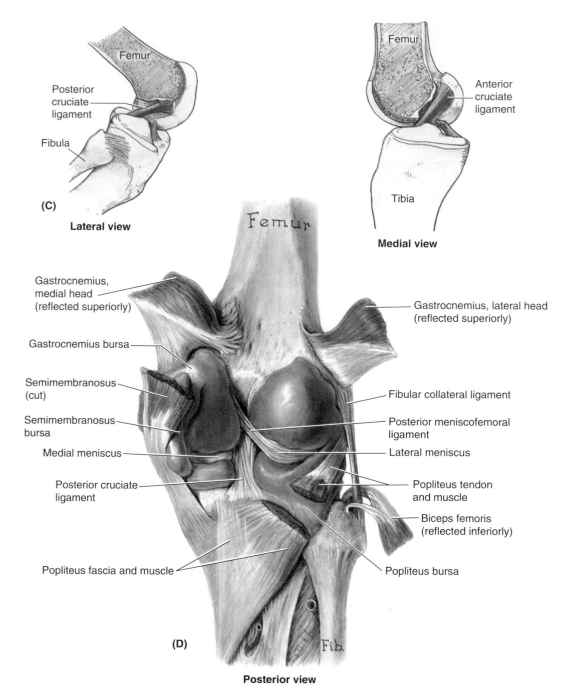

(C)
Lateral view

Femur

Posterior cruciate ligament

Fibula

Femur

Anterior cruciate ligament

Tibia

Medial view

Femur

Gastrocnemius, medial head (reflected superiorly)

Gastrocnemius bursa

Semimembranosus (cut)

Semimembranosus bursa

Medial meniscus

Posterior cruciate ligament

Popliteus fascia and muscle

Gastrocnemius, lateral head (reflected superiorly)

Fibular collateral ligament

Posterior meniscofemoral ligament

Lateral meniscus

Popliteus tendon and muscle

Biceps femoris (reflected inferiorly)

Popliteus bursa

Fib.

(D)

Posterior view

Figure 5.60. Cruciate ligaments of knee joint. (continued) C. In these lateral and medial views, the femur has been sectioned longitudinally and the near half has been removed with the proximal part of the corresponding cruciate ligament. The lateral view demonstrates how the posterior cruciate ligament resists anterior displacement of the femur on the tibial plateau. The medial view demonstrates how the anterior cruciate ligament resists posterior displacement of the femur on the tibial plateau. **D.** Both heads of the gastrocnemius are reflected superiorly, and the biceps femoris is reflected inferiorly. The articular cavity has been inflated with purple latex to demonstrate its continuity with the various bursae and the reflections and attachments of the complex synovial membrane.

(A) Superior view

Quadriceps tendon

Patellar ligament

Anterior cruciate ligament

Tibial collateral ligament

Medial meniscus

Posterior cruciate ligament

Posterior meniscofemoral ligament

Transverse ligament of knee

Lateral meniscus

Fibular collateral ligament

Anterior ligament of fibular head

Posterior ligament of fibular head

(B) Posterior view

Intercondylar notch

Medial epicondyle

Medial meniscus

Tibial collateral ligament

Posterior cruciate ligament

Popliteal surface of tibia

Anterior cruciate ligament

Lateral epicondyle

Posterior meniscofemoral ligament

Lateral meniscus

Fibular collateral ligament

Posterior tibiofibular ligaments (parts of joint capsule of proximal tibiofibular joint)

Head of fibula

(C) Coronal MRI of right knee

Femur

Tibia

(D) Anterior view of coronal section of right knee

Femur

Anterior cruciate ligament (6)

Lateral meniscus (1)

Fibular collateral ligament (2)

Superior tibiofibular joint

Head of fibula (3)

Posterior cruciate ligament (7)

Tibial collateral ligament (5)

Medial meniscus (4)

Tibia

Bursa deep to tibial collateral ligament

Figure 5.61. Menisci of knee joint. A. The quadriceps tendon is cut, and the patella and patellar ligament are reflected inferiorly and anteriorly. The menisci, their attachments to the intercondylar area of the tibia, and the tibial attachments of the cruciate ligaments are shown. **B.** The band-like tibial collateral ligament is attached to the medial meniscus. The cord-like fibular collateral ligament is separated from the lateral meniscus. The posterior meniscofemoral ligament attaches the lateral meniscus to the medial femoral condyle. **C and D.** The numbers on the MRI study refer to the structures labeled in the corresponding anatomical coronal section. (Part **C** courtesy of Dr. W. Kucharczyk, Chair of Medical Imaging, University of Toronto, and Clinical Director of Tri-Hospital Magnetic Resonance Centre, Toronto, Ontario, Canada.)

the femur (on the tendon's medial aspect) and the FCL that overlies its lateral aspect (Figs. 5.59*A* and 5.60*B* & *D*). The other, more medial part of the popliteal tendon attaches to the posterior limb of the lateral meniscus. A strong tendinous slip, the **posterior meniscofemoral ligament,** joins the lateral meniscus to the PCL and the medial femoral condyle (Figs. 5.60*D* and 5.61*B*).

Movements of the Knee Joint

Flexion and extension are the main knee movements; some rotation occurs when the knee is flexed. When the knee is fully extended with the foot on the ground, the knee passively "locks" because of medial rotation of the femoral condyles on the tibial plateau. This position makes the lower limb a solid column and more adapted for weight bearing. When the knee is "locked," the thigh and leg muscles can relax briefly without making the knee joint too unstable. To unlock the knee, the popliteus contracts, rotating the femur laterally about 5° on the tibial plateau so that flexion of the knee can occur. The main movements of the knee joint, the muscles producing them, and relevant details are provided in Table 5.16.

Movements of the Menisci. Although the rolling movement of the femoral condyles during flexion and extension is limited (converted to spin) by the cruciate ligaments, some

Table 5.16. Movements of the Knee Joint and the Muscles Producing Them

| Extension | Flexion | Medial rotation of leg, knee joint flexed | Lateral rotation of leg, knee joint flexed |

Movement	Degrees Possible	Muscles Producing Movement		Factors Limiting (Checking) Movement	Comments
		Primary	**Secondary**		
Extension		Quadriceps femoris	Weakly: tensor of fascia lata	Anterior edge of lateral meniscus contacts shallow groove between tibial and patellar surfaces of femoral condyles; anterior cruciate ligament contacts groove in intercondylar fossa	Ability of quadriceps to produce extension is most effective when hip joint is extended; flexion diminishes its efficiency
Flexion	120° (hip extended); 140° (hip flexed); 160° passively	Hamstrings (semitendinosus, semimembranosus, long head of biceps); short head of biceps	Gracilis, sartorius, gastrocnemius, popliteus	Calf of leg contacts thigh; length of hamstrings is also a factor—more knee flexion is possible when hip joint is flexed; cannot fully flex knee when hip is extended	Normally, role of gastrocnemius is minimal, but in presence of a supracondylar fracture, it rotates (flexes) distal fragment of femur
Medial rotation	10° with knee flexed; 5° with knee extended	Semitendinosus and semimembranosus when knee is flexed; popliteus when non-bearing knee is extended	Gracilis, sartorius	Collateral ligaments, loose during flexion without rotation, become taut at limits of rotation	When extended knee is bearing weight, action of popliteus laterally rotates femur; when not bearing weight, popliteus medially rotates patella
Lateral rotation	30°	Biceps femoris when knee is flexed		Collateral ligaments become taut; anterior cruciate ligament becomes wound around posterior cruciate ligament	At end of rotation, with no opposition, tensor of fascia lata can assist in maintaining position

rolling does occur, and the point of contact between the femur and the tibia moves posteriorly with flexion and returns anteriorly with extension. Furthermore, during rotation of the knee, one femoral condyle moves anteriorly on the corresponding tibial condyle while the other femoral condyle moves posteriorly, rotating about the chiasm of the cruciate ligaments. The menisci must be able to migrate on the tibial plateau as the points of contact between femur and tibia change.

Blood Supply of the Knee Joint

The arteries supplying the knee joint are the 10 vessels that form the periarticular *genicular anastomoses* around the knee: the genicular branches of the femoral, popliteal, and anterior and posterior recurrent branches of the anterior tibial recurrent and circumflex fibular arteries (Figs. 5.62 and 5.63*B*). The middle genicular branches of the popliteal artery penetrate the fibrous layer of the joint capsule and supply the cruciate ligaments, synovial membrane, and peripheral margins of the menisci.

Innervation of the Knee Joint

Reflecting Hilton's law, the nerves supplying the muscles crossing (acting on) the knee joint also supply the joint (Fig. 5.63*D*); thus articular branches from the femoral (the branches to the vasti), tibial, and common fibular nerves supply its anterior, posterior, and lateral aspects, respectively. In addition, however, the obturator and saphenous (cutaneous) nerves supply articular branches to its medial aspect.

Bursae around the Knee Joint

There are at least 12 bursae around the knee joint because most tendons run parallel to the bones and pull lengthwise across the joint during knee movements. The **subcutaneous prepatellar** and **infrapatellar bursae** are located at the convex surface of the joint, allowing the skin to be able to move freely during movements of the knee (Figs. 5.58*B* and 5.59*A*). The main bursae of the knee are illustrated and described in Table 5.17.

Four bursae communicate with the synovial cavity of the knee joint: suprapatellar bursa, popliteus bursa (deep to the distal quadriceps), anserine bursa (deep to the tendinous distal attachments of the sartorius, gracilis, and semitendinosus), and gastrocnemius bursa (Figs. 5.59*A* and 5.60*D*). The large **suprapatellar bursa** (Figs. 5.57*A* and 5.59*A*) is especially important because an infection in it may spread to the knee joint cavity. Although it develops separately from the knee joint, the bursa becomes continuous with it.

Knee Joint Injuries

Knee joint injuries are common because the knee is a low-placed, mobile, weight-bearing joint, serving as a fulcrum between two long levers (thigh and leg). Its stability depends almost entirely on its associated ligaments and surrounding muscles. The knee joint is essential for everyday activities such as standing, walking, and climbing stairs. It is also a main joint for sports that involve running, jumping, kicking, and changing directions. To perform these activities, the knee joint must be mobile; however, this mobility makes it ▶

(*cont'd on page 697*)

(A) Lateral view   **(B) Medial view**

Figure 5.62. Arterial anastomoses around knee. In addition to providing collateral circulation, the genicular arteries of the genicular anastomosis supply blood to the structures surrounding the joint as well as to the joint itself (e.g., its joint or articular capsule). Compare these views with the anterior view in Figure 5.63*B*.

Figure 5.63. Joints and neurovascular structures of leg and foot. A. The tibiofibular articulations include the synovial tibiofibular joint and the tibiofibular syndesmosis; the latter is made up of the interosseous membrane of the leg and the anterior and posterior tibiofibular ligaments. The oblique direction of the fibers of the interosseous membrane, primarily extending infero-laterally from the tibia, allows slight upward movement of the fibula but resists downward pull on it. **B.** The arterial supply of the joints of the leg and foot is demonstrated. Periarticular anastomoses surround the knee and ankle. **C.** Of the nine muscles attached to the fibula, all except one exert a downward pull on the fibula. **D.** The nerve supply of the leg and foot is demonstrated. Starting with the knee and progressing distally in the limb, cutaneous nerves become increasingly involved in providing innervation to joints, taking over completely in the distal foot and toes.

Table 5.17. Bursae about the Knee Joint

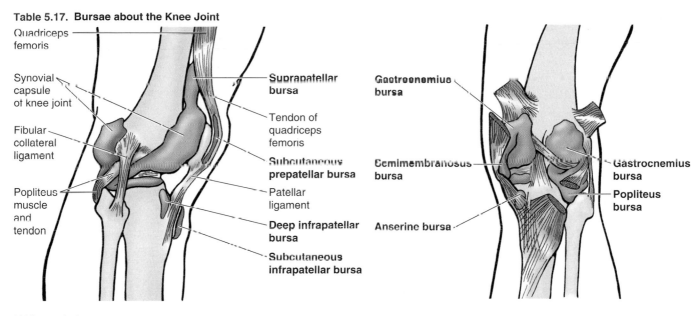

(A) Lateral view

(B) Posterior view

Bursae	Locations	Comments
Suprapatellar	Between femur and tendon of quadriceps femoris	Held in position by articularis genu muscles; communicates freely with (superior extension of) synovial cavity of knee joint
Popliteus	Between tendon of popliteus and lateral condyle of tibia	Opens into synovial cavity of knee joint inferior to lateral meniscus
Anserine	Separates tendons of sartorius, gracilis, and semitendinosus from tibia and tibial collateral ligament	Area where tendons of these muscles attach to tibia; resembles a goose's foot (L. *pes anserinus*)
Gastrocnemius	Deep to proximal attachment of tendon of medial head of gastrocnemius	An extension of synovial cavity of knee joint
Semimembranosus	Between medial head of gastrocnemius and semimembranosus tendon	Related to distal attachment of semimembranosus
Subcutaneous prepatellar	Between skin and anterior surface of patella	Allows free movement of skin over patella during movements of leg
Subcutaneous intrapatellar	Between skin and tibial tuberosity	Helps knee withstand pressure when kneeling
Deep infrapatellar	Between patellar ligament and anterior surface of tibia	Separated from knee joint by infrapatellar fat pad

susceptible to injuries. The most common knee injuries in contact sports are *ligament sprains,* which occur when the foot is fixed in the ground (Fig. B5.26A). If a force is applied against the knee when the foot cannot move, ligament injuries are likely to occur. The tibial and fibular collateral ligaments (TCL and FCL) are tightly stretched when the leg is extended, normally preventing disruption of the sides of the knee joint.

The firm attachment of the TCL to the medial meniscus is of considerable clinical significance because tearing of this ligament frequently results in concomitant tearing of the medial meniscus. The injury is frequently caused by a blow to the lateral side of the extended knee or excessive lateral twisting of the flexed knee that disrupts the TCL and concomitantly tears and/or detaches the medial meniscus from the joint capsule (Fig. B5.26A). This injury is common in athletes who twist their flexed knees while running (e.g., in basketball, the various forms of football, and volleyball). The ACL, which serves as a pivot for rotatory movements of the knee and is taut during flexion, may also tear subsequent to the rupture of the TCL, creating an "unhappy triad" of knee injuries. ▶

Twisting motion

Foot fixed

(A)

Anterior cruciate ligament (torn)

Tibial collateral ligament (torn)

Medial meniscus (torn)

"Unhappy triad" of knee injuries

(B) Anterior drawer sign (ACL)

Half of bone is removed to show ligaments

Anterior cruciate ligament (torn)

The anterior cruciate ligament prevents the femur from sliding posteriorly on the tibia and hyperextension of the knee and limits medial rotation of the femur when the foot is on the ground, and the leg is flexed.

(C) Posterior drawer sign (PCL)

Posterior cruciate ligament (torn)

The posterior cruciate ligament prevents the femur from sliding anteriorly on the tibia, particularly when the knee is flexed.

Figure B5.26

Hyperextension and severe force directed anteriorly against the femur with the knee semiflexed (e.g., a cross-body block in football) may tear the ACL. *ACL ruptures* are also common knee injuries in skiing accidents. This injury causes the free tibia to slide anteriorly under the fixed femur, known as **the anterior drawer sign** (Fig. B5.26*B*). The ACL may tear away from the femur or tibia; however, tears commonly occur in the midportion of the ligament.

Although strong, *PCL ruptures* may occur when a player lands on the tibial tuberosity with the knee flexed (e.g., when knocked to the floor in basketball). PCL ruptures usually occur in conjunction with tibial or fibular ligament tears. These injuries can also occur in head-on collisions when seat belts are not worn and the proximal end of the tibia strikes the dashboard. PCL ruptures allow the free tibia to slide posteriorly under the fixed femur, known as **the posterior drawer sign** (Fig. B5.26*C*).

Meniscal tears usually involve the medial meniscus. The lateral meniscus does not usually tear because of its mobility. *Pain on lateral rotation of the tibia* on the femur indicates injury of the lateral meniscus (Fig. B5.27*A*), whereas *pain on medial rotation of the tibia* on the femur indicates injury of the medial meniscus (Fig. B5.27*B*). Most meniscal tears occur in conjunction with TCL or ACL tears. Peripheral meniscal tears can often be repaired or may heal on their own because of the generous blood supply to this area. Meniscal tears that do not heal or cannot be repaired are usually removed (e.g., by arthroscopic surgery). Knee joints from which the menisci have been removed suffer no loss of mobility; however, the knee may be less stable and the tibial plateaus often undergo inflammatory reactions.

Arthroscopy of the Knee Joint

Arthroscopy is an endoscopic examination that allows visualization of the interior of the knee joint cavity with minimal disruption of tissue (Fig. B5.28). The arthroscope and one (or more) additional canula(e) are inserted through tiny incisions, known as *portals*. The second canula is for passage of specialized tools (e.g., manipulative probes or forceps) or equipment for trimming, shaping, or removing damaged tissue. This technique allows removal of torn menisci, loose bodies in the joint (such as bone chips), and *débridement* (the excision of devitalized articular cartilaginous material) in advanced cases of arthritis. Ligament repair or replacement may also be performed using an arthroscope. Although general anesthesia is usually preferable, knee arthroscopy can be performed using local or regional anesthesia. During arthroscopy, the articular cavity of the knee must be treated essentially as two separate (medial and lateral) femorotibial articulations owing to the imposition of the synovial fold around the cruciate ligaments. For further information see Soames (1995).

Aspiration of the Knee Joint

Fractures of the distal end of the femur or lacerations of the anterior thigh may involve the suprapatellar bursa and result in infection of the knee joint. When the knee joint is infected and inflamed, the amount of synovial fluid may increase. **Joint effusions,** the escape of fluid from blood ▶

(A)   (B)

Figure B5.27

Normal lateral meniscus of the knee

ACL graft (*black arrow*) with femoral anchoring screw visable (*white arrow*)

Trimming of a torn lateral meniscus

Figure B5.28

or lymphatic vessels, results in increased amounts of fluid in the joint cavity. Because the suprapatellar bursa communicates freely with the synovial cavity of the knee joint, fullness of the thigh in the region of the suprapatellar bursa may indicate increased synovial fluid. This bursa can be aspirated to remove the fluid for examination. Direct *aspiration of the knee joint* is usually performed with the patient sitting on a table with the knee flexed. The joint is approached laterally, using three bony points as landmarks for needle insertion: the anterolateral tibial (Gerdy) tubercle, the lateral epicondyle of the femur, and the apex of the patella. In addition to being the route for aspiration of serous and sanguineous (bloody) fluid, this triangular area also lends itself to drug injection for treating pathology of the knee joint.

Bursitis in the Knee Region

Prepatellar bursitis is caused by friction between the skin and the patella; however, the bursa may also be injured by compressive forces resulting from a direct blow or from falling on the flexed knee (Anderson et al., 2000). If the inflammation is chronic, the bursa becomes distended with fluid and forms a swelling anterior to the knee. This condition has been called "housemaid's knee" (Fig. B5.29); however, other people who work on their knees without knee pads, such as hardwood floor and rug installers, may also develop prepatellar bursitis.

Subcutaneous infrapatellar bursitis is caused by excessive friction between the skin and the tibial tuberosity; the edema occurs over the proximal end of the tibia. This condition was formerly called "clergyman's knee" because of frequent genuflecting (L. *genu,* knee); however, it occurs more commonly in roofers and floor tilers if they do not wear knee pads. *Deep infrapatellar bursitis* results in edema between the patellar ligament and the tibia, superior to the tibial tuberosity. The inflammation is usually caused by overuse and subsequent friction between the patellar ten-

Figure B5.30

don and the structures posterior to it, the infrapatellar fat-pad and tibia (Anderson et al., 2000). Enlargement of the deep infrapatellar bursa obliterates the dimples normally occurring on each side of the patellar ligament when the leg is extended.

Abrasions or penetrating wounds may result in *suprapatellar bursitis,* an infection caused by bacteria entering the bursa from the torn skin. The infection may spread to the cavity of the knee joint, causing localized redness and enlarged popliteal and inguinal lymph nodes.

Popliteal Cysts

Popliteal cysts (Baker cysts) are abnormal fluid-filled sacs of synovial membrane in the region of the popliteal fossa. A popliteal cyst is almost always a complication of chronic knee joint effusion (Slaby et al., 1994). The cyst may be a herniation of the gastrocnemius or semimembranosus bursa through the fibrous layer of the joint capsule into the popliteal fossa, communicating with the synovial cavity of the knee joint by a narrow stalk (Fig. B5.30). Synovial fluid may also escape from the knee joint (*synovial effusion*) or a bursa around the knee and collect in the popliteal fossa. Here it forms a new synovial-lined sac, or popliteal cyst. Popliteal cysts are common in children but seldom cause symptoms. In adults, popliteal cysts can be large, extending as far as the midcalf, and may interfere with knee movements.

Knee Replacement

If a person's knee is diseased, resulting from osteoarthritis, for example, an artificial knee joint may be inserted (*total knee replacement arthroplasty*) (Fig. B5.31). The artificial knee joint consists of plastic and metal components that are cemented to the femoral and tibial bone ends after removal of the defective areas. The combination of metal and plastic mimics the smoothness of cartilage on cartilage and produces good results in "low-demand" people ▶

Figure B5.29

who have a relatively sedentary life. In "high-demand" people who are active in sports, the bone–cement junctions may break down, and the artificial knee components may loosen; however, improvements in bioengineering and surgical technique have provided better results. For more information see Soames (1995). ⊕

Metal femoral component

Plastic tibial component

Metal tibial component

Figure B5.31

THE BOTTOM LINE: The knee is a hinge joint with a wide range of motion (primarily flexion and extension, with rotation increasingly possible with flexion). It is our most vulnerable joint owing to its incongruous articular surfaces and the mechanical disadvantage resulting from bearing the body's weight plus momentum while serving as a fulcrum between two long levers. Compensation is attempted by several features, including (1) strong intrinsic, extracapsular, and intracapsular ligaments; (2) splinting by many surrounding tendons (including the iliotibial tract); and (3) menisci that fill the spatial void, providing mobile articular surfaces. Of particular clinical importance are (1) collateral ligaments that are taut during (and limit) extension and are relaxed during flexion, allowing rotation for which they serve as check ligaments; (2) cruciate ligaments that maintain the joint during flexion, providing the pivot for rotation; and (3) the medial meniscus that is attached to the tibial collateral ligament and is frequently injured because of this attachment.

Tibiofibular Joints

The tibia and fibula are connected by two joints: the *superior tibiofibular joint* and the *tibiofibular syndesmosis* (inferior tibiofibular) *joint*. In addition, an *interosseous membrane* joins the shafts of the two bones (Fig. 5.63A). The fibers of the interosseous membrane and all ligaments of both tibiofibular articulations run inferiorly from the tibia to the fibula. Thus the membrane and ligaments strongly resist the downward pull placed on the fibula by eight of the nine muscles attached to it (Fig. 5.63C). However, they allow slight upward movement of the fibula that occurs when the wide (posterior) end of the trochlea of the talus is wedged between the malleoli

during dorsiflexion at the ankle. Movement at the superior tibiofibular joint is impossible without movement at the inferior tibiofibular syndesmosis.

The anterior tibial vessels pass through a hiatus at the superior end of the interosseous membrane (Fig. 5.63A & B). At the inferior end of the membrane is a smaller hiatus through which the perforating branch of the fibular artery passes.

Superior Tibiofibular Joint

The **superior tibiofibular joint** is a plane type of synovial joint between the flat facet on the fibular head and a similar articular facet located posterolaterally on the lateral tibial condyle (Figs. 5.61B & D and 5.63A). A tense joint capsule surrounds the joint and attaches to the margins of the articular surfaces of the fibula and tibia. The joint capsule is strengthened by *anterior* and *posterior tibiofibular ligaments*, which pass superomedially from the fibular head to the lateral tibial condyle (Fig. 5.61B). The joint is crossed posteriorly by the tendon of the popliteus. A pouch of synovial membrane from the knee joint, the *popliteus bursa* (Table 5.17), passes between the tendon of the popliteus and the lateral condyle of the tibia. About 20% of the time, the bursa also communicates with the synovial cavity of the tibiofibular joint, enabling transmigration of inflammatory processes between the two joints.

Movement. Slight movement of the joint occurs during dorsiflexion of the foot as a result of wedging of the trochlea of the talus between the malleoli (see "Articular Surfaces of the Ankle Joint," later in this chapter).

Blood Supply. The arteries of the superior tibiofibular joint are from the inferior lateral genicular and anterior tibial recurrent arteries (Figs. 5.62A and 5.63B).

Nerve Supply. The nerves of the tibiofibular joint are from the common fibular nerve and the nerve to the popliteus (Fig. 5.63D).

Tibiofibular Syndesmosis

The **tibiofibular syndesmosis** is a compound fibrous joint. It is the fibrous union of the tibia and fibula by means of the *interosseous membrane* (uniting the shafts) and the *anterior, interosseous* and *posterior tibiofibular ligaments* (the latter making up the **inferior tibiofibular joint,** uniting the distal ends of the bones). The integrity of the inferior tibiofibular joint is essential for the stability of the ankle joint because it keeps the lateral malleolus firmly against the lateral surface of the talus.

Articular Surfaces and Ligaments. The rough, triangular articular area on the medial surface of the inferior end of the fibula articulates with a facet on the inferior end of the tibia (Fig. 5.63A). The strong deep **interosseous tibiofibular ligament,** continuous superiorly with the interosseous membrane, forms the principal connection between the tibia and the fibula. The joint is also strengthened anteriorly and posteriorly by the strong external **anterior** and **posterior inferior tibiofibular ligaments.** The distal deep continuation of the posterior inferior tibiofibular ligament, the **inferior**

transverse (tibiofibular) ligament, forms a strong connection between the distal ends of the tibia (medial malleolus) and the fibula (lateral malleolus). It contacts the talus and forms the posterior "wall" of a square socket (with three deep walls and a shallow or open anterior wall), the **malleolar mortise,** for the trochlea of the talus. The lateral and medial walls of the mortise are formed by the respective malleoli (Fig. 5.64).

Movement. Slight movement of the joint occurs to accommodate wedging of the wide portion of the trochlea of the talus between the malleoli during dorsiflexion of the foot.

Blood Supply. The arteries are from the perforating branch of the fibular artery and from medial malleolar branches of the anterior and posterior tibial arteries (Fig. 5.63B).

Nerve Supply. The nerves to the syndesmosis are from the deep fibular, tibial, and saphenous nerves (Fig. 5.63D).

THE BOTTOM LINE: The tibiofibular joints include a superior synovial joint and the tibiofibular syndesmosis, consisting of an interosseous membrane and an inferior tibiofibular joint with anterior, interosseous, and posterior tibiofibular ligaments. Together they make up a compensatory system that allows a slight upward movement of the fibula owing to forced transverse expansion of the malleolar mortise (deep square socket) during maximal dorsiflexion of the ankle. All fibrous tibiofibular connections run downward from tibia to fibula, allowing this slight upward movement while strongly resisting the downward pull applied to the fibula by the contraction of eight of the nine muscles attached to it.

Tibia

Fibula

Epiphysial cartilage plate of distal end of fibula

Ankle joint "space"

Trochlea of talus

Epiphysial plate of distal end of fibula

Medial malleolus

Lateral malleolus

Body of talus

Posteroanterior view (slightly oblique)

Figure 5.64. Radiograph of ankle joint of a 14-year-old boy. The trochlea of the body of the talus fits into the mortise formed by the medial and lateral malleoli. Epiphysial (growth) plates are evident at this age.

Ankle Joint

The **ankle joint (talocrural articulation)** is a hinge-type synovial joint. It is located between the distal ends of the tibia and the fibula and the superior part of the talus. The ankle joint can be felt between the tendons on the anterior surface of the ankle as a slight depression, approximately 1 cm proximal to the tip of the medial malleolus.

Articular Surfaces of the Ankle Joint

The distal ends of the tibia and fibula (along with the inferior transverse part of the posterior tibiofibular ligament) (Figs. 5.63A and 5.65B) form a *malleolar mortise* into which the pulley-shaped *trochlea of the talus* fits (Fig. 5.64). The trochlea (L. pulley) is the rounded superior articular surface of the talus (Table 5.18A). The medial surface of the lateral malleolus articulates with the lateral surface of the talus. The tibia articulates with the talus in two places:

1. Its inferior surface forms the roof of the malleolar mortise, transferring the body's weight to the talus.

2. Its medial malleolus articulates with the medial surface of the talus.

The malleoli grip the talus tightly as it rocks in the mortise during movements of the joint. The grip of the malleoli on the trochlea is strongest during dorsiflexion of the foot (as when "digging in one's heels" when descending a steep slope or during tug-of-war) because this movement forces the wider, anterior part of the trochlea posteriorly between the malleoli, spreading the tibia and fibula slightly apart. This spreading is limited especially by the strong interosseous tibiofibular ligament as well as the anterior and posterior tibiofibular ligaments that unite the tibia and fibula (Figs. 5.63A and 5.65). The interosseous ligament is deeply placed between the nearly congruent surfaces of the tibia and fibula; although demonstrated in the inset for Figure 5.63A, the ligament can actually be observed only by rupturing it or in a cross section.

The ankle joint is relatively unstable during plantarflexion because the trochlea is narrower posteriorly and, therefore, lies relatively loosely within the mortise. It is during plantarflexion that most injuries of the ankle occur (usually as a result of sudden, unexpected—and therefore inadequately resisted—inversion of the foot).

Joint Capsule of the Ankle Joint

The joint capsule is thin anteriorly and posteriorly but is supported on each side by strong collateral ligaments (Figs. 5.65 and 5.66; thin areas of the capsule have been removed in Figure. 5.65, leaving only the reinforced parts—the ligaments—and a synovial fold). Its fibrous layer is attached superiorly to the borders of the articular surfaces of the tibia and the malleoli and inferiorly to the talus. The synovial membrane is loose and lines the fibrous layer of the capsule. The synovial cavity often extends superiorly between the tibia and the fibula as far as the interosseous tibiofibular ligament.

(A) Anterolateral view

Tibialis anterior (TA)
Calcaneal tendon
Anterior inferior tibiofibular ligament
Anterior talofibular ligament
Calcaneal bursa
Calcaneofibular ligament
Interosseous talocalcaneal ligament
Fibularis longus (FL)
Fibularis brevis (FB)
Synovial fold
Dorsal talonavicular ligament
Head of talus
Bifurcate ligament
Navicular band
Cuneiform bones
Dorsal calcaneocuboid ligament
Calcaneus and cuboid

(B) Posterior View

Posterior tibiofibular ligament
Inferior part of posterior inferior talofibular ligament
Talus
Lateral malleolus
Posterior talofibular ligament
Calcaneofibular ligament
Calcaneal tendon
Medial malleolus
Parts of deltoid ligament: Posterior tibiotalar, Tibiocalcanean
Groove for tendon of flexor hallucis longus
For bursa of calcaneal tendon

Figure 5.65. Dissection of ankle joint and joints of inversion and eversion. A and B. The foot has been inverted (note wedge under foot) to demonstrate the articular areas and the lateral ligaments that become taut during inversion of the foot.

Ligaments of the Ankle Joint

The ankle joint is reinforced laterally by the **lateral ligament of the ankle,** a compound structure consisting of three completely separate ligaments (Fig. 5.65A & B):

1. **Anterior talofibular ligament,** a flat, weak band that extends anteromedially from the lateral malleolus to the neck of the talus,

2. **Posterior talofibular ligament,** a thick, fairly strong band that runs horizontally medially and slightly posteriorly from the malleolar fossa to the lateral tubercle of the talus.

3. **Calcaneofibular ligament,** a round cord that passes posteroinferiorly from the tip of the lateral malleolus to the lateral surface of the calcaneus.

The joint capsule is reinforced medially by the large, strong **medial ligament of the ankle (deltoid ligament)** that attaches proximally to the medial malleolus (Fig. 5.66). The medial ligament fans out from the malleolus, attaching distally to the talus, calcaneus, and navicular via four adjacent and continuous parts: the **tibionavicular part,** the **tibiocalcaneal part,** and the **anterior** and **posterior tibiotalar parts.** The medial ligament stabilizes the ankle joint during eversion and prevents subluxation (partial dislocation) of the joint.

Table 5.18. Joints of Foot

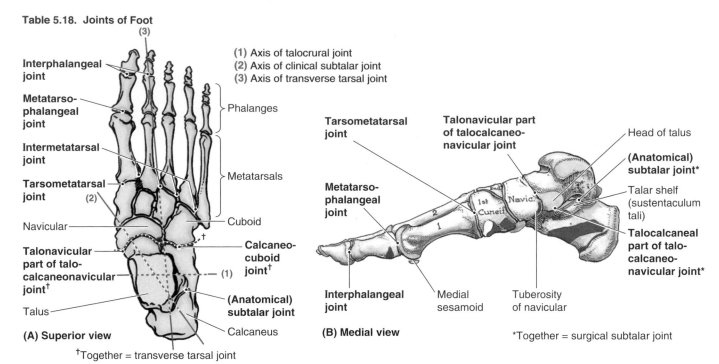

(1) Axis of talocrural joint
(2) Axis of clinical subtalar joint
(3) Axis of transverse tarsal joint

Interphalangeal joint

Metatarso-phalangeal joint

Intermetatarsal joint

Tarsometatarsal joint (2)

Navicular

Talonavicular part of talo-calcaneonavicular joint†

Talus

(A) Superior view

Phalanges

Metatarsals

Cuboid

Calcaneo-cuboid joint†

(Anatomical) subtalar joint

Calcaneus

†Together = transverse tarsal joint

Tarsometatarsal joint

Metatarso-phalangeal joint

Interphalangeal joint

(B) Medial view

Talonavicular part of talocalcaneo-navicular joint

Head of talus

(Anatomical) subtalar joint*

Talar shelf (sustentaculum tali)

Talocalcaneal part of talo-calcaneo-navicular joint*

Medial sesamoid

Tuberosity of navicular

*Together = surgical subtalar joint

Joint	Type	Articulating Surfaces	Joint Capsule	Ligaments	Movements	Blood Supply	Nerve Supply
Subtalar (talocalcaneal, anatomical subtalar joint)	Plane synovial joint	Inferior surface of body of talus (posterior calcaneal articular facet) articulates with superior surface (posterior talar articular surface) of calcaneus	Fibrous layer of joint capsule is attached to margins of articular surfaces	Medial, lateral, and posterior talocalcaneal ligaments support capsule; interosseous talocalcaneal ligament binds bones together	Inversion and eversion of foot	Posterior tibial and fibular arteries	Plantar aspect: medial or lateral plantar nerve; Dorsal aspect: deep fibular nerve
Talocalcaneonavicular	Synovial joint; talonavicular part is ball and socket type	Head of talus articulates with calcaneus and navicular bones	Joint capsule incompletely encloses joint	Plantar calcaneonavicular (spring) ligament supports head of talus	Gliding and rotatory movements possible	Anterior tibial artery via lateral tarsal artery, a branch of dorsal artery of foot	
Calcaneocuboid		Anterior end of calcaneus articulates with posterior surface of cuboid	Fibrous capsule encloses joint	Dorsal calcaneocuboid ligament, plantar calcaneocuboid, and long plantar ligaments support joint capsule	Inversion and eversion of foot; circumduction		
Cuneonavicular joint	Plane synovial joint(s)	Anterior navicular articulates with bases of meta-tarsal bones	Common capsule encloses joints	Dorsal and plantar cuneonavicular ligaments	Little movement occurs		
Tarsometatarsal		Anterior tarsal bones articulate with bases of metatarsal bones	Separate joint capsules enclose each joint	Dorsal, plantar, and interosseous tarsometatarsal ligaments bind bones together	Gliding or sliding		Deep fibular; medial and lateral plantar nerves; sural nerve

(continues)

Table 5.18. Joints of Foot *(continued)*

Joint	Type	Articulating Surfaces	Joint Capsule	Ligaments	Movements	Blood Supply	Nerve Supply
Intermetatarsal	Plane synovial joint	Bases of metatarsal bones articulate with each other		Dorsal, plantar, and interosseous tarsometatarsal ligaments bind bones together	Little individual movement occurs	Lateral metatarsal artery (a branch of dorsal artery of foot)	Digital nerves
Metatarsophalangeal	Condyloid synovial joint	Heads of metatarsal bones articulate with bases of proximal phalanges	Separate joint capsules enclose each joint	Collateral ligaments support capsule on each side; plantar ligament supports plantar part of capsule	Flexion, extension, and some abduction, adduction and circumduction		
Interphalangeal	Hinge synovial joint	Head of one phalanx articulates with base of one distal to it		Collateral and plantar ligaments support joints	Flexion and extension	Digital branches of plantar arch	

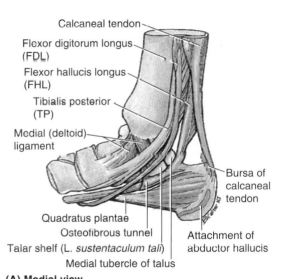

Calcaneal tendon
Flexor digitorum longus (FDL)
Flexor hallucis longus (FHL)
Tibialis posterior (TP)
Medial (deltoid) ligament
Bursa of calcaneal tendon
Quadratus plantae
Osteofibrous tunnel
Talar shelf (L. *sustentaculum tali*)
Attachment of abductor hallucis
Medial tubercle of talus

(A) Medial view

Figure 5.66. Ankle and tarsal joints. A. The flexor tendons, which descend the posterolateral aspect of the ankle region and enter the foot, are shown as is their relationship to the medial malleolus and talar shelf. Except for the part tethering the flexor hallucis longus tendon, the flexor retinaculum has been removed. **B.** This dissection of the ankle and tarsal joints demonstrates the four parts of the medial (deltoid) ligament of the ankle.

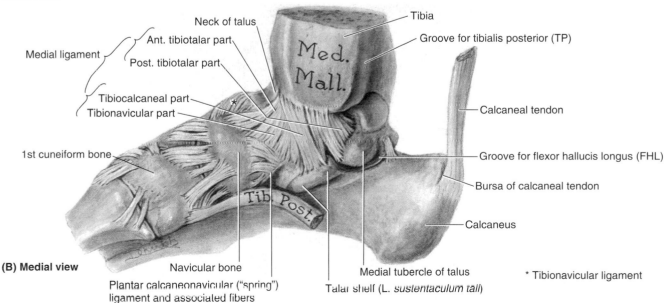

Neck of talus
Ant. tibiotalar part
Medial ligament
Post. tibiotalar part
Tibiocalcaneal part
Tibionavicular part
1st cuneiform bone
Tibia
Groove for tibialis posterior (TP)
Med. Mall.
Calcaneal tendon
Groove for flexor hallucis longus (FHL)
Tib. Post.
Bursa of calcaneal tendon
Calcaneus

(B) Medial view
Navicular bone
Plantar calcaneonavicular ("spring") ligament and associated fibers
Medial tubercle of talus
Talar shelf (L. *sustentaculum tali*)
* Tibionavicular ligament

Movements of the Ankle Joint

The main movements of the ankle joint are dorsiflexion and plantarflexion of the foot, which occur around a transverse axis passing through the talus (Table 5.18*A*). Because the narrow end of the trochlea of the talus lies loosely between the malleoli when the foot is plantarflexed, some "wobble" (small amounts of abduction, adduction, inversion, and eversion) is possible in this unstable position.

- *Dorsiflexion of the ankle* is produced by the muscles in the anterior compartment of the leg (Table 5.10). Dorsiflexion is usually limited by the passive resistance of the triceps surae to stretching and by tension in the medial and lateral ligaments.

- *Plantarflexion of the ankle* is produced by the muscles in the posterior compartment of the leg (Table 5.13). In toe dancing by ballet dancers, for example, the dorsum of the foot is in line with the anterior surface of the leg.

Blood Supply of the Ankle Joint

The arteries are derived from malleolar branches of the fibular and anterior and posterior tibial arteries (Fig. 5.63*B*).

Nerve Supply of the Ankle Joint

The nerves are derived from the tibial nerve and the deep fibular nerve, a division of the common fibular nerve (Fig. 5.63*D*).

Ankle Injuries

The ankle is the most frequently injured major joint in the body. *Ankle sprains* (torn fibers of ligaments) are most common. A sprained ankle is nearly always an *inversion injury,* involving twisting of the weight-bearing plantarflexed foot. The person steps on an uneven surface and the foot is forcibly inverted. *Lateral ligament sprains* occur in sports in which running and jumping are common, particularly basketball (70–80% of players have had at least one sprained ankle). The lateral ligament is injured because it is much weaker than the medial ligament and is the ligament that resists inversion at the talocrural joint. The *anterior talofibular ligament*—part of the lateral ligament—is most vulnerable and most commonly torn during ankle sprains, either partially or completely, resulting in instability of the ankle joint (Fig. B5.32). The *calcaneofibular ligament* may also be torn. In severe sprains, the lateral malleolus of the fibula may be fractured. *Shearing injuries fracture the lateral malleolus* at or superior to the ankle joint. *Avulsion fractures* break the malleolus inferior to the ankle joint; a fragment of bone is pulled off by the attached ligament(s).

A **Pott fracture–dislocation of the ankle** occurs when the foot is forcibly everted (Fig. B5.33). This action pulls on the extremely strong medial ligament, often tearing off the medial malleolus. The talus then moves laterally, shearing off the lateral malleolus or, more commonly, breaking the fibula superior to the tibiofibular syndesmosis. If the tibia is carried anteriorly, the posterior margin of the distal end of the tibia is also sheared off by the talus, producing a "trimalleolar fracture." In applying this term to this injury, the entire distal end of the tibia is erroneously considered to be a "malleolus."

Torn fibers of anterior talofibular ligament

Figure B5.32

Tibial Nerve Entrapment

The tibial nerve leaves the posterior compartment of the leg by passing deep to the flexor retinaculum in the interval between the medial malleolus and the calcaneus (Fig. 5.46*B*). Entrapment and compression of the tibial nerve

(*tarsal tunnel syndrome*) occurs when there is edema and tightness in the ankle involving the synovial sheaths of the tendons of muscles in the posterior compartment of the leg. The area involved is from the medial malleolus to the calcaneus, and the heel pain results from compression of the tibial nerve by the flexor retinaculum. ▶

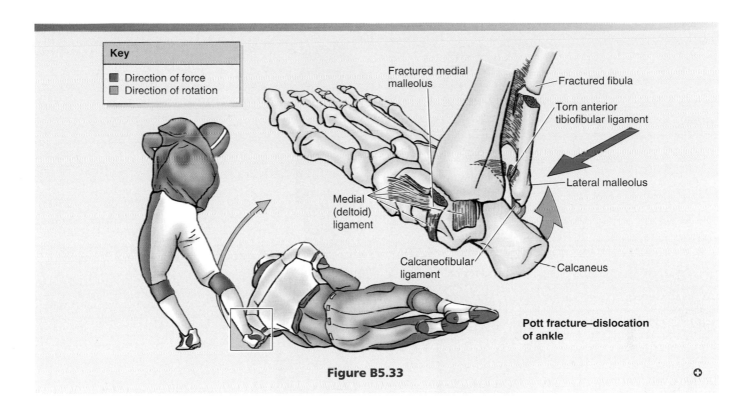

Key

☐ Direction of force
☐ Direction of rotation

Fractured medial malleolus

Fractured fibula

Torn anterior tibiofibular ligament

Lateral malleolus

Medial (deltoid) ligament

Calcaneofibular ligament

Calcaneus

Pott fracture–dislocation of ankle

Figure B5.33

THE BOTTOM LINE: The ankle (talocrural) joint is composed of a superior mortise, formed by the weight-bearing inferior surface of the tibia and the two malleoli, which receive the trochlea of the talus. The joint is maintained medially by a strong, medial (deltoid) ligament, and a much weaker lateral ligament. The lateral ligament (specifically its anterior talofibular ligament component) is the most frequently injured ligament of the body. Injury occurs primarily by inadvertent inversion of the plantarflexed, weight-bearing foot). About 70° of dorsiflexion and plantarflexion is possible at the joint, in addition to which small amounts of wobble occur in the less stable plantarflexed position.

Foot Joints

The many joints of the foot involve the tarsals, metatarsals, and phalanges (Table 5.18). The important intertarsal joints are the *subtalar (talocalcaneal) joint* and the *transverse tarsal joint (calcaneocuboid* and *talonavicular joints)*. Inversion and eversion of the foot are the main movements involving these joints. The other intertarsal joints (e.g., *intercuneiform joints*) and the *tarsometatarsal* and *intermetatarsal joints* are relatively small and are so tightly joined by ligaments that only slight movement occurs between them. In the foot, flexion and extension occurs in the forefoot at the metatarsophalangeal and interphalangeal joints (Table 5.19) Inversion is augmented by flexion of the toes (especially the great and 2nd toes), and eversion by their extension (especially of the

lateral toes). All bones of the foot proximal to the metatarsophalangeal joints are united by dorsal and plantar ligaments. The bones of the metatarsophalangeal and interphalangeal joints are united by lateral and medial collateral ligaments.

The **subtalar joint** occurs where the talus rests on and articulates with the calcaneus. The *anatomical subtalar joint* is a single synovial joint between the slightly concave posterior calcaneal articular surface of the talus and the convex posterior articular facet of the calcaneus (Table 5.18). The joint capsule is weak but is supported by medial, lateral, posterior, and interosseous *talocalcaneal ligaments* (Fig. 5.65). The **interosseous talocalcaneal ligament** lies within the *tarsal sinus*, which separates the subtalar and talocalcaneonavicular joints and is especially strong. Orthopaedic surgeons use the term *subtalar joint* for the compound functional joint consisting of the anatomical subtalar joint plus the **talocalcaneal part of the talocalcaneonavicular joint.** The two separate elements of the *clinical subtalar joint* straddle the talocalcaneal intcrosseous ligament. Structurally, the anatomical definition is logical because the anatomical subtalar joint is a discrete joint, having its own joint capsule and articular cavity. Functionally, however, the clinical definition is logical because the two parts of the compound joint function as a unit; it is impossible for them to function independently. The subtalar joint (by either definition) is where the majority of inversion and eversion occurs, around an axis that is oblique.

The **transverse tarsal joint** is a compound joint formed by two separate joints aligned transversely: the **talonavicular**

Table 5.19. Movements of the Joints of the Forefoot and the Muscles Producing Them

(A)   Flexion   **(B)   Extension**

(C)   Abduction   **(D)   Adducted (relaxed position)**

Movement	Muscles[a]	Movement	Muscles[a]
Metatarsophalangeal joints		Interphalangeal joints	
Flexion (A)	**Flexor digitorum brevis** **Lumbricals** **Interossei** **Flexor hallucis brevis** **Flexor hallucis longus** Flexor digit minimi brevis Flexor digitorum longus	Flexion (fig. A)	**Flexor hallucis longus** **Flexor digitorum longus** **Flexor digitorum brevis** Quadratus plantae
Extension (B)	**Extensor hallucis longus** **Extensor digitorum longus** **Extensor digitorum brevis**	Extension (fig. B)	**Extensor hallucis longus** **Extensor digitorum longus** **Extensor digitorum brevis**
Abduction (C)	**Abductor hallucis** **Abductor digiti minimi** **Dorsal interossei**		
Adduction (D)	**Adductor hallucis** **Plantar interossei**		

[a]Muscles in boldface are chiefly responsible for the movement; the other muscles assist them.

part of the talocalcaneonavicular joint and the calcaneocuboid joint. At this joint, the midfoot and forefoot rotate as a unit on the hindfoot around a longitudinal (AP) axis, augmenting the inversion and eversion movements occurring at the clinical subtalar joint. Transection across the transverse tarsal joint is a standard method for *surgical amputation of the foot.*

Major Ligaments of the Foot

The major ligaments of the plantar aspect of the foot (Fig. 5.67) are the:

- **Plantar calcaneonavicular ligament (spring ligament)**, which extends across and fills a wedge-shaped gap between the talar shelf and the inferior margin of the posterior ar-

Figure 5.67. Plantar ligaments. A and B. Deep dissection of the sole of the right foot showing the attachments of the ligaments and the long tendons of the long evertor and invertor muscles. The main ligaments from this view are the plantar calcaneonavicular and the long and short plantar ligaments.

Plantar views

ticular surface of the navicular (Fig. 5.67*A* & *B*). The spring ligament supports the head of the talus and plays important roles in the transfer of weight from the talus and in maintaining the longitudinal arch of the foot, of which it is the keystone (superiormost element).

- **Long plantar ligament,** which passes from the plantar surface of the calcaneus to the groove on the cuboid. Some of its fibers extend to the bases of the metatarsals, thereby forming a tunnel for the tendon of the fibularis longus (Fig. 5.67*A*). The long plantar ligament is important in maintaining the longitudinal arch of the foot.

- **Plantar calcaneocuboid ligament** (**short plantar ligament**), which is located on a plane between the plantar calcaneonavicular and the long plantar ligaments (Fig. 5.67*B*). It extends from the anterior aspect of the inferior surface of the calcaneus to the inferior surface of the cuboid. It is also involved in maintaining the longitudinal arch of the foot.

Arches of the Foot

If the feet were more rigid structures, each impact with the ground would generate extremely large forces of short duration (shocks) that would be propagated through the skeletal system. Because the foot is composed of numerous bones connected by ligaments, it has considerable flexibility that allows it to deform with each ground contact, thereby absorbing much of the shock. Furthermore, the tarsal and metatarsal bones are arranged in longitudinal and transverse arches passively supported and actively restrained by flexible tendons that add to the weight-bearing capabilities and resiliency of the foot. Thus much smaller forces of longer duration are transmitted through the skeletal system.

The arches distribute weight over the pedal platform (foot), acting not only as shock absorbers but also as springboards for propelling it during walking, running, and jumping. The resilient arches add to the foot's ability to adapt to changes in surface contour. The weight of the body is transmitted to the talus from the tibia. Then it is transmitted posteriorly to the calcaneus and anteriorly to the "ball of the foot" (the sesamoids of the 1st metatarsal and the head of the 2nd metatarsal), and that weight/pressure is shared laterally with the heads of the 3rd–5th metatarsals as necessary for balance and comfort (Fig. 5.68). Between these weight-bearing points are the relatively elastic arches of the foot, which become slightly flattened by body weight during standing. They normally resume their curvature (recoil) when body weight is removed.

The **longitudinal arch of the foot** is composed of medial and lateral parts (Fig. 5.69). Functionally, both parts act as a unit with the transverse arch of the foot, spreading the weight in all directions. The **medial longitudinal arch** is higher and more important than the lateral longitudinal arch (Fig. 5.69*A* & *D*). The medial longitudinal arch is composed of the calcaneus, talus, navicular, three cuneiforms, and three metatarsals. *The talar head is the keystone of the medial longitudinal arch.* The tibialis anterior, attaching to the 1st metatarsal and medial cuneiform, helps strengthen the medial

Plantar view

Figure 5.68. Weight-bearing areas of foot. Body weight is divided approximately equally between the hindfoot (calcaneus) and the forefoot (heads of the metatarsals). The forefoot has five points of contact with the ground: a large medial one that includes the two sesamoid bones associated with the head of the 1st metatarsal and the heads of the lateral four metatarsals. The 1st metatarsal supports the major share of the load, with the lateral forefoot providing balance.

longitudinal arch. The fibularis longus tendon, passing from lateral to medial, also helps support this arch (Fig. 5.69*A*). The *lateral longitudinal arch* is much flatter than the medial part of the arch and rests on the ground during standing (Fig. 5.69*B* & *D*). It is made up of the calcaneus, cuboid, and lateral two metatarsals.

The **transverse arch of the foot** runs from side to side (Fig. 5.69*C*). It is formed by the cuboid, cuneiforms, and bases of the metatarsals. The medial and lateral parts of the longitudinal arch serve as pillars for the transverse arch. The tendons of the fibularis longus and tibialis posterior, crossing under the sole of the foot like a stirrup (Fig. 5.69*C*), help maintain the curvature of the transverse arch. The integrity of the bony arches of the foot is maintained by both passive factors and dynamic supports (Fig. 5.69*E*).

Passive factors involved in forming and maintaining the arches of the foot include

- The shape of the united bones (both arches, but especially the transverse arch).

- Four successive layers of fibrous tissue that bowstring the longitudinal arch (superficial to deep):

  1. Plantar aponeurosis.

  2. Long plantar ligament.

  3. Plantar calcaneocuboid (short plantar) ligament.

  4. Plantar calcaneonavicular (spring) ligament.

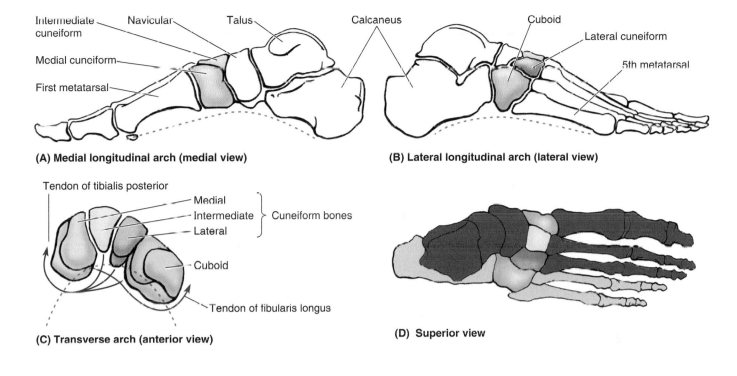

(A) **Medial longitudinal arch (medial view)**

(B) **Lateral longitudinal arch (lateral view)**

(C) **Transverse arch (anterior view)**

(D) **Superior view**

(E) **Medial longitudinal arch (medial view)**

Figure 5.69. Arches of foot. A and B. The medial longitudinal arch is higher than the lateral longitudinal arch, which may contact the ground when standing erect. **C.** The transverse arch is demonstrated at the level of the cuneiforms, receiving stirrup-like support from a major invertor (tibialis posterior) and evertor (fibularis longus). **D.** The components of the medial (*dark gray*) and lateral (*light gray*) longitudinal arches are indicated. The calcaneus (*medium gray*) is common to both. The medial arch is primarily weight bearing, whereas the lateral arch provides balance. **E.** The active (*red lines*) and passive (*gray*) supports of the longitudinal arches are represented. There are four layers of passive support (*1–4*).

Dynamic supports involved in maintaining the arches of the foot include

- Active (reflexive) bracing action of intrinsic muscles of foot (longitudinal arch).
- Active and tonic contraction of muscles with long tendons extending into foot:
  - Flexors hallucis and digitorum longus for the longitudinal arch.
  - Fibularis longus and tibialis posterior for the transverse arch.

Of these factors, the plantar ligaments and the plantar aponeurosis bear the greatest stress and are most important in maintaining the arches of the foot.

THE BOTTOM LINE: Functionally, there are three compound joints in the foot: (1) the clinical subtalar joint between the talus and the calcaneus, where inversion and eversion occur about an oblique axis; (2) the transverse tarsal joint, where the midfoot and forefoot rotate as a unit on the hindfoot around a longitudinal axis, augmenting inversion and eversion; and (3) the remaining joints of the foot, which allow the pedal platform (foot) to form dynamic longitudinal and transverse arches. The arches provide the resilience necessary for walking, running, and jumping, and are maintained by four layers of passive, fibrous support plus the dynamic support provided by the intrinsic muscles of the foot and the long fibular, tibial, and flexor tendons.

Hallux Valgus

Hallux valgus is a foot deformity caused by pressure from footwear and degenerative joint disease; it is characterized by lateral deviation of the great toe (Fig. B5.34). The **L** in valgus indicates *lateral deviation.* In some people, the painful deviation is so large that the great toe overlaps the 2nd toe (Fig. B5.34*A*), and there is a decrease in the medial longitudinal arch. Such deviation occurs especially in females, and its frequency increases with age. These individuals cannot move their 1st digit away from their 2nd digit because the sesamoids under the head of the 1st metatarsal are usually displaced and lie in the space between the heads of the 1st and 2nd metatarsals (Fig. B5.34*B*). The 1st metatarsal shifts medially and the sesamoids shift laterally. Often the surrounding tissues swell and the resultant pressure and friction against the shoe cause a subcutaneous

bursa to form; when tender and inflamed, the bursa is called a **bunion** (Fig. B5.34*A*). Often hard **corns** (inflamed areas of thick skin) also form over the proximal interphalangeal joints, especially the little toe.

Hammer Toe

Hammer toe is a foot deformity in which the proximal phalanx is permanently and markedly dorsiflexed (hyperextended) at the metatarsophalangeal joint and the middle phalanx strongly plantarflexed at the proximal interphalangeal joint. The distal phalanx of the digit is often also hyperextended. This gives the digit (usually the 2nd) a hammer-like appearance (Fig. B5.35*A*). This deformity of one or more toes may result from weakness of the lumbrical and interosseous muscles, which flex the metatarsophalangeal joints and extend the interphalangeal joints. A *callosity* ▶

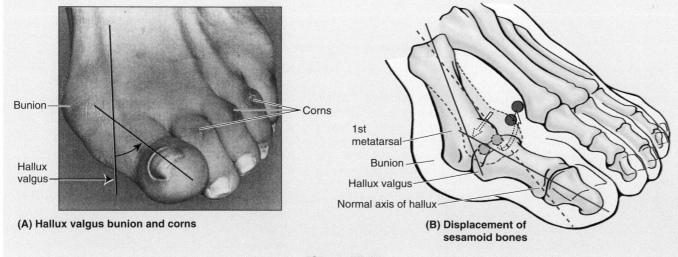

(A) Hallux valgus bunion and corns

(B) Displacement of sesamoid bones

Figure B5.34

(A) Hammer toe

(B) Claw toes

Normal footprint

Flatfoot footprint

(C) View of normal arch

(D) View of fallen arch

Figure B5.35

or *callus,* hard thickening of the keratin layer of the skin, often develops where the dorsal surface of the toe repeatedly rubs on the shoe.

Claw Toes

Claw toes are characterized by hyperextension of the metatarsophalangeal joints and flexion of the distal interphalangeal joints (Fig. B5.35*B*). Usually, the lateral four toes are involved. Callosities develop on the dorsal surfaces of the toes because of pressure of the shoe. They may also form on the plantar surfaces of the metatarsal heads and the toe tips because they bear extra weight when claw toes are present.

Pes Planus (Flatfeet)

The flat appearance of the foot before age 3 is normal and results from the thick subcutaneous fat-pad in the sole. As children get older, the fat is lost, and a normal medial longitudinal arch becomes visible (Fig. B5.35*C*). Flatfeet can either be *flexible* (flat, lacking a medial arch, when weight bearing but normal in appearance when not bearing weight [Fig. B5.35*D*]) or *rigid* (flat even when not bearing weight).

The more common *flexible flatfeet* result from loose or degenerated intrinsic ligaments (inadequate passive arch support). Flexible flatfoot is common in childhood but usually resolves with age as the ligaments grow and mature. The condition occasionally persists into adulthood and may or may not be symptomatic.

Rigid flatfeet with a history that goes back to childhood are likely to result from a bone deformity (such as a fusion of adjacent tarsal bones). *Acquired flatfeet* ("fallen arches") are likely to be secondary to dysfunction of the tibialis posterior (dynamic arch support) owing to trauma, degeneration with age, or denervation. In the absence of normal passive or dynamic support, the plantar calcaneonavicular ligament fails to support the head of the talus. Consequently, the talar head displaces inferomedially and becomes prominent (Fig. B5.35*D, red arrow*). As a result, some flattening of the medial part of the longitudinal arch occurs, along with lateral deviation of the forefoot. Flatfeet are common in older people, particularly if they undertake much unaccustomed standing or gain weight rapidly, adding stress on the muscles and increasing the strain on the ligaments supporting the arches. ▶

Clubfoot (Talipes)

Clubfoot refers to a foot that is twisted out of position. Of the several types, all are *congenital* (present at birth). *Talipes equinovarus,* the common type (2 per 1000 live births), involves the subtalar joint; boys are affected twice as often as girls. The foot is inverted, the ankle is plantarflexed, and the forefoot is adducted (turned toward the midline in an abnormal manner) (Fig. B5.36). The foot assumes the position of a horse's hoof, hence the prefix "equino" (L. *equinus,* horse). In half of those affected, both feet are malformed. A person with an uncorrected clubfoot cannot put the heel and sole flat and must bear the weight on the lateral surface of the forefoot. Consequently, walking is painful. The main abnormality is shortness and tightness of the muscles, tendons, ligaments, and joint capsules on the medial side and posterior aspect of the foot and ankle. ●

(A)

Ankle joint (plantarflexed)
Talus (deformed)
Tibionavicular ligament and tendons of extensor digitorum longus, tibialis anterior, and extensor hallucis longus tendons (note tightness)
Calcaneus (inverted)
Bones of forefoot (in extreme varus position)

(B)

Figure B5.36

Surface Anatomy of the Ankle and Foot

The surface anatomy of the bones of the foot was presented earlier in this chapter (see "Surface Anatomy of the Bones of the Foot").

If the foot is actively inverted, the **tendon of the tibialis posterior** may be palpated as it passes posterior and distal to the medial malleolus, then superior to the talar shelf, to reach its attachment to the tuberosity of the navicular. Hence the tibialis posterior tendon is the guide to the navicular. The tendon of the tibialis posterior also indicates the site for palpating the *posterior tibial pulse* (halfway between the medial malleolus and the calcaneal tendon).

The **talar shelf** (L. *sustentaculum tali*), approximately 2 cm distal to the tip of the medial malleolus, is best felt by palpating it from below where it is somewhat obscured by the **tendon of the flexor digitorum longus**, which crosses it (Fig. SA5.4*B*). On the lateral side, when the foot is inverted, the lateral margin of the **anterior surface of the calcaneus** is uncovered and palpable. This indicates the site of the *calcaneocuboid joint*. When the foot is plantarflexed, the **head of the talus** is exposed. Palpate it dorsal to where the anterior surface of the calcaneus is felt. The **calcaneal tendon** at the posterior aspect of the ankle is easily palpated and traced to its attachment to the *calcaneal tuberosity*. In the depression on each side of the tendon, the ankle joint is superficial. When the joint is overfilled with fluid, these depressions may be obliterated.

The tendons in the ankle region can be identified satisfactorily only when their muscles are acting. The tendons of the fibularis longus and brevis may be followed distally, posterior and inferior to the lateral malleolus, and then anteriorly along the lateral aspect of the foot (Fig. SA5.4*C*). The **fibularis longus tendon** can be palpated as far as the cuboid, and then it disappears as it turns into the sole. The **fibularis brevis tendon** can easily be traced to its attachment to the dorsal surface of the tuberosity on the base of the 5th metatarsal. This tuberosity is located at the middle of the lateral border of the foot. With toes actively extended, the small fleshy belly of the **extensor digitorum brevis** may be seen and palpated anterior to the lateral malleolus. Its position should be observed and palpated so that it may not be mistaken subsequently for an abnormal edema.

The **metatarsophalangeal joint of the great toe** lies distal to the knuckle formed by the head of the 1st ▶

metatarsal (Fig. SA5.4*A*). *Gout,* a metabolic disorder, commonly causes edema and tenderness of this joint, as does *osteoarthritis* (degenerative joint disease). Severe pain in the 1st metatarsophalangeal joint is called *podagra* (from G. *pous* + G. *agra,* a seizure). Often the 1st metatarsophalangeal joint is the first one affected by arthritis.

The tendons on the anterior aspect of the ankle (from medial to lateral side) are easily palpated when the foot is dorsiflexed.

- The large **tendon of the tibialis anterior** leaves the cover of the superior extensor tendon (Fig. SA5.4*A*), from which level the tendon is invested by a continuous synovial sheath; the tendon may be traced to its attachment to the 1st cuneiform and the base of the 1st metatarsal.

- The **tendon of the extensor hallucis longus**, obvious when the great toe is dorsiflexed against resistance, may be followed to its attachment to the base of the distal phalanx of the great toe.

- The **tendons of the extensor digitorum longus** may be followed easily to their attachments to the lateral four toes (Fig. SA5.4*C*).

- The **tendon of the fibularis tertius** may also be traced to its attachment to the base of the 5th metatarsal. This muscle is of minor importance and may be absent.

The *transverse tarsal joint* is indicated by a line from the posterior aspect of the tuberosity of the navicular to a point halfway between the lateral malleolus and the tuberosity of the 5th metatarsal (Table 5.18). ▶

(A)

Figure SA5.4

1 Abductor hallucis
2 Ball of foot
3 Calcaneal tendon
4 Extensor hallucis longus tendon
5 Medial malleolus
6 Medial longitudinal arch of foot
7 Navicular tuberosity
8 Talar shelf
9 Tibialis anterior tendon
10 Tibialis posterior tendon
11 Head of 1st metatarsal

(B)

Tibialis anterior

Inferior extensor retinaculum

Extensor digitorum longus andŁ
fibularis tertius (4)

Extensor hallucis longus (5)

Extensor hallucis brevis

Lateral malleolus (L)

Anterolateral view

Fibularis longus (1)

Fibularis brevis (2)

Fibularis tertius

Extensor digitorum brevis (3)

(C)

Figure SA5.4. (Continued)

Medical Imaging of the Lower Limb

Radiography

Pelvic Girdle and Hip Joint

Radiographs of the pelvis and hip show bone and joint abnormalities or malalignment. In the AP projection of the hip joint shown in Figure 5.70A, the patient is in the supine position on the radiographic table. The central X-ray beam is centered over the hip joint (see orientation figures). Superimposed on the femoral head is the posterior rim of the acetabulum (PR). At the junction of the femoral neck and shaft, the greater and lesser trochanters may be seen. Between the trochanters is an oblique line cast by the superimposed intertrochanteric line and crest (IC).

When viewing a full-size radiograph of the hip joint (i.e., on film or a monitor), observe the architecture of the trabecular bone of the head, neck, and proximal shaft of the femur. The strength of the angled bone depends on this structure. In a healthy femur without osteoporosis, the trabeculae correspond to tension and pressure lines reflecting the weight-bearing function of this bone. The dense compact bone appears transparent (white), whereas the less dense spongy bone appears dark.

Extrapolated lines and curves superimposed on the radiographic image (e.g., the Kohler, Shenton, and iliofemoral lines in Figure 5.70A) in specific views are used to assess normal alignment of bony features. Interrupted lines, irregular curve or lack of symmetry between left and right sides indicates dislocations, fractures, or slipped epiphyses. To ensure detection of a fracture of the femoral neck, several views must be obtained (Fig. 5.70B).

Knee Joint

Multiple radiographic projections (AP, lateral, and oblique) are necessary to evaluate the knee properly. In an AP projection of the knee joint (Fig. 5.71B), the person is in the supine position with the knee extended. The central X-ray beam is directed through the joint cavity. Outlines of the femoral and tibial condyles and the shadows of the patella are superimposed over the distal end of the femur. The joint cavity appears large because the menisci are not visible. The menisci can be visualized if air or opaque fluid is injected into the joint cavity. The adductor tubercle is evident just superior to the medial epicondyle of the femur. The lateral femoral epicondyle appears more prominent than the medial one. The intercondylar fossa is opposite the medial and lateral tubercles of the inter-

AP projections

Figure 5.70. Radiographs of normal hip joint. A. On the femur, observe the head, neck, greater trochanter, intertrochanteric crest (*IC*), and shaft. On the hip bone, observe the lunate surface of the acetabulum, the posterior rim of the acetabulum (*PR*), the anterior superior iliac spine (*ASIS*), the ischial spine, and the sacroiliac joint. Several different lines and curvatures are used in the detection of hip abnormalities (dislocations, fractures or slipped epiphyses). The Kohler line (*A*) is normally tangential to the pelvic inlet and the obturator foramen. The acetabular fossa should lie lateral to this line. A fossa that crosses the line suggests an acetabular fracture with inward displacement. The Shenton line (*B*) and the iliofemoral line (*C*) should appear in a normal AP radiograph as smooth, continuous lines that are bilaterally symmetrical. The Shenton line is a radiographic indication of the angle of inclination. **B.** In this view the left thigh was abducted. Observe the acetabular fossa, anterior inferior iliac spine (*AIIS*), head of the femur (*H*), neck of the femur (*N*), greater trochanter (*G*), lesser trochanter (*L*), intertrochanteric crest (*IC*), and shaft of femur (*S*).

Femur
Medial thigh
Patella
Adductor tubercle
Medial epicondyle
Lateral condyle of femur
Medial condyle of femur
Lateral condyle of tibia
Medial and lateral intercondylar tubercles of intercondylar eminence
Head of fibula
Shaft of fibula
Shaft of tibia

(A) Anterior view

(B) AP projection

Key	
- - - - -	Posterior aspect of condyles

Figure 5.71. Knee joint. A and B. The orientation drawing depicts the structures visible in the AP radiograph of the right knee joint.

condylar eminence of the proximal tibia. The articular surfaces of the condyles of the tibia are concave in an AP view.

In the lateral projection of an arthrogram of the knee joint shown in Figure 5.72, the knee is slightly flexed. A contrast medium was injected through the joint capsule to show the joint cavity and the extent of the synovial membrane. The articular cartilage on the femoral condyle is radiolucent and the fibrous layer of the joint capsule, lined with synovial membrane, is distinct. The large suprapatellar bursa is continuous with the joint cavity. Although MRI has largely replaced arthrography, it is sometimes useful for detecting loose articular bodies if the MRI is inconclusive.

Ankle Joint and Foot

The most common radiographic views of the ankle joint and foot are lateral and AP. A lateral radiograph is taken with the lateral malleolus placed against the X-ray detector (Fig. 5.73*A*). In Figure 5.73, the articulation of the convex surface of the trochlea of the talus (T) with the malleoli of the tibia and fibula is apparent, and shadows of the malleoli are visible. The neck (N) and head (H) of the talus, the disc-shaped navicular (Na), and the talonavicular joint can be seen. The calcaneus (Ca) and cuboid (C) articulate at the calcaneocuboid joint. The *tarsal sinus* (TS), the space between the calcaneus and talus, contains the interosseous talocalcaneal ligament.

Suprapatellar bursa
Patella
Joint cavity
Fibrous layer of joint capsule
Articular cartilage

Lateral projection

Figure 5.72. Arthrogram of knee joint. Contrast medium was injected into the synovial cavity. The knee is slightly flexed. The large suprapatellar bursa communicates with the knee joint cavity.

Figure 5.73. Radiographs of lower leg, ankle, and foot. A. The left foot is shown in a neutral position. **B.** The left foot, in slight plantarflexion, is shown. **C.** The left ankle is shown. *C,* cuboid; *Ca,* calcaneus; *H,* head of talus; *L,* lateral malleolus; *M,* medial malleolus; *N,* neck of talus; *Na,* navicular; *T,* talus; *TS,* tarsal sinus (tunnel). (Part **C** Courtesy of Dr. P. Bobechko and Dr. E. Becker, Department of Medical Imaging, University of Toronto, Toronto, Ontario, Canada.)

In the dorsoplantar projection, the patient is supine with the knee flexed, and the plantar surface of the foot is placed on the X-ray detector (Fig. 5.73*B*). The central X-ray beam is centered on the base of the 3rd metatarsal. This view demonstrates the phalanges and interphalangeal joints. However, because the toes are in slight flexion, the interphalangeal joints of the 2nd–5th toes are not clear. The sesamoids on the plantar surface of the head of the 1st metatarsal are evident, as is the articulation of the base of the 1st metatarsal with the medial cuneiform and the base

of the 2nd metatarsal. The bases of the 2nd–5th metatarsals overlap, so the intermetatarsal joints are easy to see. The tarsal bones overlap somewhat because of the normal curvature of the foot. Consequently, all the tarsal joints do not show clearly. Only anterior parts of the talus and calcaneus are visible because of the overlap of the malleoli.

An AP radiograph is taken with the person in the supine position with the foot dorsiflexed to a right angle and the great toe pointed slightly medially (Fig. 5.73*C*).

To visualize all the bones and joints of the ankle and foot, other projections are required.

Arteriography

Visualization of arteries by X-ray imaging after injection of a radiopaque contrast medium is a helpful way of studying selected arteries to determine the existence of abnormalities such as *popliteal aneurysm* (circumscribed dilation of the popliteal artery). In a **popliteal arteriogram** (Fig. 5.74), the radiopaque material is injected into the femoral artery and spreads through the popliteal artery and its branches, the tibial and fibular arteries.

Computed Tomography

CT uses X-rays that pass through the limb at various angles; however, the images are created by computer reconstructions of the data. CT scans can be set to display soft tissues or bone. Hypodense areas on CT scans suggest strains (swelling), and hyperdense areas suggest hematomas. CT of the knee (arthrotomography) provides a reliable assessment of the cruciate ligaments, menisci, patellar cartilage, and localizes of osteochondral defects and loose bodies.

Magnetic Resonance Imaging

MRI produces images of exquisite resolution of limbs without the use of radiation. MRI scanning requires the individual to keep the limbs motionless for 5–10 min. MRIs show much more detail in the soft tissues than do radiographs or CTs (Figs. 5.75–5.78).

Hip Joint

In Figure 5.75, observe that the joint capsule of the joint is thick near the iliofemoral ligament and thin posterior to the psoas bursa and tendon. In sections at this level, the femoral sheath, which encloses the femoral artery, vein, lymph node, lymphatic vessels, and fat, protrudes into the subcutaneous tissue. The loose connective tissue nearly surrounds it except posteriorly where, between the iliopsoas and the pectineus, it is attached to the capsule of the hip joint. The femoral artery is separated from the hip joint by the iliopsoas muscle and/or tendon. In the interval between the iliopsoas, the pectineus, and the femoral nerve, the femoral vein lies between the iliopsoas and its fascia.

Knee

MRIs are extremely helpful for determining if there are injuries to the menisci, collateral ligaments, and cruciate ligaments (Fig. 5.76). It is the procedure of choice for assessing internal derangements of the knee. ▶

Femoral artery

Medial superior genicular artery

Popliteal artery

Medial inferior genicular artery

Posterior tibial artery

Anterior tibial artery

Fibular artery

Posterior tibial artery

Lateral plantar artery

Medial plantar artery

Dorsal artery of foot

Plantar arch

Left anterior oblique view of right limb

Figure 5.74. Popliteal arteriogram. The popliteal artery begins at the site of the adductor hiatus (where it may be compressed) and then lies successively on the distal end of the femur, joint capsule of the knee joint, and popliteus muscle (not visible) before dividing into the anterior and posterior tibial arteries at the inferior angle of the popliteus fossa. Here it is subject to entrapment as it passes beneath the tendinous arch of the soleus muscle. (Courtesy of Dr. K. Sniderman, Associate Professor of Medical Imaging, University of Toronto, Toronto, Ontario, Canada)

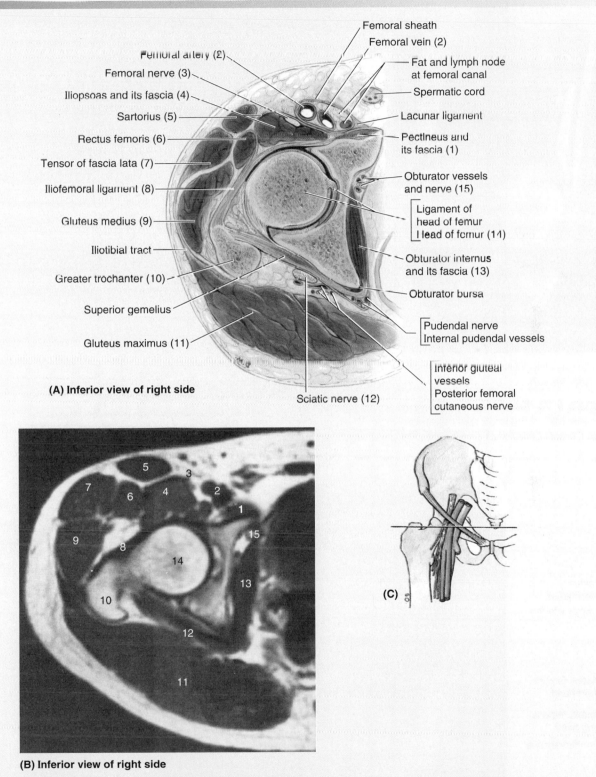

(A) Inferior view of right side

Femoral sheath
Femoral vein (2)
Femoral artery (2)
Femoral nerve (3)
Iliopsoas and its fascia (4)
Sartorius (5)
Rectus femoris (6)
Tensor of fascia lata (7)
Iliofemoral ligament (8)
Gluteus medius (9)
Iliotibial tract
Greater trochanter (10)
Superior gemelius
Gluteus maximus (11)
Sciatic nerve (12)

Fat and lymph node at femoral canal
Spermatic cord
Lacunar ligament
Pectineus and its fascia (1)
Obturator vessels and nerve (15)
Ligament of head of femur
Head of femur (14)
Obturator internus and its fascia (13)
Obturator bursa
Pudendal nerve
Internal pudendal vessels
Inferior gluteal vessels
Posterior femoral cutaneous nerve

(B) Inferior view of right side

(C)

Figure 5.75. Sectional and radiographic anatomy of gluteal region and proximal anterior thigh at level of hip joint. A and B. A descriptive drawing and transverse (axial MRI) study of an anatomical section of the thigh are shown. **C.** The orientation drawing shows the level of the section.

(A) Anterior view

(B) Anterior view

Figure 5.76. Sectional anatomy of knee joint. A and B. The orientation drawing depicts the structures visible in the coronal MRI of the knee joint. (Courtesy of Dr. W. Kucharczyk, Professor and Chair of Medical Imaging, University of Toronto, and Clinical Director of Tri-Hospital Magnetic Resonance Centre, Toronto, Ontario, Canada.)

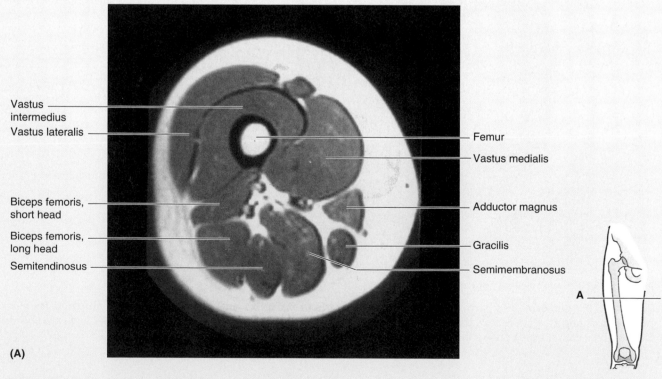

(A)

Figure 5.77. Transverse MRIs of lower limb, from below. A. Sections at the mid-thigh level (**A**) and mid-leg level (**B**) are shown.

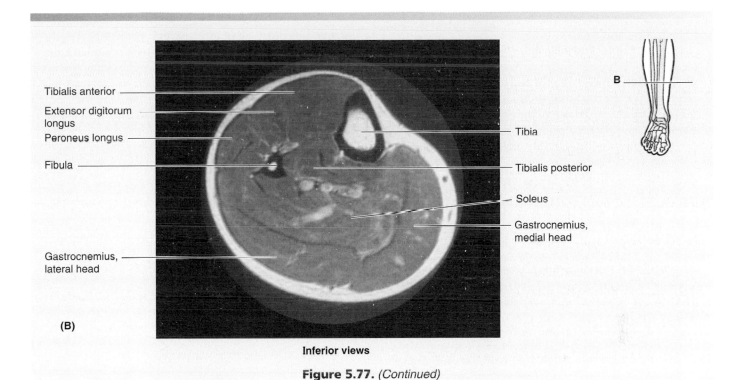

Tibialis anterior

Extensor digitorum longus

Peroneus longus

Fibula

Tibia

Tibialis posterior

Soleus

Gastrocnemius, medial head

Gastrocnemius, lateral head

B

(B)

Inferior views

Figure 5.77. *(Continued)*

Tibia

M

12

Talus

L

1

11

10   9

2

8

7

3

Calcaneus

6

5   4

(A)

Lower limit of subcutaneous fat

Medial malleolus (M)

Medial or deltoid ligament (12)

Tibialis posterior (11)

Talar shelf (9)
Flexor hallucis longus (8)

Flexor digitorum longus (10)

Abductor hallucis longus (7)

Medial plantar artery and nerve

Quadratus plantae
Lateral plantar artery and nerve

Flexor digitorum brevis
Plantar aponeurosis (6)

Talus

Calcaneus

Interosseous ligament

Lateral malleolus (L)

Posterior talofibular ligament (1)

Fibularis (peroneus) brevis (2)

Fibularis (peroneus) longus (3)

Medial tubercle

Abductor digiti minimi (4)

Encapsulated cushions of fat (5)

(B) Posterior view

Figure 5.78. Sectional anatomy of ankle region. A and B. The orientation drawing depicts the structures visible in the MRI of the ankle. (Courtesy of Dr. W. Kucharczyk, Professor and Chair of Medical Imaging, University of Toronto, and Clinical Director of Tri-Hospital Magnetic Resonance Centre, Toronto, Ontario, Canada.)

Thigh, Leg, and Ankle

MRIs are helpful for identifying the soft tissue (such as muscle) and osseous and neurovascular anatomy of the thigh and leg (Fig. 5.77). In the coronal MRI shown in Figure 5.78, the tibia rests on the talus and the talus rests on the calcaneus. Between the calcaneus and the skin, several encapsulated cushions of fat are evident. It is also clearly seen that the lateral malleolus descends much farther inferiorly than the medial malleolus. In the anatomical coronal section, the interosseous band between the talus and calcaneus separates the subtalar joint from the talocalcaneonavicular joint. Both the anatomical section and the MRI demonstrate the talar shelf acting as a pulley for the flexor hallucis longus and giving attachment to the calcaneotibial band of the medial ligament. **◉**

References and Suggested Readings

Anderson MK, Hall SJ, Martin M: *Sports Injury Management,* 2nd ed. Baltimore, Lippincott Williams & Wilkins, 2000.

Birrer RB (ed): *Sports Medicine for the Primary Care Physician,* 2nd ed. Boca Raton, FL, CRC Press, 1994.

Clay JH, Pounds DM: *Basic Clinical Message Therapy: Integrating Anatomy and Treatment.* Baltimore, Lippincott Williams & Wilkins, 2003.

Foerster O: The dermatomes in man. *Brain* 56:1, 1933.

Frick H, Leonhardt H, Starck D: *Human Anatomy 1: General Anatomy, Special Anatomy: Limbs, Trunk Wall, Head and Neck.* Stuttgart, Thieme, 1991.

Ger R, Sedlin E: The accessory soleus muscle. *Clin Orthop* 116: 200, 1976.

Gross A: Orthopedic surgery adult. *In* Gross A, Gross P, Langer B (eds): *Surgery: A Complete Guide for Patients and Their Families.* Toronto, Harper & Collins, 1989.

Hamill J, Knutzen KM: *Biomechanical Basis of Human Movement.* Baltimore, Lippincott Williams & Wilkins, 1995.

Jenkins DB: *Hollinshead's Functional Anatomy of the Limbs and Back,* 8th ed. Philadelphia, Saunders, 2002.

Kapandji IA: *The Physiology of the Joints, Vol. 2. Lower Limb,* 5th ed. Edinburgh, UK, Churchill Livingstone, 1987.

Keegan JJ, Garrett FD: The segmental distribution of the cutaneous nerves in the limbs of man. *Anat Rec* 102:409, 1948.

Lawson, JP: Clinically significant radiologic anatomic variants of the skeleton. *Am J Radiol* 163:249, 1994.

Levandowski R, Difiori JP: Thigh injuries. *In* Birrer RB (ed): *Sports Medicine for the Primary Care Physician,* 2nd ed. Boca Raton, FL, CRC Press, 1994.

Markhede G, Stener G: Function after removal of various hip and thigh muscles for extirpation of tumors. *Acta Orthop Scand* 52:373, 1981.

Middleton JA, Kolodon EL. Plantar fasciitis: Heel pain in athletes. *J Ath Train* 27:70, 1992.

Moore KL, Persaud TVN: *The Developing Human. Clinically Oriented Embryology,* 7th ed., Philadelphia, Saunders, 2003.

Palastanga N, Field D, Soames R: *Anatomy and Human Movement,* 4th ed., Oxford, UK, Butterworth-Heinemann, 2002.

Rose J, Gamble JG: *Human Walking,* 2nd ed., Baltimore, Lippincott Williams & Wilkins, 1994.

Salter RB: Orthopedic surgery pediatric. *In* Gross A, Gross P, Langer B (eds): *Surgery: A Complete Guide for Patients and Their Families.* Toronto, Harper & Collins, 1989.

Salter RB: *Textbook of Disorders and Injuries of the Musculoskeletal System,* 3rd ed. Baltimore, Lippincott Williams & Wilkins, 1999.

Slaby FJ, McCune SK, Summers RW: *Gross Anatomy in the Practice of Medicine.* Baltimore, Lea & Febiger, 1994.

Soames RW: Arthroscopy of the knee. *In* Williams PH, Bannister LH, Berry MM, Collins P, Dyson M, Dussek JE, Ferguson MWJ (eds): *Gray's Anatomy,* 38th ed. New York, Churchill Livingstone, 1995.

Soderberg GL: *Kinesiology: Application to Pathological Motion.* Baltimore: Williams & Wilkins, 1986.

Swartz MH: *Textbook of Physical Diagnosis,* 4th ed. Philadelphia, Saunders, 2002.

Williams PH, Bannister LH, Berry MM, Collins P, Dyson M, Dussek JE, Ferguson MWJ: *Gray's Anatomy,* 38th ed. New York, Churchill Livingstone, 1995.

6

Upper Limb

Overview

The upper limb is characterized by its mobility and ability to grasp, strike, and conduct fine motor skills (*manipulation*).

These characteristics are especially marked in the hand when performing manual activities such as buttoning a shirt. Synchronized interplay occurs between the joints of the upper limb to coordinate the intervening segments to perform smooth, efficient motion at the most workable distance or position required for a specific task. Efficiency of hand function results in large part from the ability to place it in the proper position by movements at the scapulothoracic, glenohumeral, elbow, radioulnar, and wrist joints.

The upper limb consists of four segments (Fig. 6.1):

1. **Shoulder:** proximal segment of the limb that overlaps parts of the trunk (thorax and back) and lower lateral neck. It includes the pectoral, scapular, and lateral supra-clavicular regions and is built on half of the pectoral girdle. The **pectoral** (shoulder) **girdle** is a bony ring, incomplete posteriorly, formed by the scapulae and clavicles and completed anteriorly by the *manubrium of the sternum* (part of the axial skeleton).

2. *Arm* (L. *brachium*): first segment of the free upper limb (more mobile part of the upper limb independent of the trunk) and the longest segment of the limb. It extends between and connects the shoulder and the elbow and is centered around the humerus.

3. *Forearm* (L. *antebrachium*): second longest segment of the limb. It extends between and connects the elbow and the wrist and contains the ulna and radius.

4. *Hand* (L. *manus*): part of the upper limb distal to the forearm that is formed around the carpus, metacarpus, and phalanges. It is composed of the wrist, palm, dorsum of hand, and fingers (including an opposable thumb) and is richly supplied with sensory endings for touch, pain, and temperature.

Upper Limb Injuries

Because the disabling effects of an injury to the upper limb, particularly the hand, are far out of proportion to the extent of the injury, a sound understanding of the structure and function of the upper limb is of the highest importance. Knowledge of its structure without an understanding of its functions is almost useless clinically because the aim of treating an injured limb is to preserve or restore its functions. ✚

Comparison of the Upper and Lower Limbs

Developing in a similar fashion (see Chapter 5), the upper and lower limbs share many common features. However, they are sufficiently distinct in structure to enable markedly different functions and abilities. Because the upper limb is not usually involved in weight bearing or motility, its stability has been sacrificed to gain mobility. The upper limb still possesses remarkable strength. And because of the hand's ability to conform to a paddle or assume a gripping or platform configuration, it may assume a role in motility in certain circumstances.

Both the upper and the lower limbs are connected to the **axial skeleton** (cranium, vertebral column, and associated thoracic cage) via the bony pectoral and pelvic girdles, respectively. The *pelvic girdle* consists of the two hip bones connected to the sacrum (see Chapter 5). The *pectoral girdle* consists of the scapulae and clavicles, connected to the manubrium of the sternum. Both girdles possess a large flat bone located posteriorly, which provides for attachment of proximal muscles and connects with its contralateral partner anteriorly via small bony braces, the pubic rami and clavicles.

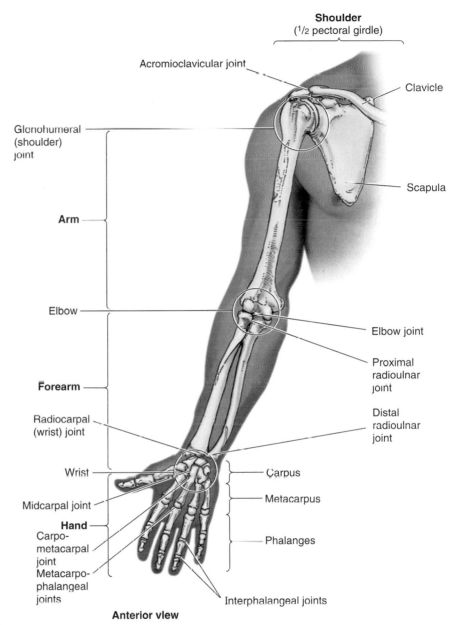

Figure 6.1. Regions and bones of upper limb. The joints divide the superior appendicular skeleton, and thus the limb itself, into four main regions: shoulder, arm, forearm, and hand.

However, the flat iliac bones of the pelvic girdle are also connected posteriorly through their primary attachment to the sacrum via the essentially rigid, weight-transferring sacroiliac joints. This posterior connection to the axial skeleton places the lower limbs inferior to the trunk, enabling them to be supportive as they function primarily in relation to the line of gravity. Furthermore, because the two sides are connected both anteriorly and posteriorly, the pelvic girdle forms a complete rigid ring that limits mobility, making the movements of one limb markedly affect the movements of the other. The pectoral girdle, however, is connected to the trunk only anteriorly via the sternum by flexible joints with 3° of freedom and is an incomplete ring because the scapulae are not connected with each other posteriorly. Thus the motion of one upper limb is independent of the other, and the limbs are able to operate effectively anterior to the body, at a distance and level that enables precise eye–hand coordination.

In both the upper and the lower limbs, the long bone of the most proximal segment is the largest and is unpaired. The long bones increase progressively in number but decrease in size in the more distal segments of the limb. The second most proximal segment of both limbs (i.e., the leg and forearm) has two parallel bones, although only in the forearm do both articulate with the bone of the proximal segment and only in the leg do both articulate directly with the distal segment. While the paired bones of both the leg and forearm flex and extend as a unit, only those of the upper limb are able to move (supinate and pronate) relative to each other, the bones of the leg being fixed in the pronated position.

The wrist and ankle have a similar number of short bones (eight and seven, respectively). Both groups of short bones interrupt a series of long bones that resumes distally with several sets of long bones of similar lengths, with a similar number of joints of essentially the same type. The digits of the upper limb (fingers including the thumb) are the most mobile parts of either limb, but all the other parts of the upper limb are more mobile than the comparable parts of the lower limb.

THE BOTTOM LINE: Although the upper and lower limbs have much in common regarding their development and structure, the upper limb has evolved into a mobile organ of manipulation that, along with the brain, allows humans not only to respond to their environments but to manipulate and control them to a large degree. The upper limb is composed of four increasingly mobile segments, the proximal three (shoulder, arm, and forearm) serving primarily to position the fourth (hand), which is for grasping, manipulation and touch. Four distinctions from the lower limbs enable the independent operation of the upper limbs, allowing the hands to be precisely positioned anterior to the body at a distance and height that enables accurate eye–hand coordination: (1) the upper limbs are not involved in weight bearing or ambulation, (2) the pectoral girdle is attached to the axial skeleton only anteriorly via a very mobile joint, (3) paired bones of the forearm are able to be moved relative to each other, and (4) the hands have long, mobile fingers and an opposable thumb.

Bones of the Upper Limb

The pectoral girdle and bones of the free part of the upper limb form the **superior appendicular skeleton** (Fig. 6.2); the pelvic girdle and bones of the free part of the lower limb form

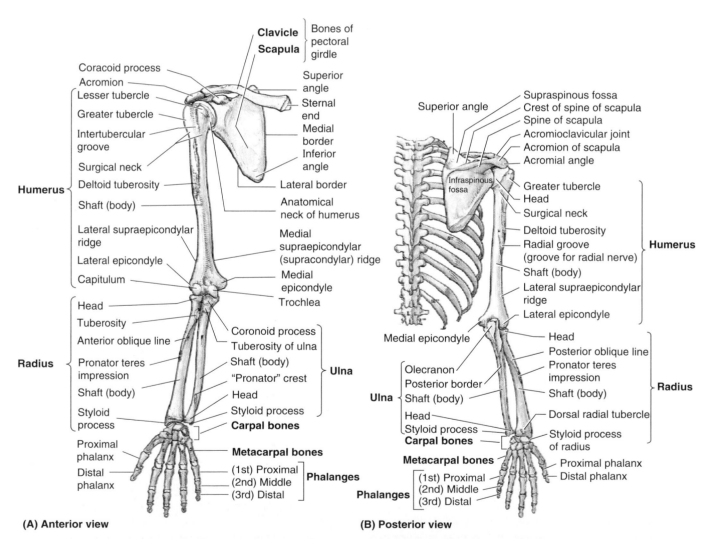

(A) Anterior view

(B) Posterior view

Figure 6.2. Bones of upper limb. A. The right superior appendicular skeleton includes the right half of the pectoral (shoulder) girdle, composed of the right clavicle and scapula, and the skeleton of the free right upper limb, formed by the remaining bones distal to the scapula. **B.** The superior appendicular and thoracic parts of the axial skeleton demonstrate that the scapula overlaps parts of the 2nd–7th ribs. Only the thin clavicle links the axial and superior appendicular skeletons. Although not a "true" anatomical joint, the scapula rests and moves on (articulates with) the posterosuperior thoracic wall via the physiological "scapulothoracic joint."

Right clavicle

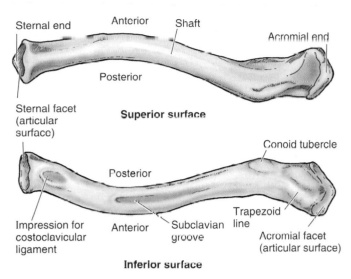

Figure 6.3. Right clavicle. Prominent features of the superior and inferior surfaces of the clavicle are shown. The bone acts as a mobile strut (supporting brace), connecting the trunk to the upper limb.

the **inferior appendicular skeleton.** The superior appendicular skeleton articulates with the axial skeleton only at the sternoclavicular joint, allowing great mobility. The clavicles and scapulae of the pectoral girdle are supported, stabilized, and moved by **axioappendicular muscles** that attach to the relatively fixed ribs, sternum, and vertebrae of the *axial skeleton.*

Clavicle

The **clavicle** (collar bone) connects the upper limb to the trunk (Fig. 6.3). The shaft of the clavicle has a double curve in a horizontal plane. Its medial half is convex anteriorly, and its **sternal end** is enlarged and triangular where it articulates with the **manubrium of the sternum** at the *sternoclavicular (SC) joint.* Its lateral half is concave anteriorly, and its **acromial end** is flat where it articulates with the *acromion of the scapula* at the *acromioclavicular (AC) joint* (Figs. 6.2*B* and 6.3). The medial two thirds of the shaft of the clavicle are convex anteriorly, whereas the lateral third is flattened and concave anteriorly. These curvatures increase the resilience of the clavicle and give it the appearance of an elongated capital *S.*

The clavicle:

- Serves as a moveable, crane-like strut (rigid support) from which the scapula and free limb are suspended, keeping

---

them away from the trunk so that the limb has maximum freedom of motion. The strut is movable and allows the scapula to move on the thoracic wall at the "scapulothoracic joint,"[1] increasing the range of motion of the limb. Fixing the strut in position, especially after its elevation, enables elevation of the ribs for deep inspiration.

- Forms one of the bony boundaries of the *cervicoaxillary canal* (passageway between the neck and the arm), affording protection to the neurovascular bundle supplying the upper limb.

- Transmits shocks (traumatic impacts) from the upper limb to the axial skeleton.

Although designated as a long bone, the clavicle has no medullary (marrow) cavity. It consists of spongy (trabecular) bone with a shell of compact bone.

The **superior surface** of the clavicle, lying just deep to the skin and platysma (G. flat plate) muscle in the subcutaneous tissue, is smooth. The **inferior surface** of the clavicle is rough because strong ligaments bind it to the 1st rib near its sternal end and suspend the scapula from its acromial end. The **conoid tubercle,** near the acromial end of the clavicle (Fig. 6.3), gives attachment to the *conoid ligament,* the medial part of the *coracoclavicular ligament* by which the remainder of the upper limb is passively suspended from the clavicle. Also, near the acromial end of the clavicle is the **trapezoid line,** to which the *trapezoid ligament* attaches; it is the lateral part of the coracoclavicular ligament. The **subclavian groove (groove for the subclavius)** in the medial third of the shaft of the clavicle is the site of attachment of the subclavius muscle. More medially is the **impression for the costoclavicular ligament,** a rough, often depressed, oval area that gives attachment to the ligament binding the 1st rib (L. *costa*) to the clavicle, limiting elevation of the shoulder.

Variations of the Clavicle

The clavicle varies more in shape than most other long bones. Occasionally, the clavicle is pierced by a branch of the supraclavicular nerve. The clavicle is thicker and more curved in manual workers, and the sites of muscular attachments are more marked. The right clavicle is usually stronger and shorter than the left clavicle.

Fracture of the Clavicle

The clavicle is one of the most frequently fractured bones. Clavicular fractures are especially common in children and are often caused by an indirect force transmitted from an outstretched hand through the bones of the forearm and arm to the shoulder during a fall. A fracture may also result from a fall directly on the shoulder. The weakest part of the clavicle is the junction of its middle and lateral thirds. ▶

After fracture of the clavicle, the sternocleidomastoid muscle elevates the medial fragment of bone (Fig. B6.1). Because of the subcutaneous position of the clavicles, the end of the superiorly directed fragment is prominent—readily palpable and/or apparent. The trapezius muscle is unable to hold the lateral fragment up owing to the weight of the upper limb, and thus the shoulder drops. The strong coracoclavicular ligament usually prevents dislocation of the AC joint. People with fractured clavicles support the sagging limb with the other limb. In addition to being de-

pressed, the lateral fragment of the clavicle may be pulled medially by the adductor muscles of the arm, such as the pectoralis major. Overriding of the bone fragments shortens the clavicle.

The slender clavicles of newborn infants may be fractured during delivery if the neonates are broad shouldered; however, the bones usually heal quickly. A fracture of the clavicle is often incomplete in younger children—that is, it is a **greenstick fracture,** in which one side of a bone is broken and the other is bent. This fracture was so named because the parts of the bone do not separate; the bone resembles a tree branch (greenstick) that has been sharply bent but not disconnected.

Ossification of the Clavicle

The clavicle is the first long bone to ossify (via *intramembranous ossification*), beginning during the 5th and 6th embryonic weeks from medial and lateral primary centers that are close together in the shaft of the clavicle. The ends of the clavicle later pass through a cartilaginous phase (*endochondral ossification*); the cartilages form growth zones similar to those of other long bones. A secondary ossification center appears at the sternal end and forms a scale-like epiphysis that begins to fuse with the shaft (diaphysis) between 18 and 25 years of age and is completely fused to it between 25 and 31 years of age. This is the last of the epiphyses of long bones to fuse. An even smaller scale-like epiphysis may be present at the acromial end of the clavicle; it must not be mistaken for a fracture.

Sometimes fusion of the two ossification centers of the clavicle fails to occur; as a result, a bony defect forms between the lateral and the medial thirds of the clavicle. Awareness of this possible congenital defect should prevent diagnosis of a fracture in an otherwise normal clavicle. When doubt exists, both clavicles are radiographed because this defect is usually bilateral (Ger et al., 1996). ●

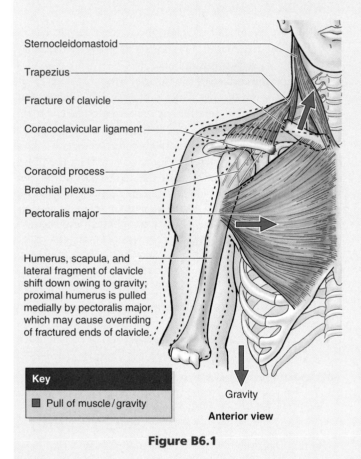

Sternocleidomastoid

Trapezius

Fracture of clavicle

Coracoclavicular ligament

Coracoid process

Brachial plexus

Pectoralis major

Humerus, scapula, and lateral fragment of clavicle shift down owing to gravity; proximal humerus is pulled medially by pectoralis major, which may cause overriding of fractured ends of clavicle.

Gravity

Anterior view

Key
■ Pull of muscle / gravity

Figure B6.1

THE BOTTOM LINE: The subcutaneous clavicle connects the upper limb (superior appendicular skeleton) to the trunk (axial skeleton). It serves as a movable crane-like strut from which the scapula and free limb are suspended at a distance from the trunk that enables freedom of motion. Shocks received by the upper limb (especially the shoulder) are transmitted through the clavicle, resulting in a fracture that most commonly occurs between its middle and lateral thirds. The clavicle is the first long bone to ossify and the last to be fully formed.

Scapula

The **scapula** (shoulder blade) is a triangular flat bone that lies on the posterolateral aspect of the thorax, overlying the 2nd–7th ribs (Fig. 6.2*B*). The convex **posterior surface** of the scapula is unevenly divided by a thick projecting ridge of bone, the **spine of the scapula,** into a small **supraspinous fossa** and a much larger **infraspinous fossa** (Fig. 6.4*A*). The concave **costal surface** of most of the scapula forms a large **subscapular fossa.** The broad bony surfaces of the three fossae provide attachments for fleshy muscles. The triangular **body of the**

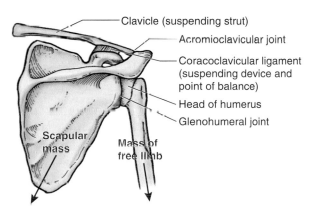

(B) Posterior view

Figure 6.4. Right scapula. A. The bony features of the costal and posterior surfaces of the scapula are demonstrated. **B.** The scapula is suspended from the clavicle by the coracoclavicular ligament, at which a balance is achieved among the weight of the scapula, its attached muscles, and the muscular activity medially and the weight of the free limb laterally. **C.** The borders and angles of the scapula are demonstrated.

scapula is thin and translucent superior and inferior to the scapular spine; although its borders, especially the lateral one, are somewhat thicker. The spine continues laterally as the flat expanded **acromion** (G. *akros,* point), which forms the subcutaneous point of the shoulder and articulates with the acromial end of the clavicle. The **deltoid tubercle of the scapular spine** is the prominence indicating the medial point of attachment of the deltoid. The spine and acromion serve as levers for the attached muscles, particularly the trapezius.

Because the acromion is a lateral extension of the scapula, the AC joint is placed lateral to the mass of the scapula and its attached muscles (Fig. 6.4*B*). The *glenohumeral* (shoulder) *joint* on which these muscles operate is almost directly inferior to the AC joint; thus the scapular mass is balanced with that of the free limb, and the suspending structure (coracoclavicular ligament) lies between the two masses.

Superolaterally, the lateral surface of the scapula has a **glenoid cavity** (G. socket), which receives and articulates with the head of the humerus at the glenohumeral joint (Fig. 6.4*A* & *B*). The glenoid cavity is a shallow, concave, oval fossa (L. *fossa ovalis*), directed anterolaterally and slightly superiorly, that is considerably smaller than the ball (head of the humerus) for which it serves as socket. The beak-like **coracoid process**

(G. *korakōdés,* like a crow's beak) is superior to the glenoid cavity and projects anterolaterally. This process also resembles in size, shape, and direction a bent finger pointing to the shoulder, the knuckle of which provides the inferior attachment for the passively supporting coracoclavicular ligament.

The scapula has medial, lateral, and superior borders and superior, lateral, and inferior angles (Fig. 6.4*C*). When the scapular body is in the anatomical position, the thin **medial border of the scapula** runs parallel to and approximately 5 cm lateral to the spinous processes of the thoracic vertebrae (Fig. 6.2*B*); hence it is often called the *vertebral border* (Fig. 6.4*C*). From the inferior angle, the **lateral border of the scapula** runs superolaterally toward the apex of the axilla; hence it is often called the *axillary border.* The lateral border is made up of a thick bar of bone that prevents buckling of this stress-bearing region of the scapula. The lateral border terminates in the truncated **lateral angle of the scapula,** the thickest part of the bone that bears the broadened **head of the scapula.** The glenoid cavity is the primary feature of the head. The shallow constriction between the head and the body defines the **neck of the scapula.** The **superior border of the scapula** is marked near the junction of its medial two thirds and lateral third by the **suprascapular notch,** which is located where the superior border joins the base of the coracoid process. The superior border is the thinnest and shortest of the three borders.

The scapula is capable of considerable movement on the thoracic wall at the physiological *scapulothoracic joint,* providing the base from which the upper limb operates. These movements, enabling the arm to move freely, are discussed later in this chapter with the muscles that move the scapula.

Fracture of the Scapula

Fracture of the scapula is usually the result of severe trauma, as occurs in pedestrian–vehicle accidents. Usually there are also fractured ribs. Most fractures require little treatment because the scapula is covered on both sides by muscles. Most fractures involve the protruding subcutaneous acromion. ✪

THE BOTTOM LINE: The scapula forms the mobile base from which the free upper limb acts. This triangular flat bone is curved to conform to the thoracic wall and provides large surface areas and edges for attachment of muscles. These muscles (1) move the scapula on the thoracic wall at the physiological scapulothoracic joint and (2) extend to the proximal humerus maintaining the integrity of—and producing motion at—the glenohumeral joint. Its spine and acromion serve as levers; the acromion enables the scapula and attached muscles to be located medially against the trunk with the AC and glenohumeral joints, thereby allowing movement lateral to the trunk. Its coracoid process is the site of attachment for the coracoclavicular ligament that passively supports the upper limb and a site for muscular (tendon) attachment.

Humerus

The **humerus** (arm bone), the largest bone in the upper limb, articulates with the scapula at the glenohumeral joint and the radius and ulna at the elbow joint (Figs. 6.1 and 6.2). The proximal end of the humerus has a head, surgical and anatomical necks, and greater and lesser tubercles. The spherical **head of the humerus** articulates with the glenoid cavity of the scapula. The **anatomical neck of the humerus** is formed by the groove circumscribing the head and separating it from the greater and lesser tubercles. It indicates the line of attachment of the glenohumeral joint capsule. The **surgical neck of the humerus,** a common site of fracture, is the narrow part distal to the head and tubercles. The junction of the head and neck with the shaft of the humerus is indicated by the greater and lesser tubercles, which provide attachment and leverage to some scapulohumeral muscles. The **greater tubercle** is at the lateral margin of the humerus, whereas the **lesser tubercle** projects anteriorly from the bone. The **intertubercular (bicipital) groove** separates the tubercles and provides protected passage for the slender tendon of the long head of the biceps muscle.

The **shaft (body) of the humerus** has two prominent features: the **deltoid tuberosity** laterally, for attachment of the deltoid muscle, and the oblique **radial groove (groove for radial nerve,** spiral groove) posteriorly, in which the radial nerve and deep artery of the arm lie as they pass anterior to the long and between the medial and lateral heads of the triceps brachii muscle. The inferior end of the humeral shaft widens as the sharp medial and lateral **supraepicondylar (supracondylar) ridges** form and then end distally in the especially prominent **medial epicondyle** and the **lateral epicondyle,** providing for muscle attachment.

The distal end of the humerus, including the trochlea; the capitulum; and the olecranon, coronoid, and radial fossae, makes up the **condyle of the humerus** (Fig. 6.5). The condyle has two articular surfaces: a lateral **capitulum** (L. lit-

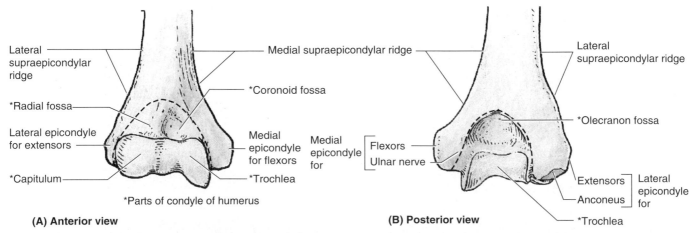

(A) Anterior view   **(B) Posterior view**

Figure 6.5. Distal end of right humerus. A and B. Anterior and posterior views illustrate the lateral and medial epicondyles, supraepicondylar ridges, and condyle of the humerus. The condyle (the boundaries of which are indicated by the *dashed line*) consists of the capitulum; the trochlea; and the radial, coronoid, and olecranon fossae.

tle head) for articulation with the head of the radius and a medial, spool-shaped or pulley-like **trochlea** (L. pulley) for articulation with the proximal end (trochlear notch) of the ulna. Two hollows or fossae occur back to back superior to the trochlea, making the condyle quite thin between the epicondyles. Anteriorly, the **coronoid fossa** receives the coronoid process of the ulna during full flexion of the elbow. Posteriorly, the **olecranon fossa** accommodates the olecranon of the ulna during full extension of the elbow. Superior to the capitulum anteriorly, a shallower **radial fossa** accommodates the edge of the head of the radius when the forearm is fully flexed.

Fractures of the Humerus

Most injuries of the proximal end of the humerus are *fractures of the surgical neck*. These injuries are especially common in elderly people with *osteoporosis,* whose demineralized bones are brittle. Humeral fractures are often result in one fragment being driven into the spongy bone of the other fragment (**impacted fracture**). The injuries usually result from a minor fall on the hand, with the force being transmitted up the forearm bones of the extended limb. Because of impaction of the fragments, the fracture site is sometimes stable and the person is able to move the arm passively with little pain.

An *avulsion fracture of the greater tubercle of the humerus* (pulling the tubercle away from the humeral head) is seen most commonly in middle-aged and elderly people (Fig. B6.2*A*). The fracture usually results from a fall on the acromion, the point of the shoulder. In younger people, an avulsion fracture of the greater tubercle usually results from a fall on the hand when the arm is abducted. Muscles (especially the subscapularis) that remain attached to the humerus pull the limb into medial rotation. ▶

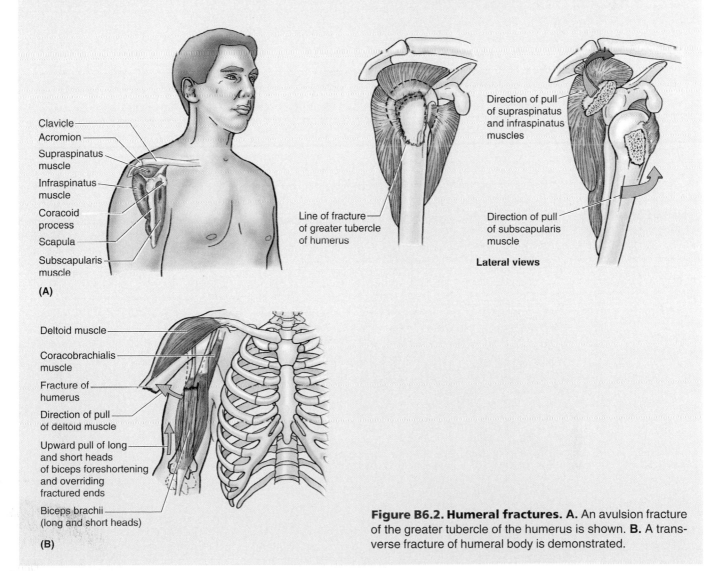

Clavicle
Acromion
Supraspinatus muscle
Infraspinatus muscle
Coracoid process
Scapula
Subscapularis muscle

(A)

Line of fracture of greater tubercle of humerus

Direction of pull of supraspinatus and infraspinatus muscles

Direction of pull of subscapularis muscle

Lateral views

Deltoid muscle
Coracobrachialis muscle
Fracture of humerus
Direction of pull of deltoid muscle
Upward pull of long and short heads of biceps foreshortening and overriding fractured ends
Biceps brachii (long and short heads)

(B)

Figure B6.2. Humeral fractures. A. An avulsion fracture of the greater tubercle of the humerus is shown. **B.** A transverse fracture of humeral body is demonstrated.

A *transverse fracture of the shaft of the humerus* frequently results from a direct blow to the arm. The pull of the deltoid muscle carries the proximal fragment laterally (Fig. B6.2*B*). Indirect injury resulting from a fall on the outstretched hand may produce a *spiral fracture of the humeral shaft.* Overriding of the oblique ends of the fractured bone may result in foreshortening. Because the humerus is surrounded by muscles and has a well-developed periosteum, the bone fragments usually unite well. An *intercondylar fracture of the humerus* results from a severe fall on the flexed elbow. The olecranon of the ulna is driven like a wedge between the medial and lateral parts of the condyle, separating one or both parts from the humeral shaft.

The following parts of the humerus are in direct contact with the indicated nerves:

- Surgical neck: axillary nerve.

- Radial groove: radial nerve.

- Distal end of humerus: median nerve.

- Medial epicondyle: ulnar nerve.

These nerves may be injured when the associated part of the humerus is fractured. These injuries are discussed later in this chapter. ❂

THE BOTTOM LINE: The long, strong humerus is a mobile strut—the first in a series of two—used to position the hand at a height (level) and distance from the trunk to maximize its efficiency. Its spherical head enables a great range of motion on the mobile scapular base, and the trochlea and capitulum at its distal end facilitate the hinge movements of the elbow and, at the same time, the pivoting of the radius. The long shaft of the humerus enables reach and makes it an effective lever for power in lifting as well as providing surface area for attachment of muscles that act primarily at the elbow. Added surface area for attachment of flexors and extensors of the wrist is provided by the epicondyles, the medial and lateral extensions of the shaft.

Bones of the Forearm

The two forearm bones serve together to form the second unit of an articulated mobile strut (the first unit being the humerus), with a mobile base formed by the shoulder, that positions the hand. However, because this unit is formed by two parallel bones, one of which (the radius) can pivot about the other (the ulna), supination and pronation are possible. This makes it possible to rotate the hand when the elbow is flexed.

Ulna

The **ulna** is the stabilizing bone of the forearm and is the medial and longer of the two forearm bones (Figs. 6.6 and 6.7).

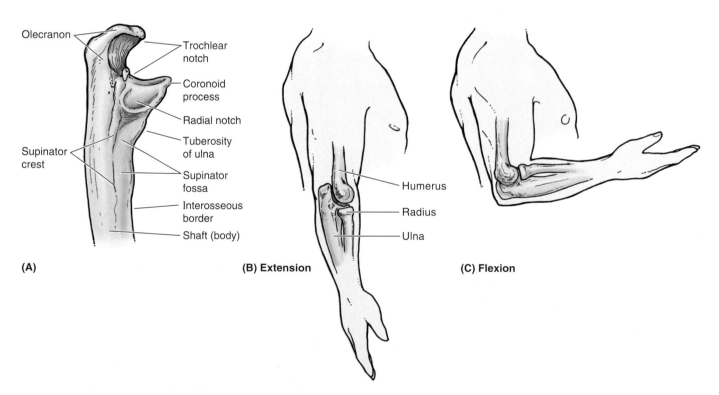

Figure 6.6. Bones of right elbow region. A. The proximal part of the ulna is shown. **B.** The bones of the elbow region are shown, demonstrating the relationship of the distal humerus and proximal ulna and radius during extension of the elbow joint. **C.** The relationship of the humerus and forearm bones during flexion of the elbow joint is demonstrated.

(A) Anterior view

(D) Posterior view

(C) Posterior view of distal end of radius

(D) Inferior view of distal ends of ulna and radius

**(E) Inferior view of cross section through shafts (bodies)
of ulna and radius and interosseous membrane**

Figure 6.7. Right radius and ulna. A and B. The radius
and ulna are shown in the articulated position, connected by
the interosseous membrane. **C and D.** The features of the distal ends of the forearm bones include grooves for tendons; a
dorsal tubercle of the radius (used as a pulley); and articular
surfaces for articulation with (1) each other (ulnar notch of radius, articular circumference of head of ulna; see part **A**), (2)
an articular disc (ulna), and (3) the proximal carpal bones (radius). **E.** In cross section, the shafts of the radius and ulna appear almost as mirror images of one another for much of the
middle and distal thirds of their lengths.

Its more massive proximal end is specialized for articulation
with the humerus proximally and the head of the radius laterally. For articulation with the humerus, it has two prominent
projections: (1) the **olecranon,** which projects proximally
from its posterior aspect (forming the point of the elbow) and
serves as a short lever for extension of the elbow, and (2) the
coronoid process, which projects anteriorly. The olecranon
and coronoid processes form the walls of the **trochlear notch,**
which in profile resembles the jaws of a crescent wrench as
it "grips" (articulates with) the trochlea of the humerus
(Fig. 6.6*B* & *C*). The articulation between the ulna and the
humerus primarily allows only flexion and extension of the elbow joint, although a small amount of abduction–adduction
occurs during pronation and supination of the forearm. Inferior to the coronoid process is the **tuberosity of the ulna** for attachment of the tendon of the brachialis muscle (Fig. 6.6*A*).

On the lateral side of the coronoid process is a smooth,
rounded concavity, the **radial notch,** which receives the broad
periphery of the head of the radius. Inferior to the radial
notch on the lateral surface of the ulnar shaft is a prominent
ridge, the **supinator crest.** Between it and the distal part of the
coronoid process is a concavity, the **supinator fossa.** The deep
part of the supinator muscle attaches to the supinator crest
and fossa.

The **shaft (body) of the ulna** is thick and cylindrical proximally; but it tapers, diminishing in diameter, as it continues
distally (Fig. 6.7*A*). At the narrow distal end of the ulna is a
small but abrupt enlargement, the disc-like **head of the ulna**
with a small, conical **ulnar styloid process.** The ulna does not
reach—and therefore does not participate in—the wrist (radiocarpal) joint.

Radius

The **radius** is the lateral and shorter of the two forearm
bones. Its proximal end includes a short head, neck, and
medially directed tuberosity (Fig. 6.7*A*). Proximally, the
smooth superior aspect of the discoid **head of the radius** is
concave for articulation with the capitulum of the humerus
during flexion and extension of the elbow joint. The head
also articulates peripherally with the radial notch of the
ulna; thus the head is covered with articular cartilage. The
neck of the radius is a constriction distal to the head. The
oval **radial tuberosity** is distal to the medial part of the neck
and demarcates the proximal end (head and neck) of the radius from the shaft.

The **shaft (body) of the radius,** in contrast to that of the
ulna, gradually enlarges as it passes distally. The distal end
of the radius is essentially four sided when sectioned transversely. Its medial aspect forms a concavity, the **ulnar notch**
(Fig. 6.7*C* & *D*), which accommodates the head of the
ulna. Its lateral aspect becomes increasingly ridge-like, terminating distally in the **radial styloid process.** Projecting
dorsally, the **dorsal tubercle of the radius** lies between otherwise shallow grooves for the passage of the tendons of
forearm muscles. The radial styloid process is larger than the
ulnar styloid process and extends farther distally. This rela-

tionship is of clinical importance when the ulna and/or the radius is fractured.

Most of the length of the shafts of the radius and ulna are essentially triangular in cross section, with a rounded, superficially directed base and an acute, deeply directed apex (Fig. 6.7*E*). The apex is formed by a section of the sharp **interosseous border of the radius or ulna** that connects to the thin, fibrous **interosseous membrane of the forearm** (Fig. 6.7*A, B, & E*). The majority of the fibers of the interosseous membrane run an oblique course, passing inferiorly from the radius as they extend medially to the ulna (Fig. 6.7*A & B*). Thus they are positioned to transmit forces received by the radius (via the hands) to the ulna for transmission to the humerus.

Fractures of the Radius and Ulna

Fractures of both the radius and the ulna are usually the result of severe injury. A direct injury usually produces transverse fractures at the same level, usually in the middle third of the bones. Isolated fractures of the radius or ulna also occur. Because the shafts of these bones are firmly bound together by the interosseous membrane, a fracture of one bone is likely to be associated with dislocation of the nearest joint.

Fracture of the distal end of the radius is a common fracture in adults > 50 years of age and occurs more frequently in women because their bones are more commonly weakened by *osteoporosis*. A complete transverse fracture of the distal 2 cm of the radius, called a **Colles fracture,** is the most common fracture of the forearm (Fig. B6.3). The distal fragment is displaced dorsally and is often **comminuted** (broken into pieces). The fracture results from forced dorsiflexion of the hand, usually as the result of trying to ease a fall by outstretching the upper limb. Often the ulnar styloid process is **avulsed** (broken off). Normally the radial styloid process projects farther distally than the ulnar styloid (Fig. B6.3*A*); consequently, when a Colles fracture occurs, this relationship is reversed because of shortening of the radius (Fig. B6.3*B*). This clinical condition is often referred to as a *dinner fork* (silver fork) *deformity* because a posterior angulation occurs in the forearm just proximal to the wrist and the normal anterior curvature of the relaxed hand. The posterior bending is produced by the posterior displacement and tilt of the distal fragment of the radius.

The typical history of a person with a Colles fracture includes slipping or tripping and, in an attempt to break the fall, landing on the outstretched limb with the forearm and hand pronated. Because of the rich blood supply to the distal end of the radius, bony union is usually good.

When the distal end of the radius fractures in children, the fracture line may extend through the distal epiphysial plate. *Epiphysial plate injuries* are common in older children because of their frequent falls in which the forces are transmitted from the hand to the radius and ulna. The healing process may result in malalignment of the epiphysial plate and disturbance of radial growth. ●

Radial styloid process

Ulnar styloid process

Palmar view
(A)

Lateral view

(B)

Avulsed ulnar styloid process

Distal fragment of radius overrides the rest of the bone

Dinner fork deformity

Palmar view

Lateral view

Figure B6.3. Right wrist. A. A normal wrist is shown. **B.** A Colles fracture with a dinner fork deformity is demonstrated.

THE BOTTOM LINE: The ulna and radius together make up the second unit of a two-unit articulated strut (the first unit being the humerus), projecting from a mobile base (shoulder) that serves to position the hand. Because the forearm unit is formed by two parallel bones, and the radius is able to pivot about the ulna, supination and pronation of the hand are possible during elbow flexion. Proximally, the larger medial ulna forms the primary articulation with the humerus, whereas distally, the shorter lateral radius forms the primary articulation with the hand via the wrist. Because the ulna does not reach the wrist, forces received by the hand are transmitted from the radius to the ulna via the interosseous membrane.

Bones of the Hand

The **wrist**, or **carpus**, is composed of eight **carpal bones** (carpals) arranged in proximal and distal rows of four (Fig. 6.8). These small bones give flexibility to the wrist. The carpus is markedly convex from side to side posteriorly and concave anteriorly. Augmenting movement at the wrist joint, the two rows of carpals glide on each other; in addition, each bone glides on those adjacent to it.

From lateral to medial, the four bones in the proximal row of carpals (purple in Fig. 6.8) are the:

- **Scaphoid** (G. *skaphé,* skiff, boat): a boat-shaped bone that articulates proximally with the radius and has a prominent **scaphoid tubercle**; it is the largest bone in the proximal row of carpals.
- **Lunate** (L. *luna,* moon): a moon-shaped bone between the scaphoid and the triquetral bones; it articulates

proximally with the radius and is broader anteriorly than posteriorly.

- **Triquetrum** (L. *triquetrus,* three-cornered): a pyramidal bone on the medial side of the carpus, it articulates proximally with the articular disc of the distal radioulnar joint.
- **Pisiform** (L. *pisum,* pea), a small, pea shaped bone that lies on the palmar surface of the triquetrum.

From lateral to medial, the four bones in the distal row of carpals (green in Fig. 6.8) are the:

- **Trapezium** (G. *trapeze,* table): a four-sided bone on the lateral side of the carpus; it articulates with the 1st and 2nd metacarpals, scaphoid, and trapezoid bones.
- **Trapezoid:** a wedge-shaped bone that resembles the trapezium; it articulates with the 2nd metacarpal, trapezium, capitate, and scaphoid bones.
- **Capitate** (L. *caput,* head): a head-shaped bone with a rounded extremity and the largest bone in the carpus; it articulates primarily with the 3rd metacarpal distally, and with the trapezoid, scaphoid, lunate, and hamate.
- **Hamate** (L. *hamulus,* a little hook): a wedge-shaped bone on the medial side of the hand; it articulates with the 4th and 5th metacarpal, capitate, and triquetral bones; it has a distinctive hooked process, the **hook of the hamate**, that extends anteriorly.

The proximal surfaces of the distal row of carpals articulate with the proximal row of carpals, and their distal surfaces articulate with the metacarpals.

The **metacarpus** forms the skeleton of the palm of the hand between the carpus and the phalanges. It is composed

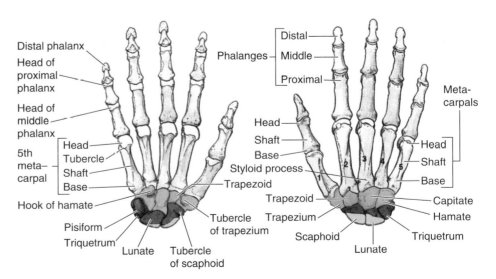

Figure 6.8. Bones of right hand. A and B. The skeleton of the hand consists of three segments: carpals of the wrist, metacarpals of the palm, and phalanges of the fingers or digits.

(A) Anterior (palmar) view   **(B) Posterior (dorsal) view**

of five **metacarpal bones** (metacarpals). Each metacarpal consists of a base, shaft, and head. The proximal **bases of the metacarpals** articulate with the carpal bones, and the distal **heads of the metacarpals** articulate with the proximal phalanges and form the knuckles. The 1st metacarpal (of the thumb) is the thickest and shortest of these bones. The 3rd metacarpal is distinguished by a **styloid process** on the lateral side of its base.

Each digit has three **phalanges** except for the first (the thumb), which has only two; however, the phalanges of the first digit are stouter than those in the other fingers. Each phalanx has a **base** proximally, a **shaft** (**body**), and a **head** distally (Fig. 6.8). The proximal phalanges are the largest, the middle ones are intermediate in size, and the distal ones are the smallest. The shafts of the phalanges taper distally. The terminal phalanges are flattened and expanded at their distal ends, which underlie the nail beds.

Fracture of the Scaphoid

The scaphoid is the most frequently fractured carpal bone. It often results from a fall on the palm when the hand is abducted, the fracture occurring across the narrow part ("waist") of the scaphoid (Fig. B6.4). Pain occurs primarily on the lateral side of the wrist, especially during dorsiflexion and abduction of the hand. Initial radiographs of the wrist may not reveal a fracture; often this injury is (mis-)diagnosed as a *severely sprained wrist.* Radiographs taken 10–14 days later reveal a fracture because bone resorption has occurred there. Owing to the poor blood supply to the proximal part of the scaphoid, union of the fractured parts may take at least 3 months. *Avascular necrosis of the proximal fragment of the scaphoid* (pathological death of bone resulting from inadequate blood supply) may occur and produce *degenerative joint disease of the wrist.* In some cases, it is necessary to fuse the carpals surgically (**arthrodesis**).

Radial artery
Palmar carpal branch
Scaphoid (fractured and necrotic)
Trapezoid
Radius
Ulna
Triquetrum
Lunate
Pisiform
Hook of hamate
Capitate
Trapezium

Figure B6.4

Fracture of the Hamate

Fracture of the hamate may result in non-union of the fractured bony parts because of the traction produced by the attached muscles. Because the ulnar nerve is close to the hook of the hamate, the nerve may be injured by this fracture, causing decreased grip strength of the hand. The ulnar artery may also be damaged when the hamate is fractured.

Fracture of the Metacarpals

The metacarpals (except the 1st) are closely bound together; hence isolated fractures tend to be stable. Furthermore, these bones have a good blood supply, and fractures usually heal rapidly. *Severe crushing injuries of the hand* may produce multiple metacarpal fractures, resulting in instability of the hand. Fracture of the 5th metacarpal, often referred to as a *boxer's fracture,* occurs when an unskilled person punches someone with a closed fist. The head of the bone rotates over the distal end of the shaft, producing a flexion deformity.

Fracture of the Phalanges

Crushing injuries of the distal phalanges are common (e.g., when a finger is caught in a car door). Because of the highly developed sensation in the fingers, these injuries are extremely painful. A *fracture of a distal phalanx* is usually comminuted, and a painful **hematoma** (local collection of blood) soon develops. Fractures of the proximal and middle phalanges are usually the result of crushing or hyperextension injuries. Because of the close relationship of phalangeal fractures to the flexor tendons, the bone fragments must be carefully realigned to restore normal function of the fingers. ⊙

THE BOTTOM LINE: Each segment of the upper limb increases the functionality of the end unit, the hand. Located on the free end of a two-unit articulated strut (arm and forearm) projecting from a mobile base (shoulder), the hand can be positioned over a wide range relative to the trunk. Its connection to the flexible strut via the multiple small bones of the wrist, combined with the pivoting of the forearm, greatly increases its ability to be placed in a particular position with the fingers able to flex (push or grip) in the necessary direction. The carpal bones are organized into two rows of four bones each, and as a group articulate with the radius proximally and the metacarpals distally. The highly flexible, elongated fingers—extending from a semirigid base (the palm)—enable the ability to grip, manipulate, or perform complex tasks involving multiple and simultaneous individual motions (e.g., when typing or playing a piano).

Surface Anatomy of the Upper Limb Bones

Most bones of the upper limb offer a palpable segment or surface (notable exceptions being the lunate and trapezoid), enabling the skilled examiner to discern abnormalities owing to trauma (fracture or dislocation) or malformation (Fig. SA6.1).

The **clavicle** is subcutaneous and can be easily palpated throughout its length. Its sternal end projects superior to the manubrium (Fig. SA6.1*A*). Between the elevated sternal ends of the clavicles is the **jugular notch** (suprasternal notch). The acromial end of the clavicle often rises higher than the acromion, forming a palpable elevation at the **acromioclavicular (AC) joint.** The acromial end can be palpated 2–3 cm medial to the lateral border of the acromion, particularly when the arm is alternately flexed and extended. Either or both ends of the clavicle may be prominent; when present, this condition is usually bilateral. Note the elasticity of the skin over the clavicle and how easily it can be pinched into a mobile fold. This property of the skin is useful when ligating the third part of the subclavian artery: the skin lying superior to the clavicle is pulled down onto the clavicle and then incised; after the incision is made, the skin is allowed to return to its position superior to the clavicle, where it overlies the artery (thus not endangering it during the incision).

The **acromion of the scapula** is easily felt and often visible. The superior surface of the acromion is subcutaneous and may be traced medially to the AC joint. The lateral ▶

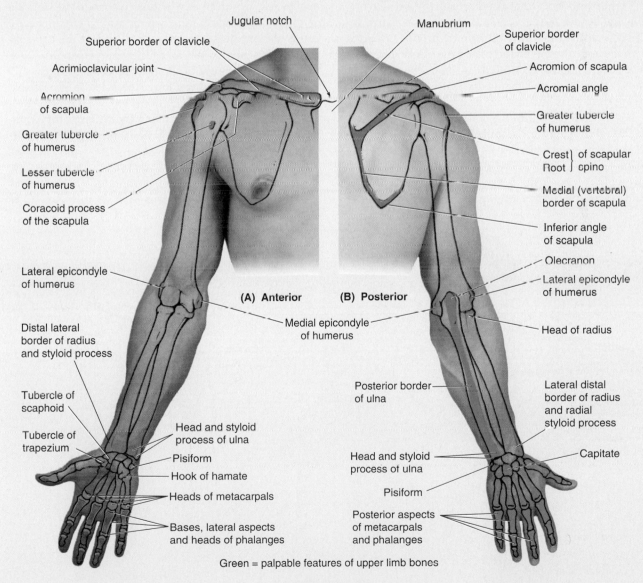

Green = palpable features of upper limb bones

Figure SA6.1.

and posterior borders of the acromion meet to form the **acromial angle** (Fig. SA6.1*B*). Inferior to the acromion, the *deltoid muscle* forms the rounded curve of the shoulder. The **crest of the scapular spine** is subcutaneous throughout and easily palpated.

When the upper limb is in the anatomical position, the:

• Superior angle of the scapula lies at the level of the T2 vertebra.

• Medial end of the root of the scapular spine is opposite the spinous process of the T3 vertebra.

• Inferior angle of the scapula lies at the level of the T7 vertebra, near the inferior border of the 7th rib and 7th intercostal space.

The **medial border of the scapula** is palpable inferior to the root of the spine of the scapula as it crosses the 3rd–7th ribs; the lateral border of the scapula is not easily palpated because it is covered by the teres major and minor muscles. When the upper limb is abducted and the hand is placed on the back of the head, the scapula is rotated, elevating the glenoid cavity such that the medial border of the scapula parallels the 6th rib and thus can be used to estimate its position and, deep to the rib, the oblique fissure of the lung. The **inferior angle of the scapula** is easily felt and is often visible. It is grasped when testing movements of the glenohumeral joint to immobilize the scapula. The **coracoid process of the scapula** can be felt by palpating deeply at the lateral side of the **clavipectoral triangle** (Fig. SA6.2).

The **head of the humerus** is surrounded by muscles, except inferiorly; consequently, it can be palpated only by pushing the fingers well up into the *axillary fossa* (armpit). The arm should not be fully abducted, otherwise the fascia in the axilla will be tense and impede palpation of the humeral head. When the arm is moved and the scapula is fixed (held in place), the head of the humerus can be palpated.

The **greater tubercle of the humerus** may be felt with the person's arm by the side on deep palpation through the deltoid, inferior to the lateral border of the acromion. In this position, the greater tubercle is the most lateral bony point of the shoulder and, along with the deltoid, gives the shoulder its rounded contour. When the arm is abducted, the greater tubercle is pulled beneath the acromion and is no longer palpable. The **lesser tubercle of the humerus** may be felt with difficulty by deep palpation through the deltoid on the anterior aspect of the arm, approximately 1 cm lateral and slightly inferior to the tip of the coracoid process. Rotation of the arm facilitates palpation of this tubercle. The location of the **intertubercular groove**, between the greater and the lesser tubercles, is identifiable during flexion and extension of the elbow joint by palpating in an upward direction along the tendon of the long head of the biceps brachii as it moves through the intertubercular groove.

The **shaft of the humerus** may be felt with varying distinctness through the muscles surrounding it. No part of the proximal part of the humeral shaft is subcutaneous. ▶

Coracoid process

Greater tubercle

Lesser tubercle

Intertubercular groove

Shaft of humerus

Clavipectoral (deltopectoral) triangle

Coracoid process

Deltoid

Pectoralis major

Anterior view

Figure SA6.2

The medial and lateral epicondyles of the humerus are subcutaneous and easily palpated on the medial and lateral aspects of the elbow region. The knob-like **medial epicondyle**, projecting posteromedially, is more prominent than the lateral epicondyle. When the elbow joint is partially flexed, the **lateral epicondyle** is visible. When the elbow joint is fully extended, the lateral epicondyle can be palpated but not seen deep to a depression on the posterolateral aspect of the elbow.

The **olecranon** of the ulna can be easily palpated (Fig. SA6.3). When the elbow joint is extended, observe that the tip of the olecranon and the humeral epicondyles lie in a straight line (Fig. SA6.3*A* & *B*). When the elbow is flexed, the olecranon descends until its tip forms the apex of an approximately equilateral triangle, of which the epicondyles form the angles at its base (Fig. SA6.3*C*). These normal relationships are important in the diagnosis of certain elbow injuries (e.g., dislocation of the elbow joint). The **posterior border of the ulna**, palpable throughout the length of the forearm, demarcates the posteromedial boundary between the flexor–pronator and the extensor–supinator compartments of the forearm. The **head of the ulna** forms a large, rounded subcutaneous prominence that can be easily seen and palpated on the medial side of the dorsal aspect of the wrist, especially when the hand is pronated. The pointed subcutaneous **ulnar styloid process** may be felt slightly distal to the rounded ulnar head when the hand is supinated.

The **head of the radius** can be palpated and felt to rotate in the depression on the posterolateral aspect of the extended elbow joint, just distal to the lateral epicondyle of the humerus. The radial head can also be palpated as it rotates during pronation and supination of the forearm. The **ulnar nerve** feels like a thick cord where it passes posterior to the medial epicondyle of the humerus; pressing the nerve here evokes an unpleasant "crazy bone" sensation.

The **radial styloid process** can be easily palpated in the **anatomical snuff box** on the lateral side of the wrist; it is larger and approximately 1 cm more distal than the ulnar styloid process. The radial styloid process is easiest to palpate when the thumb is abducted. It is overlaid by the ▶

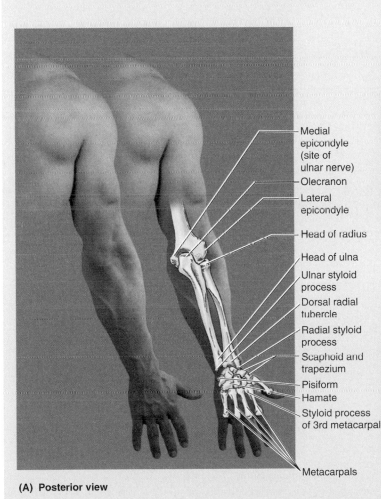

Medial epicondyle (site of ulnar nerve)
Olecranon
Lateral epicondyle
Head of radius
Head of ulna
Ulnar styloid process
Dorsal radial tubercle
Radial styloid process
Scaphoid and trapezium
Pisiform
Hamate
Styloid process of 3rd metacarpal
Metacarpals

(A) Posterior view

Posterior view

(B) Extension: condyles and olecranon aligned during extension

Posterior view   **Lateral view**

(C) Flexion: condyles form triangle and align vertically with olecranon during flexion

Figure SA6.3

tendons of the thumb muscles. Because the radial styloid process extends more distally than the ulnar styloid process, more ulnar deviation than radial deviation of the wrist is possible. The relationship of the radial and ulnar processes is important in the diagnosis of certain wrist injuries (e.g., Colles fracture). Proximal to the radial styloid process, the anterior, lateral, and posterior **surfaces of the radius** are palpable for several centimeters. The **dorsal radial tubercle** is easily felt around the middle of the dorsal aspect of the distal end of the radius. The dorsal tubercle acts as a pulley for the long extensor tendon of the thumb, which passes medial to it.

The **pisiform** can be felt on the anterior aspect of the medial border of the wrist and can be moved from side to side when the hand is relaxed. The **hook of the hamate** can be palpated on deep pressure over the medial side of the palm, approximately 2 cm distal and lateral to the pisiform. The **tubercles of the scaphoid and trapezium** can be palpated at the base and medial aspect of the **thenar eminence** (ball of thumb) when the hand is extended.

The **metacarpals**, although overlain by the long extensor tendons of the digits, can be palpated on the dorsum of the hand. The heads of these bones form the knuckles of the fist; the 3rd metacarpal head is most prominent. The **styloid process of the 3rd metacarpal** can be palpated approximately 3.5 cm from the dorsal radial tubercle. The dorsal aspects of the phalanges can also be easily palpated. The knuckles of the fingers are formed by the heads of the proximal and middle phalanges.

When measuring the upper limb, or segments of it, for comparison with the contralateral limb or with standards for normal limb growth or size, the acromial angle, lateral epicondyle of the humerus, styloid process of the radius, and tip of the third finger are most commonly used as measuring points, with the limb relaxed (dangling) but with palms directed anteriorly. ✪

THE BOTTOM LINE: The upper limb presents multiple palpable bony features that are useful (1) when diagnosing fractures, dislocations, or malformations; (2) for approximating the position of deeper structures; and (3) for precisely describing the location of incisions and sites for therapeutic puncture or of pathology or injury.

Superficial Structures of the Upper Limb

Deep to the skin is subcutaneous tissue (superficial fascia) containing fat and deep fascia surrounding the muscles. If no structure (no muscle, tendon, or bursa, for example) intervenes between the skin and the bone, the deep fascia is usually attached to bone.

Fascia of the Upper Limb

The fascia of the pectoral region is attached to the clavicle and sternum. The **pectoral fascia** invests the pectoralis major and is continuous inferiorly with the fascia of the anterior abdominal wall (Fig. 6.9). The pectoral fascia leaves the lateral border of the pectoralis major and becomes the **axillary fascia,** which forms the floor of the axilla. Deep to the pectoral fascia and the pectoralis major, another fascial layer, the **clavipectoral fascia,** descends from the clavicle, enclosing the subclavius and then the pectoralis minor, becoming continuous inferiorly with the axillary fascia. The part of the clavipectoral fascia between the pectoralis minor and the subclavius, the **costocoracoid membrane,** is pierced by the lateral pectoral nerve, which primarily supplies the pectoralis major. The part of the clavipectoral fascia inferior to the pectoralis minor, the **suspensory ligament of the axilla,** supports the axillary fascia and pulls it and the skin inferior to it upward during abduction of the arm, forming the **axillary fossa.**

The scapulohumeral muscles that cover the scapula and form the bulk of the shoulder are also ensheathed by deep fascia. The **deltoid fascia** descends over the superficial surface of the deltoid from the clavicle, acromion, and scapular spine. From the deep surface of the deltoid fascia, numerous septa penetrate between the fascicles (bundles) of the muscle. Inferiorly, the deltoid fascia is continuous with the pectoral fascia anteriorly and the dense infraspinous fascia posteriorly. The muscles that cover the anterior and posterior surfaces of the scapula are covered superficially with deep fascia, which is attached to the margins of the scapula and posteriorly to the spine of the scapula. This arrangement creates osseofibrous *subscapular, supraspinous*, and *infraspinous compartments;* the muscles in each compartment attach to (originate from) the deep surface of the overlying fascia in part, allowing the muscles to have greater bulk (mass) than would be the case if only bony attachments occurred. The **supraspinous** and **infraspinous fascia** overlying the supraspinatus and infraspinatus muscles, respectively, on the posterior aspect of the scapula are so dense and opaque that they must be removed during dissection to view the muscles.

The **brachial fascia,** a sheath of deep fascia, encloses the arm like a snug sleeve deep to the skin and subcutaneous tissue (Fig. 6.10*A* & *B*); it is continuous superiorly with the deltoid, pectoral, axillary, and infraspinous fasciae. The brachial fascia is attached inferiorly to the epicondyles of the humerus and the olecranon of the ulna and is continuous with the antebrachial fascia, the deep fascia of the forearm. Two intermuscular septa, the **medial** and **lateral intermuscular septa,** extend from the deep surface of the brachial fascia to the central shaft and medial and lateral supraepicondylar ridges of

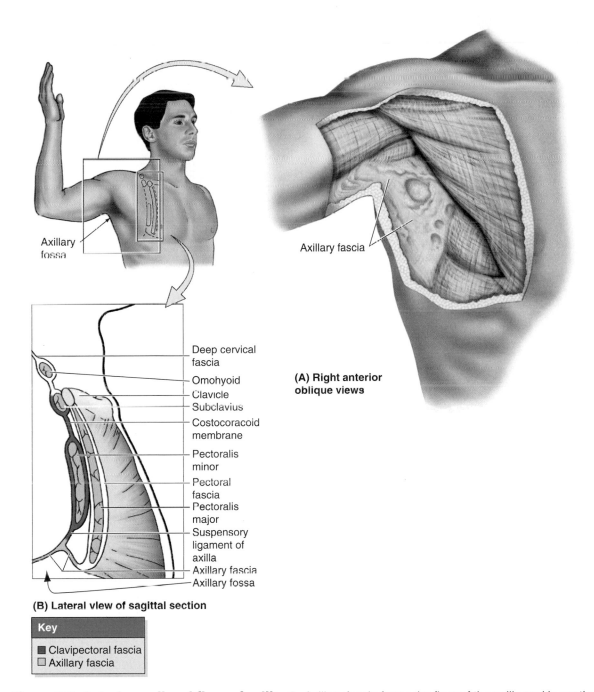

Axillary
fossa

Axillary fascia

**(A) Right anterior
oblique views**

Deep cervical
fascia
Omohyoid
Clavicle
Subclavius
Costocoracoid
membrane
Pectoralis
minor
Pectoral
fascia
Pectoralis
major
Suspensory
ligament of
axilla
Axillary fascia
Axillary fossa

(B) Lateral view of sagittal section

Key

■ Clavipectoral fascia
□ Axillary fascia

Figure 6.9. Anterior wall and floor of axilla. A. Axillary fascia forms the floor of the axilla and is continuous with the pectoral fascia. **B.** The pectoral fascia surrounds the pectoralis major, forming the anterior layer of the anterior axillary wall. The clavipectoral fascia extends between the coracoid process of the scapula, the clavicle, and the axillary fascia, enveloping the subclavius and pectoralis minor muscles and forming the posterior layer of the anterior axillary wall. The suspensory ligament of the axilla is the part of the clavipectoral, which attaches to the axillary fascia; when the arm is abducted, traction by the suspensory ligament pulls the axillary fascia superiorly, producing the hollow of the axillary fossa.

the humerus (Fig. 6.10*B*). These septa divide the arm into **anterior (flexor)** and **posterior (extensor) fascial compartments,** each of which contains muscles serving similar functions and sharing common innervation. As discussed in relation to the fascial compartments of the lower limb (see Chapter 5), the fascial compartments of the upper limb are

important clinically because they also contain and direct the spread of infection or hemorrhage in the limb.

In the forearm, similar fascial compartments are surrounded by the **antebrachial fascia** and separated by the *interosseous membrane* connecting the radius and ulna (Fig. 6.10*C*). The antebrachial fascia thickens posteriorly over the

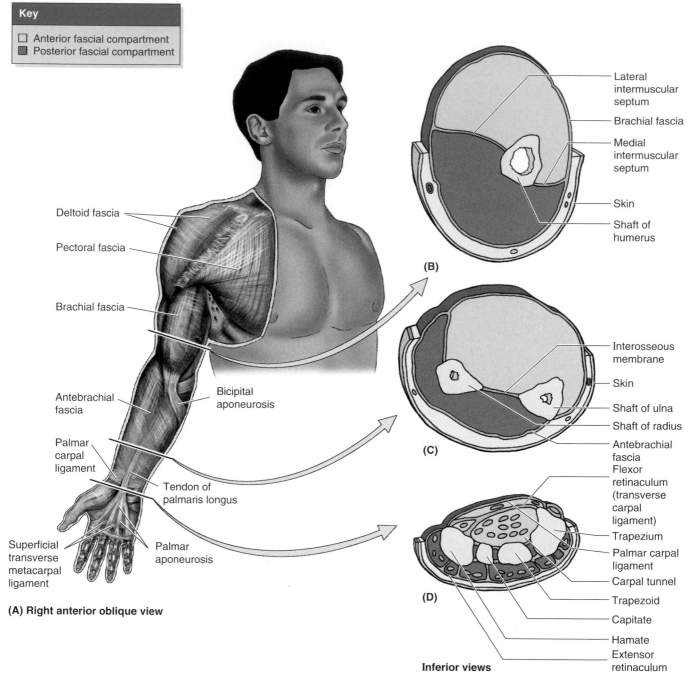

Key
☐ Anterior fascial compartment
■ Posterior fascial compartment

Deltoid fascia

Pectoral fascia

Brachial fascia

Antebrachial fascia

Bicipital aponeurosis

Palmar carpal ligament

Tendon of palmaris longus

Superficial transverse metacarpal ligament

Palmar aponeurosis

(A) Right anterior oblique view

Lateral intermuscular septum

Brachial fascia

Medial intermuscular septum

Skin

Shaft of humerus

(B)

Interosseous membrane

Skin

Shaft of ulna

Shaft of radius

Antebrachial fascia

(C)

Flexor retinaculum (transverse carpal ligament)

Trapezium

Palmar carpal ligament

Carpal tunnel

Trapezoid

Capitate

Hamate

Extensor retinaculum

(D)

Inferior views

Figure 6.10. Fascia and compartments of upper limb. A. Brachial and antebrachial fascia surround the structures of the free upper limb. **B.** The intermuscular septa and humerus divide the space inside the brachial fascia into anterior and posterior compartments, each of which contains muscles serving similar functions and the nerves and vessels supplying them. **C.** The interosseous membrane and the radius and ulna similarly separate the space inside the antebrachial fascia into anterior and posterior compartments. **D.** Continuing distal to the radius and ulna onto the carpal bones, the deep fascia of the forearm thickens to form the extensor retinaculum posteriorly and a corresponding thickening anteriorly (palmar carpal ligament). At a deeper level to the latter, a ligamentous formation, the flexor retinaculum (transverse carpal ligament) extends between the anterior prominences of the outer carpal bones, converting the anterior concavity of the carpus into an osseofibrous carpal tunnel.

distal ends of the radius and ulna to form a transverse band, the **extensor retinaculum**, which retains the extensor tendons in position. The antebrachial fascia also forms an anterior thickening, which is continuous with the extensor retinaculum but is officially unnamed; some authors identify it as the *palmar carpal ligament* (Fig. 6.10*D*). Immediately distal and at a deeper level to the latter, the antebrachial fascia is also continued as the **flexor retinaculum (transverse carpal ligament)**.[2] This fibrous band extends between the anterior prominences of the outer carpal bones and converts the anterior concavity of the carpus into a *carpal tunnel,* through which the flexor tendons and median nerve pass.

The deep fascia of the upper limb continues beyond the extensor and flexor retinacula as the *palmar fascia.* The central part of the palmar fascia, the *palmar aponeurosis,* is thick, tendinous, and triangular and it overlies the central compartment of the palm. Its apex, located proximally, is continuous with the tendon of the palmaris longus (when it is present) (Fig. 6.10*A*). The aponeurosis forms four distinct thickenings that radiate to the bases of the fingers and become continuous with the fibrous tendon sheaths of the digits. The bands are traversed distally by the **superficial transverse metacarpal ligament,** which forms the base of the palmar aponeurosis. Innumerable minute, strong *skin ligaments* (L. *retinacula cutis*) extend from the palmar aponeurosis to the skin (see the Introduction). These ligaments hold the palmar skin close to the aponeurosis, allowing little sliding movement of the skin.

THE BOTTOM LINE: The firm deep fascia of the upper limb surrounds and contains the structures of the upper limb as an expansion-limiting membrane deep to the skin and subcutaneous tissue. Its deep surface, which occasionally serves to extend the surface area available for muscular origin, is attached directly or via intermuscular septa to the enclosed bones. The deep fascia thus forms fascial compartments containing individual muscles or muscle groups of similar function and innervation. The compartments also contain or direct the spread of infection or hemorrhage.

Cutaneous Nerves of the Upper Limb

The cutaneous nerves of the upper limb follow a general pattern that is easy to understand if it is noted that developmentally the limbs grow as lateral protrusions of the trunk, with the 1st digit (thumb or great toe) located on the cranial side (thumb is directed superiorly). Thus the lateral surface of the upper limb is more cranial than the medial surface.

There are two dermatome maps in common use. One has gained popular acceptance because of its more intuitive aesthetic qualities, corresponding to concepts of limb development (Keegan and Garrett, 1948); the other is based on clinical findings and is generally preferred by neurologists (Foerster, 1933). Both maps are approximations, delineating dermatomes as distinct zones when actually there is much overlap between adjacent dermatomes and much variation (even from side to side in the same individual). In both maps, observe the progression of the segmental innervation of the various cutaneous areas around the limb when it is placed in its "initial embryonic position" (abducted with thumb directed superiorly) (Fig. 6.11*A–D*):

- C3 and C4 nerves supply the region at the base of the neck extending laterally over the shoulder.

- C5 nerve supplies the arm laterally (i.e., on the superior aspect of the abducted limb).

- C6 nerve supplies the forearm laterally and the thumb.

- C7 nerve supplies the middle and ring fingers (or middle three fingers) and the middle of the posterior surface of the limb.

- C8 nerve supplies the little finger, the medial side of the hand, and the forearm (i.e., the inferior aspect of the outstretched limb).

- T1 nerve supplies the middle of the forearm to the axilla.

- T2 nerve supplies a small part of the arm and the skin of the axilla. (This is not indicated on the Keegan and Garrett map; however, pain experienced during a heart attack, considered to be mediated by T1 and T2, is commonly described as "radiating down the medial side of the left arm").

Most cutaneous nerves of the upper limb are derived from the *brachial plexus,* a major nerve network formed by the anterior rami of the C5–T1 spinal nerves (see "Brachial Plexus," later in this chapter). The nerves to the shoulder, however, are derived from the **cervical plexus,** a nerve network consisting of a series of nerve loops formed between adjacent anterior rami of the first four cervical nerves. The cervical plexus lies deep to the sternocleidomastoid muscle on the anterolateral aspect of the neck.

The cutaneous nerves of the arm and forearm[3] are as follows (Fig. 6.11*E & F*):

- The **supraclavicular nerves** (C3, C4) pass anterior to the clavicle, immediately deep to the platysma, and supply the skin over the clavicle and the superolateral aspect of the pectoralis major.

---

[2] It is awkward that the structure officially identified as the flexor retinaculum does not correspond in position and structure to the extensor retinaculum when there is another structure (the palmar carpal ligament, currently unrecognized by *Terminologia Anatomica*) that does. The clinical community has proposed and widely adopted the use of the more structurally based term *transverse carpal ligament* to replace the term *flexor retinaculum.* The authors urge FICAT to adopt this terminology in future editions of *Terminologia Anatomica.*

[3] The preferred English-equivalent terms listed by *Terminologia Anatomica* are used here. Official alternate *TA* terms replace *of the arm* with *brachial,* and *of the forearm* with *antebrachial.*

■ Preaxial   ■ Postaxial

Figure 6.11. Segmental (dermatomal) and peripheral (cutaneous nerve) innervation of upper limb. A and B. The pattern of segmental (dermatomal) innervation of the upper limb proposed by Foerster (1933) depicts innervation of the medial aspect of the limb by upper thoracic (T1–T3) spinal cord segments, consistent with the experience of heart pain (angina pectoris) referred to that area. **C and D.** The pattern of segmental innervation proposed by Keegan and Garrett (1948) has gained popular acceptance, perhaps because of the regular progression of its stripes and correlation with developmental concepts. In both patterns, the dermatomes progress sequentially around the periphery of the outstretched limb (with the thumb directed superiorly), providing a way to approximate the segmental innervation.

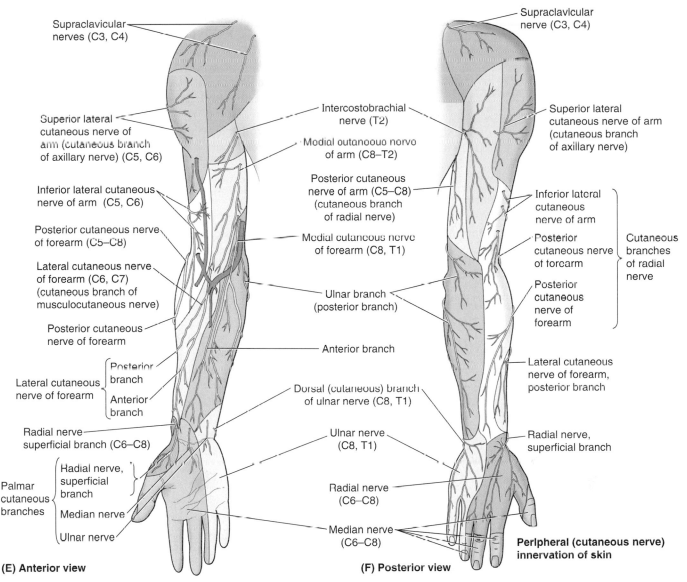

Supraclavicular nerves (C3, C4)

Supraclavicular nerve (C3, C4)

Superior lateral cutaneous nerve of arm (cutaneous branch of axillary nerve) (C5, C6)

Inferior lateral cutaneous nerve of arm (C5, C6)

Posterior cutaneous nerve of forearm (C5–C8)

Lateral cutaneous nerve of forearm (C6, C7) (cutaneous branch of musculocutaneous nerve)

Posterior cutaneous nerve of forearm

Lateral cutaneous nerve of forearm { Posterior branch, Anterior branch }

Radial nerve superficial branch (C6–C8)

Palmar cutaneous branches { Radial nerve, superficial branch, Median nerve, Ulnar nerve }

Intercostobrachial nerve (T2)

Medial cutaneous nerve of arm (C8–T2)

Posterior cutaneous nerve of arm (C5–C8) (cutaneous branch of radial nerve)

Medial cutaneous nerve of forearm (C8, T1)

Ulnar branch (posterior branch)

Anterior branch

Dorsal (cutaneous) branch of ulnar nerve (C8, T1)

Ulnar nerve (C8, T1)

Radial nerve (C6–C8)

Median nerve (C6–C8)

Superior lateral cutaneous nerve of arm (cutaneous branch of axillary nerve)

Inferior lateral cutaneous nerve of arm

Posterior cutaneous nerve of forearm

Posterior cutaneous nerve of forearm

} Cutaneous branches of radial nerve

Lateral cutaneous nerve of forearm, posterior branch

Radial nerve, superficial branch

Peripheral (cutaneous nerve) innervation of skin

(E) Anterior view

(F) Posterior view

Figure 6.11 *(Continued)* **E and F.** The distribution of the peripheral (named) cutaneous nerves in the upper limb is demonstrated. Most of the nerves are branches of nerve plexuses and therefore contain fibers from more than one spinal nerve or spinal cord segment.

- The **posterior cutaneous nerve of the arm** (C5–C8), a branch of the radial nerve, supplies the skin on the posterior surface of the arm.

- The **posterior cutaneous nerve of the forearm** (C5–C8), also a branch of the radial nerve, supplies the skin on the posterior surface of the forearm.

- The **superior lateral cutaneous nerve of the arm** (C5, C6), the terminal branch of the axillary nerve, emerges from beneath the posterior margin of the deltoid and supplies skin over the lower part of this muscle and on the lateral side of the midarm inferior to its distal attachment to the lateral side of the arm a little above its middle.

- The **inferior lateral cutaneous nerve of the arm** (C5, C6), a branch of the radial nerve, supplies the skin over the inferolateral aspect of the arm; it is frequently a branch of the posterior cutaneous nerve of the forearm.

- The **lateral cutaneous nerve of the forearm** (C6, C7), the terminal cutaneous branch of the musculocutaneous nerve, supplies the skin on the lateral side of the forearm.

- The **medial cutaneous nerve of the arm** (C8–T2) arises from the medial cord of the brachial plexus, often unites in the axilla with the lateral cutaneous branch of the 2nd intercostal nerve, and supplies the skin on the medial side of the arm.

- The **intercostobrachial nerve** (T2), a lateral cutaneous branch of the 2nd intercostal nerve, also contributes to the innervation of the skin on the medial surface of the arm.

- The **medial cutaneous nerve of the forearm** (C8, T1) arises from the medial cord of the brachial plexus and supplies the skin of the anterior and medial surfaces of the forearm.

Note that there are lateral, medial, and posterior (but no anterior) cutaneous nerves of the arm and forearm; as discussed later in this chapter, this pattern corresponds to that of the cords of the brachial plexus.

THE BOTTOM LINE: As a consequence of plexus formation, two patterns of cutaneous innervation occur in the upper limb: (1) segmental innervation (dermatomes) by spinal nerves and (2) innervation by multisegmental peripheral (named) nerves. The former pattern is easiest to visualize if

---

the limb is placed in its initial embryonic position (abducted with the thumb directed superiorly). The segments then progress in descending order around the limb (starting with C4 dermatome at the root of the neck, proceeding laterally or distally along the superior surface and then medially or proximally along the inferior surface, as the T2 dermatome continues onto the thoracic wall). Like the brachial plexus, which forms posterior, lateral, and medial (but no anterior) cords, the arm and forearm have posterior, lateral, and medial (but no anterior) cutaneous nerves.

Superficial Veins of the Upper Limb

The main superficial veins of the upper limb, the cephalic and basilic veins, originate in the subcutaneous tissue on the dorsum of the hand from the **dorsal venous network** (Fig. 6.12). **Perforating veins** form communications between the superficial and

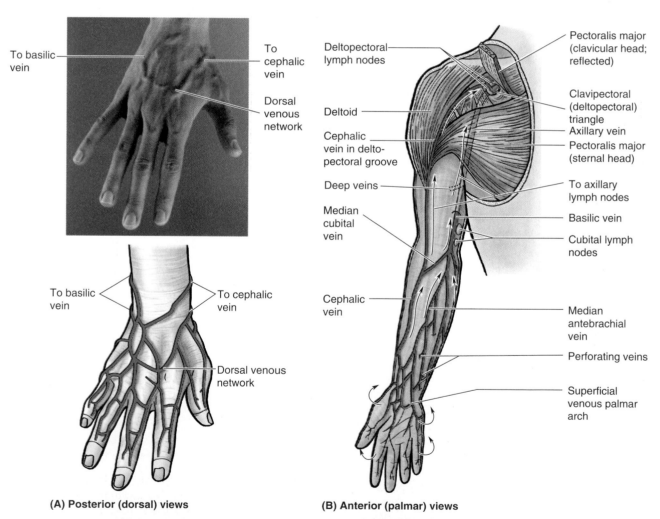

(A) Posterior (dorsal) views   **(B) Anterior (palmar) views**

Figure 6.12. Superficial veins and lymph nodes of upper limb. A. The digital veins drain into the dorsal venous network on the dorsum of the hand, which leads to two prominent superficial vessels: the cephalic and basilic veins. **B.** The basilic and cephalic veins ultimately drain into the origin and termination of the axillary vein, respectively. The median cubital vein is the communication between the basilic and the cephalic veins in the cubital fossa. Perforating veins connect the superficial veins to the deep veins. *Arrows* indicate the flow of lymph within lymphatic vessels that converge toward the vein and drain into the cubital and axillary lymph nodes.

deep veins. Like the dermatomal pattern, the logic for naming the main superficial veins of the upper limb cephalic (toward the head) and basilic (toward the base) becomes apparent when the limb is placed in its initial embryonic position.

The **cephalic vein** (G. *kephalé*, head) ascends in the subcutaneous tissue from the lateral aspect of the dorsal venous network, proceeding along the lateral border of the wrist and the anterolateral surface of the proximal forearm and arm; it is often visible through the skin. Anterior to the elbow, the cephalic vein communicates with the **median cubital vein,** which passes obliquely across the anterior aspect of the elbow in the cubital fossa (a depression in front of the elbow) and joins the basilic vein. The cephalic vein courses superiorly between the deltoid and the pectoralis major muscles along the deltopectoral groove and enters the *clavipectoral triangle* (Fig. 6.12*B*). It then pierces the costocoracoid membrane, part of the clavipectoral fascia, and joins the terminal part of the axillary vein.

The **basilic vein** ascends in the subcutaneous tissue from the medial end of the dorsal venous network along the medial side of the forearm and the inferior part of the arm; it is often visible through the skin. It then passes deeply near the junction of the middle and inferior thirds of the arm, piercing the brachial fascia and running superiorly parallel to the brachial artery and the medial cutaneous nerve of the forearm to the axilla, where it merges with the accompanying veins (L. *venae comitantes*) of the axillary artery to form the axillary vein.

The highly variable **median antebrachial vein (median vein of the forearm)** begins at the base of the dorsum of the thumb, curves around the lateral side of the wrist, and ascends in the middle of the anterior aspect of the forearm between the cephalic and the basilic veins. The median antebrachial vein sometimes divides into a median basilic vein, which joins the basilic vein, and a median cephalic vein, which joins the cephalic vein.

Lymphatic Drainage of the Upper Limb

Superficial lymphatic vessels arise from **lymphatic plexuses** in the skin of the fingers, palm, and dorsum of the hand and ascend mostly with the superficial veins, such as the cephalic and basilic veins (Fig. 6.13). Some vessels accompanying the basilic vein enter the **cubital (lymph) nodes,** located proximal to the medial epicondyle and medial to the basilic vein. Efferent vessels from these lymph nodes ascend in the arm and terminate in the **humeral (lateral) axillary lymph nodes** (see Chapter 1). Most superficial lymphatic vessels accompanying the cephalic vein cross the proximal part of the arm and the anterior aspect of the shoulder to enter the **apical axillary lymph nodes**; however, some vessels previously enter the more superficial **deltopectoral lymph nodes.** *Deep lymphatic vessels,* less numerous than superficial vessels, accompany the major deep veins in the upper limb and terminate in the humeral axillary lymph nodes. They drain lymph from the joint capsules, periosteum, tendons, nerves, and muscles and ascend with the deep veins; a few deep lymph nodes may occur along their

Anterior (palmar) view

Figure 6.13. Lymphatic drainage of upper limb. Superficial lymphatic vessels originate from the digital lymphatic vessels of the digits and lymphatic plexus of the palm; most drainage from the palm passes to the dorsum of the hand (*arrows*). The vessels ascend through the forearm and arm, converging toward the cephalic and especially the basilic veins. Some lymph following this superficial route passes through the cubital lymph nodes in the elbow region or deltopectoral nodes in the shoulder region. The superficial and deep lymphatics of the upper limb drain initially to the humeral (lateral) and apical axillary lymph nodes; axillary nodes are drained in turn by the subclavian lymphatic trunk.

course. The axillary lymph nodes are drained by the subclavian lymphatic trunk; both are discussed in greater detail with the axilla, later in this chapter.

THE BOTTOM LINE: Like the dermatomes, the pattern of the superficial veins is easy to visualize when the limb is placed in its embryonic position (abducted to 90° with the thumb directed superiorly). The cephalic vein courses along the cranial (cephalic) margin of the limb, while the basilic vein courses along the caudal (basic) margin of the limb. Both veins come from the dorsal venous network on the dorsum of the hand and drain into the beginning (basilic vein) and end (cephalic vein) of the axillary vein.

The superficial lymphatic vessels generally converge on and follow the superficial veins, whereas the deep lymphatics follow the deep veins. The lymph collected from the upper limb by both superficial and deep lymphatics drains into the axillary lymph nodes.

Anterior Axioappendicular Muscles of the Upper Limb

Four **anterior axioappendicular (thoracoappendicular or pectoral) muscles** move the pectoral girdle: pectoralis major, pectoralis minor, subclavius, and serratus anterior. The attachments, nerve supply, and main actions of these muscles are illustrated in Figure 6.14 and summarized in Table 6.1.

The **pectoralis major** is a large, fan-shaped muscle that covers the superior part of the thorax. It has **clavicular** and **sternocostal heads.** The latter head is much larger and its lateral border forms the muscular mass that makes up most of the anterior wall of the axilla. Its inferior border forms the *anterior axillary fold* (see "Axilla," later in this chapter). The pectoralis major and adjacent deltoid form the narrow **deltopectoral groove,** in which the cephalic vein runs (Fig. 6.12*B*); however, the muscles diverge slightly from each other superiorly and, along with the clavicle, form the **clavipectoral (deltopectoral) triangle** (Fig. 6.12).

Producing powerful adduction and medial rotation of the arm when acting together, the two parts of the pectoralis major can also act independently: the clavicular head flexing the humerus, and the sternocostal head extending it back from the flexed position.

To test the clavicular head of pectoralis major, the arm is abducted 90°; the individual then moves the arm anteriorly against resistance. If acting normally, the clavicular head can be seen and palpated. *To test the sternocostal head of the pectoralis major,* the arm is abducted 60° and then adducted against resistance. If acting normally, the sternocostal head can be seen and palpated.

The **pectoralis minor** lies in the anterior wall of the axilla where it is almost completely covered by the much larger pectoralis major (Fig. 6.14). The pectoralis minor is triangular in shape: Its base (proximal attachment) is formed by fleshy slips attached to the anterior ends of the 3rd–5th ribs near their costal cartilages; its apex (distal attachment) is on the coracoid process of the scapula. Variations in the costal attachments of the muscle are common. The pectoralis minor stabilizes the scapula and is used when stretching the upper limb forward to touch an object that is just out of reach. The pectoralis minor also assists in elevating the ribs for deep inspiration when the pectoral girdle is fixed or elevated. The pectoralis minor is a useful anatomical and surgical landmark for structures in the axilla (e.g., the axillary artery). With the coracoid process, the pectoralis minor forms a "bridge" under which vessels and nerves must pass to the arm.

The **subclavius** lies almost horizontally when the arm is in the anatomical position. This small, round muscle is located inferior to the clavicle and affords some protection to the subclavian vessels and the superior trunk of the brachial plexus if the clavicle fractures. The subclavius anchors and depresses the clavicle, stabilizing it during movements of the upper limb. It also helps resist the tendency for the clavicle to dislocate at the SC joint, for example, when pulling hard during a tug-of-war game.

The **serratus anterior** overlies the lateral part of the thorax and forms the medial wall of the axilla. This broad sheet of thick muscle was named because of the sawtoothed appearance of its fleshy slips or digitations (L. *serratus,* a saw). The muscular slips pass posteriorly and then medially to attach to the whole length of the anterior surface of the medial border of the scapula, including its inferior angle.

The serratus anterior is one of the most powerful muscles of the pectoral girdle. It is a strong protractor of the scapula that is used when punching or reaching anteriorly (sometimes called the "boxer's muscle"). Its strong inferior part rotates the scapula, elevating its glenoid cavity so the arm can be raised above the shoulder. It also anchors the scapula, keeping it closely applied to the thoracic wall, enabling other muscles to use it as a fixed bone for movements of the humerus. The serratus anterior holds the scapula against the thoracic wall when doing push-ups or when pushing against resistance (e.g., pushing a car).

To test the serratus anterior (or the function of the long thoracic nerve that supplies it), the hand of the outstretched limb is pushed against a wall. If the muscle is acting normally, several digitations of the muscle can be seen and palpated.

Absence of the Pectoral Muscles

Absence of part of the pectoralis major, usually its sternocostal part, is uncommon, but when it occurs, no disability usually results. However, the anterior axillary fold, formed by the skin and fascia overlying the inferior border of the pectoralis major, is absent on the affected side, and the nipple is more inferior than usual. In *Poland syndrome,* both the pectoralis major and minor are absent; breast hypoplasia and absence of two to four rib segments are also seen. ▶

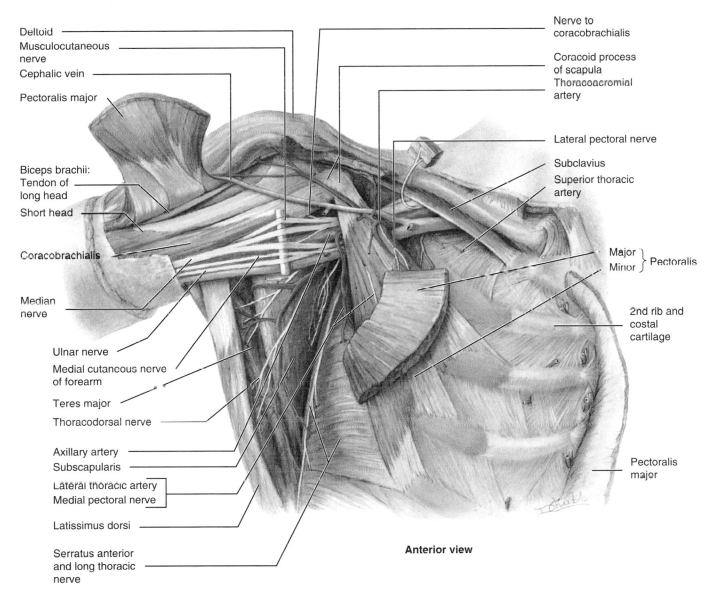

Deltoid
Musculocutaneous nerve
Cephalic vein
Pectoralis major

Biceps brachii:
Tendon of long head
Short head

Coracobrachialis

Median nerve

Ulnar nerve
Medial cutaneous nerve of forearm
Teres major
Thoracodorsal nerve

Axillary artery
Subscapularis
Lateral thoracic artery
Medial pectoral nerve

Latissimus dorsi

Serratus anterior and long thoracic nerve

Nerve to coracobrachialis
Coracoid process of scapula
Thoracoacromial artery

Lateral pectoral nerve
Subclavius
Superior thoracic artery

Major }
Minor } Pectoralis

2nd rib and costal cartilage

Pectoralis major

Anterior view

Figure 6.14. Muscular walls of the axilla. Most of the anterior wall of the axilla and the axillary fat have been removed, revealing the axilla's medial and posterior walls and neurovascular contents. Of the structures forming the anterior wall, only portions of the pectoralis major (attaching ends, a central part overlying the pectoralis minor, and a cube of muscle reflected superior to the clavicle), the pectoralis minor, and subclavius remain. All the clavipectoral fascia and axillary fat have been removed, as has the axillary sheath surrounding the neurovascular bundle. This enables observation of the medial wall of the axilla, formed by the serratus anterior overlying the lateral thoracic wall, and of the muscles forming the posterior wall.

Paralysis of the Serratus Anterior

When the serratus anterior is paralyzed owing to *injury to the long thoracic nerve* (Fig. 6.14), the medial border of the scapula moves laterally and posteriorly away from the thoracic wall, giving the scapula the appearance of a wing, especially when the person leans on a hand or presses the upper limb against a wall. When the arm is raised, the medial border and inferior angle of the scapula pull markedly away from the posterior thoracic wall, a deformation known as a **winged scapula** (Fig. B6.5). In addition, the upper limb cannot be abducted above the horizontal position because the serratus anterior is unable to rotate the glenoid cavity superiorly to allow complete abduction of the limb. Although protected when the limbs are at one's sides, the long thoracic nerve is exceptional in that ▶

Table 6.1.   Anterior Axioappendicular Muscles

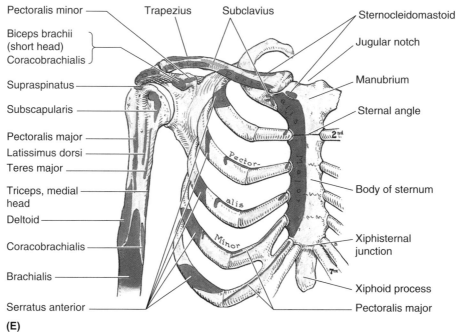

(E)

Muscle	Proximal Attachment	Distal Attachment	Innervation[a]	Main Action
Pectoralis major	Clavicular head: anterior surface of medial half of clavicle Sternocostal head: anterior surface of sternum, superior six costal cartilages, aponeurosis of external oblique muscle	Lateral lip of intertubercular groove of humerus	Lateral and medial pectoral nerves; clavicular head (C5, **C6**), sternocostal head (**C7, C8**, T1)	Adducts and medially rotates humerus; draws scapula anteriorly and inferiorly Acting alone, clavicular head flexes humerus and sternocostal head extends it from the flexed position
Pectoralis minor	3rd–5th ribs near their costal cartilages	Medial border and superior surface of coracoid process of scapula	Medial pectoral nerve (C8, T1)	Stabilizes scapula by drawing it inferiorly and anteriorly against thoracic wall
Subclavius	Junction of 1st rib and its costal cartilage	Inferior surface of middle third of clavicle	Nerve to subclavius (**C5**, C6)	Anchors and depresses clavicle
Serratus anterior	External surfaces of lateral parts of 1st–8th ribs	Anterior surface of medial border of scapula	Long thoracic nerve (C5, **C6, C7**)	Protracts scapula and holds it against thoracic wall; rotates scapula

[a] The spinal cord segmental innervation is indicated (e.g., "**C5**, C6" means that the nerves supplying the subclavius are derived from the fifth and sixth cervical segments of the spinal cord). Numbers in boldface (**C5**) indicate the main segmental innervation. Damage to one or more of the listed spinal cord segments or to the motor nerve roots arising from them results in paralysis of the muscles concerned.

it courses on the superficial aspect of the serratus anterior, which it supplies. Thus when the limbs are elevated, as in a knife fight, the nerve is especially vulnerable. Weapons, including bullets directed toward the thorax, are a common source of injury.○

Right winged scapula

Figure B6.5

Posterior Axioappendicular and Scapulohumeral Muscles

The **posterior axioappendicular muscles** (superficial and intermediate groups of extrinsic back muscles) attach the superior appendicular skeleton (of the upper limb) to the axial skeleton (in the trunk). *The intrinsic back muscles,* which maintain posture and control movements of the vertebral column, are described in Chapter 4. The posterior shoulder muscles are divided into three groups (Table 6.2):

* *Superficial posterior axioappendicular (extrinsic shoulder) muscles:* trapezius and latissimus dorsi.

* *Deep posterior axioappendicular (extrinsic shoulder) muscles:* levator scapulae and rhomboids.

* *Scapulohumeral (intrinsic shoulder) muscles:* deltoid, teres major, and the four rotator cuff muscles (supraspinatus, infraspinatus, teres minor, and subscapularis).

Superficial Posterior Axioappendicular (Extrinsic Shoulder) Muscles

The **superficial axioappendicular muscles** are the trapezius and latissimus dorsi. The attachments, nerve supply, and main actions of these muscles are given in Table 6.2.

Trapezius

The **trapezius** provides a direct attachment of the pectoral girdle to the trunk. This large, triangular muscle covers the posterior aspect of the neck and the superior half of the trunk (Fig. 6.15). It was given its name because the muscles of the two sides form a *trapezium* (G. irregular four-sided figure). The trapezius attaches the pectoral girdle to the cranium and vertebral column and assists in suspending the upper limb. The fibers of the trapezius are divided into three parts, which have different actions at the physiological scapulothoracic joint between the scapula and the thoracic wall (Table 6.3): (1) superior fibers elevate the scapula (e.g., when squaring the shoulders), (2) middle fibers retract the scapula (i.e., pull it posteriorly), and (3) inferior fibers depress the scapula and lower the shoulder.

Superior and inferior trapezius fibers act together in rotating the scapula on the thoracic wall in different directions, twisting it like a wing nut. The trapezius also braces the shoulders by pulling the scapulae posteriorly and superiorly, fixing them in position on the thoracic wall with tonic contraction; consequently, weakness of this muscle causes drooping of the shoulders.

To test the trapezius (or the function of the accessory nerve [CN XI] that supplies it), the shoulder is shrugged against resistance (the person attempts to raise the shoulders as the examiner presses down on them). If the muscle is acting normally, the superior border of the muscle can be easily seen and palpated.

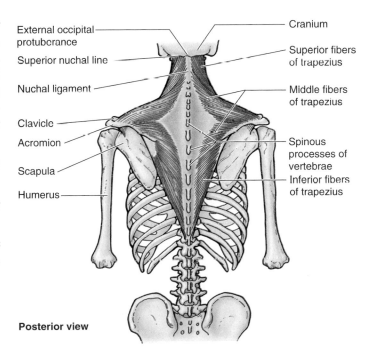

External occipital protuberance

Superior nuchal line

Nuchal ligament

Clavicle

Acromion

Scapula

Humerus

Cranium

Superior fibers of trapezius

Middle fibers of trapezius

Spinous processes of vertebrae

Inferior fibers of trapezius

Posterior view

Figure 6.15. Trapezius. This large, superficial, triangular muscle is responsible for the lateral slope between the neck and the shoulder. It assists in suspending the pectoral girdle and elevates, retracts, and rotates the scapula.

Table 6.2. Posterior Axioappendicular and Scapulohumeral Muscles

Deltoid

Trapezius

Infraspinatus

Teres minor

Triceps brachii { Long head

Lateral head }

Supraspinatus

Levator scapulae

Rhomboid minor

Infraspinatus

Rhomboid major

Teres minor

Teres major

(A) Posterior view

Superior angle

Supraspinatus

Spine of scapula

Infraspinatus

Teres minor

Teres major

Inferior angle

(B) Posterior view

Pectoralis minor

Biceps brachii (short head) and coracobrachialis

Supraspinatus

Subscapularis

Latissimus dorsi

Teres major

Pectoralis major

Subscapularis

Serratus anterior

Triceps (long head)

(C) Anterior view

Facet for articulation with the clavicle

Acromion

Capsule of shoulder joint*

Transverse humeral ligament

Tendon of long head of biceps brachii

Coracoid process   Supraspinatus

Superior angle

Subscapularis

Inferior angle

(D) Anterior view

*Musculotendinous rotator cuff

Superior trapezius

Levator scapulae

Rhomboid minor

Rhomboid major

Deltoid

Teres major

Accessory nerve

Trapezius

Latissimus dorsi

External oblique

Cutaneous branches of posterior rami

Middle trapezius

Inferior trapezius

Triangle of auscultation

Cutaneous branches of posterior rami

Thoracolumbar fascia

Cutaneous branches of posterior rami of L1, L2, and L3

(E) Posterior view

Table 6.2. Posterior Axioappendicular and Scapulohumeral Muscles *(continued)*

Muscle	Proximal Attachment	Distal Attachment	Innervation[a]	Main Action
Superficial posterior axioappendicular (extrinsic shoulder) muscles				
Trapezius	Medial third of superior nuchal line; external occipital protuberance; nuchal ligament; spinous processes of C7–C12 vertebrae	Lateral third of clavicle; acromion and spine of scapula	Accessory nerve (CN XI) (motor fibers) and C3, C4 spinal nerves (pain and proprioceptive fibers)	Descending part elevates; ascending part depresses; and middle part (or all parts together) retracts scapula; descending and ascending parts act together to rotate glenoid cavity superiorly
Latissimus dorsi	Spinous processes of inferior 6 thoracic vertebrae, thoracolumbar fascia, iliac crest, and inferior 3 or 4 ribs	Floor of intertubercular groove of humerus	Thoracodorsal nerve (**C6, C7**, C8)	Extends, adducts, and medially rotates humerus; raises body toward arms during climbing
Deep posterior axioappendicular (extrinsic shoulder) muscles				
Levator scapulae	Posterior tubercles of transverse processes of C1–C4 vertebrae	Medial border of scapula superior to root of spine	Dorsal scapular (C5) and cervical (C3, C4) nerves	Elevates scapula and tilts its glenoid cavity inferiorly by rotating scapula
Rhomboid minor and major	Minor: nuchal ligament; spinous processes of C7 and T1 vertebrae Major: spinous processes of T2–T5 vertebrae	Minor: smooth triangular area at medial end of scapular spine Major: medial border of scapula from level of spine to inferior angle	Dorsal scapular nerve (C4, **C5**)	Retract scapula and rotate it to depress glenoid cavity; fix scapula to thoracic wall
Scapulohumeral (intrinsic shoulder) muscles				
Deltoid	Lateral third of clavicle; acromion and spine of scapula	Deltoid tuberosity of humerus	Axillary nerve (**C5, C6**)	Anterior part: flexes and medially rotates arm Middle part: abducts arm Posterior part: extends and laterally rotates arm
Supraspinatus[b]	Supraspinous fossa of scapula	Superior facet of greater tubercle of humerus	Suprascapular nerve (C4, **C5**, C6)	Initiates and assists deltoid in abduction of arm and acts with rotator cuff muscles[b]
Infraspinatus[b]	Infraspinous fossa of scapula	Middle facet of greater tubercle of humerus	Suprascapular nerve (**C5**, C6)	Laterally rotate arm, help hold humeral head in glenoid cavity of scapula
Teres minor[b]	Middle part of lateral border of scapula	Inferior facet of greater tubercle of humerus	Axillary nerve (**C5**, C6)	
Teres major	Posterior surface of inferior angle of scapula	Medial lip of intertubercular groove of humerus	Lower subscapular nerve (C5, **C6**)	Adducts and medially rotates arm
Subscapularis[b]	Subscapular fossa (most of anterior surface of scapula)	Lesser tubercle of humerus	Upper and lower subscapular nerves (C5, **C6**, C7)	Medially rotates and adduct arm; helps hold humeral head in glenoid cavity

[a]The spinal cord segmental innervation is indicated (e.g., "C5, C6" means that the nerves supplying the deltoid are derived from the fifth and sixth cervical segments of the spinal cord). Numbers in boldface (**C5**) indicate the main segmental innervation. Damage to one or more of the listed spinal cord segments or to the motor nerve roots arising from them results in paralysis of the muscles concerned.

[b]Collectively, the supraspinatus, infraspinatus, teres minor, and subscapularis muscles are referred to as the rotator cuff, or SITS, muscles. Their primary function during all movements of the glenohumeral (shoulder) joint is to hold the humeral head in the glenoid cavity of the scapula.

Table 6.3. Movements of the Scapula

Elevation/Depression
Posterior view

Protraction/Retraction
Superior view of right half of pectoral girdle

Upward rotation/
Downward rotation
Posterior view

Movement of Scapula	Muscles Producing Movement[a]	Nerve to Muscles	Range of Movement (angular rotation; linear displacement)
Elevation	**Trapezius, superior part** (1) Levator scapulae (2) Rhomboids (3)	Accessory (CN XI) } Dorsal scapular	
Depression	**Gravity** (12) Pectoralis major, inferior sternocostal head (4) Latissimus dorsi (5) Trapezius, inferior part (6) Serratus anterior, inferior part (7) Pectoralis minor (8)	Pectoral nerves Thoracodorsal Accessory (CN XI) Long thoracic Medial pectoral	10–12 cm
Protraction	**Serratus anterior** (9) Pectoralis major (10) Pectoralis minor (8)	Long thoracic Pectoral nerves Medial pectoral	
Retraction	**Trapezius, middle part** (11) Rhomboids (3) Latissimus dorsi (5)	Accessory (CN XI) Dorsal scapular Thoracodorsal	40–45°; 15 cm
Upward rotation[b]	**Trapezius, superior part** (1) Trapezius, inferior part (6) **Serratus anterior, inferior part** (7)	} Accessory (CN XI) Long thoracic	
Downward rotation[c]	Gravity (12) Levator scapulae (2) Rhomboids (3) **Latissimus dorsi** (5) Pectoralis minor (8) Pectoralis major, inferior - sternocostal head (4)	} Dorsal scapular Thoracodorsal Medial pectoral Pectoral nerves	60°; inferior angle: 10–12 cm; superior angle: 5–6 cm

[a]Boldface indicates prime or essential mover(s). Numbers refer to the figure.
[b]The glenoid cavity moves superiorly, as in abduction of the arm.
[c]The glenoid cavity moves inferiorly, as in adduction of the arm.

Latissimus Dorsi

The name **latissimus dorsi** (L. widest of the back) was well chosen because the muscle covers a wide area of the back (Fig. 6.16; Table 6.2*E*). This large, fan-shaped muscle passes from the trunk to the humerus and acts directly on the glenohumeral joint and indirectly on the pectoral girdle (scapulothoracic joint). The latissimus dorsi extends, retracts, and rotates the humerus medially (e.g., when folding the arms behind the back or scratching the skin over the opposite scapula). In combination with the pectoralis major, the latissimus dorsi is a powerful adductor of the humerus, and plays a major role in downward rotation of the scapula in association with this movement (Table 6.3). It is also useful in restoring the upper limb from abduction superior to the shoulder; hence the latissimus dorsi is important in climbing. In conjunction with the pectoralis major, the latissimus dorsi raises the trunk to the arm, which occurs when performing chin-ups (hoisting oneself so the chin touches an overhead bar) or climbing a tree, for example. These movements are also used when chopping wood, paddling a canoe, and swimming (particularly during the crawl stroke).

To test the latissimus dorsi (or the function of the thoracodorsal nerve that supplies it), the arm is abducted 90° and then adducted against resistance provided by the examiner. If the muscle is normal, the anterior border of the muscle can be seen and easily palpated in the posterior axillary fold (see "Axilla," later in this chapter).

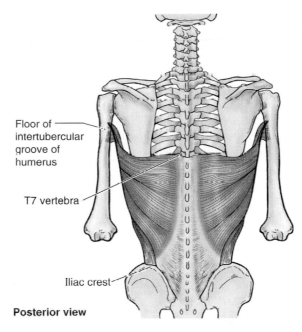

Floor of intertubercular groove of humerus

T7 vertebra

Iliac crest

Posterior view

Figure 6.16. Latissimus dorsi. This broad, triangular, mostly superficial muscle extends, adducts, and medially rotates the humerus. It is a powerful adductor and extensor of the arm and raises the body toward the arm during climbing.

Triangle of Auscultation

Near the inferior angle of the scapula is a small triangular gap in the musculature. The superior horizontal border of the latissimus dorsi, the medial border of the scapula, and the inferolateral border of the trapezius form a *triangle of auscultation* (Table 6.2*E*). This gap in the thick back musculature is a good place to examine posterior segments of the lungs with a stethoscope. When the scapulae are drawn anteriorly by folding the arms across the chest and the trunk is flexed, the auscultatory triangle enlarges and parts of the 6th and 7th ribs and 6th intercostal space are subcutaneous.

Injury of the Accessory Nerve (CN XI)

The primary clinical manifestation of *accessory nerve palsy* is a marked ipsilateral weakness when the shoulders are elevated (shrugged) against resistance. Injury of the accessory nerve is discussed in greater detail in Chapters 8 and 9.

Injury of the Thoracodorsal Nerve

Surgery in the inferior part of the axilla puts the thoracodorsal nerve (C6–C8) supplying the latissimus dorsi at risk of injury. This nerve passes inferiorly along the ▶

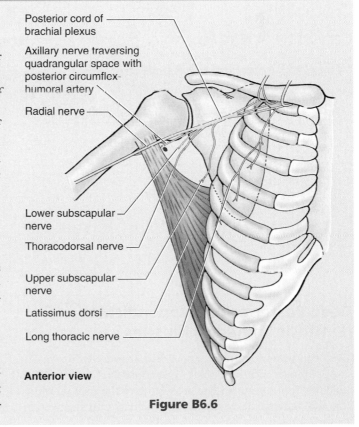

Posterior cord of brachial plexus

Axillary nerve traversing quadrangular space with posterior circumflex humoral artery

Radial nerve

Lower subscapular nerve

Thoracodorsal nerve

Upper subscapular nerve

Latissimus dorsi

Long thoracic nerve

Anterior view

Figure B6.6

posterior wall of the axilla and enters the medial surface of the latissimus dorsi close to where it becomes tendinous (Fig. B6.6). The nerve is also vulnerable to injury during surgery on scapular lymph nodes because its terminal part lies anterior to them and the subscapular artery (Fig. B6.7). The latissimus dorsi and the inferior part of the pectoralis major form an anteroposterior muscular sling between the trunk and the arm; however, the latissimus dorsi forms the more powerful part of the sling. With paralysis of the latissimus dorsi, the person is unable to raise the trunk with the upper limbs, as occurs during climbing. Furthermore, the person cannot use an axillary crutch because the shoulder is pushed superiorly by it. These are the primary activities for which active depression of the scapula is required; the passive depression provided by gravity is adequate for most activities. ⊕

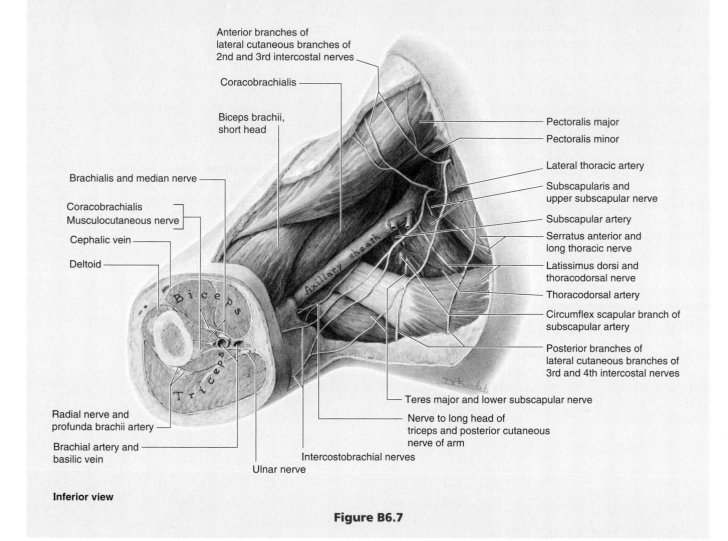

Anterior branches of lateral cutaneous branches of 2nd and 3rd intercostal nerves

Coracobrachialis

Biceps brachii, short head

Brachialis and median nerve

Coracobrachialis
Musculocutaneous nerve

Cephalic vein

Deltoid

Radial nerve and profunda brachii artery

Brachial artery and basilic vein

Ulnar nerve

Intercostobrachial nerves

Nerve to long head of triceps and posterior cutaneous nerve of arm

Teres major and lower subscapular nerve

Posterior branches of lateral cutaneous branches of 3rd and 4th intercostal nerves

Circumflex scapular branch of subscapular artery

Thoracodorsal artery

Latissimus dorsi and thoracodorsal nerve

Serratus anterior and long thoracic nerve

Subscapular artery

Subscapularis and upper subscapular nerve

Lateral thoracic artery

Pectoralis minor

Pectoralis major

Inferior view

Figure B6.7

Deep Posterior Axioappendicular (Extrinsic Shoulder) Muscles

The **deep posterior thoracoappendicular muscles** are the levator scapulae and rhomboids. These muscles provide direct attachment of the appendicular skeleton to the axial skeleton. The attachments, nerve supply, and main actions are given in Table 6.2.

Levator Scapulae

The superior third of the strap-like **levator scapulae** lies deep to the sternocleidomastoid; the inferior third is deep to the trapezius. From the transverse processes of the upper cervical vertebrae, the fibers of the levator of the scapula pass inferiorly to the superomedial border of the scapula (Fig. 6.17). True to its name, the levator scapulae acts with the descending part of the trapezius to elevate the scapula, or fix it (resists forces that would

Posterior view

Figure 6.17. Levator scapulae. This thick, strap-like muscle descends from the first four cervical vertebrae and attaches to the medial border of the superior angle of the scapula. It elevates and rotates the scapula, tilting the glenoid cavity inferiorly.

depress it, as when carrying a load). With the rhomboids and pectoralis minor, it rotates the scapula, depressing the glenoid cavity (tilting it inferiorly by rotating the scapula) (Table 6.3). Acting bilaterally (also with the trapezius), the levators extend the neck; acting unilaterally, the muscle may contribute to lateral flexion of the neck (toward the side of the active muscle).

Rhomboids

The **rhomboid major** and **rhomboid minor**, which are not always clearly separated from each other, have a rhomboid appearance—that is, they form an oblique equilateral parallelogram (Fig. 6.18). The rhomboids lie deep to the trapezius and form broad parallel bands that pass inferolaterally from the vertebrae to the medial border of the scapula. The thin, flat rhomboid major is approximately two times wider than the thicker rhomboid minor lying superior to it. The rhomboids retract and rotate the scapula, depressing its glenoid cavity (Table 6.3). They also assist the serratus anterior in holding the scapula against the thoracic wall and fixing the scapula during movements of the upper limb. The rhomboids are used when forcibly lowering the raised upper limbs (e.g., when driving a stake with a sledge hammer).

To test the rhomboids (or the function of the dorsal scapular nerve that supplies them), the individual places the hands posteriorly on the hips and pushes the elbows posteriorly against resistance provided by the examiner. If the rhomboids are acting normally, they can be palpated along the medial borders of the scapulae; because they lie deep to the trapezius, they are unlikely to be visible during testing.

Injury to the Dorsal Scapular Nerve

Injury to the dorsal scapular nerve, the nerve to the rhomboids, affects the actions of these muscles. If the rhomboids on one side are paralyzed, the scapula on the affected side is located farther from the midline than that on the normal side. ⊕

THE BOTTOM LINE: In terms of their attachments, the muscles of the proximal upper limb are axioappendicular or scapulothoracic muscles. The former consist of anterior, superficial posterior, and deep posterior groups. As a group, the axioappendicular muscles serve to position the base from which the upper limb will be extended and function relative to the trunk. The muscles work in antagonistic groups to elevate–depress and protract–retract the entire scapula or rotate it to elevate or depress the glenoid cavity and the glenohumeral joint (Table. 6.3). These movements extend the functional range of movements that occur at the glenohumeral joint. All of these movements involve both the clavicle and the scapula; the limits to all movements of the latter are imposed by the former, which provides the only attachment to the axial skeleton. Most of these movements involve the cooperation of a number of muscles with different innervations. Therefore, single nerve injuries typically weaken but do not eliminate most movements.

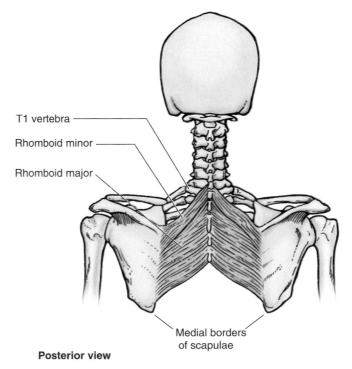

Posterior view

Figure 6.18. Rhomboids. The rhomboid muscles (major and minor) retract the scapula and rotate it to depress the glenoid cavity. They also fix the scapula to the thoracic wall.

Notable exceptions are upward rotation of the lateral angle of the scapula (superior trapezius/accessory nerve only) and lateral rotation of the inferior angle of the scapula (inferior serratus anterior/long thoracic nerve only).

Scapulohumeral (Intrinsic Shoulder) Muscles

The six **scapulohumeral muscles** (the deltoid, teres major, supraspinatus, infraspinatus, subscapularis, and teres minor) are relatively short muscles that pass from the scapula to the humerus and act on the glenohumeral joint. The attachments, nerve supply, and main actions of these intrinsic shoulder muscles are summarized in Table 6.2.

Deltoid

The **deltoid** is a thick, powerful, coarse-textured muscle covering the shoulder and forming its rounded contour (Fig. 6.19; Table 6.2*E*). As its name indicates, the deltoid is shaped like the inverted Greek letter delta (Δ). The muscle is divided into unipennate anterior and posterior parts and a multipennate middle part; the parts of the deltoid can act separately or as a whole. When all three parts contract simultaneously, the arm is abducted. The anterior and posterior parts act like guy ropes to steady the arm as it is abducted. To initiate movement during the first 15° of abduction, the deltoid is assisted by the supraspinatus (Table 6.2*B*). When the arm is fully adducted, the line of pull of the deltoid coincides with the axis of the

Figure 6.20. Testing deltoid muscle. The examiner resists the patient's abduction of the limb by the deltoid. If the deltoid is acting normally, contraction of the middle part of the muscle can be palpated.

humerus; thus it pulls directly upward on the bone and cannot initiate or produce abduction. It is, however, able to act as a shunt muscle, resisting inferior displacement of the head of the humerus from the glenoid cavity, as when lifting and carrying suitcases. From the fully adducted position, abduction must be initiated by the supraspinatus, or by leaning to the side, allowing gravity to initiate the movement. The deltoid becomes fully effective as an abductor following the initial 15° of abduction.

The anterior and posterior parts of the deltoids are used to swing the limbs during walking. The anterior part assists the pectoralis major in flexing the arm, and the posterior part assists the latissimus dorsi in extending the arm. The deltoid also helps stabilize the glenohumeral joint and hold the head of the humerus in the glenoid cavity during movements of the upper limb.

To test the deltoid (or the function of the axillary nerve that supplies it), the arm is abducted, starting from approximately 15°, against resistance (Fig. 6.20). If acting normally, the deltoid can easily be seen and palpated. The influence of gravity is avoided when the person is supine.

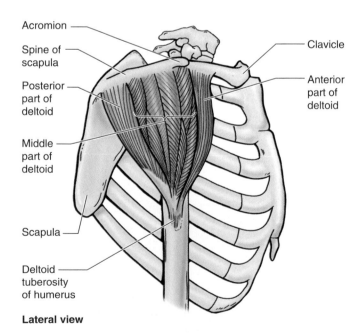

Acromion

Spine of scapula

Posterior part of deltoid

Middle part of deltoid

Scapula

Deltoid tuberosity of humerus

Clavicle

Anterior part of deltoid

Lateral view

Figure 6.19. Deltoid. This thick, coarse-textured, triangular muscle covers the glenohumeral joint and forms the rounded contour of the shoulder. The middle, multipennate part of the deltoid is the principal abductor of the arm, the anterior part flexes and medially rotates the arm, and the posterior part extends and laterally rotates the arm.

Injury to the Axillary Nerve

The deltoid atrophies when the axillary nerve (C5 and C6) is severely damaged. Because it passes inferior to the humeral head and winds around the surgical neck of the humerus, the axillary nerve is usually injured during fracture of this part of the humerus. It may also be damaged during dislocation of the glenohumeral joint and by compression from the incorrect use of crutches. As the deltoid atrophies, the rounded contour of the shoulder disappears. This gives the shoulder a flattened ▶

appearance and produces a slight hollow inferior to the acromion. In addition to atrophy of the deltoid, a loss of sensation may occur over the lateral side of the proximal part of the arm, the area supplied by the *superior lateral cutaneous nerve of the arm* (*red* in Fig. B6.8).

The deltoid is a common site for the intramuscular injection of drugs. The axillary nerve runs transversely under cover of the deltoid at the level of the surgical neck of the humerus. Awareness of its location avoids injury to it during surgical approaches to the shoulder. ✛

Figure B6.8. Area of anesthesia (*red*).

Teres Major

The **teres major** (L. *teres*, round) is a thick, rounded muscle that forms a raised oval area on the inferolateral third of the scapula when the arm is adducted against resistance (Fig. 6.21*A*; Table 6.2*B* & *E*). The inferior border of the teres major forms the inferior border of the lateral part of the posterior wall of the axilla. The teres major adducts and medially rotates the arm (Fig. 6.21*B*). It can also help extend it from the flexed position and is an important stabilizer of the humeral head in the glenoid cavity—that is, it steadies the head in its socket.

To test the teres major (or the lower subscapular nerve that supplies it), the abducted arm is adducted against resistance. If acting normally, the muscle can be easily seen and palpated in the posterior axillary fold.

Rotator Cuff Muscles

Four of the scapulohumeral muscles (intrinsic shoulder muscles)—supraspinatus, infraspinatus, teres minor, and subscapularis (referred to as the *SITS muscles*)—are called **rotator cuff muscles** because they form a musculotendinous rotator cuff around the glenohumeral joint (Fig. 6.22). All except the supraspinatus are rotators of the humerus; the supraspinatus, besides being part of the rotator cuff, initiates and assists the deltoid in the first 15° of abduction of the arm. The tendons of the SITS muscles blend with and reinforce the fibrous layer of the joint capsule of the glenohumeral joint, thus forming the rotator cuff that protects the joint and gives it stability. The tonic contraction of the contributing muscles holds the relatively large head of the humerus in the small, shallow glenoid cavity of the scapula during arm movements. The

attachments, nerve supply, and main actions of the rotator cuff muscles are given in Table 6.2.

The **supraspinatus** occupies the supraspinous fossa of the scapula. A bursa separates it from the lateral quarter of the fossa. (See "Deltoid," earlier in this chapter for discussion of this muscle's cooperative action in abducting the upper limb.)

To test the supraspinatus, abduction of the arm is attempted from the fully adducted position against resistance, while the muscle is palpated superior to the spine of the scapula.

(A) Posterior view

(B) Posterior view

Figure 6.21. Scapulohumeral muscles. A. These muscles pass from the scapula to the humerus and act on the glenohumeral joint. The surface anatomy of the scapular muscles and the latissimus dorsi are shown. **B.** The position of the scapula and humerus when the limb is abducted 90° is shown. The teres major is a thick, rounded muscle that adducts and medially rotates the arm. The latissimus dorsi and teres major form the posterior axillary fold. When the arm is adducted against resistance, this fold is accentuated.

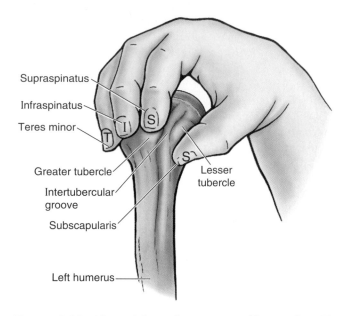

Supraspinatus
Infraspinatus
Teres minor
Greater tubercle
Intertubercular groove
Subscapularis
Left humerus
Lesser tubercle

Figure 6.22. Disposition of rotator cuff muscles. The primary combined function of the four scapulohumeral (SITS) muscles is to "grasp" and pull the relatively large head of the humerus medially, holding it against the smaller, shallow glenoid cavity of the scapula. The tendons of the muscles (represented by three fingers and the thumb) blend with the fibrous layer of the capsule of the glenohumeral joint to form a musculotendinous rotator cuff, which reinforces the capsule on three sides (anteriorly, superiorly, and posteriorly) as it provides active support for the glenohumeral joint.

The **infraspinatus** occupies the medial three quarters of the infraspinous fossa and is partly covered by the deltoid and trapezius. In addition to helping stabilize the glenohumeral joint, the infraspinatus is a powerful lateral rotator of the humerus.

To test the infraspinatus, the person flexes the elbow and adducts the arm. The arm is then laterally rotated against resistance. If acting normally, the muscle can be palpated inferior to the scapular spine. *To test the function of the suprascapular nerve,* which supplies the supraspinatus and infraspinatus, both muscles must be tested as described.

The **teres minor** is a narrow, elongate muscle that is completely hidden by the deltoid and is often not clearly delineated from the infraspinatus (Table 6.2B). The teres minor works with the infraspinatus to rotate the arm laterally and assist in its adduction. The teres minor is most clearly distinguished from the infraspinatus by its nerve supply. The teres minor is supplied by the axillary nerve, whereas the infraspinatus is supplied by the suprascapular nerve.

The **subscapularis** is a thick, triangular muscle that lies on the costal surface of the scapula and forms part of the posterior wall of the axilla. It crosses the anterior aspect of the scapulohumeral joint on its way to the humerus. The subscapularis is the primary medial rotator of the arm and also adducts it. It joins the other rotator cuff muscles in holding the head of the humerus in the glenoid cavity during all movements of the glenohumeral joint (i.e., it helps stabilize this joint during movements of the elbow, wrist, and hand).

Fracture–Dislocation of the Proximal Humeral Epiphysis

A direct blow or indirect injury of the shoulder of a child or adolescent may produce a fracture–dislocation of the proximal humeral epiphysis because the joint capsule of the glenohumeral joint, reinforced by the rotator cuff (tendons of the SITS muscles), is stronger than the epiphysial plate. In severe fractures, the shaft of the humerus is markedly displaced, but the humeral head retains its normal relationship with the glenoid cavity of the scapula (Fig. B6.9). ▶

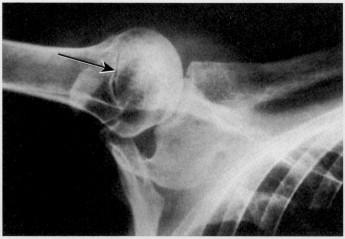

Normal epiphysis of humerus in adolescent

Separation of humeral epiphysis

Figure B6.9

Rotator Cuff Injuries and the Supraspinatus

Injury or disease may damage the musculotendinous rotator cuff, producing instability of the glenohumeral joint. Trauma may tear or rupture one or more of the tendons of the SITS muscles; that of the supraspinatus is most commonly involved (Fig. B6.10). *Degenerative tendonitis of the rotator cuff* is common, especially in older people. These syndromes are discussed in detail (later in this chapter) in relationship to the glenohumeral joint. ⊕

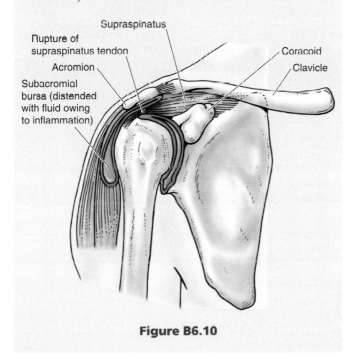

Supraspinatus

Rupture of
supraspinatus tendon

Acromion

Subacromial
bursa (distended
with fluid owing
to inflammation)

Coracoid

Clavicle

Figure B6.10

THE BOTTOM LINE: The scapulohumeral muscles (deltoid, teres major, and SITS muscles), along with certain axioappendicular muscles, act in opposing groups to position the proximal strut (humerus) of the upper limb, producing abduction–adduction, flexion–extension, medial–lateral rotation, and circumduction of the arm. This establishes the height, distance from the trunk, and direction from which the forearm and hand will operate. Essentially all movements produced by the scapulohumeral muscles at the glenohumeral joint are accompanied by movements produced by axioappendicular muscles at the sternoclavicular and scapulothoracic joints, especially beyond the initial stages of the movement. A skilled examiner, knowledgeable in anatomy, can manually fix or position the limb to isolate and test distinctive portions of specific upper limb movements. The SITS muscles contribute to the formation of the rotator cuff, which both rotates the humeral head and holds it firmly against the shallow socket of the glenoid cavity, increasing the integrity of the glenohumeral joint capsule.

Axilla

The **axilla** is the pyramidal space inferior to the glenohumeral joint and superior to the axillary fascia at the junction of the arm and thorax (Fig. 6.23). The axilla provides a passageway or "distribution center," usually protected by the adducted upper limb, for the neurovascular structures that serve the upper limb. From this distribution center, neurovascular structures pass (1) superiorly via the cervicoaxillary canal to (or from) the root of the neck, (2) anteriorly via the clavipectoral triangle to the pectoral region, (3) inferiorly and laterally into the limb itself, (4) posteriorly via the quadrangular space to the scapular region, and (5) inferiorly and medially along the thoracic wall to the inferiorly placed axioappendicular muscles (serratus anterior and latissimus dorsi). The shape and size of the axilla varies, depending on the position of the arm; it almost disappears when the arm is fully abducted—a position in which its contents are vulnerable. A "tickle" reflex causes most people to rapidly resume the protected position when invasion threatens.

The axilla has an apex, a base, and four walls, three of which are muscular:

- The *apex of axilla* is the **cervicoaxillary canal,** the passageway between the neck and the axilla, bounded by the 1st rib, clavicle, and superior edge of the scapula. The arteries, veins, lymphatics, and nerves traverse this superior opening of the axilla to pass to or from the arm (Fig. 6.23*A*).

- The *base of axilla* is formed by the concave skin, subcutaneous tissue, and axillary (deep) fascia extending from the arm to the thoracic wall (approximately the 4th rib level), forming the **axillary fossa** (armpit). The base of the axilla or axillary fossa is bounded by the anterior and posterior axillary folds, the thoracic wall, and the medial aspect of the arm (Fig. 6.23*C*).

- The *anterior wall of axilla* has two layers, formed by the pectoralis major and pectoralis minor and the pectoral and clavicopectoral fascia associated with them (Figs. 6.9*B* and 6.23*B* & *C*). The **anterior axillary fold** is the inferiormost part of the anterior wall that may be grasped between the fingers; it is formed by the pectoralis major, as it bridges from thoracic wall to humerus, and the overlying integument (Fig. 6.23*C* & *D*).

- The *posterior wall of axilla* is formed chiefly by the scapula and subscapularis on its anterior surface and inferiorly by the teres major and latissimus dorsi (Fig. 6.23*B* & *C*). The **posterior axillary fold** is the inferiormost part of the posterior wall that may be grasped. It extends farther inferiorly than the anterior wall and is formed by latissimus dorsi, teres major, and overlying integument.

(A) Anterior view

Apex of axilla
Cervicoaxillary canal
Intertubercular groove
Lateral wall
Posterior wall
Anterior wall
Base of axilla
Clavicle
1st rib
Medial wall

(B) Inferior view of transverse section

Pectoralis major — Anterior wall
Pectoralis minor
Intertubercular groove (lateral wall)
Serratus anterior — Medial wall
4th Rib
Humerus
Teres major
Latissimus dorsi
Subscapularis
Scapula
Posterior wall

(C) Lateral view of sagittal section

Brachial plexus
Subscapularis
Infraspinatus
Scapula
Teres minor
Teres major
Latissimus dorsi
Central axillary nodes
Posterior axillary fold
Axillary fascia
Trapezius
Supraspinatus
Cervicoaxillary canal
Clavicle
Subclavius
Pectoralis major
Pectoralis minor
Axillary artery and vein
Anterior axillary fold
Pectoral (anterior) axillary nodes
Axillary fat
Outline of axillary pyramid

(D) Anterior view

Supraclavicular nerves (C3 and C4)
Deltoid
Clavipectoral triangle
Cephalic vein in deltopectoral groove
Pectoralis major
Intercostobrachial nerve
Anterior and posterior branches of lateral cutaneous nerves
Serratus anterior
External oblique and nerve supply
Platysma
Skin
Subcutaneous tissue
Anterior branches of lateral cutaneous nerves
Deep (pectoral) fascia
Anterior cutaneous nerves

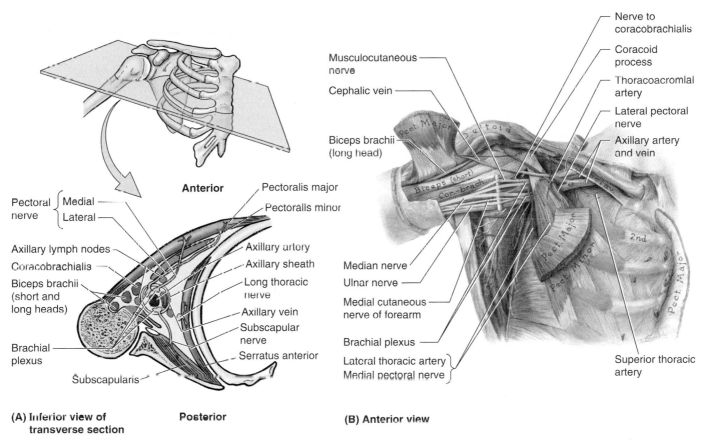

Figure 6.24. Contents of axilla. A. This cross section of the axilla demonstrates the contents of the axilla, including the axillary sheath enclosing the axillary artery and vein and the three cords of the brachial plexus. The innervation of the muscular walls of the axilla is also shown. **B.** In this dissection, most of the pectoralis major has been removed and the clavipectoral fascia, axillary fat, and axillary sheath have been completely removed. The brachial plexus of nerves surrounds the axillary artery on its lateral and medial aspects (appearing here to be its superior and inferior aspects because the limb is abducted) and on its posterior aspect (not visible from this view).

• The *medial wall of axilla* is formed by the thoracic wall (1st–4th ribs and intercostal muscles) and the overlying serratus anterior (Fig. 6.23A & B).

• The *lateral wall of axilla* is a narrow bony wall formed by the *intertubercular groove* in the humerus.

The axilla contains axillary blood vessels (axillary artery and its branches, axillary vein and its tributaries), lymphatic vessels, and several groups of *axillary lymph nodes,* all embedded in a matrix of *axillary fat* (Fig. 6.23C). The axilla also contains large nerves that make up the cords and branches of the *brachial plexus,* a network of interjoining nerves that pass from the neck to the upper limb. Proximally, these neurovascular structures are ensheathed in a sleeve-like extension of the cervical fascia, the **axillary sheath** (Fig. 6.24A).

Figure 6.23. Location, boundaries, and contents of axilla. A. The axilla is a pyramidal space inferior to the glenohumeral joint and superior to the skin of the axillary fossa at the junction of the arm and thorax. Observe its apex, base, and walls. **B.** This transverse section of the axilla illustrates its three muscular walls. The small, lateral bony wall of the axilla is the intertubercular groove of the humerus. **C.** A sagittal section of the shoulder shows the contents of the axilla and the scapular and pectoral muscles forming its posterior and anterior walls, respectively. The axilla is primarily filled with axillary fat (*yellow*), forming a matrix in which the neurovascular structures and lymph nodes are embedded. Inferiorly, the inferior border of the pectoralis major forms the anterior axillary fold, and the latissimus dorsi and teres major form the posterior axillary fold. **D.** In this superficial dissection of the pectoral region, the subcutaneous platysma muscle, which descends from the neck to the 2nd or 3rd rib, is cut short on the right side. The severed muscle is reflected superiorly on the left side, together with the supraclavicular nerves, so that the clavicular attachments of the pectoralis major and anterior deltoid can be observed.

THE BOTTOM LINE: The axilla is a pyramidal, fat-filled fascial compartment (distribution center) giving passage to or housing the major "utilities" serving (supplying, draining, and communicating with) the upper limb. Although normally protected by the arm, axillary structures are vulnerable when the arm is abducted. The "tickle" reflex causes us to recover the protected position rapidly when a threat is perceived. The structures are ensheathed in a protective wrapping (axillary sheath), embedded in a cushioning matrix (axillary fat) that allows flexibility, and are surrounded by musculoskeletal walls. From the axilla, neurovascular structures pass to and from the entire upper limb, including the pectoral, scapular, and subscapular regions as well as the free upper limb.

Axillary Artery

The **axillary artery** begins at the lateral border of the 1st rib as the continuation of the subclavian artery and ends at the inferior border of the teres major (Table 6.4). It passes posterior to the pectoralis minor into the arm and becomes the brachial artery when it passes the inferior border of the teres major, at which point it usually has reached the humerus. For descriptive purposes, the axillary artery is divided into three parts by the pectoralis minor (the part number also indicates the number of its branches):

1. The **first part of the axillary artery** is located between the lateral border of the 1st rib and the medial border of the pectoralis minor; it is enclosed in the *axillary sheath* and has one branch—the superior thoracic artery (Fig. 6.24B; Table 6.4).

2. The **second part of the axillary artery** lies posterior to pectoralis minor and has two branches—the thoracoacromial and lateral thoracic arteries—which pass medial and lateral to the muscle, respectively.

3. The **third part of the axillary artery** extends from the lateral border of pectoralis minor to the inferior border of teres major and has three branches. The subscapular artery is the largest branch of the axillary artery. Opposite the origin of this artery, the anterior circumflex humeral and posterior circumflex humeral arteries arise, sometimes by means of a common trunk.

The branches of the axillary artery are illustrated and their origin and course described in Table 6.4.

The **superior thoracic artery** is a small, highly variable vessel that arises just inferior to the subclavius. It commonly runs inferomedially posterior to the axillary vein and supplies the subclavius, muscles in the 1st and 2nd intercostal spaces, superior slips of the serratus anterior, and overlying pectoral muscles. It anastomoses with the intercostal and/or internal thoracic arteries.

The **thoracoacromial artery**, a short wide trunk, pierces the costocoracoid membrane and divides into four branches (acromial, deltoid, pectoral, and clavicular), deep to the clavicular head of the pectoralis major (Fig. 6.25).

The **lateral thoracic artery** has a variable origin. It usually arises as the second branch of the second part of the axillary artery and descends along the lateral border of the pectoralis minor, following it onto the thoracic wall (Fig. 6.24B); however, it may arise instead from the thoracoacromial, suprascapular, or subscapular arteries. The lateral thoracic artery supplies the pectoral, serratus anterior, and intercostal muscles, the axillary lymph nodes, and the lateral aspect of the breast.

The **subscapular artery**, the branch of the axillary artery with the greatest diameter but shortest length descends along the lateral border of the subscapularis on the posterior axillary wall. It soon terminates by dividing into the circumflex scapular and thoracodorsal arteries.

The **circumflex scapular artery**, often the larger terminal branch of the subscapular artery, curves posteriorly around the lateral border of the scapula, passing posteriorly between the subscapularis and the teres major to supply muscles on the dorsum of the scapula. It participates in the anastomoses around the scapula.

The **thoracodorsal artery** continues the general course of the subscapular artery to the inferior angle of the scapula and supplies adjacent muscles, principally the latissimus dorsi. It also participates in the arterial anastomoses around the scapula.

The *circumflex humeral arteries* encircle the surgical neck of the humerus, anastomosing with each other. The smaller **anterior circumflex humeral artery** passes laterally, deep to the coracobrachialis and biceps brachii. It gives off an ascending branch that supplies the shoulder. The larger **posterior circumflex humeral artery** passes medially through the posterior wall of the axilla via the **quadrangular space** with the axillary nerve to supply the glenohumeral joint and surrounding muscles (e.g., the deltoid, teres major and minor, and long head of the triceps) (Table 6.4).

Compression of the Axillary Artery

The axillary artery can be palpated in the inferior part of the lateral wall of the axilla. Compression of the third part of this artery against the humerus may be necessary when profuse bleeding occurs (e.g., resulting from a stab or bullet wound in the axilla). If compression is required at a more proximal site, the axillary artery can be compressed at its origin (as the subclavian artery crosses the 1st rib) by exerting downward pressure in the angle between the clavicle and the inferior attachment of the sternocleidomastoid. ▶

Arterial Anastomoses around the Scapula

Many arterial anastomoses (communications between arteries) occur around the scapula. Several vessels join to form networks on the anterior and posterior surfaces of the scapula: the dorsal scapular, suprascapular, and (via the circumflex scapular) subscapular arteries (Fig. B6.11). The importance of the *collateral circulation* made possible by these anastomoses becomes apparent when ligation of a lacerated subclavian or axillary artery is necessary. For example, the axillary artery may have to be ligated between the 1st rib and subscapular artery; in other cases, *vascular stenosis* (narrowing) of the axillary artery may result from an atherosclerotic lesion that causes reduced blood flow. In either case, the direction of blood flow in the subscapular artery is reversed, enabling blood to reach the third part of the axillary artery. Note that the subscapular artery receives blood through several anastomoses with the suprascapular artery, transverse cervical artery, and intercostal arteries.

Slow occlusion of the axillary artery (e.g., resulting from disease or trauma) often enables sufficient collateral circulation to develop, preventing *ischemia*. Sudden occlusion usually does not allow sufficient time for adequate collateral circulation to develop; as a result, there is an inadequate supply of blood to the arm, forearm, and hand. While potential collateral pathways (periarticular anastomoses) exist around the shoulder joint proximally and the elbow joint distally, *surgical ligation of the axillary artery* between the origins of the subscapular artery and the deep artery of the arm will cut off the blood supply to the arm because the collateral circulation is inadequate.

Aneurysm of the Axillary Artery

The first part of the axillary artery may enlarge (**aneurysm of the axillary artery**) and compress the trunks of the brachial plexus, causing pain and anesthesia (loss of sensation) in the areas of the skin supplied by the affected nerves. Aneurysm of the axillary artery may occur in baseball pitchers because of their rapid and forceful arm movements. ▶

Anterior scalene muscle

Suprascapular artery

Superficial branch of transverse cervical artery

Deep branch of transverse cervical artery

Clavicle

Superior thoracic artery

Thoracoacromial artery

Axillary artery

Ligature

Anterior and posterior circumflex humeral arteries

Lateral thoracic artery

Subscapular artery

Circumflex scapular artery

Brachial artery

Profunda brachii artery

Thoracodorsal artery

Ligature

Inferior thyroid artery

Thyrocervical artery

Vertebral artery

Subclavian artery

1st rib

Internal thoracic artery

Pectoralis minor

Dorsal scapular artery (deep branch of transverse cervical artery)

(A) Anterior view

Figure B6.11

(cont'd on page 770)

Table 6.4. Arteries of the Proximal Upper Limb (Shoulder Region and Arm)

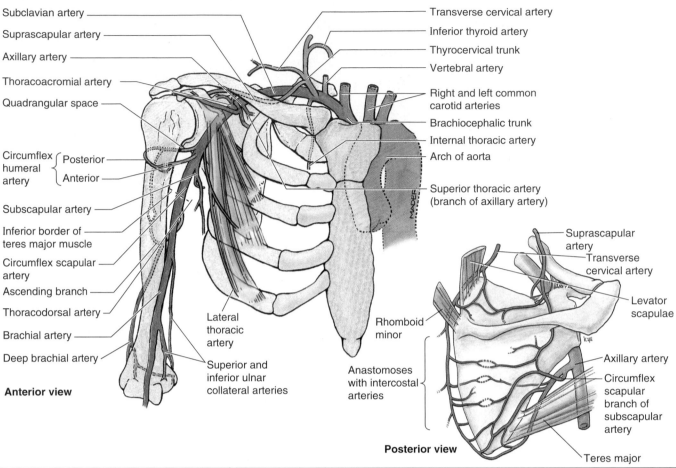

Artery	Origin			Course
Internal thoracic	Inferior surface of first part		Subclavian artery	Descends, inclining anteromedially, posterior to sternal end of clavicle and first costal cartilage; enters thorax to descend in parasternal plane; gives rise to perforating branches, anterior intercostal, musculophrenic, and superior epigastric arteries
Thyrocervical trunk	Anterior surface of first part			Ascends as a short, wide trunk, giving rise to four branches: suprascapular, transverse cervical, ascending cervical, and inferior thyroid arteries
Suprascapular	Thyrocervical (or as direct branch of subclavian artery)			Passes inferolaterally crossing anterior scalene muscle, phrenic nerve, subclavian artery, and brachial plexus, running laterally posterior and parallel to clavicle; next it passes over transverse scapular ligament to supraspinous fossa; then lateral to scapular spine (deep to acromion) to infraspinous fossa on posterior surface of scapula
Superior thoracic	First part (as only branch)		Axillary artery	Runs anteromedially along superior border of pectoralis minor; then passes between it and pectoralis major to thoracic wall; helps supply 1st and 2nd intercostal spaces and superior part of serratus anterior
Thoraco-acromial	Second part (first branch)			Curls around superomedial border of pectoralis minor; pierces costocoracoid membrane (clavipectoral fascia); divides into four branches: pectoral, deltoid, acromial, and clavicular
Lateral thoracic	Second part (second branch)			Descends along axillary border of pectoralis minor; follows it onto thoracic wall, supplying lateral aspect of breast
Circumflex humeral (anterior and posterior)	Third part (sometimes via a common trunk)			Encircle surgical neck of humerus, anastomosing with each other laterally; larger posterior branch traverses quadrangular space

Table 6.4. Arteries of the Proximal Upper Limb (Shoulder Region and Arm) *(continued)*

Subscapular	Third part of brachial artery (largest branch of any part)	Descends from level of inferior border of subscapularis along lateral border of scapula, dividing within 2–3 cm into terminal branches, the circumflex scapular and thoracodorsal arteries
Circumflex scapular	Subscapular artery	Curves around lateral border of scapula to enter infraspinous fossa, anastomosing with suprascapular artery
Thoracodorsal		Continues course of subscapular artery, descending with thoracodorsal nerve to enter apex of latissimus dorsi
Deep brachial	Near its origin	Accompanies radial nerve along radial groove of humerus, supplying posterior compartment of arm and participating in periarticular arterial anastomosis around elbow joint
Superior ulnar collateral	Near middle of arm	Accompanies ulnar nerve to posterior aspect of elbow; anastomoses with posterior ulnar recurrent artery
Inferior ulnar collateral	Superior to medial epicondyle of humerus	Passes anterior to medial epicondyle of humerus to anastomose with anterior ulnar collateral artery

(The middle column Deep brachial/Superior ulnar collateral/Inferior ulnar collateral entries are bracketed together as: Brachial artery)

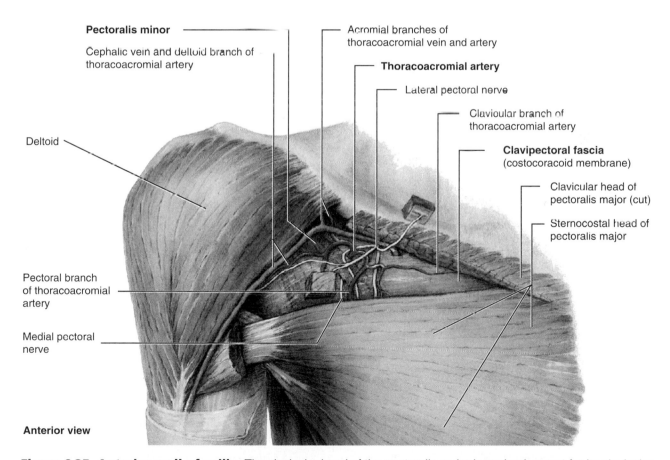

Pectoralis minor

Cephalic vein and deltoid branch of thoracoacromial artery

Acromial branches of thoracoacromial vein and artery

Thoracoacromial artery

Lateral pectoral nerve

Clavicular branch of thoracoacromial artery

Clavipectoral fascia (costocoracoid membrane)

Deltoid

Clavicular head of pectoralis major (cut)

Sternocostal head of pectoralis major

Pectoral branch of thoracoacromial artery

Medial pectoral nerve

Anterior view

Figure 6.25. Anterior wall of axilla. The clavicular head of the pectoralis major is excised except for its clavicular and humeral attaching ends and two cubes, which remain to identify its nerves. The anterior wall of the axilla is formed by the pectoralis major and minor (and the pectoral and clavipectoral fascia that envelops them). The pectoralis major covers the whole of this wall and forms the anterior axillary fold. Extending between the superior border of the pectoralis minor and the clavicle is the costocoracoid membrane (part of the clavipectoral fascia), which is perforated by the thoracoacromial artery and pectoral nerves (both exiting the axilla) and the cephalic vein (entering the axilla).

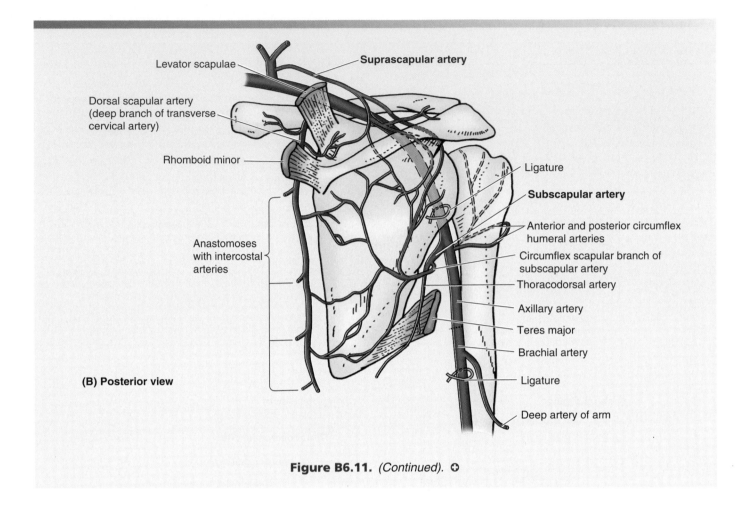

Levator scapulae

Suprascapular artery

Dorsal scapular artery
(deep branch of transverse
cervical artery)

Rhomboid minor

Ligature

Subscapular artery

Anterior and posterior circumflex
humeral arteries

Circumflex scapular branch of
subscapular artery

Thoracodorsal artery

Anastomoses
with intercostal
arteries

Axillary artery

Teres major

Brachial artery

(B) Posterior view

Ligature

Deep artery of arm

Figure B6.11. *(Continued).* ✛

Axillary Vein

The **axillary vein** lies initially (distally) on the anteromedial side of the axillary artery, with its terminal part anteroinferior to the artery (Fig. 6.26). This large vein is formed by the union of the *brachial vein* (the accompanying veins of the brachial artery) and the *basilic vein* at the inferior border of the teres major. The axillary vein is described as having three parts that correspond to the three parts of the axillary artery. Thus the initial, distal end is the third part, whereas the terminal, proximal end is the first part. The axillary vein (first part) ends at the lateral border of the 1st rib, where it becomes the **subclavian vein.** The veins of the axilla are more abundant than the arteries, are highly variable, and frequently anastomose. The axillary vein receives tributaries that generally correspond to branches of the axillary artery with a few major exceptions:

- The veins corresponding to the branches of the thoracoacromial artery do not merge to enter by a common tributary; some enter independently into the axillary vein, but others empty into the cephalic vein, which then enters the axillary vein superior to the pectoralis minor, close to its transition into the subclavian vein.

- The axillary vein receives, directly or indirectly, the *thoracoepigastric vein*(s), which is(are) formed by the anastomoses of superficial veins from the inguinal region with tributaries of the axillary vein (usually the lateral thoracic vein). These veins constitute a collateral route that enables venous return in the presence of obstruction of the inferior vena cava (see clinical correlation [blue] box "Collateral Routes for Abdominopelvic Venous Blood," in Chapter 2).

Injuries to the Axillary Vein

Wounds in the axilla often involve the axillary vein because of its large size and exposed position. When the arm is fully abducted, the axillary vein overlaps the axillary artery anteriorly. A wound in the proximal part of the axillary vein is particularly dangerous, not only because of profuse bleeding but also because of the risk of air entering it and producing *air emboli* (air bubbles) in the blood. ▶

The Role of the Axillary Vein in Subclavian Vein Puncture

Subclavian vein puncture, in which a catheter is placed into the subclavian vein, has become a common clinical procedure (see clinical correlation [blue] box "Subclavian Vein Puncture," in Chapter 8). The axillary vein becomes the subclavian vein as the first rib is crossed. Because the needle is advanced medially to enter the vein as it crosses the rib, the vein actually punctured (the point of entry) in a "subclavian vein puncture" is the terminal part of the axillary vein. However, the needle tip proceeds into the lumen of the subclavian vein almost immediately. Thus it is clinically significant that the axillary vein lies anterior and inferior (i.e., superficial) to the axillary artery and the parts of the brachial plexus that begin to surround the artery at this point. ⊙

Axillary Lymph Nodes

The fibrofatty connective tissue of the axilla (axillary fat) contains many lymph nodes. The axillary lymph nodes are arranged in five principal groups: pectoral, subscapular, humeral, central, and apical. The groups are arranged in a manner that reflects the pyramidal shape of the axilla (Fig. 6.23A). Three groups of axillary nodes are related to the triangular base, one group at each corner of the pyramid (Fig. 6.27A & B):

The **pectoral (anterior) nodes** consist of three to five nodes that lie along the medial wall of the axilla, around the lateral thoracic vein and the inferior border of the pectoralis minor. The pectoral nodes receive lymph mainly from the anterior thoracic wall, including most of the breast (especially the superolateral [upper outer] quadrant and subareolar plexus; see Chapter 1).

The **subscapular (posterior) nodes** consist of six or seven nodes that lie along the posterior axillary fold and subscapu-

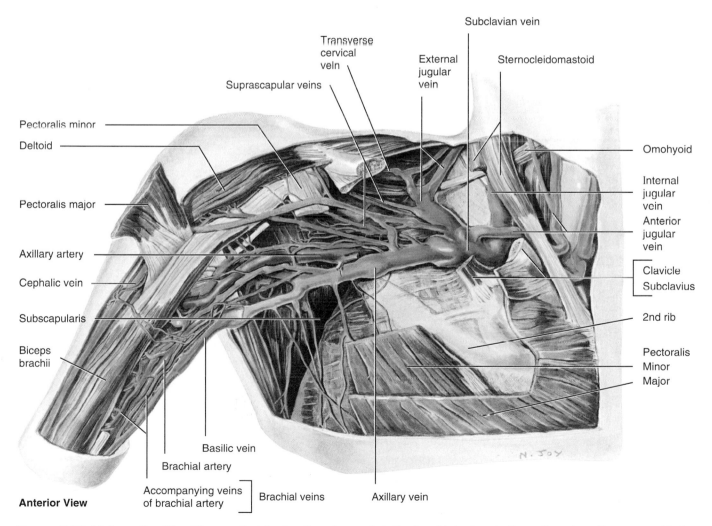

Figure 6.26. Veins of axilla. Observe that the basilic vein parallels the brachial artery to the axilla, where it merges with the accompanying veins (L. *venae comitantes*) of the axillary artery to form the axillary vein. Note the large number of highly variable veins in the axilla, which are also tributaries of the axillary vein.

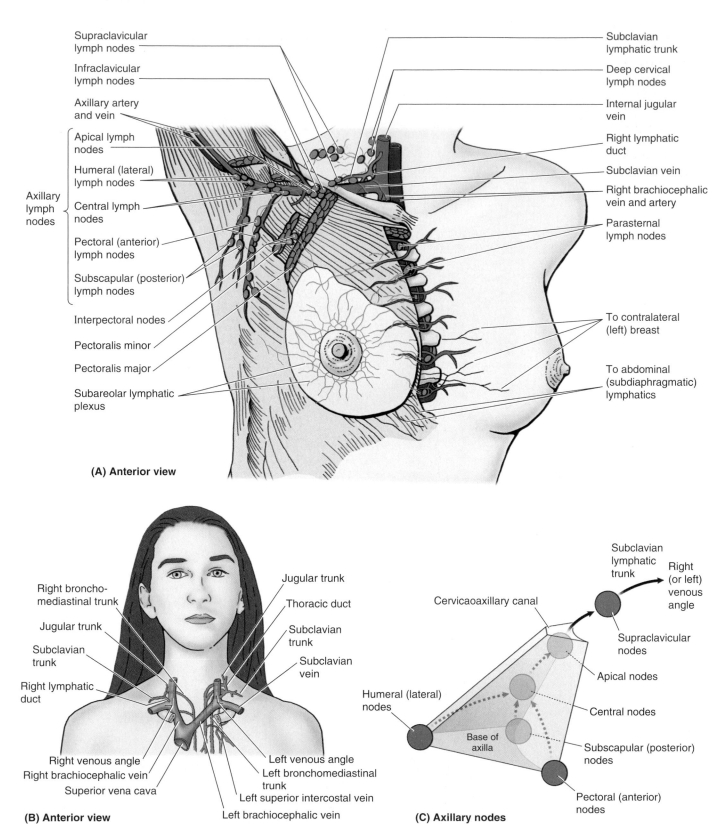

(A) Anterior view

(B) Anterior view

(C) Axillary nodes

Figure 6.27. Axillary lymph nodes and lymphatic drainage of right upper limb and breast. A. Of the five groups of axillary lymph nodes, most lymphatic vessels from the upper limb terminate in the humeral (lateral) and central lymph nodes, but those accompanying the upper part of the cephalic vein terminate in the apical lymph nodes. The lymphatics of the breast are discussed in Chapter 1. **B.** Lymph passing through the axillary nodes enters efferent lymphatic vessels that form the subclavian lymphatic trunk, which usually empties into the junctions of the internal jugular and subclavian veins (the venous angles). Occasionally, on the right side, this trunk merges with the jugular lymphatic and/or bronchomediastinal trunks to form a short right lymphatic duct; usually on the left side, it enters the termination of the thoracic duct. **C.** The positions of the five groups of axillary nodes, relative to each other and the pyramidal axilla. The typical pattern of drainage is shown.

lar blood vessels. These nodes receive lymph from the posterior aspect of the thoracic wall and scapular region.

The **humeral (lateral) nodes** consist of four to six nodes that lie along the lateral wall of the axilla, medial and posterior to the axillary vein. These nodes receive nearly all the lymph from the upper limb, except that carried by the lymphatic vessels accompanying the cephalic vein, which primarily drain directly to the apical axillary and infraclavicular nodes.

Efferent lymphatic vessels from these three groups pass to the **central nodes** (Fig. 6.27C). The central nodes are three or four large nodes situated deep to the pectoralis minor near the base of the axilla, in association with the second part of the axillary artery. Efferent vessels from the central nodes pass to the **apical nodes**. The apical nodes are located at the apex of the axilla along the medial side of the axillary vein and the first part of the axillary artery. The apical nodes receive lymph from all other groups of axillary lymph nodes as well as from lymphatics accompanying the proximal cephalic vein. Efferent vessels from the apical group of nodes traverse the *cervicoaxillary canal*. These efferent vessels ultimately unite to form the **subclavian lymphatic trunk**, although some vessels may drain en route through the **clavicular (infraclavicular and supraclavicular) nodes**. Once formed, the subclavian trunk may be joined by the jugular and bronchomediastinal trunks on the right side to form the **right lymphatic duct**, or it may enter the right venous angle independently. On the left side, the subclavian trunk most commonly joins the **thoracic duct** (Fig. 6.27A & B).

THE BOTTOM LINE: The axilla gives passage to important vascular structures passing between the neck and the upper limb. The axillary vein lies anterior and slightly inferior to the axillary artery, both being surrounded by the fascial axillary sheath. For descriptive purposes, the axillary artery and vein are assigned three parts located medial, posterior, and lateral to the pectoralis minor. Coincidentally, the first part of the artery has one branch; the second part, two branches; and the third part, three branches. The axillary lymph nodes are embedded in the axillary fat external to the axillary sheath. The axillary lymph nodes occur in groups that are arranged and receive lymph in a specific order, which is important in staging and determining appropriate treatment for breast cancer. In addition to transporting blood and lymph to and from the upper limb, the vascular structures of the axilla also serve the scapular and pectoral regions and lateral thoracic wall. The axillary lymph nodes receive lymph from the upper limb as well as the entire upper quadrant of the superficial body wall, from the level of the clavicles to the umbilicus including most from the breast.

Brachial Plexus

Most nerves in the upper limb arise from the **brachial plexus**, a major nerve network supplying the upper limb; it begins in the neck and extends into the axilla. Almost all branches of the brachial plexus arise in the axilla (after the plexus has

Enlargement of the Axillary Lymph Nodes

An infection in the upper limb can cause the axillary nodes to enlarge and become tender and inflamed, a condition called *lymphangitis* (inflammation of lymphatic vessels). The humeral group of nodes is usually the first to be involved. Lymphangitis is characterized by the development of warm, red, tender streaks in the skin of the limb. Infections in the pectoral region and breast, including the superior part of the abdomen, can also produce enlargement of axillary nodes. In metastatic cancer of the apical group, the nodes often adhere to the axillary vein, which may necessitate excision of part of this vessel. Enlargement of the apical nodes may obstruct the cephalic vein superior to the pectoralis minor.

Dissection of the Axillary Lymph Nodes

Excision and pathologic analysis of axillary lymph nodes are often necessary for *staging* and determining the ap-

propriate treatment of a cancer such as breast cancer (see Chapter 1). Because the axillary lymph nodes are arranged and receive lymph (and therefore metastatic breast cancer cells) in a specific order, removing and examining the lymph nodes in that order is important in determining the degree to which the cancer has developed and is likely to have metastasized. Lymphatic drainage of the upper limb may be impeded after the removal of the axillary nodes, resulting in **lymphedema**, swelling as a result of accumulated lymph, especially in the subcutaneous tissue.

During axillary node dissection, two nerves are at risk of injury. During surgery, the long thoracic nerve to the serratus anterior is identified and maintained against the thoracic wall. As discussed earlier in this chapter, cutting the long thoracic nerve results in a winged scapula. If the thoracodorsal nerve to the latissimus dorsi is cut, medial rotation and adduction of the arm are weakened, but deformity does not result. If the nodes around this nerve are obviously malignant, sometimes the nerve has to be sacrificed as the nodes are resected to increase the likelihood of complete removal of all malignant cells. ⊘

crossed the 1st rib). The brachial plexus is formed by the union of the anterior rami of the last four cervical (C5–C8) and the first thoracic (T1) nerves that constitute the **roots of the brachial plexus** (Fig. 6.28; Table 6.5). The roots usually pass through the gap between the anterior and the middle scalene (L. *scalenus anterior* and *medius*) muscles with the subclavian artery (Figs. 6.29 and 6.30). The sympathetic fibers carried by each root of the plexus are received from the gray rami of the middle and inferior cervical ganglia as the roots pass between the scalene muscles.

In the inferior part of the neck, the roots of the brachial plexus unite to form three trunks (Fig. 6.28):

1. A **superior trunk,** from the union of the C5 and C6 roots.

2. A **middle trunk,** which is a continuation of the C7 root.

3. An **inferior trunk,** from the union of the C8 and T1 roots.

Each trunk of the brachial plexus divides into anterior and posterior divisions as the plexus passes through the cervicoaxillary canal posterior to the clavicle. **Anterior divisions of the trunks** supply *anterior (flexor) compartments* of the upper limb, and **posterior divisions of the trunks** supply *posterior (extensor) compartments*.

The divisions of the trunks form three cords of the brachial plexus:

1. Anterior divisions of the superior and middle trunks unite to form the *lateral cord*.

2. Anterior division of the inferior trunk continues as the *medial cord*.

3. Posterior divisions of all three trunks unite to form the *posterior cord*.

The cords bear the relationship to the second part of the axillary artery that is indicated by their names. For example,

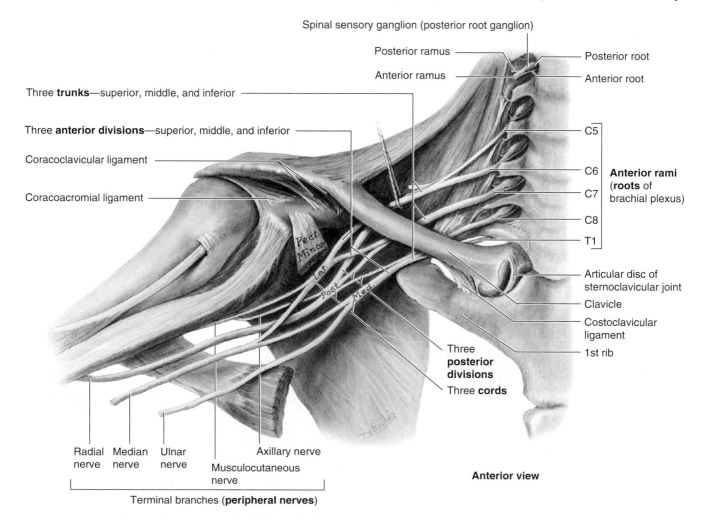

Figure 6.28. Formation of brachial plexus. This large nerve network is shown extending from the neck to the upper limb via the cervicoaxillary canal (bound by the clavicle, 1st rib, and superior scapula) to provide innervation to the upper limb and shoulder region. The brachial plexus is typically formed by the anterior rami of the C5–C8 nerves and the greater part of the anterior ramus of the T1 nerve (the *roots* of the brachial plexus). Observe the merging and continuation of certain roots of the plexus to three *trunks*, the separation of each trunk into anterior and posterior *divisions*, the union of the divisions to form three *cords*, and the derivation of the main terminal branches (*peripheral nerves*) from the cords as the products of plexus formation.

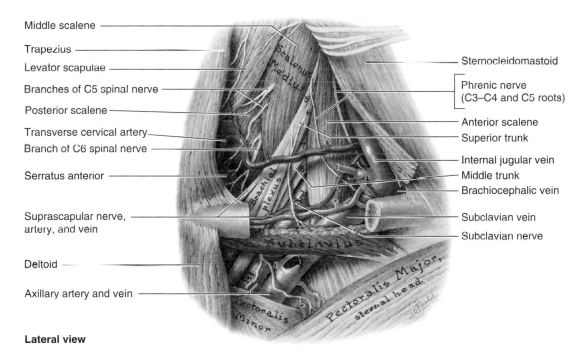

Middle scalene

Trapezius

Levator scapulae

Branches of C5 spinal nerve

Posterior scalene

Transverse cervical artery

Branch of C6 spinal nerve

Serratus anterior

Suprascapular nerve,
artery, and vein

Deltoid

Axillary artery and vein

Sternocleidomastoid

Phrenic nerve
(C3–C4 and C5 roots)

Anterior scalene

Superior trunk

Internal jugular vein

Middle trunk

Brachiocephalic vein

Subclavian vein

Subclavian nerve

Lateral view

Figure 6.29. Dissection of right lateral cervical region (posterior triangle). The brachial plexus and subclavian vessels have been dissected. The anterior rami of spinal nerves C5–C8 (plus T1, concealed here by the third part of the subclavian artery) constitute the roots of the brachial plexus (numbered). Merging and subsequent splitting of the nerve fibers conveyed by the roots form the trunks and divisions at the level shown. The subclavian artery emerges between the middle and anterior scalene muscles with the roots of the plexus. As the neurovascular structures pass posterior to the clavicle, they are traversing the cervicoaxillary canal connecting the neck and axilla. The subclavius, although not of major importance as a muscle, affords some protection to the underlying neurovascular structures when the clavicle is (commonly) fractured in its middle third.

the lateral cord is lateral to the axillary artery, although it may appear to lie superior to the artery because it is most easily seen when the limb is abducted.

The products of plexus formation are multisegmental, peripheral (named) nerves. The brachial plexus is divided into **supraclavicular** and **infraclavicular parts** by the clavicle (Fig. 6.28; Table 6.5). Four *branches of the supraclavicular part of the plexus* arise from the roots (anterior rami) and trunks of the brachial plexus (dorsal scapular nerve, long thoracic nerve, nerve to subclavius, and suprascapular nerve) and are approachable through the neck. In addition, officially unnamed *muscular branches* arise from all five roots of the plexus (anterior rami C5–T1), which supply the scaleni and longus colli muscles. The C5 root of the *phrenic nerve* (considered a branch of the cervical plexus) arises from the C5 plexus root, joining the C3–C4 components of the nerve on the anterior surface of the anterior scalene muscle (Fig 6.29). *Branches of the infraclavicular part of the plexus* arise from the cords of the brachial plexus and are approachable through the axilla. Counting side and terminal branches, three branches arise from the lateral cord, whereas the medial and posterior cords each give rise to five branches (counting the roots of the median nerve as individual branches). The branches of the supraclavicular and infraclavicular parts of the brachial plexus are listed in Table 6.5, along with the origin, course and distribution of each branch.

Variations of the Brachial Plexus

Variations in the formation of the brachial plexus are common (Bergman et al., 1988). In addition to the five anterior rami (C5–C8 and T1) that form the roots of the brachial plexus, small contributions may be made by the anterior rami of C4 or T2. When the superiormost root (anterior ramus) of the plexus is C4 and the inferiormost root is C8, it is a *prefixed brachial plexus*. Alternately, when the superior root is C6 and the inferior root is T2, it is a *postfixed brachial plexus*. In the latter type, the inferior trunk of the plexus may be compressed by the 1st rib, producing neurovascular symptoms in the upper limb. Variations may also occur in the formation of trunks, divisions, and cords; in the origin and/or combination of branches; and in the relationship to the axillary artery and scalene muscles. For example, the lateral or medial cords may receive fibers from anterior rami inferior or superior to the usual levels, respectively.

In some individuals, trunk divisions or cord formations may be absent in one or other parts of the plexus; however, the makeup of the terminal branches is unchanged. Because each peripheral nerve is a collection ▶
(cont'd on page 778)

Table 6.5. Brachial Plexus and Nerves of the Upper Limb

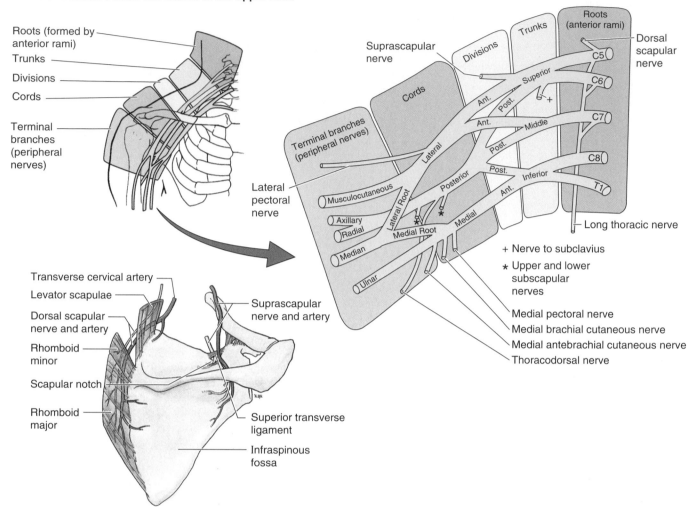

Nerve	Origin[a]	Course	Structures Innervated
Supraclavicular branches			
Dorsal scapular	Posterior aspect of anterior ramus of **C5** with a frequent contribution from C4	Pierces middle scalene; descends deep to levator scapulae and rhomboids	Rhomboids; occasionally supplies levator scapulae
Long thoracic	Posterior aspect of anterior rami of **C5, C6,** C7	Passes through cervicoaxillary canal (Fig. 6.14), descending posterior to C8 and T1 roots of plexus (anterior rami); runs inferiorly on superficial surface of serratus anterior	Serratus anterior
Suprascapular	Superior trunk, receiving fibers from **C5,** C6 and often C4	Passes laterally across lateral cervical region (posterior triangle of neck), superior to brachial plexus; then through scapular notch inferior to superior transverse cervical ligament	Supraspinatus and in-fraspinatus muscles; glenohumeral (shoulder) joint
Subclavian nerve (nerve to subclavius)	Superior trunk, receiving fibers from C5, **C6** and often C4 (Fig. 6.29)	Descends posterior to clavicle and anterior to brachial plexus and subclavian artery (Fig. 6.29); often giving an *accessory root to phrenic nerve*	Subclavius and sterno-clavicular joint (accessory phrenic root innervates di-aphragm)
Infraclavicular branches			
Lateral pectoral	Side branch of lateral cord, receiving fibers from C5, **C6,** C7	Pierces costocoracoid membrane to reach deep surface of pectoral muscles; a *communicating branch to the medial pectoral nerve* passes ante-rior to axillary artery and vein	Primarily pectoralis major; but some lateral pectoral nerve fibers pass to pec-toralis minor via branch to medial pectoral nerve (Fig. 6.30A)

Table 6.5. Brachial Plexus and Nerves of the Upper Limb *(continued)*

Nerve	Origin[a]	Course	Structures Innervated
Musculo-cutaneous	Terminal branch of lateral cord, receiving fibers from C5–C7	Exits axilla by piercing coracobrachialis (Fig. 6.28); descends between biceps brachii and brachialis (Fig. 6.31), supplying both; continues as *lateral cutaneous nerve of forearm*	Muscles of anterior compartment of arm (coracobrachialis, biceps brachii and brachialis) (Fig. 6.30*B*); skin of lateral aspect of forearm
Median	**Lateral root of median nerve** is a terminal branch of lateral cord (C6, C7); **medial root of median nerve** is a terminal branch of medial cord (C8, T1)	Lateral and medial roots merge to form median nerve lateral to axillary artery; descends through arm adjacent to brachial artery, with nerve gradually crossing anterior to artery to lie medial to artery in cubital fossa (Fig. 6.32*A*)	Muscles of anterior forearm compartment (except for flexor carpi ulnaris and ulnar half of flexor digitorum profundus), five intrinsic muscles in thenar half of palm and palmar skin (Fig. 6.30*B*)
Medial pectoral		Passes between axillary artery and vein; then pierces pectoralis minor and enters deep surface of pectoralis major; although it is called *medial* for its origin from medial cord, it lies lateral to lateral pectoral nerve	Pectoralis minor and sternocostal part of pectoralis major
Medial cutaneous nerve of arm	Side branches of medial cord, receiving fibers from C8, T1	Smallest nerve of plexus; runs along medial side of axillary and brachial veins; communicates with *intercostobrachial nerve*	Skin of medial side of arm, as far distal as medial epicondyle of humerus and olecranon of ulna
Median cutaneous nerve of forearm		Initially runs with ulnar nerve (with which it may be confused) but pierces deep fascia with basilic vein and enters subcutaneous tissue, dividing into anterior and posterior branches	Skin of medial side of forearm, as far distal as wrist
Ulnar	Larger terminal branch of medial cord, receiving fibers from C8, T1 and often C7	Descends medial arm; passes posterior to medial epicondyle of humerus; then descends ulnar aspect of forearm to hand (Figs. 6.30*C* and 6.32*A*)	Flexor carpi ulnaris and ulnar half of flexor digitorum profundus (forearm); most intrinsic muscles of hand; skin of hand medial to axial line of digit 4
Upper subscapular	Side branch of posterior cord, receiving fibers from **C5**	Passes posteriorly, entering subscapularis directly	Superior portion of subscapularis
Lower subscapular	Side branch of posterior cord, receiving fibers from **C6**	Passes inferolaterally, deep to subscapular artery and vein	Inferior portion of subscapularis and teres major
Thoracodorsal	Side branch of posterior cord, receiving fibers from C6, **C7**, C8	Arises between upper and lower subscapular nerves and runs inferolaterally along posterior axillary wall to apical part of latissimus dorsi	Latissimus dorsi
Axillary	Terminal branch of posterior cord, receiving fibers from **C5**, C6	Exits axillary fossa posteriorly, passing through quadrangular space[b] with posterior circumflex humeral artery (Fig. 6.31); gives rise to *superior lateral brachial cutaneous nerve;* then winds around surgical neck of humerus deep to deltoid (Fig. 6.30*D*)	Glenohumeral (shoulder) joint; teres minor and deltoid muscles (Fig. 6.30*D*); skin of superolateral arm (over inferior part of deltoid)
Radial	Larger terminal branch of posterior cord (largest branch of plexus), receiving fibers from C5–T1	Exits axillary fossa posterior to axillary artery; passes posterior to humerus in radial groove with deep brachial artery, between lateral and medial heads of triceps; perforates lateral intermuscular septum; enters cubital fossa, dividing into *superficial* (cutaneous) and *deep* (motor) *radial nerves* (Fig. 6.30*D*)	All muscles of posterior compartments of arm and forearm (Fig. 6.30*D*); skin of posterior and inferolateral arm, posterior forearm, and dorsum of hand lateral to axial line of digit 4

[a]Boldface (**C5**) indicates primary component of the nerve.
[b]Bounded superiorly by the subscapularis, head of humerus, and teres minor; inferiorly by the teres major; medially by the long head of the triceps; and laterally by the coracobrachialis and surgical neck of the humerus (Fig. 6.31).

of nerve fibers bound together by connective tissue, it is understandable that the median nerve, for instance, may have two medial roots instead of one (i.e., the nerve fibers are simply grouped differently). This results from the fibers of the medial cord of the brachial plexus dividing into three branches, two forming the median nerve and the third forming the ulnar nerve. Sometimes it may be more confusing when the two medial roots are completely separate; however, understand that although the median nerve may have two medial roots, the components of the nerve are the same (i.e., the impulses arise from the same place and reach the same destination whether they go through one or two roots).

Brachial Plexus Injuries

Injuries to the brachial plexus affect movements and cutaneous sensations in the upper limb. Disease, stretching, and wounds in the lateral cervical region (posterior triangle) of the neck (see Chapter 8) or in the axilla may produce brachial plexus injuries. Signs and symptoms depend on the part of the plexus involved. Injuries to the brachial plexus result in *paralysis* and *anesthesia*. Testing the person's ability to perform movements assesses the degree of paralysis. In *complete paralysis,* no movement is detectable. In *incomplete paralysis,* not all muscles are paralyzed; therefore, the person can move, but the movements are weak compared ▶

(*cont'd on page 780*)

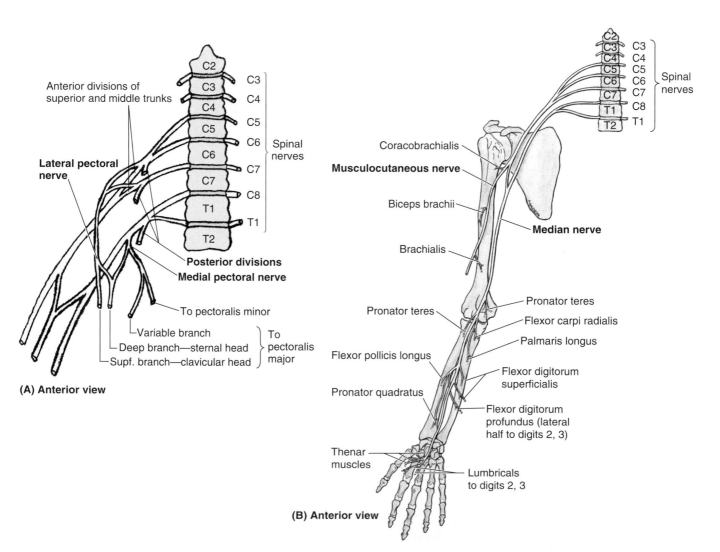

(A) Anterior view

(B) Anterior view

Figure 6.30. Summary of innervation of upper limb muscles. A. The medial and lateral pectoral nerves arise from the medial and lateral cords of the brachial plexus, respectively (or from the anterior divisions of the trunks that form them, as shown here for the lateral pectoral nerve). **B.** The courses of the median and musculocutaneous nerves and the typical pattern of branching of their motor branches are shown.

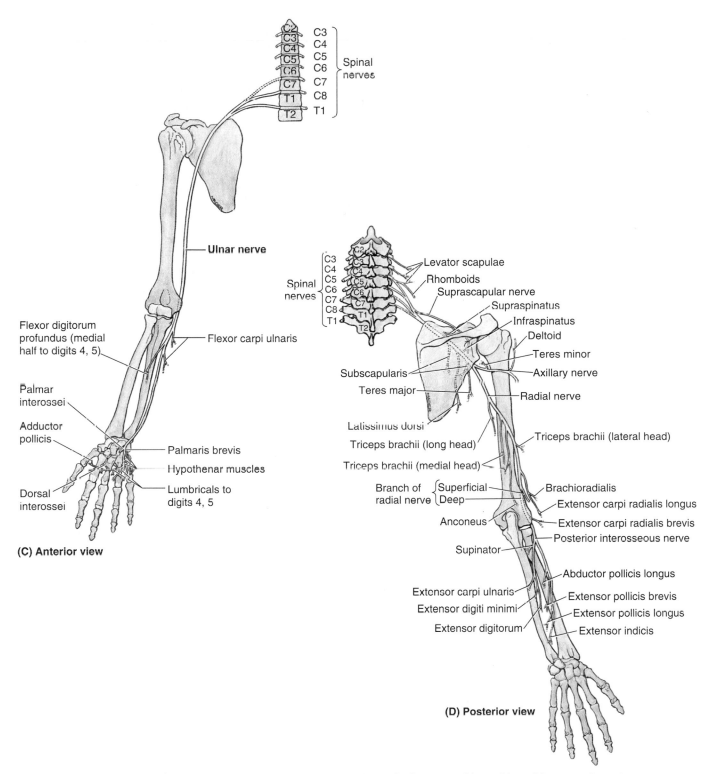

C2
C3
C4
C5
C6
C7
T1
T2

C3
C4
C5
C6
C7
C8
T1
} Spinal nerves

Ulnar nerve

Flexor digitorum profundus (medial half to digits 4, 5)

Flexor carpi ulnaris

Palmar interossei

Adductor pollicis

Palmaris brevis

Hypothenar muscles

Dorsal interossei

Lumbricals to digits 4, 5

(C) Anterior view

C3
C4
C5
C6
C7
C8
T1
Spinal nerves

C2
C3
C4
C5
C6
C7
T1
T2

Levator scapulae

Rhomboids

Suprascapular nerve

Supraspinatus

Infraspinatus

Deltoid

Teres minor

Subscapularis

Axillary nerve

Teres major

Radial nerve

Latissimus dorsi

Triceps brachii (long head)

Triceps brachii (lateral head)

Triceps brachii (medial head)

Branch of radial nerve { Superficial Deep

Brachioradialis

Extensor carpi radialis longus

Anconeus

Extensor carpi radialis brevis

Posterior interosseous nerve

Supinator

Abductor pollicis longus

Extensor carpi ulnaris

Extensor pollicis brevis

Extensor digiti minimi

Extensor pollicis longus

Extensor digitorum

Extensor indicis

(D) Posterior view

Figure 6.30. *(Continued)* **C.** The course of the ulnar nerve and the typical pattern of branching of its motor branches are shown. **D.** The courses of the axillary and radial nerves and the typical pattern of branching of their motor branches are shown. The posterior interosseous nerve is the continuation of the deep branch of the radial nerve, shown here bifurcating into two branches to supply all the muscles with fleshy bellies located entirely in the posterior compartment of the forearm. The dorsum of the hand has no fleshy muscle fibers; therefore, no motor nerves are distributed there.

with those on the normal side. Determining the ability of the person to feel pain (e.g., from a pinprick of the skin) tests the degree of anesthesia.

Injuries to superior parts of the brachial plexus (C5 and C6) usually result from an excessive increase in the angle between the neck and the shoulder. These injuries can occur in a person who is thrown from a motorcycle or a horse and lands on the shoulder in a way that widely separates the neck and shoulder (Fig. B6.12*A*). When thrown, the person's shoulder often hits something (e.g., a tree or the ground) and stops, but the head and trunk continue to move. This stretches or ruptures superior parts of the brachial plexus or **avulses** (tears) the roots of the plexus from the spinal cord. Injury to the superior trunk of the plexus is apparent by the characteristic position of the limb ("waiter's tip position"), in which the limb hangs by the side in medial rotation (Fig. B6.12*B*). *Upper brachial plexus injuries* can also occur in a newborn when excessive stretching of the neck occurs during delivery (Fig. B6.12*C*).

As a result of *injuries to the superior parts of the brachial plexus (Erb-Duchenne palsy)*, paralysis of the muscles of the shoulder and arm supplied by the C5 and C6 spinal nerves occurs: deltoid, biceps, brachialis, and brachioradialis. The usual clinical appearance is an upper limb with an adducted shoulder, medially rotated arm, and extended elbow. The lateral aspect of the upper limb also experiences loss of sensation. Chronic microtrauma to the superior trunk of the brachial plexus from carrying a heavy backpack can produce motor and sensory deficits in the distribution of the musculocutaneous and radial nerves. A *superior brachial plexus injury* may produce muscle spasms and a severe disability in hikers (*backpacker's palsy*) who carry heavy backpacks for long periods.

Acute brachial plexus neuritis (brachial plexus neuropathy) is a neurologic disorder of unknown cause that is characterized by the sudden onset of severe pain, usually around the shoulder (Rowland, 2000). Typically, the pain begins at night and is followed by muscle weakness ▶

Figure B6.12. Injuries to brachial plexus. A. Note the excessive increase in the angle between the head and the left shoulder. **B.** The waiter's tip position (left upper limb) is demonstrated. **C.** Observe the excessive increase in the angle between the head and the left shoulder during this delivery. **D and E.** Excessive increases in the angle between the trunk and the right upper limb are demonstrated. **F.** A claw hand is shown (person is attempting to assume lightly shaded "fist" position).

and sometimes muscular atrophy (*neurologic amyotrophy*). Inflammation of the brachial plexus (*brachial neuritis*) is often preceded by some event (e.g., upper respiratory infection, vaccination, or non-specific trauma). The nerve fibers involved are usually derived from the superior trunk of the brachial plexus.

Compression of cords of the brachial plexus may result from prolonged hyperabduction of the arm during performance of manual tasks over the head, such as painting a ceiling. The cords are impinged or compressed between the coracoid process of the scapula and the pectoralis minor tendon. Common neurologic symptoms are pain radiating down the arm, numbness, paresthesia (tingling), erythema (redness of the skin caused by capillary dilation), and weakness of the hands. Compression of the axillary artery and vein causes ischemia of the upper limb and distension of the superficial veins. These signs and symptoms of *hyperabduction syndrome* result from compression of the axillary vessels and nerves.

Injuries to inferior parts of the brachial plexus (Klumpke paralysis) are much less common. Inferior brachial plexus injuries may occur when the upper limb is suddenly pulled superiorly—for example, when a person grasps something to break a fall (Fig. B6.12*D*) or a baby's upper limb is pulled excessively during delivery (Fig. B6.12*E*). These events injure the inferior trunk of the brachial plexus (C8 and T1) and may avulse the roots of the spinal nerves from the spinal cord. The short muscles of the hand are affected, and a *claw hand* results (Fig. B6.12*F*).

Brachial Plexus Block

Injection of an anesthetic solution into or immediately surrounding the axillary sheath interrupts nerve impulses and produces anesthesia of the structures supplied by the branches of the cords of the plexus (Fig. 6.24*A*). Sensation is blocked in all deep structures of the upper limb and the skin distal to the middle of the arm. Combined with an occlusive tourniquet technique to retain the anesthetic agent, this procedure enables surgeons to operate on the upper limb without using a general anesthetic. The brachial plexus can be anesthetized using a number of approaches, including an interscalene, supraclavicular, and axillary approach or block (Leonard, et al., 1999). ✪

THE BOTTOM LINE: The brachial plexus is an organized intermingling of the nerve fibers of the five adjacent anterior rami (C5–T1, the roots of the plexus) innervating the upper limb. Although their segmental identity is lost in forming the plexus, the original segmental distribution to skin (dermatomes) and muscles (myotomes) remains, exhibiting a cranial to caudal distribution for the skin (see "Cutaneous Nerves of the Upper Limb," earlier in this chapter) and a proximal to distal distribution for the muscles. For example, C5 and C6 fibers primarily innervate muscles that act at the shoulder or flex the elbow; C7 and C8 fibers innervate muscles that extend the elbow or are part of the forearm; and T1 fibers innervate the intrinsic muscles of the hand.

Formation of the brachial plexus initially involves merging of the superior and inferior pairs of roots, resulting in three trunks that each divide into anterior and posterior divisions. The fibers traversing anterior divisions innervate flexors and pronators of the anterior compartments of the limb, whereas the fibers traversing posterior divisions innervate extensors and supinators of the posterior compartments of the limb. The six divisions merge to form three cords that surround the axillary artery. Two of the three cords give rise in turn to 5 nerves, and the third (lateral cord) gives rise to 3 nerves. In addition to the nerves arising from the cords, 10 more nerves arise from the various parts of the plexus. Most nerves arising from the plexus contain fibers from two or more adjacent anterior rami.

Surface Anatomy of the Pectoral and Scapular Regions

The **clavicle** is the boundary demarcating the root of the neck from the thorax. It also indicates the "divide" between the deep cervical and the axillary "lymph sheds" (like a mountain range dividing watershed areas): lymph from structures superior to the clavicles drain via the deep cervical nodes; and lymph from structures inferior to the clavicles, as far inferiorly as the umbilicus, drain via the axillary lymph nodes. As the clavicle passes laterally, its medial part can be felt to be convex anteriorly (Fig. SA6.4). The large vessels and nerves to the upper limb pass posterior to this convexity. The flattened acromial end of the clavicle does not reach the **point of the shoulder**, formed by the lateral tip of the acromion of the scapula. The **acromion** is palpable and may be obvious when the deltoid contracts against resistance.

The **infraclavicular fossa** is the depressed area just inferior to the lateral part of the clavicle. This depression overlies the *clavipectoral (deltopectoral) triangle*, bounded by the clavicle superiorly, the pectoralis major medially, and the deltoid laterally, which may be evident in the fossa in lean individuals. The *cephalic vein* ascending from the upper limb enters the clavipectoral triangle and pierces the clavipectoral fascia to enter ▶

Clavicular head of pectoralis major

Clavicular part of deltoid

Deltopectoral groove (for cephalic vein)

Anterior axillary fold

Posterior axillary fold

Sternocleidomastoid

Clavicle

Jugular notch

Superior (descending) part of trapezius

Infraclavicular fossa (overlying deltopectoral triangle)

Axillary fossa

Sternocostal head of pectoralis major

Digitations of serratus anterior

Anterior view

Figure SA6.4

the *axillary vein*. The *coracoid process* of the scapula is not subcutaneous; it is covered by the anterior border of the deltoid; however, the tip of the process can be felt on deep palpation on the lateral aspect of the clavipectoral triangle. The **coracoid process** is used as a bony landmark when performing a brachial plexus block, and its position is of importance in diagnosing shoulder dislocations. While lifting a weight, palpate the anterior sloping border of the **trapezius** and where its superior fibers attach to the lateral third of the clavicle. When the arm is abducted and then adducted against resistance, the **sternocostal part of the pectoralis major** can be seen and palpated. If the **anterior axillary fold** bounding the axilla is grasped between the fingers and thumb, the inferior border of the **sternocostal head of the pectoralis major** can be felt. Several digitations of the **serratus anterior** are visible inferior to the anterior axillary fold. The *posterior axillary fold* is composed of skin and muscular tissue (latissimus dorsi and teres major) bounding the axilla posteriorly.

The lateral border of the acromion may be followed posteriorly with the fingers until it ends at the **acromial angle** (Fig. SA6.5). Clinically, the length of the arm is measured from the acromial angle to the lateral condyle of the humerus. The **spine of the scapula** is subcutaneous throughout and is easily palpated as it extends medially and slightly inferiorly from the acromion. The **root of the scapular spine** (medial end) is located opposite the

tip of the T3 spinous process when the arm is adducted. The **medial border of the scapula** may be palpated inferior to the root of the spine as it crosses ribs 3–7 (Fig. SA6.6). It may be visible in some people, especially thin people. The **inferior angle of the scapula** is easily palpated and is usually visible. Grasp the inferior scapular angle with the thumb and fingers and move the scapula up and down. When the arm is adducted, the inferior scapular angle is opposite the tip of the T7 spinous process and lies over the 7th rib or intercostal space.

The **deltoid** covering the proximal part of the humerus forms the rounded muscular contour of the shoulder. The **greater tubercle of the humerus** is the most lateral bony point in the shoulder when the arm is adducted and may be felt on deep palpation through the deltoid inferior to the lateral border of the acromion. When the arm is abducted, observe that the greater tubercle disappears beneath the acromion and is no longer palpable. The borders and parts of the deltoid are usually visible when the arm is abducted against resistance. Loss of the rounded muscular appearance of the shoulder and the appearance of a surface depression distal to the acromion are characteristic of a *dislocated shoulder,* or dislocation of the glenohumeral joint. The depression results from displacement of the humeral head. The **teres major** is prominent when the abducted arm is adducted and medially rotated against ▶

resistance (as when an acrobat stabilizes or fixes the shoulder joint during an iron cross maneuver on the ring. [Fig. SA6.7]).

When the upper limbs are abducted, the scapulae move laterally on the thoracic wall, enabling the **rhomboids** to be palpated. Because they are deep to the *trapezius,* the rhomboids are not always visible. If the rhomboids of one side are paralyzed, the scapula on the affected side remains farther from the midline than on the normal side because the paralyzed muscles are unable to retract it. ▶

Spine of scapula

Acromial angle

Medial border

Inferior angle

Root of scapular spine

Acromion

Medial border

Inferior angle

Posterior view

Figure SA6.5

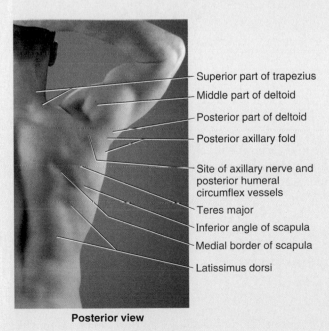

Superior part of trapezius

Middle part of deltoid

Posterior part of deltoid

Posterior axillary fold

Site of axillary nerve and posterior humeral circumflex vessels

Teres major

Inferior angle of scapula

Medial border of scapula

Latissimus dorsi

Posterior view

Figure SA6.6

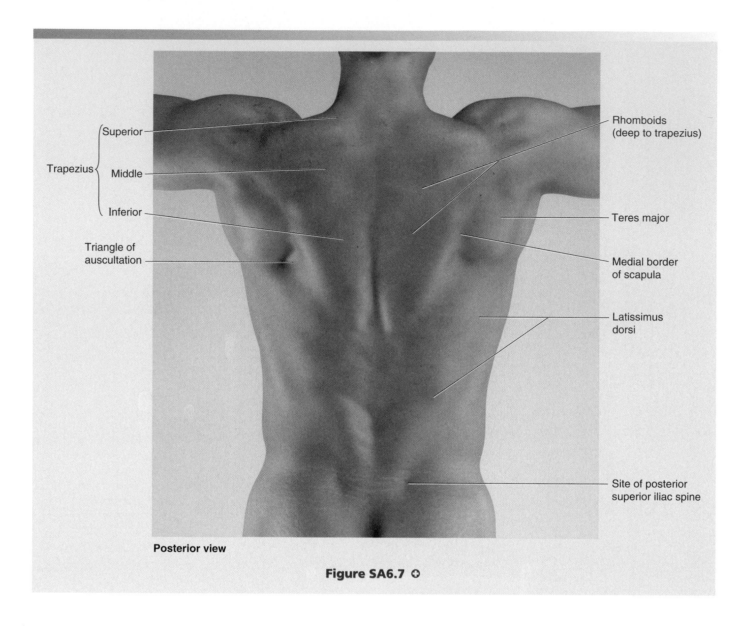

Trapezius { Superior / Middle / Inferior }

Triangle of auscultation

Rhomboids (deep to trapezius)

Teres major

Medial border of scapula

Latissimus dorsi

Site of posterior superior iliac spine

Posterior view

Figure SA6.7 ⊙

Arm

The **arm** extends from the shoulder to the elbow. Two types of movement occur between the arm and the forearm at the elbow joint: flexion–extension and pronation–supination. The muscles performing these movements are clearly divided into anterior and posterior groups. The chief action of both groups is at the elbow joint, but some muscles also act at the glenohumeral joint. The superior part of the humerus provides attachments for tendons of the shoulder muscles.

Muscles of the Arm

Of the four major arm muscles, three flexors (biceps brachii, brachialis, and coracobrachialis) are in the anterior (flexor) compartment, supplied by the musculocutaneous nerve (Figs.

6.31 and 6.32), and one extensor (triceps brachii) is in the posterior compartment, supplied by the radial nerve. A distally placed assistant to the triceps, the anconeus, also lies within the posterior compartment. The flexor muscles of the anterior compartment are almost twice as strong as the extensors in all positions; consequently, we are better pullers than pushers. It should be noted, however, that the extensors of the elbow are particularly important for raising oneself out of a chair and for wheelchair activity. Therefore, conditioning of the triceps is of particular importance in elderly or disabled persons.

The arm muscles are illustrated and their attachments, innervation, and actions are described in Table 6.6.

Biceps Brachii

As the term **biceps brachii** indicates, the proximal attachment of this fusiform muscle usually has two heads (*bi*, two + L. *caput*, head). However, approximately 10% of people have a

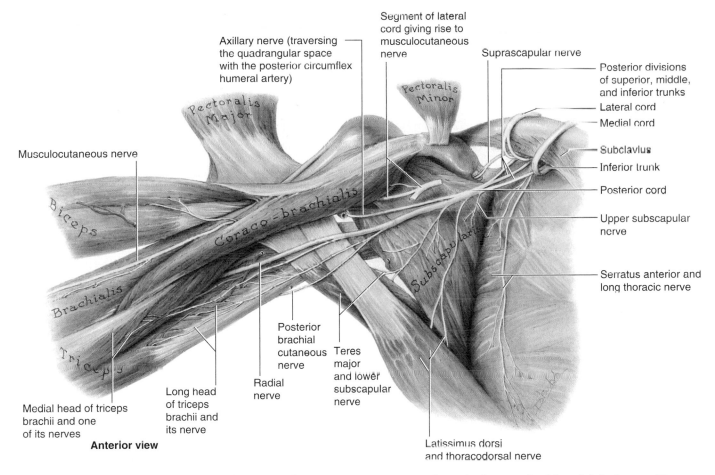

Axillary nerve (traversing the quadrangular space with the posterior circumflex humeral artery)

Segment of lateral cord giving rise to musculocutaneous nerve

Suprascapular nerve

Posterior divisions of superior, middle, and inferior trunks

Lateral cord

Medial cord

Subclavius

Inferior trunk

Posterior cord

Upper subscapular nerve

Serratus anterior and long thoracic nerve

Musculocutaneous nerve

Pectoralis Major

Pectoralis Minor

Coraco-brachialis

Biceps

Brachialis

Triceps

Subscapularis

Medial head of triceps brachii and one of its nerves

Long head of triceps brachii and its nerve

Radial nerve

Posterior brachial cutaneous nerve

Teres major and lower subscapular nerve

Latissimus dorsi and thoracodorsal nerve

Anterior view

Figure 6.31. Posterior wall of axilla, musculocutaneous nerve, and posterior cord of brachial plexus. The pectoralis major and minor muscles are reflected superolaterally, and the lateral and medial cords of the brachial plexus are reflected superomedially. All major vessels and the nerves arising from the medial and lateral cords of the brachial plexus (except for the musculocutaneous nerve from the lateral cord) are removed. The posterior cord, formed by the merging of the posterior divisions of all three trunks of the brachial plexus, gives rise to five nerves: radial, axillary, upper and lower subscapular, and thoracodorsal. Note that the musculocutaneous nerve pierces the coracobrachialis muscle and that the lower subscapular nerve supplies the teres major as well as the subscapularis.

third head to the biceps. The usual two heads of the biceps arise proximally by tendinous attachments to processes of the scapula, their fleshy bellies uniting just distal to the middle of the arm (Fig. 6.31). When present, the third head extends from the superomedial part of the brachialis (with which it is blended), usually lying posterior to the brachial artery. In either case, a single **biceps tendon** forms distally and attaches primarily to the radius.

Although the biceps is located in the anterior compartment of the arm (Fig. 6.32), it has no attachment to the humerus. The biceps is a "three-joint muscle," crossing and capable of effecting movement at the glenohumeral, elbow, and radioulnar joints, although it primarily acts at the latter two. Its action and effectiveness is markedly affected by the position of the elbow and forearm. When the elbow is extended, the bi-

ceps is a simple flexor of the forearm; however, as elbow flexion approaches 90° and more power is needed against resistance, the biceps is capable of two powerful movements, depending on the position of the forearm. When the elbow is flexed close to 90° and the forearm is supinated, the biceps is most efficient in producing flexion. Alternately, when the forearm is pronated, the biceps is the primary (most powerful) supinator of the forearm. For example, it is used when right-handed people drive a screw into hard wood and when inserting a corkscrew and pulling the cork from a wine bottle. The biceps barely operates as a flexor when the forearm is pronated, even against resistance. In the semiprone position, it is active only against resistance (Hamill and Knutzen, 2003).

Arising from the supraglenoid tubercle of the scapula and crossing the head of the humerus within the cavity of the

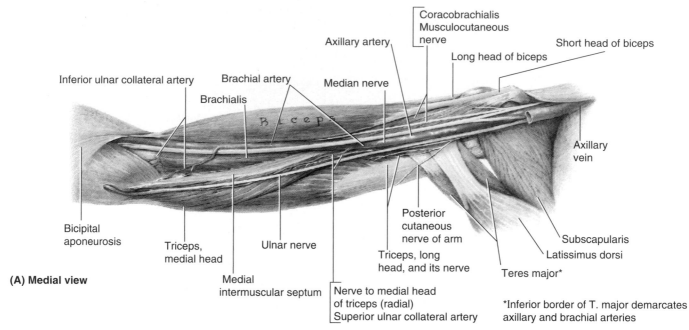

Inferior ulnar collateral artery

Brachial artery

Brachialis

Axillary artery

Median nerve

Coracobrachialis
Musculocutaneous
nerve

Long head of biceps

Short head of biceps

Axillary
vein

Bicipital
aponeurosis

Triceps,
medial head

Ulnar nerve

Posterior
cutaneous
nerve of arm

Triceps, long
head, and its nerve

Subscapularis

Latissimus dorsi

Teres major*

Medial
intermuscular septum

Nerve to medial head
of triceps (radial)

Superior ulnar collateral artery

*Inferior border of T. major demarcates
axillary and brachial arteries

(A) Medial view

Figure 6.32. Muscles, neurovascular structures, and compartments of arm. A. In this dissection of the right arm, the veins have been removed, except for the proximal part of the axillary vein. The courses of the musculocutaneous, median, and ulnar nerves and the brachial artery along the medial (protected) aspect of the arm are demonstrated. Their courses generally parallel the medial intermuscular septum that separates the anterior and posterior compartments in the distal two thirds of the arm.

glenohumeral joint, the rounded tendon of the long head of the biceps continues to be surrounded by synovial membrane as it descends in the intertubercular groove of the humerus. A broad band, the **transverse humeral ligament**, passes from the lesser to the greater tubercle of the humerus and converts the intertubercular groove into a canal (Table 6.6). The ligament holds the tendon of the long head of the biceps in the groove.

Distally, the major attachment of the biceps is to the radial tuberosity via the biceps tendon. However, a triangular membranous band, called the **bicipital aponeurosis**, runs from the biceps tendon across the cubital fossa and merges with the antebrachial (deep) fascia covering the flexor muscles in the medial side of the forearm. It attaches indirectly by means of the fascia to the subcutaneous border of the ulna. The proximal part of the bicipital aponeurosis can be easily felt where it passes obliquely over the brachial artery and median nerve (Fig. 6.33*A*). The bicipital aponeurosis affords protection for these and other structures in the cubital fossa. It also helps lessen the pressure of the biceps tendon on the radial tuberosity during pronation and supination of the forearm.

To test the biceps brachii, the elbow joint is flexed against resistance when the forearm is supinated. If acting normally, the muscle forms a prominent bulge on the anterior aspect of the arm that is easily palpated.

Bicipital Myotatic Reflex

The biceps reflex is one of several deep-tendon reflexes that are routinely tested during physical examination. The relaxed limb is passively pronated and partially extended at the elbow. The examiner's thumb is firmly placed on the biceps tendon, and the reflex hammer is briskly tapped at the base of the nail bed of the examiner's thumb (Fig. B6.13). A normal (positive) response is an involuntary contraction of the biceps, felt as a momentarily tensed tendon, usually with a brief jerk-like flexion of the elbow. A positive response ▶

Figure B6.13. Method of eliciting biceps reflex.

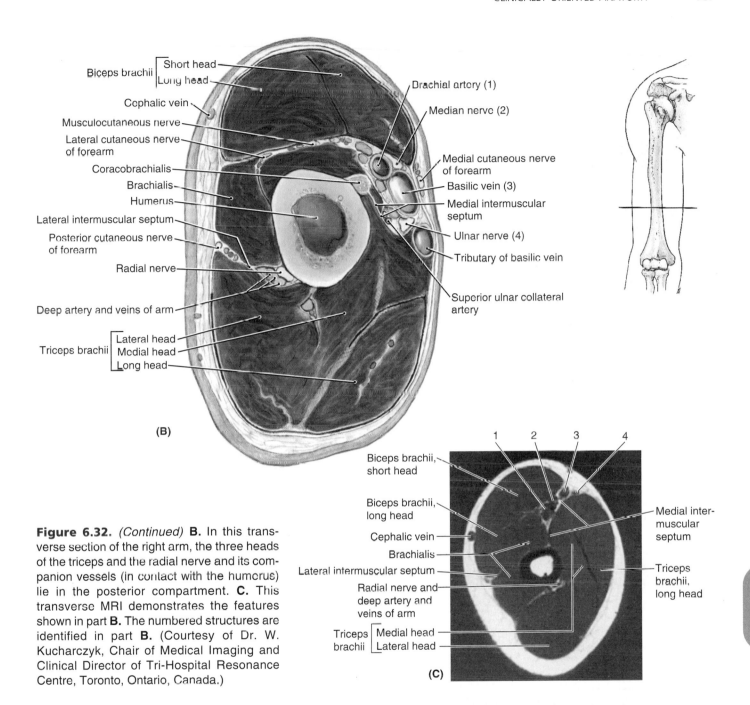

(B)

Biceps brachii { Short head / Long head
Cephalic vein
Musculocutaneous nerve
Lateral cutaneous nerve of forearm
Coracobrachialis
Brachialis
Humerus
Lateral intermuscular septum
Posterior cutaneous nerve of forearm
Radial nerve
Deep artery and veins of arm
Triceps brachii { Lateral head / Medial head / Long head

Brachial artery (1)
Median nerve (2)
Medial cutaneous nerve of forearm
Basilic vein (3)
Medial intermuscular septum
Ulnar nerve (4)
Tributary of basilic vein
Superior ulnar collateral artery

Biceps brachii, short head
Biceps brachii, long head
Cephalic vein
Brachialis
Lateral intermuscular septum
Radial nerve and deep artery and veins of arm
Triceps brachii { Medial head / Lateral head

Medial intermuscular septum
Triceps brachii, long head

(C)

Figure 6.32. *(Continued)* **B.** In this transverse section of the right arm, the three heads of the triceps and the radial nerve and its companion vessels (in contact with the humerus) lie in the posterior compartment. **C.** This transverse MRI demonstrates the features shown in part **B.** The numbered structures are identified in part **B.** (Courtesy of Dr. W. Kucharczyk, Chair of Medical Imaging and Clinical Director of Tri-Hospital Resonance Centre, Toronto, Ontario, Canada.)

confirms the integrity of the musculocutaneous nerve and the C5 and C6 spinal cord segments. Excessive, diminished, or prolonged (hung) responses may indicate central or peripheral nervous system disease or metabolic disorders (e.g., thyroid disease).

Biceps Tendinitis

The tendon of the long head of the biceps is enclosed by a synovial sheath and moves back and forth in the intertubercular groove of the humerus. Wear and tear of this mechanism can cause shoulder pain. Inflammation of the tendon (**biceps tendinitis**), usually the result of repetitive microtrauma, is common in sports involving throwing (e.g., baseball and cricket) and use of a racquet (e.g., tennis). A tight, narrow, and/or rough intertubercular groove may irritate and inflame the tendon, producing tenderness and **crepitus** (a crackling sound).

Dislocation of the Tendon of the Long Head of the Biceps

The tendon of the long head of the biceps can be partially or completely dislocated from the intertubercular ▶

Table 6.6. Muscles of the Arm

(A) Anterior views   **Biceps brachii**   **Brachialis**   **Coracobrachialis**

(B) Posterior views   **Triceps brachii**   **Anconeus**

Muscle	Proximal Attachment	Distal Attachment	Innervation[a]	Main Action
Biceps brachii	Short head: tip of coracoid process of scapula Long head: supraglenoid tubercle of scapula	Tuberosity of radius and fascia of forearm via bicipital aponeurosis	Musculocutaneous nerve[b] (C5, **C6**)	Supinates forearm and, when it is supine, flexes forearm; short head resists dislocation of shoulder
Brachialis	Distal half of anterior surface of humerus	Coronoid process and tuberosity of ulna		Flexes forearm in all positions

Table 6.6. Muscles of the Arm *(continued)*

Muscle	Proximal Attachment	Distal Attachment	Innervation[a]	Main Action
Coraco-brachialis	Tip of coracoid process of scapula	Middle third of medial surface of humerus	Musculocutaneous nerve (C5, **C6**, C7)	Helps flex and adduct arm; resists dislocation of shoulder
Triceps brachii	Long head: infraglenoid tubercle of scapula Lateral head: posterior surface of humerus, superior to radial groove Medial head: posterior surface of humerus, inferior to radial groove	Proximal end of olecranon of ulna and fascia of forearm	Radial nerve (C6, **C7**, **C8**)	Chief extensor of forearm; long head resists dislocation of humerus; especially important during abduction
Anconeus	Lateral epicondyle of humerus	Lateral surface of olecranon and superior part of posterior surface of ulna	Radial nerve (C7, C8, T1)	Assists triceps in extending forearm; stabilizes elbow joint; may abduct ulna during pronation

[a] The spinal cord segmental innervation is indicated (e.g. "C5, **C6**" means that the nerves supplying the biceps brachii are derived from the fifth and sixth cervical segments of the spinal cord). Numbers in boldface (**C6**) indicate the main segmental innervation. Damage to one or more of the listed spinal cord segments or to the motor nerve roots arising from them results in paralysis of the muscles concerned.
[b] Some of the lateral part of the brachialis is innervated by a branch of the radial nerve.

groove in the humerus. This painful condition may occur in young persons during traumatic separation of the proximal epiphysis of the humerus. The injury also occurs in older persons with a history of biceps tendinitis. Usually a sensation of popping or catching is felt during arm rotation.

Rupture of the Tendon of the Long Head of the Biceps

Rupture of the tendon usually results from wear and tear of an inflamed tendon as it moves back and forth in the intertubercular groove of the humerus. This injury usually occurs in individuals > 35 years of age. Typically, the tendon is torn from its attachment to the supraglenoid tubercle of the scapula. The rupture is commonly dramatic and is associated with a snap or pop. The detached muscle belly forms a ball near the center of the distal part of the anterior aspect of the arm (Popeye deformity) (Fig. B6.14). Rupture of the biceps tendon may result from forceful flexion of the arm against excessive resistance, as occurs in weight lifters (Anderson et al., 2000). However, the tendon ruptures more often as the result of prolonged tendinitis that weakens it. The rupture results from repetitive overhead motions, such as occurs in swimmers and baseball pitchers, which tear the weakened tendon where it passes through the intertubercular groove. ●

Rupture of biceps tendon

Figure B6.14

Anterior views

Figure 6.33. Dissections of cubital fossa. A. In this superficial dissection, the distal end of the brachial artery lies medial to the biceps tendon. During the measurement of blood pressure, a stethoscope is placed here to listen to pulsations of the brachial artery. At this level, the median nerve lies on the medial aspect of the brachial artery, and both are deep to the bicipital aponeurosis (Fig. 6.38A). **B.** In this deep dissection, part of the biceps is excised and the cubital fossa is opened widely by retracting the forearm extensor muscles laterally and the flexor muscles medially. The radial nerve, which has just left the posterior compartment of the arm by piercing the lateral intermuscular septum, emerges between the brachialis and the brachioradialis and divides into a superficial (sensory) and a deep (motor) branch (Fig. 6.39A). The superficial branch remains under the protection of the brachioradialis, but the deep branch pierces the supinator to return to the posterior aspect of the limb. The brachial artery is dividing into its terminal branches: the ulnar artery, which runs deeply, and the radial artery, which remains superficial; thus its pulsations are palpable throughout the forearm.

Brachialis

The **brachialis** is a flattened fusiform muscle that lies posterior (deep) to the biceps. Its distal attachment covers the anterior part of the elbow joint (Figs. 6.31–6.33 and 6.39A). The brachialis is the main flexor of the forearm. It is the only pure flexor, producing the greatest amount of flexion force. It flexes the forearm in all positions, not being affected by pronation and supination; during both slow and quick movements; and in the presence or absence of resistance. When the forearm is extended slowly, the brachialis steadies the movement by slowly relaxing—that is, eccentric contraction (you use it to pick up and put down a teacup carefully, for example). The brachialis always contracts when the elbow is flexed and is primarily responsible for sustaining the flexed position. Because of its important and almost constant role, it is regarded as the workhorse of the elbow flexors.

Coracobrachialis

The **coracobrachialis** is an elongated muscle in the superomedial part of the arm. It is a useful landmark for locating other structures in the arm (Figs. 6.31 and 6.32; Table 6.6). For example, the musculocutaneous nerve pierces it, and the distal part of its attachment indicates the location of the nutrient foramen of the humerus. The coracobrachialis helps flex and adduct the arm and stabilize the glenohumeral joint. With the deltoid and long head of the triceps, it serves as a *shunt muscle,* resisting downward dislocation of the head of the humerus, as when carrying a heavy suitcase. The median nerve and/or the brachial artery may run deep to the coracobrachialis and be compressed by it.

Triceps Brachii

The **triceps brachii** is a large fusiform muscle in the posterior compartment of the arm (Figs. 6.32 and 6.34; Table 6.6). As indicated by its name, the triceps has three heads: long, lateral, and medial. The triceps is the main extensor of the forearm. Because its **long head** crosses the glenohumeral joint, the triceps helps stabilize the adducted glenohumeral joint by serving as a shunt muscle, resisting inferior displacement of the head of the humerus. The long head also aids in extension and adduction of the arm, but it is actually the least active head. The **medial head** is the workhorse of forearm extension, active at all speeds and in the presence or absence of resistance. The **lateral head** is strongest but is recruited into activity primarily against resistance. (Hamill and Knutzen, 2003). Pronation and supination of the forearm do not affect triceps operation. Just proximal to the distal attachment of the tri-

ceps is a friction-reducing *subtendinous olecranon bursa,* between the triceps tendon and the olecranon.

To *test the triceps* (or to determine the level of a radial nerve lesion), the arm is abducted 90° and then the flexed forearm is extended against resistance provided by the examiner. If acting normally, the triceps can be seen and palpated. Its strength should be comparable with the contralateral muscle, given consideration for lateral dominance (right or left handedness).

Anconeus

The **anconeus** is a small, relatively unimportant triangular muscle on the posterolateral aspect of the elbow; it is usually partially blended with the triceps (Table 6.6). The anconeus helps the triceps extend the forearm and tenses of the capsule of the elbow joint, preventing its being pinched during extension. It is also said to abduct the ulna during pronation of the forearm.

Brachial Artery

The **brachial artery** provides the main arterial supply to the arm and is the continuation of the axillary artery (Fig. 6.35). It begins at the inferior border of the teres major (Figs. 6.32A and 6.35) and ends in the cubital fossa opposite the neck of the radius where, under cover of the bicipital aponeurosis, it

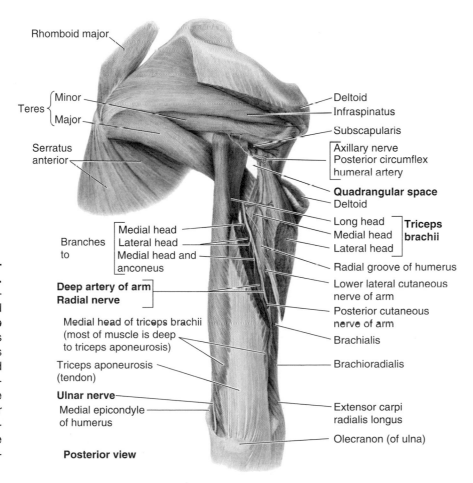

Figure 6.34. Muscles of scapular region and posterior region of arm. The lateral head of the triceps brachii is divided and displaced to show the radial nerve and the deep artery of the arm. The exposed bone of the radial groove, which is devoid of muscular attachment, separates the humeral attachments of the lateral and medial heads of the triceps (bony attachments are illustrated in Table 6.6). The structures traversing the quadrangular space and the ulnar nerve passing posterior to the medial epicondyle of the humerus (where the nerve is most commonly injured) are also demonstrated.

Teres major

Anastomotic branch

Brachial artery

Deep artery of arm

Deep artery of arm
{
Middle collateral branch

Radial collateral branch
}

Recurrent radial artery

Ulnar artery

Radial artery

Anterior view

Humeral nutrient artery

Superior ulnar collateral artery

Inferior ulnar collateral artery

Anterior
Posterior
} Ulnar recurrent arteries

Recurrent
Common
Anterior
Posterior
} Interosseous arteries

Ulnar artery

Figure 6.35. Arterial supply of arm and proximal forearm. Functionally and clinically important periarticular arterial anastomoses surround the elbow. The resulting collateral circulation allows blood to reach the forearm when flexion of the elbow compromises flow through the terminal part of the brachial artery.

sometimes double, from the radial, ulnar, and interosseous arteries, which run superiorly anterior and posterior to the elbow joint. These arteries anastomose with descending articular branches of the deep artery of the arm and the ulnar collateral arteries.

Deep Artery of the Arm

The **deep artery of the arm** (L. *arteria profunda brachii*) is the largest branch of the brachial artery and has the most superior origin. The deep artery accompanies the radial nerve along the radial groove as it passes posteriorly around the shaft of the humerus (Figs. 6.34 and 6.36). The deep artery terminates by dividing into **middle** and **radial collateral arteries** that participate in the periarticular arterial anastomoses around the elbow.

Humeral Nutrient Artery

The main **humeral nutrient artery** arises from the brachial artery around the middle of the arm (Fig. 6.35) and enters the

Musculocutaneous nerve

Radial nerve and deep artery of arm in radial groove

Lateral intermuscular septum of arm

Radial collateral artery

Middle collateral artery (posterior to humerus)

Posterior
Lateral
Medial
} Cords of brachial plexus

Axillary artery

Median nerve

Brachial artery

Radial nerve

Medial intermuscular septum of arm

Ulnar nerve (posterior to septum)

Groove for ulnar nerve (on posterior aspect)

Anterior view

Figure 6.36. Relationship of the arteries and nerves of the arm to the humerus. The cords of the brachial plexus surround the axillary artery. The radial nerve and accompanying deep artery of the arm wind posteriorly around, and directly on the surface of, the humerus in the radial groove. The radial nerve and radial collateral artery then pierce the lateral intermuscular septum to enter the anterior compartment. The ulnar nerve pierces the medial intermuscular septum to enter the posterior compartment and then lies in the groove for the ulnar nerve on the posterior aspect of the medial epicondyle of the humerus. The median nerve descends in the arm to the medial side of the cubital fossa, where it is well protected and rarely injured (Figs. 6.33 and 6.39).

divides into the radial and ulnar arteries (Figs. 6.33*B* and 6.35). The brachial artery, relatively superficial and palpable throughout its course, lies anterior to the triceps and brachialis. At first it lies medial to the humerus where its pulsations are palpable in the **medial bicipital groove** (Fig. 6.32*B*). It then passes anterior to the medial supraepicondylar ridge and trochlea of the humerus (Figs. 6.35 and 6.36). As it passes inferolaterally, the brachial artery accompanies the median nerve, which crosses anterior to the artery (Figs. 6.32*A* and 6.36). During its course through the arm, the brachial artery gives rise to many unnamed *muscular branches* and the *humeral nutrient artery* (Fig. 6.35), which arise from its lateral aspect. The unnamed muscular branches are often omitted from illustrations, but they are evident during dissection.

The main named branches of the brachial artery arising from its medial aspect are the *deep artery of the arm* and the superior and inferior *ulnar collateral arteries.* The collateral arteries help form the periarticular **arterial anastomoses of the elbow region.** Other arteries involved are recurrent branches, *nutrient canal* on the anteromedial surface of the humerus. The artery runs distally in the canal toward the elbow. Other smaller humeral nutrient arteries also occur.

Superior Ulnar Collateral Artery

The **superior ulnar collateral artery** arises from the medial aspect of the brachial artery near the middle of the arm and accompanies the ulnar nerve posterior to the medial epicondyle of the humerus (Figs. 6.32*A* and 6.35). Here it anastomoses with the posterior ulnar recurrent artery and the inferior ul-

nar collateral artery, participating in the periarticular arterial anastomoses of the elbow.

Inferior Ulnar Collateral Artery

The **inferior ulnar collateral artery** arises from the brachial artery approximately 5 cm proximal to the elbow crease (Figs. 6.32*A*, 6.33, and 6.35). It then passes inferomedially anterior to the medial epicondyle of the humerus and joins the anastomoses of the elbow region by anastomosing with the anterior ulnar recurrent artery.

Interruption of Blood Flow in the Brachial Artery

Stopping bleeding through manual or surgical control of blood flow is **hemostasis.** The best place to compress the brachial artery to control hemorrhage is medial to the humerus near the middle of the arm (Fig. B6.15). Because the arterial anastomoses around the elbow provide a functionally and surgically important collateral circulation, the brachial artery may be clamped distal to the origin of the deep artery of the arm without producing tissue damage. The anatomical basis for this procedure is that the ulnar and radial arteries will still receive sufficient blood through the anastomoses around the elbow. Although collateral pathways confer some protection against gradual temporary and partial occlusion, sudden complete occlusion or laceration of the brachial artery creates a surgical emergency because paralysis of muscles results from *ischemia of the elbow and forearm* within a few hours. Muscles and nerves can tolerate up to 6 hours of ischemia (Salter, 1999); after this, fibrous scar tissue replaces necrotic tissue and causes the involved muscles to shorten permanently, producing a flexion defor-

mity, the *ischemic compartment syndrome* (Volkmann or ischemic contracture). Contraction of the fingers and sometimes the wrist results in loss of hand power as a result of irreversible necrosis of the forearm flexor muscles.

Fracture of the Humeral Shaft

A *midhumeral fracture* may injure the radial nerve in the radial groove in the humeral shaft. When this nerve is damaged, the fracture is not likely to paralyze the triceps because of the high origin of the nerves to two of its three heads. A fracture of the distal part of the humerus, near the supraepicondylar ridges, is called a *supraepicondylar fracture* (Fig. B6.16). The distal bone fragment may be displaced anteriorly or posteriorly. The actions of the brachialis and triceps tend to pull the distal fragment over the proximal fragment, shortening the limb. Any of the nerves or branches of the brachial vessels related to the humerus may be injured by a displaced bone fragment. ☉

Shaft of humerus

Lateral supraepicondylar ridge

Medial supraepicondylar ridge

Lateral epicondyle

Medial epicondyle

Brachial artery

Figure B6.15. Compression of brachial artery.   **Figure B6.16. Supraepicondylar fracture.**

Veins of the Arm

Two sets of *veins of the arm,* superficial and deep, anastomose freely with each other. The superficial veins are in the subcutaneous tissue, and the deep veins accompany the arteries. Both sets of veins have valves, but they are more numerous in the deep veins than in the superficial veins.

Superficial Veins

The two main **superficial veins of the arm,** the *cephalic* and *basilic veins* (Figs. 6.32*B* & *C* and 6.33), are described in "Superficial Structures of the Upper Limb," earlier in this chapter.

Deep Veins

Paired deep veins, collectively constituting the **brachial vein,** accompany the brachial artery (Fig. 6.33*A*). Their frequent connections encompass the artery, forming an anastomotic network within a common vascular sheath. The pulsations of the brachial artery help move the blood through this venous network. The brachial vein begins at the elbow by union of the *accompanying veins of the ulnar and radial arteries* and end by merging with the basilic vein to form the *axillary vein.* Not uncommonly, the deep veins join to form one brachial vein during part of their course.

Nerves of the Arm

Four main nerves pass through the arm: median, ulnar, musculocutaneous, and radial (Fig. 6.36). Their origins from the brachial plexus, courses in the upper limb, and the structures innervated by them are summarized in Table 6.5. The median and ulnar nerves supply no branches to the arm.

Musculocutaneous Nerve

The **musculocutaneous nerve** begins opposite the inferior border of the pectoralis minor, pierces the coracobrachialis, and continues distally between the biceps and brachialis (Fig. 6.33*B*). After supplying all three muscles of the anterior compartment of the arm, the nerve emerges lateral to the biceps as the *lateral cutaneous nerve of the forearm.* It becomes truly subcutaneous when it pierces the deep fascia proximal to the cubital fossa to course initially with the cephalic vein in the subcutaneous tissue. After crossing the anterior aspect of the elbow, it continues to supply the skin of the lateral aspect of the forearm.

Radial Nerve in the Arm

The **radial nerve** supplies all the muscles in the posterior compartment of the arm (and forearm). The radial nerve enters the arm posterior to the brachial artery, medial to the humerus, and anterior to the long head of the triceps, where it gives branches to the long and medial heads of the triceps (Fig. 6.31). The radial nerve then descends inferolaterally with the deep brachial artery and passes around the humeral shaft in the radial groove (Figs. 6.32*B*, 6.34, and 6.36). The branch to the lateral head of the triceps arises within the radial groove. When it reaches the lateral border of the humerus, the radial nerve pierces the lateral intermuscular

septum and continues inferiorly in the anterior compartment of the arm between the brachialis and the brachioradialis to the level of the lateral epicondyle of the humerus (Fig. 6.33*B*). The radial nerve then divides into deep and superficial branches.

- The *deep branch of the radial nerve* is entirely muscular and articular in its distribution.
- The *superficial branch of the radial nerve* is entirely cutaneous in its distribution, supplying sensation to the dorsum of the hand and fingers.

Median Nerve in the Arm

The **median nerve** runs distally in the arm on the lateral side of the brachial artery until it reaches the middle of the arm, where it crosses to the medial side and contacts the brachialis (Fig. 6.36). The median nerve then descends into the cubital fossa, where it lies deep to the bicipital aponeurosis and median cubital vein (Fig. 6.33). The median nerve has no branches in the axilla or the arm, but it does supply articular branches to the elbow joint.

Ulnar Nerve in the Arm

The **ulnar nerve** passes distally from the axilla anterior to the insertion of the teres major and to the long head of the triceps, on the medial side of the brachial artery (Fig. 6.32). Around the middle of the arm it pierces the medial intermuscular septum with the superior ulnar collateral artery and descends between the septum and the medial head of the triceps (Fig. 6.36). The ulnar nerve passes posterior to the medial epicondyle and medial to the olecranon to enter the forearm (Fig. 6.30*C*). Posterior to the medial epicondyle, where the ulnar nerve is referred to in lay terms as the "crazy bone," it is superficial, easily palpable, and vulnerable to injury. Like the median nerve, the ulnar nerve has no branches in the arm, but it also supplies articular branches to the elbow joint.

Injury to the Musculocutaneous Nerve

Injury to the musculocutaneous nerve in the axilla (uncommon in this protected position) is typically inflicted by a weapon such as a knife. A musculocutaneous nerve injury results in *paralysis of the coracobrachialis, biceps, and brachialis.* Consequently, flexion of the elbow joint and supination of the forearm are greatly weakened but not lost. Weak flexion and supination are still possible, produced by the brachioradialis and supinator, respectively, both of which are supplied by the radial nerve. Loss of sensation may occur on the lateral surface of the forearm supplied by the lateral antebrachial cutaneous nerve, the continuation of the musculocutaneous nerve. ▶

Injury to the Radial Nerve in the Arm

Injury to the radial nerve superior to the origin of its branches to the triceps brachii results in *paralysis of the triceps, brachioradialis, supinator, and extensor muscles of the wrist and fingers.* Loss of sensation in areas of skin supplied by this nerve also occurs. When the nerve is injured in the radial groove, the triceps is usually not completely paralyzed but only weakened because only the medial head is affected; however, the muscles in the posterior compartment of the forearm that are supplied by more distal branches of the nerve are paralyzed. The characteristic clinical sign of radial nerve injury is **wrist-drop** (inability to extend the wrist and the fingers at the metacarpophalangeal joints (Fig. B6.17*A*). Instead, the relaxed wrist assumes a partly flexed position owing to unopposed tonus of flexor muscles and gravity (Fig. B6.17*B*). ✪

Figure B6.17. Wrist-drop.

THE BOTTOM LINE: The arm forms a column with the humerus at its center. The humerus, along with intermuscular septa in its distal two thirds, divides the arm lengthwise (or more specifically, the space inside the brachial fascia) into anterior or flexor and posterior or extensor compartments. The anterior compartment contains three flexor muscles supplied by the musculocutaneous nerve. The coracobrachialis acts (weakly) at the shoulder, and the biceps and brachialis act at the elbow. The biceps is also the primary supinator of the forearm (when the elbow is flexed). The brachialis is the primary flexor of the forearm. The posterior compartment contains a three-headed extensor muscle, the triceps, which is supplied by the radial nerve. One of the heads (the long head) acts at the shoulder, but mostly the heads work together to extend the elbow. Both compartments are supplied by the brachial artery, the posterior compartment primarily via its major branch, the deep artery of the arm. The primary neurovascular bundle is located on the medial side of the limb; thus it is usually protected by the limb it serves.

Cubital Fossa

The **cubital fossa** is seen superficially as a depression on the anterior aspect of the elbow. Deeply, it is a space filled with a variable amount of fat anterior to the most distal part of the humerus and the elbow joint. The three boundaries of the triangular cubital fossa are as follows (Figs. 6.33 and 6.37*C*):

1. Superiorly, an imaginary line connecting the medial and lateral epicondyles.

2. Medially, the mass of flexor muscles of the forearm arising from the common flexor attachment on the medial epicondyle; most specifically, the pronator teres.

3. Laterally, the mass of extensor muscles of the forearm arising from the lateral epicondyle and supraepicondylar ridge; most specifically, the brachioradialis.

The floor of the cubital fossa is formed by the brachialis and supinator muscles of the arm and forearm, respectively. The roof of the cubital fossa is formed by the continuity of brachial and antebrachial (deep) fascia reinforced by the bicipital aponeurosis (Figs. 6.38 and 6.39), subcutaneous tissue, and skin.

The contents of the cubital fossa are the (Figs. 6.33 and 6.38*A*):

- Terminal part of the brachial artery and the commencement of its terminal branches, the radial and ulnar arteries. The brachial artery lies between the biceps tendon and the median nerve.

- (Deep) accompanying veins of the arteries.

- Biceps brachii tendon.

- Median nerve.

- Radial nerve, deep between the muscles forming lateral boundary of the fossa (the brachioradialis, in particular) and the brachialis, dividing into its superficial and deep branches. The muscles must be retracted to expose the nerve.

Superficially, in the subcutaneous tissue overlying the fossa are the *median cubital vein,* lying anterior to the brachial artery, and the medial and lateral antebrachial cutaneous nerves, related to the basilic and cephalic veins.

(A) Anteroposterior view

(B) Medial view

(C) Anterior view—forearm supinated

(D) Anterosuperior view

(E) Anterior view

Figure 6.37. Bones, muscles, and compartments of forearm. A. An anteroposterior (AP) radiograph of the forearm in pronation is shown. (Courtesy of Dr. J. Heslin, Toronto, Ontario, Canada.) **B.** The bones of the forearm and the radioulnar ligaments are demonstrated. **C.** In this dissection the superficial muscles of the forearm and the palmar aponeurosis are revealed. **D.** This stepped transverse section demonstrates the compartments of the forearm. **E.** The flexor digitorum superficialis (FDS) and related structures are shown. Observe the ulnar artery descending obliquely posterior to the FDS to meet and accompany the ulnar nerve.

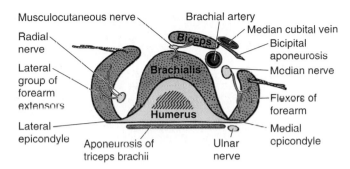

(A) Cross section of cubital fossa

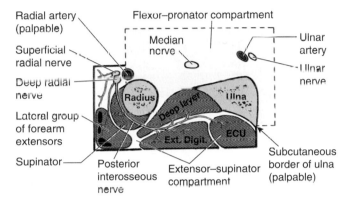

(B) Cross section of proximal forearm

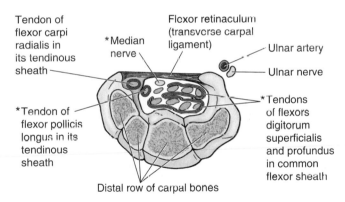

* – Structures traversing carpal tunnel

(C) Cross section of carpus (wrist)

Inferior views of transverse cross sections, right upper limb

Figure 6.38. Cross sections demonstrating relationships at level of cubital fossa, proximal forearm, and wrist. A. At the level of the cubital fossa, the flexors and extensor of the elbow occupy the anterior and posterior aspects of the humerus. Lateral and medial extensions (epicondyles and supraepicondylar ridges) of the humerus provide proximal attachment (origin) for the forearm flexors and extensors. **B.** Consequently, in the proximal forearm, the "anterior" flexor–pronator compartment actually lies anteromedially, and the "posterior" extensor–supinator compartment lies posterolaterally. The radial artery (laterally) and the sharp, subcutaneous posterior border of the ulna (medially) are palpable features separating the anterior and posterior compartments. No motor nerves cross either demarcation, making them useful for surgical approaches. *Ext. digit.,* extensor digitorum; *ECU,* extensor carpi ulnaris. **C.** At the level of the wrist, nine tendons from three muscles (and one nerve) of the anterior compartment of the forearm traverse the carpal tunnel; eight of the tendons share a common synovial flexor sheath.

Brachial fascia

Antebrachial fascia

Bicipital aponeurosis

Brachioradialis

Pronator teres

Flexor carpi radialis

Palmaris longus

Flexor carpi ulnaris

Distal thickening of fascia of forearm (palmar carpal ligament)

Pronator quadratus

Site of flexor retinaculum (transverse carpal ligament)

Thenar fascia

Palmar aponeurosis

Hypothenar fascia

Palmar fascia

Fibrous digital sheath

Anterior view

Figure 6.39. Antebrachial fascia and superficial muscles of forearm. The brachioradialis, representing the lateral group of muscles, slightly overlaps the radial artery. The four superficial muscles of the anterior (flexor–pronator) compartment of the forearm (pronator teres, flexor carpi radialis, palmaris longus, and flexor carpi ulnaris) radiate from the medial epicondyle of the humerus (Fig. 6.38C). Over the distal ends of the radius and ulna, the antebrachial fascia thickens to form the extensor retinaculum posteriorly and a corresponding thickening, the palmar carpal ligament, anteriorly. Immediately distal and at a deeper level to the latter thickening, the flexor retinaculum (also continuous with the distal part of the antebrachial fascia), retains the tendons of the flexor muscles of the hand and fingers in the carpal tunnel.

Venipuncture in the Cubital Fossa

The cubital fossa is the common site for sampling and transfusion of blood and intravenous injections because of the prominence and accessibility of veins. Usually, the median cubital vein or basilic vein is selected. The median cubital vein lies directly on the deep fascia, crossing the bicipital aponeurosis, which separates it from the underlying brachial artery and median nerve and provides some protection to the latter. Historically, during the days of bloodletting, the bicipital aponeurosis was known as the *grace Deux* (Fr. grace of God) *tendon*, by the grace of which arterial hemorrhage was usually avoided. A tourniquet is placed around the midarm to distend the veins in the cubital fossa. Once the vein is punctured, the tourniquet is removed so that when the needle is removed the vein will not bleed extensively. The cubital veins are also a site for the introduction of cardiac catheters to secure blood samples from the great vessels and chambers of the heart. These veins may also used for *cardioangiography* (see Chapter 1).

Variation of Veins in the Cubital Fossa

The pattern of veins in the cubital fossa varies greatly. In approximately 20% of people, the median antebrachial vein (median vein of the forearm) divides into a *median basilic vein,* which joins the basilic vein. and a *median cephalic vein,* which joins the cephalic vein (Fig. B6.18). In these cases, a clear *M* formation is produced by the cubital veins. It is important to observe and remember that either the median cubital vein or the median basilic vein, whichever pattern is present, crosses superficial to the brachial artery, from which it is separated by the bicipital aponeurosis. These veins are good sites for drawing blood but are not ideal for injecting an irritating drug because of the danger of injecting it into the brachial artery. In obese people, a considerable amount of fatty tissue may overlie the vein. ◐

Cephalic vein

Basilic vein

Median cephalic vein

Median basilic vein

Basilic vein

Cephalic vein

Median antebrachial vein

Figure B6.18

Surface Anatomy of the Arm and Cubital Fossa

The borders of the *deltoid* are visible when the arm is abducted against resistance. The **distal attachment of the deltoid** can be palpated on the lateral surface of the humerus (Fig. SA6.8). The **long, lateral, and medial heads of the triceps brachii** form a bulge on the posterior aspect of the arm and are identifiable when the forearm is extended from the flexed position against resistance. The **olecranon,** to which the triceps tendon attaches distally, is easily palpated. It is separated from the skin only by the *olecranon bursa,* which accounts for the mobility of the overlying skin. The **triceps tendon** is easily felt as it descends along the posterior aspect of the arm to the olecranon. The fingers can be pressed inwards on each side of the tendon, where the elbow joint is superficial. An abnormal collection of fluid in the elbow joint or in the *triceps bursa* or *subtendinous olecranon bursa* is palpable at these sites; the bursa lies deep to the triceps tendon.

The **biceps brachii** forms a bulge on the anterior aspect of the arm; its belly becomes more prominent when the elbow is flexed and supinated against resistance (Fig. SA6.9). The **biceps brachii tendon** can be palpated in the cubital fossa, immediately lateral to the midline, especially when the elbow is flexed against resistance. The proximal part of the **bicipital aponeurosis** can be palpated where it passes obliquely over the brachial artery and median nerve. Medial and lateral *bicipital grooves* separate the bulges formed by the biceps and triceps and indicate the location of the medial and lateral intermuscular septa (Fig. SA6.10). The cephalic vein runs superiorly in the lateral bicipital groove, and the basilic vein ascends in the medial bicipital groove. Deep to the latter is the main neurovascular bundle of the limb.

No part of the shaft of the humerus is subcutaneous; however, it can be palpated with varying distinctness ▶

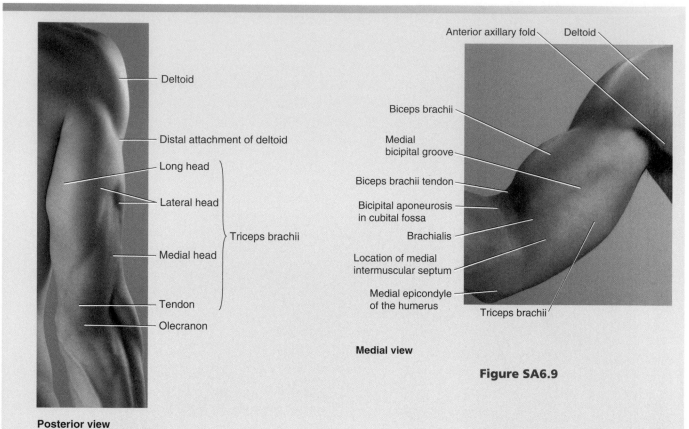

Deltoid

Distal attachment of deltoid

Long head

Lateral head

Triceps brachii

Medial head

Tendon

Olecranon

Posterior view

Figure SA6.8

Anterior axillary fold   Deltoid

Biceps brachii

Medial
bicipital groove

Biceps brachii tendon

Bicipital aponeurosis
in cubital fossa

Brachialis

Location of medial
intermuscular septum

Medial epicondyle
of the humerus

Triceps brachii

Medial view

Figure SA6.9

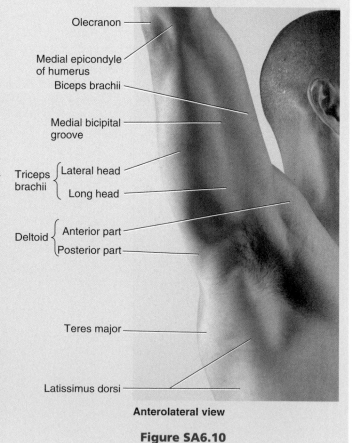

Olecranon

Medial epicondyle
of humerus

Biceps brachii

Medial bicipital
groove

Triceps
brachii { Lateral head

Long head

Deltoid { Anterior part

Posterior part

Teres major

Latissimus dorsi

Anterolateral view

Figure SA6.10

through the muscles surrounding it, especially in many elderly people. The **head of the humerus** is surrounded by muscles on all sides, except inferiorly; thus it can be palpated by pushing the fingers well up into the axilla. The arm should be close to the side so the axillary fascia is loose. The humeral head can be identified by its movements when the arm is moved and the inferior angle of the scapula is held so the scapula does not move. The *brachial artery* may be felt pulsating deep to the medial border of the biceps. The medial and lateral **epicondyles of the humerus** are subcutaneous and can be easily palpated at the medial and lateral aspects of the elbow. The medial epicondyle is more prominent.

In the cubital fossa, the *cephalic* and *basilic veins* in the subcutaneous tissue are clearly visible when a tourniquet is applied to the arm, as is the *median cubital vein*. This vein crosses the bicipital aponeurosis as it runs superomedially connecting the cephalic to the basilic vein (Figs. SA6.11 and 6.38A). If the thumb is pressed into the cubital fossa, the muscular masses of the **long flexors of the forearm** will be felt forming the medial border, the pronator teres most directly. The **lateral group of forearm extensors** (a soft mass that can be grasped separately), the brachioradialis (most medial) and the long and short extensors of the wrist, can be grasped between the fossa and the lateral epicondyle. ▶

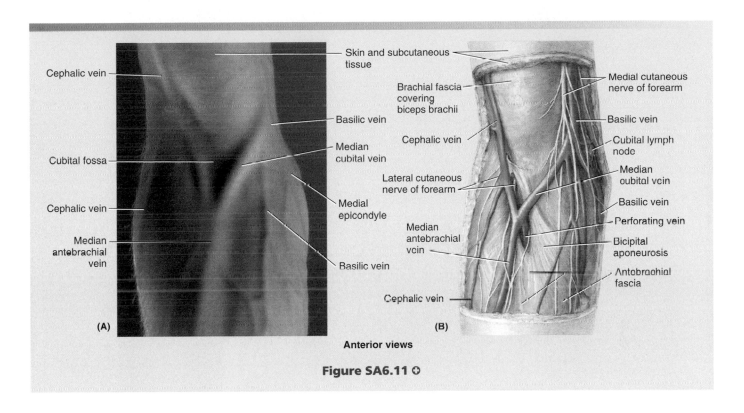

Anterior views

Figure SA6.11 ⊕

Forearm

The **forearm** is the distal unit of the articulated strut of the upper limb. It extends from the elbow to the wrist and contains two bones, the *radius* and *ulna* (Fig. 6.37*A, B,* & *D*), which are joined by an interosseous membrane. Although thin, this fibrous membrane is strong. In addition to firmly tying the forearm bones together while permitting pronation and supination, the *interosseous membrane* provides the proximal attachment for some deep forearm muscles. The head of the ulna is at the distal end of the forearm, whereas the head of the radius is at its proximal end. The role of forearm movement, occurring at the elbow and radioulnar joints, is to assist the shoulder in the application of force and in controlling the placement of the hand in space.

Compartments of the Forearm

As in the arm, the muscles of similar purpose and innervation are grouped within the same fascial compartments in the forearm. Although the proximal boundary of the forearm per se is defined by the joint plane of the elbow, functionally the forearm includes the distal humerus. For the distal forearm, wrist, and hand to have minimal bulk to maximize their functionality, they are operated by "remote control" by extrinsic muscles having their bulky, fleshy, contractile parts located proximally in the forearm, distant from the site of action. Their long, slender tendons extend distally to the operative site, like long ropes reaching to distant pulleys. Furthermore, because the structures on which the muscles and tendons act (wrist and fingers) have an extensive range of motion, a long range of contraction is needed, requiring that the muscles have long contractile parts as well as a long tendon(s).

The forearm proper is not, in fact, long enough to provide the required length and sufficient area for attachment proximally, so the proximal attachments (origins) of the muscles must occur proximal to the elbow—in the arm—and be provided by the humerus. Generally, flexors lie anteriorly and extensors posteriorly; however, the anterior and posterior aspects of the distal humerus are occupied by the chief flexors and extensors of the elbow (Fig. 6.38*A*). To provide the required attachment sites for the flexors and extensors of the wrist and fingers, medial and lateral extensions (epicondyles and supraepicondylar ridges) have developed from the distal humerus. The medial epicondyle and supraepicondylar ridge provide attachment for the forearm flexors, and the lateral formations provide attachment for the forearm extensors. Thus rather than lying strictly anteriorly and posteriorly, the proximal parts of the "anterior" (flexor–pronator) compartment of the forearm lie anteromedially, and the "posterior" (extensor–supinator) compartment lies posterolaterally (Figs. 6.37*D*, 6.38*B,* and 6.40*C*). Spiraling gradually over the length of the forearm, the compartments become truly anterior and posterior in position in the distal forearm and wrist. These fascial compartments, containing the muscles in functional groups, are demarcated by the subcutaneous border of the ulna posteriorly (in the proximal forearm) and then medially (distal forearm) and by the radial artery anteriorly and then laterally. These structures are palpable (the artery by its pulsations) throughout the forearm. Because neither boundary is crossed by motor nerves, they also provide sites for surgical incision.

(A) Posterior view

(B) Lateral view

(C) Transverse section of forearm (at level indicated in part B)

Figure 6.40. Extensor muscles of right forearm. A. The superficial layer of extensor muscles is shown. The distal extensor tendons have been removed from the dorsum of the hand without disturbing the arteries because they lie on the skeletal plane. The fascia on the posterior aspect of the forearm is thickened to form the extensor retinaculum, which is anchored on its deep aspect to the radius and ulna. **B.** The deep layer of extensor muscles is shown. Three outcropping muscles of the thumb* emerge from between the extensor carpi radialis brevis and the extensor digitorum: abductor pollicis longus, extensor pollicis brevis, and extensor pollicis longus. The furrow from which the three muscles emerge has been opened proximally to the lateral epicondyle, exposing the supinator muscle. **C.** This transverse section of the forearm shows the superficial and deep layers of muscles in the posterior compartment (*pink*), supplied by the radial nerve, and the anterior compartment (*gold*), supplied by the ulnar and median nerves. Figure 6.38*B* also demonstrates these concepts.

The flexors and pronators of the forearm are in the anterior compartment and are served mainly by the *median nerve;* the one and a half exceptions are innervated by the *ulnar nerve.* The extensors and supinators of the forearm are in the posterior compartment and are all served by the radial nerve (directly or by its deep branch). The fascial compartments of the limbs generally end at the joints; therefore, fluids and infections in compartments are usually contained and cannot readily spread to other compartments. The anterior compartment is exceptional in this regard because it communicates with the central compartment of the palm through the carpal tunnel (Fig. 6.38C).

Muscles of the Forearm

There are 17 muscles crossing the elbow joint, some of which act on the elbow joint exclusively, whereas others act at the wrist and fingers. In the proximal part of the forearm, the muscles form fleshy masses extending inferiorly from the medial and lateral epicondyles of the humerus (Figs. 6.37C and 6.38A). The tendons of these muscles pass through the distal part of the forearm and continue into the wrist, hand, and fingers (Figs. 6.37C & E and 6.38C). The flexor muscles of the anterior compartment have approximately twice the bulk and strength of the extensor muscles of the posterior compartment.

Flexor–Pronator Muscles of the Forearm

The **flexor muscles of the forearm** are in the anterior (flexor–pronator) compartment of the forearm and are separated from the **extensor muscles of the forearm** by the radius and ulna (Fig. 6.38B) and, in the distal two thirds of the forearm, by the interosseous membrane that connects them (Fig. 6.37B & D). The tendons of most flexor muscles are located on the anterior surface of the wrist and are held in place by the **palmar carpal ligament** and the *flexor retinaculum* (*transverse carpal ligament*), thickenings of the antebrachial fascia (Figs. 6.37C and 6.39). The flexor muscles are arranged in three layers or groups (Table 6.7):

1. A **superficial layer or group** of four muscles (pronator teres, flexor carpi radialis, palmaris longus, and flexor carpi ulnaris). These muscles are all attached proximally by a *common flexor tendon* to the medial epicondyle of the humerus, the *common flexor attachment.*

2. An **intermediate layer,** consisting of one muscle (flexor digitorum superficialis).

3. A **deep layer or group** of three muscles (flexor digitorum profundus, flexor pollicis longus, and pronator quadratus).

The five superficial and intermediate muscles cross the elbow joint; the three deep muscles do not. With the exception of the *pronator quadratus,* the more distally placed a muscle's distal attachment lies, the more distally and deeply placed is its proximal attachment.

All muscles in the anterior compartment of the forearm are supplied by the median and/or ulnar nerves (most by the median; only one and a half exceptions are supplied by the ulnar). Functionally, the brachioradialis is a flexor of the forearm, but it is located in the posterior (posterolateral) or extensor compartment and is thus supplied by the radial nerve. Therefore, the brachioradialis is a major exception to the rule that (1) the radial nerve supplies only extensor muscles and (2) that all flexors lie in the anterior (flexor) compartment.

The **long flexors of the digits** (flexor digitorum superficialis and flexor digitorum profundus) also flex the metacarpophalangeal and wrist joints. The flexor digitorum profundus flexes the fingers in slow action; this action is reinforced by the flexor digitorum superficialis when speed and flexion against resistance are required. When the wrist is flexed at the same time that the metacarpophalangeal and interphalangeal joints are flexed, the long flexor muscles of the fingers are operating over a shortened distance between attachments, and the action resulting from their contraction is consequently weaker. Extending the wrist increases their operating distance, and thus their contraction is more efficient in producing a strong grip (Fig. 6.48). Tendons of the long flexors of the digits pass through the distal part of the forearm, wrist, and palm and continue to the medial four fingers. The flexor digitorum superficialis flexes the middle phalanges, and the flexor digitorum profundus flexes the distal phalanges.

The attachments, innervation, and main actions of the muscles of the anterior compartment of the forearm are listed by layers, in Table 6.7. The following discussion provides additional details, beginning with the muscles of the superficial and intermediate layers.

Pronator Teres. The **pronator teres,** a fusiform muscle, is the most lateral of the superficial forearm flexors. Its lateral border forms the medial boundary of the cubital fossa.

To test the pronator teres, the person's forearm is flexed at the elbow and pronated from the supine position against resistance provided by the examiner. If acting normally, the muscle is prominent and can be palpated at the medial margin of the cubital fossa.

Flexor Carpi Radialis. The **flexor carpi radialis** (FCR) is a long fusiform muscle located medial to the pronator teres. In the middle of the forearm, its fleshy belly is replaced by a long, flattened tendon that becomes cord-like as it approaches the wrist. The FCR produces flexion (when acting with the flexor carpi ulnaris) and abduction of the wrist (when acting with the extensors carpi radialis longus and brevis). When acting alone, the FCR produces a combination of flexion and abduction simultaneously at the wrist so that the hand moves anterolaterally. To reach its distal attachment, the FCR tendon passes through a canal in the lateral part of the flexor retinaculum and through a vertical groove in the trapezium in its own synovial **tendinous sheath of the flexor carpi radialis** (Fig. 6.38C). The FCR tendon is a good guide to the radial artery, which lies just lateral to it (Fig. 6.37C).

To test the flexor carpi radialis, the person is asked to flex the wrist against resistance. If acting normally, its tendon can be easily seen and palpated.

Table 6.7. Muscles of the Anterior Compartment of the Forearm

Pronator teres
Common flexor origin
Flexor digitorum superficialis (humeroulnar head)
Pronator teres, ulnar head
Flexor digitorum superficialis (radial head)
Pronator teres
Flexor digitorum profundus
Flexor pollicis longus
Pronator quadratus
Adductor pollicis (oblique head)
Flexor carpi radialis
Flexor pollicis longus
Flexor digitorum superficialis
Flexor digitorum profundus

(A)

Flexor carpi ulnaris
Pisohamate ligament
Pisometacarpal ligament

Pronator teres
Flexor carpi radialis
Palmaris longus
Flexor carpi ulnaris (FCU)

(B) First layer

Flexor pollicis longus (FPL)
Humeroular head
Radial head
Flexor digitorum superficialis (FDS)

(C) Second layer

Flexor digitorum profundus (FDP)

(D) Third layer

Pronator quadratus

(E) Fourth layer

Anterior views

Muscle	Proximal Attachment	Distal Attachment	Innervation[a]	Main Action
Superficial (first) layer				
Pronator teres		Middle of convexity of lateral surface of radius	Median nerve (C6, **C7**)	Pronates and flexes forearm (at elbow)
Ulnar head	Coronoid process			
Humeral head				
Flexor carpi radialis (FCR)		Base of 2nd metacarpal		Flexes and abducts hand (at wrist)
Palmaris longus	Medial epicondyle of humerus (common flexor origin)	Distal half of flexor retinaculum and apex of palmar aponeurosis	Median nerve (C7, C8)	Flexes hand (at wrist) and tenses palmar aponeurosis
Flexor carpi ulnaris (FCU)				Flexes and adducts hand (at wrist)
Humeral head		Pisiform, hook of hamate, 5th metacarpal	Ulnar nerve (C7, **C8**)	
Ulnar head	Olecranon and posterior border (via aponeurosis)			
Intermediate (second) layer				
Flexor digitorum superficialis (FDS)		Shafts (bodies) of middle phalanges of medial four fingers	Median nerve (C7, C8, T1)	Flexes middle phalanges at proximal interphalangeal joints of middle four fingers; acting more strongly, it also flexes proximal phalanges at metacarpophalangeal joints
Humeroulnar head	Medial epicondyle (common flexor origin and coronoid process)			
Radial head	Superior half of anterior border			

Table 6.7. Muscles of the Anterior Compartment of the Forearm *(continued)*

Muscle	Proximal Attachment	Distal Attachment	Innervation[a]	Main Action
Deep (third) layer				
Flexor digitorum profundus (FDP)	Proximal three quarters of medial and anterior surfaces of ulna and interosseous membrane	Bases of distal phalanges of 4th and 5th fingers	Ulnar nerve (C8, **T1**)	Flexes distal phalanges 4 and 5 at distal interphalangeal joints
Medial part				
Lateral part			Anterior interosseous nerve, from median nerve (**C8**, T1)	Flexes distal phalanges 2 and 3 at distal interphalangeal joints
Flexor pollicis longus (FPL)	Anterior surface of radius and adjacent interosseous membrane	Base of distal phalanx of thumb		Flexes phalanges of 1st digit (thumb)
Pronator quadratus	Distal quarter of anterior surface of ulna	Distal quarter of anterior surface of radius		Pronates forearm; deep fibers bind radius and ulna together

[a]The spinal cord segmental innervation is indicated (o.g., "C6, **C7**" means that the nerves supplying the pronator teres are derived from the sixth and seventh cervical segments of the spinal cord). Numbers in boldface (**C7**) indicate the main segmental innervation. Damage to one or more of the listed spinal cord segments or to the motor nerve roots arising from them results in paralysis of the muscles concerned.

Palmaris Longus. The **palmaris longus,** a small fusiform muscle, is absent on one or both sides (usually the left) in approximately 14% of people, but its actions are not missed. It has a short belly and a long, cord-like tendon that passes superficial to the flexor retinaculum and attaches to it and the apex of the palmar aponeurosis (Figs. 6.37C and 6.39). The palmaris longus tendon is a useful guide to the median nerve at the wrist. The tendon lies deep and slightly medial to this nerve before it passes deep to the flexor retinaculum.

To test the palmaris longus, the wrist is flexed and the pads of the little finger and thumb are tightly pinched together. If present and acting normally, the tendon can be easily seen and palpated.

Flexor Carpi Ulnaris. The **flexor carpi ulnaris** (FCU) is the most medial of the superficial flexor muscles. The FCU simultaneously flexes and adducts the hand at the wrist if acting alone. It flexes the wrist when it acts with the FCR and adducts it when acting with the extensor carpi ulnaris. The ulnar nerve enters the forearm by passing between the humeral and the ulnar heads of its proximal attachment (Fig. 6.37C). This muscle is exceptional among muscles of the anterior compartment, being fully innervated by the ulnar nerve. The tendon of the FCU is a guide to the ulnar nerve and artery, which are on its lateral side at the wrist (Fig. 6.37C & E).

To test the flexor carpi ulnaris, the person puts the posterior aspect of the forearm and hand on a flat table and is then asked to flex the wrist against resistance while the examiner palpates the muscle and its tendon.

Flexor Digitorum Superficialis. The **flexor digitorum superficialis** (FDS) is often included with the superficial muscles of the forearm, which attach to the common flexor origin and therefore cross the elbow (Table 6.7). When considered this way, it is the largest superficial muscle in the forearm. However, the FDS actually forms an intermediate layer between the superficial and the deep groups of forearm muscles

(Fig. 6.37C & E). The median nerve and ulnar artery enter the forearm by passing between its humeroulnar and radial heads (Table 6.7A & C). Near the wrist, the FDS gives rise to four tendons, which pass deep to the flexor retinaculum through the carpal tunnel to the fingers. The four tendons are enclosed (along with the four tendons of the flexor digitorum profundus) in a synovial *common flexor sheath* (Fig. 6.38C). The FDS flexes the middle phalanges of the medial four fingers at the proximal interphalangeal joints. In continued action, the FDS also flexes the proximal phalanges at the metacarpophalangeal joints and the wrist joint. The FDS is capable of flexing each finger it serves independently.

To test the flexor digitorum superficialis, one finger is flexed at the proximal interphalangeal joint against resistance and the other three fingers are held in an extended position to inactivate the flexor digitorum profundus.

The fascial plane between the intermediate and the deep layers of muscles makes up the primary neurovascular plane of the anterior (flexor–pronator) compartment; the main neurovascular bundles exclusive to this compartment course within it.

The following three muscles form the deep layer of forearm flexor muscles.

Flexor Digitorum Profundus. The **flexor digitorum profundus** (FDP) is the only muscle that can flex the distal interphalangeal joints of the fingers (Fig. 6.37E). This thick muscle "clothes" the anterior aspect of the ulna. The FDP flexes the distal phalanges of the medial four fingers after the FDS has flexed their middle phalanges (i.e., it curls the fingers and assists with flexion of the hand, making a fist). Each tendon is capable of flexing two interphalangeal joints, the metacarpophalangeal joint and the wrist joint. The FDP divides into four parts, which end in four tendons that pass posterior to the FDS tendons and the flexor retinaculum within the common flexor sheath (Fig. 6.38*C*). The part of the muscle going to the index finger usually separates from the rest of the muscle relatively early in the distal part of the forearm and is capable of independent contraction. Each tendon enters the fibrous sheath of its digit, posterior to the FDS tendons. Unlike the FDS, the FDP can flex only the index finger independently; thus the fingers can be independently flexed at the proximal but not the distal interphalangeal joints.

To test the flexor digitorum profundus, the proximal interphalangeal joint is held in the extended position while the person attempts to flex the distal interphalangeal joint. The integrity of the median nerve in the proximal forearm can be tested by performing this test using the index finger, and that of the ulnar nerve can be assessed by using the little finger.

Flexor Pollicis Longus. The **flexor pollicis longus** (FPL), the long flexor of the thumb (L. *pollex,* thumb), lies lateral to the FDP, where it clothes the anterior aspect of the radius distal to the attachment of the supinator (Fig. 6.37*C* & *E;* Table 6.7*A* & *D*). The flat FPL tendon passes deep to the flexor retinaculum, enveloped in its own synovial **tendinous sheath of the flexor pollicis longus** on the lateral side of the common flexor sheath (Fig. 6.38*C*). The FPL primarily flexes the distal phalanx of the thumb at the interphalangeal joint and, secondarily, the proximal phalanx and 1st metacarpal at the metacarpophalangeal and carpometacarpal joints, respectively. The FPL is the only muscle that flexes the interphalangeal joint of the thumb. It also may assist in flexion of the wrist joint.

To test the flexor pollicis longus, the proximal phalanx of the thumb is held and the distal phalanx is flexed against resistance.

Pronator Quadratus. The **pronator quadratus,** as its name indicates, is quadrangular and pronates the forearm (Figs. 6.37*E* and 6.39). It cannot be palpated or observed, except in dissections, because it is the deepest muscle in the anterior aspect of the forearm. Sometimes it is considered to constitute a fourth muscle layer. The pronator quadratus clothes the distal fourth of the radius and ulna and the interosseous membrane between them (Table 6.7*A* & *E*). The pronator quadratus is the only muscle that attaches only to the ulna at one end and only to the radius at the other end. The pronator quadratus is the prime mover for pronation. The muscle initiates pronation; it is assisted by the pronator teres when more speed and power are needed. The pronator quadratus also helps the interosseous membrane hold the radius and ulna together, particularly when upward thrusts are transmitted through the wrist (e.g., during a fall on the hand).

THE BOTTOM LINE: The superficial and intermediate muscles of the anterior (flexor–pronator) compartment of the forearm are located anteromedially because they arise mainly from the common flexor attachment (medial epicondyle and supraepicondylar ridge) of the humerus. Muscles in superficial layer "bend" the wrist to position the hand (i.e., flex the wrist when acting exclusively and abduct or adduct the wrist when working with their extensor counterparts) and assist pronation. The only muscle of the intermediate layer (FDS) primarily flexes the proximal joints of 2nd–5th fingers. Muscles of the deep layer attach to the anterior aspects of the radius and ulna, flex all (but especially the distal) joints of all five digits, and pronate the forearm. The muscles of the anterior compartment are innervated mostly by the median nerve, but one and a half muscles (the FCU and ulnar half of the FDP) are innervated by the ulnar nerve. The nerves and the ulnar artery traverse the compartment in the fascial plane between the intermediate and the deep layers of muscles. Flexion of the wrist and hand is used for grasping, gripping, and drawing things toward one self. Pronation is used for positioning the hand to manipulate or pick things up. Both movements are basic protective (defensive) movements.

Extensor Muscles of the Forearm

The **extensor muscles** are in the posterior (extensor–supinator) compartment of the forearm, and all are innervated by branches of the radial nerve (Figs. 6.40 and 6.41; Table 6.8). These muscles can be organized physiologically into three functional groups:

1. Muscles that extend and abduct or adduct the hand at the wrist joint (extensor carpi radialis longus, extensor carpi radialis brevis, and extensor carpi ulnaris).

2. Muscles that extend the medial four fingers (extensor digitorum, extensor indicis, and extensor digiti minimi).

3. Muscles that extend or abduct the thumb (abductor pollicis longus, extensor pollicis brevis, and extensor pollicis longus).

The extensor tendons are held in place in the wrist region by the *extensor retinaculum,* which prevents bowstringing of the tendons when the hand is extended at the wrist joint. As the tendons pass over the dorsum of the wrist, they are provided with **synovial tendon sheaths** that reduce friction for the extensor tendons as they traverse the osseofibrous tunnels formed by the attachment of the extensor retinaculum to the distal radius and ulna (Fig. 6.41).

The extensor muscles of the forearm are organized anatomically into superficial and deep layers. Four of the *superficial extensors* (extensor carpi radialis brevis, extensor digitorum, extensor digiti minimi, and extensor carpi ulnaris) are attached proximally by a *common extensor tendon* to the lateral epicondyle (Fig. 6.40; Table 6.8). The proximal attachment of the other two muscles in the superficial group (brachioradialis and extensor carpi radialis longus) is to the lateral supraepicondylar ridge of the humerus and adjacent lateral intermuscular septum. The four flat tendons of the extensor digitorum pass deep to the extensor retinaculum to the medial four fingers. The common tendons of the index and little fingers are joined on their medial sides near the knuckles by the respective tendons of the extensor indicis and extensor digiti minimi (extensors of the index and little fingers, respectively).

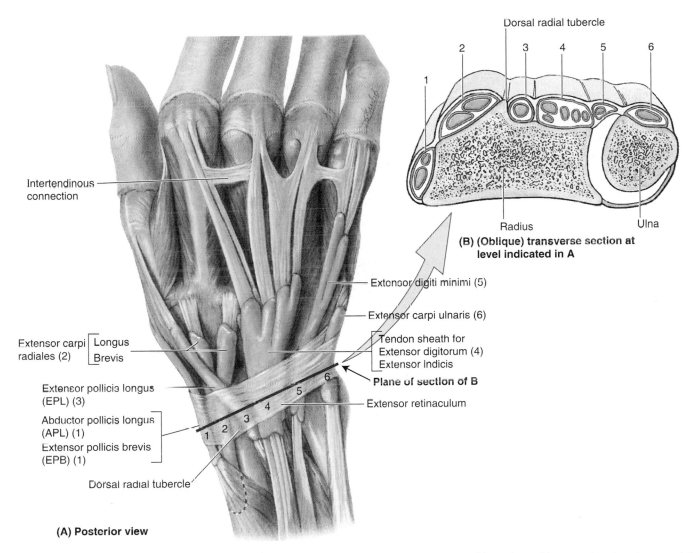

Intertendinous connection

Extensor carpi radiales (2) — Longus / Brevis

Extensor pollicis longus (EPL) (3)

Abductor pollicis longus (APL) (1)

Extensor pollicis brevis (EPB) (1)

Dorsal radial tubercle

(A) Posterior view

Extensor digiti minimi (5)

Extensor carpi ulnaris (6)

Tendon sheath for Extensor digitorum (4) Extensor indicis

Plane of section of B

Extensor retinaculum

Dorsal radial tubercle

Radius   Ulna

(B) (Oblique) transverse section at level indicated in A

Figure 6.41. Synovial sheaths and tendons on distal forearm and dorsum of hand. A. Observe that the six synovial tendon sheaths (*blue*) occupy six osseofibrous tunnels formed by attachments of the extensor retinaculum to the ulna and especially the radius, which give passage to 12 tendons of nine extensor muscles. Numbers refer to the labeled osseofibrous tunnels. **B.** This slightly oblique transverse section of the distal end of the forearm shows the extensor tendons traversing the six osseofibrous tunnels deep to the extensor retinaculum.

The attachments, innervation, and main actions of the muscles of the posterior compartment of the forearm are provided, by layer, in Table 6.8. The following discussion provides additional details.

Brachioradialis. The **brachioradialis,** a fusiform muscle, lies superficially on the anterolateral surface of the forearm (Figs. 6.39 and 6.40). It forms the lateral border of the cubital fossa (Fig. 6.38C). As mentioned previously, the brachioradialis is exceptional among muscles of the posterior (extensor) compartment in that it has rotated to the anterior aspect of the humerus and thus flexes the forearm at the elbow. It is especially active during quick movements or in the presence of resistance during flexion of the forearm (e.g., when a weight is lifted), acting as a shunt muscle resisting subluxation of the head of the radius. The brachioradialis and the supinator are the only muscles of the compartment that do not cross and

therefore are incapable of acting at the wrist. As it descends, the brachioradialis overlies the radial nerve and artery where they lie together on the supinator, pronator teres tendon, FDS, and FPL. The distal part of the tendon is covered by the abductors pollicis longus and brevis as they pass to the thumb (Fig. 6.40).

To test the brachioradialis, the elbow joint is flexed against resistance with the forearm in the midprone position. If the brachioradialis is acting normally, the muscle can be seen and palpated.

Extensor Carpi Radialis Longus. The **extensor carpi radialis longus** (ECRL), a fusiform muscle, is partly overlapped by the brachioradialis, with which it often blends (Figs. 6.40 and 6.41). As it passes distally, posterior to the brachioradialis, its tendon is crossed by the abductor pollicis brevis and extensor pollicis brevis. The ECRL is indispensable when clenching the fist.

Table 6.8. Muscles of the Posterior Compartment of the Forearm

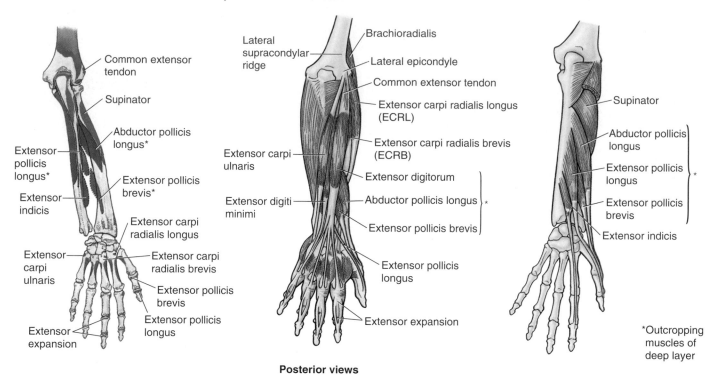

Posterior views

*Outcropping muscles of deep layer

Muscle	Proximal Attachment	Distal Attachment	Innervation[a]	Main Action
Superficial layer				
Brachioradialis	Proximal two thirds of supraepicondylar ridge of humerus	Lateral surface of distal end of radius proximal to styloid process	Radial nerve (C5, **C6**, C7)	Relatively week flexion of forearm, maximal when forearm is in midpronated position
Extensor carpi radialis longus (ECRL)	Lateral supraepicondylar ridge of humerus	Dorsal aspect of base of 2nd metacarpal	Radial nerve (C6, C7)	Extend and abduct hand at the wrist joint; ECRL active during fist clenching
Extensor carpi radialis brevis (ECRB)	Lateral epicondyle of humerus (common extensor origin)	Doral aspect of base of 3rd metacarpal	Deep branch of radial nerve (**C7**, C8)	
Extensor digitorum		Extensor expansions of medial four fingers	Posterior interosseous nerve (**C7**, C8), continuation of deep branch of radial nerve	Extends medial four fingers primarily at metacarpophalangeal joints, secondarily at interphalangeal joints
Extensor digiti minimi (EDM)		Extensor expansion of 5th finger		Extends 5th finger primarily at metacarpophalangeal joint, secondarily at interphalangeal joint
Extensor carpi ulnaris (ECU)	Lateral epicondyle of humerus; posterior border of ulna via a shared aponeurosis	Dorsal aspect of base of 5th metacarpal		Extends and adducts hand at wrist joint (also active during fist clenching)
Deep layer				
Supinator	Lateral epicondyle of humerus; radial collateral and anular ligaments; supinator fossa; crest of ulna	Lateral posterior, and anterior surfaces of proximal third of radius	Deep branch of radial nerve (C7, **C8**)	Supinates forearm; rotates radius to turn palm anteriorlyor superiorly (if elbow is flexed)

Table 6.8. Muscles of the Posterior Compartment of the Forearm *(continued)*

Muscle	Proximal Attachment	Distal Attachment	Innervation[a]	Main Action
Extensor indicis	Posterior surface of distal third of ulna and interosseous membrane	Extensor expansion of 2nd finger	Posterior interosseous nerve (C7, **C8**), continuation of deep branch of radial nerve	Extends 2nd finger (enabling its independent extension); helps extend hand at wrist
Outcropping muscles of deep layer				
Abductor pollicis longus (APL)	Posterior surface of proximal halves of ulna, radius, and interosseous membrane	Base of 1st metacarpal		Abducts thumb and extends it at carpometacarpal joint
Extensor pollicis longus (EPL)	Posterior surface of middle third of ulna and interosseous membrane	Dorsal aspect of base of distal phalanx of thumb	Posterior interosseous nerve (C7, **C8**), continuation of deep branch of radial nerve	Extends distal phalanx of thumb at interphalangeal joint; extends metacarpophalangeal and carpometacarpal joints
Extensor pollicis brevis (EPB)	Posterior surface of distal third of radius and interosseous membrane	Dorsal aspect of base of proximal phalanx of thumb		Extends proximal phalanx of thumb at metacarpophalangeal joint; extends carpometacarpal joint

[a] The spinal cord segmental innervation is indicated (e.g., "**C7**, C8" means that the nerves supplying the extensor carpi radialis brevis are derived from the seventh and eighth cervical segments of the spinal cord). Numbers in boldface (**C7**) indicate the main segmental innervation. Damage to one or more of the listed spinal cord segments or to the motor nerve roots arising from them results in paralysis of the muscles concerned.

To test the extensor carpi radialis longus, the wrist is extended and abducted with the forearm pronated. If acting normally, the muscle can be palpated inferoposterior to the lateral side of the elbow. Its tendon can be palpated proximal to the wrist.

Extensor Carpi Radialis Brevis. The **extensor carpi radialis brevis** (ECRB), as its name indicates, is a shorter muscle than the ECRL because it arises distally in the limb, yet it attaches adjacent to the ECRL in the hand (but to the base of the 3rd metacarpal rather than the 2nd). As it passes distally, it is covered by the ECRL. The ECRB and ECRL pass under the extensor retinaculum together within the **tendinous sheath of the extensor carpi radiales** (Fig. 6.41). The two muscles act together to various degrees, usually as synergists to other muscles. When the two muscles act by themselves, they abduct the hand as they extend it. Acting with the extensor carpi ulnaris, they extend the hand (the brevis is more involved in this action); acting with the FCR they produce pure abduction. Their synergistic action with the extensor carpi ulnaris is important in steadying the wrist during tight flexion of the medial four fingers (clenching a fist), a function in which the longus is more active.

Extensor Digitorum. The **extensor digitorum,** the principal extensor of the medial four fingers, occupies much of the posterior surface of the forearm (Figs. 6.40–6.42). Proximally its four tendons join the tendon of the extensor indicis to pass deep to the extensor retinaculum through the **tendinous sheath of the extensor digitorum and extensor indicis** (common extensor synovial sheath) (Fig. 6.41A & B). On the dorsum of the hand, the tendons spread out as they run toward the fingers. Adjacent tendons are linked proximal to the knuckles (metacarpophalangeal joints) by three oblique *inter-*

tendinous connections that restrict independent extension of the fingers (especially the ring finger). Consequently, normally no finger can remain fully flexed as the other ones are fully extended. Commonly, the fourth tendon is fused initially with the tendon to the ring finger and reaches the little finger by a tendinous band.

On the distal ends of the metacarpals and along the phalanges, the four tendons flatten to form **extensor expansions** (Fig. 6.42). Each extensor digital expansion (dorsal expansion or hood) is a triangular, tendinous aponeurosis that wraps around the dorsum and sides of a head of the metacarpal and proximal phalanx. The visor-like "hood" formed by the extensor expansion over the head of the metacarpal, holding the extensor tendon in the middle of the digit, is anchored on each side to the **palmar ligament** (a reinforced portion of the fibrous layer of the joint capsule of the metacarpophalangeal joints) (Fig. 6.42B & D). In forming the extensor expansion, each flexor digitorum tendon divides into a **median band,** which passes to the base of the middle phalanx, and two **lateral bands,** which pass to the base of the distal phalanx (Fig. 6.42D & E). The tendons of the interosseous and lumbrical muscles of the hand join the lateral bands of the extensor expansion (Fig. 6.42).

The **retinacular ligament** is a delicate fibrous band that runs from the proximal phalanx and fibrous digital sheath obliquely across the middle phalanx and two interphalangeal joints (Fig. 6.42C). It joins the extensor expansion to the distal phalanx. During flexion of the distal interphalangeal joint, the retinacular ligament becomes taut and pulls the proximal joint into flexion. Similarly, on extending the proximal joint, the distal joint is pulled by the retinacular ligament into nearly complete extension.

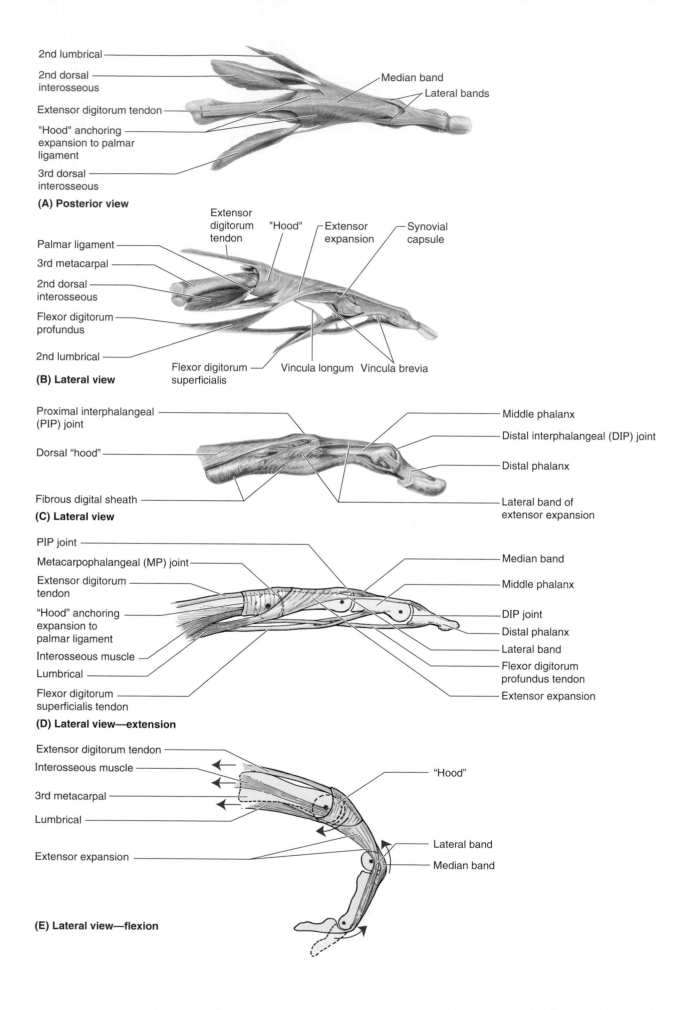

2nd lumbrical

2nd dorsal interosseous

Extensor digitorum tendon

"Hood" anchoring expansion to palmar ligament

3rd dorsal interosseous

Median band

Lateral bands

(A) Posterior view

Extensor digitorum tendon

"Hood"

Extensor expansion

Synovial capsule

Palmar ligament

3rd metacarpal

2nd dorsal interosseous

Flexor digitorum profundus

2nd lumbrical

Flexor digitorum superficialis

Vincula longum

Vincula brevia

(B) Lateral view

Proximal interphalangeal (PIP) joint

Dorsal "hood"

Fibrous digital sheath

Middle phalanx

Distal interphalangeal (DIP) joint

Distal phalanx

Lateral band of extensor expansion

(C) Lateral view

PIP joint

Metacarpophalangeal (MP) joint

Extensor digitorum tendon

"Hood" anchoring expansion to palmar ligament

Interosseous muscle

Lumbrical

Flexor digitorum superficialis tendon

Median band

Middle phalanx

DIP joint

Distal phalanx

Lateral band

Flexor digitorum profundus tendon

Extensor expansion

(D) Lateral view—extension

Extensor digitorum tendon

Interosseous muscle

3rd metacarpal

Lumbrical

Extensor expansion

"Hood"

Lateral band

Median band

(E) Lateral view—flexion

The extensor digitorum acts primarily to extend proximal phalanges and, through its collateral reinforcements, it secondarily extends the middle and distal phalanges as well. After exerting its traction on the digits, or in the presence of resistance to digital extension, it helps extend the hand at the wrist joint.

To test the extensor digitorum, the forearm is pronated and the fingers are extended. The person attempts to keep the fingers extended at the metacarpophalangeal joints as the examiner exerts pressure on the proximal phalanges by attempting to flex them. If acting normally, the extensor digitorum can be palpated in the forearm, and its tendons can be seen and palpated on the dorsum of the hand.

Extensor Digiti Minimi. The extensor digiti minimi (EDM), a fusiform slip of muscle, is a partially detached part of the extensor digitorum (Figs. 6.40 and 6.41). The tendon of this extensor of the little finger runs through a separate compartment of the extensor retinaculum, posterior to the distal radioulnar joint, within the **tendinous sheath of the extensor digiti minimi.** The tendon then divides into two slips; the lateral one is joined to the tendon of the extensor digitorum, with all three tendons attaching to the dorsal digital expansion of the little finger. After exerting its traction primarily on the 5th finger, it contributes to extension of the hand.

Extensor Carpi Ulnaris. The extensor carpi ulnaris (ECU), a long fusiform muscle located on the medial border of the forearm, has two heads: a humeral head from the common extensor tendon and an ulnar head that arises by a common aponeurosis attached to the posterior border of the ulna and shared by the FCU, FDP, and deep fascia of the forearm. Distally, its tendon runs in a groove between the ulnar head and its styloid process, through a separate compartment of the extensor retinaculum within the **tendinous sheath of the extensor carpi ulnaris.** Acting with the ECRL and ECRB, it extends the hand; acting with the FCU, it adducts the hand. Like the ECRL, it is indispensable when clenching the fist.

To test the extensor carpi ulnaris, the forearm is pronated and the fingers are extended. The extended wrist is then adducted against resistance. If acting normally, the muscle can

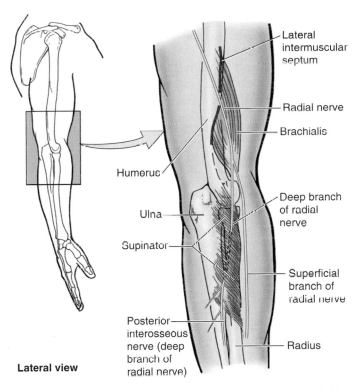

Lateral view

Figure 6.43. Relationship of radial nerve to brachialis and supinator muscles. In the cubital fossa, lateral to the brachialis, the radial nerve divides into deep (motor) and superficial (sensory) branches. The deep branch penetrates the supinator muscle and emerges in the posterior compartment of the forearm as the posterior interosseous nerve. It joins the artery of the same name to run in the plane between the superficial and the deep extensors of the forearm.

be seen and palpated in the proximal part of the forearm and its tendon can be felt proximal to the head of the ulna.

Supinator. The **supinator** lies deep in the cubital fossa and, along with the brachialis, forms its floor (Figs. 6.40 and 6.43). Spiraling medially and distally from its continuous, osseofibrous origin, this sheet-like muscle envelops the neck and proximal part of the shaft of the radius. The deep branch

Figure 6.42. Dorsal digital (extensor) apparatus of 3rd digit. The metacarpal bone and all three phalanges are shown in parts **A, B, D,** and **E;** only the phalanges are shown in part **C. A.** This posterior view shows the extensor digitorum tendon trifurcating (expanding) into three bands: two lateral bands that unite over the middle phalanx to insert into the base of the distal phalanx, and one median band that inserts into the base of the middle phalanx. **B.** Part of the tendon of the interosseous muscles attaches to the base of the proximal phalanx; the other part contributes to the extensor expansion, attaching primarily to the lateral bands, but also fans out into an aponeurosis. Some of the aponeurotic fibers fuse with the median band, and other fibers arch over it to blend with the aponeurosis arising from the other side. On the radial side of each digit, a lumbrical muscle attaches to the radial lateral band. The dorsal hood consists of a broad band of transversely oriented fibers attached anteriorly to the palmar ligaments of the metacarpophalangeal (MP) joints that encircle the metacarpal head and MP joint, blending with the extensor expansion to keep the apparatus centered over the dorsal aspect of the digit. **C.** Distally, retinacular ligaments extending from the fibrous digital sheath to the lateral bands also help keep the apparatus centered and coordinate movements at the proximal interphalangeal (PIP) and distal interphalangeal (DIP) joints. **D.** Contraction of the extensor digitorum alone results in extension at all joints (including the MP joint in the absence of action by the interossei and lumbricals). **E.** Because of the relationship of the tendons and the lateral bands to the rotational centers of the joints (*red dots* in parts **D** and **E**), simultaneous contraction of the interossei and lumbricals produces flexion at the MP joint but extension at the PIP and DIP joints (the so-called Z-movement).

of the radial nerve passes between its muscle fibers, separating them into superficial and deep parts, as it passes from the cubital fossa to the posterior part of the arm. As it exits the muscle and joins the posterior interosseous artery, it may be referred to as the posterior interosseous nerve. The supinator is the prime mover for slow, unopposed supination, especially when the forearm is extended. The biceps brachii also supinates the forearm and is the prime mover during rapid and forceful supination against resistance when the forearm is flexed (e.g., when a right-handed person drives a screw).

The **deep extensors of the forearm** act on the thumb (abductor pollicis longus, extensor pollicis longus, and extensor pollicis brevis) and the index finger (extensor indicis) (Figs. 6.40 and 6.41; Table 6.8). The three muscles acting on the thumb are deep to the superficial extensors and "crop out" (emerge) from the furrow in the lateral part of the forearm that divides the extensors. Because of this characteristic, they are referred to as *outcropping muscles* (Fig. 6.40A).

Abductor Pollicis Longus. The **abductor pollicis longus** (APL) has a long, fusiform belly that lies just distal to the supinator and is closely related to the extensor pollicis brevis. Its tendon, and sometimes its belly, is commonly split into two parts, one of which may attach to the trapezium instead of the usual site at the base of the 1st metacarpal. The APL acts with the abductor pollicis brevis during abduction of the thumb and with the extensor pollicis muscles during extension of this digit. Although deeply situated, the APL emerges at the wrist as one of the outcropping muscles. Its tendon passes deep to the extensor retinaculum with the tendon of the extensor pollicis brevis in the common synovial **tendinous sheath of the abductor pollicis longus and extensor pollicis brevis.**

To test the abductor pollicis longus, the thumb is abducted against resistance at the metacarpophalangeal joint. If acting normally, the tendon of the muscle can be seen and palpated at the lateral side of the *anatomical snuff box* and on the lateral side of the adjacent extensor pollicis brevis tendon.

Extensor Pollicis Brevis. The belly of the **extensor pollicis brevis** (EPB), the fusiform short extensor of the thumb, lies distal to the APL and is partly covered by it. Its tendon lies parallel and immediately medial to that of the APL but extends farther, reaching the base of the proximal phalanx (Fig. 6.41). In continued action after acting to flex the proximal phalanx of the thumb, or acting when that joint is fixed by its antagonists, it helps extend the 1st metacarpal and extend and abduct the hand. When the thumb is fully extended, a hollow called the *anatomical snuff box,* can be seen on the radial aspect of the wrist (Fig. 6.44).

To test the extensor pollicis brevis, the thumb is extended against resistance at the metacarpophalangeal joint. If the EPB is acting normally, the tendon of the muscle can be seen and palpated at the lateral side of the anatomical snuff box and on the medial side of the adjacent APL tendon (Figs. 6.40 and 6.41).

Extensor Pollicis Longus. The **extensor pollicis longus** (EPL) is larger and its tendon is longer than that of the EPB

(Figs. 6.40 and 6.41). The tendon passes under the extensor retinaculum in its own tunnel, within the **tendinous sheath of the extensor pollicis longus,** medial to the dorsal tubercle of the radius. It uses the tubercle as a trochlea (pulley) to change its line of pull as it proceeds to the base of the distal phalanx of the thumb. The gap thus created between the long extensor tendons of the thumb is the *anatomical snuff box.* In addition to its main actions (Table 6.8), the EPL also adducts the extended thumb and rotates it laterally.

To test the extensor pollicis longus, the thumb is extended against resistance at the interphalangeal joint. If the EPL is acting normally, the tendon of the muscle can be seen and palpated on the medial side of the anatomical snuff box.

The tendons of the APL and EPB bound the **anatomical snuff box** anteriorly, and the tendon of the EPL bounds it posteriorly (Figs. 6.40, 6.41, and 6.44). The snuff box is visible when the thumb is fully extended; this draws the tendons up and produces a triangular hollow between them. Observe that the:

- *Radial artery* lies in the floor of the snuff box.

- *Radial styloid process* can be palpated proximally and the

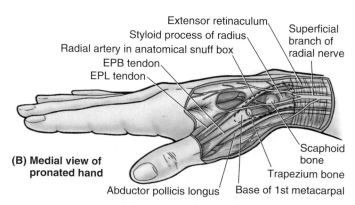

Extensor pollicis longus (EPL) tendon

(A) Medial view of pronated hand

Extensor pollicis brevis (EPB) tendon

Anatomical snuff box

Extensor retinaculum
Styloid process of radius
Radial artery in anatomical snuff box
EPB tendon
EPL tendon
Superficial branch of radial nerve

(B) Medial view of pronated hand

Abductor pollicis longus

Scaphoid bone
Trapezium bone
Base of 1st metacarpal

Figure 6.44. Anatomical snuff box. A. When the thumb is extended, a triangular hollow appears between the tendon of the extensor pollicis longus (EPL) medially and the tendons of the extensor pollicis brevis (EPB) and abductor pollicis longus (APL) laterally. **B.** The floor of the snuff box, formed by the scaphoid and trapezium bones, is crossed by the radial artery as it passes diagonally from the anterior surface of the radius to the dorsal surface of the hand.

Elbow Tendinitis or Lateral Epicondylitis

Elbow tendinitis (tennis elbow) is a painful musculoskeletal condition that may follow repetitive use of the superficial extensor muscles of the forearm. Pain is felt over the lateral epicondyle and radiates down the posterior surface of the forearm. People with elbow tendinitis often feel pain when they open a door or lift a glass. Repeated forceful flexion and extension of the wrist strain the attachment of the common extensor tendon, producing inflammation of the periosteum of the lateral epicondyle (*lateral epicondylitis*).

Mallet or Baseball Finger

Sudden severe tension on a long extensor tendon may avulse part of its attachment to the phalanx. The most common result of the injury is a *mallet or baseball finger* (Fig. B6.19*A*). This deformity results from the distal interphalangeal joint suddenly being forced into extreme flexion (hyperflexion when, for example, a baseball is miscaught or a finger is jammed into the base pad (Fig. B6.19*B*). These actions avulse the attachment of the tendon to the base of the distal phalanx. As a result, the person cannot extend the distal interphalangeal joint. The resultant deformity bears some resemblance to a mallet.

Fracture of the Olecranon

Fracture of the olecranon, called a "fractured elbow" by laypersons, is common because the olecranon is subcutaneous and protrusive. The typical mechanism of injury is a fall on the elbow combined with sudden powerful contraction of the triceps. The fractured olecranon is pulled away by the active and tonic contraction of the triceps (Fig. B6.20), and the injury is often considered to be an avulsion fracture (Salter, 1999). This is a serious fracture requiring the services of an orthopedic surgeon. Because of the traction produced by the tonus of the triceps on the olecranon fragment, pinning is usually required. Healing occurs slowly, and often a cast must be worn for nearly a year.

Synovial Cyst of the Wrist

Sometimes a non-tender cystic swelling appears on the hand, most commonly on the dorsum of the wrist (Fig. B6.21). Usually the cyst is the size of a small grape, but it varies and may be as large as a plum. The thin-walled cyst contains clear mucinous fluid. The cause of the cyst is unknown, but it may result from mucoid degeneration (Salter, 1999). Flexion of the wrist makes the cyst enlarge, and it may be painful. Clinically, this type of swelling is called a "ganglion" (G. swelling or knot). ▶

(A)

(B)

Figure B6.19. Mallet finger. The clinical appearance (**A**) and mechanism of injury (**B**) are shown.

Figure B6.20

Anatomically, a ganglion refers to a collection of nerve cells (e.g., a spinal ganglion). These synovial cysts are close to and often communicate with the synovial sheaths on the dorsum of the wrist. The distal attachment of the ECRB tendon to the base of the 3rd metacarpal is another common site for such a cyst. A cystic swelling of the common flexor synovial sheath on the anterior aspect of the wrist can enlarge enough to produce compression

of the median nerve by narrowing the carpal tunnel (*carpal tunnel syndrome*). This syndrome produces pain and paresthesia in the sensory distribution of the median nerve and clumsiness of finger movements (see clinical correlation [blue] box "Carpal Tunnel Syndrome," earlier in this chapter. ⊕

Figure B6.21

base of the 1st metacarpal can be palpated distally in the snuff box.

- *Scaphoid* and *trapezium* can be felt in the floor of the snuff box between the radial styloid process and the 1st metacarpal (see clinical correlation [blue] box "Fracture of the Scaphoid," earlier in this chapter).

Extensor Indicis. The **extensor indicis** has a narrow, elongated belly that lies medial to and alongside that of the EPL (Figs. 6.40 and 6.41). This muscle confers independence to the index finger in that the extensor indicis may act alone or together with the extensor digitorum to extend the index finger at the proximal interphalangeal joint, as in pointing. It also helps extend the hand.

THE BOTTOM LINE: Proximally, the extensor–supinator muscles are located posterolaterally. Generally, the more distal their distal attachment (insertion) the more distal and more deeply placed is their proximal attachment (origin). Thus the most proximal muscle (brachioradialis) does not cross and thus cannot act at the wrist (true also of the supinator). The next most proximal muscles act to "bend" the wrist (extend or act with their flexor counterparts to abduct and adduct). The most distal muscles, which make up the deep layer, act at the thumb and index finger. The extensors of the wrist and hand enable reach (extension),

opening of the hand in preparation for grasping, and pushing; supination enables the holding of objects and feeding. Extension is an aggressive movement (hitting, striking, pushing). Extension of the wrist, however, is also an important component of tight grip (clenching).

Arteries of the Forearm

The main arteries of the forearm are the ulnar and radial arteries, which usually arise opposite the neck of the radius in the inferior part of the cubital fossa as terminal branches of the brachial artery (Fig. 6.45). The origins and courses of the named arteries of the forearm are described in Table 6.9. The following discussion provides additional details.

Ulnar Artery

Pulsations of the **ulnar artery** can be palpated on the lateral side of the FCU tendon, where it lies anterior to the ulnar head. The ulnar nerve is on the medial side of the ulnar artery. Branches of the ulnar artery arising in the forearm participate in the periarticular anastomosis of the elbow and supply muscles of the medial and central forearm, the common flexor sheath, and the ulnar and median nerves.

- The *anterior* and *posterior ulnar recurrent arteries* anastomose with the inferior and superior ulnar collateral arteries, respectively, thereby participating in the periarticular arterial anastomoses of the elbow. The anterior and poste-

(cont'd on page 817)

Biceps
Brachial artery
Median nerve

Ulnar nerve
Triceps
Medial intermuscular septum

Pronator teres

Flexor carpi radialis

Brachioradialis

Radial nerve
Superficial branch
Deep branch

Brachialis

Radial recurrent artery

Nerve to:
Flexor carpi ulnaris
Flexor digitorum profundus

Ulnar artery

Supinator

Pronator teres

Flexor carpi ulnaris (FCU)

Radial artery

Ulnar nerve and ulnar artery

Flexor digitorum superficialis (FDS)

FDS (radial head)

Flexor digitorum profundus

Flexor pollicis longus

Pronator quadratus

Pronator quadratus

Dorsal (cutaneous) branch of ulnar nerve

Palmar carpal branch of radial artery

Dorsal carpal branch of ulnar artery

Flexor digitorum profundus

Superficial palmar branch

Persisting median artery
Median nerve

Palmar radiocarpal ligament

Flexor carpi radialis

Palmaris longus

Anterior view

Figure 6.45. Flexor digitorum superficialis and related vasculature. Three muscles of the superficial layer (pronator teres, flexor carpi radialis, and palmaris longus) have been removed, leaving only their attaching ends; the fourth muscle of the layer (the flexor carpi ulnaris) has been retracted medially. The tendinous humeral attachment of the FDS to the medial epicondyle is thick; and the linear attachment to the radius, immediately distal to the radial attachments of the supinator and pronator teres, is thin (Table 6.7). The ulnar artery and median nerve pass between the humeral and the radial heads of the FDS. The artery descends obliquely deep to the FDS to join the ulnar nerve, which descends vertically near the medial border of the FDS (exposed here by splitting a fusion of the FDS and the FCU). A (proximal) probe is elevating the FDS tendons (and median nerve and persisting median artery). A second (distal) probe is elevating all the remaining structures that cross the wrist (radiocarpal) joint anteriorly.

Table 6.9. Arteries of the Forearm and Wrist

Brachial artery
Deep artery of arm
Radial collateral artery
Radial recurrent artery
Recurrent interosseous artery
Posterior interosseous artery
Radial artery
Palmar carpal arch
Deep palmar arch

Superior ulnar collateral artery
Inferior ulnar collateral artery
Brachial artery
Anterior and posterior ulnar recurrent arteries
Common interosseous artery
Ulnar artery
Anterior interosseous artery
Palmar carpal branch of radial artery
Superficial palmar arch

Palmar view

Dorsal carpal branch of ulnar artery
Anterior interosseous artery
Posterior interosseous artery

Radial artery
Dorsal carpal arch

Posterior view

Artery	Origin	Course in Forearm
Ulnar	As larger terminal branch of brachial artery in cubital fossa	Descends inferomedially and then directly inferiorly, deep to superficial (pronator teres and palmaris longus) and intermediate (flexor digitorum superficialis) layers of flexor muscles to reach medial side of forearm; passes superficial to flexor retinaculum at wrist in ulnar (Guyon) canal to enter hand
Anterior ulnar recurrent artery	Ulnar artery just distal to elbow joint	Passes superiorly between brachialis and pronator teres, supplying both; then anastomoses with inferior ulnar collateral artery anterior to medial epicondyle
Posterior ulnar recurrent artery	Ulnar artery distal to anterior ulnar recurrent artery	Passes superiorly, posterior to medial epicondyle and deep to tendon of flexor carpi ulnaris; then anastomoses with superior ulnar collateral artery
Common interosseous	Ulnar artery in cubital fossa, distal to bifurcation of brachial artery	Passes laterally and deeply, terminating quickly by dividing into anterior and posterior interosseous arteries
Anterior interosseous	As terminal branches of common interosseous artery, between radius and ulna	Passes distally on anterior aspect of interosseous membrane to proximal border of pronator quadratus; pierces membrane and continues distally to join dorsal carpal arch on posterior aspect of interosseous membrane
Posterior interosseous		Passes to posterior aspect of interosseous membrane, giving rise to recurrent interosseous artery; runs distally between superficial and deep extensor muscles, supplying both; replaced distally by anterior interosseous artery
Recurrent interosseous	Posterior interosseous artery, between radius and ulna	Passes superiorly, posterior to proximal radioulnar joint and capitulum, to anastomose with middle collateral artery (from deep brachial artery)
Palmar carpal branch	Ulnar artery in distal forearm	Runs across anterior aspect of wrist, deep to tendons of flexor digitorum profundus, to anastomose with the palmar carpal branch of the radial artery, forming palmar carpal arch
Dorsal carpal branch	Ulnar artery, proximal to pisiform	Passes across dorsal surface of wrist, deep to extensor tendons, to anastomose with dorsal carpal branch of radial artery, forming dorsal carpal arch

Table 6.9. Arteries of the Forearm and Wrist (*continued*)

Artery	Origin	Course in Forearm
Radial	As smaller terminal branch of brachial artery in cubital fossa	Runs inferolaterally under cover of brachioradialis; lies lateral to flexor carpi radialis tendon in distal forearm; winds around lateral aspect of radius and crosses floor of anatomical snuff box to pierce first dorsal interosseous muscle
Radial recurrent	Lateral side of radial artery, just distal to brachial artery bifurcation	Ascends between brachioradialis and brachialis, supplying both (and elbow joint); then anastomoses with radial collateral artery (from deep brachial artery)
Palmar carpal branch	Distal radial artery near distal border of pronator quadratus	Runs across anterior wrist deep to flexor tendons to anastomose with the palmar carpal branch of ulnar artery to form palmar carpal arch
Dorsal carpal branch	Distal radial artery in proximal part of snuff box	Runs medially across wrist deep to pollicis and extensor radialis tendons, anastomoses with ulnar dorsal carpal branch forming dorsal carpal arch

rior arteries may be present as anterior and posterior branches of a (common) ulnar recurrent artery.

- The *common interosseous artery,* a short branch of the ulnar artery, arises in the distal part of the cubital fossa and divides almost immediately into anterior and posterior interosseous arteries.

- The *anterior interosseous artery* passes distally, running directly on the anterior aspect of the interosseous membrane with the anterior interosseous nerve, whereas the *posterior interosseous artery* courses between the superficial and the deep layers of the extensor muscles in the company of the posterior interosseous nerve. The relatively small posterior interosseous artery is the principal artery serving the structures of the middle third of the posterior compartment. Thus it is mostly exhausted in the distal forearm and is replaced by the anterior interosseous artery, which pierces the interosseous membrane near the proximal border of the pronator quadratus.

- Unnamed *muscular branches of the ulnar artery* supply muscles on the medial side of the forearm, mainly those in the flexor–pronator group.

Radial Artery

The pulsations of the **radial artery** can be felt throughout the forearm, making it useful as an anterolateral demarcation of the flexor and extensor compartments of the forearm. When the brachioradialis is pulled laterally, the entire length of the artery is visible (Fig. 6.45; Table 6.9). The radial artery lies on muscle until it reaches the distal part of the forearm. Here it lies on the anterior surface of the radius and is covered by only skin and fascia, making this an ideal location for checking the radial pulse. The course of the radial artery in the forearm is represented by a line joining the midpoint of the cubital fossa to a point just medial to the radial styloid process. The radial artery leaves the forearm by winding around the lateral aspect of the wrist and crosses the floor of the anatomical snuff box (Figs. 6.44 and 6.45).

- The *radial recurrent artery* participates in the periarticular arterial anastomoses around the elbow by anastomosing with the *radial collateral artery,* a branch of the deep artery of the arm.

- The *palmar* and *dorsal carpal branches of the radial artery* participate in the periarticular arterial anastomosis around the wrist by anastomosing with the corresponding branches of the ulnar artery and terminal branches of the anterior and posterior interosseous arteries, forming the palmar and dorsal carpal arches.

- The unnamed *muscular branches of the radial artery* supply muscles in the adjacent (anterolateral) aspects of both the flexor and the extensor compartments because the radial artery runs along (and demarcates) the anterolateral boundary between the compartments.

High Division of the Brachial Artery

Sometimes the brachial artery divides at a more proximal level than usual. In this case, the ulnar and radial arteries begin in the superior or middle part of the arm, and the median nerve passes between them (Fig. B6.22). The musculocutaneous and median nerves commonly communicate as shown in this illustration.

Superficial Ulnar Artery

In approximately 3% of people, the ulnar artery descends superficial to the flexor muscles (Fig. B6.23). Pulsations of a superficial ulnar artery can be felt and may be visible. This variation must be kept in mind when performing venesections for withdrawing blood or making intravenous injections. If an aberrant ulnar artery is mistaken for a vein, it may be damaged and ▶

Figure B6.22

Figure B6.23

A radial pulse may also be felt by pressing lightly in the anatomical snuff box.

Variations in the Origin of the Radial Artery

The origin of the radial artery may be more proximal than usual; it may be a branch of the axillary artery or the brachial artery. Sometimes the radial artery is superficial to the deep fascia instead of deep to it. When a superficial vessel is pulsating near the wrist, it is probably a superficial radial artery. The aberrant vessel is vulnerable to laceration. ⊙

produce bleeding. If certain drugs are injected into the aberrant artery, the result could be fatal.

Measuring the Pulse Rate

The common place for measuring the pulse rate is where the radial artery lies on the anterior surface of the distal end of the radius, lateral to the tendon of the FCR. Here the artery is covered by only fascia and skin. The artery can be compressed against the distal end of the radius, where it lies between the tendons of the FCR and APL. When measuring the radial pulse rate, the pulp of the thumb should not be used because it has its own pulse, which could obscure the patient's pulse. If a pulse cannot be felt, try the other wrist because an *aberrant radial artery* on one side may make the pulse difficult to palpate.

Veins of the Forearm

In the forearm, as in the arm, there are superficial and deep veins. The superficial veins ascend in the subcutaneous tissue. The deep veins accompany the deep arteries of the forearm.

Superficial Veins

The pattern, common variations, and clinical significance of the superficial veins of the upper limb were discussed earlier in this chapter.

Deep Veins

Deep veins accompanying arteries are plentiful in the forearm (Fig. 6.46). These accompanying veins (L. *venae comitantes*) arise from the anastomosing **deep venous palmar arch** in the hand. From the lateral side of the arch, paired **radial veins** arise and accompany the radial artery; from the medial side, paired **ulnar veins** arise and accompany the ulnar artery. The veins accompanying each artery anastomose freely with each other. The radial and ulnar veins drain the forearm but carry

Figure 6.46. Deep venous drainage of upper limb. The deep accompanying veins surround the arteries as their companions, with which they share names. They are relatively small, usually paired, and interconnected at intervals by transverse branches.

relatively little blood from the hand. The deep veins ascend in the forearm along the sides of the corresponding arteries, receiving tributaries from veins leaving the muscles with which they are related. Deep veins communicate with the superficial veins. The deep **interosseous veins,** which accompany the interosseous arteries, unite with the accompanying veins of the radial and ulnar arteries. In the cubital fossa the deep veins are connected to the *median cubital vein,* a superficial vein. These deep cubital veins also unite with the accompanying veins of the brachial artery.

Nerves of the Forearm

The nerves of the forearm are the median, ulnar, and radial. The median nerve is the principal nerve of the anterior (flexor–pronator) compartment of the forearm (Figs. 6.38B and 6.48). Although the radial nerve appears in the cubital region, it soon enters the posterior (extensor–supinator) compartment of the forearm. Besides the cutaneous branches, there are only two nerves of the anterior aspect of the forearm: the median and ulnar nerves. The named nerves of the

forearm are illustrated and their origins and courses are described in Table 6.10. The following discussion provides additional details and discusses unnamed branches.

Median Nerve In the Forearm
The *median nerve* is the principal nerve of the anterior compartment of the forearm (Fig. 6.47). It supplies muscular branches directly to the muscles of the superficial and intermediate layers of forearm flexors (except the FCU), and deep muscles (except for the medial [ulnar] half of the FDP) via its branch, the anterior interosseous nerve.

The median nerve has no branches in the arm other than small twigs to the brachial artery. Its major named nerve in the forearm is the anterior interosseous nerve (Table 6.10). In addition, the following unnamed branches of the median nerve arise in the forearm:

- *Articular branches.* These branches pass to the elbow joint as the median nerve passes it.

- *Muscular branches.* The *nerve to the pronator teres* usually arises at the elbow and enters the lateral border of the muscle. A broad bundle of nerves pierces the superficial flexor group of muscles and innervates the FCR, the palmaris longus, and the FDS.

- *Anterior interosseous nerve.* This branch runs distally on the interosseous membrane with the anterior interosseous branch of the ulnar artery. After supplying the deep forearm flexors (except the ulnar part of the FDP, which sends tendons to 4th and 5th fingers), it passes deep to and supplies the pronator quadratus, then ends by sending articular branches to the wrist joint.

- *Palmar cutaneous branch of the median nerve.* This branch arises in the forearm, just proximal to the flexor retinaculum, but is distributed to skin of the central part of the palm.

Median Nerve Injury

When the median nerve is severed in the elbow region, flexion of the proximal interphalangeal joints of the 1st–3rd fingers is lost and flexion of the 4th and 5th fingers is weakened. Flexion of the distal interphalangeal joints of the 2nd and 3rd fingers is also lost. Flexion of the distal interphalangeal joints of the 4th and 5th fingers is not affected because the medial part of the FDP, which produces these movements, is supplied by the ulnar nerve. The ability to flex the metacarpophalangeal joints of the 2nd and 3rd fingers is affected because the digital branches of the median nerve supply the 1st and 2nd lumbricals. Thus, when the person attempts to make a fist, the 2nd and 3rd fingers remain partially extended ("hand of benediction") (Fig. B6.24). Thenar ▶

(cont'd on page 822)

Table 6.10. Nerves of the Forearm

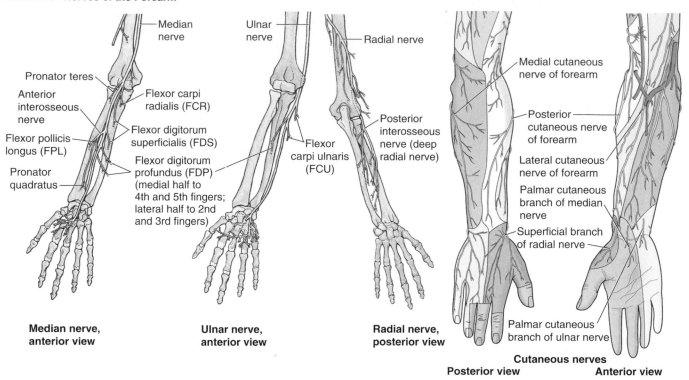

Median nerve,
anterior view

Ulnar nerve,
anterior view

Radial nerve,
posterior view

Cutaneous nerves
Posterior view   Anterior view

Nerve	Origin	Course in Forearm
Median	By union of lateral root of median nerve (C6 and C7, from lateral cord of brachial plexus) with medial root (C8 and T1) from medial cord)	Enters cubital fossa medial to brachial artery; exits by passing between heads of pronator teres; descends in fascial plane between flexors digitorum superficialis and profundus; runs deep to palmaris longus tendon as it approaches flexor retinaculum to traverse carpal tunnel
Anterior interosseous	Median nerve in distal part of cubital fossa	Descends on anterior aspect of interosseous membrane with artery of same name, between FDP and FPL, to pass deep to pronator quadratus
Palmar cutaneous branch of median nerve	Median nerve of middle to distal forearm, proximal to flexor retinaculum	Passes superficial to flexor reticulum to reach skin of central palm
Ulnar	Larger terminal branch of medial cord of brachial plexus (C8 and T1, often receives fibers from C7)	Enters forearm by passing between heads of flexor carpi ulnaris, after passing posterior to medial epicondyle of humerus; descends forearm between FCU and FDP; becomes superficial in distal forearm
Palmar cutaneous branch of ulnar nerve	Ulnar nerve near middle of forearm	Descends anterior to ulnar artery; perforates deep fascia in distal forearm; runs in subcutaneous tissue to palmar skin medial to axis of 4th finger
Dorsal cutaneous branch of ulnar nerve	Ulnar nerve in distal half of forearm	Passes posteroinferiorly between ulna and flexor carpi ulnaris; enters subcutaneous tissue to supply skin of dorsum medial to axis of 4th finger
Radial	Larger terminal branch of posterior cord of brachial plexus (C5–T1)	Enters cubital fossa between brachioradialis and brachialis; anterior to lateral epicondyle divides into terminal superficial and deep branches
Posterior cutaneous nerve of forearm	Radial nerve, as it traverses radial groove of posterior humerus	Perforates lateral head of triceps; descends along lateral side of arm and posterior aspect of forearm to wrist
Superficial branch of radial nerve	Sensory terminal branch of radial nerve, in cubital fossa	Descends between pronator teres and brachioradialis, emerging from latter to arborize over anatomical snuff box and supply skin of dorsum lateral to axis of 4th finger

Table 6.10. Nerves of the Forearm *(continued)*

Nerve	Origin	Course in Forearm
Deep branch of radial/posterior interosseous nerve	Motor terminal branch of radial nerve, in cubital fossa	Deep branch exits cubital fossa winding around neck of radius, penetrating and supplying supinator; emerges in posterior compartment of forearm as posterior interosseous; descends on membrane with artery of same name
Lateral cutaneous nerve of forearm	Continuation of musculocutaneous nerve distal to muscular branches	Emerges lateral to biceps brachii on brachialis, running initially with cephalic vein; descends along lateral border of forearm to wrist
Medial cutaneous nerve of forearm	Medial cord of brachial plexus, receiving C8 and T1 fibers	Perforates deep fascia of arm with basilic vein proximal to cubital fossa; descends medial aspect of forearm in subcutaneous tissue to wrist

Figure 6.47. Neurovascular structures in anterior aspect of forearm and wrist. A. At the elbow, the brachial artery lies between the biceps tendon and the median nerve. It bifurcates into the radial and ulnar arteries. In the forearm, the radial artery courses between the extensor and the flexor muscle groups. **B.** This deep dissection of the distal part of the forearm and proximal part of the hand shows the course of the arteries and nerves.

Figure B6.24. Medium nerve injury (palsy). A. Testing the flexion of the distal interphalangeal joint of the index finger is shown. **B.** The hand of benediction is demonstrated.

muscle function (function of the muscles at the base of the thumb) is also lost, as in carpal tunnel syndrome (see clinical correlation [blue] box "Carpal Tunnel Syndrome," later in this chapter).

Pronator Syndrome

Pronator syndrome, a nerve entrapment syndrome, is caused by compression of the median nerve near the elbow. The nerve may be compressed between the heads of the pronator teres as a result of trauma, muscular hypertrophy, or fibrous bands. Individuals with this syndrome are first seen clinically with pain and tenderness in the proximal aspect of the anterior forearm. Symptoms often follow activities that involve repeated elbow movements. ✪

Ulnar Nerve in the Forearm

Like the median nerve, the *ulnar nerve* does not give rise to branches during its passage through the arm. In the forearm it supplies only one and a half muscles, the FCU (as it enters the forearm by passing between its two heads of proximal attachment) and the ulnar part of the FDP, which sends tendons to the 4th and 5th fingers. The ulnar nerve and artery emerge from beneath the FCU tendon and become superficial just proximal to the wrist. They pass superficial to the flexor retinaculum and enter the hand by passing through a groove between the pisiform and the hook of the hamate. A band of fibrous tissue from the flexor retinaculum bridges the groove to form the small **ulnar canal** (Guyon canal) (Fig. 6.47*B*). The branches of the ulnar nerve arising in the forearm include unnamed muscular and articular branches, and cutaneous branches that pass to the hand:

- *Articular branches* pass to the elbow joint while the nerve is between the olecranon and medial epicondyle.

- *Muscular branches* supply the FCU and the medial half of the FDP.

- The *palmar* and *dorsal cutaneous branches* arise from the ulnar nerve in the forearm, but their sensory fibers are distributed to the skin of the hand.

Communications between the Median and the Ulnar Nerves

Occasionally, communications occur between the median and the ulnar nerves in the forearm. These branches are usually represented by slender nerves, but the communications are important clinically because even with a complete lesion of the median nerve, some muscles may not be paralyzed. This may lead to an erroneous conclusion that the median nerve has not been damaged.

Ulnar Nerve Injury

More than 27% of nerve lesions of the upper limb affect the ulnar nerve (Rowland, 2000). Ulnar nerve injuries usually occur in four places: (1) posterior to the medial epicondyle of the humerus, (2) in the cubital tunnel formed by the tendinous arch connecting the humeral and ulnar heads of the FCU, (3) at the wrist, and (4) in the hand.

Ulnar nerve injury occurs most commonly where the nerve passes posterior to the medial epicondyle of the humerus (Fig. B6.25). The injury results when the medial part of the elbow hits a hard surface, fracturing the medial epicondyle ("funny bone"). Compression of the ulnar nerve at the elbow (*cubital tunnel syndrome*) is also common (see clinical correlation [blue] box "Cubital Tunnel Syndrome," later in this chapter). Ulnar nerve injury usually produces numbness and tingling (*paresthesia*) of the medial part of the palm and the medial one and a half fingers (Fig. B6.26). Pluck your ulnar nerve at the posterior aspect of your elbow with your index finger and you may feel tingling in these fingers. Severe compression may also produce elbow pain that radiates distally. Uncommonly, the ulnar nerve is compressed as it passes through the ulnar canal (see clinical correlation [blue] box "Ulnar Canal Syndrome (Guyon Tunnel Syndrome)," later in this chapter).

Ulnar nerve injury can result in extensive motor and sensory loss to the hand. An injury to the nerve in the distal part of the forearm denervates most intrinsic hand muscles. Power of wrist adduction is impaired, and when an attempt is made to flex the wrist joint, the hand is drawn to the lateral side by the FCR (supplied ▶

phalangeal joints when trying to straighten the fingers. This characteristic appearance of the hand, resulting from a distal lesion of the ulnar nerve, is known as *claw hand* (*main en griffe*). The deformity results from atrophy of the interosseous muscles of the hand supplied by the ulnar nerve. The claw is produced by the unopposed action of the extensors and FDP.

Cubital Tunnel Syndrome

The ulnar nerve may be compressed (*ulnar nerve entrapment*) in the cubital tunnel formed by the tendinous arch joining the humeral and ulnar heads of attachment of the FCU (Table 6.7). The signs and symptoms of cubital tunnel syndrome are the same as an ulnar nerve lesion in the ulnar groove on the posterior aspect of the medial epicondyle of the humerus. ○

Medial epicondyle
Ulnar nerve
Posterior ulnar recurrent artery
Olecranon
Aponeurosis of flexor carpi ulnaris blended with antebrachial fascia

Triceps

Figure B6.25. Vulnerable position of ulnar nerve.

by the median nerve) in the absence of the "balance" provided by the FCU. After ulnar nerve injury, the person has difficulty making a fist because, in the absence of opposition, the metacarpophalangeal joints become hyperextended, and he or she cannot flex the 4th and 5th fingers at the distal interphalangeal joints when trying to make a fist. Furthermore, the person cannot extend the inter-

Palmar digital branches

Palmar branch

Figure B6.26. Claw hand and sensory distribution of ulnar nerve.

Radial Nerve in the Forearm

Unlike the medial and ulnar nerves, the *radial nerve* serves motor and sensory functions in both the arm and the forearm (but only sensory functions in the hand). However, its sensory and motor fibers are distributed in the forearm by two separate branches, the superficial (sensory or cutaneous) and deep radial/posterior interosseous nerve (motor). It divides into these terminal branches as it appears in the cubital fossa, anterior to the lateral epicondyle of the humerus, between the brachialis and the brachioradialis (Fig. 6.43). The two branches immediately part company, the deep branch winding laterally around the radius, piercing the supinator enroute to the posterior compartment.

The *posterior cutaneous nerve of the forearm* arises from the radial nerve in the posterior compartment of the arm, as it runs along the radial groove of the humerus. Thus it reaches

the forearm independent of the radial nerve, descending in the subcutaneous tissue of the posterior aspect of the forearm to the wrist, supplying the skin.

The *superficial branch of the radial nerve* is also a cutaneous nerve, but it gives rise to articular branches as well. It is distributed to skin on the dorsum of the hand and to a number of joints in the hand, branching soon after it emerges from the overlying brachioradialis and crosses the roof of the anatomical snuff box (Fig. 6.44).

After it pierces the supinator, the *deep branch of the radial nerve* runs in the fascial plane between superficial and deep extensor muscles in close proximity to the posterior interosseous artery; it is usually referred to as the *posterior interosseous nerve* (Fig. 6.43). It supplies motor innervation to all the muscles with fleshy bellies located entirely in the posterior compartment of the forearm (distal to the lateral epicondyle of the humerus).

Radial Nerve Injury in the Forearm

The radial nerve is usually injured in the arm by a fracture of the humeral shaft. This injury is proximal to the branches to the extensors of the wrist, and so *wrist-drop* is the primary clinical manifestation of an injury at this level (see clinical correlation [blue] box "Injury to the Radial Nerve in the Arm," earlier in this chapter). Injury to the deep branch of the radial nerve may occur when wounds of the forearm are deep (penetrating). Severance of the deep branch of the radial nerve results in an inability to extend the thumb and the metacarpophalangeal (MP) joints of the other digits. Thus the integrity of the deep radial nerve may be tested by asking the person to extend the MP joints while the examiner provides resistance (Fig. B6.27). If the nerve is intact, the long extensor tendons should appear prominently on the dorsum of the hand, confirming that the extension is occurring at the MP joints rather than at the interphalangeal joints (movements under the control of other nerves). Loss of sensation does not occur because the deep branch of the radial nerve is entirely muscular and articular in distribution. See Table 6.8 to determine the muscles that are paralyzed (e.g., extensor digitorum) when this nerve is severed.

When the superficial branch of the radial nerve, a cutaneous nerve, is severed, sensory loss is usually minimal. Commonly, a coin-shaped area of anesthesia occurs distal to the bases of the 1st and 2nd metacarpals. The reason the area of sensory loss is less than expected, given the areas highlighted in Table 6.10, is the result of the considerable overlap from cutaneous branches of the median and ulnar nerves. ●

Figure B6.27. Testing the radial nerve.

Lateral and Medial Cutaneous Nerves of Forearm

The *lateral cutaneous nerve* of the forearm (lateral antebrachial cutaneous nerve) is the continuation of the musculocutaneous nerve after its motor branches have all been given off to the muscles of the anterior compartment of the arm. The *medial cutaneous nerve of the forearm* (medial antebrachial cutaneous nerve) is an independent branch of the medial cord of the brachial plexus. With the *posterior cutaneous nerve of the forearm* from the radial nerve, each supplying the area of skin indicated by its name, these three nerves provide all the cutaneous innervation of the forearm. There is no "anterior cutaneous nerve of the forearm." (*Memory device:* This is similar to the brachial plexus, which has lateral, medial and posterior cords, but no anterior cord.)

Although the arteries, veins, and nerves of the forearm have been considered separately, it is important to place them into their anatomical context. Except for the superficial veins, which often course independently in the subcutaneous tissue, these neurovascular structures usually exist as components of neurovascular bundles. These bundles are composed of arteries, veins (in the limbs, usually in the form of accompanying veins), and nerves as well as lymphatic vessels, which are usually surrounded by a neurovascular sheath of varying density.

THE BOTTOM LINE: Well-developed subcutaneous veins course in the subcutaneous tissue of the forearm. These veins are subject to great variation. Once they have penetrated the deep fascia, cutaneous nerves run independently of the veins in the subcutaneous tissue where they remain constant in location and size, with lateral, medial, and posterior cutaneous nerves of the forearm supplying the aspects of the forearm described by their names. Three major (radial, median or middle, and ulnar) and two minor (anterior and posterior interosseous) neurovascular bundles occur deep to the antebrachial fascia.

The radial bundle—containing the radial artery, accompanying veins, and superficial radial nerve—course along and define the border between the anterior and the posterior forearm compartments (the vascular structures serving both) deep to the brachioradialis. The middle (median nerve and variable median artery and veins) and ulnar (ulnar nerve, artery, and accompanying veins) bundles course in a fascial plane between the intermediate and the deep flexor muscles. The median nerve supplies most muscles in the anterior compartment, many via its anterior interosseous branch, which courses on the interosseous membrane. The ulnar nerve supplies the one and a half exceptions (FCU and ulnar half of the FDP). The deep radial nerve penetrates the supinator to join the posterior interosseous artery in the plane between the superficial and the deep extensors. This nerve supplies all the muscles arising in the posterior compartment. The flexor muscles of the anterior compartment have approximately twice the bulk and strength of the extensor muscles of the posterior compartment. This, and the fact that the flexor aspect of the limb is the more protected aspect, accounts for the major neurovascular structures being located in the anterior compartment, with only the relatively small posterior interosseous vessels and nerve in the posterior compartment.

Surface Anatomy of the Forearm

Three bony landmarks are easily palpated at the elbow: the **medial** and **lateral epicondyles** of the humerus and the **olecranon** of the ulna (Fig. SA6.12). In the hollow located posterolaterally when the forearm is extended, the **head of the radius** can be palpated distal to the lateral epicondyle. Supinate and pronate your forearm and feel the movement of the radial head. The **posterior border of the ulna** is subcutaneous and can be palpated distally from the olecranon along the entire length of the bone. This landmark demarcates the posteromedial boundary separating the flexor–pronator (anterior) and extensor–supinator (posterior) compartments of the forearm.

The **cubital fossa,** the triangular hollow area on the anterior surface of the elbow, is bounded medially by the prominence formed by the *flexor–pronator group of muscles* that are attached to the medial epicondyle. To estimate the position of these muscles, put your thumb posterior to your medial epicondyle and then place your fingers on your forearm as shown in Figure SA6.13. The *black dot* on the dorsum of the hand indicates the position of the medial epicondyle. The cubital fossa is bounded laterally by the prominence of the *extensor–supinator group of muscles* attached to the lateral epicondyle (Fig. SA6.14). The *pulsations of the radial artery* can be palpated throughout the forearm as it runs its superficial course from the cubital fossa to the wrist (anterior to the radial styloid process), demarcating the anterolateral boundary separating the flexor–pronator and extensor–supinator compartments of the forearm.

The **head of the ulna** is at its distal end and is easily seen and palpated. It appears as a rounded prominence at the wrist when the hand is pronated. The **ulnar styloid process** can be palpated just distal to the ulnar head. The larger **radial styloid process** can be easily palpated on the ▶

Olecranon

Flexor muscles of forearm

Subcutaneous posterior border of ulna

Extensor muscles of forearm

Ulnar styloid process

Medial epicondyle

Olecranon

Lateral epicondyle

Head of radius

Head of ulna

Ulnar ⎫
      ⎬ Styloid process
Radial ⎭

Posterior view

Figure SA6.12

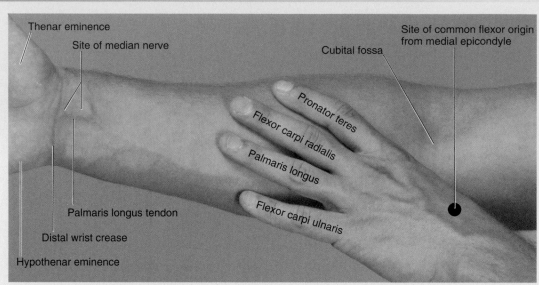

Thenar eminence

Site of median nerve

Palmaris longus tendon

Distal wrist crease

Hypothenar eminence

Cubital fossa

Site of common flexor origin
from medial epicondyle

Pronator teres

Flexor carpi radialis

Palmaris longus

Flexor carpi ulnaris

Anterior view of supinated forearm

Figure SA6.13

lateral side of the wrist when the hand is supinated, particularly when the tendons covering it are relaxed. The radial styloid process is located approximately 1 cm more distal than the ulnar styloid process. This relationship of the styloid processes is important in the diagnosis of certain injuries in the wrist region (e.g., fracture of the distal end of the radius). Proximal to the radial styloid process, the **surfaces of the radius** are palpable for a few centimeters. The lateral surface of the distal half of the radius is easy to palpate. ⊙

Dorsal venous network

Ulnar styloid process
Head of ulna

Cephalic vein

Extensor–supinator
muscles of forearm

1 cm.

**Anterior view of
pronated forearm**

Radial styloid process
Anatomical snuff box

Course of
radial artery

Flexor–pronator muscles of forearm

Cubital fossa

Figure SA6.14

Hand

The **wrist** is located at the junction of the forearm and hand, and the **hand** is the manual part of the upper limb distal to the forearm. Once positioned at the desired height and location relative to the body by movements at the shoulder and elbow, and the direction of action is established by pronation and supination of the forearm, the working position or attitude (tilt) of the hand is adjusted by movement at the wrist joint. The skeleton of the hand con-sists of *carpals* in the wrist, *metacarpals* in the hand proper, and *phalanges* in the digits. The digits are numbered from one to five, beginning with the thumb and ending with the little finger. The palmar aspect of the hand features a central concavity that, with the crease proximal to it (over the wrist bones) separates two eminences: a lateral, larger and more prominent **thenar eminence** at the base of the thumb, and a medial, smaller **hypothenar eminence** proximal to the base of the 5th finger (Fig SA6.13).

Because of the importance of manual dexterity in occupa-tional and recreational activities, a good understanding of the

(A) Lateral view

(B) Anterior view

(C) Medial view

(D) Medial view

(E) Medial view

(F) Medial view

(G) Anterior view

(H) Anterior view

Figure 6.48. Functional positions of hand. A. In the power grip, when grasping an object, the metacarpophalangeal (MP) and interphalangeal (IP) joints are flexed, but the radiocarpal and midcarpal joints are extended. "Cocking" (extension of) the wrist increases the distance over which the flexor tendons act, increasing tension of the long flexor tendons beyond that produced by maximal contraction of the muscles alone. **B.** The hook grip (flexion of the IP joints of the 2nd–4th digits) resists gravitational (downward) pull with only digital flexion. **C.** The precision grip is used when writing. **D and E.** One uses the precision grip to hold a coin to enable manipulation (**D**) and when pinching an object (**E**). **F.** Casts for fractures are applied with the hand and wrist in the resting position. Note the mild extension of the wrist. **G and H.** When gripping an unattached rod loosely (**G**) or firmly (**H**), the 2nd and 3rd carpometacarpal joints are rigid and stable, but the 4th and 5th are saddle joints permitting flexion and extension. The increased flexion changes the angle of the rod during the firm grip.

structure and function of the hand is essential for all persons involved in maintaining or restoring its activities: free motion, power grasping, precision handling, and pinching.

The **power grip** (palm grasp) refers to forcible motions of the digits acting against the palm; the fingers are wrapped around an object with counterpressure from the thumb—for example, when grasping a cylindrical structure (Fig. 6.48A). The power grip involves the long flexor muscles to the fingers (acting at the interphalangeal joints), the intrinsic muscles in the palm (acting at the metacarpophalangeal joints), and the extensors of the wrist (acting at the radiocarpal and midcarpal joints). The "cocking" of the wrist by the extensors increases the distance over which the flexors of the fingers act, producing the same result as a more complete muscular contraction. Conversely, as flexion increases at the wrist, the grip becomes weaker and more insecure.

A **hook grip** is the posture of the hand that is used when carrying a briefcase (Fig. 6.48*B*). This grip consumes less energy, involving mainly the long flexors of the fingers, which are flexed to a varying degree, depending on the size of the object that is grasped.

The **precision handling grip** involves a change in the position of a handled object that requires fine control of the movements of the fingers and thumb—for example, holding a pencil, manipulating a coin, threading a needle, or buttoning a shirt (Fig. 6.48*C* & *D*). In a precision grip, the wrist and fingers are held firmly by the long flexor and extensor muscles, and the intrinsic hand muscles perform fine movements of the digits.

Pinching refers to compression of something between the thumb and the index finger—for example, handling a teacup or holding a coin on edge (Fig. 6.48*E*)—or between the thumb and the adjacent two fingers—for example, snapping the fingers. The **position of rest** is assumed by an inactive hand—for example, when the forearm and hand are laid on a table (Fig. 6.48*F*). This position is often used when it is necessary to immobilize the wrist and hand in a cast to stabilize a fracture.

Fascia of the Palm

The **fascia of the palm** is continuous with the antebrachial fascia and the fascia of the dorsum of the hand (Fig. 6.39). The **palmar fascia** is thin over the thenar and hypothenar eminences, but it is thick centrally where it forms the fibrous palmar aponeurosis and in the fingers where it forms the digital sheaths (Figs. 6.39 and 6.49). The **palmar**

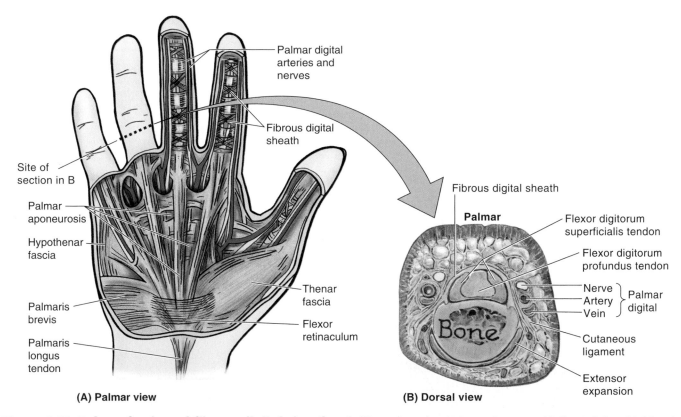

(A) Palmar view

Palmar digital arteries and nerves

Fibrous digital sheath

Site of section in B

Palmar aponeurosis

Hypothenar fascia

Palmaris brevis

Palmaris longus tendon

Thenar fascia

Flexor retinaculum

(B) Dorsal view

Fibrous digital sheath

Palmar

Flexor digitorum superficialis tendon

Flexor digitorum profundus tendon

Nerve
Artery } Palmar digital
Vein

Cutaneous ligament

Extensor expansion

Bone

Figure 6.49. Palmar fascia and fibrous digital sheaths. A. The palmar fascia is continuous with the antebrachial fascia. The thin thenar and hypothenar fascia covers the intrinsic muscles of the thenar and hypothenar eminences, respectively. Between the thenar and the hypothenar muscle masses, the central compartment of the palm is roofed by the thick palmar aponeurosis. When present (approximately 80% of the time), the distal end of the palmaris longus tendon blends with the aponeurosis superficial to the flexor retinaculum. Fibrous digital sheaths (shown here for the middle and index fingers), continuous with the longitudinal fiber bundles of the palmar aponeurosis, form the coverings of the digital portions of the tendons of the FDS and FDP. **B.** A transverse section of the 4th finger (proximal phalanx level) is shown. Within the fibrous digital sheath and proximal to its attachment to the base of the middle phalanx, the FDS tendon has split into two parts to allow continued central passage of the FDP tendon to the distal phalanx. The palmar digital nerve, artery, and vein are adjacent to the sheath, not to the phalanx (*Bone*). The dorsal digital neurovascular structures become exhausted near the midpoint of the middle phalanges; thus the palmar nerves, arteries, and veins serve all (palmar and dorsal aspects) of the digits distally.

aponeurosis, a strong, well-defined part of the deep fascia of the palm, covers the soft tissues and overlies the long flexor tendons. The proximal end or apex of the triangular palmar aponeurosis is continuous with the flexor retinaculum and the palmaris longus tendon. When the palmaris longus is present, the palmar aponeurosis is the expanded tendon of the palmaris longus. Distal to the apex, the palmar aponeurosis forms four longitudinal digital bands or rays that radiate from the apex and attach distally to the bases of the proximal phalanges and become continuous with the fibrous digital sheaths.

The **fibrous digital sheaths** are ligamentous tubes that enclose the synovial sheaths, the superficial and deep flexor tendons, and the tendon of the FPL in their passage along the palmar aspect of their respective fingers (Figs. 6.39, 6.42C, and 6.49). The flexor digital sheaths are composed of five anular and four *cruciform* (cross-shaped) parts or "pulleys."

A **medial fibrous septum** extends deeply from the medial border of the palmar aponeurosis to the 5th metacarpal (Fig.

6.50A). Medial to this septum is the medial or **hypothenar compartment** containing the hypothenar muscles. Similarly, a **lateral fibrous septum** extends deeply from the lateral border of the palmar aponeurosis to the 3rd metacarpal. Lateral to this septum is the lateral or **thenar compartment** containing the thenar muscles. Between the hypothenar and the thenar compartments is the **central compartment** containing the flexor tendons and their sheaths, the lumbricals, the superficial palmar arterial arch, and the digital vessels and nerves. The deepest muscular plane of the palm is the **adductor compartment** containing the adductor pollicis.

Between the flexor tendons and the fascia covering the deep palmar muscles are two potential spaces, the **thenar space** and the **midpalmar space** (Fig. 6.50). The spaces are bounded by fibrous septa passing from the edges of the palmar aponeurosis to the metacarpals. Between the two spaces is the especially strong lateral fibrous septum, which is attached to the 3rd metacarpal. Although most fascial compartments end at the joints, the midpalmar space is continuous with the anterior compartment of the forearm via the carpal tunnel.

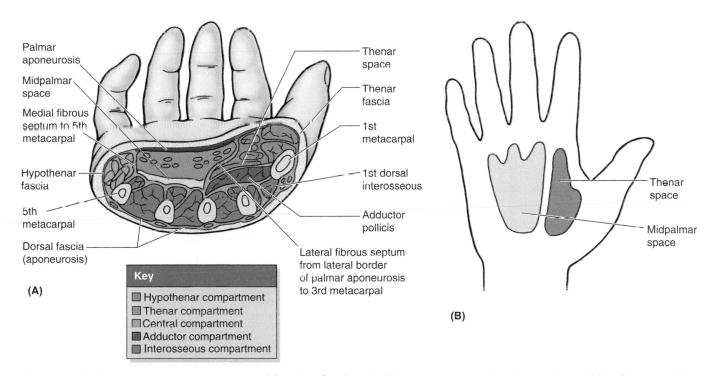

Key
- ☐ Hypothenar compartment
- ☐ Thenar compartment
- ☐ Central compartment
- ■ Adductor compartment
- ☐ Interosseous compartment

Figure 6.50. Compartments, spaces, and fascia of palm. A. This transverse section through the middle of the palm illustrates the fascial compartments of the hand. The hypothenar fascia, attached to the lateral side of the 5th metacarpal, bounds the hypothenar compartment. Similarly, the thenar fascia, attached to the palmar aspect of the 1st metacarpal, bounds (with the metacarpal) the thenar compartment. The central compartment of the palm is covered by the palmar aponeurosis and separated from the thenar and hypothenar compartments by medial and lateral fibrous septa attaching to the 5th and 3rd metacarpals, respectively. The septum attached to the 3rd metacarpal also separates the midpalmar and thenar spaces The adductor compartment contains the adductor pollicis muscle. **B.** The midpalmar space underlies the central compartment of the palm and is related distally to the synovial tendon sheaths of the 3rd–5th digits and proximally to the common flexor sheath as it emerges from the carpal tunnel. The thenar space underlies the thenar compartment and is related distally to the synovial tendon sheath of the index finger and proximally to the common flexor sheath distal to the carpal tunnel.

Dupuytren Contracture of Palmar Fascia

Dupuytren contracture is a disease of the palmar fascia resulting in progressive shortening, thickening, and fibrosis of the palmar fascia and aponeurosis. The fibrous degeneration of the longitudinal bands of the palmar aponeurosis on the medial side of the hand pulls the 4th and 5th fingers into partial flexion at the metacarpophalangeal and proximal interphalangeal joints (Fig. B6.28*A*). The contracture is frequently bilateral and is seen in some men >50 years of age. Its cause is unknown, but evidence points to a hereditary predisposition. The disease first manifests as painless nodular thickenings of the palmar aponeurosis that adhere to the skin. Gradually, progressive contracture of the longitudinal bands produces raised ridges in the palmar skin that extend from the proximal part of the hand to the base of the 4th and 5th fingers (Fig. B6.28*B*). Treatment of Dupuytren con-

tracture usually involves surgical excision of all fibrotic parts of the palmar fascia to free the fingers (Salter, 1999).

Hand Infections

Because the palmar fascia is thick and strong, swellings resulting from hand infections usually appear on the dorsum of the hand, where the fascia is thinner. The potential fascial spaces of the palm are important because they may become infected. The fascial spaces determine the extent and direction of the spread of pus formed by these infections. Depending on the site of infection, pus will accumulate in the thenar, hypothenar, or adductor compartments. Antibiotic therapy has made infections that spread beyond one of these fascial compartments rare; however, an untreated infection can spread proximally through the carpal tunnel into the forearm, anterior to the pronator quadratus and its fascia. ☉

(A)

(B)

Figure B6.28. Dupuytren contracture.

Muscles of the Hand

The intrinsic muscles of the hand are located in five compartments (Fig. 6.50):

1. Thenar muscles in the *thenar compartment:* abductor pollicis brevis, flexor pollicis brevis, and opponens pollicis.

2. Adductor pollicis in the *adductor compartment.*

3. Hypothenar muscles in the *hypothenar compartment.* abductor digiti minimi, flexor digiti minimi brevis, and opponens digiti minimi.

4. Short muscles of the hand, the lumbricals, are in the *central compartment* with the long flexor tendons.

5. The interossei lie in separate *interosseous compartments* between the metacarpals.

Thenar Muscles

The **thenar muscles** form the *thenar eminence* on the lateral surface of the palm and are chiefly responsible for opposition of the thumb. Normal movement of the thumb is important for the precise activities of the hand. The high degree of freedom of movements of the thumb results from the 1st metacarpal being independent, with mobile joints at both ends. Thus several muscles are required to control its freedom of movement:

- *Extension:* extensor pollicis longus, extensor pollicis brevis, and abductor pollicis longus.

- *Flexion:* flexor pollicis longus and flexor pollicis brevis.

- *Abduction:* abductor pollicis longus and abductor pollicis brevis.

- *Adduction:* adductor pollicis and 1st dorsal interosseous.

- *Opposition:* opponens pollicis. This movement occurs at the carpometacarpal joint and results in a "cupping" of the palm. Bringing the tip of the thumb into contact with the 5th finger or any of the other fingers involves considerably more movement than can be produced by the opponens pollicis alone. This complex movement begins with the thumb in the extended position and initially involves abduction and medial rotation of the 1st metacarpal (cupping the palm) produced by the action of the opponens pollicis at the carpometacarpal joint and then flexion at the metacarpophalangeal joint (Fig. 6.51). The reinforcing action of the adductor pollicis and FPL increases the pressure that the opposed thumb can exert on the fingertips. In pulp-to-pulp opposition, movements of the finger opposing the thumb are also involved.

The first four movements occur at the carpometacarpal and metacarpophalangeal joints.

The thenar muscles are illustrated in Figure 6.52; their attachments, innervations, and main actions are summarized in Table 6.11.

Abductor Pollicis Brevis. The abductor pollicis brevis (APB), the short abductor of the thumb, forms the anterolateral part of the thenar eminence. In addition to abducting the thumb, the APB assists the opponens pollicis during the early stages of opposition by rotating its proximal phalanx slightly medially.

To test the abductor pollicis brevis, abduct the thumb against resistance. If acting normally, the muscle can be seen and palpated.

Flexor Pollicis Brevis. The **flexor pollicis brevis** (FPB), the short flexor of the thumb, is located medial to the APB (Fig. 6.52*A*). Its two bellies, located on opposite sides of the

| Abduction | Adduction | Extension | Flexion | Opposition | Reposition |

Figure 6.51. Movements of thumb. The thumb is rotated 90° to the other digits. (This can be confirmed by noting the direction the nail of the thumb faces compared with the nails of the other fingers.) Thus abduction and adduction occur in a sagittal plane and flexion and extension occur in a coronal plane. Opposition, the action bringing the tip of the thumb in contact with the pads of the other fingers (e.g., with the little finger), is the most complex movement. The components of opposition are abduction and medial rotation at the carpometacarpal joint and flexion of the metacarpophalangeal joint.

Table 6.11. Intrinsic Muscles of the Hand

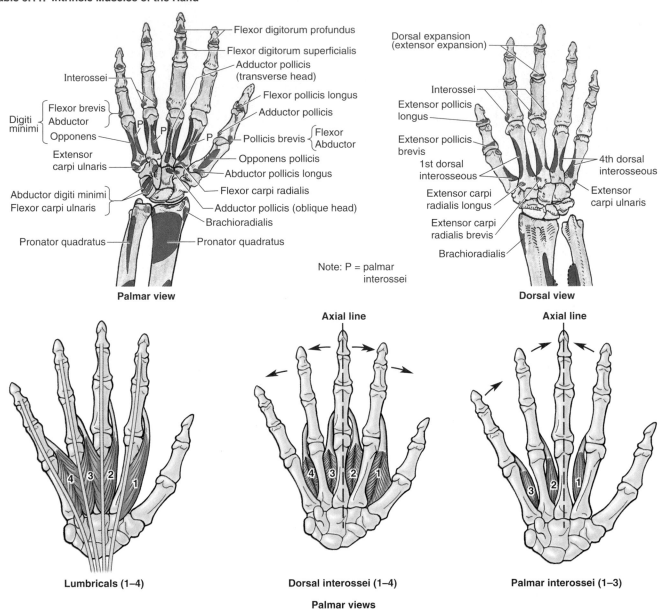

Palmar view

Note: P = palmar interossei

Dorsal view

Lumbricals (1–4)

Dorsal interossei (1–4)

Palmar interossei (1–3)

Palmar views

Muscle	Proximal Attachment	Distal Attachment	Innervation[a]	Main Action
Thenar muscles				
Opponens pollicis	Flexor retinaculum and tubercles of scaphoid and trapezium	Lateral side of 1st metacarpal	Recurrent branch of medial nerve (**C8**, T1)	To oppose thumb, it draws 1st metacarpal medially to center of palm and rotates it medially
Abductor pollicis brevis		Lateral side of base of proximal phalanx of thumb		Abducts thumb; helps oppose it
Flexor pollicis brevis				Flexes thumb
Superficial head				
Deep head			Deep branch of ulnar nerve (C8, **T1**)	
Adductor pollicis	Bases of 2nd and 3rd metacarpals, capitate, adjacent carpals	Medial side of base of proximal phalanx of thumb		Adducts thumb toward lateral border of palm
Oblique head				
Transverse head	Anterior surface of shaft of 3rd metacarpal			

Table 6.11. Intrinsic Muscles of the Hand *(continued)*

Muscle	Proximal Attachment	Distal Attachment	Innervation[a]	Main Action
Hypothenar muscles				
Abductor digiti minimi	Pisiform	Medial side of base of proximal phalanx of 5th finger	Deep branch of ulnar nerve (C8, **T1**)	Abducts 5th finger; assists in flexion of its proximal phalanx
Flexor digiti minimi brevis	Hook of hamate and flexor retinaculum			Flexes proximal phalanx of 5th finger
Opponens digiti minimi		Medial border of 5th metacarpal		Draws 5th metacarpal anterior and rotates it, bringing 5th finger into opposition with thumb
Short muscles				
Lumbricals	Lateral two tendons of flexor digitorum profundus (as unipennate muscles)	Lateral sides of extensor expansions of 2nd–5th fingers	Median nerve (C8, **T1**)	Flex metacarpophalangeal joints; extend interphalangeal joints of 2nd–5th fingers
1st and 2nd				
3rd and 4th	Medial three tendons of flexor digitorum profundus (as bipennate muscles)			
Dorsal interossei, 1st–4th	Adjacent sides of two metacarpals (as bipennate muscles)	Bases of proximal phalanges; extensor expansions of 2nd–4th fingers	Deep branch of ulnar nerve (C8, **T1**)	Abduct 2nd–4th fingers from axial line; act with lumbricals in flexing metacarpophalangeal joints and extending interphalangeal joints
Palmar interossei, 1st–3rd	Palmar surfaces of 2nd, 4th, and 5th metacarpals (as unipennate muscles)	Bases of proximal phalanges; extensor expansions of 2nd, 4th, and 5th fingers		Adduct 2nd, 4th, and 5th fingers toward axial line; assist lumbricals in flexing metacarpophalangeal joints and extending interphalangeal joints; extensor expansions of 2nd–4th fingers

[a]The spinal cord segmental innervation is indicated (e.g., "**C8**, T1" means that the nerves supplying the opponens pollicis are derived from the eighth cervical segment and first thoracic segment of the spinal cord). Numbers in boldface (**C8**) indicate the main segmental innervation. Damage to one or more of the listed spinal cord segments or to the motor nerve roots arising from them results in paralysis of the muscles concerned.

tendon of the FPL, share (with each other and often with the APB) a common, sesamoid-containing tendon at their distal attachment. The bellies usually differ in their innervation: The larger superficial head of the FPB is innervated by the recurrent branch of the median nerve, whereas the smaller deep head is usually innervated by the deep palmar branch of the ulnar nerve. The FPB flexes the thumb at the carpometacarpal and metacarpophalangeal joints and aids in opposition of the thumb.

To test the flexor pollicis brevis, flex the thumb against resistance. If acting normally, the muscle can be seen and palpated; however, keep in mind that the FPL also flexes the thumb.

Opponens Pollicis. The **opponens pollicis** is a quadrangular muscle that lies deep to the APB and lateral to the FPB (Fig. 6.52*B*). The opponens pollicis opposes the thumb, the most important thumb movement. It flexes and rotates the 1st metacarpal medially at the carpometacarpal joint during opposition; this movement occurs when picking up an object. During opposition, the tip of the thumb is brought into contact with the pad of the little finger, as shown in Figure 6.51.

Adductor Pollicis

The **adductor pollicis** is the deeply placed, fan-shaped adductor of the thumb. It is located in the adductor compartment of the hand (Figs. 6.50*A* and 6.53). The adductor pollicis has two heads of origin, which are separated by the radial artery as it enters the palm to form the deep palmar arch. Its tendon usually contains a sesamoid bone. The adductor pollicis adducts the thumb, moving the thumb to the palm of the hand (Fig. 6.51), thereby giving power to the grip (Fig. 6.48*G & H*).

Hypothenar Muscles

The **hypothenar muscles** (abductor digiti minimi, flexor digiti minimi brevis, and opponens digiti minimi) produce the *hypothenar eminence* on the medial side of the palm and move the little finger. These muscles are in the hypothenar compartment with the 5th metacarpal (Figs. 6.50*A* and 6.52). The attachments, innervations, and main actions of the hypothenar muscles are summarized in Table 6.11.

Abductor Digiti Minimi. The **abductor digiti minimi** is the most superficial of the three muscles forming the hypothenar eminence. The abductor digiti minimi abducts the 5th finger and helps flex its proximal phalanx.

(A)

Proper palmar digital arteries

Proper palmar digital nerves

Radialis indicis artery

1st lumbrical

Fibrous digital sheath

1st dorsal interosseous

Flexor digitorum superficialis

Adductor pollicis

Common palmar digital arteries and nerves

Superficial palmar arch

Flexor pollicis brevis (FPB)

Abductor digiti minimi

Recurrent branch of median nerve

Palmar aponeurosis

Abductor pollicis brevis (APB)

Site of fusion of tendon of palmaris longus and palmar aponeurosis to underlying flexor retinaculum

Palmaris brevis

Ulnar nerve and artery (in ulnar canal)

Abductor pollicis longus (APL)

Superficial palmar branch

Pisiform

Radial artery

Dorsal carpal branch

Dorsal cutaneous branch of ulnar nerve

Palmaris longus

Flexor carpi ulnaris

(B)

Ligaments of skin

Palmar digital nerve

2nd lumbrical

1st lumbrical

Digiti minimi { Abductor, Flexor brevis, Opponens

Tendon of flexor pollicis longus (FPL)

Flexor pollicis brevis (FPB)

Branches of ulnar nerve { Communicating, Superficial, Deep

Opponens pollicis

Pisiform

Flexor retinaculum

Abductor pollicis brevis (APB)

Ulnar nerve and artery

Abductor pollicis longus (APL)

Figure 6.52. Superficial dissections of right palm. The skin and subcutaneous tissue have been removed, as have most of the palmar aponeurosis and the thenar and hypothenar fasciae. **A.** The superficial palmar arch is located immediately deep to the palmar aponeurosis, superficial to the long flexor tendons. This arterial arch gives rise to the common palmar digital arteries. In the digits, a digital artery (e.g., radialis indicis) and nerve lie on the medial and lateral sides of the fibrous digital sheath. The pisiform bone protects the ulnar nerve and artery as they pass into the palm. **B.** Three thenar and three hypothenar muscles attach to the flexor retinaculum and to the four marginal carpal bones united by the retinaculum.

Figure 6.53. Muscles and arteries of distal forearm and deep palm. This deep dissection of the palm reveals the anastomosis of the palmar carpal branch of the radial artery with the palmar carpal branch of the ulnar artery to form the palmar carpal arch, and the deep palmar arch. The deep palmar arch lies at the level of the bases of the metacarpal bones, 1.5–2 cm proximal to the superficial palmar arch.

Flexor Digiti Minimi Brevis. The flexor digiti minimi brevis is variable in size; it lies lateral to the abductor digiti minimi. The flexor digiti minimi brevis flexes the proximal phalanx of the 5th finger at the metacarpophalangeal joint.

Opponens Digiti Minimi. The **opponens digiti minimi** is a quadrangular muscle that lies deep to the abductor and flexor muscles of the 5th finger. The opponens digiti minimi draws the 5th metacarpal anteriorly and rotates it laterally, thereby deepening the hollow of the palm and bringing the 5th finger into opposition with the thumb (Fig. 6.51). Like the opponens pollicis, the opponens digiti minimi acts exclusively at the carpometacarpal joint.

Palmaris Brevis. The **palmaris brevis** is a small, thin muscle in the subcutaneous tissue of the hypothenar eminence (Fig. 6.52A); it is not in the hypothenar compartment. The palmaris brevis wrinkles the skin of the hypothenar eminence and deepens the hollow of the palm, thereby aiding the palmar grip. The palmaris brevis covers and protects the ulnar nerve and artery. It is attached proximally to the medial border of the palmar aponeurosis and to the skin on the medial border of the hand.

Short Muscles of the Hand

The short muscles of the hand are the lumbricals and interossei (Table 6.11).

Lumbricals. The four slender **lumbrical muscles** were named because of their worm-like form (L. *lumbricus*, earthworm) (Fig. 6.52A & B). The lumbricals flex the fingers at the metacarpophalangeal joints and extend the interphalangeal joints.

Interossei. The four **dorsal interosseous muscles** (dorsal interossei) are located between the metacarpals; the three **palmar interosseous muscles** (palmar interossei) are on the palmar surfaces of the metacarpals in the interosseous compartment of the hand (Fig. 6.50A). The 1st dorsal interosseous muscle is easy to palpate; oppose the thumb firmly against the index finger and it can be easily felt. (Some authors describe four palmar interossei; in so doing, they are including the deep head of the FPB because of its similar innervation and placement on the thumb; Table 6.11). The four dorsal interossei abduct the fingers, and the three palmar interossei adduct them. A mnemonic device is to make acronyms of **D**orsal **AB**duct (DAB) and **P**almar **AD**uct (PAD). Acting together, the dorsal and palmar interossei and the lumbricals produce flexion at the metacarpophalangeal joints and extension of the interphalangeal joints (the so-called Z-movement). This occurs because of their attachment to the lateral bands of the extensor expansions (Fig. 6.42B). Understanding the Z-movement is useful because it is the opposite of claw hand, which occurs in ulnar paralysis when the interossei and the 3rd and 4th lumbricals are incapable of acting together to produce the Z-movement (see clinical correlation [blue] box "Ulnar Nerve Injury," earlier in this chapter).

Long Flexor Tendons and Tendon Sheaths in the Hand

The tendons of the FDS and FDP enter the **common flexor sheath** (ulnar bursa) deep to the flexor retinaculum (Fig. 6.54A). The tendons enter the central compartment of the hand and fan out to enter their respective **digital synovial sheaths.** The flexor and digital sheaths enable the tendons to slide freely over each other during movements of the fingers. Near the base of the proximal phalanx, the tendon of FDS splits and surrounds the tendon of FDP (Figs. 6.49B and 6.54B). The halves of the FDS tendon are attached to the margins of the anterior aspect of the base of the middle phalanx (Fig. 6.42D). The tendon of FDP, after passing through the split in the FDS tendon, the **tendinous chiasm,** passes distally to attach to the anterior aspect of the base of the distal phalanx.

The *fibrous digital sheaths* are the strong ligamentous tunnels containing the flexor tendons and their synovial sheaths (Figs. 6.49 and 6.54C). The sheaths extend from the heads of the metacarpals to the bases of the distal phalanges. These sheaths prevent the tendons from pulling away from the digits (bowstringing). The fibrous digital sheaths combine with the bones to form **osseofibrous tunnels** through which the tendons pass to reach the digits. The **anular** and **cruciform parts** (often referred to clinically as "pulleys") are thickened reinforcements of the fibrous digital sheaths (Fig. 6.54B).

The long flexor tendons are supplied by small blood vessels that pass within synovial folds (*vincula*) from the periosteum of the phalanges (Fig. 6.42B). The tendon of the FPL passes deep to the flexor retinaculum to the thumb within its own synovial sheath. At the head of the metacarpal, the tendon runs between two *sesamoid bones,* one in the combined tendon of the FPB and APB and the other in the tendon of the adductor pollicis.

THE BOTTOM LINE: The larger (wider range) and stronger movements of the hand and fingers (grasping, pinching, pointing, etc.) are produced by extrinsic muscles with fleshy bellies located distant from the hand (near the elbow) and long tendons passing into the hand and fingers. The shorter, more delicate and weaker movements (typing,

playing musical instruments, and writing) and positioning of the fingers for the more powerful movements are accomplished largely by the intrinsic muscles. The muscles and tendons of the hand are organized into five fascial compartments: two radial compartments (thenar and adductor) that serve the thumb; an ulnar (hypothenar) compartment that serves the little finger; and two more central compartments that serve the medial four fingers (a palmar one for the long flexor tendons and lumbricals, and a deep one between the metacarpals for the interossei).

The greatest mass of intrinsic muscles is dedicated to the highly mobile thumb. Indeed, when extrinsic muscles are also considered, the thumb has eight muscles producing and controlling the wide array of movements that distinguish the human hand. The interossei produce multiple movements: the dorsal interossei (and abductors pollicis and digiti minimi) abduct the fingers, whereas the palmar interossei (and adductor pollicis) adduct them. Both movements occur at the metacarpophalangeal joints. Acting together with the lumbricals, the interossei flex the metacarpophalangeal and extend the interphalangeal joints of the medial four fingers (the Z-movement).

Tenosynovitis

Injuries such as a puncture of a finger by a rusty nail can cause infection of the digital synovial sheaths. When inflammation of the tendon and synovial sheath occurs (**tenosynovitis**), the digit swells and movement becomes painful. Because the tendons of the 2nd, 3rd, and 4th fingers nearly always have separate synovial sheaths, the infection is usually confined to the infected finger. If the infection is untreated, however, the proximal ends of these sheaths may rupture, allowing the infection to spread to the midpalmar space (Fig. 6.51B). Because the synovial sheath of the little finger is usually continuous with the common flexor sheath (Fig. 6.54B), tenosynovitis in this finger may spread to the common sheath and thus through the palm and carpal tunnel to the anterior forearm, draining into the space between the pronator quadratus and the overlying flexor tendons (*Parona space*). Likewise, tenosynovitis in the thumb may spread via the continuous synovial sheath of the FPL (radial bursa). How far an infection spreads from the fingers depends on variations in their connections with the common flexor sheath.

The tendons of the APL and EPB are in the same tendinous sheath on the dorsum of the wrist. Excessive friction of these tendons on their common sheath results in fibrous thickening of the sheath and stenosis of the osseofibrous tunnel. The excessive friction is caused by repetitive forceful use of the hands during gripping and wringing (e.g., squeezing water out of clothes). This ▶

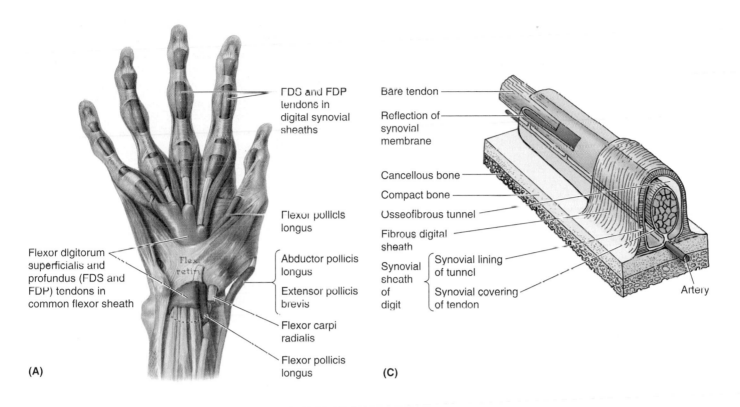

(A)

FDS and FDP tendons in digital synovial sheaths

Flexor pollicis longus

Flexor digitorum superficialis and profundus (FDS and FDP) tendons in common flexor sheath

Flex retin

Abductor pollicis longus

Extensor pollicis brevis

Flexor carpi radialis

Flexor pollicis longus

Bare tendon

Reflection of synovial membrane

Cancellous bone

Compact bone

Osseofibrous tunnel

Fibrous digital sheath

Synovial sheath of digit { Synovial lining of tunnel / Synovial covering of tendon }

Artery

(C)

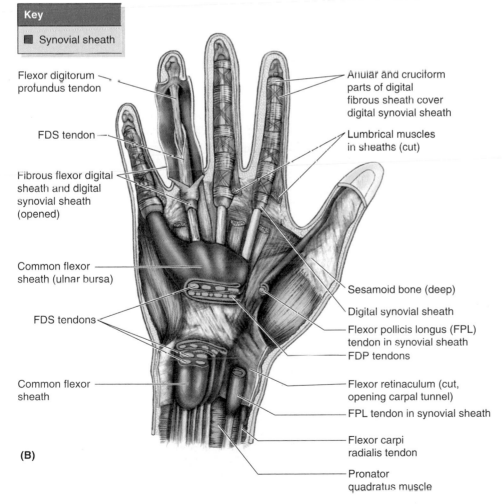

(B)

Key

■ Synovial sheath

Flexor digitorum profundus tendon

FDS tendon

Fibrous flexor digital sheath and digital synovial sheath (opened)

Common flexor sheath (ulnar bursa)

FDS tendons

Common flexor sheath

Anular and cruciform parts of digital fibrous sheath cover digital synovial sheath

Lumbrical muscles in sheaths (cut)

Sesamoid bone (deep)

Digital synovial sheath

Flexor pollicis longus (FPL) tendon in synovial sheath

FDP tendons

Flexor retinaculum (cut, opening carpal tunnel)

FPL tendon in synovial sheath

Flexor carpi radialis tendon

Pronator quadratus muscle

Figure 6.54. Flexor tendons, common flexor sheath, fibrous digital sheaths, and synovial sheaths of digits. A. This dissection of the anterior aspect of the distal forearm and hand shows the synovial sheaths of the long flexor tendons to the digits. Observe the two sets: (1) proximal or carpal, posterior to the flexor retinaculum, and (2) distal or digital, within the fibrous sheaths of the digital flexors. **B.** This dissection of the palm illustrates the tendons and fibrous digital sheaths. The fibrous sheaths of the digits attach along the borders of the proximal and middle phalanges to capsules (palmar ligaments) of the interphalangeal joints and to the surface of the distal phalanx. **C.** The structure of an osseofibrous tunnel of a finger, containing a tendon, is shown. Within the fibrous sheath, the synovial sheath consists of the (parietal) synovial lining of the tunnel and the (visceral) synovial covering of the tendon. These layers of the synovial sheath are actually separated by only a capillary layer of synovial fluid, which lubricates the synovial surfaces to facilitate gliding of the tendon (see Introduction).

condition, called **Quervain tenovaginitis stenosans,** causes pain in the wrist that radiates proximally to the forearm and distally toward the thumb. Local tenderness is felt over the common fibrous sheath on the lateral side of the wrist.

Thickening of a fibrous digital sheath on the palmar aspect of the digit produces stenosis of the osseofibrous tunnel, the result of repetitive forceful use of the fingers. If the tendons of the FDS and FDP enlarge proximal to the tunnel, the person is unable to extend the finger. When the finger is extended passively, a snap is audible. Flexion produces another snap as the thickened tendon moves. This condition is called **digital tenovaginitis stenosans** (trigger finger or snapping finger). ✪

Arteries of the Hand

Because its function requires it to be placed and held in many different positions, often while grasping or applying pressure, the hand is supplied with an abundance of highly branched and anastomosing arteries so that oxygenated blood is generally available to all parts in all positions. Furthermore, the arteries or their derivatives are relatively superficial, underlying skin capable of sweating, so that excess heat can be released. To prevent undesirable heat loss in a cold environment, the arterioles of the hands are capable of reducing blood flow to the surface and to the ends of the fingers. The ulnar and radial arteries and their branches provide all the blood to the hand. The arteries of the hand are illustrated and their origins and courses are described in Table 6.12.

Ulnar Artery

The *ulnar artery* enters the hand anterior to the flexor retinaculum between the pisiform and the hook of the hamate via the *ulnar canal* (Guyon canal) (Fig. 6.47*B*). The ulnar artery lies lateral to the ulnar nerve (Fig. 6.52*A*). The artery divides into two terminal branches, the superficial palmar arch and the deep palmar branch. The **superficial palmar arch,** the main termination of the ulnar artery, gives rise to three **common palmar digital arteries** that anastomose with the **palmar metacarpal arteries** from the deep palmar arch. Each common palmar digital artery divides into a pair of **proper palmar digital arteries** that run along the adjacent sides of the 2nd–4th fingers.

Radial Artery

The *radial artery* curves dorsally around the scaphoid and trapezium and crosses the floor of the *anatomical snuff box* (Fig. 6.44*C*). It enters the palm by passing between the heads of the 1st dorsal interosseous muscle and then turns medially, passing between the heads of the adductor pollicis. The radial artery ends by anastomosing with the deep branch of the ulnar artery to form the **deep palmar arch,** which is formed mainly by the radial artery. This arch lies across the metacarpals just distal to their bases (Fig. 6.53). The deep pal-

mar arch gives rise to three *palmar metacarpal arteries* and the *princeps pollicis artery*. The *radialis indicis* artery passes along the lateral side of the index finger. It usually arises from the radial artery, but it may originate from the princeps pollicis.

Laceration of the Palmar Arches

Bleeding is usually profuse when the palmar (arterial) arches are lacerated. It may not be sufficient to ligate only one forearm artery when the arches are lacerated, because these vessels usually have numerous communications in the forearm and hand and thus bleed from both ends. To obtain a bloodless surgical operating field for treating complicated hand injuries, it may be necessary to compress the brachial artery and its branches proximal to the elbow (e.g., using a pneumatic tourniquet). This procedure prevents blood from reaching the ulnar and radial arteries through the anastomoses around the elbow.

Ischemia of the Fingers

Intermittent bilateral attacks of *ischemia of the fingers*, marked by cyanosis and often accompanied by paresthesia and pain, is characteristically brought on by cold and emotional stimuli. The condition may result from an anatomical abnormality or an underlying disease. When the cause of the condition is idiopathic (unknown) or primary, it is called *Raynaud syndrome* (disease). The arteries of the upper limb are innervated by sympathetic nerves. Postsynaptic fibers from the sympathetic ganglia enter nerves that form the brachial plexus and are distributed to the digital arteries through branches arising from the plexus. When treating ischemia resulting from Raynaud syndrome, it may be necessary to perform a cervicodorsal *presynaptic sympathectomy* (excision of a segment of a sympathetic nerve) to dilate the digital arteries. ✪

Veins of the Hand

Superficial and *deep venous palmar arches,* associated with the superficial and deep palmar (arterial) arches, drain into the deep veins of the forearm (Fig. 6.46). The dorsal digital veins drain into three dorsal metacarpal veins, which unite to form a *dorsal venous network* (Fig. 6.12*A*). Superficial to the metacarpus, this network is prolonged proximally on the lateral side as the *cephalic vein*. The *basilic vein* arises from the medial side of the dorsal venous network.

Nerves of the Hand

The median, ulnar, and radial nerves supply the hand (Figs. 6.47, 6.52, and 6.55). These nerves and their branches in the hand are illustrated and their origins, courses, and distributions

Table 6.12. Arteries of the Hand

Anterior view

Lateral view
(isolated 3rd digit)

Posterior view

Artery	Origin	Course
Superficial palmar arch	Direct continuation of ulnar artery; arch is completed on lateral side by superficial branch of radial artery or another of its branches	Curves laterally deep to palmar aponeurosis and superficial to long flexor tendons; curve of arch lies across palm at level of distal border of extended thumb
Deep palmar arch	Direct continuation of radial artery; arch is completed on medial side by deep branch of ulnar artery	Curves medially, deep to long flexor tendons; is in contact with bases of metacarpals
Common palmar digitals	Superficial palmar arch	Pass distally on lumbricals to webbing of fingers
Proper palmar digitals	Common palmar digital arteries	Run along sides of 2nd–5th fingers
Princeps pollicis	Radial artery as it turns into palm	Descends on palmar aspect of 1st metacarpal; divides at base of proximal phalanx into two branches that run along sides of thumb
Radialis indicis	Radial artery but may arise from princeps pollicis artery	Passes along lateral side of index finger to its distal end
Dorsal carpal arch	Radial and ulnar arteries	Arches within fascia on dorsum of hand

are provided in Table 6.13. In addition, branches or communications from the lateral and posterior cutaneous nerves may contribute some fibers that supply the skin of the dorsum of the hand.

The Median Nerve in the Hand

The *median nerve* enters the hand through the carpal tunnel, deep to the flexor retinaculum, along with the nine tendons of the FDS, FDP, and FPL (Fig. 6.55). The **carpal tunnel** is the passageway deep to the flexor retinaculum between the tubercles of the scaphoid and trapezoid bones on the lateral side and the pisiform and hook of the hamate on the medial side. Distal to the carpal tunnel, the median nerve supplies two and a half thenar muscles and the 1st and 2nd lumbricals (Table 6.13). It also sends sensory fibers to the skin on the entire palmar surface, the sides of the first three digits,

the lateral half of the 4th digit, and the dorsum of the distal halves of these digits. Note, however, that the *palmar cutaneous branch of the median nerve,* which supplies the central palm, arises proximal to the flexor retinaculum and passes superficial to it (i.e., it does not pass through the carpal tunnel).

Lesions of the Median Nerve

Lesions of the median nerve usually occur in two places: the forearm and the wrist. The most common site is where the nerve passes through the carpal tunnel. ▶

Carpal Tunnel Syndrome

Carpal tunnel syndrome results from any lesion that significantly reduces the size of the carpal tunnel (Fig. B6.29A–D) or, more commonly, increases the size of some of the nine structures (or their coverings) that pass through it (e.g., inflammation of synovial sheaths). Fluid retention, infection, and excessive exercise of the fingers may cause swelling of the tendons or their synovial sheaths. The median nerve is the most sensitive structure in the carpal ▶

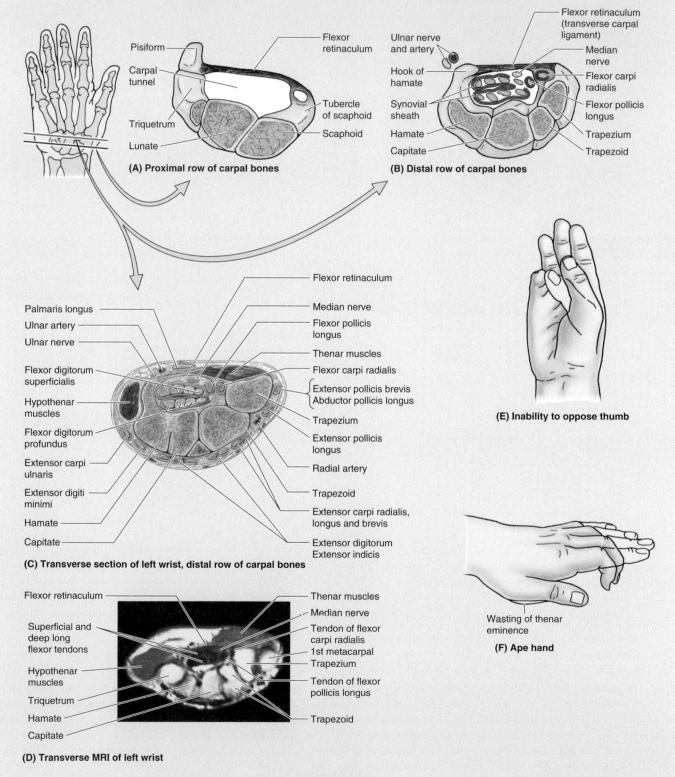

(A) Proximal row of carpal bones

Pisiform
Carpal tunnel
Triquetrum
Lunate
Flexor retinaculum
Tubercle of scaphoid
Scaphoid

(B) Distal row of carpal bones

Ulnar nerve and artery
Hook of hamate
Synovial sheath
Hamate
Capitate
Flexor retinaculum (transverse carpal ligament)
Median nerve
Flexor carpi radialis
Flexor pollicis longus
Trapezium
Trapezoid

(C) Transverse section of left wrist, distal row of carpal bones

Palmaris longus
Ulnar artery
Ulnar nerve
Flexor digitorum superficialis
Hypothenar muscles
Flexor digitorum profundus
Extensor carpi ulnaris
Extensor digiti minimi
Hamate
Capitate
Flexor retinaculum
Median nerve
Flexor pollicis longus
Thenar muscles
Flexor carpi radialis
Extensor pollicis brevis
Abductor pollicis longus
Trapezium
Extensor pollicis longus
Radial artery
Trapezoid
Extensor carpi radialis, longus and brevis
Extensor digitorum
Extensor indicis

(E) Inability to oppose thumb

(D) Transverse MRI of left wrist

Flexor retinaculum
Superficial and deep long flexor tendons
Hypothenar muscles
Triquetrum
Hamate
Capitate
Thenar muscles
Median nerve
Tendon of flexor carpi radialis
1st metacarpal
Trapezium
Tendon of flexor pollicis longus
Trapezoid

Wasting of thenar eminence

(F) Ape hand

Figure B6.29

(cont'd on page 843)

Thenar eminence

Recurrent branch of median nerve to thenar muscles

Pisiform

Flexor carpi ulnaris (FCU)

Ulnar nerve and artery

Dorsal branch of ulnar nerve

Flexor digitorum superficialis (FDS)

Palmaris longus

Tubercle of scaphoid crossed by flexor carpi radialis

Abductus pollicis longus (APL)

Level of section for B

Median nerve with palmar cutaneous branch

Flexor pollicis longus (FPL)

Radial artery with palmar carpal and superficial palmar branches

Superficial branch of radial nerve

Brachioradialis

Ulnar
←
(medial)

Radial
→
(lateral)

(A)

(C)

Flexor digitorum superficialis (FDS)

Flexor digitorum profundus (FDP)

Flexor carpi ulnaris (FCU)

Ulnar nerve and artery

Distal radioulnar joint

Extensor carpi ulnaris (ECU)

5 4 3 2

Palmaris longus tendon

Median nerve and flexor carpi radialis

Flexor pollicis longus (FPL)

Superficial palmar branch

Pronator quadratus

Brachioradialis

Abductor pollicis longus (APL)

Radial artery (aberrant)

Extensor pollicis brevis (EPB)

Extensor carpi radialis longus (ECRL)

Extensor carpi radialis brevis (ECRB)

Extensor pollicis longus (EPL)

(B)   Extensor digiti minimi   Extensor indicis   Extensor digitorum

Figure 6.55. Structures in distal forearm (wrist region). A. A distal skin incision was made along the transverse wrist crease, crossing the pisiform bone. The skin and fasciae are removed proximally, revealing the tendons and neurovascular structures. A circular incision and removal of the skin and thenar fascia reveals the recurrent branch of the median nerve to the thenar muscles, vulnerable to injury when this area is lacerated because of its subcutaneous location. **B.** This transverse section of the distal forearm demonstrates the long flexor and extensor tendons and neurovascular structures en route from forearm to hand. The ulnar nerve and artery are under cover of the flexor carpi ulnaris; therefore, the pulse of the artery cannot be easily detected here. **C.** Orientation drawing indicating the plane of the section shown in part **D.**

Table 6.13. Nerves of the Hand

(A) Palmar aspect

(B) Dorsal aspect

Nerve	Origin[a]	Course	Distribution
Median nerve	Arises by two roots, one from lateral cord of brachial plexus (C6, C7 fibers) and one from medial cord (C8, T1 fibers)	Becomes superficial proximal to wrist; passes deep to flexor retinaculum (transverse carpal ligament) as it passes through carpal tunnel to hand	Thenar muscles (except adductor pollicis and deep head of flexor pollicis brevis) and lateral lumbricals (for digits 2 and 3); provides sensation to skin of palmar and distal dorsal aspects of lateral (radial) 3½ digits and adjacent palm
Recurrent (thenar) branch of median nerve	Arises from median nerve as soon as it has passed distal to flexor retinaculum	Loops around distal border of flexor retinaculum; enters thenar muscles	Abductor pollicis brevis; opponens pollicis; superficial head of flexor pollicis brevis
Lateral branch of median nerve	Arises as lateral division of median nerve as it enters palm of hand	Runs laterally to palmar thumb and radial side of 2nd finger	1st lumbrical; skin of palmar and distal dorsal aspects of thumb and radial half of 2nd finger
Medial branch of median nerve	Arises as medial division of median nerve as it enters palm of hand	Runs medially to adjacent sides of 2nd–4th fingers	2nd lumbrical; skin of palmar and distal dorsal aspects of adjacent sides of 2nd–4th fingers
Palmar cutaneous branch of median nerve	Arisies from median nerve just proximal to flexor retinaculum	Passes between tendons of palmaris longus and flexor carpi radialis; runs superficial to flexor retinaculum	Skin of central palm

Table 6.13. Nerves of the Hand (*continued*)

Nerve	Origin*a*	Course	Distribution
Ulnar nerve	Terminal branch of medial cord of brachial plexus (C8 and T1 fibers; often also receives C7 fibers)	Becomes superficial in distal forearm, passing superficial to flexor retinaculum (transverse carpal ligament) to enter hand	The majority of intrinsic muscles of hand (hypothenar, interosseous, adductor pollicis, and deep head of flexor pollicis brevis, plus the medial lumbricals [for digits 4 and 5]); provides sensation to skin of palmar and distal dorsal aspects of medial (ulnar) 1½ digits and adjacent palm
Palmar cutaneous branch of ulnar nerve	Arises from ulnar nerve near middle of forearm	Descends on ulnar artery and perforates deep fascia in the distal third of forearm	Skin at base of medial palm, overlying the medial carpals
Dorsal branch of ulnar nerve	Arises from ulnar nerve about 5 cm proximal to flexor retinaculum	Passes distally deep to flexor carpi ulnaris, then dorsally to perforate deep fascia and course along medial side of dorsum of hand, dividing into 2 to 3 dorsal digital nerves	Skin of medial aspect of dorsum of hand and proximal portions of little and medial half of ring finger (occasionally also adjacent sides of proximal portions of ring and middle fingers)
Superficial branch of ulnar nerve	Arises from ulnar nerve at wrist as they pass between pisiform and hamate bones	Passes palmaris brevis and divides into two common palmar digital nerves	Palmaris brevis and sensation to skin of the palmar and distal dorsal aspects of digit 5 and of the medial (ulnar) side of digit 4 and proximal portion of palm
Deep branch of ulnar nerve		Passes between muscles of hypothenar eminence to pass deeply across palm with deep palmar (arterial) arch	Hypothenar muscles (abductor, flexor, and opponens digiti minimi), lumbricals of digits 4 and 5, all interossei, adductor pollicis, and deep head of flexor pollicis brevis
Radial nerve Superficial branch	Arises from radial nerve in cubital fossa	Courses deep to brachioradialis, emerging from beneath it to pierce the deep fascia lateral to distal radius	Skin of the lateral (radial half of dorsal aspect of the hand and thumb, the proximal portions of the dorsal aspects of digits 2 and 3, and of the lateral (radial) half of digit 4

tunnel (Fig. B6.29*B–D*) and therefore is the most affected. This nerve has two terminal sensory branches that supply the skin of the hand; hence, **paresthesia** (tingling), **hypoesthesia** (diminished sensation), or **anesthesia** (absence of sensation) may occur in the lateral three and a half digits. Recall, however, that the palmar cutaneous branch of the median nerve arises proximal to and does not pass through the carpal tunnel; thus sensation in the central palm remains unaffected. The nerve also has one terminal motor branch, the recurrent branch, which serves the three thenar muscles (Table 6.11).

Progressive loss of coordination and strength in the thumb (owing to weakness of the APB and opponens pollicis) may occur if the cause of compression is not alleviated.

Individuals with carpal tunnel syndrome are unable to oppose the thumb (Fig. B6.29*E*) and have difficulty buttoning a shirt or blouse as well as gripping things such as a comb. As the condition progresses, sensory changes radiate into the forearm and axilla. Symptoms of compression can be reproduced by compression of the median nerve with your finger at the wrist for approximately 30 s. To relieve both the compression and the resulting symptoms, partial or complete surgical division of the flexor retinaculum, a procedure called **carpal tunnel release,** may be necessary. The incision for carpal tunnel release is made toward the medial side of the wrist and flexor retinaculum to avoid possible injury to the recurrent branch of the median nerve. ✪

Trauma to the Median Nerve

Laceration of the wrist often causes median nerve injury because this nerve is relatively close to the surface. In attempted suicides by wrist slashing, the median nerve is commonly injured just proximal to the flexor retinaculum. This results in paralysis of the thenar muscles and the first two lumbricals. Hence, opposition of the thumb is not possible and fine control movements of the 2nd and 3rd digits are impaired. Sensation is also lost over the thumb and adjacent two and a half fingers.

Most nerve injuries in the upper limb affect opposition of the thumb. Undoubtedly, injuries to the nerves supplying the intrinsic muscles of the hand, especially the median nerve, have the most severe effects on this complex movement. If the median nerve is severed in the forearm or at the wrist, the thumb cannot be opposed; however, the APL and adductor pollicis (supplied by the posterior interosseous and ulnar nerves, respectively) may imitate opposition.

Median nerve injury resulting from a perforating wound in the elbow region results in loss of flexion of the proximal ▶

and distal interphalangeal joints of the 2nd and 3rd digits. The ability to flex the metacarpophalangeal joints of these fingers is also affected because digital branches of the median nerve supply the 1st and 2nd lumbricals. *Ape hand* (Fig. B6.29F) refers to a deformity in which thumb movements are limited to flexion and extension of the thumb in the plane of the palm.

This condition is caused by the inability to oppose and by limited abduction of the thumb. The recurrent branch of the median nerve to the thenar muscles (Fig. 6.55A) lies subcutaneously and may be severed by relatively minor lacerations of the thenar eminence. Severance of this nerve paralyzes the thenar muscles and the thumb loses much of its usefulness. ☉

The Ulnar Nerve in the Hand

The *ulnar nerve* leaves the forearm by emerging from deep to the tendon of the FCU (Figs. 6.52 and 6.55). It continues distally to the wrist via the *ulnar canal* (Fig. 6.48). Here the ulnar nerve is bound by fascia to the anterior surface of the flexor retinaculum as it passes between the pisiform (medially) and the ulnar artery (laterally). Just proximal to the wrist, the ulnar nerve gives off a *palmar cutaneous branch* that passes superficial to the flexor retinaculum and palmar aponeurosis and supplies skin on the medial side of the palm (Table 6.13). The *dorsal cutaneous branch of the ulnar nerve* supplies the medial half of the dorsum of the hand, the 5th finger, and the medial half of the 4th finger (Fig. 6.55B). The ulnar nerve ends at the distal border of the flexor retinaculum by dividing into superficial and deep branches (Fig. 6.52B). The *superficial branch of the ulnar nerve* supplies cutaneous branches to the anterior surfaces of the medial one and a half fingers. The *deep branch of the ulnar nerve* supplies the hypothenar muscles, the medial two lumbricals, the adductor pollicis, the deep head of the FPB, and all the interossei. The deep branch also supplies several joints (wrist, intercarpal, carpometacarpal, and intermetacarpal). The ulnar nerve is often referred to as the *nerve of fine movements* because it innervates most of the intrinsic muscles that are concerned with intricate hand movements (Table 6.13).

compresses their ulnar nerves. This type of nerve compression, which has been called *handlebar neuropathy,* results in sensory loss on the medial side of the hand and weakness of the intrinsic hand muscles. ☉

Radial Nerve in the Hand

The *radial nerve* supplies no hand muscles (Table 6.13). The *superficial branch of the radial nerve* is entirely sensory (Fig. 6.55A). It pierces the deep fascia near the dorsum of the wrist to supply the skin and fascia over the lateral two thirds of the dorsum of the hand, the dorsum of the thumb, and proximal parts of the lateral one and a half digits (Table 6.10).

Ulnar Canal Syndrome (Guyon Tunnel Syndrome)

Compression of the ulnar nerve may occur at the wrist where it passes between the pisiform and the hook of the hamate. The depression between these bones is converted by the pisohamate ligament into an osseofibrous tunnel, the ulnar canal (Guyon tunnel; Fig. 6.47B). **Ulnar canal syndrome** is manifest by hypoesthesia in the medial one and a half fingers and weakness of the intrinsic muscles of the hand. "Clawing" of the 4th and 5th fingers (hyperextension at the metacarpophalangeal joint with flexion at the proximal interphalangeal joint) may occur, but—in contradistinction to proximal ulnar nerve injury—their ability to flex is unaffected and there is no radial deviation of the hand.

Handlebar Neuropathy

People who ride long distances on bicycles with their hands in an extended position against the hand grips put pressure on the hooks of their hamates, which

Radial Nerve Injury and the Hand

Although the radial nerve supplies no muscles in the hand, radial nerve injury in the arm can produce serious hand disability. The characteristic handicap is inability to extend the wrist resulting from *paralysis of extensor muscles of the forearm,* all of which are innervated by the radial nerve (Fig. 6.40B; Table 6.8). The hand is flexed at the wrist and lies flaccid, a condition known as *wrist-drop* (see clinical correlation [blue] box "Injury to the Radial Nerve in the Arm," earlier in this chapter). The fingers of the relaxed hand also remain in the flexed position at the metacarpophalangeal joints. The interphalangeal joints can be extended weakly through the action of the intact lumbricals and interossei, which are supplied by the median and ulnar nerves (Table 6.11). The radial nerve has only a small area of exclusive cutaneous supply onthe hand. Thus the extent of anesthesia is minimal, even in serious radial nerve injuries, and is usually confined to a small area on the lateral part of the dorsum of the hand. ☉

THE BOTTOM LINE: The vasculature of the hand is characterized by multiple anastomoses between both radial and ulnar vessels and palmar and dorsal vessels. The arteries of the hand collectively constitute a periarticular arterial anastomosis around the collective joints of the wrist and hand. Thus blood is generally available to all parts of the hand in all positions as well as while performing functions (gripping or pressing) that might otherwise compromise especially the palmar structures. The arteries to the digits are also characterized by their ability to vasoconstrict during exposure to cold to conserve heat and to dilate (while the hand becomes sweaty) to radiate excess heat.

Unlike the dermatomes of the trunk and proximal limbs, the zones of cutaneous innervation and the roles of motor innervation are well defined, as are functional deficits. In terms of intrinsic structure, the radial nerve is only sensory via its superficial branch to the dorsum of the hand. The me-

dian nerve is most important to the function of the thumb and sensation from the lateral three and half digits and adjacent palm, whereas the ulnar nerve supplies the remainder. The intrinsic muscles of the hand constitute the T1 myotome.

The palmar nerves and vessels are dominant, supplying not only the more sensitive and functional palmar aspect but also the dorsal aspect of the distal part of the digits (nail beds). The superficial dorsal venous network is commonly used for administering intravenous fluids.

Surface Anatomy of the Hand

The *radial artery pulse*, like other palpable pulses, is a peripheral reflection of cardiac action. The radial pulse rate is measured where the radial artery lies on the anterior surface of the distal end of the radius, lateral to the FCR tendon, which serves as a guide to the artery (Fig. SA6.15). Here the artery can be felt pulsating between the tendons of the FCR and the APL and where it can be compressed against the radius. The **tendons of FCR and palmaris longus** can be palpated anterior to the wrist, a little lateral to its middle, and are usually observed by flexing the closed fist against resistance. The palmaris longus tendon is smaller than the FCR tendon and is not always present. The palmaris longus tendon serves as a guide to the median nerve, which lies deep to it (Fig. 6.55*B*). The **FCU tendon** can be palpated as it

crosses the anterior aspect of the wrist near the medial side and inserts into the pisiform. The FCU tendon serves as a guide to the ulnar nerve and artery. The **tendons of the FDS** can be palpated as the fingers are alternately flexed and extended. The ulnar pulse is often difficult to palpate. The **tendons of the APL and EPB** indicate the anterior boundary of the **anatomical snuff box** (Fig. SA6.16). The **tendon of the EPL** indicates the posterior boundary of the box. The radial artery crosses the floor of the snuff box, where its pulsations may be felt. The **scaphoid** and, less distinctly, the **trapezium** are palpable in the floor of the snuff box.

The skin covering the dorsum of the hand is thin and loose when the hand is relaxed. Prove this by pinching and pulling folds of your skin here. The looseness of the skin results from the mobility of the subcutaneous tissue and from the relatively few fibrous skin ligaments that are present. ▶

Hypothenar eminence

Location of pisiform bone

Tendon of flexor carpi ulnaris (FCU)

Tendon of palmaris longus

Thenar eminence

Tendon of abductor pollicis longus (APL)

Site for taking radial pulse

Tendon of flexor carpi radialis (FCR)

Anterolateral view   S = location of tendons of FDS

Figure SA6.15

Adductor pollicis

1st dorsal interosseous

Tendon of extensor
pollicis longus (EPL)

Anatomical snuff box

Tendon of abductor
pollicis longus (APL)
and extensor pollicis
brevis (EPB)

Tendons of extensor
digitorum

Head of ulna

Posterior view

Figure SA6.16

Hair is present in this region and on the proximal parts of the digits, especially in men. If the dorsum of the hand is examined with the wrist extended against resistance and the digits abducted, the **tendons of the extensor digitorum** to the fingers stand out, particularly in thin individuals. These tendons are not visible far beyond the knuckles because they flatten here to form the extensor expansions of the fingers (Fig. 6.42B). The knuckles that become visible when a fist is made are produced by the **heads of the metacarpals.** Under the loose subcutaneous tissue and extensor tendons on the dorsum of the hand, the metacarpals can be palpated. A prominent feature of the dorsum of the hand is the *dorsal venous network* (Fig. 6.12A).

The skin on the palm is thick because it must withstand the wear and tear of work and play (Fig. SA6.17). It is richly supplied with sweat glands but contains no hair or sebaceous glands. The *superficial palmar arch* lies across the center of the palm, level with the distal border of the fully extended thumb. The main part of the arch ends at the **thenar eminence.** The *deep palmar arch* lies approximately 1 cm proximal to the superficial palmar arch. The palmar skin presents several more or less constant *flexion creases,* where the skin is firmly bound to the deep fascia, that help locate palmar wounds and underlying structures: ▶

- **Wrist creases, proximal, middle, distal:** The distal wrist crease indicates the proximal border of the flexor retinaculum.

- **Palmar creases, transverse, longitudinal:** The longitudinal creases deepen when the thumb is opposed; the transverse creases deepen when the metacarpophalangeal joints are flexed.

    - **Radial longitudinal crease** (the "life line" of palmistry): partially encircles the *thenar eminence*, formed by the short muscles of the thumb.

    - **Proximal (transverse) palmar crease:** commences on the lateral border of the palm, superficial to the head of the 2nd metacarpal; extends medially and slightly proximally across the palm, superficial to the bodies of the 3rd–5th metacarpals.

- **Distal (transverse) palmar crease:** begins at or near the cleft between the index and the middle fingers; crosses the palm with a slight convexity, superficial to the head

of the 3rd metacarpal and then proximal to the heads of the 4th and 5th metacarpals.

Each of the medial four fingers usually has three *transverse digital flexion creases:*

- **Proximal digital crease:** located at the root of the finger, approximately 2 cm distal to the metacarpophalangeal joint.

- **Middle digital crease:** lies over the proximal interphalangeal joint.

- **Distal digital crease:** lies over or just proximal to the distal interphalangeal joint.

The thumb, having two phalanges, has only two flexion creases. The proximal digital crease of the thumb crosses obliquely, at or proximal to the 1st metacarpophalangeal joint. The **skin ridges** on the pads of the digits, forming the *fingerprints,* are used for identification because of their unique patterns. The physiological function of the skin ridges is to reduce slippage when grasping objects. ◐

Anterior view

Figure SA6.17

Dermatoglyphics

The science of studying ridge patterns of the palm, called **dermatoglyphics,** is a valuable extension of the conventional physical examination of people with certain congenital anomalies and genetic diseases (Nussbaum et al., 2004). For example, people with trisomy 21 (Down syndrome) have dermatoglyphics that are highly characteristic. In addition, they often have a single transverse palmar crease (simian crease); however, approximately 1% of the general population has this crease with no other clinical features of the syndrome.

Palmar Wounds and Surgical Incisions

The location of superficial and deep palmar arches should be kept in mind when examining wounds of the palm and when making palmar incisions. Furthermore, it is important to know that the superficial palmar arch is at the same level as the distal extremity of the common flexor sheath (Figs. 6.52 and 6.54). As mentioned previously, incisions or wounds along the medial surface of the thenar eminence may injure the recurrent branch of the median nerve to the thenar muscles (see clinical correlation [blue] box "Trauma to the Median Nerve," earlier in this chapter). ✪

Joints of the Upper Limb

Movement of the *pectoral girdle* involves the sternoclavicular, acromioclavicular, and glenohumeral joints (Fig. 6.56), usually all moving simultaneously. Functional defects in any of the joints impair movements of the pectoral girdle. Mobility of the scapula is essential for free movement of the upper limb. The clavicle forms a strut that holds the scapula, and hence the glenohumeral joint, away from the thorax so it can move freely. The clavicle establishes the radius at which the shoulder (half of the pectoral girdle and glenohumeral joint) rotates at the SC joint. The 15–20° of movement at the AC joint permits positioning of the glenoid cavity that is necessary for arm movements.

When *testing the range of motion of the pectoral girdle,* both scapulothoracic (movement of the scapula on the thoracic wall) and glenohumeral movements must be considered. Although the initial 30° of abduction may occur without scapular motion, in the overall movement of fully elevating the arm, the movement occurs in a 2:1 ratio: For every 3° of elevation, approximately 2° occurs at the glenohumeral joint and 1° at the physiological scapulothoracic

joint. In other words, when the upper limb has been elevated so that the arm is vertical at the side of the head (180° of arm abduction or flexion), 120° occurred at the glenohumeral joint and 60° occurred at the scapulothoracic joint. This is known as *scapulohumeral rhythm.* The important movements of the pectoral girdle are scapular movements (Table 6.3): elevation and depression, protraction (lateral or forward movement of the scapula) and retraction (medial or backward movement of the scapula), and rotation of the scapula.

Sternoclavicular Joint

The **sternoclavicular joint** is a saddle type of synovial joint but functions as a ball-and-socket joint. The SC joint is divided into two compartments by an *articular disc.* The disc is firmly attached to the *anterior* and *posterior sternoclavicular ligaments,* thickenings of the fibrous layer of the joint capsule, as well as the *interclavicular ligament.* The great strength of the SC joint is a consequence of these attachments. Thus, although the articular disc serves as a shock absorber of forces transmitted along the clavicle from the upper limb, dislocation of the clavicle is rare, whereas fracture of the clavicle is common. The SC joint is the only articulation between the upper limb and the axial skeleton, and it can be readily palpated because the sternal end of the clavicle lies superior to the manubrium of the sternum.

Articulation of the Sternoclavicular Joint
The sternal end of the clavicle articulates with the manubrium and the 1st costal cartilage. The articular surfaces are covered with fibrocartilage.

Joint Capsule of the Sternoclavicular Joint
The *joint capsule* surrounds the SC joint, including the epiphysis at the sternal end of the clavicle. It is attached to the margins of the articular surfaces, including the periphery of the articular disc. A *synovial membrane* lines the internal surface of the *fibrous layer* of the joint capsule, extending to the edges of the articular surfaces.

Ligaments of the Sternoclavicular Joint
The strength of the SC joint depends on ligaments and its articular disc. **Anterior** and **posterior sternoclavicular ligaments** reinforce the joint capsule anteriorly and posteriorly. The **interclavicular ligament** strengthens the capsule superiorly. It extends from the sternal end of one clavicle to the sternal end of the other clavicle. In between, it is also attached to the superior border of the manubrium. The **costoclavicular ligament** anchors the inferior surface of the sternal end of the clavicle to the 1st rib and its costal cartilage, limiting elevation of the pectoral girdle.

Movements of the Sternoclavicular Joint
Although the SC joint is extremely strong, it is significantly mobile to allow movements of the pectoral girdle and upper limb (Figs. 6.57 and 6.58C). During full elevation of the limb, the clavicle is raised to approximately a 60° angle.

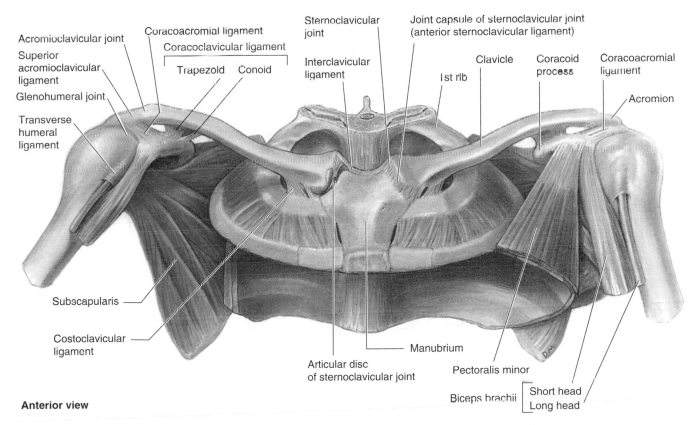

Anterior view

Figure 6.56. Pectoral girdle and associated tendons and ligaments. The pectoral (shoulder) girdle is a partial bony ring (incomplete posteriorly) formed by the manubrium of the sternum, the clavicle, and the scapulae. Joints associated with these bones are the sternoclavicular, acromioclavicular, and glenohumeral (shoulder). The girdle provides for attachment of the superior appendicular skeleton to the axial skeleton and provides the mobile base from which the upper limb operates.

Figure 6.57. Movements of upper limb at joints of pectoral girdle. A. Range of motion of lateral end of clavicle permitted by movements at the sternoclavicular joint. $A \leftrightarrow C$ = protraction/retraction; $A \leftrightarrow D$ = elevation/depression. **B–F.** Circumduction of upper limb requires coordinated movements of the pectoral girdle and glenohumeral joint. **B.** Beginning with extended limb, retracted girdle; **C.** Neutral position. **D.** Flexed limb, protracted girdle; **E.** Elevated limb and girdle.

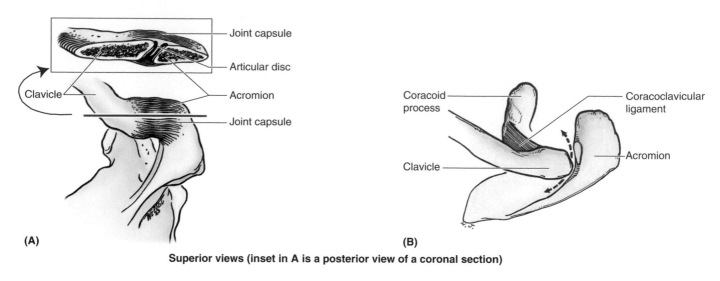

(A)   **(B)**

Superior views (inset in A is a posterior view of a coronal section)

Superior view

Figure 6.58. Acromioclavicular and sternoclavicular joints. A. This view of the right AC joint shows the joint capsule and partial disc (*inset*). **B.** The function of the coracoclavicular ligament is demonstrated. As long as this ligament is intact with the clavicle tethered to the coronoid process, the acromion cannot be driven inferior to the clavicle. The ligament, however, does permit protraction and retraction of the acromion. **C.** Clavicular movements at the SC and AC joints permit protraction and retraction of the scapula on the thoracic wall (*red and green lines*) and winging of the scapula (*blue line*). Movements of a similar scale occur during elevation, depression, and rotation of the scapula. The latter movements are shown in Table 6.3, which also indicate the muscles specifically responsible for these movements.

When elevation is achieved via flexion, it is accompanied by rotation of the clavicle around its longitudinal axis. The SC joint can also be moved anteriorly or posteriorly over a range of up to 25–30°. Although not a typical movement, except perhaps during calisthenics, it is capable of performing these movements sequentially, moving the acromial end along a circular path—a form of *circumduction*.

Blood Supply of the Sternoclavicular Joint

The SC joint is supplied by internal thoracic and suprascapular arteries (Table 6.4).

Nerve Supply of the Sternoclavicular Joint

Branches of the medial supraclavicular nerve and the nerve to the subclavius supply the SC joint (Table 6.5).

Dislocation of the Sternoclavicular Joint

The rarity of dislocation of the SC joint attests to its strength, which depends on its ligaments, its disc, and the way forces are generally transmitted along the clavicle. When a blow is received to the acromion of the scapula, or when a force is transmitted to the pectoral girdle during a fall on the outstretched hand, the force of the blow is usually transmitted along the length of the clavicle, i.e., along its long axis. The clavicle may fracture near the junction of its middle and lateral thirds, but it is rare for the SC joint to dislocate. Most dislocations of the SC joint in persons < 25 years of age result from fractures through the epiphysial plate because the epiphysis at the sternal end of the clavicle does not close until 23–25 years of age.

Ankylosis of the Sternoclavicular Joint

Movement at the SC joint is critical to movement of the shoulder. When **ankylosis** (stiffening or fixation) of the joint occurs, or is necessary surgically, a section of the center of the clavicle is removed, creating a pseudojoint or "flail" joint to permit scapular movement. ☉

Acromioclavicular Joint

The **acromioclavicular joint** (AC joint) is a plane type of synovial joint, which is located 2–3 cm from the "point" of the shoulder formed by the lateral part of the acromion (Figs. 6.56 and 6.58).

Articulation of the Acromioclavicular Joint

The acromial end of the clavicle articulates with the acromion of the scapula. The articular surfaces, covered with fibrocartilage, are separated by an incomplete wedge-shaped *articular disc.*

Joint Capsule of the Acromioclavicular Joint

The sleeve-like, relatively loose *fibrous layer of the joint capsule* is attached to the margins of the articular surfaces (Fig. 6.58A). A *synovial membrane* lines the fibrous layer. Although relatively weak, the joint capsule is strengthened superiorly by fibers of the trapezius.

Ligaments of the Acromioclavicular Joint

The **acromioclavicular ligament** is a fibrous band extending from the acromion to the clavicle that strengthens the AC joint superiorly (Figs. 6.56 and 6.59). However, the integrity of the joint is maintained by extrinsic ligaments, distant from the joint itself. The *coracoclavicular ligament* is a strong pair of bands that unite the coracoid process of the scapula to the clavicle, anchoring the clavicle to the coracoid process. The coracoclavicular ligament consists of two ligaments, the

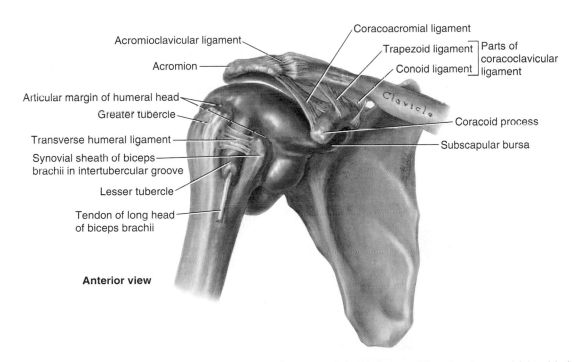

Anterior view

Labels: Acromioclavicular ligament · Acromion · Articular margin of humeral head · Greater tubercle · Transverse humeral ligament · Synovial sheath of biceps brachii in intertubercular groove · Lesser tubercle · Tendon of long head of biceps brachii · Coracoacromial ligament · Trapezoid ligament · Conoid ligament (Parts of coracoclavicular ligament) · Clavicle · Coracoid process · Subscapular bursa

Figure 6.59. Glenohumeral joint. The extent of the synovial membrane of the glenohumeral (shoulder) joint is demonstrated in this specimen in which the articular cavity has been injected with blue latex and the fibrous layer of the joint capsule has been removed. The articular cavity has two extensions: one where it forms a synovial sheath for the tendon of the long head of the biceps brachii in the intertubercular groove of the humerus, and the other inferior to the coracoid process where it is continuous with the subscapular bursa between the subscapularis tendon and the margin of the glenoid cavity. The joint capsule and intrinsic ligaments of the AC joint are also demonstrated.

conoid and trapezoid ligaments, which are often separated by a bursa. The vertical **conoid ligament** is an inverted triangle (cone), which has its apex inferiorly where it is attached to the root of the *coracoid process*. Its wide attachment (base of the triangle) is to the *conoid tubercle* on the inferior surface of the clavicle. The nearly horizontal **trapezoid ligament** is attached to the superior surface of the coracoid process and extends laterally to the trapezoid line on the inferior surface of the clavicle. In addition to augmenting the AC joint, the coracoclavicular ligament provides the means by which the scapula and free limb are (passively) suspended from the clavicular strut.

Movements of the Acromioclavicular Joint

The acromion of the scapula rotates on the acromial end of the clavicle. These movements are associated with motion at the physiological scapulothoracic joint (Figs. 6.57 and 6.58; Table 6.3). No muscles connect the articulating bones to move the AC joint; the axioappendicular muscles that attach to and move the scapula cause the acromion to move on the clavicle.

Blood Supply of the Acromioclavicular Joint

The AC joint is supplied by the suprascapular and thoracoacromial arteries (Table 6.4).

Nerve Supply of the Acromioclavicular Joint

Consistent with the Hilton law (joints are supplied by articular branches of the nerves supplying the muscles that act on the joint), the lateral pectoral and axillary nerves supply the AC joint (Table 6.5). However, consistent with the joint's subcutaneous location and the fact that no muscles connect the articulating bones, innervation is also provided to the AC joint by the subcutaneous lateral supraclavicular nerve, an occurrence more typical of the distal limb.

Dislocation of the Acromioclavicular Joint

Although its extrinsic coracoclavicular ligament is strong, the AC joint itself is weak and easily injured by a direct blow (Fig. B6.30). In contact sports such as football, soccer, hockey, or the martial arts, it is not uncommon for *dislocation of the AC joint* to result from a hard fall on the shoulder or on the outstretched upper limb. Dislocation of the AC joint can also occur when a hockey player is driven into the boards or when a person receives a severe blow to the superolateral part of the back. An AC joint dislocation, ▶

Prominence of dislocated clavicle
Clavicle
Torn coracoclavicular ligament
Torn acromioclavicular ligament
Acromion
Coraco-acromial ligament
Coracoid process
Scapula
Humerus
(C)

(A) Dislocation of acromioclavicular joint without ligament rupture

(B) Dislocation of acromioclavicular joint and rupture of coracoclavicular ligament

Figure B6.30

often called a "shoulder separation," is severe when both the AC and the coracoclavicular ligaments are torn. When the coracoclavicular ligament tears, the shoulder separates from the clavicle and falls because of the weight of the upper limb. *Rupture of the coracoclavicular ligament* allows the fibrous layer of the joint capsule to be torn so that the acromion can pass inferior to the acromial end of the clavicle. Dislocation of the AC joint makes the acromion more prominent, and the clavicle may move superior to this process. ○

Glenohumeral Joint

The **glenohumeral (shoulder) joint** is a ball-and-socket type of synovial joint that permits a wide range of movement; however, its mobility makes the joint relatively unstable.

Articulation of the Glenohumeral Joint

The large, round *humeral head* articulates with the relatively shallow *glenoid cavity* of the scapula (Figs. 6.60 and 6.61), which is deepened slightly but effectively by the ring-like, fibrocartilaginous **glenoid labrum** (L. lip). Both articular surfaces are covered with hyaline cartilage. The glenoid cavity accepts little more than a third of the humeral head, which is

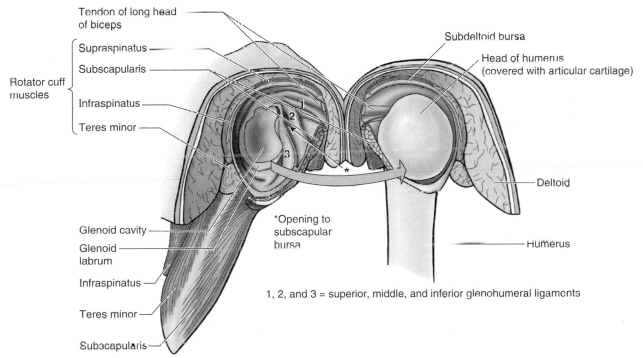

(A) Anterolateral view of glenoid cavity; posteromedial view of humerus

1, 2, and 3 = superior, middle, and inferior glenohumeral ligaments

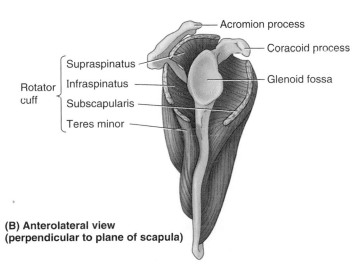

(B) Anterolateral view (perpendicular to plane of scapula)

Figure 6.60. Rotator cuff and glenohumeral joint. A. In this dissection of the glenohumeral joint, the joint capsule was sectioned and the joint opened from its posterior aspect as if it were a book. Four short SITS muscles (supraspinatus, infraspinatus, teres minor, and subscapularis) cross and surround the joint, blending with its capsule. The anterior, internal surface demonstrates the glenohumeral ligaments, which were incised to open the joint. **B.** The SITS muscles of the left rotator cuff are shown as they relate to the scapula and its glenoid cavity. The prime function of these muscles and the musculotendinous rotator cuff is to hold the relatively large head of the humerus in the much smaller and shallow glenoid cavity of the scapula.

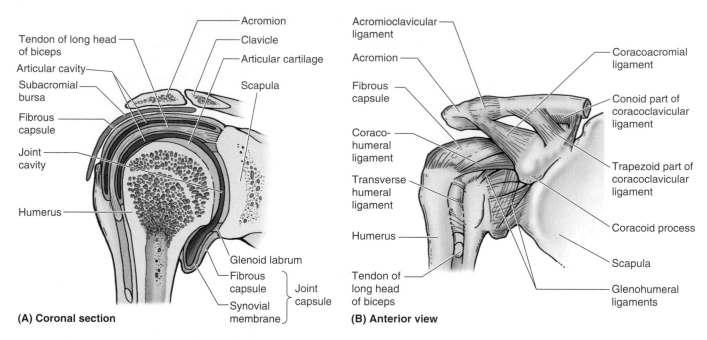

(A) Coronal section

Labels (A): Tendon of long head of biceps; Articular cavity; Subacromial bursa; Fibrous capsule; Joint cavity; Humerus; Acromion; Clavicle; Articular cartilage; Scapula; Glenoid labrum; Fibrous capsule; Synovial membrane; Joint capsule

(B) Anterior view

Labels (B): Acromioclavicular ligament; Acromion; Fibrous capsule; Coracohumeral ligament; Transverse humeral ligament; Humerus; Tendon of long head of biceps; Coracoacromial ligament; Conoid part of coracoclavicular ligament; Trapezoid part of coracoclavicular ligament; Coracoid process; Scapula; Glenohumeral ligaments

(C)

Figure 6.61. Capsules and ligaments of glenohumeral and acromioclavicular joints. A. The bones, articular surfaces, joint capsule, cavity of the joints, the subacromial bursa are shown. **B.** The acromioclavicular, coracohumeral, and glenohumeral ligaments are demonstrated. Although shown on the external aspect of the joint capsule, the glenohumeral ligaments are actually a feature observed from the internal aspect of the joint (as in Fig. 6.60A). These ligaments strengthen the anterior aspect of the capsule of the glenohumeral joint, and the coracohumeral ligament strengthens the capsule superiorly. **C.** This coronal MRI shows the right glenohumeral and AC joints. *A,* acromion; *C,* clavicle; *G,* glenoid cavity; *Gr,* greater tubercle of humerus; *H,* head of humerus; *N,* surgical neck of humerus. (Courtesy of Dr. W. Kucharczyk, Chair of Medical Imaging and Clinical Director of Tri-Hospital Resonance Centre, Toronto, Ontario, Canada.)

held in the cavity by the tonus of the musculotendinous rotator cuff, or SITS, muscles (supraspinatus, infraspinatus, teres minor, and subscapularis) (Table 6.2).

Joint Capsule of the Glenohumeral Joint

The loose fibrous layer of the joint capsule surrounds the glenohumeral joint and is attached medially to the margin of the glenoid cavity and laterally to the anatomical neck of the humerus (Fig. 6.61A & B). Superiorly, this part of the joint capsule encroaches on the root of the coracoid process so that the fibrous layer of the joint capsule encloses the proximal attachment of the long head of the biceps brachii to the supraglenoid tubercle of scapula within the joint. The joint capsule has two apertures: (1) an opening between the tubercles of the humerus for passage of the tendon of the long head of the biceps brachii (Fig. 6.59) and (2) an opening situated anteriorly, inferior to the coracoid process that allows communication between the *subscapular bursa* and the synovial cavity of the joint. The inferior part of the joint capsule, the only part not reinforced by the rotator cuff muscles, is its weakest area. Here the capsule is particularly lax and lies in folds when the arm is adducted; however, it becomes taut when the arm is abducted.

The *synovial membrane* lines the internal surface of the fibrous layer of the joint capsule and reflects from it onto the glenoid labrum and the humerus, as far as the articular margin of the head (Figs. 6.59, 6.60A, and 6.61). The synovial membrane also forms a tubular sheath for the tendon of the long head of the biceps brachii, where it lies in the intertubercular groove of the humerus and passes into the joint cavity, extending as far as the surgical neck of the humerus (Fig. 6.59).

Ligaments of the Glenohumeral Joint

The glenohumeral ligaments, which strengthen the anterior aspect of the joint capsule of the joint, and the coracohumeral ligament, which strengthens the capsule superiorly, are intrinsic ligaments—that is, part of the fibrous layer of the joint capsule (Figs. 6.60A and 6.61B). The **glenohumeral ligaments** are three fibrous bands, evident only on the internal aspect of the capsule, that reinforce the anterior part of the joint capsule. These ligaments radiate laterally and inferiorly from the glenoid labrum at the supraglenoid tubercle of the scapula and blend distally with the fibrous layer of the capsule as it attaches to the anatomical neck of the humerus. The **coracohumeral ligament** is a strong broad band that passes from the base of the coracoid process to the anterior aspect of the greater tubercle of the humerus (Fig. 6.61B). The *transverse humeral ligament* is a broad fibrous band that runs more or less obliquely from the greater to the lesser tubercle of the humerus, bridging over the intertubercular groove (Figs. 6.59 and 6.62B). The ligament converts the groove into a canal, which holds the synovial sheath and tendon of the biceps brachii in place during movements of the glenohumeral joint.

The **coracoacromial arch** is an extrinsic, protective structure formed by the smooth inferior aspect of the *acromion* and the *coracoid process* of the scapula, with the **coracoacromial ligament** spanning between them (Fig. 6.61B). This osseoligamentous structure forms a protective arch that overlies the humeral head, preventing its superior displacement from the glenoid cavity. The coracoacromial arch is so strong that a forceful superior thrust of the humerus will not fracture it; the humeral shaft or clavicle fractures first. Transmitting force superiorly along the humerus (e.g., when standing at a desk and partly supporting the body with the outstretched limbs), the humeral head presses against the coracoacromial arch. The supraspinatus muscle passes under this arch and lies deep to the deltoid as its tendon blends with the joint capsule of the glenohumeral joint as part of the rotator cuff (Fig. 6.60A & B). Movement of the supraspinatus tendon, passing to the greater tubercle of the humerus, is facilitated as it passes under the arch by the *subacromial bursa* (Fig. 6.61A), which lies between the arch superiorly and the tendon and tubercle inferiorly.

Movements of the Glenohumeral Joint

The glenohumeral joint has more freedom of movement than any other joint in the body. This freedom results from the laxity of its joint capsule and the large size of the humeral head compared with the small size of the glenoid cavity. The glenohumeral joint allows movements around three axes and permits flexion–extension, abduction–adduction, rotation (medial and lateral) of the humerus, and circumduction. Lateral rotation of the humerus increases the range of abduction. When the arm is abducted without rotation, available articular surface is exhausted and the greater tubercle contacts the *coracoacromial arch,* preventing further abduction. If the arm is then laterally rotated 180°, the tubercles are rotated posteriorly and more articular surface becomes available to continue elevation. *Circumduction* at the glenohumeral joint is an orderly sequence of flexion, abduction, extension, and adduction—or the reverse (Fig. 6.57). Unless performed over a

small range, these movements do not occur at the glenohumeral joint in isolation; they are accompanied by movements at the two other joints of the pectoral girdle (SC and AC). Stiffening or fixation of the joints of the pectoral girdle (*ankylosis*) results in a much more restricted range of movement, even if the glenohumeral joint is normal.

Muscles Moving the Glenohumeral Joint

The movements of the glenohumeral joint and muscles that produce them—the *axioappendicular muscles*, which may act indirectly on the joint (i.e., act on the pectoral girdle), and the *scapulohumeral muscles,* which act directly on the glenohumeral joint (Tables 6.2 and 6.3)—are listed in Table 6.14. Other muscles that serve the glenohumeral joint as shunt muscles, acting to resist dislocation without producing movement at the joint (e.g., when carrying a heavy suitcase), or that maintain the large head of the humerus in the relatively shallow glenoid cavity are also listed.

Blood Supply of the Glenohumeral Joint

The glenohumeral joint is supplied by the *anterior* and *posterior circumflex humeral arteries* and branches of the *suprascapular artery* (Table 6.4).

Innervation of the Glenohumeral Joint

The suprascapular, axillary, and lateral pectoral nerves supply the glenohumeral joint (Table 6.5).

Bursae around the Glenohumeral Joint

Several **bursae** (sac-like cavities) containing capillary films of *synovial fluid* (secreted by the synovial membrane) are situated near the glenohumeral joint. Bursae are located where tendons rub against bone, ligaments, or other tendons and where skin moves over a bony prominence. The bursae around the glenohumeral joint are of special clinical importance because some of them communicate with the articular (joint) cavity (e.g., the subscapular bursa). Consequently, opening a bursa may mean entering the cavity of the glenohumeral joint.

Subscapular Bursa. The **subscapular bursa** is located between the tendon of the subscapularis and the neck of the scapula (Fig. 6.59). The bursa protects the tendon where it passes inferior to the root of the coracoid process and over the neck of the scapula. It usually communicates with the cavity of the glenohumeral joint through an opening in the fibrous layer of the joint capsule (Fig. 6.60A); thus it is really an extension of the glenohumeral joint cavity.

Subacromial Bursa. Sometimes referred to as the *subdeltoid bursa,* the **subacromial bursa** is located between the acromion, coracoacromial ligament and deltoid superiorly and the supraspinatus tendon and joint capsule of the glenohumeral joint inferiorly (Fig. 6.61A). Thus it facilitates movement of the supraspinatus tendon under the coracoacromial arch and of the deltoid over the joint capsule of the glenohumeral joint and the greater tubercle of the humerus. Its size varies, but it does not normally communicate with the cavity of the glenohumeral joint.

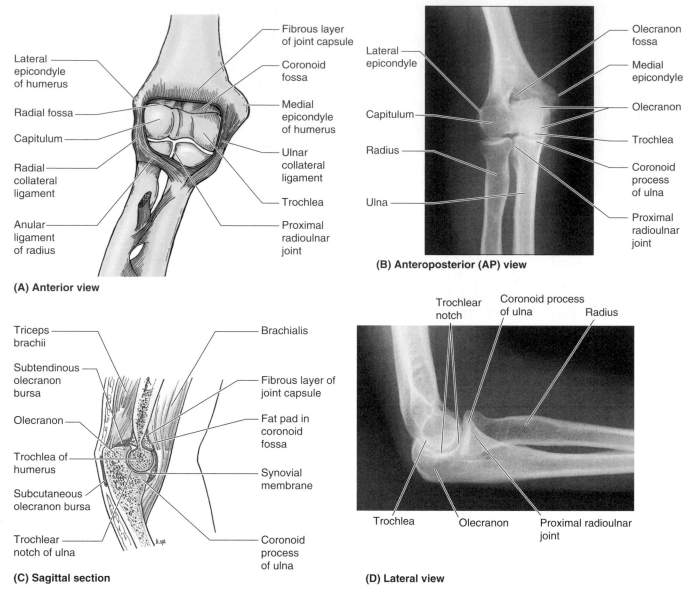

Figure 6.62. Elbow and proximal radioulnar joints. A. The thin anterior aspect of the joint capsule has been removed to reveal the articulating surfaces of the bones inside. The strong collateral ligaments were left intact. **B.** This anteroposterior radiograph shows the extended elbow joint. **C.** The fibrous layer and synovial membrane of the joint capsule, the subtendinous and subcutaneous olecranon bursae, and humeroulnar articulation of the elbow joint are demonstrated. **D.** This lateral radiograph shows the flexed elbow joint. (Parts **B** and **D** courtesy of Dr. E. Becker, Associate Professor of Medical Imaging, University of Toronto, Toronto, Ontario, Canada.)

Calcific Supraspinatus Tendinitis

Inflammation and calcification of the subacromial bursa result in pain, tenderness, and limitation of movement of the glenohumeral joint. This condition is also known as *calcific scapulohumeral bursitis.* Deposition of calcium in the supraspinatus tendon is common. This causes increased local pressure that often causes excruciating pain during abduction of the arm; the pain may radiate as far as the hand.

The calcium deposit may irritate the overlying subacromial bursa, producing an inflammatory reaction known as *subacromial bursitis.* As long as the glenohumeral joint is adducted, no pain usually results because in this position the painful lesion is away from the inferior surface of the acromion. In most people, the pain occurs during 50–130° of abduction (*painful arc syndrome*) because during this arc the supraspinatus tendon is in intimate contact with the inferior surface of the acromion. The pain usually ▶

Table 6.14. Movements of the Glenohumeral (Shoulder) Joint

Movement (function)	Prime Mover(s) (from pendent position)	Synergists	Notes
Flexion	Pectoralis major (clavicular head); deltoid (anterior part)	Coracobrachialis (assisted by biceps)	From fully extended position to its own (coronal) plane, sternocostal head of pectoralis major is major force
Extension	Deltoid (posterior part)	Teres major	Latissimus dorsi, sternocostal head of pectoralis major, and long head of triceps act from fully flexed position to their own (coronal) planes
Abduction	Deltoid (as a whole, but especially central part)	Supraspinatus	Supraspinatus is particularly important in initiating movement; also, upward rotation of scapula occurs throughout movement, making a significant contribution
Adduction	Pectoralis major; latissimus dorsi	Subscapularis; infraspinatus; teres minor	In upright position and in absence of resistance, gravity is prime mover
Medial rotation	Subscapularis	Pectoralis major; deltoid (anterior fibers); latissimus dorsi	With arm elevated, "synergists" become more important than prime movers
Lateral rotation	Infraspinatus	Teres minor; deltoid (posterior fibers)	
Tensors of articular capsule (to hold head of humerus against glenoid cavity)	Supscapularis; infraspinatus (simultaneously)	Supraspinatus; teres minor	Rotator cuff (SITS) muscles acting together; when "resting," their tonus adequately maintains integrity of joint
Resisting downward dislocation (shunt muscles)	Deltoid (as a whole)	Long head of triceps; coracobrachialis; short head of biceps	Used especially when carrying heavy objects (suitcases, buckets)

develops in males 50 years of age and older after unusual or excessive use of the glenohumeral joint.

Rotator Cuff Injuries

The musculotendinous rotator cuff is commonly injured during repetitive use of the upper limb above the horizontal (e.g., during throwing and racquet sports, swimming, and weightlifting). Recurrent inflammation of the rotator cuff, especially the relatively avascular area of the supraspinatus tendon, is a common cause of shoulder pain and results in tears of the musculotendinous rotator cuff. Repetitive use of the rotator cuff muscles (e.g., by baseball pitchers) may allow the humeral head and rotator cuff to impinge on the coracoacromial arch, producing irritation of the arch and inflammation of the rotator cuff. As a result, *degenerative tendonitis of the rotator cuff* develops. Attrition of the supraspinatus tendon also occurs (Fig. B6.31).

To test for degenerative tendonitis of the rotator cuff, the person is asked to lower the fully abducted limb slowly and smoothly. From approximately 90° abduction, the limb will suddenly drop to the side in an uncontrolled manner if the rotator cuff (especially the supraspinatus part) is diseased and/or torn.

Rotator cuff injuries can also occur during a sudden strain of the muscles, for example, when an older person strains to lift something, such as a window sash that is stuck, a previously degenerated musculotendinous rotator cuff may rupture. A fall on the shoulder may also tear a previously degenerated rotator cuff. Often the intracapsular part of the tendon of the long head of the biceps brachii becomes frayed (even worn away) leaving it adherent to the intertubercular groove. As a result, shoulder stiffness occurs. Because they fuse, the integrity of the fibrous layer of the joint capsule of the glenohumeral joint is usually compromised when the rotator cuff is injured. As a result, the articular cavity communicates with the ▶

subacromial bursa. Because the supraspinatus muscle is no longer functional with a complete tear of the rotator cuff, the person cannot initiate abduction of the upper limb. If the arm is passively abducted 15° or more, the person can usually maintain or continue the abduction using the deltoid.

Dislocation of the Glenohumeral Joint

Because of its freedom of movement and instability, the glenohumeral joint is commonly dislocated by direct or indirect injury. Because the presence of the coracoacromial arch and the support of the rotator cuff are effective in preventing upward dislocation, most dislocations of the humeral head occur in the downward (inferior) direction. However, they are described clinically as anterior or (more rarely) posterior dislocations, indicating whether the humeral head has descended anterior or posterior to the infraglenoid tubercle and the long head of the triceps. The head ends up lying anterior or posterior to the glenoid cavity.

Anterior dislocation of the glenohumeral joint occurs most often in young adults, particularly athletes. It is usually caused by excessive extension and lateral rotation of the humerus (Fig. B6.32). The head of the humerus is driven inferoanteriorly, and the fibrous layer of the joint capsule and glenoid labrum may be stripped from the anterior aspect of the glenoid cavity in the process. A hard blow to the humerus when the glenohumeral joint is fully abducted tilts the head of the humerus inferiorly onto the inferior weak part of the joint capsule. This may tear the capsule and dislocate the shoulder so that the humeral head comes to lie inferior to the glenoid cavity and anterior to the infraglenoid tubercle. The strong flexor and adductor muscles of the glenohumeral joint usually subsequently pull the humeral head anterosuperiorly into a subcoracoid position. Unable to use the arm, the person commonly supports it with the other hand. *Inferior dislocation of the glenohumeral joint* often occurs after an avulsion fracture of the greater tubercle, owing to the absence of the upward and medial pull produced by the muscles attaching to the tubercle.

Axillary Nerve Injury

The axillary nerve may be injured when the glenohumeral joint dislocates because of its close relation to the inferior part of the joint capsule of this joint. The subglenoid displacement of the head of the humerus into the quadrangular space damages the axillary nerve. Axillary nerve injury is indicated by paralysis of the deltoid (manifest as an ▶

Superiorly reflected flap including deltoid and superficial portion of synovial membrane of subacromial bursa

Perforation

Supraspinatus tendon blended with fibrous capsule of glenohumeral joint

Perforation

Teres minor

Coracoid process

Tendon of long head of biceps brachii seen through perforation

Cut edge of subacromial bursa

Tendon of long head of biceps brachii

Lateral view

Figure B6.31. Attrition of the supraspinatus tendon.

inability to abduct the arm to or above the horizontal level) and loss of sensation in a small area of skin covering the central part of the deltoid.

Glenoid Labrum Tears

Tearing of the fibrocartilaginous glenoid labrum commonly occurs in athletes who throw a baseball or football and in those who have shoulder instability and subluxation (partial dislocation) of the glenohumeral joint. The tear often results from sudden contraction of the biceps or forceful subluxation of the humeral head over the glenoid labrum. Usually a tear occurs in the anterosuperior part of the labrum. The typical symptom is pain while throwing, especially during the acceleration phase, but a sense of popping or snapping may be felt in the glenohumeral joint during abduction and lateral rotation of the arm.

Adhesive Capsulitis of the Glenohumeral Joint

Adhesive fibrosis and scarring between the inflamed joint capsule of the glenohumeral joint, rotator cuff, subacromial bursa, and deltoid usually cause **adhesive capsulitis** ("frozen shoulder"), a condition seen in individuals 40–60 years of age. A person with this condition has difficulty abducting the arm and can obtain an apparent abduction of up to 45° by elevating and rotating the scapula. Because of the lack of movement of the glenohumeral joint, strain is placed on the AC joint, which may be painful during other movements (e.g., elevation, or shrugging, of the shoulder). Injuries that may initiate acute capsulitis are glenohumeral dislocations, calcific supraspinatus tendinitis, partial tearing of the rotator cuff, and bicipital tendinitis (Salter, 1999). ☉

Figure B6.32. Dislocation of glenohumeral joint.

Lateral rotation

Excessive extension

THE BOTTOM LINE: The joints of the pectoral girdle are accessory to the glenohumeral joint in positioning the upper limb. The SC joint links the appendicular skeleton to the axial skeleton. The SC and AC joints enable the movement at the physiological scapulothoracic joint, where approximately 1° of movement occurs for every 3° of arm movement (scapulohumeral rhythm). In turn, approximately two thirds of the movement at the scapulothoracic joint result from motion at the SC joint, and one third is from motion at the AC joint. The strength and integrity of the joints of the shoulder complex do not depend on congruity of the articular surfaces. The integrity of the SC and AC joints results from intrinsic and extrinsic ligaments and the SC articular disc, whereas that of the glenohumeral joint is maintained by the tonic and active contraction of the muscles acting across it, particularly the SITS (rotator cuff) muscles.

Elbow Joint

The **elbow joint**, a hinge type of synovial joint, is located 2–3 cm inferior to the epicondyles of the humerus (Fig. 6.62).

Articulation of the Elbow Joint

The spool-shaped *trochlea* and spheroidal *capitulum* of the humerus articulate with the *trochlear notch* of the ulna and the slightly concave superior aspect of the *head of the radius,* respectively; therefore, there are humeroulnar and humeroradial articulations. The articular surfaces, covered with hyaline cartilage, are most fully congruent (in contact) when the forearm is in a position midway between pronation and supination and is flexed to a right angle.

Joint Capsule of the Elbow Joint

The *fibrous layer of the joint capsule* surrounds the elbow joint (Fig. 6.62A & C). It is attached to the humerus at the margins of the lateral and medial ends of the articular surfaces of the capitulum and trochlea. Anteriorly and posteriorly it is carried superiorly, proximal to the coronoid and olecranon fossae. The *synovial membrane* lines the internal surface of the fibrous layer of the capsule and the intracapsular non-articular parts of the humerus. It is also continuous inferiorly with the synovial membrane of the proximal radioulnar joint. The joint capsule is weak anteriorly and posteriorly but is strengthened on each side by collateral ligaments.

Ligaments of the Elbow Joint

The collateral ligaments of the elbow joint are strong triangular bands that are medial and lateral thickenings of the fibrous layer of the joint capsule (Figs. 6.62A and 6.63). The lateral, fan-like **radial collateral ligament** extends from the lateral epicondyle of the humerus and blends distally with the **anular ligament of the radius,** which encircles and holds the head of the radius in the radial notch of the ulna, forming the proximal radioulnar joint and permitting pronation and supination of the forearm. The medial, triangular **ulnar collateral ligament** extends from the medial epicondyle of the humerus to the coronoid process and olecranon of the ulna and consists of three bands: (1) the *anterior cord-like band* is the strongest, (2) the *posterior fan-like band* is the weakest, and (3) the slender *oblique band* deepens the socket for the trochlea of the humerus.

Movements of the Elbow Joint

Flexion and extension occur at the elbow joint. The long axis of the fully extended ulna makes an angle of approximately 170° with the long axis of the humerus. This angle, called the **carrying angle** (Fig. 6.64), is named for the way the forearm angles away from the body when something is carried, such as a pail of water. The obliquity of the ulna and thus of the carrying angle is more pronounced (the angle is approximately

10° more acute) in women than in men. It is teleologically said to enable the swinging limbs to clear the wide female pelvis when walking. In the anatomical position, the elbow is against the waist. The carrying angle disappears when the forearm is pronated.

Muscles Moving the Elbow Joint

A total of 17 muscles cross the elbow and extend to the forearm and hand, most of which have some potential to affect elbow movement. In turn, their function and efficiency in the other movements they produce are affected by elbow position. However, the *chief flexors of the elbow joint* are the brachialis and biceps brachii (Fig. 6.65). The brachioradialis can produce rapid flexion in the absence of resistance (even when the chief flexors are paralyzed). Normally, in the pres-

(A) Lateral view

(B) Medial view

Figure 6.63. Collateral ligaments of elbow joint A. The fan-like radial collateral is attached to the anular ligament of the radius, but its superficial fibers continue on to the ulna. **B.** The ulnar collateral ligament has a strong, round, cord-like anterior band (part), which is taut when the elbow joint is extended, and a weak, fan-like posterior band, which is taut when the joint is flexed. The oblique fibers merely deepen the socket for the trochlea of the humerus.

ence of resistance, the brachioradialis and pronator teres assist the chief flexors in producing slower flexion. The *chief extensor of the elbow joint* is the triceps brachii, especially the medial head, weakly assisted by the anconeus.

Blood Supply of the Elbow Joint
The arteries supplying the elbow joint are derived from the anastomosis around the elbow joint (Fig. 6.35).

Nerve Supply of the Elbow Joint
The elbow joint is supplied by the musculocutaneous, radial, and ulnar nerves (Table 6.10).

Bursae around the Elbow Joint
Only some of the bursae around the elbow joint are clinically important. The *three olecranon bursae* are (Figs. 6.62C and 6.66) the:

1. **Intratendinous olecranon bursa,** which is sometimes present in the tendon of triceps brachii.

2. **Subtendinous olecranon bursa,** which is located between the olecranon and the triceps tendon, just proximal to its attachment to the olecranon.

3. **Subcutaneous olecranon bursa,** which is located in the subcutaneous connective tissue over the olecranon.

The **bicipitoradial bursa** (biceps bursa) separates the biceps tendon from, and reduces abrasion against, the anterior part of the radial tuberosity

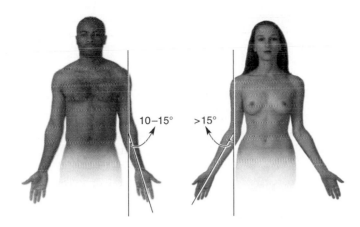

Figure 6.64. Carrying angle of elbow joint. This angle is made by the axes of the arm and forearm when the elbow is fully extended. Note that the forearm diverges laterally, forming an angle that is greater in the woman. Teleologically, this is said to allow for clearance of the wider female pelvis as the limbs swing during walking; however, no significant difference exists regarding the function of the elbow.

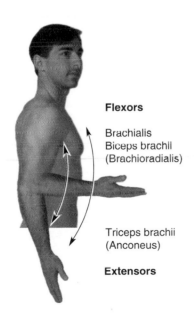

Figure 6.65. Flexor and extensor muscles of elbow joint. During slow flexion or maintenance of flexion against gravity, the brachialis and biceps brachii are mainly involved. With increasing speed, the brachioradialis becomes involved. In the absence of resistance, the brachioradialis can flex the elbow when the other flexors are paralyzed. The triceps brachii is the main extensor of the forearm at the elbow joint. The anconeus muscle and gravity assist the triceps in extending the elbow joint.

Figure 6.66. Bursae around elbow joint. Of the several bursae around the elbow joint, the olecranon bursae are most important clinically. Trauma of these bursae may produce bursitis (inflammation of the bursae).

Figure B6.33

Bursitis of the Elbow

The subcutaneous olecranon bursa is exposed to injury during falls on the elbow and to infection from abrasions of the skin covering the olecranon. Repeated excessive pressure and friction, as occurs in wrestling, for example, may cause this bursa to become inflamed, producing a friction *subcutaneous olecranon bursitis* (e.g., "student's elbow") (Fig. B6.33). This type of bursitis is also known as "dart thrower's elbow" and "miner's elbow." Occasionally, the bursa becomes infected and the area over the bursa becomes inflamed.

Subtendinous olecranon bursitis is much less common. It results from excessive friction between the triceps tendon and olecranon, for example, resulting from repeated flexion–extension of the forearm as occurs during certain assembly-line jobs. The pain is most severe during flexion of the forearm because of pressure exerted on the inflamed subtendinous olecranon bursa by the triceps tendon.

Bicipitoradial bursitis (*biceps bursitis*) results in pain when the forearm is pronated because this action compresses the bicipitoradial bursa against the anterior half of the tuberosity of the radius.

Avulsion of the Medial Epicondyle

Avulsion of the medial epicondyle in children can result from a fall that causes severe abduction of the extended elbow, an abnormal movement of this articulation. The resulting traction on the ulnar collateral ligament pulls the medial epicondyle distally (Fig. B6.34). The anatomical basis of avulsion of the epicondyle is that the epiphysis for the medial epicondyle may not fuse with the distal end of the humerus until up to age 20. Usually fusion is complete radiographically at age 14 in females and age 16 in males. *Traction injury of the ulnar nerve* is a frequent complication of the abduction type of avulsion of the medial epicondyle. The anatomical basis for this stretching of the ulnar nerve is that it passes posterior to the medial epicondyle before entering the forearm.

Dislocation of the Elbow Joint

Posterior dislocation of the elbow joint may occur when children fall on their hands with their elbows flexed. Dislocations of the elbow may result from hyperextension or a blow that drives the ulna posterior or posterolateral (Anderson et al., 2000). The distal end of the humerus is driven through the weak anterior part of the fibrous layer of the joint capsule as the radius and ulna dislocate posteriorly (Fig. B6.35). The ulnar collateral ligament is often torn, and an associated fracture of the head of the radius, coronoid process, or olecranon process of the ulna may occur. Injury to the ulnar nerve may occur, resulting in numbness of the little finger and weakness of flexion and adduction of the wrist. ▶

Ulnar nerve

Fracture of medial epicondyle

Flexor muscles

Ulnar collateral ligament

Figure B6.34

Figure B6.35 Dislocation of elbow. ○

Proximal Radioulnar Joint

The **proximal (superior) radioulnar joint** is a pivot type of synovial joint that allows movement of the head of the radius on the ulna (Figs. 6.62*A*, *B*, & *D* and 6.67).

Articulation of the Proximal Radioulnar Joint
The head of the radius articulates with the radial notch of the ulna. The radial head is held in position by the *anular ligament of the radius.*

Joint Capsule of the Proximal Radioulnar Joint
The *fibrous layer of the joint capsule* encloses the joint and is continuous with that of the elbow joint. The *synovial membrane* lines the deep surface of the fibrous layer and non-articulating aspects of the bones. The synovial membrane is an inferior prolongation of the synovial membrane of the elbow joint.

Ligaments of the Proximal Radioulnar Joint
The strong *anular ligament,* attached to the ulna anterior and posterior to its radial notch, surrounds the articulating bony surfaces and forms a collar that, with the radial notch, creates a ring that completely encircles the head of the radius (Figs. 6.67, 6.68 and 6.69). The deep surface of the anular ligament is lined with synovial membrane, which continues distally as a **sacciform recess of the proximal radioulnar joint** on the neck of the radius. This arrangement allows the radius to rotate within the anular ligament without binding, stretching, or tearing the synovial membrane.

Movements of the Proximal Radioulnar Joint
During pronation and supination of the forearm, the head of the radius rotates within the collar formed by the anular ligament and the radial notch of the ulna. **Supination** turns the

palm anteriorly, or superiorly when the forearm is flexed (Figs. 6.37*A* & *C*, 6.68 and 6.70). **Pronation** turns the palm posteriorly, or inferiorly when the forearm is flexed. The axis for these movements passes proximally through the center of the head of the radius and distally through the site of attachment of the apex of the articular disc to the head (styloid process) of the ulna. During pronation and supination, it is the radius that rotates; its head rotates within the cup-shaped collar formed by the anular ligament and the radial notch on the ulna. Distally, the end of the radius rotates around the head of the ulna. Almost always, supination and pronation are accompanied by synergistic movements of the glenohumeral and elbow joints that produce simultaneous movement of the ulna, except when the elbow is flexed.

Muscles Moving the Proximal Radioulnar Joint
Supination is produced by the supinator (when resistance is absent) and biceps brachii (when power is required because of resistance), with some assistance from the EPL and ECRL (Fig. 6.68*C*). *Pronation* is produced by the pronator quadratus (primarily) and pronator teres (secondarily), with some assistance from the FCR, palmaris longus, and brachioradialis (when the forearm is in the midpronated position).

Blood Supply of the Proximal Radioulnar Joint
The proximal radioulnar joint is supplied by the radial portion of the *periarticular arterial anastomosis of the elbow joint* (radial and middle collateral arteries anastomosing with the

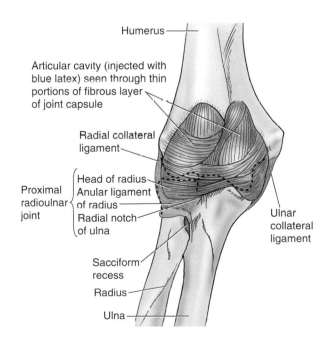

Figure 6.67. Proximal radioulnar joint The anular ligament attaches to the radial notch of the ulna, forming a collar around the head of the radius (Fig. 6.68*A*), creating a pivot type of synovial joint. The articular cavity of the joint is continuous with that of the elbow joint, as demonstrated by the blue latex injected into that space and seen through the thin parts of the fibrous layer of the capsule.

(A) Superior view of transverse section of proximal radioulnar joint

Anular ligament

Head of radius

Radial notch of ulna

Olecranon (cut)

Trochlear articulating surface

Axis of rotary movement

Anular ligament of radius

Proximal radioulnar joint

Radius

Distal radioulnar joint

Ulna

Proximal radioulnar joint

Ulna

Radius

Distal radioulnar joint

Supination

Pronation

(B) Anterior views

Radius

Supinator m.

Biceps brachii m.

Bursa

Supinator crest

Ulna

(C) Transverse section (inferior view)

Figure 6.68. Supination and pronation of forearm. A. The head of the radius rotates in the "socket" formed by the anular ligament and radial notch of the ulna. **B.** Supination is the movement of the forearm that rotates the radius laterally around its longitudinal axis so that the dorsum of the hand faces posteriorly and the palm faces anteriorly. Pronation is the movement of the forearm that rotates the radius medially around its longitudinal axis so that the palm of the hand faces posteriorly and its dorsum faces anteriorly (Fig. 6.77). **C.** The actions of the biceps brachii and supinator in producing supination from the pronated position at the radioulnar joints are shown.

radial and recurrent interosseous arteries, respectively) (Fig. 6.34; Table 6.9).

Innervation of the Proximal Radioulnar Joint

The proximal radioulnar joint is supplied mainly by the musculocutaneous, median, and radial nerves. Pronation is essentially a function of the median nerve, whereas supination is a function of the musculocutaneous and radial nerves.

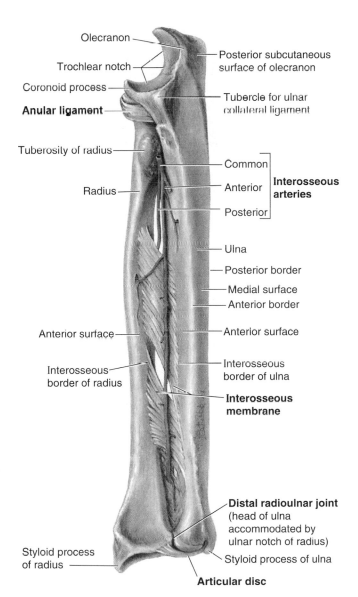

Medial view with radius in "resting (midprone) position" (midway between pronation and supination) so that the palm is directed toward the body

Figure 6.69. Radioulnar ligaments and interosseous arteries. The ligament of the proximal radioulnar joint is the anular ligament. The ligament of the distal radioulnar joint is the articular disc. The interosseous membrane connects the interosseous margins of the radius and ulna, forming the radioulnar syndesmosis. The general direction of the fibers of the interosseous membrane is such that a superior thrust to the hand is received by the radius and is transmitted to the ulna.

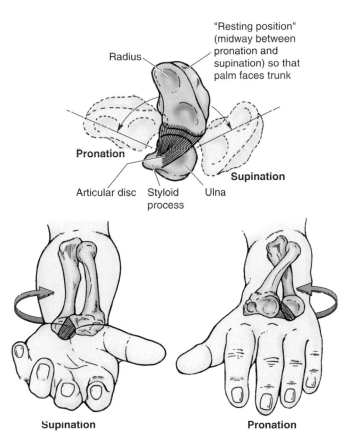

Figure 6.70. Movements of distal radioulnar joint during supination and pronation of forearm. The distal radioulnar joint is the pivot type of synovial joint between the head of the ulna and the ulnar notch of the radius. The inferior end of the radius moves around the relatively fixed end of the ulna during supination and pronation of the hand. The two bones are firmly united distally by the articular disc, referred to clinically as the triangular ligament of the distal radioulnar joint. It has a broad attachment to the radius but a narrow attachment to the styloid process of the ulna, which serves as the pivot point for the rotary movement.

Subluxation and Dislocation of Radial Head

Preschool children, particularly girls, are vulnerable to transient subluxation (incomplete temporary dislocation) of the head of the radius (also called "nursemaid's elbow" and "pulled elbow"). The history of these cases is typical. The child is suddenly lifted (jerked) by the upper limb while the forearm is pronated (e.g., lifting a child into a bus) (Fig. B6.36). The child may cry out, refuse to use the limb, protects the limb by holding it with the elbow flexed and the forearm pronated. The sudden pulling of the upper limb tears the distal ▶

Figure B6.36

attachment of the anular ligament, where it is loosely attached to the neck of the radius. The radial head then moves distally, partially out of the anular ligament. The proximal part of the torn ligament may become trapped between the head of the radius and the capitulum of the humerus. The source of pain is the pinched anular ligament. Treatment of the subluxation consists of supination of the child's forearm while the elbow is flexed (Salter, 1999). The tear in the anular ligament soon heals when the limb is placed in a sling for 2 weeks. ✪

Distal Radioulnar Joint

The **distal (inferior) radioulnar joint** is a pivot type of synovial joint (Fig. 6.69). The radius moves around the relatively fixed distal end of the ulna.

Articulation of the Distal Radioulnar Joint

The rounded head of the ulna articulates with the ulnar notch on the medial side of the distal end of the radius. A fibrocartilaginous **articular disc of the distal radioulnar joint** (sometimes referred to by clinicians as the "triangular ligament")

binds the ends of the ulna and radius together and is the main uniting structure of the joint (Figs. 6.70, 6.71 and 6.72*B*). The base of the articular disc is attached to the medial edge of the ulnar notch of the radius, and its apex is attached to the lateral side of the base of the styloid process of the ulna. The proximal surface of this triangular disc articulates with the distal aspect of the head of the ulna. Hence, the joint cavity is L-shaped in a coronal section; the vertical bar of the *L* is between the radius and the ulna, and the horizontal bar is between the ulna and the articular disc (Figs. 6.71*B* & *C* and

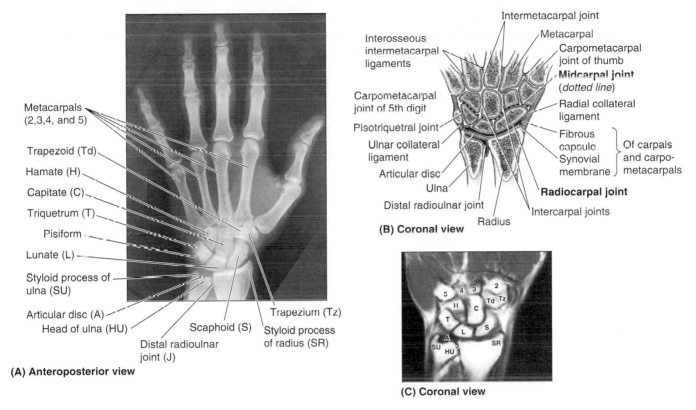

(A) Anteroposterior view

Metacarpals (2,3,4, and 5)
Trapezoid (Td)
Hamate (H)
Capitate (C)
Triquetrum (T)
Pisiform
Lunate (L)
Styloid process of ulna (SU)
Articular disc (A)
Head of ulna (HU)
Distal radioulnar joint (J)
Scaphoid (S)
Trapezium (Tz)
Styloid process of radius (SR)

(B) Coronal view

Interosseous intermetacarpal ligaments
Carpometacarpal joint of 5th digit
Pisotriquetral joint
Ulnar collateral ligament
Articular disc
Ulna
Distal radioulnar joint
Radius
Intermetacarpal joint
Metacarpal
Carpometacarpal joint of thumb
Midcarpal joint (*dotted line*)
Radial collateral ligament
Fibrous capsule
Synovial membrane
Of carpals and carpo-metacarpals
Radiocarpal joint
Intercarpal joints

(C) Coronal view

Figure 6.71. Bones of wrist and hand. A. In radiographs of the wrist and hand the "joint space" at the distal end of the ulna appears wide because of the radiolucent articular disc. (Courtesy of Dr. E. L. Lansdown, Professor of Medical Imaging, University of Toronto, Toronto, Ontario, Canada.) **B.** This coronal section of the right hand demonstrates the distal radioulnar, wrist, intercarpal, carpometacarpal, and intermetacarpal joints. Although they appear to be continuous when viewed radiographically in parts **A** and **C**, the articular cavities of the distal radioulnar and wrist joints are separated by the articular disc of the distal radioulnar joint. **C.** This coronal MRI shows the wrist. Structures are identified in part **A.** (Courtesy of Dr. W. Kucharczyk, Chair of Medical Imaging and Clinical Director of Tri-Hospital Magnetic Resonance Centre, Toronto, Ontario, Canada.)

6.72A). The articular disc separates the cavity of the distal radioulnar joint from the cavity of the wrist joint.

Joint Capsule of the Distal Radioulnar Joint

The *fibrous layer of the joint capsule* encloses the distal radioulnar joint but is deficient superiorly. The *synovial membrane* extends superiorly between the radius and the ulna to form the **sacciform recess of the distal radioulnar joint** (Fig. 6.72A). This redundancy of the synovial capsule accommodates the twisting of the capsule that occurs when the distal end of the radius travels around the relatively fixed distal end of the ulna during pronation of the forearm.

Ligaments of the Distal Radioulnar Joint

Anterior and posterior ligaments strengthen the fibrous layer of the joint capsule of the distal radioulnar joint. These relatively weak transverse bands extend from the radius to the ulna across the anterior and posterior surfaces of the joint.

Movements of the Distal Radioulnar Joint

During pronation of the forearm and hand, the distal end of the radius moves (rotates) anteriorly and medially, crossing over the ulna anteriorly (Fig. 6.70). During supination, the

radius uncrosses from the ulna, its distal end moving (rotating) laterally and posteriorly so the bones become parallel.

Muscles Moving the Distal Radioulnar Joint

The muscles producing movements of the distal radioulnar joint are discussed with the proximal radioulnar joint.

Blood Supply of the Distal Radioulnar Joint

The anterior and posterior *interosseous arteries* supply the distal radioulnar joint (Fig. 6.69).

Innervation of the Distal Radioulnar Joint

The anterior and posterior *interosseous nerves* supply the distal radioulnar joint.

THE BOTTOM LINE: Although the elbow joint appears simple because of its primary function as a hinge joint, the fact that it involves the articulation of a single bone proximally with two bones distally, one of which rotates, confers surprising complexity on this compound (three-part) joint. The hinge movement, the ability to transmit forces, and the high degree of stability of the joint primarily re-

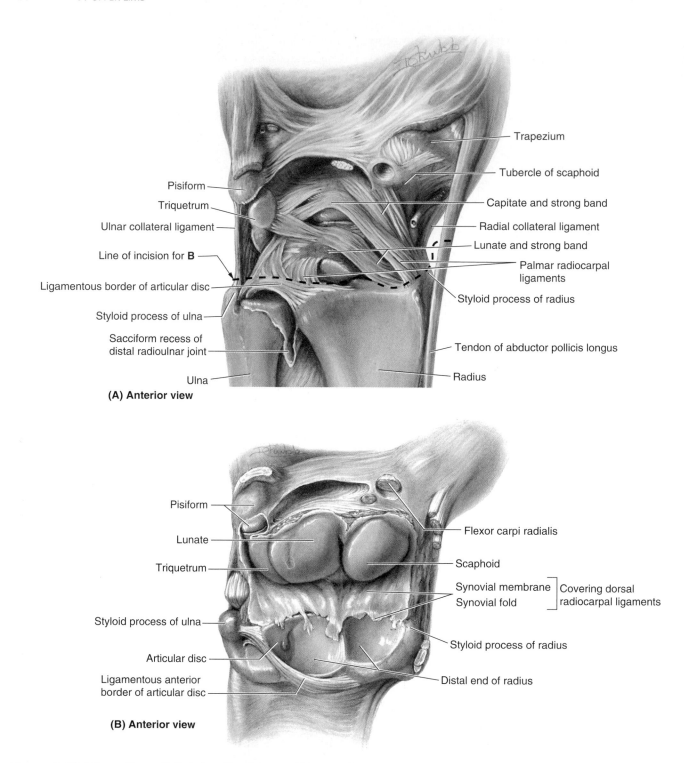

Pisiform

Triquetrum

Ulnar collateral ligament

Line of incision for **B**

Ligamentous border of articular disc

Styloid process of ulna

Sacciform recess of
distal radioulnar joint

Ulna

(A) Anterior view

Trapezium

Tubercle of scaphoid

Capitate and strong band

Radial collateral ligament

Lunate and strong band

Palmar radiocarpal
ligaments

Styloid process of radius

Tendon of abductor pollicis longus

Radius

Pisiform

Lunate

Triquetrum

Styloid process of ulna

Articular disc

Ligamentous anterior
border of articular disc

(B) Anterior view

Flexor carpi radialis

Scaphoid

Synovial membrane
Synovial fold

Covering dorsal
radiocarpal ligaments

Styloid process of radius

Distal end of radius

Figure 6.72. Dissection of distal radioulnar, radiocarpal, and intercarpal joints. A. The ligaments of these joints are shown. The hand is forcibly extended but the joint is intact. Observe the palmar radiocarpal ligaments, passing from the radius to the two rows of carpal bones. These strong ligaments are directed so that the hand follows the radius during supination. **B.** The joint is opened anteriorly, with the dorsal radiocarpal ligaments serving as a hinge. Observe the nearly equal proximal articular surfaces of the scaphoid and lunate and that the lunate articulates with both the radius and the articular disc. Only during adduction of the wrist does the triquetrum articulate with the disc.

sult from the conformation of the articular surfaces of the humeroulnar joint (i.e., of the trochlear notch of the ulna to the trochlea of the humerus). The integrity and functions of the humeroradial joint–proximal radioulnar joint complex depends primarily on the combined radial collateral and anular ligaments. The combined synovial proximal and distal radioulnar joints plus the interosseous membrane enable pronation and supination of the forearm. The anular ligament of the proximal joint, articular disc of the distal joint, and interosseous membrane not only hold the two bones together while permitting the necessary motion between them, but they (especially the membrane) also transmit forces received from the hand by the radius to the ulna for subsequent transmission to the humerus and pectoral girdle.

Wrist Joint

The *wrist* (*carpus*), the proximal segment of the hand, is a complex of eight carpal bones, articulating proximally with the forearm via the wrist joint and distally with the five metacarpals. The **wrist** (**radiocarpal**) **joint** is a condyloid (ellipsoid) type of synovial joint. The position of the joint is indicated approximately by a line joining the styloid processes of the radius and ulna, or by the proximal wrist crease (Figs. 6.71, 6.72A & B, and SA6.17).

Articulation of the Wrist Joint

The ulna does not participate in the wrist joint. The distal end of the radius and the articular disc of the distal radioulnar joint articulate with the proximal row of carpal bones, except for the pisiform. The latter bone acts primarily as a sesamoid bone, increasing the leverage of the FCU. It lies in a plane anterior to the other carpal bones, articulating with only the triquetrum.

Joint Capsule of the Wrist Joint

The *fibrous layer of the joint capsule* surrounds the wrist joint and is attached to the distal ends of the radius and ulna and the proximal row of carpals (scaphoid, lunate, and triquetrum). The *synovial membrane* lines the internal surface of the fibrous layer of the joint capsule and is attached to the margins of the articular surfaces (Fig. 6.72B). Numerous synovial folds are present.

Ligaments of the Wrist Joint

The fibrous layer of the joint capsule is strengthened by strong dorsal and palmar radiocarpal ligaments. The **palmar radiocarpal ligaments** pass from the radius to the two rows of carpals (Fig. 6.72A). They are strong and directed so that the hand follows the radius during supination of the forearm. The **dorsal radiocarpal ligaments** take the same direction so that the hand follows the radius during pronation of the forearm. The joint capsule is also strengthened medially by the **ulnar collateral ligament**, which is attached to the ulnar styloid

process and triquetrum (Figs. 6.71B and 6.72A). The joint capsule is also strengthened laterally by the **radial collateral ligament**, which is attached to the radial styloid process and scaphoid.

Movements of the Wrist Joint

The movements at the wrist joint may be augmented by additional smaller movements at the intercarpal and midcarpal joints (Fig. 6.73). The movements are flexion–extension, abduction–adduction (radial deviation–ulnar deviation), and circumduction. The hand can be flexed on the forearm more than it can be extended; these movements are accompanied (actually, are initiated) by similar movements at the midcarpal joint between the proximal and the distal rows of carpal bones. Adduction of the hand is greater than abduction (Fig. 6.73B). Most adduction occurs at the wrist joint. Abduction from the neutral position occurs at the midcarpal joint. Circumduction of the hand consists of successive flexion, adduction, extension, and abduction.

Muscles Moving the Wrist Joint

Movement at the wrist is produced primarily by the "carpi" muscles of the forearm, the tendons of which extend along the four corners of the wrist (comparing a cross-section of the wrist to a rectangle [Fig. 6.73C]) to attach to the bases of the metacarpals. The FCU does so via the **pisohamate ligament**, a continuation of the FCU tendon if the pisiform is considered a sesamoid bone within the continuous tendon.

- *Flexion of the wrist* is produced by the FCR and FCU, with assistance from the flexors of the fingers and thumb, the palmaris longus and the APL.

- *Extension of the wrist* is produced by the ECRL, ECRB, and ECU, with assistance from the extensors of the fingers and thumb.

- *Abduction of the wrist* is produced by the APL, FCR, ECRL, and ECRB; it is limited to approximately 15° because of the projecting radial styloid process.

- *Adduction of the wrist* is produced by simultaneous contraction of the ECU and FCU.

Most activities require a small amount of wrist flexion; however, tight grip (clenching of the fist) requires extension at the wrist. The mildly extended position is also the most stable and the "resting position."

Blood Supply of the Wrist Joint

The arteries supplying the wrist joint are branches of the dorsal and palmar carpal arches (Figs. 6.40A and 6.46A).

Innervation of the Wrist Joint

The nerves to the wrist joint are derived from the anterior interosseous branch of the *median nerve,* the posterior interosseous branch of the *radial nerve,* and the dorsal and deep branches of the *ulnar nerve* (Tables 6.10 and 6.13).

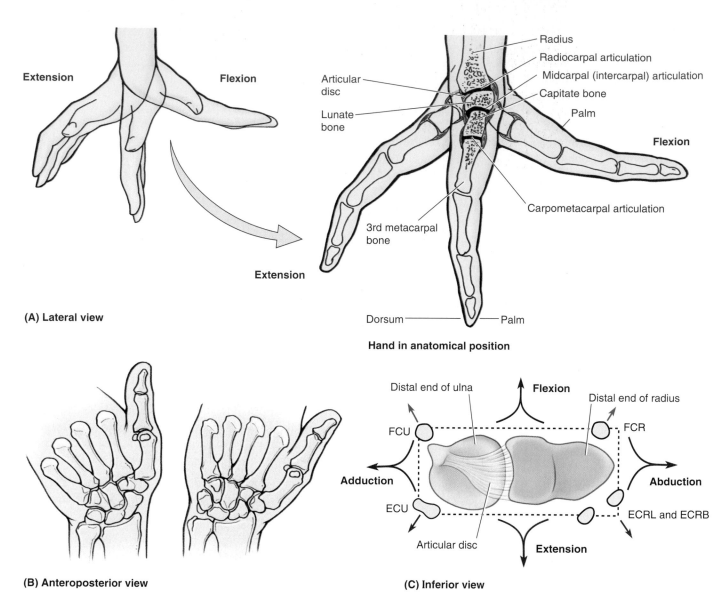

(A) Lateral view

Hand in anatomical position

(B) Anteroposterior view

(C) Inferior view

Figure 6.73. Movements of wrist. A. In this sagittal section of the wrist and hand during extension and flexion, observe the radiocarpal, midcarpal, and carpometacarpal articulations. Most movement occurs at the radiocarpal joint, with additional movement taking place at the midcarpal joint during full flexion and extension. **B.** Movement at the radiocarpal and midcarpal joints during adduction and abduction is demonstrated as seen in posteroanterior radiography. **C.** This view of the proximal articular surface of the radiocarpal joint indicates the position of the tendons of the primary ("carpi") muscles acting at the ("four corners" of the) joint and the movements produced by their combined activity. The carpi muscles include the flexor carpi ulnaris (*FCU*), extensor carpi ulnaris (*ECU*), flexor carpi radialis (*FCR*), extensor carpi radialis longus (*ECRL*), and extensor carpi radialis brevis (*ECRB*).

Wrist Fractures

Fracture of the distal end of the radius (*Colles fracture*), the most common fracture in people >50 years of age, is discussed in the clinical correlation (blue) box "Fractures of the Radius and Ulna," earlier in this chapter. *Fracture of the scaphoid,* relatively common in young adults, is discussed in the clinical correlation (blue) box "Fracture of the Scaphoid," earlier in this chapter.

Anterior dislocation of the lunate is an uncommon but serious injury that usually results from a fall on the dorsiflexed wrist (Fig. B6.37*A*). The lunate is pushed out of its place in the floor of the carpal tunnel toward the palmar surface of the wrist. The displaced lunate may compress the median nerve and lead to *carpal tunnel syndrome* (discussed earlier in this chapter). Because of its poor blood supply, *avascular necrosis of the lunate* may occur. In some cases, excision of the lunate may be required. ▶

Posterolateral view of pronated
limb with wrist extended

AP view (B)   (C)   Lateral view

Figure B6.37. Wrist fractures. A. Dislocation of lunate is shown. **B.** This radiograph of a young person shows a normal epiphyseal plate (*arrow*). *E*, distal radial epiphysis (*R*); *U*, ulna. **C.** A fracture–separation of the distal radial epiphysis is shown.

In *degenerative joint disease of the wrist,* surgical fusion of carpals (**arthrodesis**) may be necessary to relieve the severe pain.

Fracture–separation of the distal radial epiphysis is common in children because of frequent falls in which forces are transmitted from the hand to the radius (Fig. B6.37*B* & *C*). In a lateral radiograph of a child's wrist, dorsal displacement of the distal radial epiphysis is obvious (Fig. B6.37*C*). A small fracture of the shaft of the radius is also visible (not obvious). When the epiphysis is placed in its normal position during reduction, the prognosis for normal bone growth is good. ⊕

Intercarpal Joints

The **intercarpal** (IC) **joints,** interconnecting the carpal bones, are plane synovial joints (Fig. 6.71), which may be summarized as:

- Joints between the carpal bones of the proximal row.

- Joints between the carpal bones of the distal row.

- The **midcarpal joint,** a complex joint between the proximal and distal rows of carpal bones.

- The **pisotriquetral joint,** formed from the articulation of the pisiform with the palmar surface of the triquetrum.

Joint Capsule of the Intercarpal Joints

A continuous, common articular cavity is formed by the IC and carpometacarpal joints, with the exception of the

carpometacarpal joint of the thumb, which is independent. The wrist joint is also independent. The continuity of the articular cavities, or the lack of it, is significant in relation to the spread of infection and to arthroscopy, in which a flexible fiberoptic scope is inserted into the articular cavity to view its internal surfaces and features. The *fibrous layer of the joint capsule* surrounds these joints, which helps unite the carpals. The *synovial membrane* lines the fibrous layer and is attached to the margins of the articular surfaces of the carpals.

Ligaments of the Intercarpal Joints

The carpals are united by anterior, posterior, and interosseous ligaments (Figs. 6.72 and 6.74*A*).

Movements at the Intercarpal Joints

The gliding movements possible between the carpals occur concomitantly with movements at the wrist (radiocarpal) joint, augmenting them and increasing the overall range of movement. Flexion and extension of the hand are actually initiated at the *midcarpal joint,* between the proximal and the distal rows of carpals (Figs. 6.71*B* and 6.73). Investigators disagree regarding the amount of movement occurring at the wrist vs. the midcarpal joints. Most state that flexion and adduction occur mainly at the wrist joint whereas extension and abduction occur primarily at the midcarpal joint. Movements at the other IC joints are small, with the proximal row being more mobile than the distal row.

Blood Supply of the Intercarpal Joints

The arteries supplying the IC joints are derived from the dorsal and palmar carpal arches.

Innervation of the Intercarpal Joints

The IC joints are supplied by the anterior interosseous branch of the median nerve and the dorsal and deep branches of the ulnar nerve.

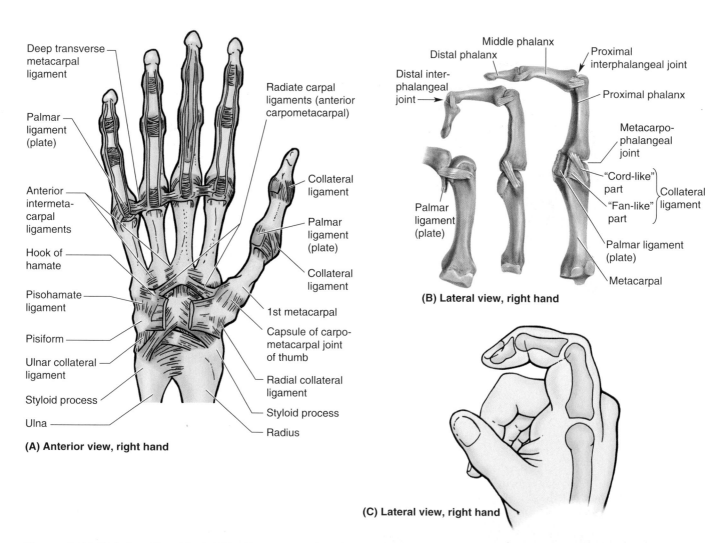

Figure 6.74. Joints of hand. A. This dissection of the hand shows the palmar ligaments of the radioulnar, radiocarpal, intercarpal, carpometacarpal, and interphalangeal joints. **B.** A dissection showing the metacarpophalangeal and interphalangeal joints. The palmar ligaments (plates) are modifications of the anterior aspect of the MP and IP joint capsules. **C.** The flexed index finger demonstrates its phalanges and the position of the MP and IP joints. The knuckles are formed by the heads of the bones, with the joint plane lying distally.

Carpometacarpal and Intermetacarpal Joints

The **carpometacarpal** (CMC) and **intermetacarpal** (IM) joints are the plane type of synovial joint, except for the **CMC joint of the thumb**, which is a saddle joint (Fig. 6.71).

Articulations of the Carpometacarpal and Intermetacarpal Joints

The distal surfaces of the carpals of the distal row articulate with the carpal surfaces of the bases of the metacarpals at the CMC joints. The important CMC joint of the thumb is between the trapezium and the base of the 1st metacarpal and has a separate articular cavity. Like the carpals, adjacent metacarpals articulate with each other; IM joints occur between the radial and the ulnar aspects of the bases of the metacarpals.

Joint Capsule of the Carpometacarpal and Intermetacarpal Joints

The medial four CMC joints and three IM joints are enclosed by a common joint capsule on the palmar and dorsal surfaces. A common synovial membrane lines the internal surface of the fibrous layer of the joint capsule, surrounding a common articular cavity.

The fibrous layer of the CMC joint of the thumb surrounds the joint and is attached to the margins of the articular surfaces. The synovial membrane lines the internal surface of the fibrous layer. The looseness of the capsule facilitates free movement of the joint.

Ligaments of the Carpometacarpal and Intermetacarpal Joints

The bones are united in the region of the joints by **palmar** and **dorsal CMC** and **IM ligaments** (Fig. 6.74A) and by **interosseous IM ligaments** (Fig. 6.71B). In addition, the *superficial* and *deep transverse metacarpal ligaments* (the former part of the palmar aponeurosis), associated with the distal ends of the metacarpals, play a role in limiting movement at the CMC and IM joints as they limit separation of the metacarpal heads.

Movements at the Carpometacarpal and Intermetacarpal Joints

The CMC joint of the thumb permits angular movements in any plane (flexion–extension, abduction–adduction, or circumduction) and a restricted amount of axial rotation. Most important, the movement essential to opposition of the thumb occurs here. Although the opponens pollicis is the prime mover, all of the hypothenar muscles contribute to opposition. Almost no movement occurs at the CMC joints of the 2nd and 3rd fingers, that of the 4th finger is slightly mobile, and that of the 5th finger is moderately mobile, flexing and rotating slightly during a tight grasp (Fig. 6.48G & H). When the palm of the hand is "cupped," (as during pad-to-pad opposition of thumb and little finger), two thirds of the movement occur at the CMC joint of the thumb, and one third occurs at the CMC and IC joints of the 4th and 5th fingers.

Blood Supply of the Carpometacarpal and Intermetacarpal Joints

The CMC and IM joints are supplied by *periarticular arterial anastomoses of the wrist and hand* (dorsal and palmar carpal arches, deep palmar arch, and metacarpal arteries) (Fig. 6.79).

Innervation of the Carpometacarpal and Intermetacarpal Joints

The CMC and IM joints are supplied by the anterior interosseous branch of the *median nerve*, posterior interosseous branch of the *radial nerve*, and dorsal and deep branches of the *ulnar nerve*.

Metacarpophalangeal and Interphalangeal Joints

The **metacarpophalangeal joints** are the condyloid type of synovial joint that permit movement in two planes: flexion–extension and adduction–abduction. The **interphalangeal joints** are the hinge type of synovial joint and permit flexion–extension only (Fig. 6.74B).

Articulations of the Metacarpophalangeal and Interphalangeal Joints

The heads of the metacarpals articulate with the bases of the proximal phalanges in the MP joints, and the heads of the phalanges articulate with the bases of more distally located phalanges in the IP joints.

Joint Capsule of the Metacarpophalangeal and Interphalangeal Joints

A *joint capsule* encloses each MC and IP joint with a *synovial membrane* lining a *fibrous layer* that is attached to the margins of each joint.

Ligaments of the Metacarpophalangeal and Interphalangeal Joints

The fibrous layer of each MC and IP joint capsule is strengthened by two (medial and lateral) **collateral ligaments**. These ligaments have two parts: (1) denser *cord-like parts* that pass distally from the heads of the metacarpals and phalanges to the bases of the phalanges (Fig. 6.74A & B), and (2) thinner *fan-like parts* that pass anteriorly to attach to thick, densely fibrous or fibrocartilaginous plates, the *palmar ligaments* (plates), which form the palmar aspect of the joint capsule. The fan-like parts of the collateral ligaments cause the palmar ligaments to move like a visor over the underlying metacarpal or phalangeal heads. The strong cord-like parts of the collateral ligaments of the MP joint, being eccentrically attached to the metacarpal heads are slack during extension and taut during flexion. As a result, the fingers cannot usually be spread (abducted) when the MP joints are fully flexed. The interphalangeal joints have corresponding ligaments but the distal ends of the proximal and middle phalanges, being flattened anteroposteriorly and having two small condyles, permit neither adduction or abduction.

The palmar ligaments blend with the fibrous digital sheaths and provide a smooth, longitudinal groove that allows the long flexor ligaments to glide and remain centrally placed as they cross the convexities of the joints. The palmar ligaments of the 2nd–5th MP joints are united by **deep transverse metacarpal ligaments** that hold the heads of the metacarpals together. In addition, the dorsal hood of each extensor apparatus attaches anteriorly to the sides of the palmar plates of the MP joints.

Movements of the Metacarpophalangeal and Interphalangeal Joints

Flexion–extension, abduction–adduction, and circumduction of the 2nd–5th digits occur at the 2nd–5th MP joints. Movement at the MP joint of the thumb is limited to flexion–extension. Only flexion and extension occur at the IP joints.

Blood Supply of the Metacarpal and Interphalangeal Joints

Deep digital arteries that arise from the superficial palmar arches supply the MC and IP joints (Fig. 6.79).

Innervation of the Metacarpal and Interphalangeal Joints

Digital nerves arising from the ulnar and median nerves supply the MC and IP joints.

THE BOTTOM LINE: Motion at the wrist moves the entire hand, making a dynamic contribution to a skill or movement, or allowing it to be stabilized in a particular position to maximize the effectiveness of the hand and fingers in manipulating and holding objects. Complexity as well as flexibility of the wrist results from the number of bones involved. Extension–flexion, abduction–adduction, and circumduction occur. Overall, most wrist movement occurs at the wrist (radiocarpal) joint between the radius and articular disc of the distal radioulnar joint and the proximal row of carpal bones (primarily the scaphoid and lunate). However, concomitant movement at the IC joints (especially the midcarpal IC joint) augments these movements. The CMC joints of the four medial fingers, which share a common articular cavity, have limited motion (especially those of the 2nd and 3rd digits), contributing to the stability of the palm as a base from and against which the fingers operate. Motion occurs at the CMC joints for the 3rd and 4th digits, mostly in association with a tight grip or cupping of the palm, as during opposition. However, the great mobility of the CMC joint of the thumb, a saddle joint, provides the digit with the major portion of its range of motion and specifically enables opposition. Therefore it is key to the effectiveness of the human hand. In contrast to the CMC joints, the MP joints of the medial four fingers offer considerable freedom of movement (flexion–extension and abduction–adduction), whereas that of the thumb is limited to flexion–extension, as are all IP joints.

Bull Rider's Thumb

Bull rider's thumb refers to a sprain of the radial collateral ligament and an avulsion fracture of the lateral part of the proximal phalanx of the thumb. This injury is common in individuals who ride mechanical bulls.

Skier's Thumb

Skier's thumb (historically, game-keeper's thumb) refers to the rupture or chronic laxity of the collateral ligament of the 1st MP joint (Fig. B6.38). The injury results from hyperabduction of the MP joint of the thumb, which occurs when the thumb is held by the ski pole while the rest of the hand hits the ground or enters the snow. In severe injuries, the head of the metacarpal has an avulsion fracture. **☉**

Skier's thumb

Figure B6.38

Medical Imaging of the Upper Limb

Radiography

Radiographs are often taken when an injury produces bone tenderness, angulation, rotation, or instability. Anteroposterior (AP), lateral, axial, and oblique views are usually sufficient to detect bony and other injuries. Radiological examinations of the upper limb focus mainly on bony structures, because muscles, tendons, and nerves are not well visualized. When examining radiographs of the upper limb, it is essential to know the ▶

median times of appearance of postnatal ossification centers and when fusion of epiphyses is radiographically complete in males and females. Without such knowledge, an epiphysial line could be mistaken for a fracture.

Pectoral Girdle and Joints

The usual radiograph is an AP view with the humerus laterally rotated so that its epicondyles are parallel with the X-ray film cassette (Figs. 6.77A and 6.76A). Because some obliquity of the glenoid cavity occurs normally, it appears oval in shape. In this view, the lateral two thirds of the clavicle is visible. The articulation of the acromial end of the clavicle with the acromion of the scapula at the *AC joint* is apparent. This is a frequent site of subluxation of the joint. The surgical neck of the humerus, approximately 2.5 cm distal to the greater and lesser tubercles, is a common site of fracture. The axillary nerve is in contact with the surgical neck and vulnerable to injury. Examination of the humerus reveals dense cortical bone along the shaft, which thins out proximally and becomes extremely thin over the head of the bone. The radial nerve runs inferolaterally in the radial groove on the posterior surface of the humerus and is vulnerable to injury in a midhumeral fracture.

An axial projection of the shoulder provides an essential additional view of the AC and glenohumeral joints. To obtain an axial projection, the person is asked to abduct the arm and extend the shoulder over the X-ray film cassette. In Figure 6.75B, the acromion, glenoid cavity, humeral head, coracoid process, and suprascapular notch are visible.

Elbow Joint

In an AP projection, the extended elbow is placed on the X-ray film cassette with the forearm supinated. The X-ray beam is directed perpendicular to the cassette and at the elbow joint. Figure 6.76A shows the distal end of the humerus as it flares out and ends as the prominent medial epicondyle and the more flattened lateral epicondyle. The ulnar nerve is in contact with the medial epicondyle and may be injured when it is fractured or its epiphysis is dislocated. Distal to the epicondyles are the convex capitulum and pulley-shaped trochlea. Between the epicondyles is a radiolucent area representing the superimposed olecranon and coronoid fossae. The disc-shaped radial head and its concave articular surface, distal to the capitulum, is apparent.

Fractures of the radial head are relatively common in young adults after a fall on the hand. The radial notch in the ulna is overlapped by the medial aspect of the radial head where they are in contact, forming the proximal radioulnar joint. The olecranon of the ulna is superimposed on the distal end of the humerus where it lies in the olecranon fossa. Just distal to the trochlea of the humerus is the coronoid process of the ulna.

In a lateral projection of the elbow (Fig. 6.76B), the elbow is flexed 90°, and the arm and forearm are placed on the X-ray film cassette with the thumb extended. In this projection, the epicondyles, capitulum, and trochlea are superimposed. The superimposed supraepicondylar ridges form a dense radiopaque shadow. The coronoid process of the ulna is partly obscured by the radial head.

Forearm

To obtain the AP view shown in Figure 6.77A, the forearm is positioned so that it is supinated and the elbow joint is fully extended. Note that both the elbow and wrist joints are shown. Observe the translucent area between the capitulum and the radial head and between the trochlea and the coronoid process. This area is where the articular cartilages of the articulating bones are located. The radius and ulna bow (are outwardly convex) as they extend distally from the elbow. The bones become increasingly separated from each other in their distal two thirds, coming into contact more abruptly distally. The interosseous membrane is *radiolucent* (invisible to radiographic study). To detect fractures and verify their correct *reduction* (restoration to the normal position), keep in mind that the radial styloid process normally ends 1 cm distal to the ulnar styloid process. In Figure 6.77B, the way in which the radius crosses the ulna during forearm pronation is demonstrated.

Wrist and Hand

Radiographs of the wrist and hand are commonly used to assess skeletal age. For clinical studies, the radiographs are compared with a series of standards in a radiographic atlas of skeletal development to determine the age of the child. *Epiphysial fractures* are more common in young children than in adolescents because tight fusion of the epiphyses with the bodies of the bones has not occurred. Fusion of the distal radial and ulnar epiphyses is complete radiographically at age 16 in females and at age 18 in males. The carpal bones are superimposed on each other; however, when compared with a skeleton of the wrist and hand, the bones can be identified. A lateral projection of the wrist and hand is of great importance because certain fractures may be revealed only in this projection (Fig. 6.78A).

A fall on the outstretched hand may result in *fracture of the scaphoid,* generally across its narrow part. A radiologist looks for a scaphoid fracture if the physician reported tenderness over the scaphoid in the anatomical snuff box; however, it may not be detectable even in several oblique views until approximately 2 weeks after the injury (see clinical correlation [blue] box "Fracture of the Scaphoid." earlier in this chapter).

Each carpal usually ossifies from one center postnatally. The centers for the capitate and hamate appear first. ▶

(cont'd on page 880)

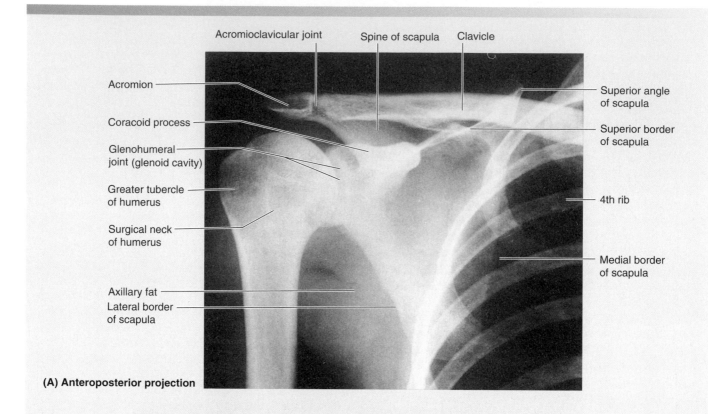

Acromioclavicular joint   Spine of scapula   Clavicle

Acromion

Coracoid process

Glenohumeral
joint (glenoid cavity)

Greater tubercle
of humerus

Surgical neck
of humerus

Axillary fat
Lateral border
of scapula

Superior angle
of scapula

Superior border
of scapula

4th rib

Medial border
of scapula

(A) Anteroposterior projection

Shaft of humerus

Body of scapula

Acromion

Suprascapular notch

Glenoid cavity

Head of humerus

Clavicle

Coracoid process

X-ray film
or detector

(B) Axial projection   X-ray beam

Figure 6.75. Radiographs of glenohumeral joint. A. The head of the humerus and the glenoid cavity overlap, obscuring the joint plane because the scapula does not lie in the coronal plane (therefore the glenoid cavity is oblique, not in a sagittal plane, which is especially evident in part **B**). (Courtesy of Dr. E. L. Lansdown, Professor of Medical Imaging, University of Toronto, Toronto, Ontario, Canada) **B.** The orientation drawing shows how the axial projection radiograph was taken.

(A) Anteroposterior view

Lateral
supraepicondylar
ridge

Lateral
epicondyle

Capitulum

Of
radius
{ Head
Neck
Tuberosity }

Medial
supraepicondylar
ridge

Coracoid and
olecranon fossa
(superimposed)

Medial
epicondyle

Olecranon

Trochlea

Coronoid
process
of ulna

Proximal
radioulnar
joint

Radial
notch
in ulna

Ulna

(B) Lateral view

Coronoid fossa

Supraepicondylar ridge

Of radius

Head   Neck   Tuberosity

Of
humerus
{ Olecranon
fossa }

Capitulum and
trochlea
(superimposed)   Olecranon

Trochlear
notch

Site of
radial
notch

Coronoid
process

Of ulna

Figure 6.76. Radiographs of elbow joint. A. The joint planes (occupied by radiolucent articular cartilage) are especially evident in the extended joint. **B.** The elbow is flexed to a 90° angle. The spherical nature of the capitulum, around which the superior surface of the radius glides, is especially evident. The head of the radius and the radial notch of the ulna overlap at the proximal radioulnar joint. (Courtesy of Dr. E. Becker, Associate Professor of Medical Imaging, University of Toronto, Toronto, Ontario, Canada.)

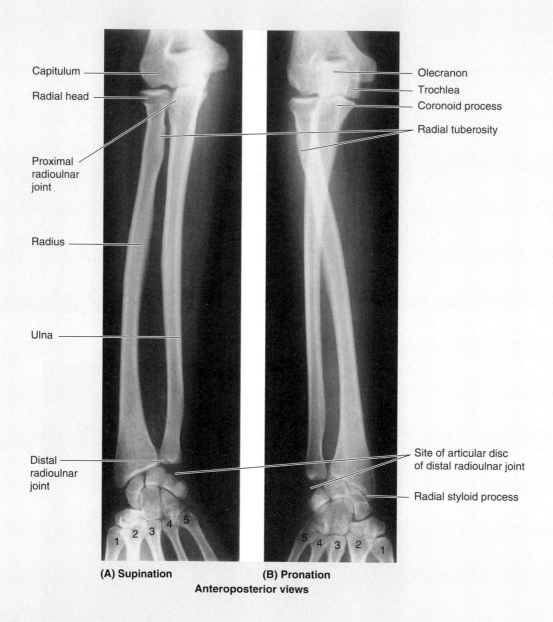

Capitulum

Radial head

Proximal
radioulnar
joint

Radius

Ulna

Distal
radioulnar
joint

Olecranon

Trochlea

Coronoid process

Radial tuberosity

Site of articular disc
of distal radioulnar joint

Radial styloid process

(A) Supination   **(B) Pronation**
Anteroposterior views

Figure 6.77. Radiographs of radioulnar joints. A. In the supinated position, the radius and ulna are parallel. **B.** During pronation, the inferior end of the radius moves anteriorly and medially around the inferior end of the ulna, carrying the hand with it; thus in the pronated position, the radius crosses the ulna anteriorly. *1–5,* the metacarpals. (Courtesy of Dr. J. Heslin, Toronto, Ontario, Canada.)

Distal phalanx
of thumb

Interphalangeal
joint of thumb

Proximal
phalanx
of thumb

1st metacarpo-
phalangeal joint

Sesamoid bones

1st metacarpal

Trapezium

Scaphoid

Lunate

Radius

3rd metacarpophalangeal joint

Head of 5th metacarpal

Intercarpal (midcarpal) joint

Radiocarpal (wrist) joint

Ulna

(A) Lateral view

Figure 6.78. Radiographs of right wrist and hand. A. This lateral view shows the adult hand. (Courtesy of Dr. E. L. Lansdown, Professor of Medical Imaging, University of Toronto, Toronto, Ontario, Canada.)

(B) Anteroposterior view

(C) Anteroposterior view

Figure 6.78. *(Continued)* **B.** The distal end of the forearm and the hand of a 2.5-year-old child are shown. Ossification centers of only four carpal bones are visible. Observe the distal radial epiphysis (*R*). *C,* capitate; *H,* hamate; *L,* lunate; *Tq,* triquetrum. **C.** The inferior end of the forearm and hand of an 11-year-old child are shown. Ossification centers of all carpal bones are visible. The *arrow* indicates the pisiform lying on the anterior surface of the triquetrum. The distal epiphysis of the ulna (*U*) has ossified but all epiphyseal plates (lines) "remain open" (i.e., they are still unossified). *S,* scaphoid; *Td,* trapezoid; *Tz,* trapezium. (Courtesy of Dr. D. Armstrong, Associate Professor of Medical Imaging, University of Toronto, Toronto, Ontario, Canada.)

Ossification centers are usually obvious during the 1st year; however, they may appear before birth. *Accessory ossicles* (small bones) are sometimes observed between the usual carpals; their possible occurrence should be kept in mind when examining radiographs of the carpus. *Carpal fusions* (e.g., between the lunate and the triquetrum) may occur and should be regarded as variations.

Except for the thumb, the metacarpals and phalanges of the fingers are superimposed, and little information can be obtained by examining them in this view (Fig. 6.78*A*). If a particular finger is injured and suspected of having a fracture, it is viewed laterally with the other fingers flexed. The shaft of each metacarpal begins to ossify during fetal life, and ossification centers appear postnatally in the heads of the four medial metacarpals and in the base of the 1st metacarpal (Fig. 6.78*B*). By age 11, ossification centers of all carpal bones are visible (Fig. 6.78*C*). *Pseudoepiphyses* (accessory centers) are occasionally seen in the head of the 1st metacarpal and in the base of the 2nd metacarpal.

Ultrasonography

Ultrasonography is highly accurate for rotator cuff tears (Halpern, 2004). *Doppler ultrasound* is used to visualize blood flowing through the vessels of the limbs and to mea-

sure its velocity. *Color Doppler ultrasound* technology allows red and blue colors to be superimposed on the standard gray-scale images.

Arteriography

Arteriography (visualization of arteries) is used to detect vascular injuries, ischemia, and variations of arteries. *Arteriograms* are produced by injecting a dye into an artery as a radiograph is taken (Fig. 6.79). When interest is in a specific artery, the dye is injected directly into it, usually through a catheter. Arteriography may be used to determine the patency of arteries before and after surgical procedures in the upper limb to repair injuries resulting from trauma.

Computed Tomography

CT scans of the upper limb are produced by X-rays, but the anatomical images are created by computer reconstructions of the electronic data. The reconstructed images look like cross sections of the limb, and they can be reconstructed in the coronal and sagittal planes. Because the person must be in the CT scanner for only brief periods, fast (2-s) scans can be produced; consequently, involuntary ▶

Proper palmar
digital arteries

Common palmar
digital arteries

Superficial palmar arch

Deep palmar branch
of ulnar artery

Ulnar artery

Radialis indicis
artery

Princeps pollicis
artery

Palmar metacarpal
arteries

Deep palmar arch

Radial artery

Figure 6.79. Angiogram of hand. The superficial palmar arch, formed primarily by the ulnar artery, is usually completed by the superficial palmar branch of the radial artery. In this teenage hand, the carpal bones are fully ossified, but the epiphyseal lines of the long bones (e.g., radius and ulna) are still open. Closure occurs when growth is complete, usually at the end of the teenage years. (Courtesy of Dr. D. Armstrong, University of Toronto, Toronto, Ontario, Canada)

movement produces minimal distortion of the images. For example, *arthrotomography* enhanced by CT is able to demonstrate subtle fractures (e.g., of the rim of the glenoid cavity) and reactive bone changes around a recurrently dislocating glenohumeral joint (Halpern, 2004).

Magnetic Resonance Imaging

MRI produces images with good resolution of the various soft tissues of the limbs because adults can keep their limbs motionless for the 5–10 min required for scanning. This technique produces cross-sectional, coronal, and sagittal images and has the advantage that it does not involve the use of X-rays. Because MRI requires the person to remain still for several minutes, this technique is difficult to use with children. In Figure 6.80, observe the good resolution of the muscles, bones, and joints. MRI is helpful in the diagnosis of subluxation, dislocation, impingement of nerves, cartilage tears, and rotator cuff tears of the glenohumeral joint (Halpern, 2004). Coronal MRIs are helpful in demonstrating ruptured tendons in the shoulder, elbow, hand, and wrist regions. ▶

(A) Coronal view

Acromioclavicular joint

Deltoid muscle

Subcutaneous tissue

Quadrangular space

Subclavius

Coracoclavicular (trapezoid) ligament

Articulating surfaces of glenohumeral joint

Subscapularis

1st rib

Axillary vein

Intercostal muscle

Lung

Axillary fat

Long head of triceps

(B) Sagittal view

Triceps brachii

Subcutaneous tissue (fat) of cubital fossa

Olecranon fossa of humerus

Brachialis

Olecranon of ulna

Trochlea of humerus

Trochlear notch of ulna

Coronoid process of ulna

Superficial flexors

Ulna

Flexor digitorum profundus

Figure 6.80. MRI studies of upper limb. A. The glenohumeral and acromioclavicular joints are shown. The "white" (signal-intense) parts of the identified bones are the fatty matrix of cancellous bone; the thin black outlines (absence of signal) of the bones are the compact bone that forms their outer surfaces. *A,* acromion; *C,* clavicle; *G,* glenoid cavity; *Gr,* greater tubercle of humerus; *H,* head of humerus; *N,* surgical neck of humerus. **B.** The elbow region is shown.

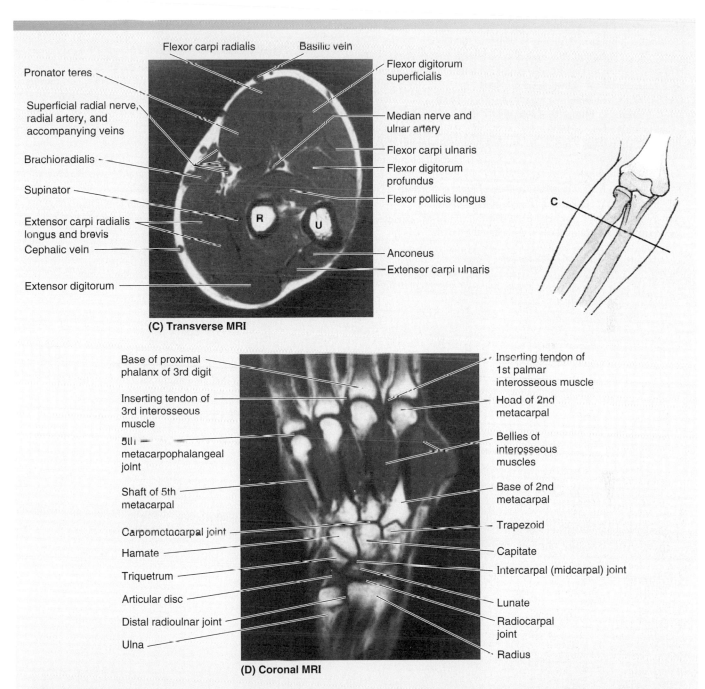

Flexor carpi radialis   Basilic vein

Pronator teres

Superficial radial nerve,
radial artery, and
accompanying veins

Brachioradialis

Supinator

Extensor carpi radialis
longus and brevis

Cephalic vein

Extensor digitorum

Flexor digitorum
superficialis

Median nerve and
ulnar artery

Flexor carpi ulnaris

Flexor digitorum
profundus

Flexor pollicis longus

Anconeus

Extensor carpi ulnaris

R

U

C

(C) Transverse MRI

Base of proximal
phalanx of 3rd digit

Inserting tendon of
3rd interosseous
muscle

5th
metacarpophalangeal
joint

Shaft of 5th
metacarpal

Carpometacarpal joint

Hamate

Triquetrum

Articular disc

Distal radioulnar joint

Ulna

Inserting tendon of
1st palmar
interosseous muscle

Head of 2nd
metacarpal

Bellies of
interosseous
muscles

Base of 2nd
metacarpal

Trapezoid

Capitate

Intercarpal (midcarpal) joint

Lunate

Radiocarpal
joint

Radius

(D) Coronal MRI

Figure 6.80. *(Continued)* **C.** The proximal part of the forearm is shown. The orientation drawing shows the plane of the MRI. The subcutaneous border of the ulna (*U*) and the radial artery demarcate the anteromedial flexor and posterolateral extensor compartments. *R,* radius. **D.** In this image of the wrist and hand, the bones, joints, and interosseous muscles can be observed. (Courtesy of Dr. W. Kucharczyk, Professor and Chair of Medical Imaging, University of Toronto, and Clinical Director of Tri-Hospital Magnetic Resonance Centre, Toronto, Ontario, Canada.) ✪

References and Suggested Readings

Anderson MK, Hall SJ, Martin, M: *Sports Injury Management,* 2nd ed. Baltimore, Lippincott Williams & Wilkins, 2000.

Bergman RA, Thompson SA, Afifi AK, Saadeh FA: *Compendium of Human Anatomic Variation: Text, Atlas and World Literature.* Baltimore, Urban & Schwarzenberg, 1988.

Foerster O: The dermatomes in man. *Brain* 56:1, 1933.

Ger R, Abrahams P, Olson T: *Essentials of Clinical Anatomy,* 3rd ed. New York, Parthenon, 1996.

Halpern BC: Shoulder injuries. *In* Birrer RB, O'Connor FG (eds): *Sports Medicine for the Primary Care Physician,* 3rd ed. Boca Raton, FL, CRC Press, 2004.

Hamill J, Knutzen KM: *Biomechanical Basis of Human Movement,* 2nd ed. Baltimore, Lippincott Williams & Wilkins, 2003.

Keegan JJ, Garrett FD: The segmental distribution of the cutaneous nerves in the limbs of man. *Anat Rec* 102:409, 1948.

Leonard LJ (Chair), Educational Affairs Committee, American Association of Clinical Anatomists: The clinical anatomy of several invasive procedures. *Clin Anat* 12:43, 1999.

Moore KL, Persaud TVN: *The Developing Human: Clinically Oriented Embryology,* 7th ed. Philadelphia, Saunders, 2003.

Nussbaum RL, McInnes RR, Willard HF: *Thompson & Thompson Genetics in Medicine,* 6th ed., Philadelphia, Saunders, 2004.

Rowland LP (ed): *Merritt's Textbook of Neurology,* 10th ed. Baltimore: Lippincott Williams & Wilkins, 2000.

Sabiston DC Jr, Lyerly HK: *Sabiston Essentials of Surgery,* 2nd ed. Philadelphia, Saunders, 1994.

Salter RB: *Textbook of Disorders and Injuries of the Musculoskeletal System,* 3rd ed. Baltimore, Lippincott Williams & Wilkins, 1999.

Williams PL, Bannister LH, Berry MM, Collins P, Dyson M, Dussek JE, Fergusson MWJ (eds): *Gray's Anatomy,* 38th ed. Edinburgh, UK, Churchill Livingstone, 1995.

7

Head

Overview

The **head** is the superior part of the body that is attached to the trunk by the neck.

It is the control and communications center as well as the "loading dock" for the body. It houses the brain and therefore is the site of our consciousness: ideas, creativity, imagination, responses, decision making, and memory. It includes special sensory receivers (eyes, ears, mouth, and nose), broadcast devices for voice and expression, and portals for the intake of fuel (food), water, and oxygen and the exhaust of carbon dioxide.

The head consists of the *brain* and its protective coverings, the *ears,* and the *face.* The face includes openings and passageways, with lubricating glands and valves (seals) to close some of them, the masticatory (chewing) devices, and the orbits that house the visual apparatus. The face also provides our identity as individuals. Disease, malformation, or trauma of structures in the head form the bases of many specialties, including dentistry, maxillofacial surgery, neurology, neuroradiology, neurosurgery, ophthalmology, oral surgery, otology, rhinology, and psychiatry.

Head Injuries

Head injuries are a major cause of death and disability. The complications of head injuries include hemorrhage, infection, and injury to the brain and cranial nerves. Disturbance in the level of consciousness (LOC) is the most common symptom of head injury. Almost 10% of all deaths in the United States are caused by head injuries, and approximately half of traumatic deaths involve the brain (Rowland, 2000). Head injuries occur mostly in young persons between the ages of 15 and 24 years. The major cause of brain injury varies but motor vehicle and motorcycle accidents are prominent. Men are affected three to four times as often as women.

Headaches and Facial Pain

Few complaints are more common than *headaches* and *facial pain.* Although usually benign and frequently associated with tension, fatigue, or mild fever, headaches may indicate a serious intracranial problem such as a brain tumor, subarachnoid hemorrhage, or meningitis. *Neuralgias* (G. *algos,* pain) are characterized by severe throbbing or stabbing pain in the course of a nerve caused by a demyelinating lesion. They are a common cause of facial pain. Terms such as *facial neuralgia* describe diffuse painful sensations. Localized aches have specific names, such as *earache* (otalgia) and *toothache* (odontalgia). A sound knowledge of the anatomy of the head helps in understanding the causes of headaches and facial pain. ✪

Cranium

The **cranium** (skull) is the skeleton of the head (Fig. 7.1*A*). A series of bones form its two parts, the neurocranium and viscerocranium (Fig. 7.1*B*). The **neurocranium** (cranial vault) is the bony covering (case) of the brain and its membranous coverings, the cranial meninges. It also contains proximal parts of the cranial nerves and the vasculature of the brain. The neurocranium has a dome-like roof, the **calvaria** (skullcap), and a floor or **cranial base** (basicranium). The neurocranium in adults is formed by a series of eight bones: four singular bones centered on the midline (*frontal, ethmoidal, sphenoidal,* and *occipital*) and two sets of bones occurring as bilateral pairs (*temporal* and *parietal*) (Fig. 7.1*A* & *D*).

The bones forming the calvaria are primarily flat bones (frontal, temporal, and parietal) formed by intramembranous ossification of head mesenchyme from the neural crest. The bones contributing to the cranial base are primarily irregular bones with substantial flat portions (sphenoidal and

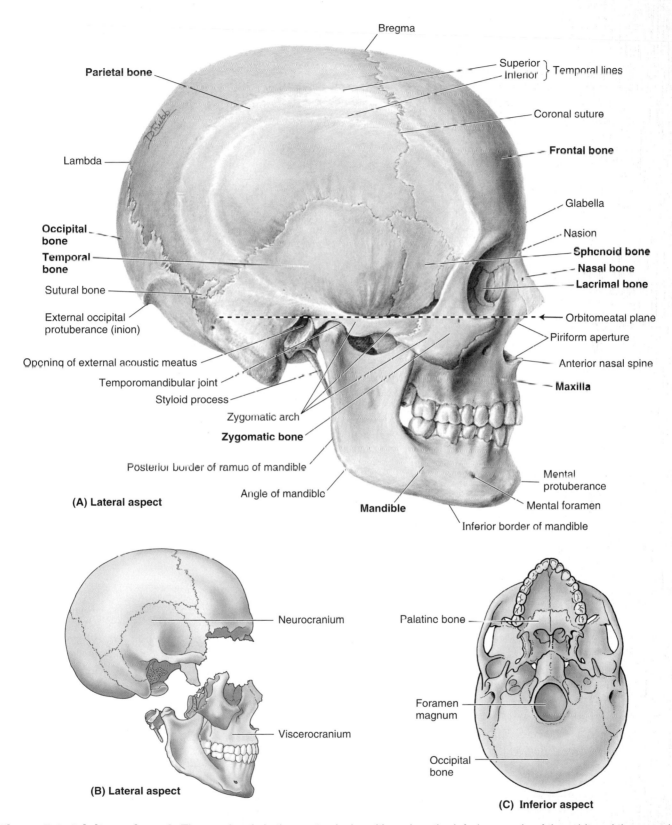

Figure 7.1. Adult cranium. A. The cranium is in the anatomical position when the inferior margin of the orbit and the superior margin of the external acoustic meatus lie in the same horizontal orbitomeatal or Frankfort horizontal plane, a standard craniometric reference. The temporal fossa is the region of the lateral aspect of the cranium superior to the zygomatic arch and inferior to the temporal lines. **B.** The neurocranium and viscerocranium are the two primary functional parts of the cranium. **C.** The irregularly shaped palatine bone contributes to the formation of the nasal cavity, the hard palate, and a small part of the orbit. The spinal cord is continuous with the brain through the foramen magnum, the large opening in the basal part of the occipital bone.

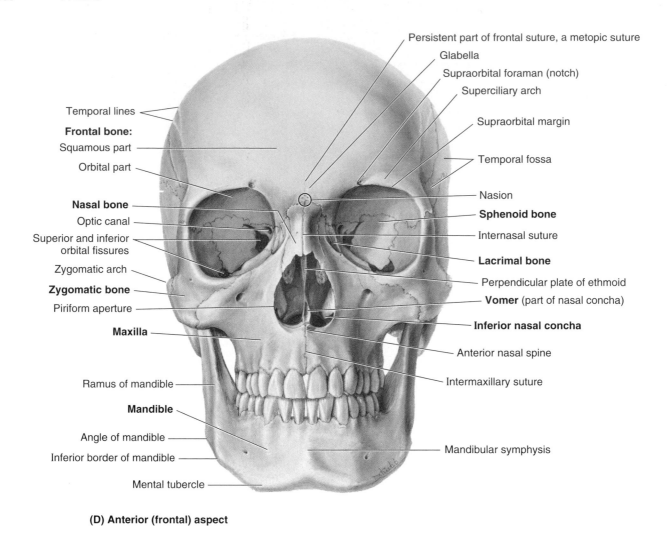

Temporal lines

Frontal bone:

Squamous part

Orbital part

Nasal bone

Optic canal

Superior and inferior orbital fissures

Zygomatic arch

Zygomatic bone

Piriform aperture

Maxilla

Ramus of mandible

Mandible

Angle of mandible

Inferior border of mandible

Mental tubercle

Persistent part of frontal suture, a metopic suture

Glabella

Supraorbital foraman (notch)

Superciliary arch

Supraorbital margin

Temporal fossa

Nasion

Sphenoid bone

Internasal suture

Lacrimal bone

Perpendicular plate of ethmoid

Vomer (part of nasal concha)

Inferior nasal concha

Anterior nasal spine

Intermaxillary suture

Mandibular symphysis

(D) Anterior (frontal) aspect

Figure 7.1. *(Continued)* **D.** The supraorbital notch, the infraorbital foramen, and the mental foramen are approximately in a vertical line.

temporal) formed by endochondral ossification of cartilage (chondrocranium) or from more than one type of ossification. The *ethmoid bone* is an irregular bone that makes a relatively minor midline contribution to the neurocranium but is primarily part of the viscerocranium. The "flat" bones and "flat" portions of the bones forming the neurocranium are actually curved, with convex external and concave internal surfaces.

Most calvarial bones are united by fibrous interlocking *sutures;* however, during childhood, some bones (sphenoid and occipital) are united by hyaline cartilage (*synchondroses*). The spinal cord is continuous with the brain through the *foramen magnum,* a large opening in the cranial base (Fig. 7.1*C*).

The **viscerocranium** (facial skeleton) comprises the facial bones that mainly develop in the mesenchyme of the embryonic pharyngeal arches (Moore and Persaud, 2003). The viscerocranium forms the anterior part of the cranium and consists of the bones surrounding the mouth (upper and lower jaws), nose/nasal cavity, and most of the *orbits* (eye sockets or orbital cavities). It consists of 15 irregular bones: three singular bones centered on or lying in the midline (*mandible, ethmoid,* and *vomer*) and 6 bones occurring as bilateral pairs (*maxillae; inferior nasal conchae;* and *zygomatic, palatine, nasal,* and *lacrimal bones*) (Fig. 7.1*A, C,* & *D*). The maxillae and mandible house the teeth—that is, they provide the sockets and supporting bone for the maxillary and mandibular teeth. The maxillae contribute the greatest part of the upper facial skeleton, forming the skeleton of the upper jaw, which is fixed to the cranial base. The mandible forms the skeleton of the lower jaw, which is movable because it articulates with the cranial base at the *temporomandibular joints* (TMJs).

Several bones of the cranium (frontal, temporal, sphenoid, and ethmoid bones) are **pneumatized bones,** which contain air spaces (*air cells* or larger *sinuses*), presumably to decrease their weight. The total volume of the air spaces in these bones increases with age.

In the *anatomical position,* the cranium is oriented so that the inferior margin of the orbit and the superior margin of the external acoustic opening of the external acoustic meatus of both sides lie in the same horizontal plane (Fig. 7.1*A*). This standard craniometric reference is the **orbitomeatal plane** (Frankfort horizontal plane).

Facial Aspect of the Cranium

Features of the anterior or **facial (frontal) aspect of the cranium** (L. *norma facialis* or *frontalis*) are the frontal and zygomatic bones, orbits, nasal region, maxillae, and mandible (Fig. 7.1*D*).

The **frontal bone,** specifically its **squamous** (flat) **part,** forms the skeleton of the forehead, articulating inferiorly with the nasal and zygomatic bones. In some adults a remnant of the frontal suture, the **metopic suture,** is visible in the midline of the **glabella,** the smooth, slightly depressed area between the superciliary arches. The **frontal suture** divides the frontal bones of the fetal cranium (see clinical correlation [blue] box "Development of the Cranium," later in this chapter). The intersection of the frontal and nasal bones is the **nasion** (L. *nasus,* nose), which in most people is related to a distinctly depressed area (bridge of the nose). The frontal bone also articulates with the lacrimal, ethmoid, and sphenoids, and a horizontal portion of bone (the **orbital part)** forms both the roof of the orbit and part of the floor of the anterior part of the cranial cavity.

The **supraorbital margin** of the frontal bone, the angular boundary between the squamous and the orbital parts, has a **supraorbital foramen** or **notch** in some crania for passage of the supraorbital nerve and vessels. Just superior to the supraorbital margin is a ridge, the **superciliary arch,** that extends laterally on each side from the glabella. The prominence of this ridge, deep to the eyebrows, is generally greater in males. Within the orbits are the superior and inferior orbital fissures and optic canals.

The **zygomatic bones** (cheek bones, malar bones), forming the prominences of the cheeks, lie on the inferolateral sides of the orbits and rest on the maxillae. The anterolateral rims, walls, floor, and much of the infraorbital margins of the orbits are formed by these quadrilateral bones. A small **zygomaticofacial foramen** pierces the lateral aspect of each bone (Fig. 7.2*A* & *B*). The zygomatic bones articulate with the frontal, sphenoid, and temporal bones and the maxillae. Inferior to the nasal bones is the pear-shaped **piriform aperture,** the anterior nasal opening in the cranium (Fig. 7.1*A* & *D*). The bony **nasal septum** can be observed through this aperture, dividing the nasal cavity into right and left parts. On the lateral wall of each nasal cavity are curved bony plates, the **nasal conchae** (Figs. 7.1*D* and 7.2*A*).

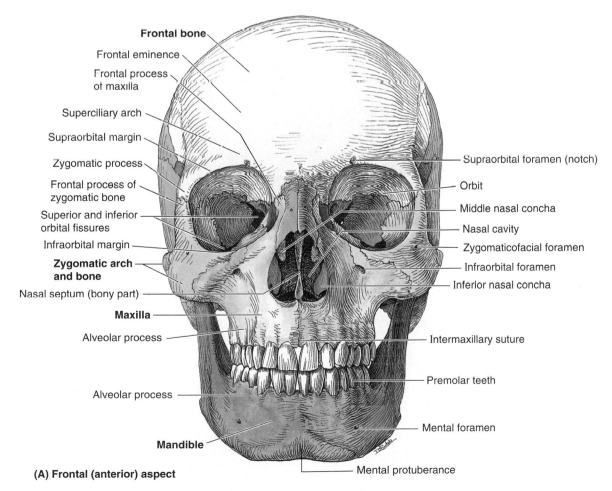

(A) Frontal (anterior) aspect

Figure 7.2. Bones of adult cranium. A. The forehead, the orbits, the bony part of the external nose, and the upper (maxilla) and lower (mandible) jaws are shown.

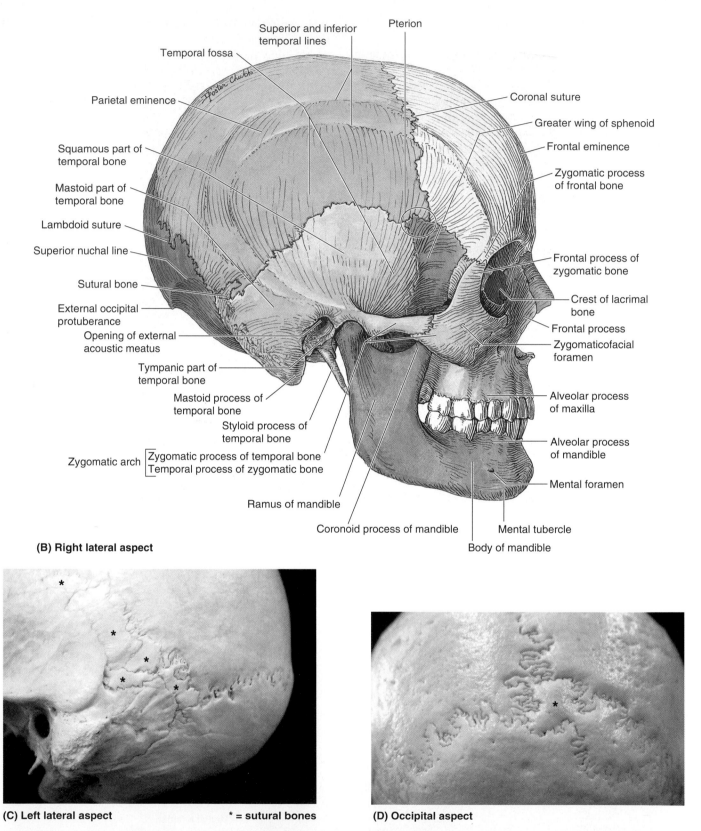

(B) Right lateral aspect

(C) Left lateral aspect   * = sutural bones   **(D) Occipital aspect**

Figure 7.2. *(Continued)* **B.** Within the temporal fossa, the pterion is a craniometric point at the junction of the greater wing of the sphenoid, the squamous temporal bone, the frontal, and the parietal bones. **C and D.** Sutural bones occurring along the temporoparietal (**C**) and lambdoid (**D**) sutures are shown.

The **maxillae** form the upper jaw; their **alveolar processes** include the tooth sockets (alveoli) and constitute the supporting bone for the **maxillary teeth**. The maxillae surround most of the piriform aperture and form the infraorbital margins medially. They have a broad connection with the zygomatic bones laterally and an **infraorbital foramen** inferior to each orbit for passage of the infraorbital nerve and vessels (Fig. 7.2*A*). The two maxillae are united at the **intermaxillary suture** in the median plane (Fig. 7.2*A*).

The **mandible** is a U-shaped bone with an alveolar process that supports the **mandibular teeth**. It consists of a horizontal part, the **body**, and a vertical part, the **ramus** (Fig. 7.2*B*). Inferior to the second premolar teeth are the **mental foramina** for the mental nerves and vessels (Fig. 7.2*A*). The **mental protuberance**, forming the prominence of the chin, is a triangular bony elevation inferior to the **mandibular symphysis** (L. *symphysis menti*), the osseous union where the halves of the infantile mandible fuse (Fig. 7.1*D*).

Injury to the Superciliary Arches

The superciliary arches are relatively sharp bony ridges; consequently, a blow to them (e.g., during boxing) may lacerate the skin and cause bleeding. Bruising of the skin surrounding the orbit causes tissue fluid and blood to accumulate in the surrounding connective tissue, which gravitates into the superior (upper) eyelid and around the eye ("black eye").

Malar Flush

The zygomatic bone was once called the malar bone; consequently, you will hear the clinical term *malar flush*. This redness of the skin covering the zygomatic prominence (malar eminence) is associated with a rise in temperature in various fevers occurring with certain diseases, such as *tuberculosis* and *systemic lupus erythematosus disease* (SLE).

Fractures of the Maxillae and Associated Bones

Dr. Léon-Clement Le Fort (Paris surgeon and gynecologist, 1829–1893) classified three common variants of fractures of the maxillae (Fig. B7.1):

- **Le Fort I fracture:** wide variety of horizontal fractures of the maxillae, passing superior to the maxillary alveolar process (i.e., to the roots of the teeth), crossing the bony nasal septum and possibly the pterygoid plates of the sphenoid.

- **Le Fort II fracture:** passes from the posterolateral parts of the maxillary sinuses (cavities in the maxillae) superomedially through the infraorbital foramina, lacrimals, or ethmoids to the bridge of the nose. As a result, the entire central part of the face, including the hard palate and alveolar processes, is separated from the rest of the cranium.

- **Le Fort III fracture:** horizontal fracture that passes through the superior orbital fissures and the ethmoid and nasal bones and extends laterally through the greater wings of the sphenoid and the frontozygomatic

Le Fort I

Le Fort II

Le Fort III

Figure B7.1

sutures. Concurrent fracturing of the zygomatic arches causes the maxillae and zygomatic bones to separate from the rest of the cranium.

Fractures of the Mandible

A fracture of the mandible usually involves two fractures, which frequently occur on opposite sides of the mandible; thus if one fracture is observed, a search should be made for another. For example, a hard blow to the jaw often fractures the neck of the mandible and its body in the region of the opposite canine tooth. *Fractures of the coronoid process* are uncommon and usually single (Fig. B7.2, line A). *Fractures of the neck of the mandible* are often transverse and may be associated with dislocation of the TMJ on the same side (Fig. B7.2, line B). *Fractures of the angle of the mandible* are usually oblique and may involve the bony socket or ▶

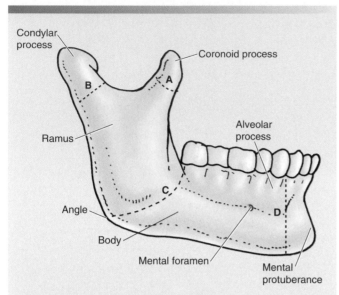

Figure B7.2. Fractures of mandible. *A,* Fracture of the coronoid process; *B,* fracture of the neck of the mandible; *C,* fracture of the angle of the mandible; *D,* fracture of the body of the mandible.

alveolus of the 3rd molar tooth (Fig. B7.2, line C). *Fractures of the body of the mandible* frequently pass through the socket of a canine tooth (Fig. B7.2, line D).

Resorption of Alveolar Bone

Extraction of teeth causes the alveolar bone to resorb in the affected region(s) (Fig. B7.3). Following complete loss or extraction of maxillary teeth, the sockets begin to fill in with bone and the alveolar process begins to resorb. Similarly, extraction of mandibular teeth causes the bone to resorb. Gradually, the mental foramen lies near the superior border of the body of the mandible. In some cases, the mental foramina disappear, exposing the mental nerves to injury. *Pressure from a dental prosthesis* (e.g., a denture resting on an exposed mental nerve) may produce pain during eating. Loss of all the teeth results in a decrease in the vertical facial dimension and *mandibular prognathism* (overclosure). Deep creases in the facial skin also appear that pass posteriorly from the corners of the mouth. ✛

Figure B7.3. Resorption of edentulous alveolar bone.

Lateral Aspect of the Cranium

The **lateral aspect of the cranium** (L. *norma lateralis*) is formed by both the neurocranium and the viscerocranium (Figs. 7.1*B* and 7.2*B*). The main features of the neurocranial part include the *temporal fossa,* the *external acoustic opening,* and the *mastoid process of the temporal bone.* The main features of the viscerocranial part include the *infratemporal fossa, zygomatic arch,* and lateral aspects of the maxilla and mandible. The **temporal fossa** (Fig. 7.1*D*) is bounded superiorly and

Table 7.1. Craniometric Points of the Cranium

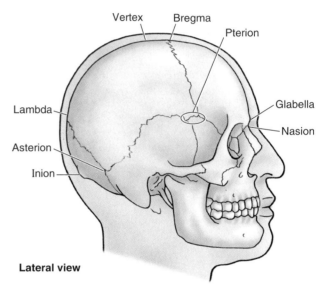

Lateral view

Landmark	Shape and Location
Pterion (G. wing)	Junction of the greater wing of the sphenoid, squamous temporal, frontal, and parietal bones; overlies course of anterior division of middle meningeal artery
Lambda (G. the letter *L*)	Point on calvaria at junction of lambdoid and sagittal sutures
Bregma (G. forepart of head)	Point on calvaria at junction of coronal and sagittal sutures
Vertex (L. whirl, whorl)	Superior point of neurocranium, in the middle with the cranium oriented in anatomical (orbitomeatal or Frankfort) plane
Asterion (G. *asterios,* starry)	Star shaped; located at junction of three sutures: parietomastoid, occipitomastoid, and lambdoid
Glabella (L. smooth, hairless)	Smooth prominence; most marked in males; on the frontal bones superior to root of nose; most anterior projecting part of forehead
Inion (G. back of head)	Most prominent point of external occipital protuberance
Nasion (L. nose)	Point on cranium where frontonasal and internasal sutures meet

posteriorly by the **superior** and **inferior temporal lines**, anteriorly by the frontal and zygomatic bones, and inferiorly by the zygomatic arch (Fig. 7.2*A* & *B*). The superior border of this arch corresponds to the inferior limit of the cerebral hemisphere of the brain. The **zygomatic arch** is formed by the union of the **temporal process of the zygomatic bone** and the **zygomatic process of the temporal bone.**

In the anterior part of the temporal fossa, 3–4 cm superior to the midpoint of the zygomatic arch, is a clinically important area of bone junctions: the **pterion** (G. *pteron,* wing) (Fig. 7.2*B*; Table 7.1). It is usually indicated by an H-shaped formation of

sutures that unite the frontal, parietal, sphenoid (greater wing), and temporal bones. Less commonly, the frontal and temporal bones articulate; sometimes all four bones meet at a point.

The **external acoustic opening** is the entrance to the **external acoustic meatus** (canal), which leads to the tympanic membrane (eardrum). The **mastoid process** of the temporal bone is posteroinferior to the external acoustic pore. Anteromedial to the mastoid process is the **styloid process** of the temporal bone, a slender needle-like, pointed projection. The *infratemporal fossa* is an irregular space inferior and deep to the zygomatic arch and the mandible and posterior to the maxilla.

Fractures of the Calvaria

The convexity of the calvaria distributes and thereby usually minimizes the effects of a blow to the head. However, hard blows in thin areas of the calvaria are likely to produce *depressed fractures*, in which a bone fragment is depressed inward, compressing and/or injuring the brain (Fig. B7.4). *Linear calvarial fractures*, the most frequent type, usually occur at the point of impact; but fracture lines often radiate away from it in two or more directions. In *comminuted fractures*, the bone is broken into several pieces. If the area of the calvaria is thick at the site of impact, the bone may bend inward without fracturing; however, a fracture may occur some distance from the site of direct trauma where the calvaria is thinner. In a *contrecoup (counterblow) fracture*, no fracture occurs at the point of impact, but one occurs on the opposite side of the cranium.

Fracture of the Pterion

Fracture of the pterion can be life-threatening because it overlies the anterior branches of the middle meningeal vessels, which lie in grooves on the internal aspect of the lateral wall of the calvaria (Fig. 7.2*B*). The pterion is two fingers' breadth superior to the zygomatic arch and a thumb's breadth posterior to the frontal process of the zygomatic bone (Fig. B7.5*A*). A hard blow to the side of the head may fracture the thin bones forming the pterion (Fig. 7.2*A*), producing a rupture of the anterior branch of the middle meningeal artery crossing the pterion (Fig. B7.5*B*). The resulting *hematoma* exerts pressure on the underlying cerebral cortex. An untreated *middle meningeal artery hemorrhage* may cause death in a few hours. ▶

Depressed fracture

Comminuted fracture

Linear fracture

Basilar fracture

Median View

Figure B7.4. Fractures of calvaria

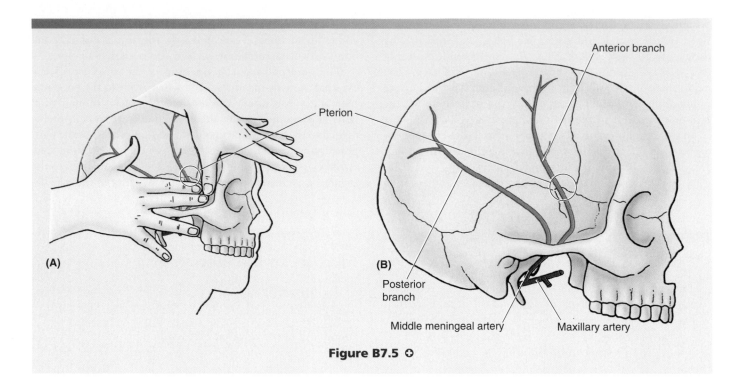

Figure B7.5 ⊕

Occipital Aspect of the Cranium

The posterior or **occipital aspect of the cranium** (L. *norma occipitalis*) is composed of the **occiput** (L. back of head, the convex posterior protuberance of the occipital bone), parts of the parietal bones, and mastoid parts of the temporal bones (Fig. 7.3*A*). The **external occipital protuberance** (Table 7.1), is usually easily palpable in the median plane; however, occasionally (especially in females) it may be inconspicuous. A craniometric point (a point used in making cranial measurements and comparisons) defined by the tip of the external protuberance is the **inion** (G. nape of neck).

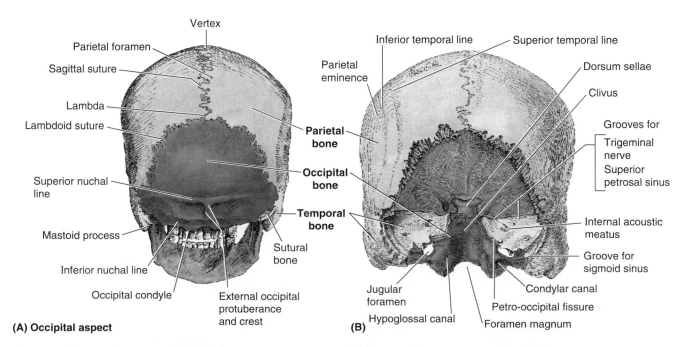

(A) Occipital aspect

(B)

Figure 7.3. Occiput of adult cranium. A. The posterior aspect of the cranium, or occiput, is composed of parts of the parietal bones, the occipital bone, and the mastoid parts of the temporal bones. The sagittal and lambdoid sutures meet at lambda, which can often be felt as a depression in living persons. **B.** The squamous part of the occipital bone has been removed to expose the anterior part of the anterior cranial fossa.

The **external occipital crest** descends from the protuberance toward the *foramen magnum,* the large opening in the basal part of the occipital bone (Figs. 7.1*C* and 7.3*B*). The **superior nuchal line,** marking the superior limit of the neck, extends laterally from each side of the protuberance; the **inferior nuchal line** is less distinct. In the center of the occiput, the **lambda** indicates the junction of the sagittal and lambdoid sutures (Fig. 7.3*A;* Table 7.1). The lambda can sometimes be felt as a depression. One or more **sutural bones** (accessory bones) may be located at the lambda or near the mastoid process (Fig. 7.2*B–D*).

Superior Aspect of the Cranium

The **superior (vertical) aspect** of the cranium (L. *norma superioris* or *verticalis*), usually somewhat oval in form, broadens posterolaterally at the **parietal eminences** (Figs. 7.2*B* and 7.3*B*). In some people, **frontal eminences** are also visible, giving the calvaria an almost square appearance. The **coronal suture** separates the frontal and parietal bones (Figs. 7.4*A* & *B*), the **sagittal suture** separates the parietal bones, and the **lambdoid suture** separates the parietal and temporal bones from the occipital bone (Figs. 7.3*A* and 7.4*C*). The **bregma** is the landmark formed by the intersection of the sagittal and coronal sutures (Fig. 7.4*A;* Table 7.1). The **vertex,** the most superior point of the calvaria, is near the midpoint of the sagittal suture.

The **parietal foramen** is a small, inconstant aperture located posteriorly in the parietal bone near the sagittal suture (Fig. 7.4*C*); paired parietal foramina may be present. Most irregular, highly variable foramina that occur in the neurocranium are *emissary foramina* that transmit *emissary veins,* veins connecting scalp veins to the venous sinuses of the dura mater (see "Structure of the Scalp," later in this chapter) (Fig 7.4*B*).

External Surface of the Cranial Base

The cranial base (basicranium) is the inferior portion of the neurocranium (floor of the cranial cavity) and viscerocranium minus the mandible (Fig. 7.5*A–C*). The **external surface of the cranial base** (L. *basis cranii externa*) features the **alveolar arch of the maxillae** (the free border of the alveolar processes surrounding and supporting the maxillary teeth); the palatine processes of the maxillae; and the palatine, sphenoid, vomer, temporal, and occipital bones (Fig. 7.5*A* & *B*). The *hard palate* (bony palate) is formed by the **palatine processes of the maxillae** anteriorly and the **horizontal plates of the palatine bones** posteriorly. The free posterior border of the hard palate projects posteriorly in the median plane as the **posterior nasal spine.** Posterior to the central incisor teeth is the **incisive fossa,** a depression in the midline of the bony palate into which the incisive canals open.

The right and left nasopalatine nerves pass from the nose through a variable number of incisive canals and foramina (they may be bilateral or merged into a single formation). Posterolaterally are the **greater** and **lesser palatine foramina.** Superior to the posterior edge of the palate are two large openings: the **choanae** (posterior nasal apertures), which are separated from each other by the **vomer** (L. *plowshare*), a flat unpaired bone of trapezoidal shape that forms a major part of the bony nasal septum.

Wedged between the frontal, temporal, and occipital bones is the **sphenoid,** an irregular unpaired bone that consists of a body and three pairs of processes: greater wings, lesser wings, and pterygoid processes. The **greater** and **lesser wings** of the sphenoid spread laterally from the lateral aspects of the body of the bone (Fig. 7.5*C*). The **pterygoid processes,** consisting of **lateral** and **medial pterygoid plates,** extend inferiorly on each side of the sphenoid from the junction of the body and greater wings. The *groove for the cartilaginous part of the pharyngotympanic (auditory) tube* lies medial to the **spine** of the

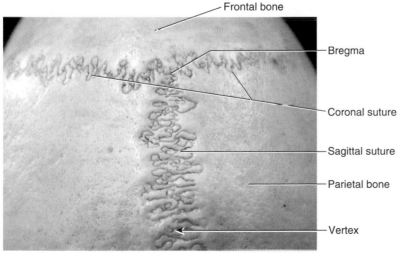

(A) Superior (vertical) aspect

Figure 7.4. Anterior part of adult calvaria. A. The external aspect demonstrates the bregma, where the coronal and sagittal sutures meet, and the vertex, the superiormost point of the cranium.

(B) Inferior view

Coronal suture

M

D

Sagittal suture

Groove for superior sagittal sinus

FC

Parietal foramen

Sagittal suture

Lambda

Lambdoid suture

(C) Posterosuperior view

Figure 7.4. *(Continued)* **B.** The internal aspect of the calvaria reveals the pits (granular foveolae; *dotted lines*) in the frontal and parietal bones, which are produced by enlarged arachnoid granulations or clusters of smaller ones (Fig. 7.7). Multiple small emissary veins pass between the superior sagittal sinus and veins in the diploë (*D*) and scalp through the emissary foramina (*arrows*) located on each side of the sagittal suture. The spongy diploë of cancellous bone contains red marrow in life. The sinuous vascular groove (*M*) on the lateral wall is formed by the frontal branch of the middle meningeal artery. The cerebral falx, a short process of dura mater (the outermost covering of the brain), attaches to the frontal crest (*FC*). **C.** This external view demonstrates a prominent, unilateral parietal foramen. Although emissary foramina often occur in this general location, there is much variation. They may be bilateral but are more commonly absent.

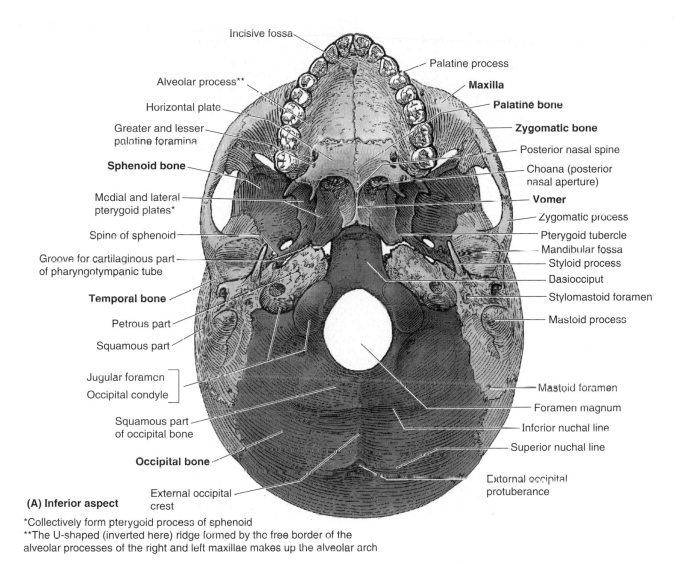

Incisive fossa

Palatine process

Alveolar process**

Maxilla

Horizontal plate

Palatine bone

Greater and lesser
palatine foramina

Zygomatic bone

Sphenoid bone

Posterior nasal spine

Choana (posterior
nasal aperture)

Medial and lateral
pterygoid plates*

Vomer

Zygomatic process

Spine of sphenoid

Pterygoid tubercle

Mandibular fossa

Groove for cartilaginous part
of pharyngotympanic tube

Styloid process

Basiocciput

Temporal bone

Stylomastoid foramen

Petrous part

Mastoid process

Squamous part

Jugular foramen

Occipital condyle

Mastoid foramen

Foramen magnum

Squamous part
of occipital bone

Inferior nuchal line

Superior nuchal line

Occipital bone

External occipital
protuberance

(A) Inferior aspect   External occipital
crest

*Collectively form pterygoid process of sphenoid
**The U-shaped (inverted here) ridge formed by the free border of the
alveolar processes of the right and left maxillae makes up the alveolar arch

Figure 7.5. Cranial base. A. The external aspect demonstrates the contributing bones. The inferior surface is formed posteriorly by the occipital bone, which becomes continuous anteriorly with the sphenoid bone following synostosis.

sphenoid, inferior to the junction of the greater wing of the sphenoid and the **petrous** (L. rock-like) **part of the temporal bone.** Depressions in the **squamous** (L. flat) **part of the temporal bone,** called the **mandibular fossae** (Fig. 7.5*B*), accommodate the mandibular condyles when the mouth is closed. The cranial base is formed posteriorly by the occipital bone, which articulates with the sphenoid anteriorly.

The four parts of the **occipital bone** are arranged around the **foramen magnum,** the most conspicuous feature of the cranial base. The major structures passing through this large foramen are the *spinal cord* (where it becomes continuous with the medulla oblongata of the brain), the *meninges* (coverings) of the brain and spinal cord, the *vertebral arteries,* the anterior and posterior *spinal arteries,* and the *accessory nerve* (CN XI). On the lateral parts of the occipital bone are two large protuberances, the **occipital condyles,** by which the cranium articulates with the vertebral column (Fig. 7.5*B*).

The large opening between the occipital bone and the petrous part of the temporal bone is the **jugular foramen,** from which the internal jugular vein (IJV) and several cranial nerves (CN IX–CN XI) emerge from the cranium (Fig. 7.5*C*). Superolateral to the jugular foramen is the *internal acoustic meatus,* a passage for CN VII and CN VIII. The entrance to the **carotid canal** for the internal carotid artery is just anterior to the jugular foramen (Fig. 7.5*B*). The *mastoid processes* provide for muscle attachments. The **stylomastoid foramen,** transmitting the facial nerve (CN VII) and stylomastoid artery, lies posterior to the base of the styloid process.

Internal Surface of the Cranial Base

The **internal surface of the cranial base** (L. *basis cranii interna*) has three large depressions that lie at different levels: the *anterior, middle,* and *posterior cranial fossae* (Fig. 7.5*D*), which form the bowl-shaped floor of the cranial cavity. The

Incisive fossa

Greater and lesser
palatine foramina

Medial pterygoid
plate

Foramen spinosum
Spine of sphenoid

Mandibular fossa
Tympanic plate

Styloid process
Stylomastoid foramen

Mastoid process

Groove for
occipital artery

Inferior nuchal line

(B) Inferior aspect

Palatine process of maxilla ⎤ Hard palate
Horizontal plate of palatine ⎦
bone

Posterior nasal spine ⎤
Vomer
Choana ⎦

Zygomatic arch

Lateral pterygoid plate ⎤
Foramen ovale ⎦

Bony part of pharyngotympanic
tube

Foramen lacerum ⎤
Pharyngeal tubercle ⎦

Carotid canal ⎤
Jugular foramen ⎦

Stylomastoid foramen

Groove for digastric muscle,
posterior belly

Occipital condyle

External occipital crest

External occipital protuberance

Foramen cecum
Crista galli of ethmoid bone

Ethmoidal ⎡ Anterior
foramina ⎣ Posterior

Ethmoidal spine
Sphenoidal limbus
Prechiasmatic sulcus
Tuberculum sellae†

Greater wing of sphenoid bone

Hypophysial fossa†

Posterior clinoid process†

Dorsum sellae†

Foramen lacerum

Clivus

Petrous ridge

Groove for sigmoid sinus

Jugular foramen

Groove for transverse sinus

Cerebellar fossa

(C) Superior view, internal surface of cranial base

Frontal crest
External table of compact bone
Diploë
Internal table of compact bone
Orbital part of frontal bone
Cribriform plate of ethmoid bone
Lesser wing of sphenoid bone
Optic canal
Sphenoidal crest
Superior orbital fissure*
Anterior clinoid process
Foramen rotundum*
Carotid groove
Foramen ovale*
Foramen spinosum*
Groove for greater petrosal nerve
Internal acoustic meatus
Hypoglossal canal
Foramen magnum
Internal occipital crest
Internal occipital protuberance

† Collectively form sella turcica
* Form crescent of four foramina

Figure 7.5. *(Continued)* **B.** Features of external cranial base are shown. The foramen magnum is located midway between and on a level with the mastoid processes. The hard palate forms both a part of the roof of the mouth and the floor of the nasal cavity. The large choanae on each side of the vomer are the posterior entrance to the nasal cavities. **C.** The internal aspect demonstrates the contributing bones and features.

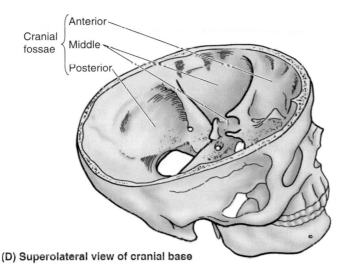

Cranial fossae
- Anterior
- Middle
- Posterior

(D) Superolateral view of cranial base

Figure 7.5. *(Continued)* **D.** The floor of the cranial cavity is divisible into three levels (steps): the anterior, middle, and posterior cranial fossae.

anterior cranial fossa is at the highest level, and the posterior cranial fossa is at the lowest level.

Anterior Cranial Fossa

The inferior and anterior parts of the frontal lobes of the brain occupy the **anterior cranial fossa**, the shallowest of the three cranial fossae (Fig. 7.5*D*). The fossa is formed by the frontal bone anteriorly, the ethmoid bone in the middle, and the body and lesser wings of the sphenoid posteriorly (Fig. 7.5*C*; Table 7.2). The greater part of the fossa is formed by the **orbital parts of the frontal bone**, which support the frontal lobes of the brain and form the roofs of the orbits. This surface shows sinuous impressions (*brain markings*) of the orbital gyri (ridges) of the frontal lobes (Table 7.2). The **frontal crest** is a median bony extension of the frontal bone. At its base is the **foramen cecum of the frontal bone**, which gives passage to vessels during fetal development but is insignificant postnatally. The **crista galli** (L. cock's comb) is a thick, median ridge of bone posterior to the foramen cecum, which projects superiorly from the ethmoid. On each side of this ridge is the sieve-like **cribriform plate of the ethmoid** (Fig. 7.5*C*). Its numerous tiny foramina transmit the olfactory nerves (CN I) from the olfactory areas of the nasal cavities to the olfactory bulbs of the brain, which lie on this plate (see Chapter 9).

Middle Cranial Fossa

The butterfly-shaped **middle cranial fossa** has a *central part* composed of the *sella turcica* on the body of the sphenoid and large, depressed *lateral parts* on each side. The middle cranial fossa is posteroinferior to the anterior cranial fossa, separated from it by the sharp *sphenoidal crests* laterally and the *sphenoidal limbus* centrally. The **sphenoidal crests** are formed mostly by the sharp posterior borders of the *lesser wings of the sphenoid bones*, which overhang the lateral parts of the fossae anteriorly. The sphenoidal crests end medially in two sharp

bony projections, the *anterior clinoid processes*. A variably prominent ridge, the **sphenoid limbus** forms the anterior boundary of the transversely oriented **prechiasmatic sulcus** extending between the right and the left *optic canals*. The bones forming the lateral parts of the fossa are the greater wings of the sphenoid and squamous parts of the temporal bones laterally and the petrous parts of the temporal bones posteriorly (Fig. 7.5*C*; Table 7.2). The lateral parts of the middle cranial fossa support the temporal lobes of the brain. The boundary between the middle and the posterior cranial fossae is the **superior border of the petrous part of the temporal bone** laterally and a flat plate of bone, the *dorsum sellae of the sphenoid*, medially.

The **sella turcica** (L. Turkish saddle) is the saddle-like bony formation on the upper surface of the body of the sphenoid, which is surrounded by the **anterior** and **posterior clinoid processes** (Fig. 7.5*C*). *Clinoid* means "bedpost," and the four processes (two anterior and two posterior) surround the hypophysial fossa, the "bed" of the pituitary gland, like the posts of a four-poster bed. The sella turcica is composed of three parts:

1. The **tuberculum sellae** (horn of the saddle): a variable slight to prominent median elevation forming the posterior boundary of the *prechiasmatic sulcus* and the anterior boundary of the hypophysial fossa.

2. The **hypophysial fossa** (pituitary fossa): a median depression (seat of the saddle) in the body of the sphenoid that accommodates the *pituitary gland* (L. *hypophysis*).

3. The **dorsum sellae** (back of the saddle): a square plate of bone projecting superiorly from the body of the sphenoid. It forms the posterior boundary of the sella turcica, and its prominent superolateral angles make up the **posterior clinoid processes**.

On each side of the body of the sphenoid a *crescent of four foramina* perforate the roots of the greater wings of the sphenoids (Fig. 7.5*C*; Table 7.2):

1. **Superior orbital fissure:** Located between the greater and lesser wings, it communicates with the orbit and transmits the ophthalmic veins and nerves (CN III, CN IV, CN V$_1$, CN VI, and sympathetic fibers) entering the orbit.

2. **Foramen rotundum** (round foramen): Located posterior to the medial end of the superior orbital fissure, it transmits the maxillary nerve (CN V$_2$) that supplies the skin, teeth, and mucosa related to the maxilla (i.e., lining the upper jaw and maxillary sinus).

3. **Foramen ovale** (oval foramen): A large foramen posterolateral to the foramen rotundum, it opens inferiorly into the infratemporal fossa and transmits the mandibular nerve (CN V$_3$) and a small accessory meningeal artery.

Table 7.2. Foramina and Other Apertures of the Cranial Fossae and Contents

Foramina/Apertures	Contents
Anterior cranial fossa	
Foramen cecum	Nasal emissary vein (1% of population)
Cribriform foramina in cribriform plate	Axons of olfactory cells in olfactory epithelium that form olfactory nerves
Anterior and posterior ethmoidal foramina	Vessels and nerves with same names
Middle cranial fossa	
Optic canals	Optic nerves (CN II) and ophthalmic arteries
Superior orbital fissure	Ophthalmic veins; ophthalmic nerve (CN V_1); CN III, IV, and VI; and sympathetic fibers
Foramen rotundum	Maxillary nerve (CN V_2)
Foramen ovale	Mandibular nerve (CN V_3) and accessory meningeal artery
Foramen spinosum	Middle meningeal artery and vein and meningeal branch of CN V_3
Foramen lacerum[a]	Internal carotid artery and its accompanying sympathetic and venous plexuses[a]
Groove or hiatus of greater petrosal nerve	Greater petrosal nerve and petrosal branch of middle meningeal artery
Posterior cranial fossa	
Foramen magnum	Medulla and meninges, vertebral arteries, CN XI, dural veins, anterior and posterior spinal arteries
Jugular foramen	CN IX, X, and XI; superior bulb of internal jugular vein; inferior petrosal and sigmoid sinuses; and meningeal branches of ascending pharyngeal and occipital arteries
Hypoglossal canal	Hypoglossal nerve (CN XII)
Condylar canal	Emissary vein that passes from sigmoid sinus to vertebral veins in neck
Mastoid foramen	Mastoid emissary vein from sigmoid sinus and meningeal branch of occipital artery

[a]Structures actually pass horizontally *across* (rather than vertically through) the area of the foramen lacerum, an artifact of dry skulls, which is closed by cartilage in life.

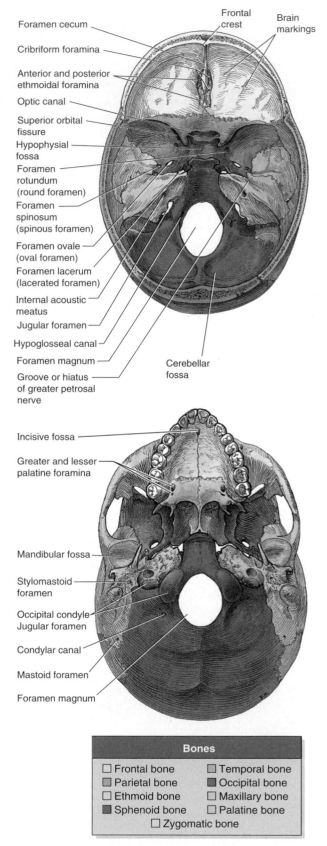

Frontal crest
Brain markings
Foramen cecum
Cribriform foramina
Anterior and posterior ethmoidal foramina
Optic canal
Superior orbital fissure
Hypophysial fossa
Foramen rotundum (round foramen)
Foramen spinosum (spinous foramen)
Foramen ovale (oval foramen)
Foramen lacerum (lacerated foramen)
Internal acoustic meatus
Jugular foramen
Hypoglosseal canal
Foramen magnum
Groove or hiatus of greater petrosal nerve
Cerebellar fossa

Incisive fossa
Greater and lesser palatine foramina
Mandibular fossa
Stylomastoid foramen
Occipital condyle
Jugular foramen
Condylar canal
Mastoid foramen
Foramen magnum

Bones	
☐ Frontal bone	☐ Temporal bone
☐ Parietal bone	☐ Occipital bone
☐ Ethmoid bone	☐ Maxillary bone
☐ Sphenoid bone	☐ Palatine bone
☐ Zygomatic bone	

4. **Foramen spinosum** (spinous foramen): Located posterolateral to the foramen ovale, it transmits the middle meningeal vessels and the meningeal branch of the mandibular nerve.

The **foramen lacerum** (lacerated or torn foramen) is not part of the crescent of foramina. This ragged foramen lies posterolateral to the hypophysial fossa and is an artifact of a dried cranium. In life, it is closed by a cartilage plate. Only some meningeal arterial branches and small veins are transmitted vertically through the cartilage, completely traversing this foramen. The internal carotid artery and its accompanying sympathetic and venous plexuses pass across the superior aspect of the cartilage (i.e., pass over the foramen), and some nerves traverse it horizontally, passing to a foramen in its anterior boundary. Extending posteriorly and laterally from the foramen lacerum is a narrow **groove for the greater petrosal nerve** on the anterosuperior surface of the petrous part of the temporal bone. There is also a small groove for the lesser petrosal nerve.

Posterior Cranial Fossa

The **posterior cranial fossa**, the largest and deepest of the three cranial fossae, lodges the cerebellum, pons, and medulla oblongata (Fig. 7.5C & D). The posterior cranial fossa is formed mostly by the occipital bone, but the *dorsum sellae of the sphenoid* marks its anterior boundary centrally and the petrous and mastoid parts of the temporal bones contribute its anterolateral "walls" (Fig. 7.5C; Table 7.2). From the dorsum sellae there is a marked incline, the **clivus**, in the center of the anterior part of the fossa leading to the *foramen magnum*. Posterior to this large opening, the posterior cranial fossa is partly divided by the **internal occipital crest** into bilateral large concave impressions, the **cerebellar fossae**. The internal occipital crest ends in the **internal occipital protuberance** formed in relationship to the *confluence of the sinuses*, a merging of dural venous sinuses (discussed later in this chapter). Broad grooves show the horizontal course of the *transverse sinus* and the S-shaped *sigmoid sinus*. At the base of the petrous ridge of the temporal bone is the *jugular foramen*, which transmits several cranial nerves in addition to the sigmoid sinus that exits the cranium as the IJV. Anterosuperior to the jugular foramen is the *internal acoustic meatus* for the facial and vestibulocochlear nerves (CN VIII) and the labyrinthine artery. The **hypoglossal canal** for the hypoglossal nerve (CN XII) is superior to the anterolateral margin of the foramen magnum.

Walls of the Cranial Cavity

The **walls of the cranial cavity** vary in thickness in different regions. They are usually thinner in females than in males and are thinner in children and elderly people. The bones tend to be thinnest in areas that are well covered with muscles, such as the squamous part of the temporal bone (Fig. 7.2B). Thin areas of bone can be seen by holding a dried cranium up to a bright light. Most bones of the calvaria consist of **internal** and

external tables of compact bone, separated by **diploë** (Fig. 7.5C). The diploë is cancellous bone containing red bone marrow during life, through which run canals formed by diploic veins. The diploë in a dried calvaria is not red because the protein was removed during preparation of the cranium. The internal table of bone is thinner than the external table and in some areas there is only a thin plate of compact bone with no diploë.

The bony substance of the cranium is unequally distributed. Relatively thin (but mostly curved) flat bones provide the necessary strength to maintain cavities and protect their contents. However, in addition to housing the brain, the bones of the neurocranium (and processes from them) provide proximal attachment for the strong muscles of mastication that attach distally to the mandible; consequently, high traction forces occur across the nasal cavity and orbits that are sandwiched between. Thus thickened portions of the cranial bones form stronger pillars or buttresses that transmit forces, bypassing the orbits and nasal cavity. The main buttresses are the **frontonasal buttress,** extending from the region of the canine teeth between the nasal and the orbital cavities to the central frontal bone, and the *zygomatic arch*–**lateral orbital margin buttress** from the region of the molars to the lateral frontal and temporal bones (Fig. 7.6). Similar buttresses transmit forces received lateral to the foramen magnum from the vertebral column. Perhaps to compensate for the denser bone required for these buttresses, some areas of the cranium not as mechanically stressed become pneumatized ("air filled").

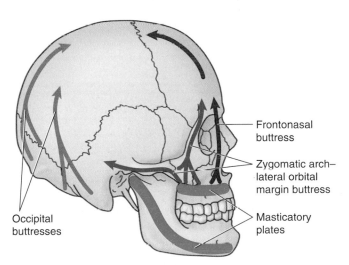

Lateral aspect

Figure 7.6. Buttresses of cranium. The strong muscles of mastication extending between the neurocranium and mandible produce high traction forces across the nasal cavity and orbits. Thickened portions of the bones of the cranium form stronger pillars or buttresses that transmit forces, bypassing the orbits and nasal cavity. Occipital buttresses transmit forces received lateral to the foramen magnum from the vertebral column.

Development of the Cranium

The bones of the calvaria and some parts of the cranial base develop by *intramembranous ossification;* most parts of the cranial base develop by *endochondral ossification.* At birth, the bones of the calvaria are smooth and unilaminar; no diploë is present. The frontal and parietal eminences are especially prominent (Fig. B7.6). The cranium of a newborn infant is disproportionately large compared to other parts of the skeleton; however, the facial aspect is small compared to the calvaria, which forms approximately one eighth of the cranium. In the adult, the facial skeleton forms one third of the cranium. The large size of the cal-

varia in infants results from precocious growth and development of the brain and eyes. The rudimentary development of the face makes the orbits appear relatively large (Fig. B7.6A). The smallness of the face results from the rudimentary development of the maxillae, mandible, and paranasal sinuses (air-filled bone cavities), the absence of erupted teeth, and the small size of the nasal cavities.

The halves of the frontal bone in the newborn are separated by the *frontal suture,* the frontal and parietal bones are separated by the *coronal suture,* and the maxillae and mandibles are separated by the *intermaxillary suture* and *mandibular symphysis* (secondary cartilaginous joint), respectively. There are no mastoid and styloid processes ▶

Figure B7.6. Cranial development. A and B. Anterior and lateral aspects of an infant's cranium are shown. **C.** This anterosuperior view shows a persistent frontal suture.

(Fig. B7.6*B*). Because there are no mastoid processes at birth, the facial nerves are close to the surface when they emerge from the stylomastoid foramina. As a result, the facial nerves may be injured by forceps during a difficult delivery or later by an incision posterior to the auricle of the external ear (as for the surgical treatment of mastoiditis or middle ear problems). The mastoid processes form gradually during the 1st year as the sternocleidomastoid muscles complete their development and pull on the petromastoid parts of the temporal bones.

The bones of the calvaria of a newborn infant are separated by membranous intervals; the largest occur between the angles (corners) of the flat bones (Fig. B7.6*A* & *B*). They include the *anterior* and *posterior fontanelles* and the paired *sphenoidal* and *mastoid fontanelles*. Palpation of the fontanelles during infancy, especially the anterior and posterior ones, enables physicians to determine the:

- Progress of growth of the frontal and parietal bones.

- Degree of hydration of an infant (a depressed fontanelle indicates dehydration).

- Level of intracranial pressure (a bulging fontanelle indicates increased pressure on the brain).

The **anterior fontanelle,** the largest one, is diamond or star shaped; it is bounded by the halves of the frontal bone anteriorly and the parietal bones posteriorly. Thus it is located at the junction of the sagittal, coronal, and frontal sutures, the future site of the *bregma* (Table 7.1). By 18 months of age, the surrounding bones have fused and the anterior fontanelle is no longer clinically palpable. Union of the halves of the frontal bone begins in the 2nd year. In most cases, the *frontal suture* is obliterated by the 8th year. However, in approximately 8% of people, a remnant of it, the **metopic suture,** persists (Fig. 7.1*D*); and much less frequently, the entire suture remains (Fig. B7.6*C*). A persistent suture must not be interpreted as a fracture in a radiograph or other medical image.

The **posterior fontanelle** is triangular and bounded by the parietal bones anteriorly and the occipital bone posteriorly. It is located at the junction of the lambdoid and sagittal sutures, the future site of *lambda* (Fig. 7.3*A* and 7.4*C*). The posterior fontanelle begins to close during the first few months after birth; and by the end of the 1st year, it is small and no longer clinically palpable.

The **sphenoidal** and **mastoid fontanelles,** overlain by the temporal (L. *temporalis*) muscle, fuse during infancy and are less important clinically than the midline fontanelles. The halves of the mandible fuse early in the 2nd year. The two maxillae and nasal bones usually do not fuse.

The softness of the cranial bones in infants and their loose connections at the sutures and fontanelles enable the shape of the calvaria to change (*mold*) during birth

Figure B7.7. Molding of calvaria.

(Fig. B7.7). During passage of the fetus through the birth canal, the halves of the frontal bone become flat, the occipital bone is drawn out, and one parietal bone slightly overrides the other. Within a few days after birth, the shape of the calvaria returns to normal. The resilience of the cranial bones of infants allows them to resist forces that would produce fractures in adults. The fibrous sutures of the calvaria also permit the cranium to enlarge during infancy and childhood. The increase in the size of the calvaria is greatest during the first 2 years, the period of most rapid brain development. The calvaria normally increases in capacity for 15–16 years. After this, the calvaria usually increases slightly in size for 3–4 years as a result of bone thickening.

Age Changes in the Face

The mandible is the most dynamic of our bones; its size and shape and the number of teeth it normally bears undergo considerable change with age. In the newborn, the mandible consists of two halves united in the median plane by a cartilaginous joint, the *mandibular symphysis*. Union between the halves of the mandible is effected by means of fibrocartilage; this union begins during the 1st year and the halves are fused by the end of the 2nd year.

The body of the mandible in newborn infants is a mere shell lacking an alveolar process, each half enclosing five deciduous (primary) teeth. These teeth usually begin to erupt in infants at approximately 6 months of age. The body of the mandible elongates, particularly posterior to the mental foramen, to accommodate this development and later eight permanent (secondary) teeth, which ▶

Figure B7.8. Left lateral view of dentition. *Arrows,* unerupted secondary teeth.

begin to erupt during the 6th year of life (Fig. B7.8). Eruption of the permanent teeth is not complete until early adulthood. Rapid growth of the face during infancy and early childhood coincides with the eruption of deciduous teeth. Vertical growth of the upper face results mainly from dentoalveolar development. These changes are more marked after the permanent teeth erupt.

Concurrent enlargement of the frontal and facial regions is associated with the increase in the size of the *paranasal sinuses,* the air-filled extensions of the nasal cavities in certain cranial bones (Fig. B7.9). Most paranasal si-

nuses are rudimentary or absent at birth. Growth of the paranasal sinuses is important in altering the shape of the face and in adding resonance to the voice.

Obliteration of the Cranial Sutures

The obliteration of sutures between the bones of the calvaria usually begins between the ages of 30 and 40 years on the internal surface and approximately 10 years later on the external surface (Fig. B7.10; compare with Fig. 7.4A). Obliteration of sutures usually begins at the bregma and continues sequentially in the sagittal, coronal, and lambdoid sutures.

Age Changes in the Cranium

As people age, the cranial bones normally become progressively thinner and lighter, and the diploë gradually become filled with a gray gelatinous material. In these individuals, the bone marrow has lost its blood cells and fat, giving it a gelatinous appearance.

Craniosynostosis and Cranial Malformations

Premature closure of the cranial sutures (*primary craniosynostosis*) results in several cranial malformations (Fig. B7.11). The incidence of primary craniosynostosis is approximately 1 per 2000 births (Behrman et al., 2004). The cause of craniosynostosis is unknown, but genetic factors appear to be important. The prevailing hypothesis is that abnormal development of the cranial base creates ▶

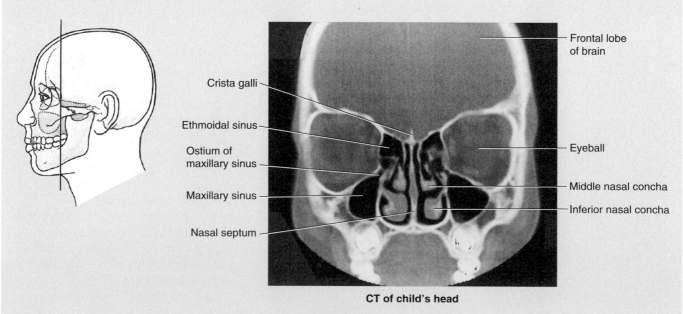

Crista galli

Ethmoidal sinus

Ostium of maxillary sinus

Maxillary sinus

Nasal septum

Frontal lobe of brain

Eyeball

Middle nasal concha

Inferior nasal concha

CT of child's head

Figure B7.9

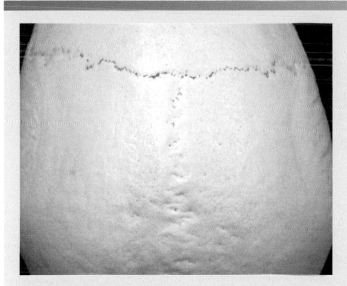

Figure B7.10. Obliteration (synostosis) of cranial sutures.

exaggerated forces on the *dura mater* (outer covering membrane of the brain) that disrupt normal cranial sutural development. These malformations are more common in males than in females and are often associated with other skeletal anomalies. The type of malformed cranium that forms depends on which sutures close prematurely.

Premature closure of the sagittal suture, in which the anterior fontanelle is small or absent, results in a long, narrow, wedge-shaped cranium, a condition called *scaphocephaly* (Fig. B7.11*A*). When *premature closure of the coronal or the lambdoid suture* occurs on one side only, the cranium is twisted and asymmetrical, a condition known as *plagio-*

cephaly (Fig. B7.11*B*). *Premature closure of the coronal suture* results in a high, tower-like cranium, called *oxycephaly* or *turricephaly* (Fig. B7.11*C*). The latter type of cranial malformation is more common in females. Premature closure of sutures usually does not affect brain development. ●

(A)

(B)   (C)

Figure B7.11. Scaphocephaly (A), plagiocephaly (B), and oxycephaly (C).

THE BOTTOM LINE: The cranium is the skeleton of the head, an amalgamation of functional components united to form a single skeletal formation. The basic functional components include the neurocranium, the container of the brain and internal ears, and viscerocranium, providing paired orbits, nasal cavities and teeth-bearing plates (alveolar processes) of the oral cavity. Although some mobility between cranial bones is advantageous during birth, they become fixed together by essentially immovable joints (sutures), allowing independent movement of only the mandible. Abundant fissures and foramina facilitate communication and passage of neurovascular structures between functional components. The bony substance of the cranium is unequally distributed. Relatively thin (but mostly curved) flat bones provide the necessary strength to maintain cavities and protect contents. However, the bones and processes of the neurocranium also provide proximal attachment for the strong muscles of mastication that attach

distally to the mandible. The high traction forces generated across the nasal cavity and orbits sandwiched between the muscle attachments are resisted by thickened portions of the bones forming stronger pillars or buttresses.

The mostly superficial surface of the cranium provides both visible and palpable landmarks. Internal features of the cranial base reflect the major formations of the brain that rest on it. Bony ridges radiating from the centrally located sella turcica or hypophysial fossa divide it into three cranial fossae. The frontal lobes of the brain lie in the anterior cranial fossa. The temporal lobes lie in the middle cranial fossa. The hindbrain, consisting of the pons, cerebellum, and medulla, occupies the posterior cranial fossa, with the medulla continuing through the foramen magnum where it is continuous with the spinal cord.

The complex construction of the cranium can be observed radiographically, facilitating the diagnosis of pathology and trauma involving the head.

Structure of the Scalp

The **scalp** consists of skin (normally hair bearing) and subcutaneous tissue, which cover the neurocranium, from the superior nuchal lines on the occipital bone to the supraorbital margins of the frontal bone. Laterally, the scalp extends over the temporal fascia to the zygomatic arches. The discussion of the scalp has been divided into two parts. Because the scalp must be reflected or removed to enter the cranial cavity and because the layered pattern evident in the scalp continues deeply with the laminae of the cranium and the meninges, the structure of the scalp is presented before that of the cranial meninges and brain. The neurovascular structures of the scalp will be discussed with those of the face, to which they are most directly related.

The scalp is composed of five layers, the first three of which are connected intimately and move as a unit (e.g., when wrinkling the forehead and moving the scalp). Each letter in the word *scalp* serves as a memory key for one of its five layers (Fig. 7.7*A*):

1. Skin: thin, except in the occipital region, containing many sweat and sebaceous glands and hair follicles. It has an abundant arterial supply and good venous and lymphatic drainage.

2. Connective tissue: forms the thick, dense, richly vascularized subcutaneous layer that is well supplied with cutaneous nerves.

3. Aponeurosis (**epicranial aponeurosis**): the broad, strong, tendinous sheet that covers the calvaria and serves as the attachment for muscle bellies converging from the forehead and occiput (the **occipitofrontalis muscle**) (Fig. 7.7*B*) and from the temporal bones on each side (the **temporoparietalis** and **superior auricular muscles**). Collectively, these structures constitute the musculoaponeurotic **epicranius.** The frontal belly of the occipitofrontalis pulls the scalp anteriorly, wrinkles the forehead, and elevates the eyebrows; the occipital belly of the occipitofrontalis pulls the scalp posteriorly, smoothing the skin of the forehead. The superior auricular muscle (actually a specialized posterior part of the temporoparietalis) elevates the auricle of the external ear. All parts of the epicranius are innervated by the facial nerve.

4. Loose areolar tissue: a sponge-like layer including potential spaces that may distend with fluid as a result of injury or infection. This layer allows free movement of the **scalp proper** (the first three layers—skin, connective tissue, and epicranial aponeurosis) over the underlying calvaria.

5. Pericranium: a dense layer of connective tissue that forms the external periosteum of the neurocranium. It is firmly attached but can be stripped fairly easily from the crania of living persons, except where the pericranium is continuous with the fibrous tissue in the cranial sutures.

Scalp Wounds

The epicranial aponeurosis is clinically important. Because of the strength of this aponeurosis, *superficial scalp wounds* do not gape and the margins of the wound are held together. Furthermore, deep sutures are not necessary when suturing superficial wounds because the epicranial aponeurosis does not allow wide separation of the skin. *Deep scalp wounds* gape widely when the epicranial aponeurosis is lacerated in the coronal plane because of the pull of the frontal and occipital bellies of the occipitofrontalis muscle in opposite directions (anteriorly and posteriorly).

Scalp Infections

The loose connective tissue layer (layer four) of the scalp is the *danger area of the scalp* because pus or blood spreads easily in it. Infection in this layer can also pass into the cranial cavity through *emissary veins,* which pass through parietal foramina in the calvaria, and reach intracranial structures such as the meninges (Fig. 7.4*C*). An infection cannot pass into the neck because the occipital bellies of the occipitofrontalis muscle attach to the occipital bone and mastoid parts of the temporal bones. Neither can a scalp infection spread laterally beyond the zygomatic arches because the epicranial aponeurosis is continuous with the temporal fascia that attaches to these arches. An infection or fluid (e.g., pus or blood) can enter the eyelids and the root of the nose because the frontalis inserts into the skin and subcutaneous tissue and does not attach to the bone. Consequently, "black eyes" can result from an injury to the scalp and/or the forehead (Fig. B7.12). *Ecchymosis,* or purple patches, develop as a result of extravasation of blood into the subcutaneous tissue and skin of the eyelids and surrounding regions.

Sebaceous Cysts

The ducts of sebaceous glands associated with hair follicles in the scalp may become obstructed, resulting in the retention of secretions and the formation of *sebaceous cysts* (wens). Because they are in the skin, sebaceous cysts move with the scalp.

Cephalhematoma

Sometimes after a difficult birth, bleeding occurs between the baby's pericranium and calvaria, usually over one parietal bone. Blood becomes trapped in this area, causing a *cephalhematoma.* This benign condition frequently results from birth trauma that ruptures multiple, minute periosteal arteries that nourish the bones of the calvaria. ▶

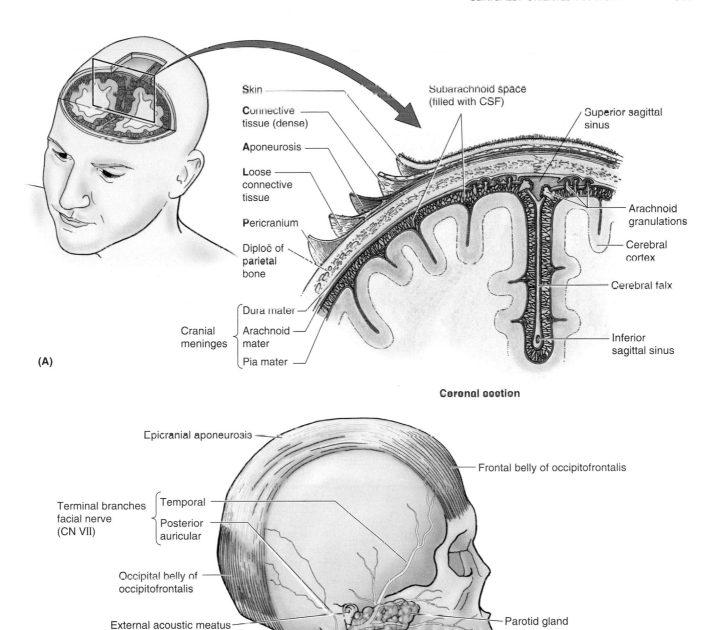

(A)

Skin

Connective tissue (dense)

Aponeurosis

Loose connective tissue

Pericranium

Diploë of parietal bone

Cranial meninges { Dura mater
Arachnoid mater
Pia mater

Subarachnoid space (filled with CSF)

Superior sagittal sinus

Arachnoid granulations

Cerebral cortex

Cerebral falx

Inferior sagittal sinus

Coronal section

(B) Lateral view

Epicranial aponeurosis

Frontal belly of occipitofrontalis

Terminal branches facial nerve (CN VII) { Temporal
Posterior auricular

Occipital belly of occipitofrontalis

External acoustic meatus

Parotid gland

Figure 7.7. Layers of scalp, cranium, and meninges. A. The skin is bound tightly to the epicranial aponeurosis, which moves freely over the pericranium and cranium because of the intervening loose connective tissue. The aponeurosis is the flat intermediate tendon of the occipitofrontalis muscle. The cranial meninges and the subarachnoid (leptomeningeal) space are shown. *CSF,* cerebrospinal fluid. **B.** The occipitofrontalis muscle, including its occipital and frontal bellies, and the epicranial aponeurosis. Innervation of the two bellies by the posterior auricular and temporal branches of the facial nerve is also demonstrated.

Figure B7.12. Ecchymosis.

Bone Flaps

Because the adult pericranium has poor osteogenic (bone-forming) properties, little regeneration occurs after bone loss (e.g., when pieces of bone are removed during repair of a comminuted cranial fracture). *Surgically produced bone flaps* are put back into place and wired to other parts of the calvaria. ✪

THE BOTTOM LINE: The scalp is the somewhat mobile soft tissue mantle covering the calvaria. The primary subcutaneous component of the scalp is the musculoaponeurotic epicranius to which the overlying skin is firmly attached but is separated from the outer periosteum (pericranium) of the cranium by loose areolar tissue. The areolar layer enables the mobility of the scalp over the calvaria and permits traumatic separation of the scalp from the cranium. Attachment of the skin to the epicranial aponeurosis keeps the edges of superficial wounds together, but a wound that also penetrates the epicranial aponeurosis gaps widely. Blood may collect in the areolar space deep to the aponeurosis after a head injury.

Cranial Meninges

The **cranial meninges** are coverings of the brain that lie immediately internal to the cranium (Figs. 7.7*A* and 7.8). The cranial meninges:

- Protect the brain.

- Form the supporting framework for arteries, veins, and venous sinuses.

- Enclose a fluid-filled cavity, the subarachnoid space, which is vital to the normal function of the brain.

The meninges are composed of three membranous connective tissue layers:

1. *Dura mater (dura):* tough, thick external fibrous layer.

2. *Arachnoid mater (arachnoid):* thin intermediate layer.

3. *Pia mater (pia):* delicate internal vasculated layer.

The intermediate and internal layers (arachnoid and pia) are continuous membranes that collectively make up the **leptomeninx** (G. slender membrane). The arachnoid is separated from the pia by the **subarachnoid (leptomeningeal) space,** which contains **cerebrospinal fluid** (CSF). This fluid-filled space helps maintain the balance of extracellular fluid in the brain. CSF is a clear liquid similar to blood in constitution; it provides nutrients but has less protein and a different ion concentration. CSF is formed by the *choroid plexuses* of the four ventricles of the brain (Fig. 7.8). This fluid leaves the ventricular system and enters the subarachnoid space between the arachnoid and the pia mater, where it cushions and nourishes the brain.

Dura Mater

The **dura mater,** a bilaminar membrane, is also called the **pachymeninx** (G. *pachy,* thick + G. *menix,* membrane) (Figs. 7.8 and 7.9). It is adherent to the internal table of the calvaria. The two layers of the cranial dura mater are an *external periosteal layer,* formed by the periosteum covering the internal surface of the calvaria, and an *internal meningeal layer,* a strong fibrous membrane that is continuous at the foramen magnum with the spinal dura mater covering the spinal cord.

The external **periosteal layer of the dura mater** adheres to the internal surface of the cranium; its attachment is tenacious along the suture lines and in the cranial base (Haines, 2002). The external periosteal layer is continuous at the cranial foramina with the periosteum on the external surface of the calvaria (Fig. 7.8*C*). This outer layer is not continuous with the dura mater of the spinal cord, which consists of only a meningeal layer. Except where the dural sinuses and infoldings occur (Fig. 7.8*B*), the internal meningeal layer is intimately fused with the periosteal layer and cannot be separated from it (Fig. 7.8*B* & *C*). The fused external and internal layers of dura over the calvaria can be easily stripped from the cranial bones (e.g., when the calvaria is removed at autopsy). In the cranial base, the two dural layers are firmly attached and difficult to separate from the bones. In life, such separation at the dural–cranial interface occurs only pathologically, creating an actual (blood- or fluid-filled) epidural space.

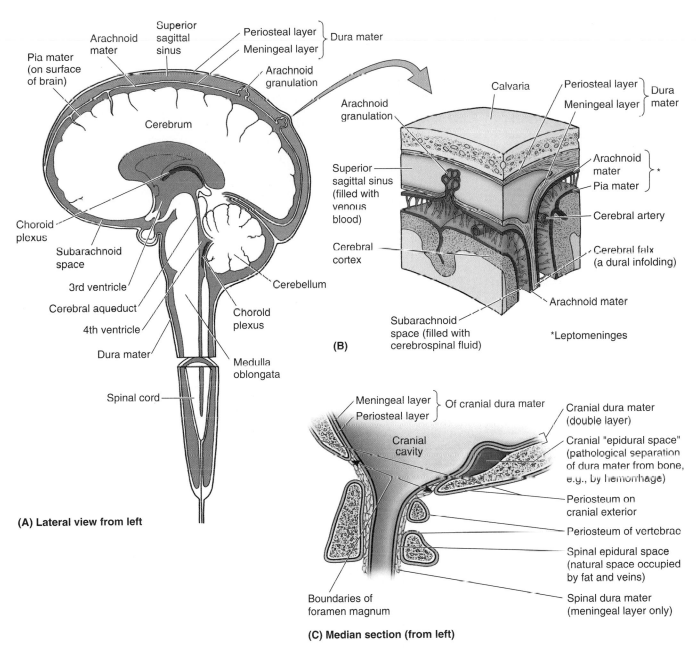

(A) Lateral view from left

(B)

*Leptomeninges

(C) Median section (from left)

Figure 7.8. Meninges and their relationship to calvaria, brain, and spinal cord. A. The dura mater and subarachnoid space (*purple*) surround the brain and are continuous with that around the spinal cord. **B.** The two layers of dura separate to form dural venous sinuses, such as the superior sagittal sinus. Arachnoid granulations protrude through the meningeal layer of the dura into the dural venous sinuses and effect transfer of cerebrospinal fluid to the venous system. **C.** The normal fat- and vein-filled spinal epidural (extradural) space is not continuous with the potential or pathological cranial epidural space. Cranial dura mater has two layers, whereas spinal dura mater consists of a single layer.

Dural Infoldings or Reflections

The internal **meningeal layer of dura mater** is a sustentacular (supporting) layer that reflects away from the external periosteal layer of dura to form dural infoldings (reflections) (Figs. 7.8*B* and 7.10). The dural infoldings divide the cranial cavity into compartments, forming partial partitions (dural septa) between certain parts of the brain and providing

support for other parts. The dural infoldings include the:

- Cerebral falx (L. *falx cerebri*).
- Cerebellar tentorium (L. *tentorium cerebelli*).
- Cerebellar falx (L. *falx cerebelli*).
- Sellar diaphragm (L. *diaphragma sellae*).

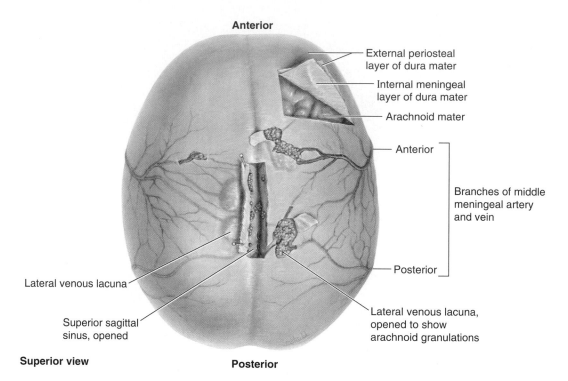

Figure 7.9. External surface of dura mater and arachnoid granulations. The calvaria is removed. In the median plane, a part of the thick roof of the superior sagittal sinus has been incised and retracted; laterally, parts of the thin roof of two lateral lacunae are reflected to demonstrate the abundant arachnoid granulations, which are responsible for absorption of CSF. On the right, an angular flap of dura is turned anteriorly; the convolutions of the cerebral cortex are visible through the arachnoid mater.

Figure 7.10. Dural infoldings and dural venous sinuses. The left side of the bisected head is shown. **A.** The two sickle-shaped dural folds (septae), the cerebral falx and cerebellar falx, are vertically oriented in the median plane. The two roof-like folds, the cerebellar tentorium and the small sellar diaphragm, lie horizontally. The left members of the paired arteries that supply the brain, the internal carotid and vertebral arteries, are shown.

Figure 7.10. *(Continued)* **B.** Venous sinuses of the dura mater and their communications are demonstrated. Cavernous sinuses lie on each side of the body of the sphenoid. These sinuses communicate anteriorly with the facial vein through the superior and inferior ophthalmic veins. The cavernous sinus also communicate inferiorly with the pterygoid venous plexus and posteriorly with the basilar plexus, which in turn communicates with the internal vertebral venous plexus.

The **cerebral falx** (L. *falx,* a sickle-shaped structure), the largest dural infolding, lies in the **longitudinal cerebral fissure** that separates the right and left *cerebral hemispheres.* The cerebral falx attaches in the median plane to the internal surface of the calvaria, from the *frontal crest* of the frontal bone and crista galli of the ethmoid bone anteriorly to the *internal occipital protuberance* posteriorly (Figs. 7.10A and 7.11). It ends by becoming continuous with the cerebellar tentorium.

The **cerebellar tentorium,** the second largest dural infolding, is a wide crescentic septum that separates the occipital lobes of the cerebral hemispheres from the cerebellum. The cerebellar tentorium attaches rostrally to the clinoid processes of the sphenoid, rostrolaterally to the petrous part of the temporal bone, and posterolaterally to the internal surface of the occipital bone and part of the parietal bone. The cerebral falx attaches to the cerebellar tentorium and holds it up, giving it a tent-like appearance (L. *tentorium,* tent). The cerebellar tentorium divides the cranial cavity into *supratentorial* and *infratentorial compartments.* The supratentorial compartment is divided into right and left halves by the cerebral falx. The concave anteromedial border of the cerebellar tentorium is free, producing a gap called the **tentorial notch** through which the brainstem (midbrain, pons, and medulla oblon-

gata) extends from the posterior into the middle cranial fossa (Fig. 7.12A & B).

The **cerebellar falx** is a vertical dural infolding that lies inferior to the cerebellar tentorium in the posterior part of the posterior cranial fossa (Figs. 7.10A & B and 7.11). It is attached to the internal occipital crest and partially separates the cerebellar hemispheres.

The **sellar diaphragm,** the smallest dural infolding, is a circular sheet of dura that is suspended between the clinoid processes forming a partial roof over the hypophysial fossa in the sphenoid (Fig. 7.10A). The sellar diaphragm covers the pituitary gland in this fossa and has an aperture for passage of the infundibulum and hypophysial veins.

Blunt Trauma to the Head

A blow to the head can detach the periosteal layer of dura mater from the calvaria without fracturing the cranial bones. In the cranial base the two dural layers are firmly attached and difficult to separate from the bones. Consequently, a fracture of the cranial base usually tears the ▶

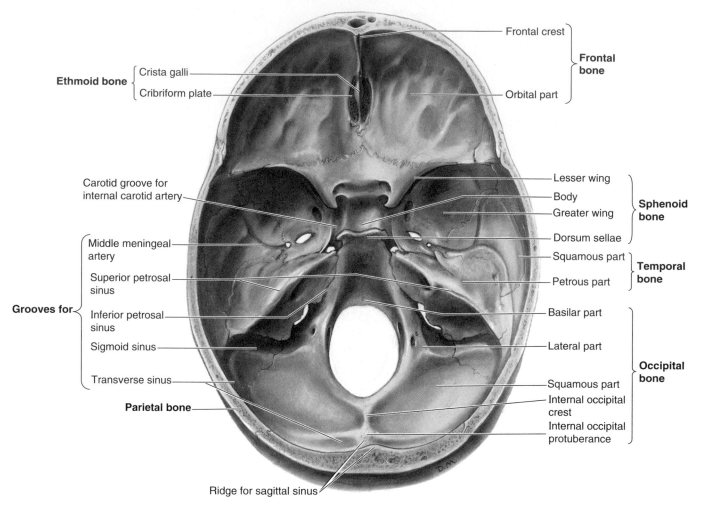

Ethmoid bone {
Crista galli
Cribriform plate

Frontal crest
Frontal bone

Orbital part

Carotid groove for internal carotid artery

Lesser wing
Body
Greater wing
Sphenoid bone

Dorsum sellae

Grooves for {
Middle meningeal artery
Superior petrosal sinus
Inferior petrosal sinus
Sigmoid sinus
Transverse sinus

Squamous part
Temporal bone
Petrous part

Basilar part

Lateral part
Occipital bone

Squamous part

Internal occipital crest
Internal occipital protuberance

Parietal bone

Ridge for sagittal sinus

Superior view of internal surface of cranial base

Figure 7.11. Interior of base of cranium. The internal occipital protuberance is formed in relationship to the confluence of sinuses (Fig. 7.12*A*), and grooves are formed in the cranial base by the dural venous sinuses (e.g., the sigmoid sinus). The cerebellar tentorium is attached along the lengths of the transverse and superior petrosal sinuses.

dura and results in leakage of CSF. The innermost part of the dura, *the dural border cell layer,* is composed of flattened fibroblasts that are separated by large extracellular spaces. This layer constitutes a plane of structural weakness at the dura–arachnoid junction (Haines, 2002).

Tentorial Herniation

The tentorial notch is the opening in the cerebellar tentorium for the brainstem, which is slightly larger than is necessary to accommodate the midbrain. Hence *space-occupying lesions,* such as tumors in the supratentorial compartment, produce increased intracranial pressure and may cause part of the adjacent temporal lobe of the brain to herniate through the tentorial notch. During *tentorial herniation,* the temporal lobe may be lacerated by the tough cerebellar tentorium and the oculomotor nerve (CN III) may be stretched, compressed, or both. *Oculomotor lesions* may produce paralysis of the extrinsic eye muscles supplied by CN III.

Bulging of the Sellar Diaphragm

Pituitary tumors may extend superiorly through the aperture in the sellar diaphragm or cause it to bulge. These tumors often expand the sellar diaphragm, producing disturbances in endocrine function early or late (i.e., before or after enlargement of the sellar diaphragm). Superior extension of a tumor may cause visual symptoms owing to pressure on the optic chiasm (L. *chiasma opticum*), the place where the optic nerve fibers cross. ✛

(A) Superolateral view

Inferior sagittal sinus
Cavernous sinus
Superior sagittal sinus
Sigmoid sinus
Cerebral falx
Great cerebral vein
Intercavernous sinus
Transverse sinus
Infundibulum
Straight sinus
Supraorbital vein
Confluence of sinuses
Superior ophthalmic vein
Cerebellar tentorium
Edge of tentorial notch
Facial vein
Inferior petrosal sinus
Superior petrosal sinus
Inferior ophthalmic vein

(B) Superior view

Superior ophthalmic vein
Sphenoparietal sinus
Intercavernous sinus
Cavernous sinus
Site of section for **C**
Superior petrosal sinus
End of sigmoid sinus; beginning of internal jugular vein
Inferior petrosal sinus
Great cerebral vein
Sigmoid sinus
Tentorial notch
Straight sinus
Cerebellar tentorium
Superior sagittal sinus
Inferior sagittal sinus
Right transverse sinus

(C) Posterior view of coronal section of right cavernous sinus

Hypophysial fossa (pituitary fossa)
Ophthalmic artery
Optic canal
Anterior clinoid process
Oculomotor nerve
Cerebral | Parts of internal
Cavernous | carotid artery
Trochlear nerve
Abducent nerve
Ophthalmic nerve
Cavernous sinus
Sphenoidal sinus
Maxillary nerve
Body of sphenoid
*Intercavernous sinus

Figure 7.12. Venous sinuses of dura mater. Blood from the brain drains into the sinuses within the dura. **A.** The brain and part of the calvaria are removed to demonstrate the sinuses related to the cerebral falx and cerebellar tentorium. **B.** This view of the interior of the base of the cranium demonstrates the most communications of the cavernous sinuses (the interior communication with the pterygoid venous plexus is a notable exception) and drainage of the confluence of sinuses. The ophthalmic veins drain into the cavernous sinus. **C.** The orientation and placement of this section of the right cavernous sinus and the body of the sphenoid are indicated in parts **A** and **B**. The cavernous sinus is situated bilaterally at the lateral aspect of the hollow body of the sphenoid and the hypophysial fossa. The internal carotid artery, having made an acute bend, is cut twice. Inferiorly, the cavernous part of the artery is sectioned as it passes anteriorly along the carotid groove toward the acute bend of the artery (radiologists refer to the bend as the "carotid siphon"); superiorly, the cerebral part of the artery is sectioned as it passes posteriorly from the bend to join the cerebral arterial circle. The ophthalmic artery has just arisen from the latter.

Dural Venous Sinuses

The **dural venous sinuses** are endothelium-lined spaces between the periosteal and the meningeal layers of the dura. They form where the dural septa attach along the free edge of the falx cerebri and in relation to formations of the cranial floor (Figs. 7.10, 7.12, and 7.13). Large veins from the surface of the brain empty into these sinuses and most of the blood from the brain ultimately drains through them into the IJVs (Fig. 7.13).

The **superior sagittal sinus** lies in the convex attached border of the cerebral falx (Fig. 7.10). It begins at the crista galli and ends near the internal occipital protuberance (Fig. 7.11)

at the **confluence of sinuses,** a meeting place of the superior sagittal, straight, occipital, and transverse sinuses (Fig. 7.13). The superior sagittal sinus receives the superior cerebral veins and communicates on each side through slit-like openings with the **lateral venous lacunae,** lateral expansions of the superior sagittal sinus (Fig. 7.9).

Arachnoid granulations (collections of arachnoid villi) are tufted prolongations of the arachnoid that protrude through the meningeal layer of the dura mater into the dural venous sinuses, especially the lateral lacunae, and effect transfer of CSF to the venous system. Enlarged arachnoid

(A) Anteroposterior view   **(B) Lateral view**

Figure 7.13. Venograms of dural sinuses. A and B. Radiopaque dye injected into the arterial system has circulated through the capillaries of the brain and collected in the dural venous sinuses, as shown in these radiographic studies. *C*, confluence of sinuses; *I*, internal jugular vein; *S*, sigmoid sinus; *T*, transverse sinus. In the AP view (**A**), notice the left-sided dominance in the drainage of the confluence of sinuses. (Courtesy of Dr. D. Armstrong, Associate Professor of Medical Imaging, University of Toronto, Toronto, Ontario, Canada.)

granulations (often called *pacchionian bodies*) may erode bone, forming pits called **granular foveolae** in the calvaria (Fig. 7.4*B*). They are usually observed in the vicinity of the superior sagittal, transverse, and some other dural venous sinuses. Arachnoid granulations are structurally adapted for the transport of CSF from the subarachnoid space to the venous system (see "Subarachnoid Cisterns," later in this chapter).

The **inferior sagittal sinus** is much smaller than the superior sagittal sinus (Fig. 7.10). It runs in the inferior concave free border of the cerebral falx and ends in the straight sinus.

The **straight sinus** (L. *sinus rectus*) is formed by the union of the inferior sagittal sinus with the *great cerebral vein*. It runs inferoposteriorly along the line of attachment of the cerebral falx to the cerebellar tentorium, where it joins the confluence of sinuses.

The **transverse sinuses** pass laterally from the confluence of sinuses, forming a groove in the occipital bones and the posteroinferior angles of the parietal bones (Figs. 7.11–7.13). The transverse sinuses course along the posterolateral attached margins of the cerebellar tentorium and then become the sigmoid sinuses as they approach the posterior aspect of the petrous temporal bones. Blood received by the *confluence of sinuses* is drained by the transverse sinuses, but rarely equally. Usually the left sinus is dominant (larger).

The **sigmoid sinuses** follow S-shaped courses in the posterior cranial fossa, forming deep grooves in the temporal and occipital bones. Each sigmoid sinus turns anteriorly and then continues inferiorly as the IJV after traversing the jugular foramen.

The **occipital sinus** lies in the attached border of the cerebellar falx and ends superiorly in the confluence of sinuses (Fig. 7.10*B*). The occipital sinus communicates inferiorly with the internal vertebral venous plexus.

The **cavernous sinus** is located on each side of the sella turcica on the upper surface of the body of the sphenoid, which contains the sphenoid (air) sinus (Figs. 7.10*B* and 7.12). The cavernous sinus consists of a venous plexus of extremely thin-walled veins that extends from the superior orbital fissure anteriorly to the apex of the petrous part of the temporal bone posteriorly. It receives blood from the superior and inferior ophthalmic veins, superficial middle cerebral vein, and sphenoparietal sinus. The venous channels in these sinuses communicate with each other through venous channels anterior and posterior to the stalk of the pituitary gland—the **intercavernous sinuses** (Fig. 7.12*A* & *B*)—and sometimes through veins inferior to the pituitary gland. The cavernous sinuses drain posteroinferiorly through the superior and inferior petrosal sinuses and emissary veins to the *pterygoid plexuses* (Figs. 7.10*B* and 7.13*B*).

Inside each cavernous sinus is the **internal carotid artery** with its small branches, surrounded by the carotid plexus of sympathetic nerve(s), and the abducent nerve (CN VI) (Fig. 7.13*C*). The oculomotor (CN III) and trochlear (CN IV) nerves, plus two of the three divisions of the trigeminal nerve (CN V) are embedded in the lateral wall of the sinus. The artery, carrying warm blood from the body's core, traverses the sinus filled with cooler blood returning from the capillaries of the body's periphery, allowing for heat exchange to conserve energy or cool the arterial blood. This does not appear to be as important in humans as it is in running animals (e.g., horses and cheetahs) in which the carotid artery runs a longer, more tortuous course through the cavernous sinuses, allowing cooling of blood before it enters the brain. Pulsations of the artery within the cavernous sinus are said to promote propulsion of venous blood from the sinus, as does gravity (Williams et al., 1995).

The **superior petrosal sinuses** run from the posterior ends of the veins making up the cavernous sinus to the transverse sinuses at the site where these sinuses curve inferiorly to form the sigmoid sinuses (Fig. 7.13*B*). Each superior petrosal sinus lies in the anterolateral attached margin of the cerebellar tentorium, which attaches to the superior border (crest) of the petrous part of the temporal bone (Fig. 7.11).

The **inferior petrosal sinuses** also commence at the posterior end of the cavernous sinus inferiorly (Fig. 7.13*B*). Each inferior petrosal sinus runs in a groove between the petrous part of the temporal bone and the basilar part of the occipital bone (Fig. 7.12). The inferior petrosal sinuses

drain the veins of the lateral cavernous sinus directly into the origin of the IJVs.

The **basilar plexus** connects the inferior petrosal sinuses and communicates inferiorly with the internal vertebral venous plexus (Fig. 7.10*B*).

Emissary veins connect the dural venous sinuses with veins outside the cranium. Although they are valveless and blood may flow in both directions, flow in the emissary veins is usually away from the brain. The size and number of emissary veins vary; many small ones are unnamed. A **frontal emissary vein** is present in children and some adults. It passes through the foramen cecum of the cranium, connecting the superior sagittal sinus with veins of the frontal sinus and nasal cavities. A **parietal emissary vein**, which may be paired bilaterally, passes through the parietal foramen in the calvaria, connecting the superior sagittal sinus with the veins external to it, particularly those in the scalp (Fig. 7.4*C*). A **mastoid emissary vein** passes through the mastoid foramen and connects each sigmoid sinus with the occipital or posterior auricular vein (Fig. 7.14). A **posterior condylar emissary vein** may also be present, passing through the condylar canal, connecting the sigmoid sinus with the suboccipital plexus of veins.

Occlusion of Cerebral Veins and Dural Venous Sinuses

Occlusion of cerebral veins and dural venous sinuses may result from thrombi (clots), thrombophlebitis (venous inflammation), or tumors (e.g., meningiomas). The dural sinuses most frequently thrombosed are the transverse, cavernous, and superior sagittal sinuses (Fishman, 2000a).

The facial veins make clinically important connections with the cavernous sinus through the superior ophthalmic veins (Fig. 7.10*B*). *Cavernous sinus thrombosis* usually results from infections in the orbit, nasal sinuses, and superior part of the face (the danger triangle). In persons with *thrombophlebitis of the facial vein*, pieces of an infected thrombus may extend into the cavernous sinus, producing *thrombophlebitis of the cavernous sinus*. The infection usually involves only one sinus initially but may spread to the opposite side through the intercavernous sinuses. Thrombophlebitis of the cavernous sinus may affect the abducent nerve as it traverses the sinus (see Chapter 9) and may also effect the nerves embedded within the lateral wall of the sinus (Fig. 7.12*C*). Septic thrombosis of the cavernous sinus often results in the development of *acute meningitis*.

Metastasis of Tumor Cells to the Dural Sinuses

The basilar and occipital sinuses communicate through the foramen magnum with the internal vertebral venous plexuses (Fig. 7.10*B*). Because these venous channels are valveless, compression of the thorax, abdomen, or pelvis, as occurs during heavy coughing and straining, may force venous blood from these regions into the internal vertebral venous system and from it into the dural venous sinuses. As a result, pus in abscesses and tumor cells in these regions may spread to the vertebrae and brain.

Fractures of the Cranial Base

In fractures of the cranial base, the internal carotid artery may be torn, producing an *arteriovenous fistula* within the sinus. Arterial blood rushes into the cavernous sinus, enlarging it and forcing retrograde blood flow into its venous tributaries, especially the ophthalmic veins. As a result, the eyeball protrudes (*exophthalmos*) and the conjunctiva becomes engorged (*chemosis*). The protruding eyeball pulsates in synchrony with the radial pulse, a phenomenon known as *pulsating exophthalmos*. Because CN III, CN IV, CN V_1, CN V_2, and CN VI lie in or close to the lateral wall of the cavernous sinus, these nerves may also be affected when the sinus is injured (Fig. 7.12*C*). ✛

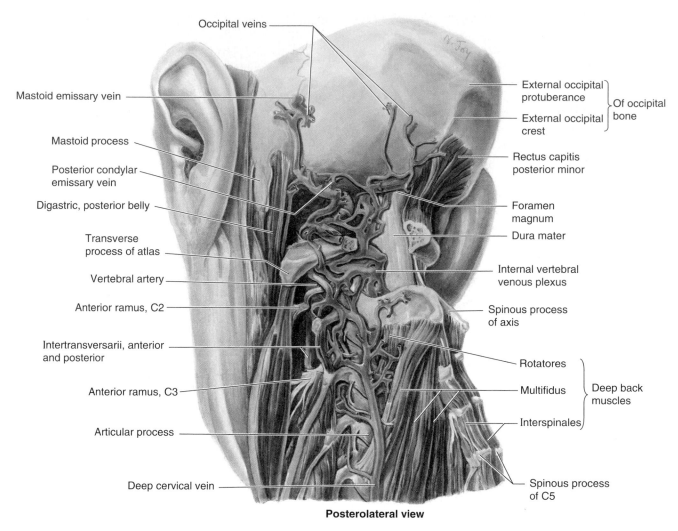

Occipital veins

Mastoid emissary vein

Mastoid process

Posterior condylar emissary vein

Digastric, posterior belly

Transverse process of atlas

Vertebral artery

Anterior ramus, C2

Intertransversarii, anterior and posterior

Anterior ramus, C3

Articular process

Deep cervical vein

External occipital protuberance
External occipital crest
} Of occipital bone

Rectus capitis posterior minor

Foramen magnum

Dura mater

Internal vertebral venous plexus

Spinous process of axis

Rotatores

Multifidus

Interspinales

} Deep back muscles

Spinous process of C5

Posterolateral view

Figure 7.14. Deep dissection of suboccipital region. The external vertebral venous system has numerous intercommunications and connections, some of which are shown here. Superiorly, the system communicates with the veins of the scalp and the intracranial venous sinuses via the foramen magnum, the mastoid foramina, and the condylar canals. Anteromedially, it passes between the laminae and through the intervertebral foramina to communicate with the internal vertebral venous plexus and veins around the vertebral artery. Inferiorly, it drains via the deep cervical vein.

Vasculature of the Dura Mater

The **arteries of the dura** supply more blood to the calvaria than to the dura. The largest of these vessels, the **middle meningeal artery,** is a branch of the maxillary artery (Fig. 7.9). It enters the floor of the middle cranial fossa through the *foramen spinosum,* runs laterally in the fossa, and turns superoanteriorly on the greater wing of the sphenoid, where it divides into anterior and posterior branches. The **anterior branch** of the middle meningeal artery runs superiorly to the pterion and then curves posteriorly to ascend toward the vertex of the cranium. The **posterior branch** of the middle meningeal artery runs posterosuperiorly and ramifies (breaks up into distributing branches) over the posterior aspect of the cranium. Small areas of dura are supplied by other arteries: meningeal branches of the ophthalmic arteries, branches of the occipital arteries, and small branches of the vertebral arteries.

The **veins of the dura** accompany the meningeal arteries, often in pairs (Fig. 7.9). The **middle meningeal veins** accompany the middle meningeal artery, leave the cranial cavity through the foramen spinosum or foramen ovale, and drain into the *pterygoid plexus* (Fig. 7.10B).

Nerve Supply of the Dura Mater

The dura of the floors of the anterior and middle cranial fossa and the roof of the posterior cranial fossa is innervated by meningeal branches arising directly or indirectly from the trigeminal nerve (CN V) (Fig. 7.15). There are three divisions of CN V (CN V_1, CN V_2, and CN V_3), each of which contributes a meningeal branch or branches. The **anterior meningeal branches of the ethmoidal nerves** (CN V_1) and the **meningeal branches of the maxillary** (CN V_2) and **mandibular** (CN V_3) **nerves** supply the dura of the anterior cranial fossa. The latter two nerves also supply the dura of the middle cranial fossa (Fig. 7.15B). The meningeal branches of CN V$_2$ and CN V$_3$ are distributed as periarterial plexuses accompanying the branches of the middle meningeal artery (Fig. 7.15A, inset).

The dura forming the roof of the posterior cranial fossa (tentorium cerebelli) and posterior part of the cerebral falx is supplied by the **tentorial nerve** (a branch of the ophthalmic nerve), whereas the anterior cerebral falx is innervated by ascending branches of the anterior meningeal branches (Fig. 7.15A). The dura of the floor of the posterior cranial fossa receives sensory fibers from the spinal ganglia of C2 and C3 carried by those spinal nerves or by fibers transferred to and traveling centrally with the vagus (CN X) and hypoglossal (CN XII) nerves. Sensory endings are more numerous in the dura along each side of the superior sagittal sinus and in the cerebellar tentorium than they are in the floor of the cranium. Pain fibers are most numerous where arteries and veins course in the dura. Pain arising from the dura is generally referred, perceived as a headache arising in cutaneous or mucosal regions supplied by the involved cervical nerve or division of the trigeminal nerve.

Dural Origin of Headaches

The dura is sensitive to pain, especially where it is related to the dural venous sinuses and meningeal arteries. Consequently, pulling on arteries at the cranial base or veins near the vertex where they pierce the dura causes pain. Distension of the scalp or meningeal vessels (or both) is believed to be one cause of headache (Raskin, 2000). Many headaches appear to be dural in origin, such as the headache occurring after a lumbar spinal puncture for removal of CSF (see Chapter 4). These headaches are thought to result from stimulation of sensory nerve endings in the dura. When CSF is removed, the brain sags slightly, pulling on the dura; this may also cause a headache. For this reason, patients are asked to keep their heads down after a lumbar puncture to minimize the pull on the dura, reducing the chances of getting a headache. ✪

Leptomeninx (Arachnoid Mater and Pia Mater)

The **arachnoid mater** and **pia mater** (arachnoid–pia) develop from a single layer of mesenchyme surrounding the embryonic brain, becoming the parietal part (arachnoid mater) and visceral part (pia mater) of the *leptomeninx*. CSF-filled spaces form within this layer and coalesce to form the *subarachnoid or leptomeningeal space* (Fig. 7.16). The derivation of the arachnoid–pia from a single embryonic layer is indicated in the adult by the numerous web-like **arachnoid trabeculae** passing between the arachnoid and the pia, which give the arachnoid its name (G. *arachnē*, spider, cobweb + G. *eidos*, resemblance). The trabeculae are composed of flattened, irregularly shaped fibroblasts that bridge the subarachnoid space (Haines, 2002). The arachnoid and pia are in continuity immediately proximal to the exit of each cranial nerve from the dura mater.

The *arachnoid mater* contains fibroblasts, collagen fibers, and some elastic fibers. Although thin, the arachnoid is thick enough to be manipulated with forceps. The avascular arachnoid, although closely applied to the meningeal layer of the dura, is not attached to the dura; it is held against the inner surface of the dura by the pressure of the CSF.

The *pia mater* is an even thinner membrane that is highly vascularized by a network of fine blood vessels. The pia is difficult to see, but it gives the surface of the brain a shiny appearance. The pia adheres to the surface of the brain and follows all its contours. When the cerebral arteries penetrate the cerebral cortex, the pia follows them for a short distance, forming a pial coat and a periarterial space (Fig. 7.16).

Meningeal Spaces

Of the three meningeal "spaces" commonly mentioned in relation to the cranial meninges, only one exists as a space in the absence of pathology:

- The **dura–cranial interface** (extradural or epidural "space") is not a natural space between the cranium and the external periosteal layer of the dura because the dura is attached to the bones. It becomes a space only pathologically, for example, when blood from torn meningeal vessels pushes the periosteum away from the cranium (Fig. 7.8C). The potential or pathological cranial epidural space is not continuous with the *spinal epidural space* (a natural space occupied by epidural fat and a venous plexus) because the former is external to the periosteum lining the cranium and the latter is internal to the periosteum covering the vertebrae.

- The **dura–arachnoid junction** or interface ("subdural space") is likewise not a natural space between the dura and the arachnoid. A space may develop in the dural border cell layer as the result of trauma, such as after a blow to the head (Haines, 2002).

- The *subarachnoid space,* between the arachnoid and the pia, is a real space that contains CSF, trabecular cells, arteries, and veins.

Although it is commonly stated that the brain "floats" in CSF, the brain is suspended in the CSF-filled subarachnoid space by the arachnoid trabeculae.

Tentorial nerves (meningeal branches of ophthalmic nerve)

Infundibulum

Internal carotid artery

Anterior meningeal branches (of anterior ethmoidal nerve)

Anterior clinoid process

Tentorial nerve

Oculomotor nerve

Trochlear nerve

Abducent nerve

CN V$_1$

CN V$_2$

CN V$_3$

Trigeminal nerve

Mandibular nerve

Meningeal branches of mandibular nerve

Nervus spinosus and sympathetic plexus

Middle meningeal artery

Ophthalmic nerve

Maxillary nerve

Meningeal branch of maxillary nerve

(A)

Key

☐ Area innervated by ophthalmic nerve (CN V$_1$)

☐ Area innervated by maxillary nerve (CN V$_2$)

☐ Area innervated by mandibular nerve (CN V$_3$)

☐ Area innervated by cervical spinal nerves (C2, C3)

Anterior meningeal branches of ethmoidal nerve

Anterior ethmoidal nerve

Meningeal branch of maxillary nerve

Posterior ethmoidal nerve

C2, C3 fibers

C2, C3 fibers distributed by CN XII

To floor of posterior cranial fossa

Meningeal branches of mandibular nerve (including nervus spinosus)

C2 fibers distributed by CN X

Tentorial nerve (recurrent meningeal branch of ophthalmic nerve)

(B)

Figure 7.15. Innervation of dura mater. The dura of the floor of the anterior and middle cranial fossa and the roof of the posterior cranial fossa is innervated by meningeal branches arising directly or indirectly from the trigeminal nerve (CN V). **A.** The right side of the calvaria and brain is removed and CN V is dissected. The cerebral falx is innervated by the ophthalmic nerve (CN V$_1$), through anterior meningeal branches of the ethmoid nerves and the tentorial nerve. The meningeal branches of the maxillary (CN V$_2$) and mandibular (CN V$_3$) nerves are distributed to the dura of the lateral part of the anterior and the middle cranial fossae as periarterial plexuses that accompany the branches of the middle meningeal artery along with vasomotor sympathetic nerve fibers from the superior cervical ganglion (*inset*). The dura of the cranial base is most sensitive in the region of the arterial branches and the superior sagittal sinus. **B.** The internal aspect of the cranial base shows innervation of the dura by branches of the trigeminal and sensory fibers of cervical spinal nerves (C2, C3) passing directly from those nerves or via meningeal branches of the vagus (CN X) and hypoglossal (CN XII) nerves.

Leptomeningitis

Leptomeningitis is an inflammation of the leptomeninges resulting from pathogenic microorganisms. The infection and inflammation are usually confined to the subarachnoid space and the arachnoid–pia (Miller and Jubelt, 2000). The bacteria may enter the subarachnoid space through the blood (*septicemia,* or "blood poisoning") or spread from an infection of the heart, lungs, or other viscera. Microorganisms may also enter the subarachnoid space from a compound cranial fracture or a fracture of the nasal sinuses. *Acute purulent meningitis* can result from infection with almost any pathogenic bacteria (e.g., *meningococcal meningitis*).

Head Injuries and Intracranial Hemorrhage

Extradural or *epidural hemorrhage* is arterial in origin. Blood from torn branches of a middle meningeal artery collects between the external periosteal layer of the dura and the calvaria, usually following a hard blow to the head, and forms an *extradural* or *epidural hematoma* (Fig. B7.13*A*). Typically, a brief *concussion* (loss of consciousness) occurs, followed by a lucid interval of some hours. Later, drowsiness and coma (profound unconsciousness) occur. Compression of the brain occurs as the blood mass increases, necessitating evacuation of the blood and occlusion of the bleeding vessels.

A *dural border hematoma* is classically called a *subdural hematoma* (Fig. B7.13*B*); however, this term is a misnomer because there is no naturally occurring space at the dura–arachnoid junction. Hematomas at this junction are usually caused by extravasated blood that splits open the dural border cell layer. The blood does not collect within a pre-existing space, but rather creates a space at the dura–arachnoid junction (Haines, 2002). *Dural border hemorrhage* usually follows a blow to the head that jerks the brain inside the cranium and injures it. The precipitating trauma may be trivial or forgotten. Dural border ▶

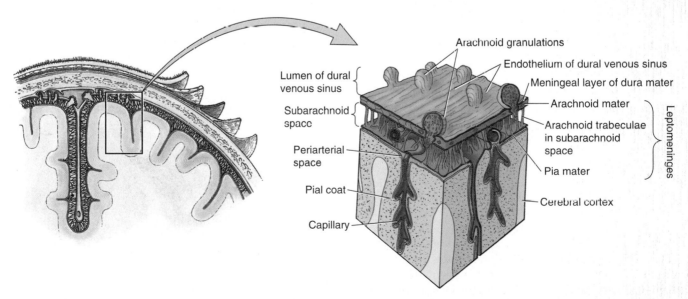

Figure 7.16. Section of scalp, calvaria, and cranial meninges. The coronal section (*left*) indicates the site of the tissue block (*right*). The subarachnoid space separates the arachnoid mater and pia mater. The main site of absorption of CSF into the venous system is through the arachnoid granulations projecting into the dural venous sinuses, especially the superior sagittal sinus and adjacent venous lacunae (Fig. 7.9).

Figure B7.13. **Intercranial hemorrhages. A.** An extradural (epidural) hemorrhage is shown. **B.** A dural border (subdural) hematoma is shown. **C.** A subarachnoid hemorrhage is shown.

hemorrhage is typically venous in origin and commonly results from tearing a superior cerebral vein as it enters the superior sagittal sinus (Fig. 7.10*B*) (Haines et al., 1993).

Subarachnoid hemorrhage is an extravasation (escape) of blood, usually arterial, into the subarachnoid space (Fig. B7.13*C*). Most subarachnoid hemorrhages result from *rupture of a saccular aneurysm* (sac-like dilation on the side of an artery), such as an aneurysm of the internal carotid artery (see clinical correlation [blue] box "Strokes," later in this chapter). Some subarachnoid hemorrhages are associated with head trauma involving cranial fractures and cerebral lacerations. Bleeding into the subarachnoid space results in meningeal irritation, a severe headache, stiff neck, and often loss of consciousness. ✪

THE BOTTOM LINE: The meninges consist of three intracranial layers: a substantial, fibrous bilaminar outer layer—the dura mater—and two continuous, delicate, membranous inner layers—the arachnoid mater and pia mater. The outer (periosteal) lamina of the dura mater is continuous with the external periosteum of the cranium and is intimately applied to the internal surface of the cranial cavity. The inner (meningeal) lamina is a sustentacular (supporting) layer that more closely reflects the contours of the brain. It leaves the outer layer in certain locations to form dural folds or reflections that penetrate the large fissures between parts of the brain, partially subdividing the cranial cavity into smaller compartments that prevent inertial brain movement. In separating from the periosteal lamina, intralaminar spaces are created that accommodate the dural venous sinuses, which receive the venous drainage of the brain and mainly drain, in turn, to the IJV.

The arachnoid and pia are the continuous parietal and visceral layers, respectively, of the leptomeninx that surround the CSF-filled subarachnoid space. They are connected by fine trabeculae that traverse the space. The subarachnoid space of the cranial cavity is continuous with that of the vertebral canal. The arachnoid is normally applied to the internal surface of the dura by CSF pressure. The pia intimately invests the neural tissue and its surface vasculature, coursing deeply along the vessels as they enter or exit the central nervous system.

The cranial meninges receive blood primarily from the middle meningeal branches of the maxillary arteries. The dura receives sensory innervation from meningeal branches of all three divisions of the trigeminal nerve and fibers from the C2 spinal ganglion.

Brain

Because the brain is usually studied in detail in a separate neuroanatomy course, the brain is covered by only a superficial survey of the gross structure in the typical anatomy course, with attention primarily concerned with the relationship between the brain and its environment—that is, its meningeal coverings, the CSF-filled subarachnoid space, and internal features of its bony encasement (the neurocranium). Because of their role in the production of CSF, the ventricles of the brain and the CSF-producing choroid plexuses found there are also covered. Furthermore, 11 of 12 cranial nerves arise from the brain (see Chapter 9).

Parts of the Brain

The brain is composed of the cerebrum, cerebellum, and brainstem (Fig. 7.17). When the calvaria and dura are removed, **gyri** (folds), **sulci** (grooves), and **fissures** (clefts) of the cerebral cortex are visible through the delicate arachnoid–pia layer. Whereas the gyri and sulci demonstrate much variation, the other features of the brain, including overall brain size, are remarkably consistent from individual to individual.

- The **cerebrum** (L. *brain*) includes the cerebral hemispheres and basal ganglia. The **cerebral hemispheres**, separated by the cerebral falx within the *longitudinal cerebral fissure*, are the dominant features of the brain (Fig. 17.7A & B). Each cerebral hemisphere is divided for descriptive purposes into four lobes, each of which is related to, but the boundaries of which do not correspond to, the overlying bones of the same name. From a superior view, the cerebrum is essentially divided into quarters by the median longitudinal cerebral fissure and the coronal **central sulcus**. The central sulcus separates **frontal lobes** (anteriorly) from **parietal lobes** (posteriorly). In a lateral view, these lobes lie superior to the transverse **lateral sulcus** and the temporal lobe inferior to it. The posteriorly placed **occipital lobes** are separated from the parietal and temporal lobes by the plane of the **parieto-occipital sulcus**, visible on the medial surface of the cerebrum in a hemisected brain (Fig. 7.17C). The anteriormost points of the anteriorly projecting frontal and temporal lobes are the **frontal** and **temporal poles.** The posteriormost point of the posteriorly project

ing occipital lobe is the **occipital pole.** The hemispheres occupy the entire supratentorial cranial cavity. The frontal lobes occupy the anterior cranial fossae, the temporal lobes occupy the lateral parts of the middle cranial fossae, and the occipital lobes extend posteriorly over the cerebellar tentorium.

- The **diencephalon** is composed of the epithalamus, dorsal thalamus, and hypothalamus and forms the central core of the brain.

- The **midbrain,** the rostral part of the brainstem, lies at the junction of the middle and posterior cranial fossae. CN III and IV are associated with the midbrain.

- The **pons** is the part of the brainstem between the midbrain rostrally and the medulla oblongata caudally; it lies in the anterior part of the posterior cranial fossa. CN V is associated with the pons (Fig. 7.17A & C).

- The **medulla oblongata (medulla)** is the most caudal subdivision of the brainstem that is continuous with the spinal cord; it lies in the posterior cranial fossa. CN IX, X, and XII are associated with the medulla, whereas CN VI–VIII are associated with the junction of pons and medulla.

- The **cerebellum** is the large brain mass lying posterior to the pons and medulla and inferior to the posterior part of the cerebrum. It lies beneath the cerebellar tentorium in the posterior cranial fossa. It consists of two lateral hemispheres that are united by a narrow middle part, the **vermis.**

Cerebral Injuries

Cerebral concussion is an abrupt, brief loss of consciousness immediately after a head injury. Consciousness may be lost for only 8–10 sec, as occurs in a knockdown during boxing. With a more severe injury, such as that resulting from an automobile accident, consciousness may be lost for hours and even days. If a person recovers consciousness within 6 hr, the long-term outcome is excellent (Rowland, 2000). If the coma lasts longer than 6 hr, brain tissue injury usually occurs. Professional boxers are especially at risk for *chronic traumatic encephalopathy,* or *punchdrunk syndrome,* a brain injury characterized by weakness in the lower limbs, unsteady gait, slowness of muscular movements, tremors of the hands, hesitancy of speech, and slow cerebration (use of one's brain). The injuries result from acceleration and deceleration of the head that shears or stretches axons (*diffuse axonal injury*). The sudden stopping of the moving head results in the brain hitting the suddenly stationary cranium.

Cerebral contusion results from brain trauma in which the pia is stripped from the injured surface of the ▶

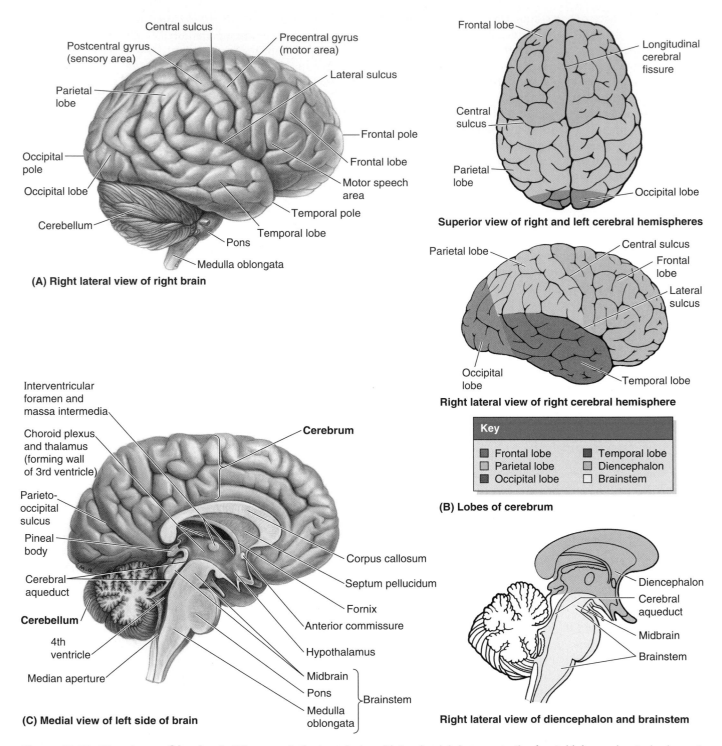

(A) Right lateral view of right brain

Superior view of right and left cerebral hemispheres

Right lateral view of right cerebral hemisphere

Key	
■ Frontal lobe	■ Temporal lobe
□ Parietal lobe	□ Diencephalon
■ Occipital lobe	□ Brainstem

(B) Lobes of cerebrum

(C) Medial view of left side of brain

Right lateral view of diencephalon and brainstem

Figure 7.17. Structure of brain. A. Whereas distinct central and lateral sulci demarcate the frontal lobe and anterior boundaries of the parietal and temporal lobes of the cerebrum, the demarcation of the posterior boundaries of the latter and the occipital lobe is less distinct externally. The cerebral surface has gyri (folds) and sulci (grooves). **B.** The lobes of the cerebrum are color coded. **C.** The medial surface of the cerebrum and deeper parts of the brain (diencephalon and brainstem) are shown after bisection of the brain. The parieto-occipital sulcus demarcating the parietal and occipital lobes can be seen on the medial aspect of the cerebrum.

brain and may be torn, allowing blood to enter the sub-arachnoid space. The bruising results either from the sudden impact of the still-moving brain against the suddenly stationary cranium or from the suddenly moving cranium against the still-stationary brain. Cerebral contusion may result in an extended loss of consciousness, but if there is no diffuse axonal injury, brain swelling, or secondary hemorrhage, recovery from a contusion may be excellent (Rowland, 2000).

Cerebral lacerations are often associated with depressed cranial fractures or gunshot wounds. Lacerations result in rupture of blood vessels and bleeding into the brain and subarachnoid space, causing increased intracranial pressure and cerebral compression. *Cerebral compression* may be produced by:

- Intracranial collections of blood.

- Obstruction of CSF circulation or absorption.

- Intracranial tumors or abscesses.

- Brain swelling caused by *brain edema,* an increase in brain volume resulting from an increase in water and sodium content (Fishman, 2000b). **◐**

Ventricular System of the Brain

The ventricular system of the brain consists of two lateral ventricles and the midline 3rd and 4th ventricles connected by the cerebral aqueduct (Fig. 7.18). CSF, largely secreted by the choroid plexuses of the ventricles, fills these brain cavities and the subarachnoid space of the brain and spinal cord.

Ventricles of the Brain
The **lateral ventricles,** the 1st and 2nd ventricles, are the largest cavities of the ventricular system and occupy large areas of the cerebral hemispheres. Each lateral ventricle opens through an **interventricular foramen** into the 3rd ventricle. The **3rd ventricle,** a slit-like cavity between the right and the left halves of the diencephalon, is continuous posteroinferiorly with the **cerebral aqueduct,** a narrow channel in the midbrain connecting the 3rd and 4th ventricles (Fig. 7.18*B*). The pyramid-shaped **4th ventricle** in the posterior part of the pons and medulla extends inferoposteriorly. Inferiorly, it tapers to a narrow channel that continues into the cervical region of the spinal cord as the central canal (Fig. 7.18*A*). CSF drains into the subarachnoid space from the 4th ventricle through a single **median aperture** and paired **lateral apertures.** These apertures are the only means by which CSF enters the subarachnoid space. If they are blocked, CSF accumulates and the ventricles distend, producing compression of the substance of the cerebral hemispheres.

Subarachnoid Cisterns
Although it is not accurate to say that the brain "floats" in the CSF, the brain actually has minimal attachment to the neurocranium. At certain areas on the base of the brain, the arachnoid and pia are widely separated by subarachnoid cisterns (Fig. 7.18*B*), which contain CSF, and soft tissue structures that "anchor" the brain, such as the arachnoid trabeculae, vasculature, and in some cases, cranial nerve roots. The cisterns are usually named according to the structures related to them. The cisterns are usually named according to the structures related to them.

Major intracranial subarachnoid cisterns include the:

- **Cerebellomedullary cistern:** The largest of the subarachnoid cisterns, located between the cerebellum and the medulla, and receives CSF from the apertures of the 4th ventricle. It is divided into the **posterior cerebellomedullary cistern** (L. *cisterna magna*) and the **lateral cerebellomedullary cistern.**

- **Pontocerebellar cistern** (pontine cistern): An extensive space ventral to the pons, continuous inferiorly with the spinal subarachnoid space.

- **Interpeduncular cistern** (basal cistern): Located in the interpeduncular fossa between the cerebral peduncles of the midbrain.

- **Chiasmatic cistern:** Inferior and anterior to *optic chiasm,* the point of crossing or decussation of optic nerve fibers.

- **Quadrigeminal cistern** (cistern of the great cerebral vein): Located between the posterior part of the corpus callosum and the superior surface of the cerebellum. It contains parts of the great cerebral vein.

- **Ambient cistern** (L. *cisterna ambiens*): Located on the lateral aspect of the midbrain and continuous posteriorly with the quadrigeminal cistern.

Secretion of Cerebrospinal Fluid
CSF is secreted (at the rate of 400–500 mL daily) by choroidal epithelial cells (modified ependymal cells) of the **choroid plexuses** in the lateral, 3rd, and 4th ventricles (Figs. 7.17*C* and 7.18). The choroid plexuses consist of vascular fringes of pia mater (tela choroidea) covered by cuboidal epithelial cells. They are invaginated into the roofs of the 3rd and 4th ventricles and on the floors of the bodies and inferior horns of the lateral ventricles.

Circulation of Cerebrospinal Fluid
CSF leaves the lateral ventricles through the *interventricular foramina* and enters the 3rd ventricle (Fig. 7.18*A*). From here, CSF passes through the *cerebral aqueduct* into the 4th ventricle. Some CSF leaves this ventricle through its *median* and *lateral apertures* and enters the *subarachnoid space,* which is continuous around the spinal cord and posterosuperiorly over the cerebellum. However, most CSF flows into the interpeduncular and quadrigeminal cisterns. CSF from the various subarachnoid cisterns flows superiorly through the sulci and fissures on the medial and superolateral

Arachnoid granulations

Superior sagittal sinus

Lateral ventricles

Inter-ventricular foramen

3rd ventricle

Communication via lateral apertures

Subarachnoid space containing CSF

Choroid plexus of the lateral ventricle

Cerebral aqueduct

4th ventricle

Choroid plexus of the 4th ventricle

Median aperture

Central canal of cervical spinal cord

(A) Median section with ventricles viewed from the left

Cerebral subarachnoid space

Body of corpus callosum

3rd ventricle

Optic chiasm

Chiasmatic cistern

Interpeduncular cistern

Pontocerebellar cistern

Spinal subarachnoid space

Septum pellucidum

Choroid plexus

Pineal body

Quadrigeminal cistern

Cerebral aqueduct

Choroid plexus

Posterior cerebello-medullary cistern

(B) Medial view, right half of hemisected brain

Figure 7.18. Ventricles, subarachnoid spaces, and cisterns. A. The ventricular system and circulation of the CSF are shown. The production of CSF is mainly by the choroid plexuses of the lateral, 3rd, and 4th ventricles. The plexuses of the lateral ventricles are the largest and most important. CSF is absorbed into the venous system through the arachnoid granulations that project into the superior sagittal sinus and its lateral lacunae. **B.** The subarachnoid cisterns, expanded regions of the subarachnoid space, contain more substantial amounts of CSF.

surfaces of the cerebral hemispheres. CSF also passes into the extensions of the subarachnoid space around the cranial nerves, the most important of which are those surrounding the optic nerves.

Absorption of Cerebrospinal Fluid

The main site of CSF absorption into the venous system is through the *arachnoid granulations* (Figs. 7.16 and 7.18*A*), especially those that protrude into the superior sagittal sinus and its lateral lacunae (Fig. 7.9). The subarachnoid space containing CSF extends into the cores of the arachnoid granulations. CSF enters the venous system through two routes: (1) most CSF enters the venous system by transport through the cells of the arachnoid granulations into the dural venous sinuses; (2) some CSF moves between the cells making up the arachnoid granulations (Corbett et al., 2002).

Functions of Cerebrospinal Fluid

Along with the meninges and calvaria, CSF protects the brain by providing a cushion against blows to the head. The CSF in the subarachnoid space provides the buoyancy that prevents the weight of the brain from compressing the cranial nerve roots and blood vessels against the internal surface of the cranium. Because the brain is slightly heavier than the CSF, the gyri on the basal surface of the brain are in contact with the cranial fossae in the floor of the cranial cavity when a person is standing erect. In many places at the base of the brain, only the cranial meninges intervene between the brain and the cranial bones. In the erect position, the CSF is in the subarachnoid cisterns and sulci on the superior and lateral parts of the brain; therefore, CSF and dura normally separate the superior part of the brain from the calvaria.

Small, rapidly recurring changes take place in *intracranial pressure* owing to the beating heart; slow recurring changes result from unknown causes. Momentarily large changes in pressure occur during coughing and straining and during changes in position (erect vs. supine). Any change in the volume of the intracranial contents (e.g., a brain tumor, an accumulation of ventricular fluid caused by blockage of the cerebral aqueduct, or blood from a ruptured aneurysm) will be reflected by a change in intracranial pressure. This rule is called the **Monro-Kellie doctrine**, which states that the cranial cavity is a closed rigid box and that a change in the quantity of intracranial blood can occur only through the displacement or replacement of CSF.

Cisternal Puncture

CSF may be obtained from the posterior cerebellomedullary cistern through a *cisternal puncture* for diagnostic or therapeutic purposes. The needle is carefully inserted through the posterior atlanto-occipital membrane into the cistern. The subarachnoid space or the ventricular system may also be entered for measuring or monitoring CSF pressure, injecting antibiotics, or administering contrast media for medical imaging. The cerebellomedullary cistern is the site of choice in infants and young children; the lumbar cistern is used most frequently in adults (see Chapter 4).

Hydrocephalus

Overproduction of CSF, obstruction of CSF flow, or interference with CSF absorption results in excess fluid in the cerebral ventricles and enlargement of the head, a condition called *obstructive hydrocephalus* (Fig. B7.14*A*). The excess CSF dilates the ventricles, thins the cerebral cortex, and separates the bones of the calvaria in infants. Although an obstruction can occur any place, the blockage usually occurs in the cerebral aqueduct (Fig. B7.14*B*) or an interventricular foramen. *Aqueductal stenosis* (narrow aqueduct) may be caused by a nearby tumor in the midbrain or by cellular debris following intraventricular hemorrhage or bacterial and fungal infections of the central nervous system (Corbett et al., 2002).

Blockage of CSF circulation results in dilation of the ventricles superior to the point of obstruction and in pressure on the cerebral hemispheres. This condition squeezes the brain between the ventricular fluid and the calvarial bones. In infants, the internal pressure results in expansion of the brain and calvaria because the sutures and fontanelles are still open. It is possible to produce an artificial drainage system to bypass the blockage and allow CSF to escape, thereby lessening damage to the brain.

In *communicating hydrocephalus*, the flow of CSF through the ventricles and into the subarachnoid space is not impaired; however, movement of CSF from this space into the venous system is partly or completely blocked. The blockage may be caused by the congenital absence of arachnoid granulations, or the granulations may be blocked by red blood cells as the result of a subarachnoid hemorrhage (Corbett et al., 2002).

Leakage of Cerebrospinal Fluid

Fractures in the floor of the middle cranial fossa may result in CSF leakage from the external acoustic meatus (*CSF otorrhea*) if the meninges superior to the middle ear are torn and the tympanic membrane is ruptured. Fractures in the floor of the anterior cranial fossa may involve the cribriform plate of the ethmoid, resulting in CSF leakage through the nose (*CSF rhinorrhea*). CSF can be distinguished from mucus by testing its glucose level; the glucose level of the CSF reflects that of the blood. CSF otorrhea and rhinorrhea may be the primary indications of a cranial base fracture and increase the risk of meningitis because an infection could spread to the meninges from the ear or nose (Rowland, 2000). ▶

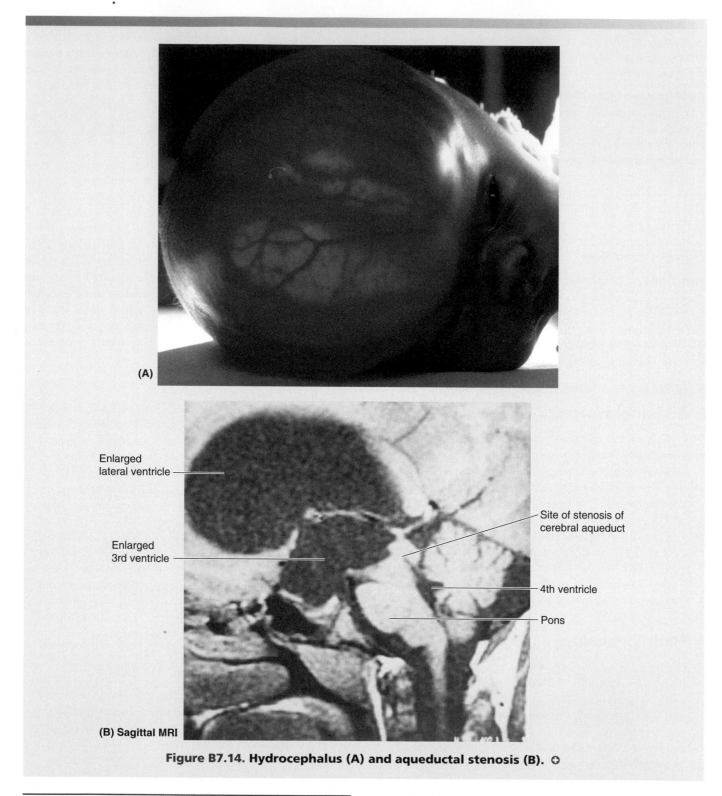

(A)

(B) Sagittal MRI

Enlarged lateral ventricle

Enlarged 3rd ventricle

Site of stenosis of cerebral aqueduct

4th ventricle

Pons

Figure B7.14. Hydrocephalus (A) and aqueductal stenosis (B). ⊙

THE BOTTOM LINE: The two hemispheres of the cerebral cortex, separated by the cerebral falx, are the dominant features of the human brain. Although the pattern of gyri and sulci are highly variable, other features of the brain, including overall brain size, are remarkably consistent from individual to individual. Each cerebral hemisphere is divided for descriptive purposes into four lobes that are related to, but the boundaries of which do not correspond to, the overlying bones of the same name.

The diencephalon forms the central core of the brain, with the midbrain, pons, and medulla oblongata making the brainstem; the medulla is continuous with the spinal cord. The cerebellum is the subtentorial brain mass occupying the posterior cranial fossa.

Each cerebral hemisphere includes a lateral ventricle in its core; otherwise, the ventricular system of the brain is an unpaired, median formation that communicates with the subarachnoid space that surrounds brain and spinal cord. Choroid plexuses secrete CSF into the ventricles, which flows out of them into the subarachnoid space. CSF is absorbed into the venous system, normally at the same rate at which it is produced, by the arachnoid granulations related to the superior sagittal sinus.

Arterial Blood Supply of the Brain

Although it accounts for only about 2.5% of body weight, the brain receives about one sixth of the cardiac output and one fifth of the oxygen consumed by the body at rest. The blood supply to the brain is derived from the internal carotid and vertebral arteries (Figs. 7.19–7.21; Table 7.3), which lie in the subarachnoid space. Venous drainage occurs via cerebral and cerebellar veins that drain to the adjacent dural venous sinuses.

Internal Carotid Arteries

The **internal carotid arteries** arise in the neck from the common carotid arteries. The cervical part of the artery ascends vertically through the neck, without branching, to the cranial base. Each internal carotid artery enters the cranial cavity through the *carotid canals* in the petrous part of the temporal bones. The intracranial course of the internal carotid artery is illustrated and described in Figure 7.19 and demonstrated radiographically in Figure 7.20. In addition to the carotid ar-

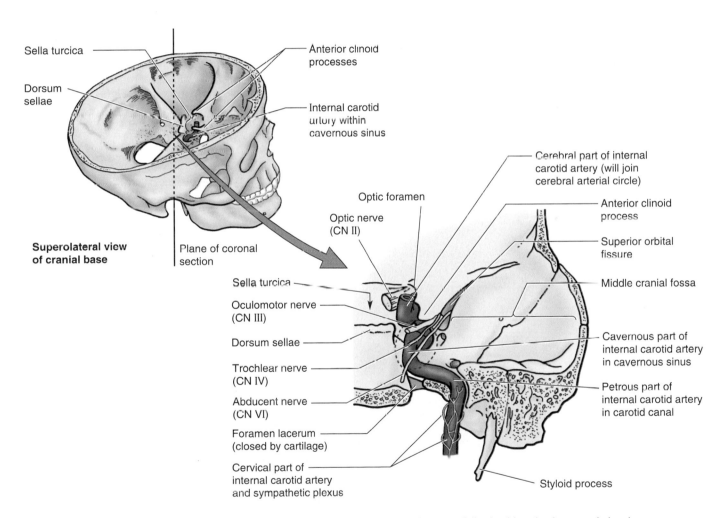

Figure 7.19. Course of internal carotid artery. The orientation drawing (*left*) indicates the plane of the coronal section that intersects the carotid canal (*right*). The cervical part of the internal carotid artery ascends vertically in the neck to the entrance of the carotid canal in the petrous temporal bone. The petrous part of the artery turns horizontally and medially in the carotid canal, toward the apex of the petrous temporal bone. It emerges from the canal superior to the foramen lacerum, closed in life by a cartilage plate, and enters the cranial cavity. The artery runs anteriorly across the cartilaginous plate; then the cavernous part of the artery runs along the carotid grooves on the lateral side of the body of the sphenoid, traversing the cavernous sinus. Inferior to the anterior clinoid process, the artery makes a 180° turn, its cerebral part heading posteriorly to join the cerebral arterial circle (Fig. 7.21).

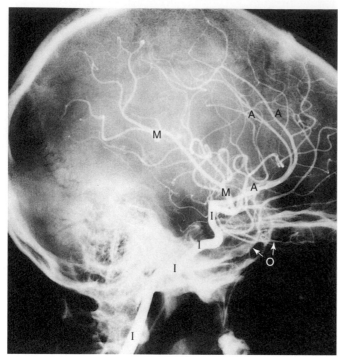

Lateral view

Figure 7.20. Carotid arteriogram. Radiopaque dye was injected into the carotid arterial system before the radiograph was taken. The four parts of the internal carotid artery (*I*), from inferior to superior, are the cervical part (in the neck), the petrous part (in the carotid canal of the petrous temporal bone), the cavernous part (in the cavernous sinus), and the cerebral part (in the cranial subarachnoid space). *A*, anterior cerebral artery and its branches; *M*, middle cerebral artery and its branches; *O*, ophthalmic artery. See also Figure 7.83. (Courtesy of Dr. D. Armstrong, Associate Professor of Medical Imaging, University of Toronto, Ontario, Canada.)

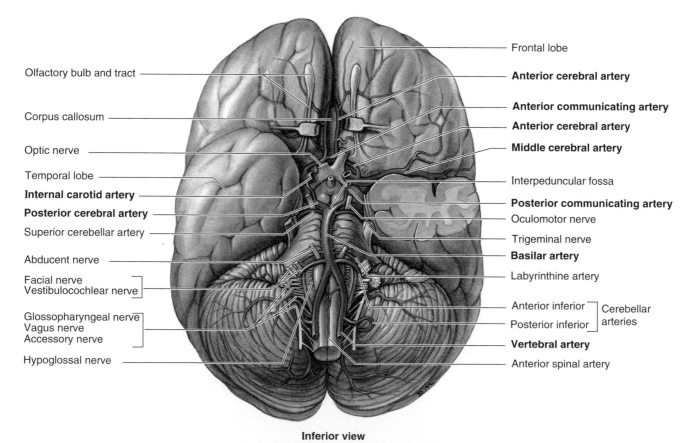

Inferior view

Figure 7.21. Base of brain with cerebral arterial circle. The three arteries that converge and anastomose to supply the brain are the right and left internal carotid arteries and the basilar artery; the latter is formed by the union of the two vertebral arteries. The three arteries form the arterial circle (of Willis) through the linkages provided by the anterior communicating artery and the two posterior communicating arteries. The cerebellum is mainly supplied by branches from the vertebral and basilar arteries. The left temporal pole is removed to show the middle cerebral artery in the lateral sulcus of the brain. The frontal lobes are separated to expose the anterior cerebral arteries.

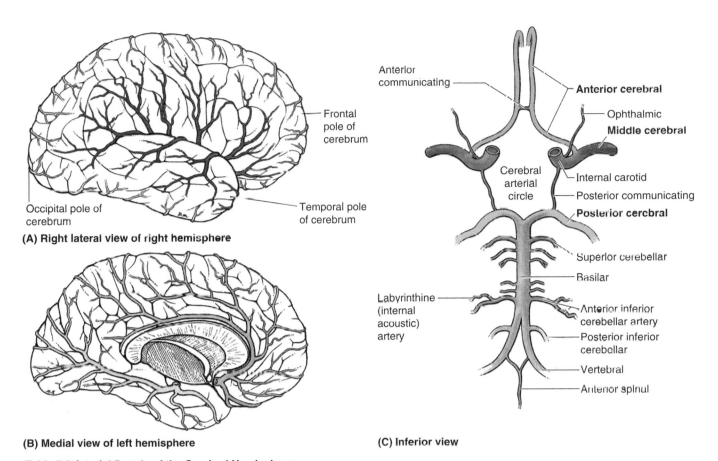

(A) Right lateral view of right hemisphere

Frontal pole of cerebrum

Occipital pole of cerebrum

Temporal pole of cerebrum

(B) Medial view of left hemisphere

Anterior communicating

Anterior cerebral

Ophthalmic

Middle cerebral

Cerebral arterial circle

Internal carotid

Posterior communicating

Posterior cerebral

Superior cerebellar

Basilar

Labyrinthine (internal acoustic) artery

Anterior inferior cerebellar artery

Posterior inferior cerebellar

Vertebral

Anterior spinal

(C) Inferior view

Table 7.3 Arterial Supply of the Cerebral Hemispheres

Artery	Origin	Distribution
Internal carotid	Common carotid artery at superior border of thyroid cartilage	Gives branches to walls of cavernous sinus, pituitary gland, and trigeminal ganglion; provides primary supply to brain
Anterior cerebral	Internal carotid artery	Cerebral hemispheres, except for occipital lobes
Anterior communicating	Anterior cerebral artery	Cerebral arterial circle (of Willis)
Middle cerebral	Continuation of internal carotid artery distal to anterior cerebral artery	Most of lateral surface of cerebral hemispheres
Vertebral	Subclavian artery	Cranial meninges and cerebellum
Basilar	Formed by union of vertebral arteries	Brainstem, cerebellum, and cerebrum
Posterior cerebral	Terminal branch of basilar artery	Inferior aspect of cerebral hemisphere and occipital lobe
Posterior communicating	Posterior cerebral artery	Optic tract, cerebral peduncle, internal capsule, and thalamus

teries, the carotid canals contain venous plexuses and *carotid plexuses of sympathetic nerves.* The internal carotid arteries course anteriorly through the *cavernous sinuses,* with the abducent nerves (CN VI) and in close proximity to the oculomotor (CN III) and trochlear (CN IV) nerves, running in the carotid groove on the side of the body of the sphenoid (Fig. 7.12). The terminal branches of the internal carotids are

the **anterior** and **middle cerebral arteries** (Figs. 7.20 and 7.21; Table 7.3).

Clinically, the internal carotids and their branches are often referred to as the *anterior circulation of the brain.* The anterior cerebral arteries are connected by the **anterior communicating artery.** Near their termination, the internal carotid arteries are joined to the posterior cerebral arteries by the **posterior communicating arteries,** completing the *cerebral arterial circle* around the *interpeduncular fossa,* the deep depression on the inferior surface of the midbrain between the cerebral peduncles.

Vertebral Arteries

The **vertebral arteries** begin in the root of the neck (the **prevertebral parts** of the vertebral arteries) as the first branches of the first part of the subclavian arteries. The two vertebral arteries are usually unequal in size, the left being larger than the right. The **cervical parts** of the vertebral arteries ascend through the *transverse foramina* of the first six cervical vertebrae. The **atlantic parts** of the vertebral arteries (parts related to the atlas, vertebra C1) perforate the dura and arachnoid and pass through the foramen magnum (Fig. 7.10*A*). The **intracranial parts** of the vertebral arteries unite at the caudal border of the pons to form the *basilar artery* (Fig. 7.20; Table 7.3). The vertebrobasilar arterial system and its branches are often referred to clinically as the *posterior circulation of the brain.*

The **basilar artery,** so-named because of its close relationship to the cranial base, ascends the *clivus,* the sloping surface from the dorsum sellae to the foramen magnum, through the pontocerebellar cistern to the superior border of the pons. It ends by dividing into the two **posterior cerebral arteries.**

Cerebral Arteries

In addition to supplying branches to deeper parts of the brain, the cortical branches of each cerebral artery supply a surface and a pole of the cerebrum (Table 7.3). The cortical branches of the:

- *Anterior cerebral artery* supply most of the medial and superior surfaces of the brain and the *frontal pole.*

- *Middle cerebral artery* supply the lateral surface of the brain and the *temporal pole.*

- **Posterior cerebral artery** supply the inferior surface of the brain and the *occipital pole.*

Anastomoses of Cerebral Arteries and Cerebral Embolism

Branches of the three cerebral arteries anastomose with each other on the surface of the brain; however, if a cerebral artery is obstructed by a *cerebral embolism* (e.g., a blood clot), these microscopic anastomoses are not capable of providing enough blood for the area of cerebral cortex concerned. Consequently, *cerebral ischemia* and *infarction* occur and an area of necrosis results. Large cerebral emboli occluding major cerebral vessels may cause severe neurologic problems and death (Haines, 2002; Rowland, 2000). ✪

Cerebral Arterial Circle

The **cerebral arterial circle** (of Willis) is a roughly pentagon-shaped circle of vessels on the ventral surface of the brain. It is an important anastomosis at the base of the brain between the four arteries (two vertebral and two internal carotid arteries) that supply the brain (Fig. 7.20; Table 7.3). The arterial circle is formed sequentially in an anterior to posterior direction by the:

- Anterior communicating artery.

- Anterior cerebral arteries.

- Internal carotid arteries.

- Posterior communicating arteries.

- Posterior cerebral arteries.

The various components of the cerebral arterial circle give numerous small branches to the brain.

Variations of the Cerebral Arterial Circle

Variations in the size of the vessels forming the cerebral arterial circle are common. The posterior communicating arteries are absent in some individuals; in others there may be two anterior communicating arteries. In approximately 1 in 3 persons, one posterior cerebral artery is a major branch of the internal carotid artery. One of the anterior cerebral arteries is often small in the proximal part of its course; the anterior communicating artery is larger than usual in these individuals.

Strokes

An *ischemic stroke* denotes the sudden development of focal neurological deficits that are usually related to *impaired cerebral blood flow.* An ischemic stroke is generally caused by an embolism in a major cerebral artery. Strokes are the most common neurologic disorders affecting adults in the United States (Sacco, 2000); they are more often disabling than fatal. The cardinal feature of a stroke is the sudden onset of neurological symptoms.

The cerebral arterial circle is an important means of collateral circulation in the event of gradual obstruction of one of the major arteries forming the circle. Sudden occlusion, even if only partial, results in neurological deficits. In elderly persons, the anastomoses of the arterial circle are often inadequate when a large artery (e.g., the internal carotid) is occluded, even if the occlusion is gradual (in which case function is impaired at least to some degree). The most common causes of strokes are *spontaneous cerebrovascular accidents,* such as cerebral thrombosis, cerebral hemorrhage, cerebral embolism, and subarachnoid hemorrhage (Rowland, 2000). ▶

Hemorrhagic stroke follows the rupture of an artery or a *saccular aneurysm*, a sac-like dilation on a weak part of the arterial wall (Fig. B7.15*A*). The most common type of saccular aneurysm is a *berry aneurysm*, occurring in the vessels of or near the cerebral arterial circle and the medium arteries at the base of the brain (Fig. B7.15*B*). Aneurysms also occur at the bifurcation of the basilar artery into the posterior cerebral arteries. In time, especially in individuals with *hypertension* (high blood pressure), the weak part of the wall of the aneurysm expands and may rupture (Fig. B7.15*C*), allowing blood to enter the subarachnoid space. Sudden *rupture of an aneurysm* usually produces a severe, almost unbearable headache and a stiff neck. These symptoms result from gross bleeding into the subarachnoid space.

Brain Infarction

An *atherosclerotic plaque* at a bend of an artery (e.g., at the bifurcation of a common carotid artery) results in progressive narrowing (*stenosis*) of the artery, producing increasingly severe neurologic deficits (Fig. B7.16). An *embolus* separates from the plaque and is carried in the blood until it lodges in an artery, usually an intracranial branch that is too small to allow its passage. This event usually results in *acute cortical infarction*, a sudden insufficiency of arterial blood to the brain (e.g., of the left parietal lobes). An interruption of blood supply for 30 sec alters a person's brain metabolism. After 1–2 min, neural function may be lost; after 5 min, lack of oxygen (*anoxia*) can result in cerebral infarction. Quickly restoring oxygen to the blood supply may reverse the brain damage (Sacco, 2000).

Figure B7.15

Transient Ischemic Attacks

Transient ischemic attacks (TIAs) refer to neurologic symptoms resulting from *ischemia*. Most TIAs last only a few minutes, but some persist for up to an hour. With major *carotid* or *vertebrobasilar stenosis*, the TIA tends to last longer and causes distal closure of intracranial vessels. The symptoms of TIA may be ambiguous: staggering, dizziness, light-headedness, fainting, and *paresthesias*. Persons with TIAs are at increased risk for myocardial infarction and ischemic stroke (Brust, 2000).

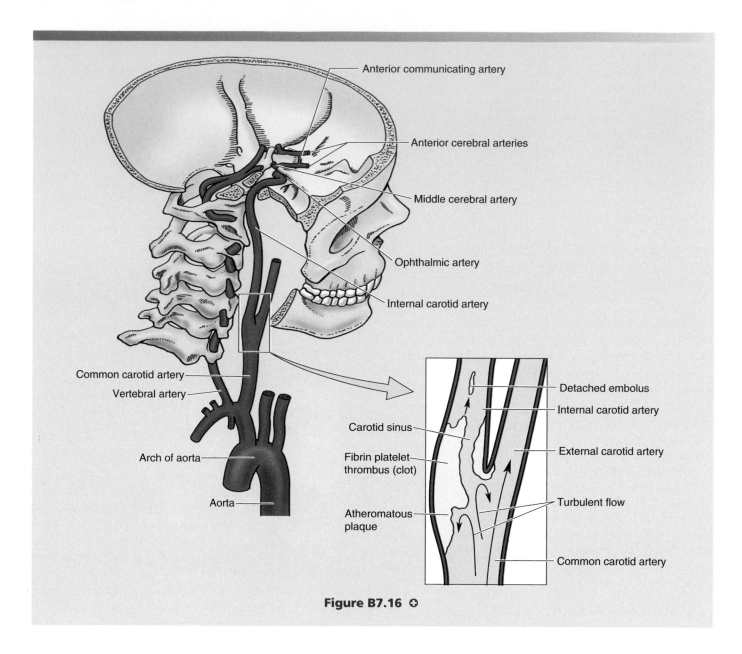

Anterior communicating artery

Anterior cerebral arteries

Middle cerebral artery

Ophthalmic artery

Internal carotid artery

Common carotid artery

Vertebral artery

Arch of aorta

Aorta

Carotid sinus

Fibrin platelet thrombus (clot)

Atheromatous plaque

Detached embolus

Internal carotid artery

External carotid artery

Turbulent flow

Common carotid artery

Figure B7.16 ◉

Venous Drainage of the Brain

The thin-walled, valveless veins draining the brain pierce the arachnoid and meningeal layer of dura to end in the nearest dural venous sinuses (Figs. 7.9–7.11), which ultimately drain for the most part into the IJVs. The **superior cerebral veins** on the superolateral surface of the brain drain into the superior sagittal sinus; **inferior** and **superficial middle cerebral veins** from the inferior, posteroinferior, and deep aspects of the cerebral hemispheres drain into the straight, transverse, and superior petrosal sinuses. The **great cerebral vein** (of Galen) is a single, midline vein formed inside the brain by the union of two internal cerebral veins; it ends by merging with the inferior sagittal sinus to form the straight sinus (Figs. 7.10 and 7.13A & B). The cerebellum is drained by **superior**

and **inferior cerebellar veins,** draining the respective aspect of the cerebellum into the transverse and sigmoid sinuses.

THE BOTTOM LINE: A continuous supply of oxygen and nutrients is essential for brain function. The brain receives a dual blood supply from the cerebral branches of the bilaterally paired internal carotid and vertebral arteries. Anastomoses between these arteries form the cerebral arterial circle. Anastomoses also occur between the branches of the three cerebral arteries on the surface of the brain. In adults, if one of the four arteries delivering blood to the brain is blocked, the remaining three are not usually capable of providing adequate collateral circulation; consequently, impaired cerebral blood flow (ischemia) and an ischemic stroke result. Venous drainage from the brain occurs via the dural venous sinuses and internal jugular veins.

Face

The **face** is the anterior aspect of the head from the forehead to the chin and from one ear to the other. The face provides our identity as an individual human. Thus defects (malformations, scarring, or other alterations resulting from pathology or trauma) have marked consequences beyond their physical effects. The basic shape of the face is determined by the underlying bones. The individuality of the face results primarily from anatomical variation: variations in the shape and relative prominence of the features of the underlying cranium; in the deposition of fatty tissue; in the color and effects of aging on the overlying skin; and in the abundance, nature, and placement of hair on the face and scalp.

The relatively large size of the **buccal fat-pads** in infants prevents collapse of the cheeks during sucking and produces their chubby-cheeked appearance. Growth of the facial bones takes longer than those of the calvaria. The ethmoid bone, orbital cavities, and superior parts of the nasal cavities have nearly completed their growth by the 7th year. Expansion of the orbits and growth of the nasal septum carry the maxillae inferoanteriorly. Considerable facial growth occurs during childhood as the paranasal sinuses develop and the permanent teeth erupt.

The face plays an important role in communication. Our interactions with others take place largely via the face (including the ears); hence the term "interface" for a site of interactions. Whereas the shape and features of the face provide our identity, much of our effect on others and their perceptions about us result from the way we use facial muscles to make the slight alterations in those features that constitute facial expression.

Muscles of the Face and Scalp

The facial muscles (muscles of facial expression) are in the subcutaneous tissue of the anterior and posterior scalp, face, and neck. They move the skin and change facial expressions to convey mood. Most muscles attach to bone or fascia and produce their effects by pulling the skin. The muscles of the scalp and face are illustrated and their attachments and actions are provided in Table 7.4. Certain muscles and/or muscle groups will be discussed in further detail.

All muscles of facial expression develop from mesoderm in the second pharyngeal arches. A subcutaneous muscular sheet forms during embryonic development that spreads over the neck and face, carrying branches of the nerve of the arch (the facial nerve, CN VII) with it to supply all the muscles formed from the arch (Moore and Persaud, 2003). The muscular sheet differentiates into muscles that surround the facial orifices (mouth, eyes, and nose), serving as sphincter and dilator mechanisms that also produce

facial expressions (Fig. 7.22). Because of their common embryological origin, the platysma and facial muscles are often fused, and their fibers are frequently intermingled.

Muscles of the Scalp, Forehead, and Eyebrows

The *occipitofrontalis* is a flat digastric muscle, with **occipital** and **frontal bellies** that share a common tendon, the *epicranial aponeurosis* (Fig. 7.22; Table 7.4A & B). Because the aponeurosis is a layer of the scalp, independent contraction of the occipital belly retracts the scalp and contraction of the frontal belly protracts it. Acting simultaneously, the occipital belly, with bony attachments, works as a synergist with the frontal belly, which has no bony attachments, to elevate the eyebrows and produce transverse wrinkles across the forehead. This gives the face a surprised look.

Muscles of the Mouth, Lips, and Cheeks

The lips and the shape and degree of opening of the mouth are important for clear speech. In addition, we add emphasis to our vocal communication with our facial expressions. Several muscles alter the shape of the mouth and lips during speaking as well as during such activities as singing, whistling, and mimicry. The shape of the mouth and lips is controlled by a complex three-dimensional group of muscular slips, which include the following:

- Elevators, retractors, and evertors of the upper lip.
- Depressors, retractors, and evertors of the lower lip.
- The orbicularis oris, the sphincter around the mouth.
- The buccinator in the cheek.

At rest, the lips are in gentle contact and the teeth are close together.

Table 7.4. Muscles of the Scalp and Face

(A) Lateral view

Muscle[a]	Origin	Insertion	Main Action(s)
Occipitofrontalis Frontal belly[1]	Epicranial aponeurosis	Skin and subcutaneous tissue of eyebrows and forehead	Elevates eyebrows and wrinkles skin of forehead; protracts scalp (indicating surprise or curiosity)
Occipital belly[a]	Lateral two thirds of superior nuchal line	Epicranial aponeurosis	Retracts scalp; increasing effectiveness of frontal belly
Orbicularis oculi (orbital sphincter)[1,2]	Medial orbital margin; medial palpebral ligament; lacrimal bone	Skin around margin of orbit; superior and inferior tarsal plates	Closes eyelids: palpebral part does so gently; orbital part tightly (winking)
Corrugator supercilii[1]	Medial end of superciliary arch	Skin superior to middle of supraorbital margin and superciliary arch	Draws eyebrow medially and inferiorly, creating vertical wrinkles above nose (demonstrating concern or worry)
Procerus plus transverse part of nasalis[3]	Fascia aponeurosis covering nasal bone and lateral nasal cartilage	Skin of inferior forehead, between eyebrows	Depresses medial end of eyebrow; wrinkles skin over dorsum of nose (conveying disdain or dislike)
Alar part of nasalis plus levator labii superioris alaeque nasii[3]	Frontal process of maxilla (inferomedial margin of orbit)	Major alar cartilage	Depresses ala laterally, dilating anterior nasal aperture (i.e., "flaring nostrils," as during anger or exertion)
Orbicularis oris (oral sphincter)[3]	Medial maxilla and mandible; deep surface of perioral skin; angle of mouth (modiolus)	Mucous membrane of lips	Tonus closes rima oris; phasic contraction compresses and protrudes lips (kissing) or resists distension (when blowing)
Levator labii superioris[3]	Infraorbital margin (maxilla)	Skin of upper lip	Part of dilators of mouth; retract (elevate) and/or evert upper lip; deepen nasolabial sulcus (showing sadness)
Zygomaticus minor[3]	Anterior aspect, zygomatic bone		

[a]All facial muscles are innervated by the facial nerve (CN VII) via its posterior auricular (*pa*) branch or via the temporal (*1*), zygomatic (*2*), buccal (*3*), marginal mandibular (*4*), or cervical (*5*) branches of the parotid plexus.

Table 7.4. Muscles of the Scalp and Face *(Continued)*

Epicranial aponeurosis**

Frontal belly of occipitofrontalis**

Procerus

Orbicularis oculi
{ Orbital part
  Palpebral part }

Nasalis

Levator labii superioris

Zygomaticus minor

Zygomaticus major

Orbicularis oris

Risorius

Depressor anguli oris

Depressor labii inferioris

Platysma

Temporal*

Corrugator supercilii

Orbicularis oculi

Levator labii superioris (cut)

Zygomaticus minor and major (cut)

Buccinator

Masseter*

Orbicularis oris

Depressor labii inferioris (cut)

Mentalis

Platysma (cut)

Sternocleidomastoid*

(B) Anterior view

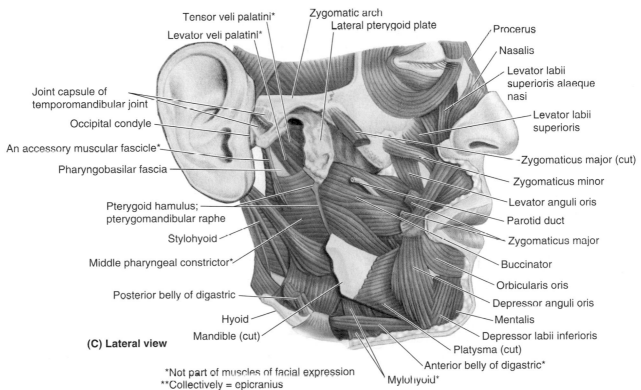

Tensor veli palatini*

Levator veli palatini*

Joint capsule of temporomandibular joint

Occipital condyle

An accessory muscular fascicle*

Pharyngobasilar fascia

Pterygoid hamulus; pterygomandibular raphe

Stylohyoid

Middle pharyngeal constrictor*

Posterior belly of digastric

Hyoid

Mandible (cut)

Zygomatic arch

Lateral pterygoid plate

Procerus

Nasalis

Levator labii superioris alaeque nasi

Levator labii superioris

Zygomaticus major (cut)

Zygomaticus minor

Levator anguli oris

Parotid duct

Zygomaticus major

Buccinator

Orbicularis oris

Depressor anguli oris

Mentalis

Depressor labii inferioris

Platysma (cut)

Anterior belly of digastric*

Mylohyoid*

(C) Lateral view

*Not part of muscles of facial expression
**Collectively = epicranius

Table 7.4. Muscles of the Scalp and Face *(Continued)*

Muscle[a]	Origin	Insertion	Main Action(s)
Buccinator (cheek muscle)[3]	Mandible, alveolar processes of maxilla and mandible, pterygomandibular raphe	Angle of mouth (modiolus); orbicularis oris	Presses cheek against molar teeth; works with tongue to keep food between occlusal surfaces and out of oral vestibule; resists distension (when blowing)
Zygomaticus major[3]	Lateral aspect of zygomatic bone	Angle of mouth (modiolus)	Part of dilators of mouth; elevate labial commissure—bilaterally to smile (happiness); unilaterally to sneer (disdain)
Levator anguli oris[3]	Infraorbital maxilla (canine fossa)		
Risorius[3]	Parotid fascia and buccal skin (highly variable)		Part of dilators of mouth; widens rima oris, as when grinning or grimacing
Depressor anguli oris[4]	Anterolateral base of mandible		Part of dilators of mouth; depresses labial commissure bilaterally to frown (sadness)
Depressor labii inferioris[4]	Platysma and anterolateral body of mandible	Skin of lower lip	Part of dilators of mouth; retracts (depresses) and/or everts lower lip (pouting, sadness)
Mentalis[4]	Body of mandible (anterior to roots of inferior incisors)	Skin of chin (mentolabial sulcus)	Elevates and protrudes lower lip; elevates skin of chin (showing doubt)
Platysma[5]	Subcutaneous tissue of infraclavicular and supraclavicular regions	Base of mandible; skin of cheek and lower lip; angle of mouth (modiolus); orbicularis oris	Depresses mandible (against resistance); tenses skin of inferior face and neck (conveying tension and stress)

[a]All facial muscles are innervated by the facial nerve (CN VII) via its posterior auricular (*pa*) branch or via the temporal (*1*), zygomatic (*2*), buccal (*3*), marginal mandibular (*4*), or cervical (*5*) branches of the parotid plexus.

The **orbicularis oris,** the first of the series of sphincters associated with the alimentary system (digestive tract), encircles the mouth within the lips, controlling entry and exit through the **oral fissure** (L. *rima oris,* the opening between the lips). The orbicularis oris is important during articulation (speech).

The **buccinator** (L. trumpeter) is a thin, flat, rectangular muscle that attaches laterally to the alveolar processes of the maxillae and mandible, opposite the molar teeth, and to the **pterygomandibular raphe,** a tendinous thickening of the buccopharyngeal fascia separating and giving origin to the superior pharyngeal constrictor posteriorly (Table 7.4C). It occupies a deeper, more medially placed plane than the other facial muscles, passing deep to the mandible so that it is more closely related to the buccal mucosa than the skin of the face. The buccinator, active in smiling, also keeps the cheek taut, thereby preventing it from folding and being injured during chewing.

Anteriorly, the fibers of the buccinator mingle medially with those of the orbicularis oris, and the tonus of the two muscles compresses the cheeks and lips against the teeth and gums. The tonic contraction of the buccinator and especially of the orbicularis oris, provides a gentle but continual resistance to the tendency of the teeth to tilt in an outward direction. In the presence of a short upper lip, or retractors that remove this force, crooked or protrusive ("buck") teeth develop.

The orbicularis oris (from the labial aspect) and buccinator (from the buccal aspect) work with the tongue (from the lingual aspect) to keep food between the occlusal surfaces of the teeth during mastication (chewing) and to prevent food from accumulating in the oral vestibule. The buccinator also helps the cheeks resist the forces generated by whistling and sucking. The buccinator was given its name because it compresses the cheeks during blowing (e.g., when a musician plays a wind instrument). Some trumpeters (notably the late Dizzy Gillespie) stretch their buccinators and other cheek muscles so much that their cheeks balloon out when they blow forcibly on their instruments.

Several dilator muscles radiate from the lips and angles of the mouth, somewhat like the spokes of a wheel, retracting the various borders of the *oral fissure* collectively, in groups, or individually. Lateral to the angles of the mouth or **labial commissures** (the junctions of the upper and lower lips) fibers of as many as nine facial muscles interlace or merge in a highly variable and multiplanar formation called the **modiolus,** which is largely responsible for the occurrence of dimples in many individuals.

The **platysma** (G. flat plate) is a broad, thin sheet of muscle in the subcutaneous tissue of the neck. The anterior borders of the two muscles decussate over the chin and blend with the facial muscles. Acting from its superior attachment,

Occipitofrontalis

Corrugator supercilii

Procerus + transverse
part of nasalis

Orbicularis oculi

Lev. labii sup. alaeque nasi +
alar part of nasalis

Buccinator + orbicularis oris

Zygomaticus major + minor

Risorius

Risorius + depressor
labii inferioris

Levator labii superioris +
depressor labii

Dilators of mouth:
Risorius plus levator labii superioris
+ depressor labii inferioris

Orbicularis oris

Depressor anguli oris

Mentalis

Platysma

Figure 7.22. Muscles of facial expression in action. These muscles are superficial sphincters and dilators of the orifices of the head. The facial muscles, supplied by the facial nerve (CN VII), are attached to and move the skin of the face, producing many facial expressions.

the platysma tenses the skin, producing vertical skin ridges, conveying great stress, and releasing pressure on the superficial veins. Acting from its inferior attachment, the platysma helps depress the mandible and draw the corners of the mouth inferiorly, as in a grimace.

Muscles of the Orbital Opening

The function of the eyelids (L. *palpebrae*) is to protect the eyeballs from injury and excessive light. The eyelids also keep the cornea moist by spreading the tears.

The **orbicularis oculi** closes the eyelids and wrinkles the forehead vertically (Fig. 7.23; Table 7.4*A* &*B*). Its fibers sweep in concentric circles around the orbital margin

and eyelids. Contraction of these fibers narrows the **palpebral fissure** (aperture between the eyelids) and assists the flow of lacrimal fluid (tears) by bringing the lids together laterally first, closing the palpebral fissure in a lateral to medial direction. The orbicularis oculi consists of three parts:

1. *Palpebral part:* arising from the **medial palpebral ligament** and mostly located within the eyelids, gently closes the eyelids (as in blinking or sleep) to keep the cornea from drying.

2. *Lacrimal part:* passing posterior to the *lacrimal sac*, draws the eyelids medially, aiding drainage of tears.

(A)   (B)   (C)

Figure 7.23. Disposition and actions of orbicularis oculi muscle. A. The orbital (*O*) and palpebral (*P*) parts of the orbicularis oculi are demonstrated. **B.** The palpebral part gently closes the eyelids. **C.** The orbital part tightly closes the eyelids.

3. *Orbital part:* overlying the orbital rim and attached to the frontal bone and maxilla medially, tightly closes the eyelids (as in winking or squinting) to protect the eyeballs against glare and dust.

When all three parts of the orbicularis oculi contract, the eyes are firmly closed (Figs. 7.22 and 7.23*C*).

Muscles of the Nose and Ears

As demonstrated in the clinical correlation (blue) box "Flar-

ing of the Nostrils" (below), the muscles of the nose may provide evidence of breathing behaviors. Otherwise, although these muscles are functionally important in certain mammals (elephants, tapirs, rabbits, and some diving mammals). They are relatively unimportant in humans except in terms of facial expression and in the specialized field of aesthetic plastic surgery. The muscles of the ears, important in animals capable of cocking or directing the ears toward the sources of sounds, are even less critical in humans.

Flaring of the Nostrils

The actions of the nasalis muscles have generally been held as insignificant; however, observant clinicians study their action because of their diagnostic value. For example, true *nasal breathers* can flare their nostrils distinctly. Habitual mouth breathing, caused by chronic nasal obstruction, for example, diminishes and sometimes eliminates the ability to flare the nostrils. Children who are chronic *mouth breathers* often develop dental malocclusion (improper bite) because the alignment of the teeth is maintained to a large degree by normal periods of occlusion and labial closure. Antisnoring devices have been developed that attach to the nose to flare the nostrils and maintain a more patent air passageway.

Paralysis of Facial Muscles

Injury to the facial nerve (CN VII) or its branches produces paralysis of some or all facial muscles on the affected side (Bell palsy). The affected area sags and facial expression is distorted, making it appear passive or sad. The loss of tonus of the orbicularis oculi causes the inferior eyelid to evert (fall away from the surface of the eyeball). As a result, lacrimal fluid is not spread over the cornea, preventing adequate lubrication, hydration, and flushing of the surface of the cornea. This makes it vulnerable to ulceration. A resulting corneal scar can impair vision. If the injury weakens or paralyzes the buccinator and orbicularis oris, food will accumulate in the oral vestibule during

chewing, usually requiring continual removal with a finger. When the sphincters or dilators of the mouth are affected, displacement of the mouth (drooping of its corner) is produced by contraction of unopposed contralateral facial muscles and gravity, resulting in food and saliva dribbling out of the side of the mouth, a sad look when the face is relaxed (Fig. B7.17), and a markedly contorted smile. Weakened lip muscles affect speech as a result of an impaired ability to produce ▶

Figure B7.17

labial (*B*, *M*, *P*, or *W*) sounds. Affected persons cannot whistle or blow a wind instrument. They frequently dab their eyes and mouth with a handkerchief to wipe the fluid (tears and saliva), which runs from the drooping lid and mouth; the fluid and constant wiping may result in localized skin irritation. ○

THE BOTTOM LINE: The face provides our identity as an individual human. Thus congenital or acquired defects have consequences beyond their physical effects. The individuality of the face results primarily from anatomical variation. The way in which the facial muscles alter the basic features is critical to communication. Lips and the shape and degree of opening of the mouth are important components of speech, but emphasis and subtleties of meaning are provided by our facial expressions. The facial muscles play important roles as the dilators and sphincters of the portals of the digestive, respiratory, and visual systems (oral and palpebral fissures and nostrils), controlling what enters and some of what exits from our bodies. Other facial muscles assist the muscles of mastication by keeping food between the teeth during chewing. Fleshy portions of the face (eyelids, cheeks) form dynamic containing walls for the orbits and oral cavity. Facial muscles are all derived from the second pharyngeal arch and are therefore supplied by the nerve of this arch, the facial nerve (CN VII). Facial muscles are subcutaneous, most having a skeletal origin and a cutaneous insertion. The face lacks the deep fascia present elsewhere in the body.

Nerves of the Face

Cutaneous (sensory) innervation of the face is provided primarily by the *trigeminal nerve* (CN V), whereas motor innervation to the facial muscles is provided by the *facial nerve* (CN VII).

Cutaneous Nerves of the Face

The cutaneous nerves of the neck overlap those of the face. Cutaneous branches of cervical nerves from the *cervical plexus* extend over the posterior aspect of the neck and scalp. The *great auricular nerve* in particular innervates the inferior aspect of the auricle and much of the parotid region of the face (the area overlying the angle of the jaw).

The **trigeminal nerve** (CN V) originates from the lateral surface of the pons of the midbrain by two roots: motor and sensory. These roots are comparable to the motor (anterior) and sensory (posterior) roots of spinal nerves. The sensory root consists of the central processes of pseudounipolar neurons located in a sensory ganglion (the **trigeminal ganglion**) at the distal end of the root, which is bypassed by the multipolar neuronal axons making up the motor root. CN V is the sensory nerve for the face and the motor nerve for the muscles of mastication and several small muscles (Fig. 7.24).

The peripheral processes of the neurons of the trigeminal ganglion constitute three divisions of the nerve: the *ophthalmic nerve* (CN V_1), the *maxillary nerve* (CN V_2), and the sensory component of the *mandibular nerve* (CN V_3). These nerves are named according to their main areas of termination: the eye, maxilla, and mandible, respectively. The first two divisions (ophthalmic and maxillary nerves) are wholly sensory. The mandibular nerve is largely sensory but it also receives the motor fibers (axons) from the motor root of CN V that mainly supply the muscles of mastication. The cutaneous nerves derived from each division of CN V are illustrated and the origin, course and distribution of each nerve are listed and mapped in Table 7.5.

Ophthalmic Nerve

The **ophthalmic nerve** (CN V_1), the superior division of the trigeminal nerve, is the smallest of the three divisions of CN V. It arises from the trigeminal ganglion as a wholly sensory nerve and supplies the area of skin derived from the embryonic *frontonasal prominence* (Moore and Persaud, 2003). As CN V_1 enters the orbit through the *superior orbital fissure*, it trifurcates into the frontal, nasociliary, and lacrimal nerves (Fig. 7.24). Except for the external nasal nerve, the cutaneous branches of CN V_1 reach the skin of the face via the orbital opening (Fig. 7.25).

The **frontal nerve**, the largest branch produced by the trifurcation of CN V_1, runs along the roof of the orbit toward the orbital opening, bifurcating approximately midway into the cutaneous **supraorbital** and **supratrochlear nerves**, distributed to the forehead and scalp (Fig. 7.26).

The **nasociliary nerve**, the intermediate branch of the CN V_1 trifurcation, supplies branches to the eyeball and divides within the orbit into the posterior ethmoidal, anterior ethmoidal, and infratrochlear nerves. The *posterior* and *anterior ethmoidal nerves* leave the orbit, the latter running a circuitous course passing through the cranial and nasal cavities. Its terminal branch, the **external nasal nerve**, is a cutaneous nerve supplying the external nose. The **infratrochlear nerve** is a terminal branch of the nasociliary nerve and its main cutaneous branch.

The **lacrimal nerve**, the smallest branch from the trifurcation of CN V_1, is primarily a cutaneous branch, but it also conveys some secretomotor fibers, sent via a communicating branch, from a ganglion associated with the maxillary nerve for innervation of the lacrimal gland.

Maxillary Nerve

The *maxillary nerve* (CN V_2), the intermediate division of the trigeminal nerve, also arises as a wholly sensory nerve (Fig. 7.24). CN V_2 passes anteriorly from the trigeminal ganglion and leaves the cranium through the *foramen rotundum* in the base of the greater wing of the sphenoid (Fig. 7.5C). It enters the *pterygopalatine fossa*, where it gives off branches to the *pterygopalatine ganglion* and continues anteriorly, entering the orbit through the inferior orbital fissure (Fig. 7.24). It gives off the zygomatic nerve and passes anteriorly into the infraorbital groove as the infraorbital nerve.

Table 7.5. Cutaneous Nerves of the Face and Scalp

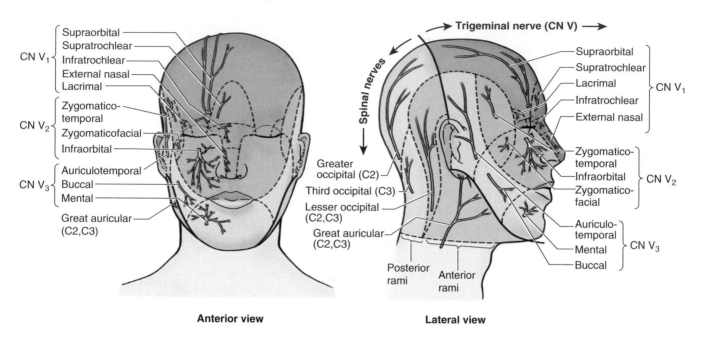

Anterior view   Lateral view

Nerve	Origin	Course	Distribution
Cutaneous nerves derived from ophthalmic nerve (CN V₁)			
Supraorbital	Largest branch from bifurcation of *frontal nerve,* approximately in middle of orbital roof	Continues anteriorly along roof of orbit, emerging via supraorbital notch or foramen; ascends forehead, breaking into branches	Mucosa of *frontal sinus;* skin and conjunctiva of middle of *superior eyelid;* skin and pericranium of *anterolateral forehead and scalp* to vertex (interauricular line)
Supratrochlear	Smaller branch from bifurcation of *frontal nerve,* approximately in middle of orbital roof	Continues anteromedially along roof of orbit, passing lateral to trochlea and ascending forehead	Skin and conjunctive of medial aspect of *superior eyelid;* skin and pericranium of *anteromedial forehead*
Lacrimal	Smallest branch from trifurcation of *CN V₁* proximal to superior orbital fissure	Runs superolaterally through orbit, receiving secretomotor fibers via a communicating branch from the zygomaticotemporal nerve	*Lacrimal gland* (secretomotor fibers); small area of skin and conjunctiva of *lateral part of superior eyelid*
Infratrochlear	Terminal branch (with anterior ethmoidal nerve) of *nasociliary nerve*	Follows medial wall of orbit, passing inferior to trochlea	Skin lateral to *root of nose;* skin and conjunctiva of *eyelids adjacent to medial canthus, lacrimal sac,* and *lacrimal caruncle*
External nasal	Terminal branch of *anterior ethmoidal nerve*	Emerges from nasal cavity by passing between nasal bone and lateral nasal cartilage	Skin of nasal *ala, vestibule,* and *dorsum of nose,* including *apex*
Cutaneous nerves derived from maxillary nerve (CN V₂)			
Infraorbital	Continuation of *CN V₂* distal to its entrance into the orbit via the inferior orbital fissure	Traverses infraorbital groove and canal in orbital floor, giving rise to superior alveolar branches; then emerges via infraorbital foramen, immediately dividing into inferior palpebral, internal and external nasal, and superior labial branches	Mucosa of *maxillary sinus;* premolar, canine, and incisor *maxillary teeth;* skin and conjunctiva of *inferior eyelid;* skin of *cheek, lateral nose,* and anteroinferior *nasal septum;* skin and oral mucosa of *superior lip*

Table 7.5. Cutaneous Nerves of the Face and Scalp *(continued)*

Nerve	Origin	Course	Distribution
Zygomaticofacial	Smaller terminal branch (with zygomaticotemporal nerve) of *zygomatic nerve*	Traverses zygomaticofacial canal in zygomatic bone at inferolateral angle of orbit	Skin on prominence of *cheek*
Zygomaticotemporal	Larger terminal branch (with zygomaticofacial nerve) of *zygomatic nerve*	Sends communicating branch to lacrimal nerve in orbit; then passes to temporal fossa via zygomaticotemporal canal in zygomatic bone	Hairless skin *anterior part of temporal fossa*
Cutaneous nerves derived from mandibular nerve (CN V₃)			
Auriculotemporal	In infratemporal fossa via two roots from *posterior trunk of CN V₃* that encircle middle meningeal artery	Passes posteriorly deep to ramus of mandible and superior deep part of parotid gland, emerging posterior to temporomandibular joint	Skin anterior to auricle and posterior two thirds of *temporal region*; skin of tragus and adjacent helix of *auricle*; skin of roof of *external acoustic meatus*; and skin of superior *tympanic membrane*
Buccal	In infratemporal fossa as sensory branch of *anterior trunk of CN V₃*	Passes between two parts of lateral pterygoid muscle, emerging anteriorly from cover of ramus of mandible and masseter, uniting with buccal branches of facial nerve	Skin and oral mucosa of *cheek* (overlying and deep to anterior part of buccinator); *buccal gingivae* (gums) adjacent to second and third molars
Mental	Terminal branch of *inferior alveolar nerve (CN V₃)*	Emerges from mandibular canal via mental foramen in anterolateral aspect of body of mandible	Skin of *chin* and skin; oral mucosa of *inferior lip*
Cutaneous nerves derived from anterior rami of cervical spinal nerves			
Greater auricular	Spinal nerves C2 and C3 via cervical plexus	Ascends vertically across sternocleidomastoid, posterior to external jugular vein	Skin overlying angle of mandible and inferior lobe of auricle; parotid sheath
Lesser occipital		Follows posterior border of sternocleidomastoid; then ascends posterior to auricle	Scalp posterior to auricle
Cutaneous nerves derived from posterior rami of cervical spinal nerves			
Greater occipital nerve	As medial branch of posterior ramus of spinal nerve C2	Emerges between axis and obliquus capitis inferior; then pierces trapezius	Scalp of occipital region
Third occipital nerve	As lateral branch of posterior ramus of spinal nerve C3	Pierces trapezius	Scalp of lower occipital and suboccipital regions

The **zygomatic nerve** runs to the lateral wall of the orbit, giving rise to two of the three cutaneous branches of CN V₂, the **zygomaticofacial** and **zygomaticotemporal nerves**. The latter sends a communicating branch conveying secretomotor fibers to the lacrimal nerve. En route to the face, the **infraorbital nerve** gives off palatine branches, branches to the mucosa of the maxillary sinus, and branches to the posterior teeth. It reaches the skin of the face by traversing the *infraorbital foramen* on the infraorbital surface of the maxilla. The three cutaneous branches of the maxillary nerve supply the area of skin derived from the embryonic *maxillary prominences*.

Mandibular Nerve

The *mandibular nerve* (CN V₃), the inferior and largest division of the trigeminal nerve, is formed by the union of sensory fibers from the sensory ganglion and the motor root of CN V in the *foramen ovale* in the greater wing of the sphenoid through which CN V₃ emerges from the cranium (Fig. 7.24). CN V₃ has three sensory branches that supply the area of skin derived from the embryonic *mandibular prominence*. It also supplies motor fibers to the muscles of mastication (Fig. 7.24C). CN V₃ is the only division of CN V that carries motor fibers. The major cutaneous branches of CN V₃ are the

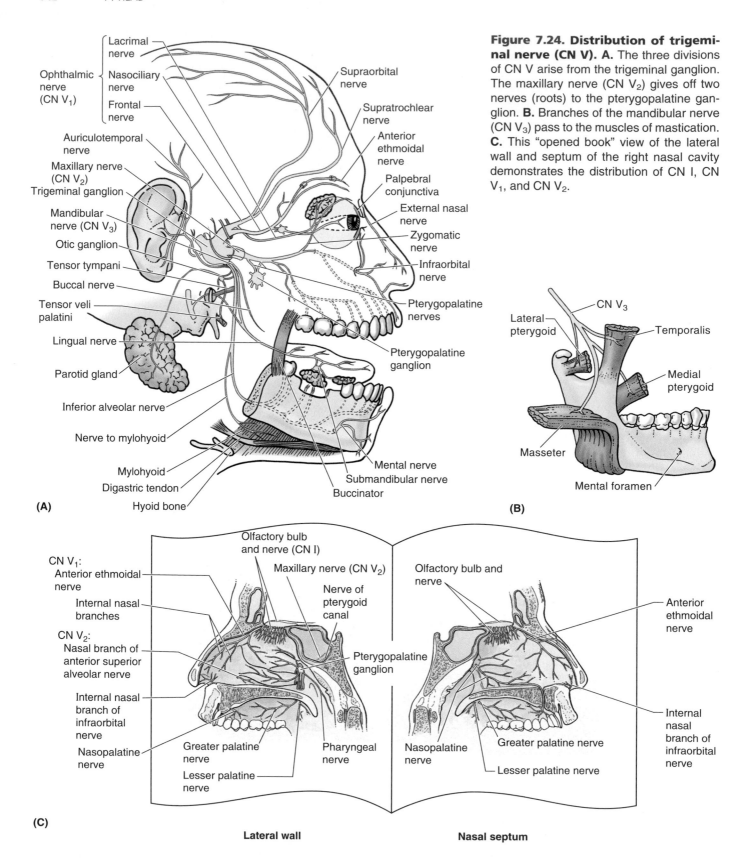

(A)

Ophthalmic nerve (CN V₁)
- Lacrimal nerve
- Nasociliary nerve
- Frontal nerve

Auriculotemporal nerve
Maxillary nerve (CN V₂)
Trigeminal ganglion
Mandibular nerve (CN V₃)
Otic ganglion
Tensor tympani
Buccal nerve
Tensor veli palatini
Lingual nerve
Parotid gland
Inferior alveolar nerve
Nerve to mylohyoid
Mylohyoid
Digastric tendon
Hyoid bone

Supraorbital nerve
Supratrochlear nerve
Anterior ethmoidal nerve
Palpebral conjunctiva
External nasal nerve
Zygomatic nerve
Infraorbital nerve
Pterygopalatine nerves
Pterygopalatine ganglion
Mental nerve
Submandibular nerve
Buccinator

(B)

CN V₃
Lateral pterygoid
Temporalis
Medial pterygoid
Masseter
Mental foramen

(C)

CN V₁:
- Anterior ethmoidal nerve
- Internal nasal branches

CN V₂:
- Nasal branch of anterior superior alveolar nerve
- Internal nasal branch of infraorbital nerve
- Nasopalatine nerve

Olfactory bulb and nerve (CN I)
Maxillary nerve (CN V₂)
Nerve of pterygoid canal
Pterygopalatine ganglion
Greater palatine nerve
Lesser palatine nerve
Pharyngeal nerve

Olfactory bulb and nerve
Anterior ethmoidal nerve
Internal nasal branch of infraorbital nerve
Nasopalatine nerve
Greater palatine nerve
Lesser palatine nerve

Lateral wall   **Nasal septum**

Figure 7.24. Distribution of trigeminal nerve (CN V). A. The three divisions of CN V arise from the trigeminal ganglion. The maxillary nerve (CN V₂) gives off two nerves (roots) to the pterygopalatine ganglion. **B.** Branches of the mandibular nerve (CN V₃) pass to the muscles of mastication. **C.** This "opened book" view of the lateral wall and septum of the right nasal cavity demonstrates the distribution of CN I, CN V₁, and CN V₂.

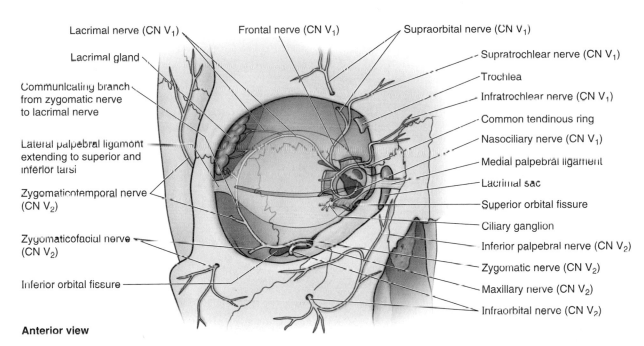

Lacrimal nerve (CN V₁)
Lacrimal gland
Communicating branch
from zygomatic nerve
to lacrimal nerve
Lateral palpebral ligament
extending to superior and
inferior tarsi
Zygomaticotemporal nerve
(CN V₂)
Zygomaticofacial nerve
(CN V₂)
Inferior orbital fissure

Frontal nerve (CN V₁)

Supraorbital nerve (CN V₁)
Supratrochlear nerve (CN V₁)
Trochlea
Infratrochlear nerve (CN V₁)
Common tendinous ring
Nasociliary nerve (CN V₁)
Medial palpebral ligament
Lacrimal sac
Superior orbital fissure
Ciliary ganglion
Inferior palpebral nerve (CN V₂)
Zygomatic nerve (CN V₂)
Maxillary nerve (CN V₂)
Infraorbital nerve (CN V₂)

Anterior view

Figure 7.25. Innervation of eyelids. The cutaneous nerves serving the orbital region are shown in relation to the skeleton of the eyelids. This skeleton is formed by the superior and inferior tarsi and their attachments, the medial and lateral palpebral ligaments, and the orbital septum. The fan-shaped aponeurosis of the levator palpebrae superioris is attached to the superior tarsus. The skin of the superior eyelid is supplied by branches of the ophthalmic nerve (CN V₁), whereas the inferior eyelid is supplied mainly by branches of the maxillary nerve (CN V₂).

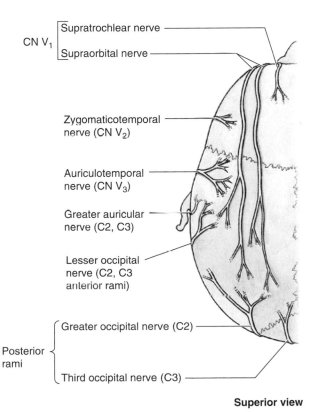

CN V₁ {
Supratrochlear nerve
Supraorbital nerve
}

Zygomaticotemporal
nerve (CN V₂)

Auriculotemporal
nerve (CN V₃)

Greater auricular
nerve (C2, C3)

Lesser occipital
nerve (C2, C3
anterior rami)

Posterior
rami {
Greater occipital nerve (C2)
Third occipital nerve (C3)
}

Superior view

Figure 7.26. Nerves of scalp. The nerves appear in sequence: CN V₁, CN V₂, CN V₃, anterior rami of C2 and C3, and posterior rami of C2 and C3.

auriculotemporal, buccal, and **mental nerves** En route to the skin, the auriculotemporal nerve passes deep to the parotid gland, conveying secretomotor fibers to it from a ganglion associated with this division of CN V.

Nerves of the Scalp

Innervation of the scalp anterior to the auricles is through branches of all three divisions of CN V, the *trigeminal nerve* (Fig. 7.26). Posterior to the auricles, the nerve supply is from spinal cutaneous nerves (C2 and C3).

Infraorbital Nerve Block

For treating wounds of the upper lip and cheek or, more commonly, for repairing the maxillary incisor teeth, local anesthesia of the inferior part of the face is achieved by infiltration of the infraorbital nerve with an anesthetic agent. The injection is made in the region of the infraorbital foramen, by elevating the upper lip and passing the needle through the junction of the oral mucosa and gingiva at the superior aspect of the oral vestibule. To determine where the infraorbital nerve emerges, pressure is exerted on the maxilla in the region of the infraorbital foramen. Too much pressure on the nerve causes considerable pain. Because companion ▶

infraorbital vessels leave the infraorbital foramen with the nerve, aspiration of the syringe during injection prevents inadvertent injection of anesthetic fluid into a blood vessel. Because the orbit is located just superior to the injection site, a careless injection could result in passage of anesthetic fluid into the orbit, causing temporary paralysis of the extraocular muscles.

Mental and Incisive Nerve Blocks

Occasionally, it is desirable to anesthetize one side of the skin and mucous membrane of the lower lip and the skin of the chin (e.g., to suture a severe laceration of the lip). Injection of an anesthetic agent into the mental foramen blocks the mental nerve that supplies the skin and mucous membrane of the lower lip from the mental foramen to the midline, including the skin of the chin.

Buccal Nerve Block

To anesthetize the skin and mucous membrane of the cheek (e.g., to suture a knife wound), an anesthetic injection can be made into the mucosa covering the *retromolar fossa,* located posterior to the 3rd mandibular molar between the anterior border of the ramus and the temporal crest.

Trigeminal Neuralgia

Trigeminal neuralgia (*tic douloureux*) is a sensory disorder of the sensory root of CN V that occurs most often in middle-aged and elderly persons. It is characterized by sudden attacks of excruciating, lightening-like jabs of facial pain. A *paroxysm* (sudden sharp pain) can last for 15 min or more. The pain may be so intense that the person winces; hence the common term *tic* (twitch). In some cases, the pain may be so severe that psychological changes occur, leading to depression and even suicide attempts. CN V$_2$ is most frequently involved, then CN V$_3$, and least frequently, CN V$_1$. The paroxysms of sudden stabbing pain are often set off by touching the face, brushing the teeth, shaving, drinking, or chewing. The pain is often initiated by touching an especially sensitive *trigger zone,* frequently located around the tip of the nose or the cheek (Haines, 2002).

The cause of trigeminal neuralgia is unknown; however, some investigators believe that most affected persons have an anomalous blood vessel that compresses the nerve (Lange et al., 2000). Often, when the aberrant artery is moved away from the sensory root of CN V, the symptoms disappear. Other scientists believe the condition is caused by a pathological process affecting neurons in the trigeminal ganglion; still others believe that neurons in the nucleus of the spinal tract may be involved (see Chapter 9).

Medical or surgical treatment or both are used to alleviate the pain. In cases involving the CN V$_2$, attempts have been made to block the infraorbital nerve at the infraorbital foramen by using alcohol. This treatment usually relieves pain temporarily. The simplest surgical procedure is avulsion or cutting of the branches of the nerve at the infraorbital foramen. Other treatments have used *radiofrequency selective ablation of parts of the trigeminal ganglion* by a needle electrode passing through the cheek and the foramen ovale. In some cases, it is necessary to section the sensory root for relief of the pain. To prevent regeneration of nerve fibers, the sensory root of the trigeminal nerve may be partially cut between the ganglion and the brainstem (*rhizotomy*). Although the axons may regenerate, they do not do so within the brainstem. Surgeons attempt to differentiate and cut only the sensory fibers to the division of CN V involved.

The same result may be achieved by sectioning the spinal tract of CN V (*tractotomy*). After this operation, the sensation of pain, temperature, and simple (light) touch is lost over the area of skin and mucous membrane supplied by the affected component of the CN V. This loss of sensation may annoy the patient, who may not recognize the presence of food on the lip and cheek or feel it within the mouth on the side of the nerve section, but these disabilities are usually preferable to excruciating pain

Lesions of the Trigeminal Nerve

Lesions of the entire trigeminal nerve cause widespread anesthesia involving the:

- Corresponding anterior half of the scalp.

- Face, except for an area around the angle of the mandible, the cornea, and conjunctiva.

- Mucous membranes of the nose, mouth, and anterior part of the tongue.

Paralysis of the muscles of mastication also occurs.

Herpes Zoster Infection of the Trigeminal Ganglion

A *herpes zoster virus infection* may produce a lesion in the cranial ganglia. Involvement of the trigeminal ganglion occurs in approximately 20% of cases (Bernardini, 2000). The infection is characterized by an eruption of groups of vesicles following the course of the affected nerve (e.g., *ophthalmic herpes zoster*). Any division of CN V may be involved, but the ophthalmic division is most commonly affected. Usually, the cornea is involved, often resulting in painful *corneal ulceration* and subsequent *scarring of the cornea.* ▶

Testing the Sensory Function of CN V

The sensory function of the trigeminal nerve is tested by asking the person to close his or her eyes, and respond when types of touch are felt. For example, a piece of dry gauze is gently stroked across the skin of one side of the face and then to the corresponding position on the other side. The test is then repeated until the skin of the forehead (CN V₁), cheek (CN V₂), and lower jaw (CN V₃) have been tested. The person is asked if one side feels the same as or different from the other side. The testing may then be repeated using warm or cold instruments and the gentle touch of a sharp pin, again alternating sides (Fig. B7.18). ○

A   **B**   **Figure B7.18**

Motor Nerves of the Face

The motor nerves of the face are the *facial nerve* to the muscles of facial expression and the *motor root of the trigeminal nerve/mandibular nerve* to the muscles of mastication (masseter, temporal, medial, and lateral pterygoids). These nerves also supply some more deeply placed muscles (described later in this chapter in relation to the mouth, middle ear, and neck) (Fig. 7.24A).

Facial Nerve

CN VII, the facial nerve, has both a motor root and a sensory/parasympathetic root (the latter being the *intermediate nerve*). The **motor root of CN VII** supplies the muscles of facial expression, including the superficial muscle of the neck (platysma), auricular muscles, scalp muscles, and certain other muscles derived from mesoderm in the embryonic second pharyngeal arch (Fig. 7.27). Following a circuitous route through the temporal bone, CN VII emerges from the cranium through the *stylomastoid foramen* located between the mastoid and the styloid processes (Fig. 7.5A). It immediately gives off the **posterior auricular nerve**, which passes posterosuperior to the auricle of the ear to supply the auricularis posterior and occipital belly of the occipitofrontalis muscle (Fig. 7.27). The main trunk of CN VII runs anteriorly and is engulfed by the parotid gland, in which it forms the **parotid plexus**, which gives rise to the five terminal branches of the facial nerve: *temporal, zygomatic, buccal, marginal mandibular,* and *cervical.* The names of the branches refer to the regions they supply. Specific muscles supplied by each branch are identified in Table 7.4.

The **temporal branch** of CN VII emerges from the superior border of the parotid gland and crosses the zygomatic arch to supply the auricularis superior and auricularis anterior; the frontal belly of the occipitofrontalis; and, most important, the superior part of the orbicularis oculi (Fig. 7.27A; Table 7.4).

The **zygomatic branch** of CN VII passes via two or three branches superior and mainly inferior to the eye to supply the inferior part of the orbicularis oculi and other facial muscles inferior to the orbit.

The **buccal branch** of CN VII passes external to the buccinator to supply this muscle and muscles of the upper lip (upper parts of orbicularis oris and inferior fibers of levator labii superioris).

The **marginal mandibular branch** of CN VII supplies the risorius and muscles of the lower lip and chin. It emerges from the inferior border of the parotid gland and crosses the inferior border of the mandible deep to the platysma to reach the face. In approximately 20% of people, this branch passes inferior to the angle of the mandible.

The **cervical branch** of CN VII passes inferiorly from the inferior border of the parotid gland and runs posterior to the mandible to supply the platysma (Fig. 7.27B).

Injuries to the Facial Nerve

Injury to branches of the facial nerve causes paralysis of the facial muscles (Bell palsy), with or without loss of taste on the anterior two thirds of the tongue or altered secretion of the lacrimal and salivary glands (see clinical correlation [blue] box "Paralysis of Facial Muscles," ▶

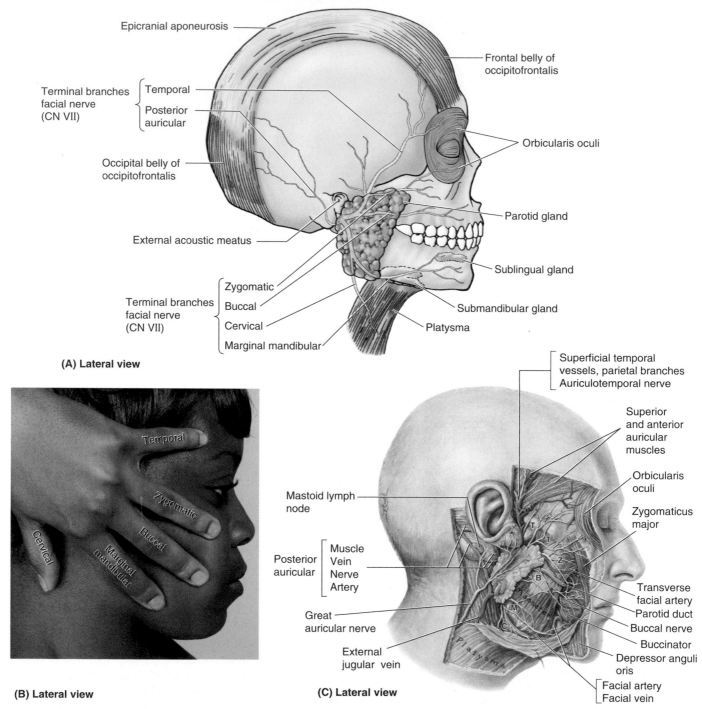

(A) Lateral view

(B) Lateral view

(C) Lateral view

Figure 7.27. Branches of facial nerve (CN VII). A. The terminal branches of CN VII arise from the parotid plexus within the parotid gland. They emerge from the gland under cover of its lateral surface and radiate in a generally anterior direction across the face. Although intimately related to the parotid gland (and often contacting the submandibular gland via one or more of its lower branches), CN VII does not send nerve fibers to the salivary glands. Two muscles representing the extremes of the distribution of CN VII, the occipitofrontalis and platysma, are also shown. **B.** A simple method for demonstrating and remembering the general course of the five terminal branches of CN VII to the face and neck. **C.** Dissection of the right side of the head showing the great auricular nerve (C2 and C3), which supplies the parotid sheath and skin over the angle of the mandible, and terminal branches of the facial nerve, which supply the muscles of facial expression. *B,* buccal; *C,* cervical; *M,* marginal mandibular; *T,* temporal; *Z,* zygomatic.

earlier in this chapter). Lesions near the origin of CN VII from the pons of the brain or proximal to the origin of the greater petrosal nerve (in the region of the geniculate ganglion), result in loss of motor, gustatory (taste), and autonomic functions. Lesions distal to the geniculate ganglion, but proximal to the origin of the chorda tympani nerve, produce the same dysfunction, except that lacrimal secretion is not affected. Lesions near the stylomastoid foramen result in loss of motor function only (i.e., facial paralysis).

Facial nerve palsy has many causes. The most common non-traumatic cause of facial paralysis is *inflammation of the facial nerve* near the stylomastoid foramen, probably as a result of a viral infection. This produces edema (swelling) and compression of the nerve in the facial canal. Injury of the facial nerve often results from *fracture of the temporal bone;* facial paralysis is evident soon after the injury. If the nerve is completely sectioned, the chances of complete or even partial recovery are remote. Muscular movement usually improves when the nerve damage is associated with blunt head trauma; however, recovery may not be complete (Rowland, 2000). Facial nerve palsy may be idiopathic, occurring without a known cause (e.g., Bell palsy); but it often follows exposure to cold, as occurs when riding in a car or sleeping with a window open.

Facial paralysis may be a complication of surgery; consequently, identification of the facial nerve is essential during surgery (e.g., *parotidectomy,* removal of a parotid gland). The facial nerve is most distinct as it emerges from the stylomastoid foramen; if necessary, electrical stimulation may be used for confirmation. Facial nerve palsy may also be associated with dental manipulation, vaccination, pregnancy, HIV infection, Lyme disease (inflammatory disorder causing headache and stiff neck), and infections of the middle ear (otitis media).

Because the branches of the facial nerve are superficial, they are subject to injury by stab and gunshot wounds, cuts, and injury at birth:

- A *lesion of the zygomatic branch* of CN VII causes paralysis, including loss of tonus of the orbicularis oculi in the inferior eyelid.
- *Paralysis of the buccal branch* of CN VII causes paralysis of the buccinator and superior portion of the orbicularis oris and upper lip muscles.
- *Paralysis of the marginal mandibular branch* of CN VII may occur when an incision is made along the inferior border of the mandible. Injury to this branch (e.g., during a surgical approach to the submandibular gland) causes paralysis of the inferior portion of the orbicularis oris and lower lip muscles.

The consequences of such paralyses are discussed in clinical correlation (blue) box "Paralysis of Facial Muscles." ○

THE BOTTOM LINE: The face is highly sensitive. It receives sensory innervation from the three divisions of the trigeminal nerve (CN V). The major terminal branches of each division reach the subcutaneous tissue of each side of the face via three foramina that are aligned vertically. Each division supplies a distinct sensory zone, similar to a dermatome but without the overlapping of adjacent nerves; therefore, injuries result in distinct and defined areas of paresthesia. The divisions of CN V supply sensation not only to the superficial skin of the face but also to deep mucosal surfaces of the conjunctival sacs, cornea, nasal cavity and paranasal sinuses, and the oral cavity and vestibule. The skin covering the angle of the mandible is innervated by the great auricular nerve, a branch of the cervical plexus. The facial nerve (CN VII) is the motor nerve of the face, supplying all the muscles of facial expression, including the platysma, occipital belly of the occipitofrontalis, and auricular muscles that are not part of the face per se. The muscles receive innervation from CN VII primarily via five branches of the parotid (nerve) plexus. Eight nerves supply sensation to the scalp via branches arising from all three divisions of CN V anterior to the auricle of the ear and branches of cervical spinal nerves posterior to the auricle.

Superficial Vasculature of the Face and Scalp

The face is richly supplied by with superficial arteries and external veins, as is evident in blushing and blanching. The terminal branches of both arteries and veins anastomose freely, including anastomoses across the midline with contralateral partners. Most arteries of the face are branches or derivatives of branches of the *external carotid artery;* the origin, course, and distribution of these arteries are presented in Table 7.6. Most external facial veins are drained by veins that accompany the arteries of the face. As with most superficial veins, they are subject to many variations; a common pattern is shown in Table 7.7. The venous return from the face is normally superficial, but anastomoses with deep veins, a dural sinus, and venous plexus can provide deep drainage for the valveless veins.

Superficial Arteries of the Face

The superficial arteries of the face are illustrated and their origins, courses, and distributions are listed in Table 7.6. The **facial artery** provides the major arterial supply to the face. It arises from the external carotid artery and winds its way to the inferior border of the mandible, just anterior to the masseter

Table 7.6. Superficial Arteries of the Face and Scalp

(A) Superior view

(B) Lateral view

*Source = internal carotid artery; all other labeled
arteries are from external carotid

Artery	Origin	Course	Distribution
Facial	External carotid artery	Ascends deep to submandibular gland; winds around inferior border of mandible and enters face	Muscles of facial expression and face
Inferior labial	Facial artery near angle of mouth	Runs medially in lower lip	Lower lip
Superior labial		Runs medially in upper lip	Upper lip and ala (side) and septum of nose
Lateral nasal	Facial artery as it ascends alongside nose	Passes to ala of nose	Skin on ala and dorsum of nose
Angular	Terminal branch of facial artery	Passes to medial angle (canthus) of eye	Superior part of cheek and inferior eyelid
Occipital	External carotid artery	Passes medial to posterior belly of digastric and mastoid process; accompanies occipital nerve in occipital region	Scalp of back of head, as far as vertex
Posterior auricular		Passes posteriorly, deep to parotid gland, along styloid process between mastoid process and ear	Scalp posterior to auricle and auricle
Superficial temporal	Smaller terminal branch of external carotid artery	Ascends anterior to ear to temporal region and ends in scalp	Facial muscles and skin of frontal and temporal regions
Transverse facial	Superficial temporal artery within parotid gland	Crosses face superficial to masseter and inferior to zygomatic arch	Parotid gland and duct, muscles and skin of face
Mental	Terminal branch of inferior alveolar artery	Emerges from mental foramen and passes to chin	Facial muscles and skin of chin
Supraorbital[a]	Terminal branch of ophthalmic artery, a branch of internal carotid artery	Passes superiorly from supraorbital foramen	Muscles and skin of forehead and scalp
Supratrochlear[a]		Passes superiorly from supratrochlear notch	Muscles and skin of scalp

[a]Source is internal carotid artery.

Table 7.7. Veins of the Face and Scalp

Parietal tributary of superficial temporal vein
Cavernous sinus
Superficial temporal vein
Middle temporal vein
Pterygoid venous plexus
Maxillary vein
Retromandibular vein
Posterior auricular vein
Communicating branch
External jugular vein
Internal jugular vein
Subclavian vein

Frontal tributary of superficial temporal vein
Superior and inferior ophthalmic veins
Supratrochlear vein
Supraorbital vein
Superior and inferior palpebral veins
Angular vein
External nasal vein
Superior labial vein
Inferior labial vein
Deep facial vein
Submental vein
Facial vein
Common facial vein
Brachiocephalic vein

Lateral view

Vein	Origin	Course	Termination	Area Drained
Supratrochlear	Begins from venous plexus on forehead and scalp, through which it communicates with frontal branch of superficial temporal vein, its contralateral partner, and supraorbital vein	Descends near midline of forehead to root of nose, where it joins supraorbital vein	Angular vein at root of nose	Anterior part of scalp and forehead
Supraorbital	Begins in the forehead by anastomosing with frontal tributary of superficial temporal vein	Passes medially superior to orbit; joins supratrochlear vein; a branch passes through supraorbital notch and joins with superior ophthalmic vein		
Angular	Begins at root of nose by union of supratrochlear and supraorbital veins	Descends obliquely along root and side of nose to inferior orbital margin	Becomes facial vein at inferior margin of orbit	Anterior part of scalp and forehead; superior and inferior eyelids and conjunctiva; may receive drainage from cavernous sinus
Facial	Continuation of angular vein past inferior margin of orbit	Descends along lateral border of nose, receiving external nasal and inferior palpebral veins; then passes obliquely across face to cross inferior border of mandible; receives communication from retromandibular vein (after which, it is sometimes called common facial vein)	Internal jugular vein opposite or inferior to level of hyoid bone	Anterior scalp and forehead; eyelids; external nose; anterior cheek; lips; chin; and submandibular gland

Table 7.7. Veins of the Face and Scalp *(continued)*

Vein	Origin	Course	Termination	Area Drained
Deep facial	Pterygoid venous plexus	Runs anteriorly on maxilla superior to buccinator and deep to masseter, emerging medial to anterior border of masseter onto face	Enters posterior aspect of facial vein	Infratemporal fossa (most areas supplied by maxillary artery)
Superficial temporal	Begins from widespread plexus of veins on side of scalp and along zygomatic arch	Frontal and parietal tributaries unite anterior to the auricle; crosses temporal root of zygomatic arch to pass from temporal region and enter substance of the parotid gland	Joins maxillary vein posterior to neck of mandible to form retromandibular vein	Side of scalp; superficial aspect of temporal muscle; and external ear
Retromandibular	Formed anterior to ear by union of superficial temporal and maxillary veins	Runs posterior and deep to ramus of mandible through substance of parotid gland; communicates at inferior end with facial vein	Unites with posterior auricular vein to form external jugular vein	Parotid gland and masseter muscle

(Fig. 7.27*C*). The artery lies superficially here, immediately deep to the platysma. The facial artery crosses the mandible, buccinator, and maxilla as it courses over the face to the medial angle (canthus) of the eye, where the superior and inferior eyelids meet. The facial artery lies deep to the zygomaticus major and levator labii superioris muscles. Near the termination of its sinuous course through the face, the facial artery passes approximately a finger's breadth lateral to the angle of the mouth. It sends branches to the upper and lower lips (the **superior** and **inferior labial arteries**), ascends along the side of the nose, and anastomoses with the dorsal nasal branch of the ophthalmic artery. Distal to the **lateral nasal artery** at the side of the nose, the terminal part of the facial artery is called the **angular artery.**

The **superficial temporal artery** is the smaller terminal branch of the external carotid artery; the other branch is the *maxillary artery.* The superficial temporal artery emerges on the face between the TMJ and the auricle, enters the temporal fossa, and ends in the scalp by dividing into *frontal* and *parietal branches.* These arterial branches accompany or run in close proximity to the corresponding branches of the auriculotemporal nerve.

The **transverse facial artery** arises from the superficial temporal artery within the parotid gland and crosses the face superficial to the masseter (Fig. 7.27*C*), approximately a finger's breadth inferior to the zygomatic arch. It divides into numerous branches that supply the parotid gland and duct, the masseter, and the skin of the face. It anastomoses with branches of the facial artery.

In addition to the superficial temporal arteries, several other arteries accompany cutaneous nerves in the face. **Supraorbital** and **supratrochlear arteries,** branches of the ophthalmic artery, accompany nerves of the same name across the eyebrows and forehead. The supraorbital artery continues and supplies the anterior scalp to the vertex. The

mental artery, the only superficial branch derived from the maxillary artery, accompanies the nerve of the same name in the chin.

Arteries of the Scalp

The scalp has a rich blood supply (Table 7.6). The arteries course within layer two of the scalp, the subcutaneous connective tissue layer between the skin and the epicranial aponeurosis. They anastomose freely with one another. The arterial walls are firmly attached to the dense connective tissue in which they are embedded, limiting their ability to constrict when cut. Consequently, bleeding from scalp wounds is profuse. The arterial supply is from the **external carotid arteries** through the *occipital, posterior auricular,* and *superficial temporal arteries* and from the *internal carotid arteries* through the *supratrochlear* and *supraorbital arteries.* The arteries of the scalp supply little blood to the neurocranium, which is supplied primarily by the middle meningeal artery.

Compression of the Facial Artery

The facial artery can be occluded by pressure against the mandible where the vessel crosses it. Because of the numerous anastomoses between the branches of the facial artery and other arteries of the face, compression of the facial artery on one side does not stop all bleeding from a lacerated facial artery or one of its branches. In lacerations of the lip, pressure must be applied on both sides of the cut to stop the bleeding. In general, facial wounds bleed freely and heal quickly. ▶

Pulses of the Arteries of the Face

The pulses of the superficial temporal and facial arteries can be used for taking the pulse. For example, anesthesiologists at the head of the operating table often take the *temporal pulse* anterior to the auricle where the superficial temporal artery crosses the zygomatic process just anterior to the auricle. Clench your teeth and feel the *facial pulse* as the facial artery crosses the inferior border of the mandible immediately anterior to the masseter muscle.

Stenosis of the Internal Carotid Artery

At the medial angle of the eye, an anastomosis occurs between the facial artery, a branch of the external carotid artery, and the cutaneous branches of the internal carotid artery. With advancing age, the internal carotid artery may become narrow (stenotic) owing to atherosclerotic thickening of the intima of the arteries. Because of the arterial anastomosis, intracranial structures such as the brain can receive blood from the connection of the facial artery to the dorsal nasal branch of the ophthalmic artery.

Scalp Lacerations

Scalp lacerations are the most common type of head injury requiring surgical care. These wounds bleed profusely because the arteries entering the periphery of the scalp bleed from both ends owing to abundant anastomoses. The arteries do not retract when lacerated because they are held open by the dense connective tissue in layer two of the scalp. Spasms of the occipitofrontalis can increase gaping of scalp wounds. Bleeding from scalp lacerations can be fatal if not controlled (e.g., by sutures).

Scalp Injuries

Because the scalp arteries arising at the sides of the head are well protected by dense connective tissue and anastomose freely, a *partially detached scalp* may be replaced with a reasonable chance of healing as long as one of the vessels supplying the scalp remains intact. During an *attached craniotomy* (surgical removal of a segment of the calvaria with a soft tissue scalp flap to expose the cranial cavity) the incisions are usually made convex upward, and the superficial temporal artery is included in the tissue flap. The *scalp proper,* the first three layers of the scalp, is often regarded clinically as a single layer because they remain together when a scalp flap is made during a craniotomy and when part of the scalp is torn off (e.g., during industrial accidents). Nerves and vessels of the scalp enter inferiorly and ascend through layer two to the skin. Consequently, surgical pedicle scalp flaps are made so that they remain attached inferiorly to preserve the nerves and vessels, thereby promoting good healing. The arteries of the scalp supply little blood to the calvaria, which is supplied by the middle meningeal arteries. Therefore, loss of the scalp does not produce necrosis of the calvarial bones. ✪

External Veins of the Face

The major external veins of the head and face are illustrated and their origins, courses, terminations, and the areas drained by each are provided in Table 7.7. Like veins elsewhere, they are highly variable and have abundant anastomoses that allow drainage to occur by alternate routes during periods of temporary compression. The alternate routes include both superficial pathways (via the facial and retromandibular/external jugular veins) and deep drainage (via the anastomoses with the cavernous sinus, pterygoid venous plexus, and the internal jugular vein).

The **facial veins,** coursing with or parallel to the facial arteries, are valveless veins that provide the primary superficial drainage of the face. Tributaries of the facial vein include the **deep facial vein,** which drains the *pterygoid venous plexus* of the infratemporal fossa. Inferior to the margin of the mandible, the facial vein is joined by the anterior (communicating) branch of the retromandibular vein. The facial vein drains directly or indirectly into the *IJV.* At the medial angle of the eye, the facial vein communicates with the *superior ophthalmic vein,* which drains into the *cavernous sinus.*

The **retromandibular vein,** formed by the union of the superficial temporal and maxillary veins, is a deep vein of the face formed by the union of the superficial temporal vein and the maxillary vein, the latter draining the pterygoid plexus. The retromandibular vein runs posterior to the ramus of the mandible within the substance of the parotid gland, superficial to the external carotid artery and deep to the facial nerve. As it emerges from the inferior pole of the gland, the retromandibular vein divides into an anterior branch that unites with the facial vein and a posterior branch that joins the posterior auricular vein inferior to the parotid gland to form the **external jugular vein.** This vein passes inferiorly and superficially in the neck to empty into the subclavian vein.

Veins of the Scalp

The venous drainage of superficial parts of the scalp is through the accompanying veins of the scalp arteries, the **supraorbital** and **supratrochlear veins** (Table 7.7). The **superficial temporal veins** and **posterior auricular veins** drain the scalp anterior and posterior to the auricles, respectively. The posterior auricular vein often receives a *mastoid emissary vein* from the sigmoid sinus, a dural venous sinus. The **occipital veins** drain the occipital region of the scalp. Venous drainage of deep parts of the scalp in the temporal region is through **deep temporal veins,** which are tributaries of the pterygoid venous plexus.

Thrombophlebitis of the Facial Vein

The facial vein makes clinically important connections with the cavernous sinus, a venous sinus of the dura mater, through the superior ophthalmic vein, and the pterygoid plexus, a network of small veins within the infratemporal fossa, through the inferior ophthalmic and deep facial veins (Fig. 7.12; Table 7.7). Because of these connections, an infection of the face may spread to the cavernous sinus and pterygoid venous plexus.

Blood from the medial angle of the eye, nose, and lips usually drains inferiorly through the facial vein, especially when a person is erect. Because the facial vein has no valves, blood may pass through it in the opposite direction; consequently, venous blood from the face may enter the cavernous sinus. In individuals with *thrombophlebitis of the facial vein,* inflammation of the facial vein with secondary thrombus (clot) formation, pieces of an infected clot may extend into the intracranial venous system and produce *thrombophlebitis of the cavernous sinus.* Infection of the facial veins spreading to the dural venous sinuses may result from lacerations of the nose or be initiated by squeezing pustules (pimples) on the side of the nose and upper lip. Consequently, the triangular area from the upper lip to the bridge of the nose is considered the *danger triangle of the face* (Fig. B7.19). ⊕

Figure B7.19

Lymphatic Drainage of the Face and Scalp

There are no lymph nodes in the scalp and except for the parotid/buccal region, there are no lymph nodes in the face. Lymph from the scalp, face, and neck drains into the *superficial ring* (pericervical collar) *of lymph nodes*—submental, submandibular, parotid, mastoid, and occipital—located at the junction of the head and neck (Fig. 7.28A). The lymphatic vessels of the face accompany other facial vessels. Superficial lymphatic vessels accompany veins, and deep lymphatics ac-

company arteries. All lymphatic vessels from the head and neck drain directly or indirectly into the *deep cervical lymph nodes* (Fig. 7.28B), a chain of nodes mainly located along the IJV in the neck. Lymph from these deep nodes passes to the **jugular lymphatic trunk,** which joins the *thoracic duct* on the left side and the IJV or **brachiocephalic vein** on the right side. A summary of the lymphatic drainage of the face follows.

- Lymph from the lateral part of the face and scalp, including the eyelids, drains to the superficial **parotid lymph nodes.**

- Lymph from the deep parotid nodes drains to the **deep cervical lymph nodes.**

- Lymph from the upper lip and lateral parts of the lower lip drains to the **submandibular lymph nodes.**

- Lymph from the chin and central part of the lower lip drains to the **submental lymph nodes.**

Squamous Cell Carcinoma of the Lip

Squamous cell carcinoma (cancer) of the lip usually involves the lower lip (Fig. B7.20). Overexposure to sunshine over many years, is a common factor in these cases. Chronic irritation from pipe smoking is also a contributing cause. Cancer cells from the central part of the lower lip, the floor of the mouth, and the apex of the tongue spread to the submental lymph nodes, whereas cancer cells from lateral parts of the lower lip drain to the submandibular lymph nodes. ⊕

Figure B7.20

THE BOTTOM LINE: The face and scalp are highly vascular. The terminal branches of the arteries of the face anastomose freely (including anastomoses across the midline with their contralateral partners); thus bleeding from facial lacerations may be diffuse, with the lacerated vessel bleeding from both ends. Most arteries of the face are branches or derivatives of branches of the external carotid artery; the arteries arising from the internal carotid that supply the

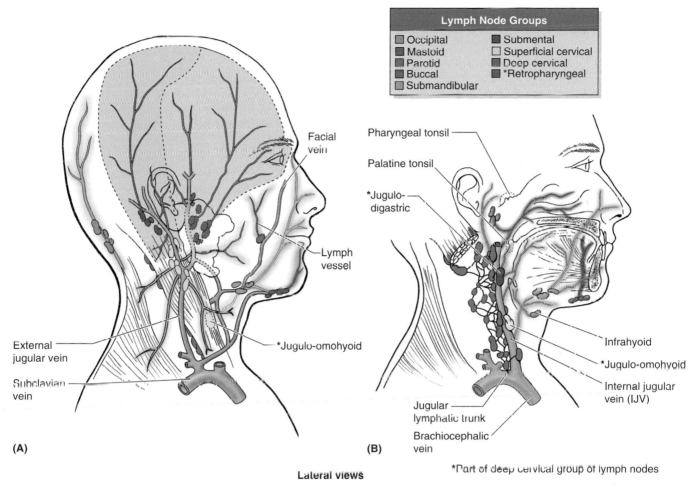

Lymph Node Groups

☐ Occipital	■ Submental
■ Mastoid	☐ Superficial cervical
■ Parotid	■ Deep cervical
■ Buccal	■ *Retropharyngeal
■ Submandibular	

Facial vein

Lymph vessel

External jugular vein

Subclavian vein

*Jugulo-omohyoid

(A)

Pharyngeal tonsil

Palatine tonsil

*Jugulo-digastric

Infrahyoid

*Jugulo-omohyoid

Internal jugular vein (IJV)

Jugular lymphatic trunk

Brachiocephalic vein

(B)

Lateral views

*Part of deep cervical group of lymph nodes

Figure 7.28. Lymphatic drainage of face and scalp. A. The superficial drainage is shown. A pericervical collar of superficial lymph nodes is formed at the junction of the head and neck by the submental, submandibular, parotid, mastoid, and occipital nodes. These nodes initially receive most of the lymph drainage from the face and scalp. **B.** The deep drainage is shown. All lymphatic vessels from the head and neck ultimately drain into the deep cervical lymph nodes, either directly from the tissues or indirectly after passing through an outlying group of nodes.

forehead are exceptions. The main artery to the face is the facial artery. The arteries of the scalp are firmly embedded in the dense connective tissue overlying the epicranial aponeurosis. Thus, when lacerated, the arteries bleed from both ends, like those of the face, but are less able to constrict or retract than other superficial vessels; therefore, profuse bleeding results. The veins of the face and scalp generally accompany arteries, providing a primarily superficial venous drainage. However, they also anastomose with the pterygoid venous plexus and with dural venous sinuses via emissary veins, which provides a potentially dangerous route for the spread of infection. Most nerves and vessels of the scalp run vertically toward the vertex; thus a horizontal laceration may produce more neurovascular damage than a vertical one.

The lymphatic drainage of most of the face follows the venous drainage to lymph nodes around the base of the anterior part of the head (submandibular, parotid, and superficial cervical nodes). An exception to this pattern is the lymph drainage of the central part of the lip and chin, which initially drains to the submental lymph nodes. All these nodes drain in turn to the deep cervical lymph nodes.

Parotid Gland

The parotid gland is the largest of three paired salivary glands. From a functional viewpoint, it would seem logical to discuss all three glands simultaneously in association with the anatomy of the mouth. However, from an anatomical viewpoint, particularly in dissection courses, the parotid gland is usually examined with or immediately subsequent to the dissection of the face to expose the facial nerve. Dissection of the parotid region must be completed before dissection of the infratemporal region and muscles of mastication or the carotid triangle of the neck. The submandibular gland is encountered primarily during dissection of the submandibular triangle of the neck, and the sublingual glands when dissecting the floor of the mouth.

The parotid gland is enclosed within a tough fascial capsule, the **parotid sheath,** derived from the *investing layer of deep cervical fascia* (Fig. 7.29). The parotid gland has an irregular shape because the area occupied by the gland, the **parotid bed,** is anteroinferior to the external acoustic meatus, where it is wedged between the ramus of the mandible and the mastoid process (Fig. 7.27*A*). Fatty tissue between the lobes of the gland confers the flexibility the gland must have to accommodate the motion of the mandible. The apex of the parotid gland is posterior to the angle of the mandible, and its base is related to the zygomatic arch. The subcutaneous lateral surface of the parotid gland is almost flat. The **parotid duct** passes horizontally from the anterior edge of the gland (Fig. 7.29). At the anterior border of the masseter, the duct turns medially, pierces the buccinator, and enters the oral cavity through a small orifice opposite the 2nd maxillary molar tooth. Embedded within the substance of the parotid gland, from superficial to deep, are the *parotid plexus of the facial nerve* (CN VII) and its branches (Figs. 7.27*A* & *C* and 7.29), the *retromandibular vein,* and the *external carotid artery.* On the parotid sheath and within the gland are *parotid lymph nodes* (Figs. 7.28*A* and 7.29).

Innervation of Parotid Gland and Related Structures

Although the parotid plexus of CN VII is embedded within it, the CN VII does not provide innervation to the gland. The *auriculotemporal nerve,* a branch of CN V$_3$, is closely related to the parotid gland and passes superior to it with the superficial temporal vessels. The **great auricular nerve,** a branch of the cervical plexus composed of fibers from C2 and C3 spinal nerves, innervates the parotid sheath (Fig. 7.29) as well as the overlying skin. The parasympathetic component of the **glossopharyngeal nerve** (CN IX) supplies presynpatic secretory fibers to the *otic ganglion.* The postsynaptic parasympathetic fibers are conveyed from the ganglion to the gland by the auriculotemporal nerve (Fig. 7.24*A*). Stimulation of the parasympathetic fibers produces a thin, watery saliva. Sympathetic fibers are derived from the cervical ganglia through the **external carotid nerve plexus** on the external carotid artery (Fig. 7.29). The vasomotor activity of these fibers may reduce secretion from the gland. Sensory nerve fibers pass to the gland through the great auricular and auriculotemporal nerves.

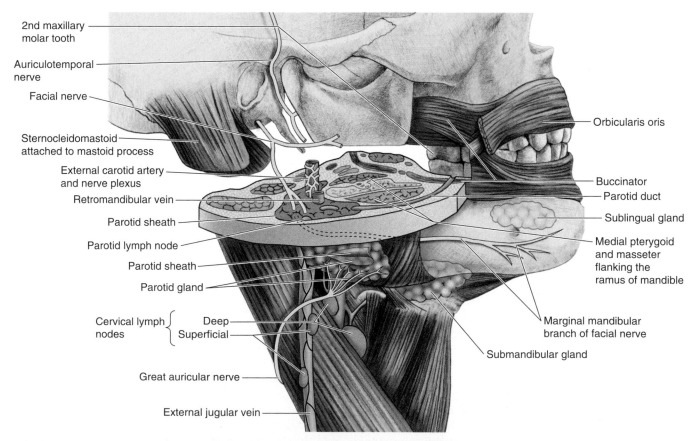

Figure 7.29. Relationships of parotid gland. A transverse slice through the bed of the parotid gland demonstrates the relationship of the gland to surrounding structures. The gland passes deeply between the ramus of the mandible, flanked by the muscles of mastication anteriorly and the mastoid process and sternocleidomastoid muscle posteriorly. The dimensions of the parotid bed change with movements of the mandible. The external carotid artery and periarterial plexus, retromandibular vein, and parotid plexus of the facial nerve (CN VII) are embedded within the gland itself. The parotid duct turns medially at the anterior border of the masseter muscle and pierces the buccinator.

Parotidectomy

About 80% of salivary gland tumors occur in the parotid glands. Most tumors of the parotid glands are benign, but most salivary gland cancer begins in the parotid. Surgical excision of the parotid gland (*parotidectomy*) is often performed as part of the treatment. Because the parotid plexus of CN VII is embedded in the parotid gland, the plexus and its branches are in jeopardy during surgery. An important step in parotidectomy is the identification, dissection, isolation, and preservation of the facial nerve. A superficial portion of the gland (often erroneously referred to as a "lobe") is removed, after which the parotid plexus, which occupies a distinct plane within the gland, can be retracted to enable dissection of the deep portion of the gland.

The parotid gland makes a substantial contribution to the posterolateral contour of the face, the extent of its contribution being especially evident after it has been surgically removed. See clinical correlation (blue) box "Paralysis of Facial Muscles," earlier in this chapter, for a discussion of the functional consequences of injury to the facial nerve.

Infection of the Parotid Gland

The parotid gland may become infected by infectious agents that pass through the bloodstream, as occurs in *mumps*, an acute communicable viral disease. Infection of the gland causes inflammation (*parotiditis*) and swelling of the gland. Severe pain occurs because the parotid sheath limits swelling. Often the pain is worse during chewing because the enlarged gland is wrapped around the posterior border of the ramus of the mandible and is compressed against the mastoid process of the temporal bone when the mouth is opened. The mumps virus may also cause *inflammation of the parotid duct,* producing *redness of the parotid papilla,* the small projection at the opening of the duct into the superior oral vestibule. Because the pain produced by mumps may be confused with a toothache, redness of the papilla is often an early sign that the disease involves the gland and not a tooth.

Parotid gland disease often causes pain in the auricle, external acoustic meatus, temporal region, and TMJ because the auriculotemporal nerve, from which the parotid gland and sheath receive sensory fibers, also supplies sensory fibers to the skin over the temporal fossa and auricle.

Abscess in the Parotid Gland

A bacterial infection localized in the parotid gland usually produces an abscess. The infection could result from extremely poor dental hygiene and spread to the gland through the parotid ducts. Physicians and dentists must determine whether a swelling of the cheek results from infection of the parotid gland or from an abscess of dental origin.

Sialography of the Parotid Duct

A radiopaque fluid can be injected into the duct system of the parotid gland through a cannula inserted through the orifice of the parotid duct in the mucous membrane of the cheek. This technique *(sialography)* is followed by radiography of the gland. *Parotid sialograms* (G. *sialon*, saliva + G. *grapho*, to write) demonstrate parts of the parotid duct system that may be displaced or dilated by disease.

Blockage of the Parotid Duct

The parotid duct may be blocked by a calcified deposit, called a *sialolith* or *calculus* (L. pebble). The resulting pain in the parotid gland is made worse by eating. Sucking a lemon slice is painful because of the buildup of saliva in the proximal part of the blocked duct.

Accessory Parotid Gland

Sometimes an accessory parotid gland lies on the masseter muscle between the parotid duct and the zygomatic arch. Several ducts open from this accessory gland into the parotid duct. ✚

THE BOTTOM LINE: The largest of the salivary glands, the parotid gland makes a substantial contribution to the contour of the face. Occupying a complex space anterior to the auricle, the gland straddles most of the posterior aspect of the ramus of the mandible. Fatty tissue in the gland gives it flexibility to accommodate the motion of the mandible. The parotid duct passes anteriorly across the masseter, parallel and about a finger's breadth inferior to the zygomatic arch, and then turns medially to enter the superior oral vestibule opposite the 2nd maxillary molar. Parotid fascia, continuous with the investing layer of deep cervical fascia, invests the gland as the parotid sheath. The sheath is innervated by the great auricular nerve, but the gland receives parasympathetic secretomotor innervation from the glossopharyngeal nerve via a complex route involving the otic ganglion.

Surface Anatomy of the Head

Regions of the Head

To allow clear communications regarding the location of structures, injuries, or pathologies, the head is divided into regions (Fig. SA7.1). The large number of regions into which the relatively small area of the face is divided (eight) is a reflection of both its functional complexity and personal importance, as are annual expenditures for elective aesthetic surgery. With the exception of the **auricular region**, which includes the external ear, the names of the regions of the neurocranial portion of the head correspond to the underlying bones or bony features: **frontal, parietal, occipital, temporal,** and **mastoid regions.** The viscerocranial portion includes the **facial region**, which is divided into five bilateral and three median regions related to superficial features (**oral** and **buccal regions**), to deeper soft tissue formations (**parotid region**), and to skeletal features (**orbital, infraorbital, nasal, zygomatic,** and **mental regions**). The remainder of this chapter discusses several of these regions in detail as well as some deep regions not represented on the surface (for example, the infratemporal region and the pterygopalatine fossa). The surface anatomy of these regions will be discussed with the description of each region.

Surface Anatomy of the Face

Despite the apparently infinite variations that enable people to be identified as individuals, the features that the human face bears are constant (Fig. SA7.2). The **eyebrows** (L. *supercilia*) are linear growths of hair overlying the **superior orbital margin.** The hairless region between the eyebrows overlies the **glabella,** and the prominent ridges that extend laterally on each side above the eyebrows are the **superciliary arches.** The **eyelids** (L. *palpebrae*) are mobile, musculofibrous folds that overlie the eyeball. They are joined at each end of the **palpebral fissure** between them at the **medial** and **lateral angles** (canthi) of the eye. The **epicanthal fold (epicanthus)** is a fold of skin that covers the medial angle of the eye in some people, chiefly Asians. The depressions superior and inferior to the lids are the **suprapalpebral** and **infrapalpebral sulci.**

The external nose presents a prominent **apex** (tip), and is continuous with the forehead at the **root of the nose** (bridge). The rounded anterior border between the root and apex is the **dorsum of the nose.** Inferior to the apex, the nasal cavity of each side opens anteriorly by a **naris** (pleural = nares), bounded medially by the **nasal septum** and laterally by an **ala** (wing) **of the nose.**

The lips surround the opening of the mouth, the **oral fissure.** The **vermillion border** of the lip marks the beginning of the **transitional zone** (commonly referred ▶

Figure SA7.1

Regions of the Head

1. Frontal region
2. Parietal region
3. Occipital region
4. Temporal region
5. Auricular region
6. Mastoid region

Facial region:

7. Orbital region
8. Infraorbital region
9. Buccal region
10. Parotid region
11. Zygomatic region
12. Nasal region
13. Oral region
14. Mental region

Regions of the Neck

Anterior region (triangle):

15. Submandibular triangle
16. Carotid triangle
17. Muscular triangle
18. Submental triangle
19. Sternocleidomastoid region
20. Lesser supraclavicular fossa
21. Lateral region (post. triangle)
22. Omoclavicular triangle
23. Suboccipital region
24. Posterior cervical region

to as the lip) between the skin and the mucous membrane of the lip. The skin of the transitional zone is hairless and thin, increasing its sensitivity and causing its color to be different (because of underlying capillary beds) from that of the adjacent skin of the face. The lateral junction of the lips is the **labial commissure;** the angle between the lips, medial to the commissure, that increases as the mouth opens and decreases as it closes is the **angle of the mouth.** The median part of the upper lip features a **tubercle,** superior to which is a shallow groove, the **philtrum** (G. love charm), extending to the nasal septum.

The musculofibrous folds of the lips continue laterally as the **cheek,** which also contains the buccinator and buccal fat-pad. The cheek is separated from the lips by the **nasolabial sulcus,** which runs obliquely between the ala of the nose and the angle of the mouth. These grooves are easiest to observe during smiling. The lower lip is separated from the **mental protuberance** (chin) by the **mentolabial sulcus.** The lips, cheeks, and chin of the mature male grow hair as part of the secondary sex characteristics, the **beard.** ⊙

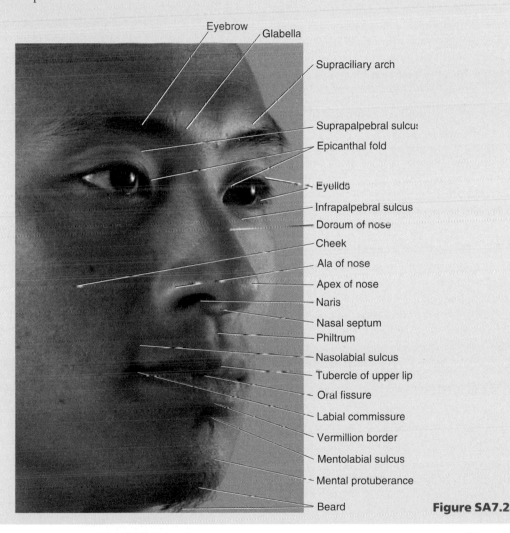

Eyebrow   Glabella

Supraciliary arch

Suprapalpebral sulcus

Epicanthal fold

Eyelids

Infrapalpebral sulcus

Dorsum of nose

Cheek

Ala of nose

Apex of nose

Naris

Nasal septum

Philtrum

Nasolabial sulcus

Tubercle of upper lip

Oral fissure

Labial commissure

Vermillion border

Mentolabial sulcus

Mental protuberance

Beard

Figure SA7.2

Orbit, Orbital Region, and Eyeball

The **orbits** are bony cavities in the facial skeleton that resemble hollow quadrangular pyramids with their bases directed anterolaterally and their apices, posteromedially (Fig. 7.30*A*). The medial walls of the two orbits, separated by the ethmoidal sinuses and the upper parts of the nasal cavity, are parallel, whereas their lateral walls are nearly at a right (90°) angle. Consequently, the axes of the orbits diverge at approx-

imately 45°. The optical axes (axes of gaze, the direction or line of sight) for the two eyeballs, are parallel, however. The orbits contain and protect the *eyeballs* (globes of eyes) and **accessory visual structures,** which include the:

- *Eyelids,* which bound the orbits anteriorly, controlling exposure of the anterior eyeball.

- *Extraocular muscles,* which position the eyeballs and raise the superior eyelids.

- Nerves and vessels in transit to the eyeballs and muscles.

- *Orbital fascia* surrounding the eyeballs and muscles.

- Mucous membrane (*conjunctiva*) lining the eyelids and anterior aspect of the eyeballs and most of the *lacrimal apparatus,* which lubricates it.

All space within the orbits not occupied by the above structures is filled with **orbital fat;** thus it forms a matrix in which the structures of the orbit are embedded.

The pyramidal orbit has a base, four walls, and an apex (Fig. 7.30*B*):

- The **base** of the orbit is outlined by the **orbital margin** that surrounds the **orbital opening.** The bone forming the orbital margin is reinforced to afford protection to the orbital contents and provides attachment for the **orbital septum,** an interrupted fibrous sheet that extends into the eyelids.

- The **superior wall** (roof) is approximately horizontal and is formed mainly by the **orbital part of the frontal bone,** which separates the orbital cavity from the anterior cranial fossa. Near the apex of the orbit, the superior wall is formed by the lesser wing of the sphenoid. Anterolaterally, a shallow depression in the orbital part of the frontal bone, called the **fossa for the lacrimal gland** (lacrimal fossa), accommodates the lacrimal gland.

- The **medial walls** of the contralateral orbits are essentially parallel and are formed primarily by the **ethmoid bone,** along with contributions from the frontal, lacrimal, and sphenoids. Anteriorly, the medial wall is indented by the **lacrimal groove** and **fossa for the lacrimal sac.** Much of the bone forming the medial wall is paper thin; the ethmoid bone is highly pneumatized with ethmoidal cells, often visible through the bone of a dried cranium.

- The **inferior wall** (floor) is formed mainly by the maxilla and partly by the zygomatic and palatine bones. The thin inferior wall is shared by the orbit and maxillary sinus. It slants inferiorly from the apex to the inferior orbital margin. The inferior wall is demarcated from the lateral wall of the orbit by the **inferior orbital fissure.**

- The **lateral wall** is formed by the frontal process of the zygomatic bone and the greater wing of the sphenoid. This is the strongest and thickest wall, which is important because it is most exposed and vulnerable to direct trauma. Its posterior part separates the orbit from the temporal and middle cranial fossae. The lateral walls of the contralateral orbits are nearly perpendicular to each other.

- The **apex of the orbit** is at the **optic canal** in the lesser wing of the sphenoid just medial to the *superior orbital fissure.*

The widest part of the orbit corresponds to the **equator of the eyeball,** an imaginary line encircling the eyeball equidistant from its anterior and posterior poles.

The bones forming the orbit are lined with **periorbita** (periosteum of orbit). The periorbita is continuous at the *optic canal* and *superior orbital fissure* with the periosteal layer of the dura mater. The periorbita is also continuous over the orbital margins and through the *inferior orbital fissure* with the periosteum covering the external surface of the cranium (pericranium), and with the orbital septa at the orbital margins, with the fascial sheaths of the extraocular muscles, and with orbital fascia that forms the **fascial sheath of the eyeball** (Fig. 7.31*A*).

Periorbital Ecchymosis

The skin of the eyelid is the thinnest of the body and is delicate and sensitive. Because of the loose nature of the subcutaneous tissue within the eyelids, even a relatively slight injury or inflammation may result in an accumulation of fluid, causing the eyelids to swell. Blows to the periorbital region usually produce soft tissue damage because the tissues are crushed against the strong and relatively sharp margin. Significant swelling and hemorrhage into the eyelids and extravasation of blood into the periorbital skin (*ecchymosis*) occur. This type of injury is common in boxers.

Fractures of the Orbit

The orbital margin is strong to protect the orbital content. However, when the blows are powerful enough and the impact is directly on the bony rim, the resulting fractures usually occur at the sutures between the bones forming the orbital margin. Because of the thinness of the medial and inferior walls of the orbit, a blow to the eye may fracture the orbital walls while the margin remains intact. Indirect traumatic injury that displaces the orbital walls is called a "blowout" fracture. Fractures of the medial wall may involve the ethmoidal and sphenoidal sinuses, whereas fractures of the inferior wall may involve the maxillary sinus. Although the superior wall is stronger than the medial and inferior walls, it is thin enough to be translucent and may be readily penetrated. Thus a sharp object may pass through it and enter the frontal lobe of the brain.

Orbital fractures often result in intraorbital bleeding, which exerts pressure on the eyeball, causing *exophthalmos* (protrusion of the eyeball). Any trauma to the eye may affect adjacent structures—for example bleeding into the maxillary sinus, displacement of maxillary teeth, and fracture of nasal bones resulting in hemorrhage, airway obstruction, and infection that could spread to the cavernous sinus through the ophthalmic vein. ▶

(cont'd on page 961)

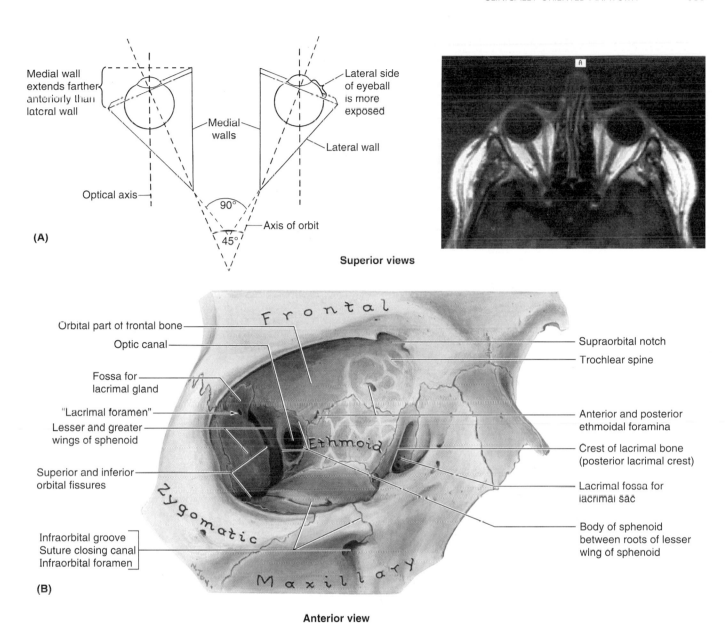

(A)

Medial wall extends farther anteriorly than lateral wall

Medial walls

Lateral side of eyeball is more exposed

Lateral wall

Optical axis

90°

Axis of orbit

45°

Superior views

(B)

Orbital part of frontal bone

Optic canal

Fossa for lacrimal gland

"Lacrimal foramen"

Lesser and greater wings of sphenoid

Superior and inferior orbital fissures

Infraorbital groove
Suture closing canal
Infraorbital foramen

Frontal

Ethmoid

Zygomatic

Maxillary

Supraorbital notch

Trochlear spine

Anterior and posterior ethmoidal foramina

Crest of lacrimal bone (posterior lacrimal crest)

Lacrimal fossa for lacrimal sac

Body of sphenoid between roots of lesser wing of sphenoid

Anterior view

Figure 7.30. Orbits. A. The diagram and MRI study demonstrate the orbits' disposition relative to each other, and to the optical axes (line of gaze). The orbits are separated by ethmoidal cells and the upper nasal cavity and septum. **B.** The bony walls of the orbit are shown. The word *ethmoid* is printed directly on the thin orbital plate of the ethmoid bone that separates the orbit from the ethmoidal sinuses. The optic canal is situated at the apex (deepest part) of the pyramidal orbital cavity, where it passes between the body of and the two roots of the lesser wing of the sphenoid. A straight probe must pass along the lateral wall of the cavity if it is to traverse the canal.

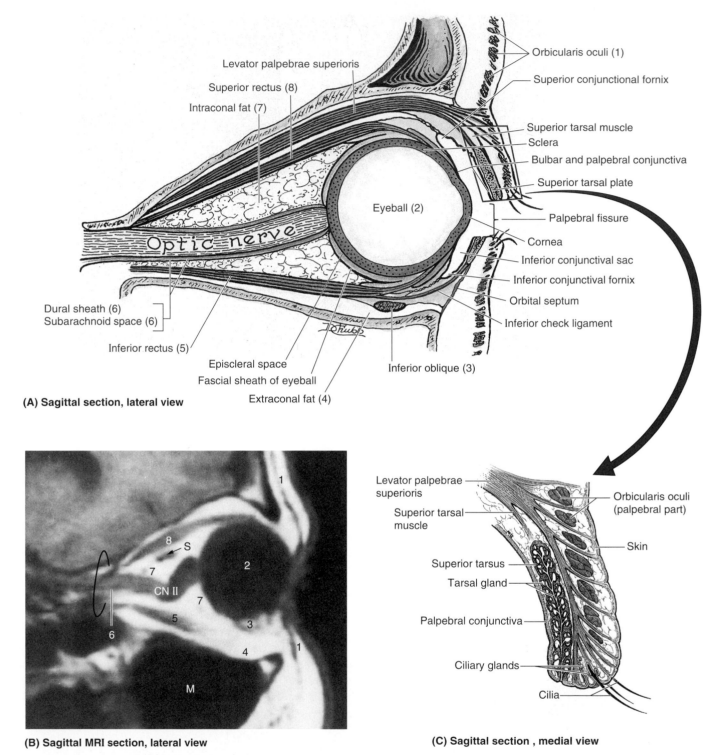

(A) Sagittal section, lateral view

Levator palpebrae superioris

Superior rectus (8)

Intraconal fat (7)

Optic nerve

Eyeball (2)

Orbicularis oculi (1)

Superior conjunctional fornix

Superior tarsal muscle

Sclera

Bulbar and palpebral conjunctiva

Superior tarsal plate

Palpebral fissure

Cornea

Inferior conjunctival sac

Inferior conjunctival fornix

Orbital septum

Inferior check ligament

Dural sheath (6)

Subarachnoid space (6)

Inferior rectus (5)

Episcleral space

Fascial sheath of eyeball

Extraconal fat (4)

Inferior oblique (3)

(B) Sagittal MRI section, lateral view

(C) Sagittal section , medial view

Levator palpebrae superioris

Superior tarsal muscle

Orbicularis oculi (palpebral part)

Skin

Superior tarsus

Tarsal gland

Palpebral conjunctiva

Ciliary glands

Cilia

Figure 7.31. Orbit, eyeball, and eyelids. A. The contents of the orbit are shown. The subarachnoid space around the optic nerve is continuous with the space between the arachnoid and the pia covering the brain. The numbers refer to structures labeled in part **C. B.** This MRI study shows a sagittal section through the optic nerve (*CN II*) and eyeball. *M,* maxillary sinus; *S,* superior ophthalmic vein; *arc,* optic canal. **C.** This detail shows the superior eyelid. The tarsus forms the skeleton of the eyelid and contains tarsal glands. (Part **B** courtesy of Dr. W. Kucharczyk, Chair of Medical Imaging, University of Toronto, and Clinical Director of Tri-Hospital Resonance Centre, Toronto, Ontario, Canada.)

Orbital Tumors

Because of the closeness of the optic nerve to the sphenoidal and posterior ethmoidal sinuses, a malignant tumor in these sinuses may erode the thin bony walls of the orbit and compress the optic nerve and orbital contents. Tumors in the orbit produce *exophthalmos*. The easiest entrance to the orbital cavity for a tumor in the middle cranial fossa is through the superior orbital fissure; tumors in the temporal or infratemporal fossa gain access to this cavity through the inferior orbital fissure. Although the lateral wall of the orbit is nearly as long as the medial wall because it extends laterally and anteriorly, it does not reach as far anteriorly as the medial wall does, which occupies essentially a sagittal plane (Fig. 7.30*A*). Thus nearly 2.5 cm of the eyeball is exposed when the pupil is turned medially as far as possible. This is why the lateral side affords a good approach for operations on the eyeball. ☉

THE BOTTOM LINE: The orbits are pyramidal cavities, with bases directed anteriorly and apices posteriorly, that house the eyeballs and accessory visual structures. The medial walls of the contralateral orbits are parallel, and the lateral walls are perpendicular to each other. The margins and lateral walls of the orbits, being most vulnerable to direct trauma, are strong. The superior wall (roof) and inferior wall (floor) are shared with the anterior cranial fossa and the maxillary sinus, respectively, and much of the paper-thin medial wall is common to the ethmoidal cells. The medial wall and floor are thus vulnerable to the spread of disease processes from the paranasal sinuses and to blowout fractures when blunt force is applied to the orbital contents, suddenly increasing intraorbital pressure. The optic canal and superior orbital fissure at the apex of the orbit are the primary paths by which structures enter and exit the orbits.

Eyelids and Lacrimal Apparatus

The eyelids and lacrimal fluid, secreted by the lacrimal glands, protect the cornea and eyeball from injury and irritation (e.g., by dust and small particles).

Eyelids

When closed, the **eyelids** cover the eyeball anteriorly, thereby protecting it from injury and excessive light. They also keep the cornea moist by spreading the lacrimal fluid. The eyelids are movable folds that are covered externally by thin skin and internally by transparent mucous membrane, the **palpebral conjunctiva** (Fig. 7.31*A* & *C*). This part of the conjunctiva is reflected onto the eyeball, where it is continuous with the **bulbar conjunctiva.** This part of the conjunctiva is thin and transparent and attaches loosely to the anterior surface of the eyeball. The bulbar conjunctiva, loose and wrinkled over the sclera (where it contains small, visible blood vessels), is adherent to the periphery of the cornea (Fig. 7.32*A*).

The lines of reflection of the palpebral conjunctiva onto the eyeball form deep recesses, the **superior** and **inferior conjunctival fornices** (Fig. 7.31*A*). The **conjunctival sac** is the space bound by the palpebral and bulbar conjunctivae; it is a closed space when the eyelids are closed, but opens via an anterior aperture, the *palpebral fissure* (L. *rima palpebrae,* the gap between the eyelids), when the eye is "open" (eyelids are parted). The conjunctival sac is a specialized form of mucosal "bursa" that enables the eyelids to move freely over the surface of the eyeball as they open and close.

The superior (upper) and inferior (lower) eyelids are strengthened by dense bands of connective tissue, the **superior** and **inferior tarsi** (sing. **tarsus**) which form the "skeleton" of the eyelids (Figs. 7.31*C* and 7.33*A*). Fibers of the palpebral portion of the *orbicularis oculi* (the sphincter of the palpebral fissure) are in the connective tissue superficial to these tarsi and deep to the skin of the eyelids. Embedded in the tarsi are **tarsal glands,** the lipid secretion of which lubricates the edges of the eyelids and prevents them from sticking together when they close. The lipid secretion also forms a barrier that lacrimal fluid does not cross when produced in normal amounts. When production is excessive, it spills over the barrier onto the cheeks as tears.

The **eyelashes** (L. *cilia*) are in the margins of the lids. The large sebaceous glands associated with the eyelashes are **ciliary glands.** The junctions of the superior and inferior eyelids make up the **medial** and **lateral palpebral commissures,** defining the **angles of the eye** (G. *kanthos,* corner of eye). Thus each eye has medial and lateral angles, or *canthi* (Fig. 7.33*B*).

Between the nose and the medial angle of the eye is the *medial palpebral ligament,* which connects the tarsi to the medial margin of the orbit (Fig. 7.33*A*). The orbicularis oculi originates and inserts onto this ligament. A similar **lateral palpebral ligament** attaches the tarsi to the lateral margin of the orbit but does not provide for direct muscle attachment. The *orbital septum* is a weak membrane that spans from the tarsi to the margins of the orbit, where it becomes continuous with the periosteum. It keeps the orbital fat contained and can limit the spread of infection to and from the orbit.

Lacrimal Apparatus

The lacrimal apparatus (Fig. 7.33*B*) consists of the:

- **Lacrimal glands:** secrete **lacrimal fluid,** a watery physiological saline containing the bacteriocidal enzyme lysozyme. The fluid moistens and lubricates the surfaces of the conjunctiva and cornea and provides some nutrients and dissolved oxygen to the cornea; when produced in excess, it constitutes tears.

- **Lacrimal ducts:** convey lacrimal fluid from the lacrimal glands to the conjunctival sac.

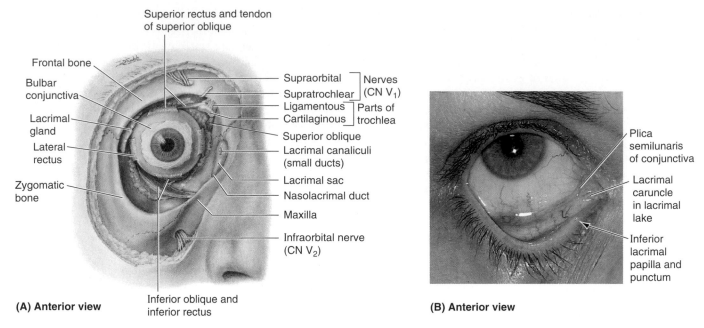

Figure 7.32. Orbit and eyeball. A. In this anterior approach dissection of the orbit, the eyelids, orbital septum, levator palpebrae superioris, and some fat have been removed. Part of the lacrimal gland is seen between the bony orbital wall laterally and the eyeball and lateral rectus muscle medially. **B.** The surface features of the eye are shown. The fibrous outer coat of the eyeball includes the tough white sclera and the central transparent cornea, through which the pigmented iris with its aperture, the pupil, can be seen. The inferior eyelid has been everted to show the reflection of conjunctiva from the anterior surface of the eyeball to the inner surface of the eyelid. *Arrow,* the inferior lacrimal punctum (opening) of the lacrimal canaliculi. The semilunar fold is a vertical fold of conjunctiva near the medial angle, at the lacrimal caruncle.

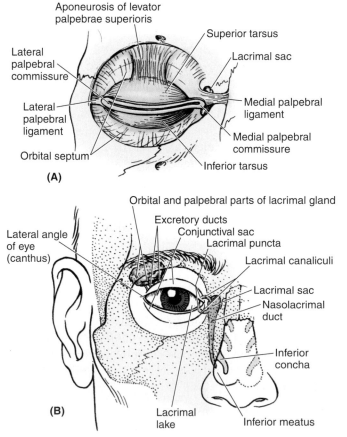

Figure 7.33. Skeleton of eyelids and lacrimal apparatus. A. The superior and inferior tarsi and their attachments are shown. Their ciliary margins are free but they are attached peripherally to the orbital septum (palpebral fascia in the eyelid). The angles are anchored by medial and lateral palpebral ligaments. The fan-shaped aponeurosis of the levator palpebrae superioris is attached to the anterior surface and superior edge of the superior tarsus. **B.** The components of the lacrimal apparatus, by which tears flow from the superolateral aspect of the conjunctival sac to the nasal cavity, are demonstrated.

- **Lacrimal canaliculi** (L. small canals): commence at a **lacrimal punctum** (opening) on the **lacrimal papilla** near the medial angle of the eye and drain lacrimal fluid from the **lacrimal lake** (L. *lacus lacrimalis;* a triangular space at the medial angle of the eye where the tears collect) to the **lacrimal sac** (the dilated superior part of the nasolacrimal duct).

- **Nasolacrimal duct:** conveys the lacrimal fluid to the *inferior nasal meatus.*

The *lacrimal gland*, almond shaped and approximately 2 cm long, lies in the *fossa for the lacrimal gland* in the superolateral part of each orbit (Figs. 7.30*B*, 7.32*A*, and 7.33*A*). The gland is divided into superior (orbital) and inferior (palpebral) parts by the lateral expansion of the tendon of the **levator palpebrae superioris** (Fig. 7.33*A*). *Accessory lacrimal glands* are also present; they are more numerous in the superior eyelid than in the inferior eyelid.

Production of lacrimal fluid is stimulated by parasympathetic impulses from CN VII. It is secreted through 8–12 **excretory ducts** that open into the lateral part of the *superior conjunctival fornix* of the conjunctival sac. The fluid flows inferiorly within the sac under the influence of gravity. When the cornea becomes dry, the eye blinks. The eyelids come together in a lateral to medial sequence pushing a film of fluid

medially over the cornea, somewhat like windshield wipers when washing the car windshield. In this way, lacrimal fluid containing foreign material such as dust is pushed toward the medial angle of the eye, accumulating in the lacrimal lake from which they drain by capillary action through the lacrimal puncta and lacrimal canaliculi to the lacrimal sac. From this sac, the tears pass to the inferior nasal meatus of the nasal cavity through the nasolacrimal duct. They drain posteriorly across the floor of the nasal cavity to the nasopharynx and are eventually swallowed. In addition to cleansing particles and irritants from the conjunctival sac, lacrimal fluid provides the cornea with nutrients and oxygen.

The **nerve supply of the lacrimal gland** is both sympathetic and parasympathetic. The presynaptic parasympathetic secretomotor fibers are conveyed from the facial nerve by the *greater petrosal nerve* and then by the *nerve of the pterygoid canal* to the *pterygopalatine ganglion,* where they synapse with the cell body of the postsynaptic fiber. Vasoconstrictive, postsynaptic sympathetic fibers, brought from the *superior cervical ganglion* by the *internal carotid plexus* and deep petrosal nerve, join the parasympathetic fibers to form the nerve of the pterygoid canal and traverse the pterygopalatine ganglion. The zygomatic nerve (from the maxillary nerve) brings both types of fibers to the lacrimal branch of the ophthalmic nerve, by which they enter the gland.

Injury to the Nerves Supplying the Eyelids

Because it supplies the levator palpebrae superioris, a lesion of the oculomotor nerve causes paralysis of the muscle, and the superior eyelid droops *(ptosis).* Damage to the facial nerve involves paralysis of the orbicularis oculi, preventing the eyelids from closing fully. Normal rapid protective blinking of the eye is also lost. The loss of tonus of the muscle in the inferior eyelid causes the lid to fall away (evert) from the surface of the eyeball, leading to drying of the cornea. This leaves the eyeball unprotected from dust and small particles. Thus irritation of the unprotected eyeball results in excessive but inefficient lacrimation (tear formation). Excessive lacrimal fluid also forms when the lacrimal drainage apparatus is obstructed, thereby preventing the fluid from reaching the inferior part of the eyeball. People often dab their eyes constantly to wipe the tears, resulting in further irritation.

Inflammation of the Palpebral Glands

Any of the glands in the eyelid may become inflamed and swollen from infection or obstruction of their ducts. If the ducts of the ciliary glands are obstructed, a painful red sup-

purative (pus-producing) swelling, a *sty (hordeolum),* develops on the eyelid. *Cysts of the sebaceous glands* of the eyelid, called *chalazia,* may also form. Obstruction of a tarsal gland produces inflammation, a *tarsal chalazion,* that protrudes toward the eyeball and rubs against it as the eyelids blink. Chalazia are usually more painful than sties.

Hyperemia of the Conjunctiva

The conjunctiva is colorless, except when its vessels are dilated and congested ("bloodshot eyes"). Hyperemia of the conjunctiva is caused by local irritation (e.g., from dust, chlorine, or smoke). An inflamed conjunctiva, *conjunctivitis* ("pinkeye"), is a common contagious infection of the eye.

Subconjunctival Hemorrhages

Subconjunctival hemorrhages are common and are manifested by bright or dark red patches deep to and within the bulbar conjunctiva. The hemorrhages may result from injury or inflammation. A blow to the eye, excessively hard blowing of the nose, and paroxysms of coughing or violent sneezing can cause hemorrhages resulting from rupture of small subconjunctival capillaries. ○

THE BOTTOM LINE: The eyelids and lacrimal apparatus are protective devices for the eyeball. The conjunctival sac is a special form of mucosal bursa, which enables the eyelids to move over the surface of the eyeball as they open and close, spreading the moistening and lubricating film of lacrimal fluid within the sac. The fluid is secreted into the lateral superior fornix of the sac and is spread by gravity and blinking across the anterior eyeball, cleansing and providing the cornea with nutrients and oxygen as it is pushed toward the medial angle of the eye. The fluid and contained irritants accumulate in the lacrimal lake. They are drained from here by capillary action through superior and inferior lacrimal puncta into lacrimal canaliculi that pass to the lacrimal sac. The sac drains via the nasolacrimal duct into the nasal cavity, where the fluid flows posteriorly and is eventually swallowed. Although the conjunctival sac opens anteriorly via the palpebral fissure, the watery lacrimal fluid will not cross the lipid barrier secreted by the tarsal glands onto the margins of the fissure unless it is produced in excess, as in crying.

The Eyeball

The **eyeball** contains the optical apparatus of the visual system and occupies most of the anterior portion of the orbit. All anatomical structures within the eyeball have a circular or spherical arrangement. The eyeball proper has three layers; however, there is an additional loose connective tissue layer that surrounds the eyeball, allowing its movement within the orbit. The loose connective tissue layer is composed posteriorly of **bulbar fascia,** which forms the true socket for the eyeball, and anteriorly of bulbar conjunctiva. The three layers of the eyeball are the (Fig. 7.34):

1. **Fibrous layer** (outer coat), consisting of the sclera and cornea.

2. **Vascular layer** (middle coat), consisting of the choroid, ciliary body, and iris.

3. **Inner layer** (inner coat), consisting of the retina that has both optic and non-visual parts.

Fibrous Layer of the Eyeball

The **sclera** is the tough opaque part of the fibrous layer (coat) of the eyeball covering the posterior five sixths of the eyeball. It is the fibrous skeleton of the eyeball, providing shape and resistance as well as attachment for both the extrinsic (extraocular) and the intrinsic muscles of the eye. The anterior part of the sclera is visible through the transparent bulbar conjunctiva as "the white of the eye." The *cornea* is the transparent part of the fibrous coat covering the anterior one sixth of the eyeball. The two parts differ primarily in terms of the regularity of the arrangement of the collagen fibers of which they are composed and the degree of hydration of each.

Vascular Layer of the Eyeball

The vascular layer of the eyeball (also called the **uvea** or **uveal tract**) consists of the choroid, ciliary body, and iris. The **choroid,** a dark reddish brown layer between the sclera and the retina, forms the largest part of the vascular layer of the eyeball and lines most of the sclera. Within this pigmented and dense vascular bed, larger vessels of the *vascular lamina* are located externally (near the sclera). The finest vessels (the **capillary lamina of the choroid** or *choriocapillaris,* an extensive capillary bed) are innermost, adjacent to the avascular light-sensitive layer of the retina, which it supplies with oxygen and nutrients. Engorged with blood in life, this layer is responsible for the "red eye" reflection that occurs in flash photography. The choroid is continuous anteriorly with the ciliary body. The choroid attaches firmly to the pigment layer of the retina, but it can easily be stripped from the sclera.

The **ciliary body,** which is muscular as well as vascular, connects the choroid with the circumference of the iris. The ciliary body provides attachment for the lens; contraction and relaxation of the smooth muscle of the ciliary body controls thickness (and therefore the focus) of the lens. Folds on the internal surface of the ciliary body, the **ciliary processes,** secrete *aqueous humor,* which fills the anterior and posterior chambers of the eye (Fig. 7.34*B*). The **anterior chamber of the eye** is the space between the cornea anteriorly and the iris/pupil posteriorly. The **posterior chamber of the eye** is between the iris/pupil anteriorly and the lens and ciliary body posteriorly.

The **iris,** which literally lies on the anterior surface of the lens, is a thin contractile diaphragm with a central aperture, the **pupil,** for transmitting light. When a person is awake, the size of the pupil varies continually to regulate the amount of light entering the eye. Two involuntary muscles control the size of the pupil: the parasympathetically stimulated *sphincter pupillae* closes the pupil, and the sympathetically stimulated *dilator pupillae* opens it. The nature of the pupillary responses is paradoxical: sympathetic responses usually occur immediately, yet it may take up to 20 min for the pupil to dilate in response to low lighting, as in a darkened theater. Parasympathetic responses are typically slower than sympathetic responses, yet parasympathetically stimulated papillary constriction is normally instantaneous.

Pupillary Light Reflex

The **pupillary light reflex** is tested using a penlight during a neurological examination. This reflex, involving CN II (afferent limb) and CN III (efferent limb), is the rapid constriction of the pupil in response to light. When light enters one eye, both pupils constrict because each retina sends fibers into the optic tracts of both sides. The sphincter pupillae muscle is innervated ▶

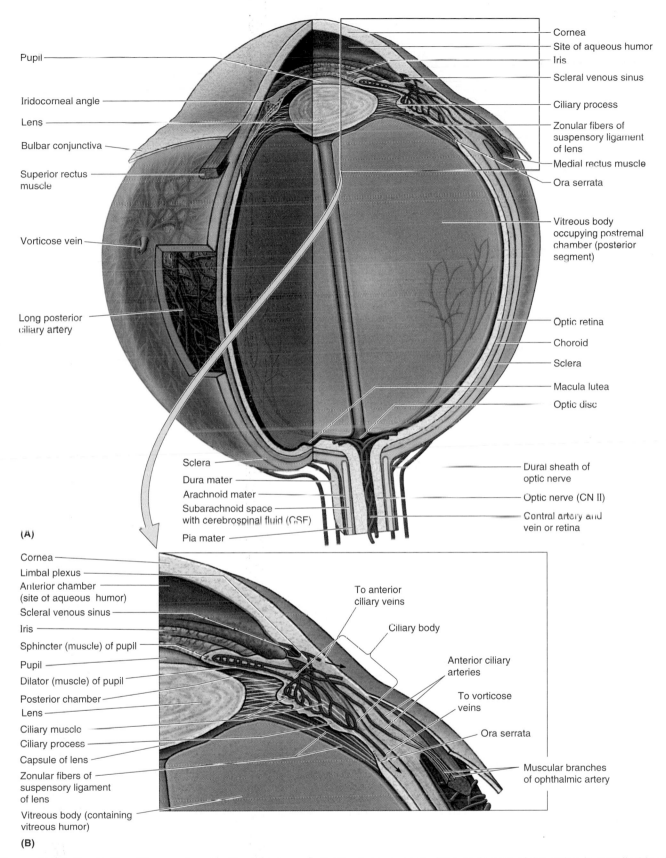

Pupil

Iridocorneal angle

Lens

Bulbar conjunctiva

Superior rectus muscle

Vorticose vein

Long posterior ciliary artery

Cornea

Site of aqueous humor

Iris

Scleral venous sinus

Ciliary process

Zonular fibers of suspensory ligament of lens

Medial rectus muscle

Ora serrata

Vitreous body occupying postremal chamber (posterior segment)

Optic retina

Choroid

Sclera

Macula lutea

Optic disc

Sclera

Dura mater

Arachnoid mater

Subarachnoid space with cerebrospinal fluid (CSF)

Pia mater

Dural sheath of optic nerve

Optic nerve (CN II)

Central artery and vein or retina

(A)

Cornea

Limbal plexus

Anterior chamber (site of aqueous humor)

Scleral venous sinus

Iris

Sphincter (muscle) of pupil

Pupil

Dilator (muscle) of pupil

Posterior chamber

Lens

Ciliary muscle

Ciliary process

Capsule of lens

Zonular fibers of suspensory ligament of lens

Vitreous body (containing vitreous humor)

To anterior ciliary veins

Ciliary body

Anterior ciliary arteries

To vorticose veins

Ora serrata

Muscular branches of ophthalmic artery

(B)

Figure 7.34. Eyeball with quarter section removed. A. The inner aspect of the optic part of the retina is supplied by the central artery of the retina, whereas the outer, light sensitive aspect is nourished by the capillary lamina of the choroid (Fig. 7.38). The central artery courses through the optic nerve and divides at the optic disc into superior and inferior branches. The branches of the central artery are end arteries that do not anastomose with each other or any other vessel. **B.** The structural details of the ciliary region are shown. The ciliary body is both muscular and vascular, as is the iris, the latter including two muscles: the sphincter pupillae and dilator pupillae muscles. Venous blood from this region, as well as the aqueous humor in the anterior chamber, drain into the scleral venous sinus.

by parasympathetic fibers; consequently, interruption of these fibers causes dilation of the pupil because of the unopposed action of the sympathetically innervated dilator pupillae muscle. The first sign of *compression of the oculomotor nerve* is ipsilateral slowness of the pupillary response to light.

Uveitis

Uveitis, inflammation of the vascular layer of the eyeball (uvea), may progress to severe visual impairment and blindness. ⊕

Inner Layer of the Eyeball

The inner layer of the eyeball is the **retina.** Grossly, the retina consists of two functional parts with distinct locations: an optic part and a non-visual retina. The **optic part** of the retina is sensitive to visual light rays and has two layers: a neural layer and pigment cell layer. The *neural layer* is light receptive. The *pigment cell layer* consists of a single layer of cells that reinforces the light-absorbing property of the choroid in reducing the scattering of light in the eyeball. The **non-visual retina** is an anterior continuation of the pigment cell layer and a layer of supporting cells over the ciliary body (**ciliary part** of the retina) and the posterior surface of the iris (**iridial part** of the retina), respectively.

The **fundus** is the posterior part of the eyeball. It has a circular depressed area called the **optic disc** (optic papilla) where the sensory fibers and vessels conveyed by the optic nerve enter the eyeball (Fig. 7.34*A*). Because it contains no photoreceptors, the optic disc is insensitive to light. Consequently, this part of the retina is commonly called the *blind spot.* Just lateral to the optic disc is the **macula lutea** (L. yellow spot). The yellow color of the macula is apparent only when the retina is examined with red-free light. The macula lutea is a small oval area of the retina with special photoreceptor cones that is specialized for acuity of vision. It is not normally observed with an *ophthalmoscope* (a device for viewing the interior of the eyeball through the pupil). At the center of the macula lutea is a depression, the **fovea centralis** (L. central pit), the area of most acute vision. The fovea is approximately 1.5 mm in diameter; its center, the **foveola,** does not have the capillary network visible elsewhere deep to the retina.

The functional optic part of the retina terminates anteriorly along the **ora serrata** (L. serrated edge), an irregular border slightly posterior to the ciliary body. The ora serrata marks the anterior termination of the light-receptive part of the retina. Except for the cones and rods of the neural layer, the retina is supplied by the **central artery of the retina,** a branch of the ophthalmic artery. The cones and rods of the

outer neural layer receive nutrients from the *capillary lamina of the choroid,* or choriocapillaris (discussed in "Vasculature of the Orbit," later in this chapter). It has the finest vessels of the inner surface of the choroid, against which the retina is pressed. A corresponding system of retinal veins unites to form the **central vein of the retina.**

Development of the Retina

The retina and optic nerve develop from the **optic cup,** an outgrowth of the embryonic forebrain, the **optic vesicle.** As it evaginates from the brain, the optic vesicle carries the developing meninges with it (Moore and Persaud, 2003). Hence the optic nerve is invested with cranial meninges and an extension of the subarachnoid space. The central artery and vein of the retina cross the subarachnoid space and run within the distal part of the optic nerve. The pigment cell layer of the retina develops from the outer layer of the optic cup, and the neural layer develops from the inner layer of the cup.

Ophthalmoscopy

Physicians use an *ophthalmoscope* (funduscope) to view the fundus (posterior part) of the eye (Fig. B7.21*A*). The retinal arteries and veins radiate over the fundus from the optic disc. The pale, oval disc appears on the medial side with the retinal vessels radiating from its center in the ophthalmoscopic view of the retina shown in Figure B7.21*A*. Pulsation of the retinal arteries is usually visible. Centrally, at the posterior pole of the eyeball, the macula appears darker than the reddish hue of surrounding areas of the retina because the black melanin pigment in the choroid and pigment cell layer is not screened by capillary blood.

Retinal Detachment

The layers of the developing retina are separated in the embryo by an intraretinal space. During the early fetal period, the embryonic layers fuse, obliterating this space. Although the pigment cell layer becomes firmly fixed to the choroid, its attachment to the neural layer is not firm. Consequently, detachment of the retina may follow a blow to the eye (Fig. B7.21*B*). A detached retina usually results from seepage of fluid between the neural and pigment cell layers of the retina, perhaps days or even weeks after trauma to the eye. Persons with a retinal detachment may complain of flashes of light or specks floating in front of the eye (Anderson et al., 2000). ▶

Branches of retinal vessels

Macula

Optic disc

(A)

(B)

Figure B7.21. Ophthalmoscopic photograph of normal fundus (A) and retinal detachment (B).

Papilledema

An increase in CSF pressure slows venous return from the retina, causing *edema of the retina* (fluid accumulation). The edema is viewed during ophthalmoscopy as swelling of the optic disc, a condition called **papilledema**. Normally, the disc is flat and does not form a papilla. Papilledema results from increased intracranial pressure and increased CSF pressure in the extension of the subarachnoid space around the optic nerve (Fig. 7.34A). A sudden reduction of pressure in the spinal subarachnoid space, as might occur with lumbar puncture, could result in a potentially fatal herniation of brain tissue into the vertebral canal if performed when intracranial pressure is elevated. ○

Refractive Media of the Eyeball

On their way to the retina, lightwaves pass through the refractive media of the eyeball: cornea, aqueous humor, lens, and vitreous humor (Fig. 7.34).

The **cornea** is the circular area of the anterior part of the outer fibrous layer of the eyeball; it is largely responsible for refraction of the light that enters the eye. It is transparent, owing to the extremely regular arrangement of its collagen fibers and its dehydrated state. The cornea is sensitive to touch; its innervation is provided by the ophthalmic nerve (CN V_1). It is avascular. Its nourishment is derived from the capillary beds at its periphery, the aqueous humor, and lacrimal fluid. The latter also provides oxygen absorbed from the air.

The **aqueous humor** in the anterior and posterior chambers of the eye is produced in the posterior chamber by the *ciliary processes* of the ciliary body. This clear watery solution provides nutrients for the avascular cornea and lens. After passing through the pupil into the anterior chamber, the aqueous humor drains into the **scleral venous sinus** (L. *sinus venosus sclerae,* canal of Schlemm) at the **iridocorneal angle.**

The humor is removed by the **limbal plexus,** a network of scleral veins close to the limbus, which drain in turn into both tributaries of the *vorticose* and the *anterior ciliary veins* (Fig. 7.34B).

The **lens** is posterior to the iris and anterior to the vitreous humor of the vitreous body. It is a transparent, biconvex structure enclosed in a capsule. The highly elastic **capsule of the lens** is anchored by the **zonular fibers** (suspensory ligament of the lens) to the ciliary body and encircled by the ciliary processes. Although most refraction is produced by the cornea, the convexity of the lens, particularly its anterior surface, constantly varies to fine-tune the focus of near or distant objects on the retina. The **ciliary muscle** in the ciliary body changes the shape of the lens; in this way the isolated unattached lens assumes a nearly spherical shape. Stretched within the circle of the relaxed ciliary body, the attachments around its periphery pull the lens relatively flat so that its refraction enables far vision. When parasympathetic stimulation causes the smooth muscle of the circular ciliary body to contract, the circle, like a sphincter, becomes smaller in size and the tension on the lens is reduced, allowing the lens to round up. The increased convexity makes its refraction suitable for near vision. In the absence of parasympathetic stimulation, the ciliary muscles relax again and the lens is pulled into its flatter, far-vision shape.

The **vitreous humor** is a watery fluid enclosed in the meshes of the **vitreous body**, a transparent jelly-like substance in the posterior four fifths of the eyeball posterior to the lens (**postremal** or **vitreous chamber,** or posterior segment). In addition to transmitting light, the vitreous humor holds the retina in place and supports the lens.

Corneal Abrasions and Lacerations

Foreign objects such as sand or metal filings (particles) produce *corneal abrasions* that cause sudden, stabbing pain in the eyeball and tears. Opening and closing the eyelids is also painful. *Corneal lacerations* are caused by sharp objects such as fingernails or the corner of a page of a book.

Presbyopia and Cataracts

As people age, their lenses become harder and more flattened. These changes gradually reduce the focusing power of the lenses, a condition known as *presbyopia* (G. *presbyos,* old). Some people also experience a loss of transparency (cloudiness) of the lens from areas of opaqueness *(cataracts). Cataract extraction* is a common operation.

Hemorrhage into the Anterior Chamber

Hemorrhage within the anterior chamber of the eyeball (*hyphema* or *hyphemia*) usually results from blunt trauma to the eyeball, such as from a squash or racquet ball or a hockey stick (Fig. B7.22). Initially, the anterior chamber is tinged red but blood soon accumulates in this chamber. The initial hemorrhage usually stops in a few days and recovery is usually good. ✚

Figure B7.22. Hyphema.

THE BOTTOM LINE: The eyeball contains the optical apparatus of the visual system. It has a trilaminar construction, with (1) a supporting outer fibrous layer, consisting of the opaque sclera and transparent anterior cornea; (2) a middle vascular layer, consisting of the choroid (largely concerned with providing nourishment to the cones and rods of the retina), the ciliary body (producer of the aqueous humor and adjuster of the lens), and the iris (protector of the retina); and (3) an inner layer, consisting of optic and nonvisual parts of the retina. The cornea is the major refractive component of the eyeball, with focusing adjustments made by the lens. Parasympathetic stimulation of the ciliary body reduces tension on the lens, allowing it to thicken for near vision. Relaxation of the ciliary body in the absence of stimulation stretches the lens, making it thinner for far vision. Parasympathetic stimulation also constricts the sphincter of the iris, which closes the pupil in response to bright light. Sympathetic stimulation of the dilator of the iris opens the pupil to admit more light. The anterior segment of the eyeball is filled with aqueous humor, produced by the ciliary processes in the posterior chamber. The humor passes through the pupil into the anterior chamber and is absorbed into the venous circulation at the scleral venous sinus. The postremal or vitreous chamber is filled with vitreous humor, which maintains the shape of the eye, transmits light, and holds the retina in place against the choroid.

Extraocular Muscles of the Orbit

The extraocular muscles of the orbit are the levator palpebrae superioris, four recti (superior, inferior, medial, and lateral), and two obliques (superior and inferior). These muscles work together to move the superior eyelids and eyeballs. They are illustrated in Figures 7.35–7.37 and Table 7.8. The attachments, nerve supply, and main actions of the orbital muscles, beginning from the primary position, are described in Table 7.8. Additional details concerning some of the extraocular muscles are provided in the following text. Although actions of the muscles are described separately, in fact extraocular muscles rarely act independently; synergistic and antagonistic activity occurs between muscles most of the time. Muscles that are synergistic for one action may be antagonistic for another.

Levator Palpebrae Superioris

The *levator palpebrae superioris* broadens into a wide bilaminar aponeurosis as it approaches its distal attachments. The superficial lamina attaches to the skin of the superior eyelid and the deep lamina to the superior tarsus (Fig. 7.33*A*). This muscle is opposed most of the time by gravity and is the antagonist of the superior half of the orbicularis oculi, the sphincter of the palpebral fissure. The deep lamina includes smooth muscle fibers, the **superior tarsal muscle,** that produce additional widening of the palpebral fissure during a sympathetic response (e.g., fright).

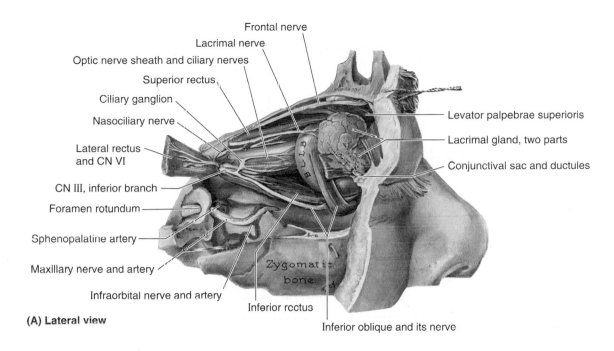

Frontal nerve

Lacrimal nerve

Optic nerve sheath and ciliary nerves

Superior rectus

Ciliary ganglion

Nasociliary nerve

Lateral rectus and CN VI

CN III, inferior branch

Foramen rotundum

Sphenopalatine artery

Maxillary nerve and artery

Infraorbital nerve and artery

Inferior rectus

Inferior oblique and its nerve

Levator palpebrae superioris

Lacrimal gland, two parts

Conjunctival sac and ductules

Zygomatic bone

(A) Lateral view

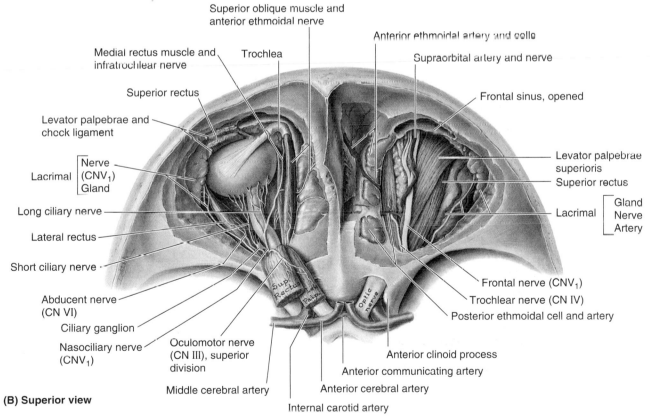

Superior oblique muscle and anterior ethmoidal nerve

Medial rectus muscle and infratrochlear nerve

Trochlea

Anterior ethmoidal artery and cells

Supraorbital artery and nerve

Superior rectus

Levator palpebrae and check ligament

Frontal sinus, opened

Lacrimal { Nerve (CNV₁) / Gland }

Long ciliary nerve

Lateral rectus

Short ciliary nerve

Abducent nerve (CN VI)

Ciliary ganglion

Nasociliary nerve (CNV₁)

Oculomotor nerve (CN III), superior division

Middle cerebral artery

Levator palpebrae superioris

Superior rectus

Lacrimal { Gland / Nerve / Artery }

Frontal nerve (CNV₁)

Trochlear nerve (CN IV)

Posterior ethmoidal cell and artery

Anterior clinoid process

Anterior communicating artery

Anterior cerebral artery

Internal carotid artery

(B) Superior view

Figure 7.35. Dissections of orbit. A. The lateral approach is shown. The ciliary ganglion receives sensory fibers from the nasociliary branches of CN V₁, sympathetic fibers from the internal carotid plexus traveling around the ophthalmic artery, and parasympathetic fibers (which synapse in the ganglion) from the inferior branch of the oculomotor nerve (CN III). Between 8 and 10 short ciliary nerves pass from the ganglion to the eyeball. **B.** In this superior approach, the orbital part of the frontal bone has been removed. Observe the three nerves applied to the roof of the orbital cavity: trochlear, frontal, and lacrimal.

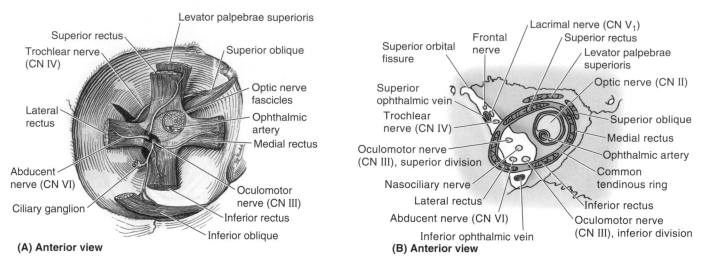

(A) Anterior view

(B) Anterior view

Figure 7.36. Nerves of orbit. *A.* After enucleation (excision) of the eyeball, structures near the apex of the orbit can be seen, including the common tendinous ring and the motor nerves of the orbit. The four rectus muscles arise from the common tendinous ring. This ring encircles the dural sheath of the optic nerve (CN II), the abducent nerve (CN VI), and the superior and inferior divisions of the oculomotor nerve (CN III). **B.** Structures in the apex of the orbit are shown. Nerves entering the orbit through the superior orbital fissure supply the muscles of the eyeball: oculomotor (CN III), trochlear (CN IV), and abducent (CN VI).

Recti and Oblique Muscles

The four **recti muscles** (L. *rectus,* straight) arise from a fibrous cuff, the **common tendinous ring,** that surrounds the optic canal and part of the superior orbital fissure (Fig. 7.36*B*). Structures that enter the orbit through this canal and the adjacent part of the fissure lie at first in the cone of recti (Fig. 7.35*A*). The lateral and medial recti lie in the same horizontal plane, and the superior and inferior recti lie in the same vertical plane (Fig. 7.36*A*).

Neither the superior rectus nor the inferior rectus pulls directly parallel to the long axis of the eyeball (neutral axis of gaze) (Table 7.8). As a result, from the primary position both recti tend to move the pupil medially (adduction). This medial pull of the superior and inferior recti is normally balanced by a similar tendency of the **oblique muscles** to move the pupil laterally (abduction). From the primary position, the **inferior oblique** directs the pupil laterally and superiorly; therefore, when the superior rectus and inferior

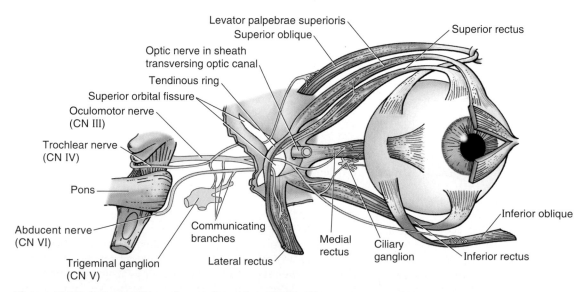

Figure 7.37. Innervation of muscles of eyeball. The oculomotor (CN III), trochlear (CN IV), and abducent (CN VI) nerves are distributed to the muscles of the eyeball. The nerves enter the orbit through the superior orbital fissure. CN IV supplies the superior oblique, CN VI supplies the lateral rectus, and CN III supplies the remaining five muscles.

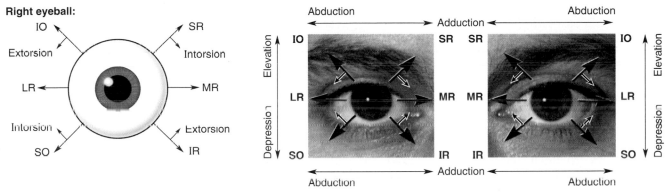

(A) Arrows, direction pupil moves when the indicated muscle acts[a]

(B) Anterolateral view from right

Individual anatomical actions of muscles as studied anatomically

Table 7.8. Extraocular Muscles of the Orbit

Muscle	Origin	Insertion	Innervation	Main Action[a]
Levator palpebrae superioris	Lesser wing of sphenoid bone, superior and anterior to optic canal	Superior tarsus and skin of superior eyelid	Oculomotor nerve; deep layer (superior tarsal muscle) is supplied by sympathetic fibers	Elevates superior eyelid
Superior oblique	Body of sphenoid bone	Its tendon passes through a fibrous ring or trochlea, changes its direction, and inserts into sclera deep to superior rectus muscle	Trochlear nerve (CN IV)	Abducts, depresses, and medially rotates eyeball
Inferior oblique	Anterior part of floor of orbit	Sclera deep to lateral rectus muscle	Oculomotor nerve (CN III)	Abducts, elevates, and laterally rotates eyeball
Superior rectus	Common tendinous ring	Sclera just posterior to corneoscleral junction		Elevates, adducts, and rotates eyeball medially
Inferior rectus				Depresses, adducts, and rotates eyeball medially
Medial rectus				Adducts eyeball
Lateral rectus			Abducent nerve (CN VI)	Abducts eyeball

[a]It is essential to appreciate that all muscles are continuously involved in eyeball movements; thus the individual actions are not usually tested clinically. *SR*, superior rectus (CN III); *LR*, lateral rectus (CN VI); *IR*, inferior rectus (CN III); *IO*, inferior oblique (CN III); *MR*, medial rectus (CN III); *SO*, superior oblique (CN IV).

oblique work synergistically, pure elevation of the eyeball occurs. Similarly, the **superior oblique** directs the pupil inferiorly and laterally; therefore, when the superior oblique works synergistically with the inferior rectus, pure depression results. When the pupil is already in the adducted position (as in the convergence involved in close reading), the oblique muscles are responsible for elevation (inferior oblique) and depression (superior oblique), moving the gaze up or down the page. Elevation and depression in the adducted position is the primary function of the oblique muscles.

In addition to these four movements around the horizontal and vertical axes, the superior and inferior recti and obliques cause rotation of the eyeball around an anteroposterior axis. Medial movement of the superior pole of the eyeball is **intorsion;** lateral movement of the superior pole is **extorsion.** These movements accommodate changes in the tilt of the head. Absence of these movements resulting from nerve lesions contributes to double vision.

To direct the gaze, coordination of both eyes must be accomplished by the paired action of contralateral *yoke muscles.* For example, in directing the gaze to the right, the right lateral rectus and left medial rectus act as yoke muscles.

Fascial Sheath of the Eyeball

The *fascial sheath of the eyeball* (L. *fascia bulbi,* Tenon capsule) envelops the eyeball from the optic nerve nearly to the corneoscleral junction, forming the actual socket for the eyeball (Fig. 7.31*A*). The fascial sheath is pierced by the tendons of the extraocular muscles and is reflected onto each of them as a tubular *muscle sheath.* The muscle sheaths of the levator and superior rectus muscles are fused; thus, when the gaze is directed superiorly, the superior eyelid is further elevated out of the line of vision.

Triangular expansions from the sheaths of the medial and lateral rectus muscles, called the medial and lateral **check ligaments,** are attached to the lacrimal and zygomatic bones, respectively. These ligaments limit abduction and adduction. A blending of the check ligaments with the fascia of the inferior rectus and inferior oblique muscles forms a hammock-like sling, the **suspensory ligament of the eyeball.** A potential **episcleral space** between the eyeball and the fascial sheath allows the eyeball to move inside the cup-like sheath. A similar check ligament from the fascial sheath of the inferior rectus retracts the inferior eyelid when the gaze is directed downward.

Nerves of the Orbit

In addition to the *optic nerve* (CN II), the nerves of the orbit include those that enter through the *superior orbital fissure* and supply the ocular muscles: oculomotor (CN III); trochlear (CN IV); and abducent (CN VI) nerves (Figs. 7.35 and 7.36; Table 7.8). A memory device for the innervation of the extraocular muscles moving the eyeball is similar to a chemical formula: $LR_6SO_4AO_3$ (lateral rectus, CN **VI;** superior oblique, CN **IV;** all others, CN **III**).

The three terminal branches of the *ophthalmic nerve,* CN V_1 (the frontal, nasociliary, and lacrimal nerves), pass through the superior orbital fissure and supply structures related to the anterior orbit (e.g., lacrimal gland and eyelids), face, and scalp. The cutaneous branches of CN V_1 (lacrimal, frontal and infratrochlear nerves) were described under "Cutaneous Nerves of the Face," earlier in this chapter, and in Table 7.5.

The **ciliary ganglion** is a small group of postsynaptic parasympathetic nerve cell bodies associated with CN V_1. It is located between the optic nerve and the lateral rectus toward the posterior limit of the orbit (Fig. 7.35*B*). The ganglion receives nerve fibers from three sources:

- Sensory fibers from CN V_1 via the **communicating branch of the nasociliary nerve** (the **sensory** or **nasociliary root of the ciliary ganglion**).

- Presynaptic parasympathetic fibers from CN III via the **parasympathetic** or **oculomotor root of the ciliary ganglion.**

- Postsynaptic sympathetic fibers from the *internal carotid plexus* via the **sympathetic root of the ciliary ganglion.**

The **short ciliary nerves** arise from the ciliary ganglion and are considered to be branches of CN V_1. They carry parasympathetic and sympathetic fibers to the ciliary body and iris. The short ciliary nerves consist of postsynaptic parasympathetic fibers originating in the ciliary ganglion, afferent fibers from the nasociliary nerve that pass through the ganglion, and postsynaptic sympathetic fibers that also pass through it. **Long ciliary nerves,** branches of the nasociliary nerve (CN V_1) that pass to the eyeball, bypassing the ciliary ganglion, convey postsynaptic sympathetic fibers to the dilator pupillae and afferent fibers from the iris and cornea. The *posterior* and *anterior ethmoidal nerves,* branches of the nasociliary nerve arising in the orbit, exit via openings in the lateral wall of the orbit to supply the mucous membrane of the sphenoidal and ethmoidal sinuses and the nasal cavities as well as the dura of the anterior cranial fossa.

Artificial Eye

The fascial sheath of the eyeball forms a socket for an artificial eye when the eyeball has to be removed (*enucleated*). After this operation, the eye muscles cannot retract too far because their fascial sheaths remain attached to the fascial sheath of the eyeball. Thus some coordinated movement of a properly fitted artificial eyeball is possible. Because the suspensory ligament supports the eyeball, it is preserved when surgical removal of the bony floor of the orbit is performed (e.g., during the removal of a tumor). ✪

Corneal Reflex

During a neurological examination, the examiner touches the cornea with a wisp of cotton. A normal (positive) response is a blink. Absence of a blink response suggests a lesion of CN V$_1$; a lesion of CN VII (the motor nerve to the orbicularis oculi) may also impair this reflex. The examiner must be certain to touch the cornea (not just the sclera) to evoke the reflex. The presence of a contact lens may hamper or abolish the ability to evoke this reflex.

Corneal Ulcers and Transplants

Damage to the sensory innervation of the cornea from CN V$_1$ leaves the cornea vulnerable to injury by foreign particles. People with scarred or opaque corneas may receive *corneal transplants* from donors. Corneal implants of non-reactive plastic material are also used.

Oculomotor Nerve Palsy

Complete oculomotor nerve palsy affects most of the ocular muscles, the levator palpebrae superioris, and the sphincter pupillae. The superior eyelid droops and cannot be raised voluntarily because of the unopposed activity of the orbicularis oculi (supplied by the facial nerve). The pupil is also fully dilated and non-reactive because of the unopposed dilator pupillae. The pupil is fully abducted and depressed ("down and out") because of the unopposed activity of the lateral rectus and superior oblique, respectively.

Horner Syndrome

Horner syndrome results from interruption of a cervical sympathetic trunk and is manifest by the absence of sympathetically stimulated functions on the ipsilateral side of the head. The syndrome includes the following signs: constriction of the pupil (miosis), drooping of the superior eyelid (ptosis), redness and increased temperature of the skin (vasodilation), and absence of sweating (anhydrosis). Constriction of the pupil occurs because the parasympathetically stimulated sphincter of the pupil is unopposed. The ptosis is a consequence of the paralysis of the smooth muscle fibers interdigitated with the aponeurosis of the levator palpebrae superioris that collectively constitute the superior tarsal muscle, supplied by sympathetic fibers.

Paralysis of the Extraocular Muscles

One or more extraocular muscles may be paralyzed by disease in the brainstem or by a head injury, resulting in *diplopia* (double vision). Paralysis of a muscle is apparent by the limitation of movement of the eyeball in the field of action of the muscle and by the production of two images when one attempts to use the muscle. When the abducent nerve (CN VI) supplying only the lateral rectus is paralyzed, the individual cannot abduct the pupil on the affected side. The pupil is fully adducted by the unopposed pull of the medial rectus. ✪

THE BOTTOM LINE: There are seven extraocular muscles: four recti, two obliques, and a levator of the superior eyelid. Six originate from the apex of the orbit, and the four rectus muscles arise from a common tendinous ring. Only the inferior oblique arises anteriorly in the orbit. The levator palpebrae superioris elevates the superior eyelid. Associated smooth muscle (superior tarsal muscle) widens the palpebral fissure even more during sympathetic responses; ptosis results from the absence of sympathetic innervation to the head (Horner syndrome). When the eyes are adducted (converged) as for close reading, the superior and inferior obliques produce depression and elevation, respectively, directing the gaze down or up the page. Coordination of the contralateral extraocular muscles as yoke muscles is necessary to direct the gaze in a particular direction.

All muscles of the orbit are supplied by CN III, except for the superior oblique and lateral rectus, which are supplied by CN IV and VI, respectively. (*Memory device:* LR$_6$SO$_4$AO$_3$; lateral rectus, CN VI; superior oblique, CN IV; all others, CN III.)

Vasculature of the Orbit

Arteries of the Orbit

The blood supply of the orbit is mainly from the **ophthalmic artery**, a branch of the internal carotid artery; the **infraorbital artery**, from the external carotid artery, also contributes blood to structures related to the orbital floor (Figs. 7.35 and 7.36; Table 7.9 and 7.10).

The *central artery of the retina*, a branch of the ophthalmic artery arising inferior to the optic nerve, runs within the dural sheath of the optic nerve until it approaches the eyeball (Fig. 7.38). The central artery pierces the optic nerve and runs within it, emerging at the optic disc. Its branches spread over the internal surface of the retina. The terminal branches are *end arteries*, which provide the only blood supply to the internal aspect of the retina. The external aspect of the retina is also supplied by the *capillary lamina of the choroid* (*choriocapillaris*). Of the eight or so *posterior ciliary arteries* (also branches of the ophthalmic artery), six **short posterior ciliary arteries** directly supply the choroid, which nourishes the outer non-vascular

Table 7.9. Arteries of the Orbit

(A) Superior view

(B) Transverse section of optic nerve

Artery	Origin	Course and Distribution
Ophthalmic	Internal carotid artery	Traverses optic foramen to reach orbital cavity
Central artery of retina	Ophthalmic artery	Runs in dural sheath of optic nerve and pierces nerve near eyeball; appears at center of optic disc; supplies optic retina (except cones and rods)
Supraorbital		Passes superiorly and posteriorly from supraorbital foramen to supply forehead and scalp
Supratrochlear		Passes from supraorbital margin to forehead and scalp
Lacrimal		Passes along superior border of lateral rectus muscle to supply lacrimal gland, conjunctiva, and eyelids
Dorsal nasal		Courses along dorsal aspect of nose and supplies its surface
Short posterior ciliaries		Pierce sclera at periphery of optic nerve to supply choroid, which in turn supplies cones and rods of optic retina
Long posterior ciliaries		Pierce sclera to supply ciliary body and iris
Posterior ethmoidal		Passes through posterior ethmoidal foramen to posterior ethmoidal cells
Anterior ethmoidal		Passes through anterior ethmoidal foramen to anterior cranial fossa; supplies anterior and middle ethmoidal cells, frontal sinus, nasal cavity, and skin on dorsum of nose
Anterior ciliary	Muscular (rectus) branches of ophthalmic artery	Pierces sclera at attachments of rectus muscles and forms network in iris and ciliary body
Infraorbital	Third part of maxillary artery	Passes along infraorbital groove and foramen to face

layer of the retina. Two **long posterior ciliary arteries,** one on each side of the eyeball, pass between the sclera and the choroid to anastomose with the **anterior ciliary arteries** (continuations of the **muscular branches of the ophthalmic artery** to the rectus muscles) to supply the ciliary plexus.

Veins of the Orbit

Venous drainage of the orbit is through the **superior** and **inferior ophthalmic veins,** which pass through the superior orbital fissure and enter the cavernous sinus (Fig. 7.39). The *central vein of the retina* (Fig. 7.38) usually enters the cavernous sinus directly, but it may join one of the ophthalmic veins. The vortex or **vorticose veins** from the vascular layer of the eyeball drain into the inferior ophthalmic vein. The *scleral venous sinus* is a vascular structure encircling the anterior chamber of the eyeball through which the aqueous humor is returned to the blood circulation.

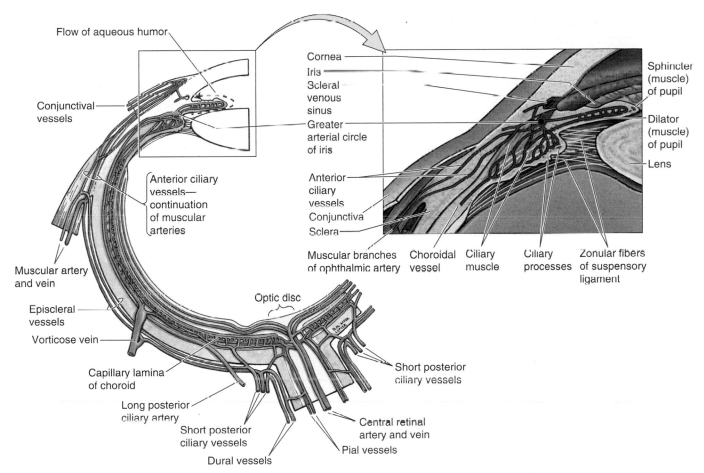

Figure 7.38. Partial horizontal section of right eyeball. The artery supplying the inner part the retina (central retinal artery) and the choroid, which in turn nourishes the outer non-vascular layer of the retina, are shown. The choroid is arranged so that the supplying vessels and larger choroidal vessels are externally placed and the smallest vessels (the capillary lamina) are most internal, adjacent to the non-vascular layer of the retina. The vorticose vein (one of four to five) drains venous blood from the choroid into the posterior ciliary and ophthalmic veins. The scleral venous sinus returns the aqueous humor, secreted into the anterior chamber by the ciliary processes, to the venous circulation.

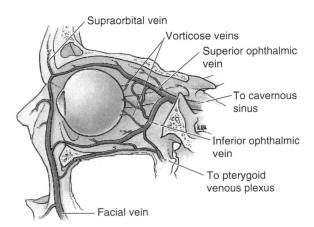

Figure 7.39. Ophthalmic veins. The superior ophthalmic vein empties into the cavernous sinus, and the inferior ophthalmic vein empties into the pterygoid venous plexus. They communicate with the facial and supraorbital veins anteriorly and each other posteriorly. The superior ophthalmic vein accompanies the ophthalmic artery and its branches.

Glaucoma

When drainage of aqueous humor through the scleral venous sinus into the blood circulation decreases significantly, pressure builds up in the anterior and posterior chambers of the eye, a condition called *glaucoma*. Blindness can result from compression of the inner layer of the eyeball (retina) and the retinal arteries if aqueous humor production is not reduced to maintain normal intraocular pressure.

Blockage of the Central Artery of the Retina

Because terminal branches of the central artery of the retina are end arteries, obstruction of them by an embolus results in instant and total blindness. Blockage of the artery is usually unilateral and occurs in older people. ▶

Blockage of the Central Vein of the Retina

Because the central vein of the retina enters the cavernous sinus, *thrombophlebitis* of this sinus may result in the passage of a thrombus to the central retinal vein and produce a blockage in one of the small retinal veins. Occlusion of a branch of the central vein of the retina usually results in slow, painless loss of vision. ✪

THE BOTTOM LINE: Extraocular circulation is provided mainly by the ophthalmic (internal carotid) and infraorbital (external carotid) arteries, the latter supplying structures near the orbital floor. Superior and inferior ophthalmic veins drain anteriorly to the facial vein, posteriorly to the cavernous sinus, and inferiorly to the pterygoid venous plexus. Intraocular circulation is exclusively from the ophthalmic artery, with the central retinal artery supplying all of the retina except the layer of cones and rods, which is nourished by the capillary lamina of the choroid. The ciliary-iridial structures receive blood from anterior ciliary arteries (from the rectus muscle branches of the ophthalmic artery) and two long posterior ciliary arteries. Multiple short posterior ciliary arteries supply the choroid. Superior and inferior vorticose veins drain the eyeballs to the respective ophthalmic veins.

Temporal Region

The **temporal region** includes the temporal and infratemporal fossae, superior and inferior to the zygomatic arch, respectively (Fig. 7.40).

Temporal Fossa

The *temporal fossa*, in which the *temporal muscle* (L. *temporalis*) is located, is bounded (Fig. 7.40*A*):

- Posteriorly and superiorly by the temporal lines.
- Anteriorly by the frontal and zygomatic bones.
- Laterally by the zygomatic arch.
- Inferiorly by the infratemporal crest (Fig. 7.40*B*).

Surface Anatomy of the Eyeball and Lacrimal Apparatus

For a description of the surface anatomy of the eyelids, see "Surface Anatomy of the Face," earlier in this chapter.

The anterior part of the **sclera** (the "white" of the eye) is covered by the transparent **bulbar conjunctiva**, which contains minute but apparent conjunctival blood vessels (Fig. SA7.3*A* & *B*). When irritated, the vessels may enlarge noticeably, and the bulbar conjunctiva may take on a distinctly pink appearance when inflamed ("red" eyes). The normal tough, opaque sclera often appears slightly blue in infants and children and commonly has a yellow hue in many older people.

The anterior transparent part of the eye is the **cornea**, which is continuous with the sclera at its margins. In a lateral view (Fig. SA7.3*A*), most of the visible part of the eyeball protrudes slightly through the **palpebral fissure**. It is apparent that the cornea has a greater curvature (convexity) than that of the rest of the eyeball (the part covered by sclera); thus a shallow angle occurs at the **sclerocorneal junction**, or *corneal limbus* (Fig. SA7.3*B*). The prominence of the cornea also makes movements of the eyeball apparent when the eyelids are closed.

The dark circular opening through which light enters the eyeball, the **pupil**, is surrounded by the **iris** (plural = irides), a circular pigmented diaphragm. The relative sizes of the pupil and iris varies with the brightness of the entering light; however, the size of the contralateral pupils and irides should be uniform.

Normally, when the eyes are open and the gaze is directed anteriorly, the superior part of the cornea and iris are covered by the edge of the **superior eyelid,** and the inferior part of the cornea and iris are fully exposed above the **inferior eyelid,** usually exposing a narrow rim of sclera. Even slight variations in the position of the eyeballs are noticeable, causing a change in facial expression to a surprised look when the superior eyelid is elevated (as occurs in *exophthalmos,* or protrusion of the eyeballs, caused by hyperthyroidism), or a sleepy appearance (as occurs when the superior eyelid droops, *ptosis,* owing to an absence of sympathetic innervation in Horner syndrome).

The **bulbar conjunctiva** is reflected from the sclera onto the deep surface of the eyelid. The **palpebral conjunctiva** is normally red and vascular and, with experience, can provide some assessment of hemoglobin levels. It is commonly examined in cases of suspected *anemia*, a blood condition commonly manifested by pallor (paleness) of the mucous membranes. When the superior eyelid is everted, the size and extent of the enclosed **superior tarsus** can be appreciated, and commonly the **tarsal glands** can be

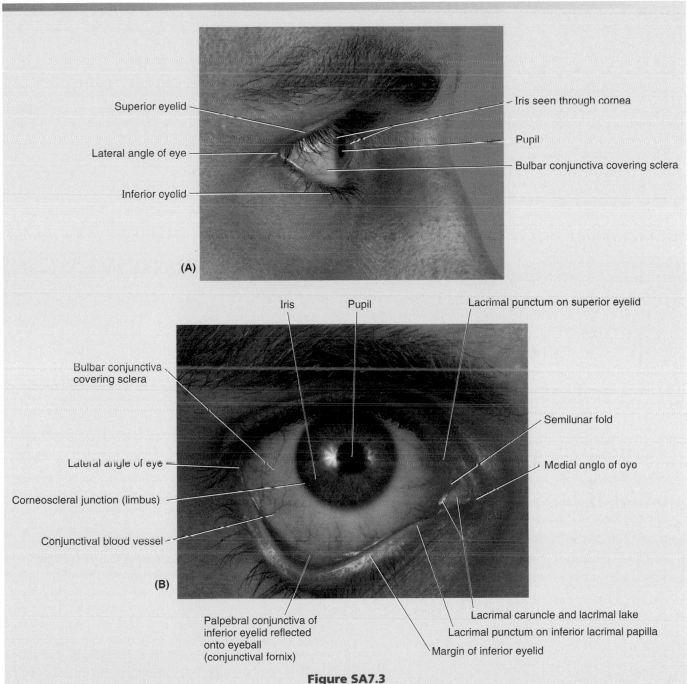

Figure SA7.3

distinguished through the palpebral conjunctiva as slightly yellow vertical stripes. Under close examination, the openings of these glands (approximately 20 per eyelid) can be seen on the margins of the eyelids, posterior to the two to three rows of emerging cilia or **eyelashes.** As the bulbar conjunctiva is continuous with the anterior epithelium of the cornea and the palpebral conjunctiva, it forms the **conjunctival sac.** The **palpebral fissure** is the "mouth," or anterior aperture, of the conjunctival sac.

In the **medial angle of the eye,** a reddish shallow reservoir of tears, the **lacrimal lake,** can be observed. Within the lake is the **lacrimal caruncle,** a small mound of moist modified skin. Lateral to the caruncle is a **semilunar conjunctival fold,** which slightly overlaps the eyeball. The semilunar fold is a rudiment of the nictitating membrane of birds and reptiles. When the edges of the eyelids are everted, a small pit, the **lacrimal punctum,** is visible at its medial end on the summit of a small elevation, the **lacrimal papilla.** ⊙

The **floor** of the temporal fossa is formed by parts of the four bones that form the *pterion:* frontal, parietal, temporal, and greater wing of the sphenoid. The fan-shaped *temporal muscle* arises from the bony floor and the overlying **temporal fascia** (Fig. 7.41), which forms the **roof** of the temporal fossa. This tough fascia covers the temporal muscle, attaching superiorly to the *superior temporal line.* Inferiorly, the fascia splits into two layers, which attach to the lateral and medial surfaces of the zygomatic arch. The temporal fascia also tethers the zygomatic arch superiorly. When the powerful masseter muscle, which is attached to the inferior border of the arch, contracts and exerts a strong downward pull on the arch, the temporal fascia provides resistance.

Infratemporal Fossa

The **infratemporal fossa** is an irregularly shaped space deep and inferior to the zygomatic arch, deep to the ramus of the mandible and posterior to the maxilla (Fig. 7.40*B*). It communicates with the temporal fossa through the interval between (deep to) the zygomatic arch and (superficial to) the cranial bones.

Boundaries of the Infratemporal Fossa
The boundaries of the infratemporal fossa are as follows (Fig. 7.40*A* & *B*):

- Laterally: the ramus of the mandible.

- Medially: the lateral pterygoid plate.

- Anteriorly: the posterior aspect of the maxilla.

- Posteriorly: the tympanic plate and the mastoid and styloid processes of the temporal bone.

- Superiorly: the inferior (infratemporal) surface of the greater wing of the sphenoid.

- Inferiorly: where the medial pterygoid muscle attaches to the mandible near its angle.

Contents of the Infratemporal Fossa
The infratemporal fossa contains the (Fig. 7.41):

- Inferior part of the temporal muscle.

- Lateral and medial pterygoid muscles.

- Maxillary artery.

- Pterygoid venous plexus.

- Mandibular, inferior alveolar, lingual, buccal, and chorda tympani nerves and the otic ganglion.

The temporal and pterygoid muscles are described with the muscles of mastication.

The **maxillary artery** is the larger of the two terminal branches of the external carotid artery (Table 7.10). It arises posterior to the neck of the mandible and is divided into three parts based on its relation to the lateral pterygoid muscle (Figs. 7.41*B* & *C* and 7.42). The courses of the three parts of the maxillary artery are illustrated and described and their branches and distributions are listed in Table 7.10.

The **pterygoid venous plexus** is located partly between the temporal and the pterygoid muscles (Table 7.7). It is the venous equivalent of most of the maxillary artery—that is, most of the veins that accompany the branches of the maxillary artery drain into this plexus. The plexus anastomoses anteriorly with the facial vein via the deep facial vein and superiorly with the cavernous sinus via emissary veins. The extensive nature and volume of this plexus is difficult to appreciate in the cadaver, in which it is usually drained of blood.

The *mandibular nerve* descends through the foramen ovale into the infratemporal fossa and divides into sensory and motor branches (Fig. 7.42). The branches of CN V$_3$ are the auriculotemporal, inferior alveolar, lingual, and buccal nerves. Branches of the CN V$_3$ also supply the four muscles of mastication but not the buccinator, which is supplied by the facial nerve.

The **otic ganglion** (parasympathetic) is located in the infratemporal fossa, just inferior to the foramen ovale, medial to CN V$_3$ and posterior to the medial pterygoid muscle. Presynaptic parasympathetic fibers, derived mainly from the glossopharyngeal nerve, synapse in the otic ganglion. Postsynaptic parasympathetic fibers, which are secretory to the parotid gland, pass from the otic ganglion to this gland through the auriculotemporal nerve.

The *auriculotemporal nerve* encircles the middle meningeal artery and divides into numerous branches, the largest of which passes posteriorly, medial to the neck of the mandible, and supplies sensory fibers to the auricle and temporal region. The auricotemporal nerve also sends articular fibers to the TMJ and parasympathetic secretomotor fibers to the parotid gland.

The **inferior alveolar nerve** enters the mandibular foramen and passes through the mandibular canal, forming the *inferior dental plexus,* which sends branches to all mandibular teeth on its side. Another branch of the plexus, the *mental nerve,* passes through the mental foramen and supplies the skin and mucous membrane of the lower lip, the skin of the chin, and the vestibular gingiva of the mandibular incisor teeth.

The **lingual nerve** lies anterior to the inferior alveolar nerve (Figs. 7.41*B* & *C* and 7.42). It is sensory to the anterior two thirds of the tongue, the floor of the mouth, and the lingual gingivae. It enters the mouth between the medial pterygoid muscle and the ramus of the mandible and passes anteriorly under cover of the oral mucosa, just inferior to the 3rd molar tooth.

The **chorda tympani nerve**, a branch of CN VII carrying taste fibers from the anterior two thirds of the tongue, joins the lingual nerve in the infratemporal fossa (Fig. 7.41*C*). The chorda tympani also carries secretomotor fibers for the submandibular and sublingual salivary glands.

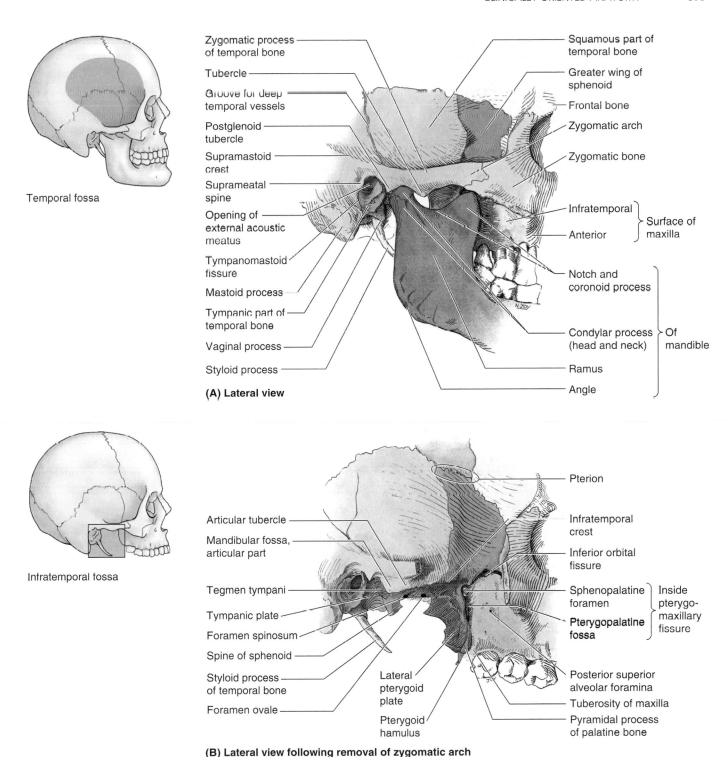

Temporal fossa

Zygomatic process of temporal bone

Tubercle

Groove for deep temporal vessels

Postglenoid tubercle

Supramastoid crest

Suprameatal spine

Opening of external acoustic meatus

Tympanomastoid fissure

Mastoid process

Tympanic part of temporal bone

Vaginal process

Styloid process

Squamous part of temporal bone

Greater wing of sphenoid

Frontal bone

Zygomatic arch

Zygomatic bone

Infratemporal ⎱ Surface of
Anterior ⎰ maxilla

Notch and coronoid process

Condylar process (head and neck) ⎱ Of
Ramus ⎰ mandible
Angle

(A) Lateral view

Infratemporal fossa

Articular tubercle

Mandibular fossa, articular part

Tegmen tympani

Tympanic plate

Foramen spinosum

Spine of sphenoid

Styloid process of temporal bone

Foramen ovale

Lateral pterygoid plate

Pterygoid hamulus

Pterion

Infratemporal crest

Inferior orbital fissure

Sphenopalatine ⎱ Inside
foramen ⎰ pterygo-
maxillary
Pterygopalatine ⎰ fissure
fossa

Posterior superior alveolar foramina

Tuberosity of maxilla

Pyramidal process of palatine bone

(B) Lateral view following removal of zygomatic arch and ramis of mandible

Figure 7.40. Bony boundaries of temporal and infratemporal fossae. A. The lateral wall of the infratemporal fossa is formed by the ramus of the mandible. The space is deep to the zygomatic arch and is traversed by the temporal muscle and the deep temporal nerves and vessels. Through this interval, the temporal fossa communicates inferiorly with the infratemporal fossa. **B.** The roof and three walls of the infratemporal fossa are shown. The fossa is an irregularly shaped space posterior to the maxilla (anterior wall). The roof of the fossa is formed by the infratemporal surface of the greater wing of the sphenoid. The medial wall is formed by the lateral pterygoid plate; and the posterior wall is formed by the tympanic plate, styloid process, and mastoid process of the temporal bone. The infratemporal fossa communicates with the pterygopalatine fossa through the pterygomaxillary fissure.

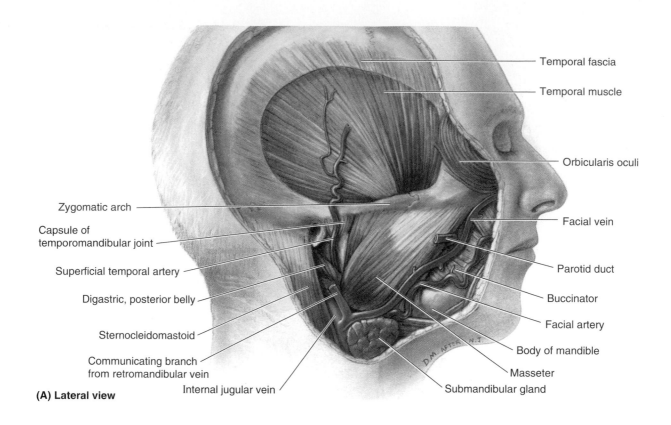

(A) Lateral view

Temporal fascia

Temporal muscle

Orbicularis oculi

Facial vein

Parotid duct

Buccinator

Facial artery

Body of mandible

Masseter

Submandibular gland

Zygomatic arch

Capsule of temporomandibular joint

Superficial temporal artery

Digastric, posterior belly

Sternocleidomastoid

Communicating branch from retromandibular vein

Internal jugular vein

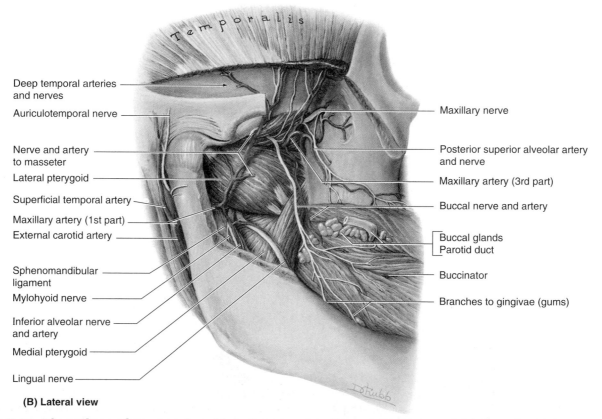

(B) Lateral view

Deep temporal arteries and nerves

Auriculotemporal nerve

Nerve and artery to masseter

Lateral pterygoid

Superficial temporal artery

Maxillary artery (1st part)

External carotid artery

Sphenomandibular ligament

Mylohyoid nerve

Inferior alveolar nerve and artery

Medial pterygoid

Lingual nerve

Maxillary nerve

Posterior superior alveolar artery and nerve

Maxillary artery (3rd part)

Buccal nerve and artery

Buccal glands
Parotid duct

Buccinator

Branches to gingivae (gums)

Figure 7.41. Dissections of temporal and infratemporal regions. A. In this superficial dissection of the great muscles on the side of the cranium, the parotid gland and most of the temporal fascia have been removed. The temporal and masseter muscles are both supplied by the trigeminal nerve (CN V) and both close the jaw. The facial artery passes deep to the submandibular gland, whereas the facial vein passes superficial to it. **B.** In this superficial dissection of the infratemporal region, most of the zygomatic arch and attached masseter, the coronoid process and adjacent parts of the ramus of the mandible, and the inferior half of the temporal muscle have been removed. The first part of the maxillary artery, the larger of the two end branches of the external carotid, run anteriorly, deep to the neck of the mandible and then pass deeply between the lateral and the medial pterygoid muscles.

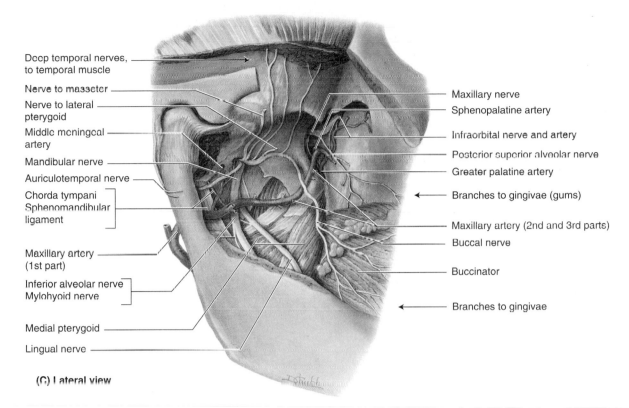

Deep temporal nerves, to temporal muscle

Nerve to masseter

Nerve to lateral pterygoid

Middle meningeal artery

Mandibular nerve

Auriculotemporal nerve

Chorda tympani
Sphenomandibular ligament

Maxillary artery (1st part)

Inferior alveolar nerve
Mylohyoid nerve

Medial pterygoid

Lingual nerve

(C) Lateral view

Maxillary nerve
Sphenopalatine artery
Infraorbital nerve and artery
Posterior superior alveolar nerve
Greater palatine artery
Branches to gingivae (gums)
Maxillary artery (2nd and 3rd parts)
Buccal nerve
Buccinator
Branches to gingivae

Figure 7.41. *(Continued)* **C.** In this deep dissection of the infratemporal region, more of the ramus of the mandible, the lateral pterygoid muscle, and most branches of the maxillary artery have been removed. Branches of the mandibular nerve (CN V₃), including the auriculotemporal nerve, and the second part of the maxillary artery pass between the sphenomandibular ligament and the neck of the mandible.

Mandibular Nerve Block

To produce a mandibular nerve block, an anesthetic agent is injected near the mandibular nerve where it enters the infratemporal fossa. In the extraoral approach, the needle passes through the mandibular notch of the ramus of the mandible into the infratemporal fossa. The injection usually anesthetizes the auriculotemporal, inferior alveolar, lingual, and buccal branches of CN V₃.

Inferior Alveolar Nerve Block

An inferior alveolar nerve block anesthetizes the inferior alveolar nerve, a branch of CN V₃. The site of the anesthetic injection is around the *mandibular foramen*, the opening into the mandibular canal on the medial aspect of the ramus of the mandible. This canal gives passage to the inferior alveolar nerve, artery, and vein. When this nerve block is successful, all mandibular teeth are anesthetized to the median plane. The skin and mucous membrane of the lower lip, the labial alveolar mucosa and gingivae, and the skin of the chin are also anesthetized because they are supplied by the mental nerve, a branch of the inferior alveolar nerve. ✪

Temporomandibular Joint

The TMJ is a modified hinge type of synovial joint (Fig. 7.43). The articular surfaces involved are the condyle of the mandible, the articular tubercle of the temporal bone, and the mandibular fossa. The joint capsule of the TMJ is loose. The fibrous layer of the capsule attaches to the margins of the articular area on the temporal bone and around the neck of the mandible (Fig. 7.43A & C). The joint has two synovial membranes: the *superior synovial membrane* lines the fibrous layer of the capsule superior to the articular disc, and the *inferior synovial membrane* lines the fibrous layer of the capsule inferior to the articular disc (Fig. 7.43A & E–G).

The **articular disc** divides the TMJ into two separate compartments. The gliding movements of protrusion and retrusion (translation) occur in the superior compartment; the hinge movements of depression and elevation occur in the inferior compartment. The thick part of the joint capsule forms the intrinsic **lateral ligament** (temporomandibular ligament), which strengthens the TMJ laterally and, with the postglenoid tubercle, acts to prevent posterior dislocation of the joint.

Two extrinsic ligaments and the lateral ligament connect the mandible to the cranium. The **stylomandibular ligament,** which is actually a thickening of the fibrous capsule of the parotid gland, runs from the styloid process to the angle of
(cont'd on page 986)

Table 7.10. Parts and Branches of the Maxillary Artery

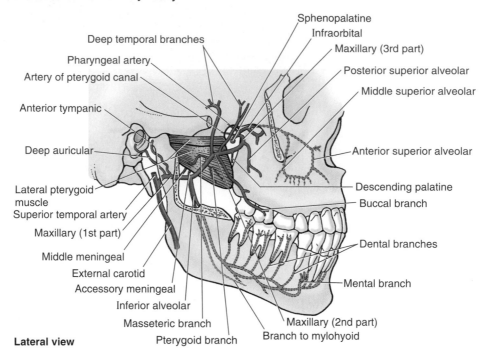

Deep temporal branches
Pharyngeal artery
Artery of pterygoid canal
Anterior tympanic
Deep auricular
Lateral pterygoid muscle
Superior temporal artery
Maxillary (1st part)
Middle meningeal
External carotid
Accessory meningeal
Inferior alveolar
Masseteric branch
Pterygoid branch

Sphenopalatine
Infraorbital
Maxillary (3rd part)
Posterior superior alveolar
Middle superior alveolar
Anterior superior alveolar
Descending palatine
Buccal branch
Dental branches
Mental branch
Maxillary (2nd part)
Branch to mylohyoid

Lateral view

Part	Course	Branches	Distribution
First (mandibular) part	Proximal (posterior) to lateral pterygoid muscle; runs horizontally, deep (medial) to neck of condylar process of mandible and lateral to stylomandibular ligament	Deep auricular artery	Supplies external acoustic meatus, external tympanic membrane, and temporomandibular joint
		Anterior tympanic artery	Supplies internal aspect of tympanic membrane
		Middle meningeal artery	Enters cranial cavity via foramen spinosum to supply periosteum, bone, red bone marrow, dura mater of lateral wall and calvaria of neurocranium, trigeminal ganglion, facial nerve and geniculate ganglion, tympanic cavity, and tensor tympani muscle
		Accessory meningeal artery	Enters cranial cavity via foramen ovale; its distribution is mainly extracranial to muscles of infratemporal fossa, sphenoid bone, mandibular nerve, and otic ganglion
		Inferior alveolar artery	Descends to enter mandibular canal of mandible via mandibular foramen; supplies mandible, mandibular teeth, chin, mylohyoid
Second (pterygoid) part	Adjacent (superficial or deep) to lateral pterygoid muscle; ascends obliquely anterosuperiorly, medial to temporal muscle	Masseteric artery	Traverses mandibular notch, supplying temporomandibular joint and masseter
		Deep temporal arteries	Anterior and posterior arteries ascend between temporal muscle and bone of temporal fossa, supplying mainly muscle
		Pterygoid branches	Irregular in number and origin; supply pterygoid muscle
		Buccal artery	Runs anteroinferiorly with buccal nerve to supply buccal fat-pad, buccinator, and buccal oral mucosa
Third (pterygo-palatine) part	Distal (anteromedial) to lateral pterygoid muscle; passes between heads of lateral pterygoid and through pterygo-maxillary fissure into pterygopalatine fossa	Posterior superior alveolar artery	Descends on maxilla's infratemporal surface with branches traversing alveolar canals to supply maxillary molar and premolar teeth, adjacent gingiva, and mucous membrane of maxillary sinus
		Infraorbital artery	Traverses inferior orbital fissure, infraorbital groove, canal, and foramen; supplies inferior oblique and rectus muscles, lacrimal sac, maxillary canines and incisors teeth, mucous membrane of the maxillary sinus, and skin of infraorbital region of face
		Artery of pterygoid canal	Passes posteriorly through pterygoid canal; supplies mucosa of upper pharynx, pharyngotympanic tube, and tympanic cavity
		Pharyngeal branch	Passes through palatovaginal canal to supply mucosa of nasal roof, nasopharynx, sphenoidal air sinus, and pharyngotympanic tube
		Descending palatine artery	Descends through palatine canal, dividing into greater and lesser palatine arteries to mucosa and glands of hard and soft palate
		Sphenopalatine artery	Terminal branch of maxillary artery, traverses sphenopalatine foramen to supply walls and septum of nasal cavity; frontal, ethmoidal, sphenoid, and maxillary sinuses; and anteriormost palate

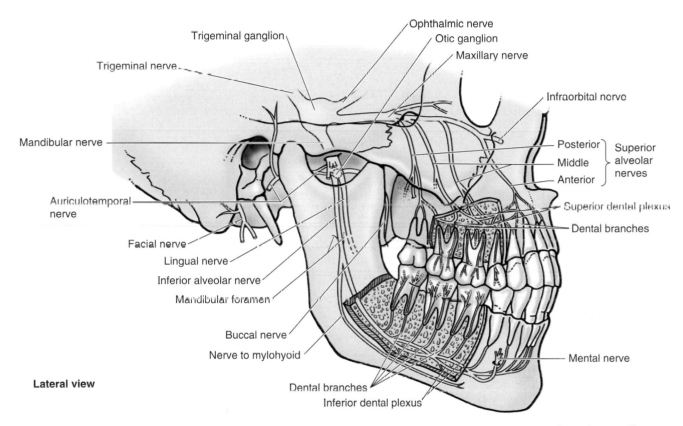

Lateral view

Figure 7.42. Innervation of teeth. The upper teeth are innervated by the superior alveolar nerves from the maxillary nerve (CN V₂). These nerves form a superior dental plexus within the upper jaw, which sends dental branches to the roots of each maxillary tooth. The posterior and middle alveolar nerves arising from the maxillary nerve and the anterior alveolar nerve from the infraorbital nerve supply the maxillary molar teeth. The lower teeth are innervated by the inferior alveolar branch of the mandibular nerve (CN V₃), the nerve entering the mandibular foramen on the medial surface of the ramus of the mandible. As in the upper jaw, an inferior dental plexus is formed, which sends dental branches to the roots of each mandibular tooth.

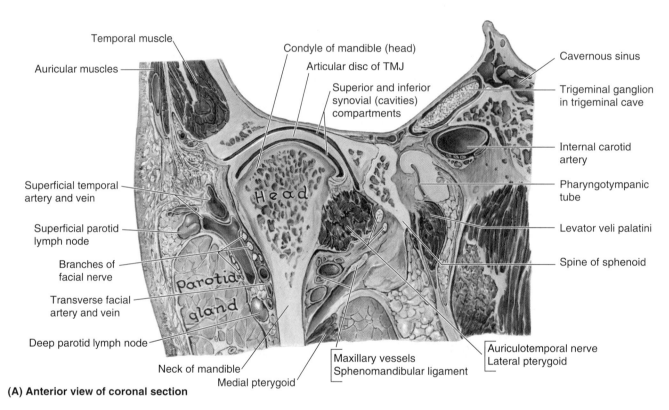

Temporal muscle

Auricular muscles

Condyle of mandible (head)

Articular disc of TMJ

Superior and inferior synovial (cavities) compartments

Cavernous sinus

Trigeminal ganglion in trigeminal cave

Internal carotid artery

Superficial temporal artery and vein

Superficial parotid lymph node

Branches of facial nerve

Transverse facial artery and vein

Deep parotid lymph node

Pharyngotympanic tube

Levator veli palatini

Spine of sphenoid

Head

Parotid gland

Neck of mandible

Medial pterygoid

Maxillary vessels
Sphenomandibular ligament

Auriculotemporal nerve
Lateral pterygoid

(A) Anterior view of coronal section

Figure 7.43. Temporomandibular joint. A. This coronal section of the right TMJ demonstrates that the articular disc divides the joint cavity into superior and inferior compartments.

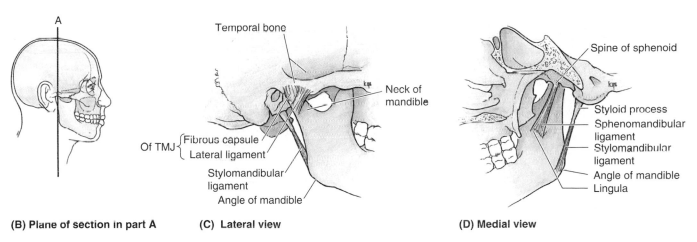

A

Temporal bone

Neck of mandible

Of TMJ { **Fibrous capsule**
{ **Lateral ligament**

Stylomandibular ligament

Angle of mandible

Spine of sphenoid

Styloid process
Sphenomandibular ligament
Stylomandibular ligament
Angle of mandible
Lingula

(B) Plane of section in part A

(C) Lateral view

(D) Medial view

Postglenoid tubercle
Mandibular fossa
Articular disc
Head of mandible
Articular tubercle
Pterygoid fovea of neck of mandible

Incus

Superior and inferior heads of lateral pterygoid

Mandible

Styloid process

(E) Sagittal section

Mandibular fossa } Of temporal
Articular tubercle } bone

Head of mandible

Articular disc

(F) Lateral view of sagittal section

(G) Sagittal MRI

Figure 7.43. *(Continued)* **B.** This orientation drawing shows the plane of the coronal section in part **A**. **C and D.** The TMJ and the extrinsic sty-lomandibular and sphenomandibular ligaments are shown. The sphe-nomandibular ligament passively bears the weight of the lower jaw and is the "swinging hinge" of the mandible, permitting protrusion and retru-sion as well as elevation and depression. **E.** The right TMJ and related structures are shown. The tendon from the upper belly of the lateral pterygoid muscle is attached to the anterior aspect of the articular disc and fibrous layer of the joint capsule (not shown); the lower belly at-taches to a depression, the pterygoid fovea of the neck of the mandible. **F and G.** The position of the TMJ with the mouth open is demonstrated. Note the position of the articular disc (*D*) and the head of the mandible (*H*) in relation to the mandibular fossa (*F*) and the articular tubercle of the temporal bone. (Part **G** courtesy of Dr. W. Kucharczyk, Chair of Medical Imaging, University of Toronto, and Clinical Director of Tri-Hos-pital Resonance Centre, Toronto, Ontario, Canada.)

the mandible (Fig. 7.43*C* & *D*). It does not contribute significantly to the strength of the joint. The **spheno-mandibular ligament** runs from the spine of the sphenoid to the lingula of the mandible (Fig. 7.43*A* & *D*). It is the primary passive support of the mandible, although the tonus of the muscles of mastication usually bears the mandible's weight. However, the ligament does serve as a "swinging hinge" for the mandible, serving both as a fulcrum and as a check ligament for the movements of the mandible at the TMJs.

The movements of the mandible at the TMJs and the muscles (or forces) producing them are summarized in Table 7.11. To enable more than a small amount of depression of the mandible—that is, to open the mouth wider than just to separate the upper and lower teeth—the head of the mandible and articular disc must move anteriorly on the articular surface until the head lies inferior to the articular tubercle (a movement

referred to as "translation" by dentists) (Fig. 7.43*E* & *F*). If this anterior gliding occurs unilaterally, the head of the contralateral mandible rotates (pivots) on the inferior surface of the articular disc, permitting simple side-to-side chewing or grinding movements over a small range. During protrusion and retrusion of the mandible, the head and articular disc slide anteriorly and posteriorly on the articular surface of the temporal bone, with both sides moving together.

TMJ movements are produced chiefly by the **muscles of mastication.** These four muscles (**temporal, masseter,** and **medial** and **lateral pterygoid muscles**) develop from the mesoderm of the embryonic first pharyngeal (mandibular) arch; consequently, they are all innervated by the nerve of that arch, the (motor root) of the mandibular nerve (CN V₃). The muscles of mastication are illustrated and their attachments, details concerning their innervation, and their main actions are described in Table 7.12. In addition to the movements listed, studies indicate that the upper head of the lateral pterygoid muscle is active during the retraction movement produced by the posterior fibers of the temporal muscle. Traction is applied to the articular disc so that it is not pushed posteriorly ahead of the retracting mandible.

Generally, depression of the mandible is produced by gravity. The *suprahyoid* and *infrahyoid muscles* are strap-like muscles on each side of the neck that are primarily used to raise and depress the hyoid bone and larynx, respectively—for example, during swallowing (see Chapter 8). Indirectly they can also help depress the mandible, especially when opening the mouth suddenly or against resistance. The platysma can be similarly used.

Table 7.11. Movements of the Temporamandibular Joint

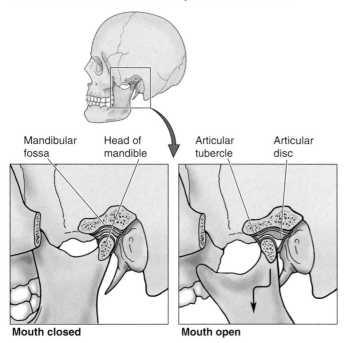

Mandibular fossa   Head of mandible   Articular tubercle   Articular disc

Mouth closed   **Mouth open**

Movements	Muscle(s)
Elevation (close mouth)	Temporal, masseter, and medial pterygoid
Depression (open mouth)	Lateral pterygoid and suprahyoid and infrahyoid muscles[a]
Protrusion (protrude chin)	Lateral pterygoid, masseter, and medial pterygoid[b]
Retrusion (retrude chin)	Temporal (posterior oblique and near horizontal fibers) and masseter
Lateral movements (grinding and chewing)	Temporal of same side, pterygoids of opposite side, and masseter

[a] The prime mover is normally gravity; these muscles are mainly active against resistance.
[b] The lateral pterygoid is the prime mover here, with minor secondary roles played by the masseter and medial pterygoid.

Dislocation of the TMJ

Sometimes during yawning or taking a large bite, excessive contraction of the lateral pterygoids may cause the heads of the mandible to dislocate anteriorly (pass anterior to the articular tubercles) (Fig. B7.23). In this position, the mandible remains wide open and the person is unable to close it. Most commonly, a sideways blow to the chin when the mouth is open dislocates the TMJ on the side that received the blow. Dislocation of the TMJ may also accompany fractures of the mandible. Posterior dislocation is uncommon, being resisted by the presence of the postglenoid tubercle and the strong intrinsic lateral ligament. Usually in falls on or direct blows to the chin, the neck of the mandible fractures before dislocation occurs. Because of the close relationship of the facial and auriculotemporal nerves to the TMJ, care must be taken during surgical procedures to preserve both the branches of the facial nerve overlying it and the articular branches of the auriculotemporal nerve that enter the posterior part of the joint. Injury to articular branches of the ▶

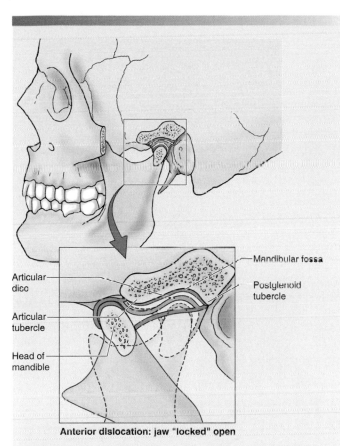

Articular disc

Articular tubercle

Head of mandible

Mandibular fossa

Postglenoid tubercle

Anterior dislocation: jaw "locked" open

Figure B7.23. Dislocation of temporomandibular joint.

auriculotemporal nerve supplying the TMJ, associated with traumatic dislocation and rupture of the articular capsule and lateral ligament, leads to laxity and instability of the TMJ.

Arthritis of the TMJ

The TMJ may become inflamed from degenerative arthritis, for example. Abnormal function of the TMJ may result in structural problems such as dental occlusion and joint clicking (*crepitus*). The clicking is thought to result from delayed anterior disc movements during mandibular depression and elevation. ○

THE BOTTOM LINE: The temporal fossa and its inferior continuation deep to the zygomatic arch and ramus of the mandible, the infratemporal fossa, are largely occupied by derivatives of the embryonic first pharyngeal arch: three of the four muscles of mastication (the temporal muscle and two pterygoid muscles) and the nerve that conveys motor fibers to them, the mandibular nerve (CN V₃). Although not part of the fossae per se, it is convenient to consider the TMJ and the fourth muscle of mastication (the masseter) at

the same time. Also contained in the infratemporal fossa is the second part of the maxillary artery and its venous equivalent, the pterygoid venous plexus. Adjacent cranial compartments communicate with the fossae, and neurovascular structures pass to and from the fossae via bony passages, including the oval foramen (through which the mandibular nerve enters from the middle cranial fossa), the foramen spinosum (through which the middle meningeal artery enters and the meningeal branch of CN V₃ returns to the middle cranial fossa), the pterygomaxillary fissure (through which the maxillary artery passes into the pterygopalatine fossa for further distribution), the inferior orbital fissure (through which the inferior ophthalmic veins drain to the pterygoid venous plexus), and the mandibular foramen (through which the inferior alveolar nerve passes to mandibular canal for distribution to lower jaw and teeth).

Oral Region

The **oral region** includes the oral cavity, teeth, gingivae, tongue, palate, and the region of the palatine tonsils. The oral cavity is where food is ingested and prepared for digestion in the stomach and small intestine. Food is chewed by the teeth, and saliva from the salivary glands facilitates the formation of a manageable *food bolus* (L. lump). *Deglutition* (swallowing) is voluntarily initiated in the oral cavity. The voluntary phase of the process pushes the bolus from the oral cavity into the pharynx, the expanded part of the alimentary (digestive) system, where the automatic phase of swallowing occurs.

Oral Cavity

The **oral cavity** consists of two parts: the *oral vestibule* and the *oral cavity proper* (Fig. 7.44). It is in the oral cavity that food and drinks are tasted and savored and where mastication and lingual manipulation of food occur. The **oral vestibule** is the slit-like space between the teeth and buccal gingiva and the lips and cheeks. The vestibule communicates with the exterior through the **mouth.** The size of the **oral fissure** (the oral opening; L. *rima oris*) is controlled by the circumoral muscles, such as the orbicularis oris (the sphincter of the oral fissure), the buccinator, risorius, and depressors and elevators of the lips (dilators of the fissure). The **oral cavity proper** is the space between the upper and the lower **dental arches** or **arcades** (maxillary and mandibular alveolar arches and the teeth they bear). It is limited laterally and anteriorly by the maxillary and mandibular alveolar arches housing the teeth. The roof of the oral cavity is formed by the palate. Posteriorly, the oral cavity communicates with the oropharynx (oral part of the pharynx). When the mouth is closed and at rest, the oral cavity is fully occupied by the tongue.

Table 7.12. Muscles Acting on the Mandible/Temporomandibular Joint (TMJ)

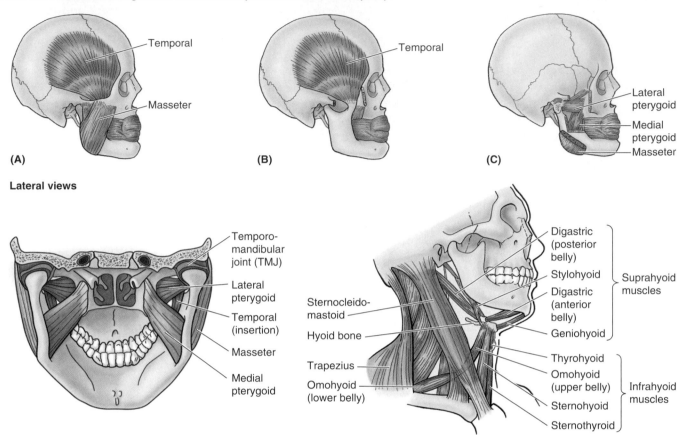

(A) **(B)** **(C)**

Lateral views

(D) Posterior view of viscerocranium **(E) Anterolateral view with head rotated slightly to left**

Muscle(s)	Proximal Attachment	Distal Attachment	Innervation		Action on Mandible
Muscles of mastication					
Temporal	Triangular muscle with broad attachment to floor of temporal fossa and deep surface of temporal fascia	Narrow attachment to tip and medial surface of coronoid process and anterior border of ramus of mandible	Anterior trunk of mandibular nerve (CN V$_3$)	Via deep temporal branches	Elevates mandible, closing jaws; posterior, more horizontal fibers are 1° retractors of mandible
Masseter	Quadrate muscle attaching to inferior border and medial surface of maxillary process of zygomatic bone and the zygomatic arch	Angle and lateral surface of ramus of mandible		Via masseteric nerve	Elevates mandible, closing jaws; superficial fibers make limited contribution to protrusion of mandible
Lateral pterygoid	Triangular two-headed muscle from (1) infratemporal surface and crest of greater wing of sphenoid and (2) lateral surface of lateral pterygoid plate	Upper head attaches primarily to joint capsule and articular disc of TMJ; inferior head attaches primarily to pterygoid fovea on anteromedial aspect of neck of condyloid process of mandible		Via lateral pterygoid nerves	Acting bilaterally, protracts mandible and depresses chin; acting unilaterally, swings jaw toward contralateral side; alternate unilateral contraction produces larger lateral chewing movements
Medial pterygoid	Quadrangular two-headed muscle from (1) medial surface of lateral pterygoid plate and pyramidal process of palatine bone and (2) tuberosity of maxilla	Medial surface of ramus of mandible, inferior to mandibular foramen; in essence, a "mirror image" of the ipsilateral masseter, the two muscles flanking the ramus		Via medial pterygoid nerve	Acts synergistically with masseter to elevate mandible; contributes to protrusion; alternate unilateral activity produces smaller grinding movements

Table 7.12. Muscles Acting on the Mandible/Temporomandibular Joint (TMJ) *(Continued)*

Muscle(s)	Proximal Attachment	Distal Attachment	Innervation	Action on Mandible
Suprahyoid muscles				
Digastric	Base of cranium	Hyoid bone	Facial and mandibular nerves	Depresses mandible against resistance when infrahyoid muscles fix or depress hyoid bone
Stylohyoid	Styloid process		Facial nerve	
Mylohyoid	Medial body of mandible		Mandibular nerve	
Geniohyoid	Anterior body of mandible		Nerve to geniohyoid (C1–2)	
Infrahyoid muscles				
Omohyoid	Scapula	Hyoid bone	Ansa cervicalis from cervical plexus (C1–3)	Fixes or depresses hyoid bone
Sternohyoid	Manubrium of sternum			
Sternothyroid and thyrohyoid	Manubrium of sternum and thyroid cartilage			
Muscle of facial expression				
Platysma	Subcutaneous tissue of infraclavicular and supraclavicular regions	Base of mandible, skin of cheek and lower lip, angle of mouth (modiolus), and orbicularis oris	Cervical branch of facial nerve (CN VII)	Depresses mandible against resistance

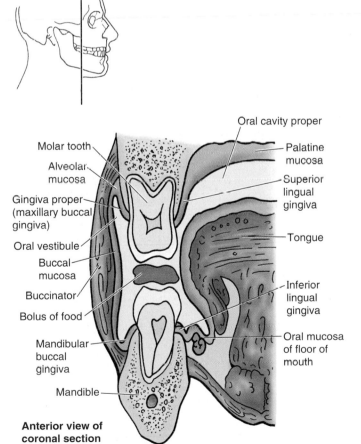

Figure 7.44. Coronal section of mouth region. The orientation drawing shows the plane of the section. During chewing, the tongue (centrally), the buccinator (laterally), and the orbicularis oris (anteriorly) work together to retain the bolus of food between the occlusive surfaces of the molar teeth.

Lips, Cheeks, and Gingivae

Lips and Cheeks

The **lips** are mobile, musculofibrous folds surrounding the mouth, extending from the *nasolabial sulci* and *nares* laterally and superiorly to the *mentolabial sulcus* inferiorly (Fig. 7.45). They contain the orbicularis oris and superior and inferior labial muscles, vessels, and nerves. The lips are covered externally by skin and internally by mucous membrane. The lips function as the valves of the *oral fissure,* containing the sphincter (orbicularis oris) that controls entry and exit from the mouth and upper alimentary and respiratory tracts. The lips are used for grasping food, sucking liquids, keeping food out of the oral vestibule, forming speech, and osculation (kissing). The *transitional zone of the lips* (commonly considered by itself to be the lip), ranging from brown to red, continues into the oral cavity where it is continuous with the mucous membrane. This membrane covers the intraoral, vestibular part of the lips (Fig. 7.46). The **labial frenula** (Mod. L. bridle) are free-edged folds of mucous membrane in the midline, extending from the vestibular gingiva to the mucosa of the upper and lower lips; the one extending to the lower lip is smaller. Other smaller frenula sometimes appear laterally in the premolar vestibular regions.

The *superior* and *inferior labial arteries,* branches of the facial arteries, anastomose with each other in the lips to form an arterial ring (Table 7.6). The pulse of these arteries may be palpated by grasping the upper or lower lip lightly between the first two digits. The upper lip is supplied by superior labial branches of the *facial* and *infraorbital arteries.* The lower lip is supplied by inferior labial branches of the *facial* and *mental arteries.* The upper lip is supplied by the superior labial branches of the *infraorbital nerves* (of CN V_2), and the lower lip is supplied by the inferior labial

branches of the mental nerves (of CN V_3). Lymph from the upper lip and lateral parts of the lower lip passes primarily to the *submandibular lymph nodes* (Fig. 7.45), whereas lymph from the medial part of the lower lip passes initially to the *submental lymph nodes.*

Cleft Lip

Cleft lip (*harelip*) is a congenital anomaly (usually of the upper lip) that occurs in 1 of 1000 births (Moore and Persaud, 2003); 60–80% of affected infants are males. The clefts vary from a small notch in the transitional zone and vermilion border to a notch that extends through the lip into the nose (Fig. B7.24). In severe cases, the cleft extends deeper and is continuous with a cleft in the palate. Cleft lip may be unilateral or bilateral.

Cyanosis of the Lips

The lips, like the fingers, have an abundant, relatively superficial blood flow. Because of this, they can lose a disproportionate amount of body heat when exposed to a cold environment. Both are provided with sympathetically innervated arteriovenous anastomoses, capable of redirecting a considerable portion of the blood back to the body core, reducing heat loss while producing cyanosis of the lips and fingers. *Cyanosis,* a dark bluish or purplish coloration of the lips and mucous membranes, results from deficient oxygenation of capillary blood and is a sign of many pathologic conditions. The common blue discoloration of the lips ▶

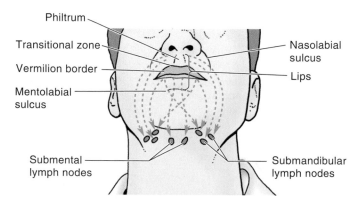

Anterior view

Figure 7.45. Lymphatic drainage of lips. Lymph from the upper lip and lateral parts of the lower lip drains to the submandibular nodes. Lymph from the middle part of the lower lip drains to the submental nodes.

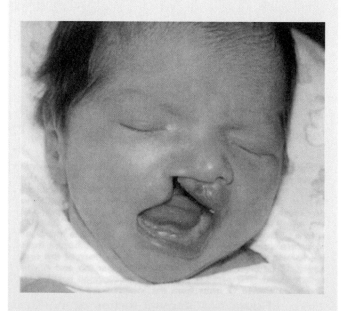

Figure B7.24. Unilateral cleft lip.

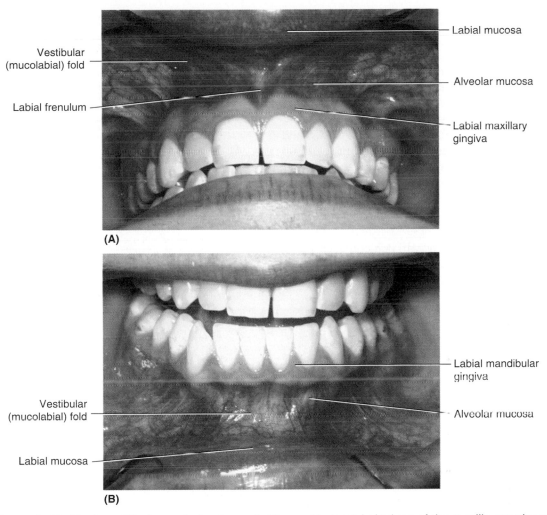

Labial mucosa

Vestibular (mucolabial) fold

Alveolar mucosa

Labial frenulum

Labial maxillary gingiva

(A)

Labial mandibular gingiva

Vestibular (mucolabial) fold

Alveolar mucosa

Labial mucosa

(B)

Figure 7.46. Oral vestibule and gingivae. A. The vestibule and gingivae of the maxilla are shown. **B.** The vestibule and gingivae of the mandible are shown. As the alveolar mucosa approaches the necks of the teeth, it changes in texture and color to become the gingiva proper. (Courtesy of Dr. B. Liebgott, Professor, Division of Anatomy, Department of Surgery, University of Toronto, Toronto, Ontario, Canada.)

owing to cold exposure does not indicate pathology; instead, it results from the decreased blood flow in the capillary beds supplied by the superior and inferior labial arteries and the increased extraction of oxygen. Simple warming restores the normal coloring of the lips.

Large Labial Frenula

Excessively large superior labial frenula in children may cause a space between the central incisor teeth. Resection of the frenulum and the underlying connective tissue (**frenulectomy**) between the incisors allows approximation of the teeth, which may require an orthodontic appliance ("brace"). Large lower labial frenula in adults may pull on the labial gingiva and contribute to *gingival recession,* which results in abnormal exposure of the roots of the teeth. ○

The **cheeks** (L. *buccae*) have essentially the same structure as the lips with which they are continuous. The cheeks form the movable walls of the oral cavity. Anatomically, the external aspect of the cheeks constitutes the *buccal region,* bounded anteriorly by the *oral* and *mental regions* (lips and chin), superiorly by the *zygomatic region,* posteriorly by the *parotid region,* and inferiorly by the inferior border of the *mandible* (Fig. SA7.1). The *prominence of the cheek* occurs at the junction of the zygomatic and buccal regions. The zygomatic bone underlying the prominence and the zygomatic arch that continues posteriorly are commonly referred to as the "cheek bone." Lay persons consider the zygomatic and parotid regions also to be part of the cheek. The principal muscles of the cheeks are the buccinators (Fig. 7.44). Numerous small buccal glands lie between the mucous membrane and the buccinators. Superficial to the buccinators are encapsulated collections of fat; these *buccal fat-pads* are proportionately much larger in infants, presumably to reinforce the cheeks and keep them from collapsing during sucking. The cheeks are supplied by buccal branches of the maxillary artery and innervated by buccal branches of the mandibular nerve.

THE BOTTOM LINE: The mouth is the primary portal of the alimentary system and a secondary portal for the respiratory system, especially important for speech in the latter case. The oral cavity extends from the oral fissure to the oropharyngeal isthmus. It is divided by the upper and lower jaws and their dental arcades into a superficial oral vestibule (between the lips and cheeks and the gingival and teeth) and a deeper oral cavity proper (internal to the jaws and dental arcades). The oral cavity (and specifically the oral vestibule) is bounded by the lips and cheeks, which are flexible dynamic musculofibrous folds containing muscles, neurovasculature, and mucosal glands, covered superficially with skin and deeply with oral mucosa. The cheeks also include buccal fat-pads.

Gingivae

The **gingivae** (gums) are composed of fibrous tissue covered with mucous membrane. The **gingiva proper** (attached gingiva) is firmly attached to the alveolar processes of the jaws and the necks of the teeth (Figs. 7.44 and 7.46). The gingiva proper is normally pink, stippled, and keratinizing. The **alveolar mucosa** (unattached gingiva) is normally shiny red and non-keratinizing. The nerves and vessels supplying the gingiva, underlying alveolar bone, and *periodontium* (which surrounds the root[s] of a tooth, anchoring it to the tooth socket), are presented in Table 7.13.

Gingivitis

Improper oral hygiene results in food and bacterial deposits in tooth and gingival crevices that may cause inflammation of the gingivae *(gingivitis)*. The gingivae swell and redden as a result. If untreated, the disease spreads to other supporting structures, including alveolar bone, producing *periodontitis* (inflammation and destruction of the bone and the periodontium). *Dentoalveolar abscesses* (collections of pus resulting from death of inflamed tissues) may drain to the oral cavity and lips. ⊕

Teeth

The chief functions of the teeth are to:

- Incise, reduce, and mix food material with saliva during mastication (chewing).

- Help sustain themselves in the tooth sockets by assisting the development and protection of the tissues that support them.

- Participate in articulation (distinct connected speech).

Table 7.13. Nerves and Vessels of Gingiva and Teeth

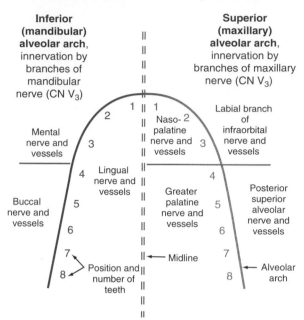

Nerves and vessels of gingiva, alveolar bone, and periodontium

Maxillary nerve (CN V$_2$)		
Posterior superior alveolar nerve and vessels	Middle superior alveolar nerve and vessels	Anterior superior alveolar nerve and vessels

	Posterior superior	Middle superior	Anterior superior
Maxillary (upper) teeth	8 7 6	5 4 3	2 1
Mandibular (lower) teeth	8 7 6	5 4 3	2 1

Inferior alveolar nerve and vessels
Mandibular nerve (CN V$_3$)

Nerves and vessels of teeth

The teeth are set in the *tooth sockets* and are used in mastication and in assisting in articulation. A tooth is identified and described on the basis of whether it is **deciduous** (primary) or **permanent** (secondary), the type of tooth, and its proximity to the midline or front of the mouth (e.g., medial and lateral incisors; the 1st molar is anterior to the 2nd). Children have 20 deciduous teeth; adults normally have 32 permanent teeth (Fig. 7.47*A* & *C*). The usual ages of the eruption ("cutting") of these teeth are given in Table 7.14. Before eruption, the developing teeth reside in the alveolar arches as **tooth buds** (Fig. 7.47*B*).

The types of teeth are identified by their characteristics: **incisors**, thin cutting edges; **canines**, single prominent cones; **premolars** (bicuspids), two cusps; and **molars**, three or more cusps. The **vestibular surface** (labial or buccal) of each tooth is directed outwardly, and the **lingual surface** is directed inwardly. As used in clinical (dental) practice, the **mesial (proximal) surface** of a tooth is directed toward the median

(A) Right anterolateral view

(B) Left anterolateral view

(C) Panoramic view

Figure 7.47. Secondary dentition. A. The teeth are shown in occlusion. There is a supernumerary midline tooth (mesodont) in this specimen (*). **B.** Maxillary and mandibular jaws of a child acquiring secondary dentition are shown. The alveolar processes are carved to reveal the roots of the teeth and tooth buds. **C.** A pantomographic radiograph of an adult mandible and maxilla is shown. The left lower 3rd molar is not present. I, incisor; *C,* canine; *PM,* premolar; *M1, M2,* and *M3,* 1st, 2nd, and 3rd molars. (Part **C** courtesy of M. J. Pharoah, Associate Professor of Dental Radiology, Faculty of Dentistry, University of Toronto, Toronto, Ontario, Canada.)

plane of the facial part of the cranium. The **distal surface** is directed away from this plane; both mesial and distal surfaces are *contact surfaces*—that is, surfaces that contact adjacent teeth. The masticatory surface is the **occlusal surface**.

Parts and Structure of the Teeth

A tooth has a crown, neck, and root (Fig. 7.48). The **crown** projects from the gingiva. The **neck** is between the crown and the root. The **root** is fixed in the tooth socket by the *periodontium;* the number of roots varies. Most of the tooth is composed of **dentin** (L. *dentinium*), which is covered by **enamel** over the crown and **cement** (L. *cementum*) over the root. The **pulp cavity** contains connective tissue, blood

vessels, and nerves. The **root canal** (pulp canal) transmits the nerves and vessels to and from the pulp cavity through the **apical foramen.**

The **tooth sockets** are in the *alveolar processes* of the maxillae and mandible and are the skeletal features that display the greatest change during a lifetime (Fig. 7.47B). Adjacent sockets are separated by **interalveolar septa;** within the socket, the roots of teeth with more than one root are separated by **interradicular septa.** The bone of the socket has a thin cortex separated from the adjacent labial and lingual cortices by a variable amount of trabeculated bone. The labial wall of the socket is particularly thin over the incisor teeth; the reverse is true for the molars, where the lingual wall is thinner. Thus the

Table 7.14. Primary (Deciduous) and Secondary Teeth

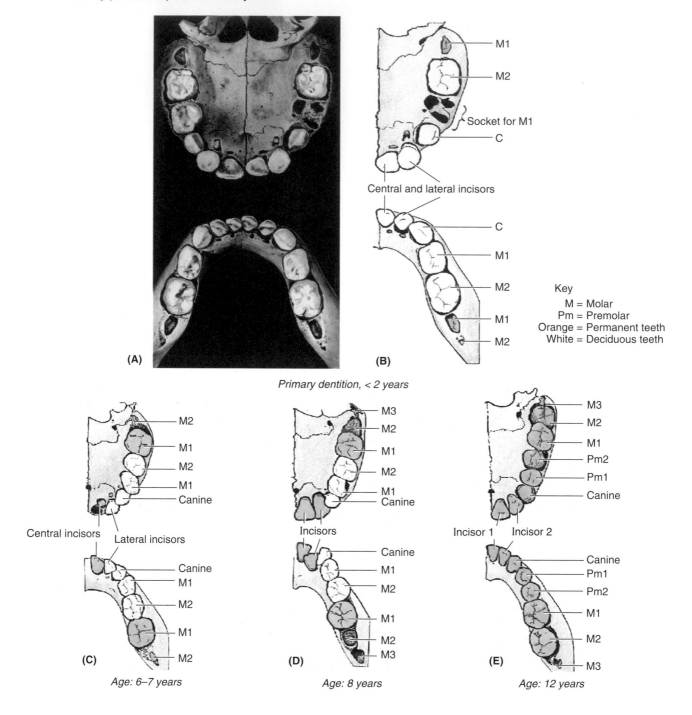

(A)

(B)

Primary dentition, < 2 years

Key
M = Molar
Pm = Premolar
Orange = Permanent teeth
White = Deciduous teeth

(C) *Age: 6–7 years*

(D) *Age: 8 years*

(E) *Age: 12 years*

Deciduous Teeth	Central Incisor	Lateral Incisor	Canine	1st Molar	2nd Molar
Eruption (months)[a]	6–8	8–10	16–20	12–16	20–24
Shedding (years)	6–7	7–8	10–12	9–11	10–12

[a]In some normal infants, the first teeth (medial incisors) may not erupt until 12–13 months of age.

Permanent Teeth	Central Incisor	Lateral Incisor	Canine	1st Premolar	2nd Premolar	1st Molar	2nd Molar	3rd Molar
Eruption (years)	7–8	8–9	10–12	10–11	11–12	6–7	12	13–25

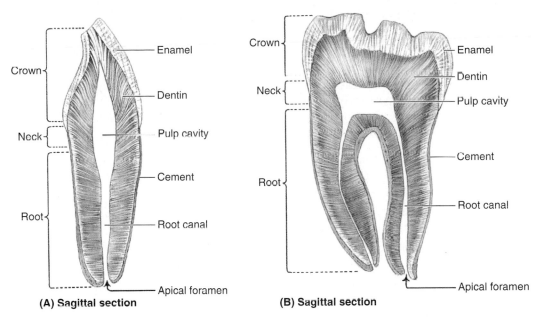

Crown
Enamel
Dentin
Neck
Pulp cavity
Root
Cement
Root canal
Apical foramen

(A) Sagittal section

Crown
Enamel
Dentin
Neck
Pulp cavity
Root
Cement
Root canal
Apical foramen

(B) Sagittal section

Figure 7.48. Sections of teeth. A. An incisor tooth is shown. **B.** A molar tooth is shown. In living people, the pulp cavity is a hollow space within the crown and neck of the tooth containing connective tissue, blood vessels, and nerves. The cavity narrows down to the root canal in a single-rooted tooth or to one canal per root of a multirooted tooth. The vessels and nerves enter or leave through the apical foramen.

labial surface commonly is broken to extract incisors and the lingual surface is broken to extract molars.

The roots of the teeth are connected to the bone of the alveolus by a springy suspension forming a special type of fibrous joint called a **dento-alveolar syndesmosis** or **gomphosis**. The **periodontium** (periodontal membrane) is composed of collagenous fibers that extend between the cement of the root and the periosteum of the alveolus. It is abundantly supplied with tactile, pressoreceptive nerve endings, lymph capillaries, and glomerular blood vessels that act as hydraulic cushioning to curb axial masticatory pressure. *Pressoreceptive nerve endings* are capable of receiving changes in pressure as stimuli.

Vasculature of the Teeth

The **superior** and **inferior alveolar arteries,** branches of the maxillary artery, supply the maxillary and mandibular teeth, respectively (Fig. 7.41B; Table 7.10). **Alveolar veins** with the same names and distribution accompany the arteries. **Lymphatic vessels** from the teeth and gingivae pass mainly to the *submandibular lymph nodes* (Fig. 7.45).

Innervation of the Teeth

The nerves supplying the teeth are illustrated in Figure 7.42 and listed in Table 7.13. The named branches of the *superior* (CN V$_2$) and *inferior* (CN V$_3$) *alveolar nerves* give rise to **dental plexuses** that supply the maxillary and mandibular teeth. The lingual nerve is closely related to the medial aspect of the 3rd molars; therefore, caution is taken to avoid injuring this nerve during their extraction.

Dental Caries, Pulpitis, and Tooth Abscesses

Decay of the hard tissues of a tooth results in the formation of *dental caries (cavities)*. Treatment involves removal of the decayed tissue and restoration of the anatomy of the tooth with a dental material. Neglected dental caries eventually invade and inflame tissues in the pulp cavity. Invasion of the pulp by a deep carious lesion results in infection and irritation of the tissues *(pulpitis)*. Because the pulp cavity is a rigid space, the swollen tissues cause considerable pain *(toothache)*. If untreated, the small vessels in the root canal may die from the pressure of the swollen tissue, and the infected material may pass through the apical canal and foramen into the periodontal tissues. An infective process develops and spreads through the root canal to the alveolar bone, producing an *abscess*. Pus from an abscess of a maxillary molar tooth may extend into the nasal cavity or the maxillary sinus. The roots of the maxillary molar teeth are closely related to the floor of this sinus. As a consequence, infection of the pulp cavity may also cause sinusitis or sinusitis may stimulate nerves entering the teeth and simulate a toothache. ▶

Extraction of the Teeth

Sometimes it is not practical to restore a tooth because of extreme tooth destruction. The only alternative is tooth extraction. A tooth may lose its blood supply as a result of trauma. The blow to the tooth disrupts the blood vessels entering and leaving the apical foramen. It is not always possible to save the tooth. *Unerupted 3rd molars* are common dental problems; these teeth are the last to erupt, usually when people are in their late teens or early 20s. Often there is not enough room for these molars to erupt, and they become lodged (impacted) under or against the 2nd molars (Fig. B7.25, *insets*). If impacted 3rd molars become painful, they are usually removed. When doing so, the surgeon takes care not to injure the alveolar nerves. ○

Figure B7.25. Superior view of normal adult mandible with full dentition. *Insets:* impacted 3rd molars.

THE BOTTOM LINE: The strong alveolar parts of the maxilla and mandible bear, in sequence, two sets of teeth (20 deciduous and 32 permanent teeth). The crowns of the teeth project from the gingiva, and the roots are anchored in tooth sockets by periodontium. The upper jaw, its teeth, gingivae, and adjacent vestibule are supplied by branches of the maxillary nerve (CN V$_2$), an artery and accompanying veins. The same features of the lower jaw are supplied by the mandibular nerve (CN V$_3$) and inferior alveolar vessels.

Palate

The **palate** forms the arched roof of the mouth and the floor of the nasal cavities (Figs. 7.49–7.51). It separates the oral cavity from the nasal cavities and the nasopharynx, the part of the pharynx superior to the soft palate. The superior (nasal) surface of the palate is covered with respiratory mucosa, and the inferior (oral) surface is covered with oral mucosa, densely packed with glands (Fig. 7.51B). The palate consists of two regions: the hard palate anteriorly and the soft palate posteriorly.

Hard Palate

The **hard palate** is vaulted (concave); this space is mostly filled by the tongue when it is at rest (Fig. 7.49). The anterior two thirds of the palate has a bony skeleton formed by the palatine processes of the maxillae and the horizontal plates of the palatine bones (Fig. 7.50A). The *incisive fossa* is a depression in the midline of the bony palate posterior to the central incisor teeth into which the incisive canals open. The nasopalatine nerves pass from the nose through a variable number of incisive canals and foramina that open into the incisive fossa (Fig. 7.50B). Medial to the 3rd molar tooth, the *greater palatine foramen* pierces the lateral border of the bony palate (Fig. 7.50A). The *greater palatine vessels and nerve* emerge from this foramen and run anteriorly on the palate. The *lesser palatine foramina* posterior to the greater palatine foramen pierce the pyramidal process of the palatine bone. These foramina transmit the *lesser palatine nerves and vessels* to the soft palate and adjacent structures (Fig. 7.52A & B).

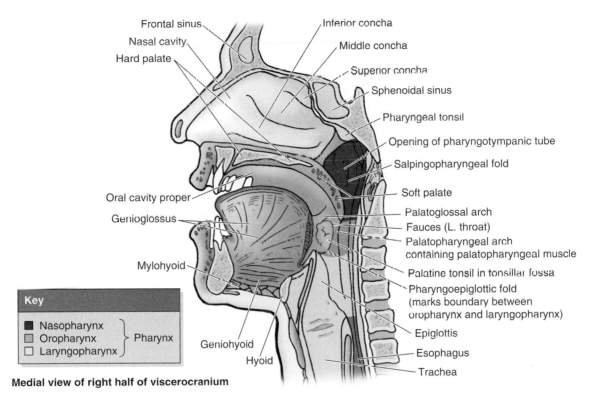

Frontal sinus
Nasal cavity
Hard palate
Oral cavity proper
Genioglossus
Mylohyoid
Geniohyoid
Hyoid

Inferior concha
Middle concha
Superior concha
Sphenoidal sinus
Pharyngeal tonsil
Opening of pharyngotympanic tube
Salpingopharyngeal fold
Soft palate
Palatoglossal arch
Fauces (L. throat)
Palatopharyngeal arch
containing palatopharyngeal muscle
Palatine tonsil in tonsillar fossa
Pharyngoepiglottic fold
(marks boundary between
oropharynx and laryngopharynx)
Epiglottis
Esophagus
Trachea

Key

■ Nasopharynx
□ Oropharynx   } Pharynx
□ Laryngopharynx

Medial view of right half of viscerocranium

Figure 7.49. Median section of head and neck. The airway and food passageways cross in the pharynx. The soft palate acts as a valve, elevating to seal the pharyngeal isthmus connecting the nasal cavity and nasopharynx with the oral cavity and oropharynx.

Soft Palate

The **soft palate** is the movable posterior third of the palate and is suspended from the posterior border of the hard palate. The soft palate has no bony skeleton; however, it has an anterior *aponeurotic part,* the **palatine aponeurosis,** which attaches to the posterior edge of the hard palate, and a posterior *muscular part* (Fig. 7.50B). The soft palate extends posteroinferiorly as a curved free margin from which hangs a conical process, the **uvula** (Figs. 7.50B and 7.51B). The soft palate is strengthened by the palatine aponeurosis, formed by the expanded tendon of the tensor veli palatini muscle (Fig. 7.50B). The aponeurosis is thick anteriorly and thin posteriorly.

When a person swallows, the soft palate initially is tensed to allow the tongue to press against it, squeezing the bolus of food to the back of the mouth. The soft palate is then elevated posteriorly and superiorly against the wall of the pharynx, thereby preventing passage of food into the nasal cavity.

Laterally, the soft palate is continuous with the wall of the pharynx and is joined to the tongue and pharynx by the **palatoglossal** and **palatopharyngeal arches,** respectively (Figs. 7.49 and 7.51B). A few taste buds are located in the epithelium covering the oral surface of the soft palate, the posterior wall of the oropharynx, and the epiglottis.

The **fauces** (L. the throat) is the space between the cavity of the mouth and the pharynx. The fauces is bounded superiorly by the soft palate, inferiorly by the root of the tongue, and laterally by the **pillars of the fauces,** the palatoglossal and palatopharyngeal arches (Fig. 7.49). The **isthmus of the fauces** is the short constricted space that establishes the connection between the oral cavity proper and the oropharynx. The isthmus is bounded anteriorly by the palatoglossal folds and posteriorly by the palatopharyngeal folds.

The **palatine tonsils,** often referred to as "the tonsils," are masses of lymphoid tissue, one on each side of the oropharynx. Each tonsil is in a **tonsillar sinus (fossa),** bounded by the palatoglossal and palatopharyngeal arches and the tongue.

Superficial Features of the Palate

The mucosa of the hard palate is tightly bound to the underlying bone (Fig. 7.51); consequently, submucous injections here are extremely painful. The *lingual gingiva,* the part of the gingiva covering the lingual surface of the teeth and the alveolar process, is continuous with the mucosa of the palate; therefore, injection of an anesthetic agent into the gingiva of a tooth anesthetizes the adjacent palatal mucosa. Deep to the mucosa are mucus-secreting **palatine glands** (Fig. 7.51B). The orifices of the ducts of these glands give the palatine mucosa a pitted (orange-peel) appearance. In the midline, posterior to the maxillary incisor teeth, is the **incisive papilla.** This elevation of the mucosa lies directly anterior to the underlying *incisive fossa.*

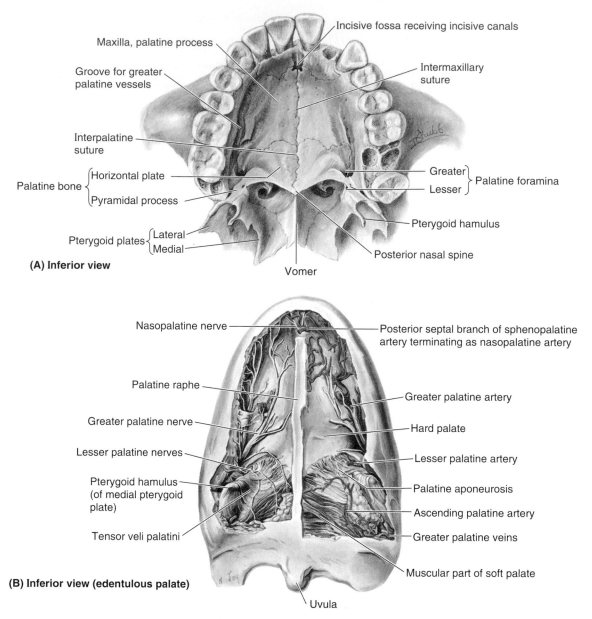

(A) Inferior view

Incisive fossa receiving incisive canals

Maxilla, palatine process

Groove for greater palatine vessels

Intermaxillary suture

Interpalatine suture

Palatine bone { Horizontal plate / Pyramidal process

Greater } Palatine foramina
Lesser

Pterygoid hamulus

Pterygoid plates { Lateral / Medial

Posterior nasal spine

Vomer

(B) Inferior view (edentulous palate)

Nasopalatine nerve

Posterior septal branch of sphenopalatine artery terminating as nasopalatine artery

Palatine raphe

Greater palatine artery

Greater palatine nerve

Hard palate

Lesser palatine nerves

Lesser palatine artery

Pterygoid hamulus (of medial pterygoid plate)

Palatine aponeurosis

Ascending palatine artery

Tensor veli palatini

Greater palatine veins

Muscular part of soft palate

Uvula

Figure 7.50. Palate. A and B. The bones of the hard palate and nerves and vessels of the edentulous palate are shown. The palate has bony, aponeurotic, and muscular parts. The mucosa has been removed on each side of the palatine raphe, demonstrating a branch of the greater palatine nerve on each side and the artery on the lateral side. There are four palatine arteries, two on the hard palate (greater palatine and the terminal branch of posterior nasal septal/sphenopalatine artery) and two on the soft palate (lesser palatine and ascending palatine).

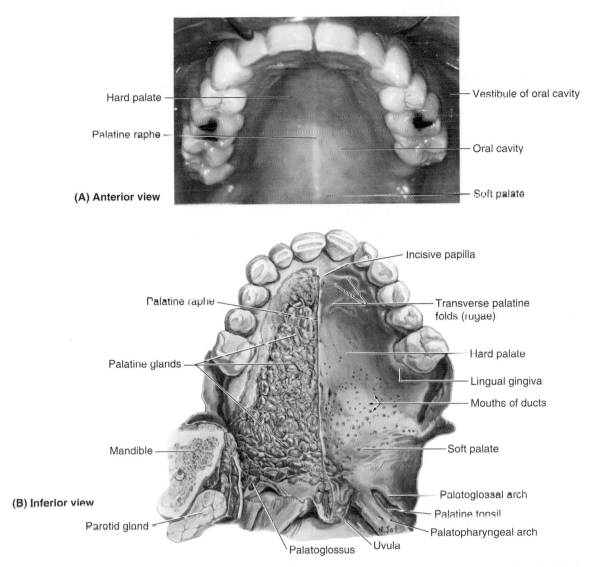

(A) Anterior view

Hard palate

Palatine raphe

Vestibule of oral cavity

Oral cavity

Soft palate

Incisive papilla

Palatine raphe

Transverse palatine folds (rugae)

Palatine glands

Hard palate

Lingual gingiva

Mouths of ducts

Mandible

Soft palate

(B) Inferior view

Palatoglossal arch

Palatine tonsil

Parotid gland

Palatopharyngeal arch

Palatoglossus

Uvula

Figure 7.51. Maxillary teeth and palate. A. The maxillary teeth and the mucosa covering the hard palate in a living person are shown. (Courtesy of Dr. B. Liebgott, Professor, Division of Anatomy, Department of Surgery, University of Toronto, Toronto, Ontario, Canada.) **B.** The mucous membrane and glands of the palate are demonstrated. The orifices of the ducts of the palatine glands give the mucous membrane an orange-skin appearance. The palatine glands form a thick layer in the soft palate, a thin one in the hard palate, and are absent in the region of the incisive fossa and the anterior part of the palatine raphe.

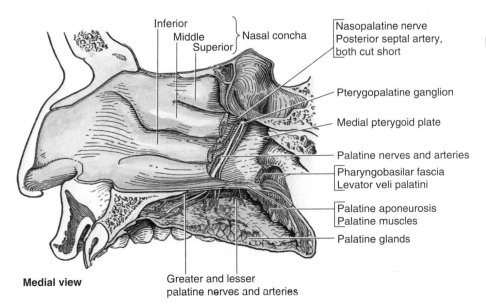

Inferior

Middle

Nasal concha

Superior

Nasopalatine nerve
Posterior septal artery, both cut short

Pterygopalatine ganglion

Medial pterygoid plate

Palatine nerves and arteries

Pharyngobasilar fascia
Levator veli palatini

Palatine aponeurosis
Palatine muscles

Palatine glands

Medial view

Greater and lesser palatine nerves and arteries

Figure 7.52. Nerves and vessels of palate. In this dissection of the posterior part of the lateral wall of the nasal cavity and the palate, the mucous membrane of the palate, containing a layer of mucous glands, has been separated from the hard and soft regions of the palate by blunt dissection. The posterior ends of the middle and inferior nasal conchae are cut through; these and the mucoperiosteum are pulled off the side wall of the nose as far as the posterior border of the medial pterygoid plate. The perpendicular plate of the palatine bone is broken through to expose the palatine nerves and arteries descending from the pterygopalatine fossa in the palatine canal.

The incisive foramina are the openings of the incisive canals that transmit the nasopalatine nerves and vessels (Fig. 7.50*A*).

Radiating laterally from the incisive papilla are several parallel **transverse palatine folds** or rugae (Fig. 7.51*A* & *B*). These folds assist with manipulation of food during mastication. Passing posteriorly in the midline of the palate from the incisive papilla is a narrow whitish streak, the **palatine raphe.** It may present as a ridge anteriorly and a groove posteriorly. The palatine raphe marks the site of fusion of the embryonic palatine processes (palatal shelves) (Moore and Persaud, 2003). You can feel the transverse palatine folds and the palatine raphe with your tongue.

Muscles of the Soft Palate

The five muscles of the soft palate arise from the base of the cranium and descend to the palate. The soft palate may be elevated so that it is in contact with the posterior wall of the pharynx. This closes the pharyngeal isthmus, requiring that one breathes through the mouth. The soft palate may also be drawn inferiorly so that it is in contact with the posterior part of the tongue. This closes the isthmus of the fauces, so that expired air passes through the nose (even when the mouth is open) and prevents substances in the oral cavity from passing to the pharynx. Tensing the soft palate pulls it tight at an intermediate level so that the tongue may push against it, compressing masticated food and propelling it into the pharynx for swallowing.

The muscles of the soft palate are illustrated and their attachments, nerve supply, and actions are described in Table 7.15. Note that the direction of pull of the belly of the *tensor veli palatini* is redirected approximately 90° because its tendon uses the pterygoid hamulus as a pulley or trochlea, allowing it to pull horizontally on the aponeurosis.

Vasculature and Innervation of the Palate

The palate has a rich blood supply, chiefly from the **greater palatine artery** on each side, a branch of the descending palatine artery (Figs. 7.50*B* and 7.52). The greater palatine artery passes through the greater palatine foramen and runs anteromedially. The **lesser palatine artery,** a smaller branch of the descending palatine artery, enters the palate through the lesser palatine foramen and anastomoses with the **ascending palatine artery,** a branch of the facial artery (Fig. 7.50*B*). The **veins of the palate** are tributaries of the *pterygoid venous plexus.*

The sensory nerves of the palate are branches of the maxillary nerve (CNV$_2$) that branch from the *pterygopalatine ganglion* (Fig. 7.52). The **greater palatine nerve** supplies the gingivae, mucous membrane, and glands of most of the hard palate. The **nasopalatine nerve** supplies the mucous membrane of the anterior part of the hard palate. The **lesser palatine nerves** supply the soft palate. The palatine nerves accompany the arteries through the greater and lesser palatine foramina, respectively. Except for the tensor veli palatini supplied by CN V$_2$, all muscles of the soft palate are supplied through the *pharyngeal plexus of nerves* (see Chapter 8).

Nasopalatine Block

The nasopalatine nerves can be anesthetized by injecting anesthetic into the incisive fossa in the hard palate. The needle is inserted immediately posterior to the incisive papilla. Both nerves are anesthetized by the same injection where they emerge through the incisive fossa (Fig. 7.50). The affected tissues are the palatal mucosa, the lingual gingivae and alveolar bone of the six anterior maxillary teeth, and the hard palate.

Greater Palatine Block

The greater palatine nerve can be anesthetized by injecting anesthetic into the greater palatine foramen. The nerve emerges between the 2nd and the 3rd molar teeth. This nerve block anesthetizes all the palatal mucosa and lingual gingivae posterior to the maxillary canine teeth and the underlying bone of the palate. Branches of the greater palatine arteries should be avoided. The anesthetic should be injected slowly to prevent stripping of the mucosa from the hard palate.

Cleft Palate

Cleft palate, with or without cleft lip, occurs in approximately 1 of 2500 births and is more common in females than in males (Moore and Persaud, 2003). The cleft may involve only the uvula, giving it a fishtail appearance, or it may extend through the soft and hard regions of the palate (Fig B7.26). In severe cases associated with cleft lip, the cleft palate extends through the alveolar processes of the maxillae and the lips on both sides. The embryological basis of cleft palate is failure of mesenchymal masses in the lateral palatine processes to meet and fuse with each other, with the nasal septum, and/or with the posterior margin of the median palatine process. ✪

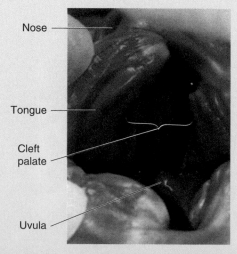

Figure B7.26. Intra-oral view of bilateral cleft palate.

Table 7.15. Muscles of the Soft Palate

Inferior view

Posterior view

Tensor veli palatini
Levator veli palatini
Palatoglossus
Palatopharyngeus
Musculus uvulae

Base of cranium
Nasal choanae
Pterygoid hamulus
Pharyngotympanic tube
Levator veli palatini
Tensor veli palatini
Palatopharyngeus
Superior constrictor (of pharynx)
Musculus uvulae
Root of tongue
Epiglottis

Muscle	Superior Attachment	Inferior Attachment	Innervation	Main Action
Tensor veli palatini	Scaphoid fossa of medial pterygoid plate, spine of sphenoid bone, and cartilage of pharyngotympanic tube	Palatine aponeurosis	Medial pterygoid nerve (a branch of mandibular nerve, CN V₃) via otic ganglion	Tenses soft palate and opens mouth of pharyngotympanic tube during swallowing and yawning
Levator veli palatini	Cartilage of pharyngotympanic tube and petrous part of temporal bone		Pharyngeal branch of vagus nerve (CN X) via pharyngeal plexus	Elevates soft palate during swallowing and yawning
Palatoglossus	Palatine aponeurosis	Side of tongue		Elevates posterior part of tongue and draws soft palate onto tongue
Palatopharyngeus	Hard palate and palatine aponeurosis	Lateral wall of pharynx		Tenses soft palate and pulls walls of pharynx superiorly, anteriorly, and medially during swallowing
Musculus uvulae	Posterior nasal spine and palatine aponeurosis	Mucosa of uvula		Shortens uvula and pulls it superiorly

THE BOTTOM LINE: The roof of the oral cavity proper is formed by the hard (anterior two thirds) and soft (posterior one third) palates, the latter being a controlled flap that allows or limits communication with the nasal cavity. The mucosa of the hard palate includes abundant palatine glands. Branches of the maxillary (greater and lesser palatine arteries) and facial (ascending palatine artery) arteries supply the palate, its venous blood draining to the pterygoid plexus. The palate receives sensory innervation from the maxillary nerve (CN V$_2$); the muscles of the soft palate receive motor innervation from the pharyngeal plexus (CN X) plus a branch from the mandibular nerve (CN V$_3$) for the tensor veli palatini.

Tongue

The **tongue** (L. *lingua;* G. *glossa*) is a mobile muscular organ that can assume a variety of shapes and positions. It is partly in the oral cavity and partly in the oropharynx. The tongue is involved with mastication, taste, deglutition (swallowing), articulation, and oral cleansing; however, its main functions are forming words during speaking and squeezing food into the oropharynx when swallowing.

Parts and Surfaces of the Tongue

The tongue has a root, a body, an apex, a curved dorsum, and an inferior surface (Fig. 7.53). The **root** of the tongue is the part of the tongue that rests on the floor of the mouth. It is usually defined as the *posterior third of the tongue.* The **body** of the tongue is the anterior two thirds of the tongue. The **apex** (**tip**) of the tongue is the anterior end of the body, which rests against the incisor teeth. The body and apex of the tongue are extremely mobile.

The **dorsum** (**dorsal surface**) of the tongue is the postero-superior surface, which is located partly in the oral cavity and partly in the oropharynx. It is characterized by a V-shaped groove, the **terminal sulcus** or **groove** (L. *sulcus terminalis*), the angle of which points posteriorly to the *foramen cecum.* This small pit, frequently absent, is the non-functional remnant of the proximal part of the embryonic thyroglossal duct from which the thyroid gland developed (Moore and Persaud, 2003). The terminal sulcus divides the dorsum of the tongue into the anterior (oral) part in the oral cavity proper and the posterior (pharyngeal) part in the oropharynx. The margin of the tongue is related on each side to the lingual gingivae and lateral teeth. The mucous membrane on the anterior part of the tongue is rough because of the presence of numerous small **lingual papillae:**

- **Vallate papillae:** Large and flat topped, they lie directly anterior to the terminal sulcus and are arranged in a V-shaped row. They are surrounded by deep moat-like trenches, the walls of which are studded with *taste buds.* The ducts of the serous glands of the tongue open into the trenches.

- **Foliate papillae:** Small lateral folds of the lingual mucosa. They are poorly developed in humans.

- **Filiform papillae:** Long and numerous, they contain afferent nerve endings that are sensitive to touch. These scaly, conical projections are pinkish gray and are arranged in V-shaped rows that are parallel to the terminal sulcus, except at the apex, where they tend to be arranged transversely.

- **Fungiform papillae:** Mushroom shaped pink or red spots, they are scattered among the filiform papillae but are most numerous at the apex and margins of the tongue.

The vallate, foliate, and most of the fungiform papillae contain taste receptors in the **taste buds.**

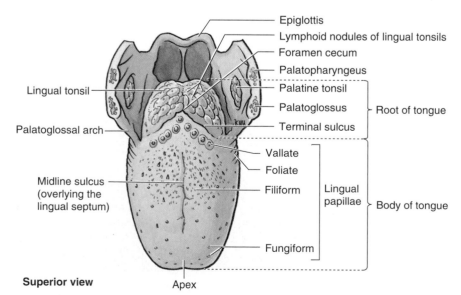

Superior view   Apex

Labels: Epiglottis, Lymphoid nodules of lingual tonsils, Foramen cecum, Palatopharyngeus, Palatine tonsil, Palatoglossus, Terminal sulcus — Root of tongue; Lingual tonsil, Palatoglossal arch, Midline sulcus (overlying the lingual septum); Vallate, Foliate, Filiform, Fungiform — Lingual papillae — Body of tongue.

Figure 7.53. Features of dorsum of tongue. The parts of the tongue (body and root) are separated by the terminal sulcus (groove) and foramen cecum. The arms of the V-shaped terminal sulcus diverge from the foramen, demarcating the posterior third of the tongue from the anterior two thirds. *Brackets* indicate the parts of the tongue and do not embrace specific labels.

Alveolar mucosa

Sublingual caruncle and opening of submandibular duct

Mandibular lingual gingiva

Frenulum of tongue

Sublingual fold (plica)

Gingiva proper (mandibular buccal gingiva)

Superior view

Figure 7.54. Floor of mouth and oral vestibule. The tongue is elevated and retracted superiorly. (Courtesy of Dr. B. Liebgott, Professor, Division of Anatomy, Department of Surgery, University of Toronto, Toronto, Ontario, Canada.)

The mucous membrane over the anterior part of the dorsum of the tongue is thin and closely attached to the underlying muscle. A shallow **midline groove of the tongue** divides the tongue into right and left halves. The groove also indicates the site of fusion of the embryonic distal tongue buds (Moore and Persaud, 2003).

The mucous membrane of the posterior part of the tongue is thick and freely movable. It has no lingual papillae, but the underlying **lymphoid nodules** give this part of the tongue an irregular, cobblestone appearance. The lymphoid nodules are known collectively as the **lingual tonsil.** The pharyngeal part of the tongue constitutes the anterior wall of the oropharynx and can be inspected only with a mirror or downward pressure on the tongue with a tongue depressor.

The **inferior surface of the tongue** is covered with a thin, transparent mucous membrane through which one can see the underlying veins. This surface is connected to the floor of the mouth by a midline fold called the **frenulum of the tongue** (Fig. 7.54). The frenulum allows the anterior part of the tongue to move freely. On each side of the frenulum, a deep lingual vein is visible through the thin mucous membrane. A **sublingual caruncle** (papilla) is present on each side of the base of the lingual frenulum that includes the *opening of the submandibular duct* from the submandibular salivary gland.

Muscles of the Tongue

The tongue is essentially a mass of muscles that is mostly covered by mucous membrane (Fig. 7.53; Table 7.16). Although it is traditional to do so, providing descriptions of the actions of tongue muscles ascribing (1) a single action to a specific muscle, or (2) implying that a particular movement is the consequence of a single muscle acting, greatly oversimplifies the actions of the tongue and is misleading. The muscles of the tongue do not act in isolation and some muscles perform multiple actions; parts of a single muscle are capable of acting independently, producing different, even antagonistic actions. In general, however, *extrinsic muscles alter the position of the tongue* while *intrinsic muscles alter its shape.* The four intrinsic and four extrinsic muscles in each half of the tongue are separated by a median fibrous **lingual septum,** which merges posteriorly with the lingual aponeurosis.

Extrinsic Muscles of the Tongue. The extrinsic muscles (genioglossus, hyoglossus, styloglossus, and palatoglossus) originate outside the tongue and attach to it. They mainly move the tongue but they can alter its shape as well. They are illustrated and their shape, position, attachments, and main actions are described in Table 7.16.

Intrinsic Muscles of the Tongue. The superior and inferior longitudinal, transverse, and vertical muscles are confined to the tongue. They have their attachments entirely within the tongue and are not attached to bone. They are illustrated and their shape, position, attachments, and main actions are described in Table 7.16. The superior and inferior longitudinal muscles act together to make the tongue short and thick and to retract the protruded tongue. The transverse and vertical muscles act simultaneously to make the tongue long and narrow, which may push the tongue against the incisor teeth or protrude the tongue from the open mouth (especially when acting with the posterior inferior part of the genioglossus).

Innervation of the Tongue

All muscles of the tongue, except the *palatoglossus* (actually a palatine muscle supplied by the *pharyngeal plexus*), receive motor innervation from CN XII, the **hypoglossal nerve** (Fig. 7.55). For general sensation (touch and temperature), the mucosa of the anterior two thirds of the tongue is supplied by the *lingual nerve,* a branch of CN V$_3$ (Fig. 7.42). For special

Table 7.16. Muscles of the Tongue

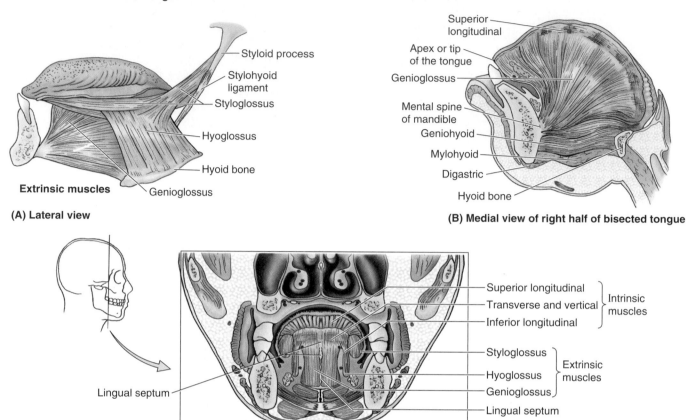

Extrinsic muscles

(A) Lateral view

Styloid process
Stylohyoid ligament
Styloglossus
Hyoglossus
Hyoid bone
Genioglossus

(B) Medial view of right half of bisected tongue

Superior longitudinal
Apex or tip of the tongue
Genioglossus
Mental spine of mandible
Geniohyoid
Mylohyoid
Digastric
Hyoid bone

Superior longitudinal — Intrinsic muscles
Transverse and vertical
Inferior longitudinal
Styloglossus — Extrinsic muscles
Hyoglossus
Genioglossus
Lingual septum

Lingual septum

(C) Anterior view of coronal section of mouth

Muscle	Shape and Position	Proximal Attachment	Distal Attachment	Main Action(s)
Extrinsic muscles of the tongue				
Genioglossus	Fan-shaped muscle; constitutes bulk of tongue	Via a short tendon from superior part of mental spine of mandible	Entire dorsum of tongue; inferior most and posterior most fibers attach to body of hyoid bone	Bilateral activity depresses tongue, especially central part, creating a longitudinal furrow; posterior part pulls tongue anteriorly for protrusion;[a] most anterior part retracts apex of protruded tongue; unilateral contraction deviates ("wags") tongue to contralateral side
Hyoglossus	Thin, quadrilateral muscle	Body and greater horn of hyoid bone	Inferior aspects of lateral part of tongue	Depresses tongue, especially pulling its sides inferiorly; helps shorten (retrude) tongue
Styloglossus	Small, short triangular muscle	Anterior border of distal styloid process; stylohyoid ligament	Sides of tongue posteriorly, interdigitating with hyoglossus	Retrudes tongue and curls (elevates) its sides, working with genioglossus to form a central trough during swallowing
Palatoglossus	Narrow crescent-shaped palatine muscle; forms posterior column of isthmus of fauces	Palatine aponeurosis of soft palate	Enters posterolateral tongue transversely, blending with intrinsic transverse muscles	Capable of elevating posterior tongue or depressing soft palate; most commonly acts to constrict isthmus of fauces
Intrinsic muscles of tongue				
Superior longitudinal	Thin layer deep to mucous membrane of dorsum	Submucous fibrous layer and median fibrous septum	Margins of tongue and mucous membrane	Curls tongue longitudinally upward, elevating apex and sides of tongue; shortens (retrudes) tongue
Inferior longitudinal	Narrow band close to inferior surface	Root of tongue and body of hyoid bone	Apex of tongue	Curls tongue longitudinally downward, depressing apex; shortens (retrudes) tongue
Transverse	Deep to superior longitudinal muscle	Median fibrous septum	Fibrous tissue at lateral lingual margins	Narrows and elongates (protrudes) tongue[a]
Vertical	Fibers intersect transverse muscle	Submucous fibrous layer of dorsum of tongue	Inferior surface of borders of tongue	Flattens and broadens tongue[a]

[a]Act simultaneously to protrude tongue.

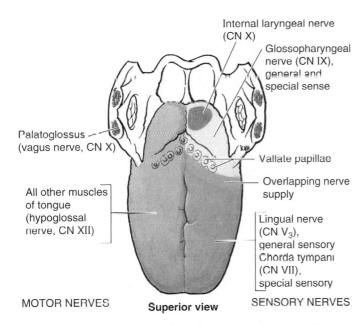

Figure 7.55. Nerve supply of tongue. The anterior two thirds of the tongue are supplied by the lingual nerve (CN V₃) for general sensation and by the chorda tympani, a branch of the facial nerve (CN VII) transferring nerve fibers to the lingual nerve, for taste. The posterior third of the tongue and the vallate papillae are supplied by the lingual branch of the glossopharyngeal nerve (CN IX) for both general sensation and taste. Another contribution is made by the internal laryngeal branch of the vagus (CN X) for general sensation and taste. Hence CN VII, CN IX, and CN X provide nerve fibers for taste; those from CN VII are ultimately conveyed by CN V₃.

sensation (taste), this part of the tongue, except for the vallate papillae, is supplied through the *chorda tympani nerve,* a branch of CN VII (Fig. 7.41*C*). The chorda tympani joins the lingual nerve and runs anteriorly in its sheath. The mucous membrane of the posterior third of the tongue and the vallate papillae are supplied by the lingual branch of the *glossopharyngeal nerve* (CN IX) for both general and special sensation. Twigs of the **internal laryngeal nerve,** a branch of the vagus nerve (CN X), supply mostly general but some special sensation to a small area of the tongue just anterior to the epiglottis. These mostly sensory nerves also carry **parasympathetic secretomotor fibers** to serous glands in the tongue. Parasympathetic fibers from the chorda tympani nerve travel with the lingual nerve to the submandibular and sublingual salivary glands. These nerve fibers synapse in the *submandibular ganglion,* which hangs from the lingual nerve (Fig. 7.59*A*).

There are four basic taste sensations: *sweet, salty, sour,* and *bitter.* Sweetness is detected at the apex, saltiness at the lateral margins, and sourness and bitterness at the posterior part of the tongue. All other "tastes" expressed by gourmets are olfactory (smell and aroma).

Vasculature of the Tongue

The **arteries of the tongue** are derived from the **lingual artery,** which arises from the *external carotid artery* (Fig. 7.56). On entering the tongue, the lingual artery passes deep to the hyoglossus muscle. The **dorsal lingual arteries** supply the posterior part (root); the **deep lingual arteries** supply the anterior part. The deep lingual arteries communicate with each other near the apex of the tongue. The dorsal lingual

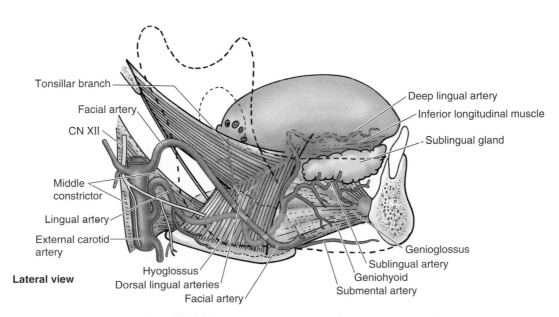

Figure 7.56. Blood supply of tongue. The main artery to the tongue is the lingual, a branch of the external carotid artery. The dorsal lingual arteries provide the blood supply to the root of the tongue and a branch to the palatine tonsil. The deep lingual arteries supply the body of the tongue. The sublingual arteries provide the blood supply to the floor of the mouth, including the sublingual glands.

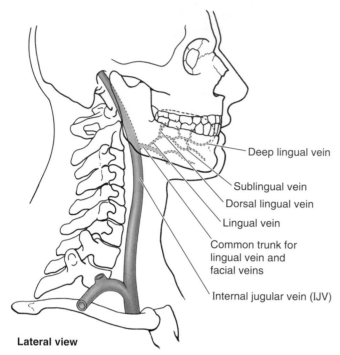

Lateral view

Figure 7.57. Venous drainage of tongue. The deep lingual vein runs posteriorly and visibly deep to the mucous membrane of the underside of the tongue at the side of the lingual frenulum. It unites with the sublingual vein from the floor of the mouth and the sublingual salivary gland and then receives the dorsal lingual veins. All these veins drain directly or indirectly into the internal jugular vein.

arteries are prevented from communicating by the *lingual septum* (Table 7.16*C*).

The **veins of the tongue** are the **dorsal lingual veins**, which accompany the lingual artery; the **deep lingual veins**, which begin at the apex of the tongue, run posteriorly beside the lingual frenulum to join the **sublingual vein** (Fig. 7.57). The sublingual veins in elderly people are often varicose (enlarged and tortuous). All these lingual veins terminate, directly or indirectly, in the IJV.

The **lymphatic drainage of the tongue** is exceptional. Most of the lymphatic drainage converges toward and follows the venous drainage; however, lymph from the tip of the tongue, frenulum, and central lower lip runs an independent course. Lymph from the tongue takes four routes (Fig. 7.58):

1. Lymph from the *posterior third* drains into the *superior deep cervical lymph nodes*.

2. Lymph from the *medial part* of the anterior two thirds drains directly to the *inferior deep cervical lymph nodes*.

3. Lymph from the lateral parts of the anterior two thirds drains to the *submandibular lymph nodes*.

4. The apex and frenulum drain to the *submental lymph nodes*.

The posterior third and the medial part of the anterior two thirds drain bilaterally.

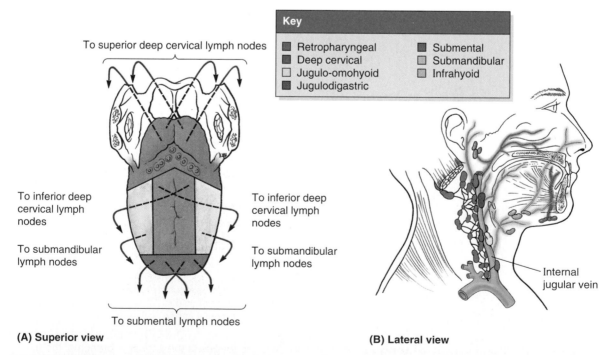

(A) Superior view

(B) Lateral view

Figure 7.58. Lymphatic drainage of tongue. A. The dorsum of the tongue is shown. **B.** Lymph drains to the submental, submandibular, and superior and inferior deep cervical lymph nodes, including the jugulodigastric and jugulo-omohyoid nodes. Extensive communications occur across the midline of the tongue

Gag Reflex

It is possible to touch the anterior part of the tongue without feeling discomfort; however, when the posterior part is touched, the individual gags. CN IX and CN X are responsible for the muscular contraction of each side of the pharynx. Glossopharyngeal branches provide the afferent limb of the gag reflex.

Paralysis of the Genioglossus

When the genioglossus muscle is paralyzed, the tongue has a tendency to fall posteriorly, obstructing the airway and presenting the risk of suffocation. Total relaxation of the genioglossus muscles occurs during general anesthesia; therefore, an airway is inserted in an anesthetized person to prevent the tongue from relapsing.

Injury to the Hypoglossal Nerve

Trauma, such as a fractured mandible, may injure the hypoglossal nerve (CN XII), resulting in paralysis and eventual atrophy of one side of the tongue. The tongue deviates to the paralyzed side during protrusion because of the action of the unaffected genioglossus muscle on the other side.

Sublingual Absorption of Drugs

For quick absorption of a drug, for instance, when nitroglycerin is used as a vasodilator in *angina pectoris,* the pill or spray is put under the tongue where it dissolves and enters the deep lingual veins in <1 min (Fig. B7.27).

Lingual Carcinoma

A *lingual carcinoma* in the posterior part of the tongue metastasizes to the superior deep cervical lymph nodes on both sides, whereas a tumor in the anterior part usually does not metastasize to the inferior deep cervical lymph nodes until late in the disease. Because these nodes are closely related to the IJV, metastases from the tongue may be widely distributed through the submental and submandibular regions and along the IJVs in the neck.

Frenectomy

An overly large lingual frenulum (tongue-tie) interferes with tongue movements and may affect speech. In unusual cases, a *frenectomy* (cutting the frenulum) in infants may be necessary to free the tongue for normal movement and speech.

Thyroglossal Duct Cyst

A cystic remnant of the thyroglossal duct, associated with development of the thyroid gland (Moore and Persaud, 2003), may be found in the root of the tongue and be connected to a sinus that opens at the foramen cecum. Surgical excision of the cyst may be necessary. Most *thyroglossal duct cysts* are in the neck, close or just inferior to the body of the hyoid bone (Fig. B7.28).

Aberrant Thyroid Gland

Aberrant thyroid glandular tissue may be found anywhere along the path of the embryonic thyroglossal duct. Although uncommon, the thyroglossal duct carrying thyroid-forming tissue at its distal end may fail to descend to its definitive position in the neck. Aberrant thyroid tissue may be in the root of the tongue, just posterior to the ▶

Palatopharyngeal arch
Uvula
Palatine tonsil
Mucosal fold over pterygomandibular raphe
Palatoglossal arch
Apex of tongue
Body of tongue
Deep lingual vein
Frenulum of tongue
Sublingual carunculae with openings of submandibular ducts

Figure B7.27

Thyroglossal duct cyst

Figure B7.28

foramen cecum, or in the neck (Fig. B7.29*A*). Cystic remnants of the thyroglossal duct may be differentiated from an undescended thyroid by radioisotope scanning (Fig. B7.29*B*). An aberrant thyroid gland may be the only thyroid tissue the person has; if so, removal will require the person be continually medicated with thyroid hormone. ⊕

Figure B7.29

THE BOTTOM LINE: The tongue is a mass of striated muscle, innervated by CN XII and covered with a specialized mucosa textured with lingual papillae. It occupies most of the oral cavity when the mouth is closed. Its extrinsic muscles primarily control its placement, whereas its intrinsic muscles primarily control its shape, for manipulation of food during chewing, swallowing, and speech. It is highly

sensitive, with four cranial nerves contributing sensory fibers to it. The terminal sulcus divides it into an anterior two thirds, receiving general sensation from the lingual nerve (CN V₃) and taste fibers from CN VII, and a posterior third receiving all sensory innervation from CN IX. Adjacent to the epiglottis, CN X provides general and special sensory innervation.

Salivary Glands

The **salivary glands** are the parotid, submandibular, and sublingual glands. The clear, tasteless, odorless viscid fluid, **saliva,** secreted by these glands and the mucous glands of the oral cavity:

- Keeps the mucous membrane of the mouth moist.

- Lubricates the food during mastication.

- Begins the digestion of starches.

- Serves as an intrinsic "mouthwash."

- Plays significant roles in the prevention of tooth decay and in the ability to taste.

In addition to the main salivary glands, small **accessory salivary glands** are scattered over the palate, lips, cheeks, tonsils, and tongue.

The *parotid glands,* the largest of the three paired salivary glands, were discussed earlier in this chapter (see "Parotid Gland").

Submandibular Glands

The **submandibular glands** lie along the body of the mandible, partly superior and partly inferior to the posterior half of the mandible, and partly superficial and partly deep to the mylohyoid muscle (Fig. 7.59). The **submandibular duct,** approximately 5 cm long, arises from the portion of the gland that lies between the mylohyoid and the hyoglossus muscles. Passing from lateral to medial, the *lingual nerve* loops under the duct that runs anteriorly, opening by one to three orifices on a small sublingual papilla beside the base of the lingual frenulum. The orifices of the submandibular ducts are visible, and saliva can often be seen trickling from them (or spraying from them during yawning).

The **arterial supply of the submandibular glands** is from the **submental arteries** (Fig. 7.56). The **veins** accompany the arteries. The submandibular glands are supplied by presynaptic parasympathetic secretomotor fibers conveyed from the facial nerve to the lingual nerve by the chorda tympani nerve, which synapse with postsynaptic neurons in the *submandibular ganglion* (Fig. 7.59*A*). The latter fibers accompany arteries to reach the gland, along with vasoconstrictive postsynaptic sympathetic fibers from the superior cervical ganglion. The **lymphatic vessels** of the glands end in the *deep cervical lymph nodes,* particularly the *jugulo-omohyoid node* (Fig. 7.58*B*).

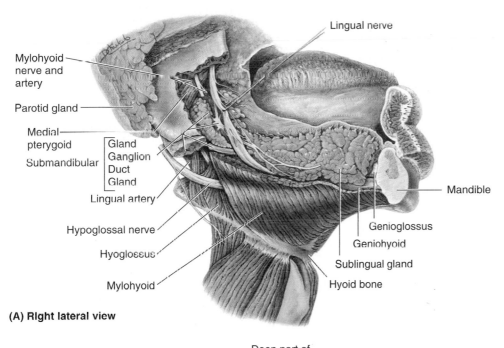

Mylohyoid nerve and artery

Parotid gland

Medial pterygoid

Submandibular

Gland
Ganglion
Duct
Gland

Lingual artery

Hypoglossal nerve

Hyoglossus

Mylohyoid

Lingual nerve

Mandible

Genioglossus

Geniohyoid

Sublingual gland

Hyoid bone

(A) Right lateral view

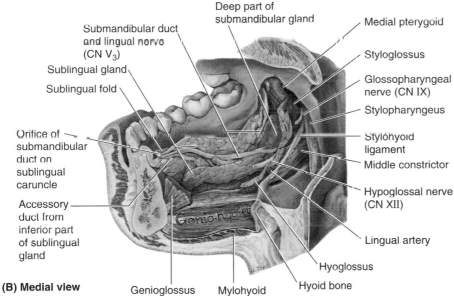

Submandibular duct and lingual nerve (CN V₃)

Sublingual gland

Sublingual fold

Orifice of submandibular duct on sublingual caruncle

Accessory duct from inferior part of sublingual gland

Deep part of submandibular gland

Medial pterygoid

Styloglossus

Glossopharyngeal nerve (CN IX)

Stylopharyngeus

Stylohyoid ligament

Middle constrictor

Hypoglossal nerve (CN XII)

Lingual artery

Genio-hyoid

Genioglossus   Mylohyoid   Hyoglossus   Hyoid bone

(B) Medial view

Figure 7.59. Parotid, submandibular, and sublingual salivary glands. A. The body and parts of the ramus of the mandible have been removed. The parotid gland contacts the deep part of the submandibular gland posteriorly. Fine ducts passing from the superior border of the sublingual gland open on the sublingual fold. **B.** The right sublingual and submandibular glands and the floor of the mouth are shown; the tongue has been excised. The orifice of the duct of the submandibular gland is visible at the anterior end of the sublingual fold. The submandibular duct adheres to the medial side of the sublingual gland; here it is receiving, as it sometimes does, a large accessory duct from the inferior part of the sublingual gland.

Sublingual Glands

The **sublingual glands** are the smallest and most deeply situated of the salivary glands (Fig. 7.59). Each almond-shaped gland lies in the floor of the mouth between the mandible and the genioglossus muscle. The glands from each side unite to form a horseshoe-shaped mass around the connective tissue core of the lingual frenulum. Numerous small **sublingual ducts** open into the floor of the mouth along the sublingual folds.

The **arterial supply of the sublingual glands** is from the *sublingual* and *submental arteries,* branches of the lingual and facial arteries, respectively (Fig. 7.56). The **nerves of the glands** accompany those of the submandibular gland. Presynaptic parasympathetic secretomotor fibers are conveyed by the facial, chorda tympani, and lingual nerves to synapse in the submandibular ganglion (Fig. 7.59*A*).

Excision of the Submandibular Gland and Removal of a Calculus

Excision of a submandibular gland because of a calculus (stone) in its duct or a tumor in the gland is not uncommon. The skin incision is made at least 2.5 cm inferior to the angle of the mandible to avoid injury to the marginal mandibular branch of the facial nerve. Caution must also be taken not to injure the lingual nerve when incising the duct. The submandibular duct passes directly over the nerve inferior to the neck of the 3rd molar tooth (Fig. 7.59). ▶

Sialography of the Submandibular Ducts

The submandibular salivary glands may be examined radiographically after injection of a contrast medium into their ducts. This special type of radiograph (*sialogram*) demonstrates the salivary ducts and some secretory units. Because of the small size of the ducts of the sublingual glands and their multiplicity, one cannot usually inject contrast medium into these ducts. ○

THE BOTTOM LINE: Salivary glands secrete saliva to initiate digestion by facilitating chewing and swallowing. The parotid gland, the largest, was discussed earlier in this chapter. It receives parasympathetic innervation from CN XI via the otic ganglion. The submandibular and sublingual glands receive parasympathetic innervation from CN VII by way of the chorda tympani nerve, lingual nerve, and submandibular ganglion. Their ducts open into the oral cavity under the tongue.

Pterygopalatine Fossa

The **pterygopalatine fossa** is a small pyramidal space inferior to the apex of the orbit (Fig. 7.60). It lies between the pterygoid process of the sphenoid posteriorly and the posterior aspect of the maxilla anteriorly. The fragile perpendicular plate of the palatine bone forms its medial wall. The incom-

plete **roof** of the pterygopalatine fossa is formed by the *greater wing of the sphenoid*. The **floor** of the pterygopalatine fossa is formed by the *pyramidal process of the palatine bone*. Its superior larger end opens into the *inferior orbital fissure;* its inferior end is closed except for the palatine foramina. The pterygopalatine fossa communicates:

- Laterally with the *infratemporal fossa* through the *pterygomaxillary fissure.*
- Medially with the nasal cavity through the *sphenopalatine foramen.*
- Anterosuperiorly with the orbit through the *inferior orbital fissure.*
- Posterosuperiorly with the middle cranial fossa through the *foramen rotundum* and *pterygoid canal* (Fig. 7.61).

The **contents of the pterygopalatine fossa** (Fig. 7.62A–C) are the:

- Terminal (pterygopalatine or third) part of the maxillary artery and the initial parts of its branches.
- Maxillary nerve, with which are associated the:
  - Nerve of the pterygoid canal.
  - Pterygopalatine ganglion.

Pterygopalatine Part of the Maxillary Artery

The maxillary artery, a terminal branch of the external carotid artery, passes anteriorly and traverses the infratemporal fossa.

Infratemporal fossa

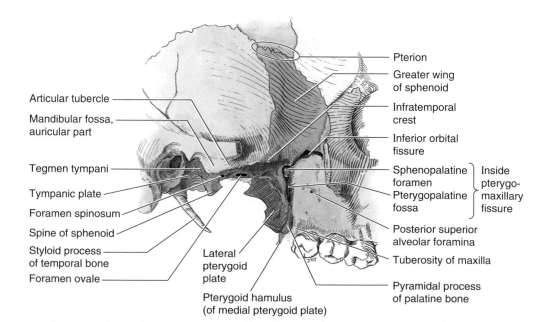

Articular tubercle
Mandibular fossa, auricular part
Tegmen tympani
Tympanic plate
Foramen spinosum
Spine of sphenoid
Styloid process of temporal bone
Foramen ovale
Lateral pterygoid plate
Pterygoid hamulus (of medial pterygoid plate)
Pterion
Greater wing of sphenoid
Infratemporal crest
Inferior orbital fissure
Sphenopalatine foramen
Pterygopalatine fossa
Inside pterygomaxillary fissure
Posterior superior alveolar foramina
Tuberosity of maxilla
Pyramidal process of palatine bone

Figure 7.60. Temporal, infratemporal, and pterygopalatine fossae. The pterygopalatine fossa is a small pyramidal space housing the pterygopalatine ganglion (Fig. 7.52). The fossa is seen through the pterygomaxillary fissure between the pterygoid process and the maxilla. The sphenopalatine foramen is an opening into the nasal cavity at the top of the palatine bone.

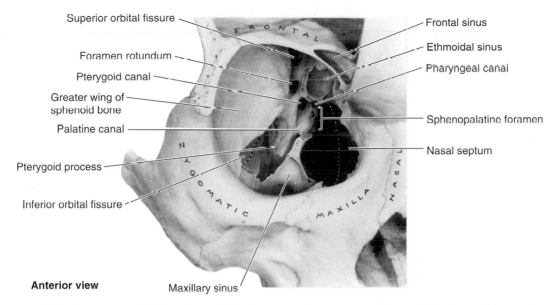

Superior orbital fissure

Foramen rotundum

Pterygoid canal

Greater wing of sphenoid bone

Palatine canal

Pterygoid process

Inferior orbital fissure

Frontal sinus

Ethmoidal sinus

Pharyngeal canal

Sphenopalatine foramen

Nasal septum

Anterior view

Maxillary sinus

Figure 7.61. Pterygopalatine fossa. The fossa has been exposed through the floor of the orbit and maxillary sinus. The foramen rotundum, pterygoid canal, and pharyngeal canal are openings in the posterior wall of the pterygopalatine fossa.

It passes over the lateral pterygoid muscle and enters the pterygopalatine fossa. The **pterygopalatine part of the maxillary artery**, its third part, passes through the *pterygomaxillary fissure* and enters the pterygopalatine fossa, where it lies anterior to the *pterygopalatine ganglion* (Figs. 7.60 and 7.62*A* & *B*). The artery gives rise to branches that accompany all nerves in the fossa with the same names. The six terminal branches of the pterygopalatine part of the maxillary artery are illustrated in Figs. 7.50*B*, 7.52, and 7.62*A* and are illustrated and listed in Table 7.10.

Maxillary Nerve

The maxillary nerve enters the pterygopalatine fossa through the *foramen rotundum* and runs anterolaterally in the posterior part of the fossa (Figs. 7.61 and 7.62). Within the pterygopalatine fossa, the maxillary nerve gives off the *zygomatic nerve*, which divides into zygomaticofacial and zygomaticotemporal nerves (Fig. 7.62*B* & *C*). These nerves emerge from the zygomatic bone through cranial foramina of the same name and supply general sensation to the lateral region of the cheek and temple. The *zygomaticotemporal nerve* also gives rise to a communicating branch, which conveys parasympathetic secretomotor fibers to the lacrimal gland by way of the heretofore purely sensory lacrimal nerve from CN V$_1$ (Fig. 7.24*A*).

While in the pterygopalatine fossa, the maxillary nerve also gives off the two *pterygopalatine nerves* that suspend the parasympathetic *pterygopalatine ganglion* in the superior part of the pterygopalatine fossa (Fig. 7.62*B* & *C*). The pterygopalatine nerves convey general sensory fibers of the maxillary nerve, which pass through the pterygopalatine ganglion without synapsing and supply the nose, palate, tonsil, and

gingivae. The maxillary nerve leaves the pterygopalatine fossa through the inferior orbital fissure, after which it is known as the *infraorbital nerve.*

The **parasympathetic fibers to the pterygopalatine ganglion** come from the facial nerve by way of its first branch, the *greater petrosal nerve* (Fig. 7.62*C*). This nerve joins the *deep petrosal nerve* as it passes through the foramen lacerum to form the **nerve of the pterygoid canal,** which passes anteriorly through this canal to the pterygopalatine fossa. The parasympathetic fibers of the greater petrosal nerve synapse in the pterygopalatine ganglion.

The **deep petrosal nerve** is a sympathetic nerve arising from the *internal carotid plexus* as the artery exits the carotid canal. It conveys postsynaptic fibers from nerve cell bodies in the *superior cervical sympathetic ganglion* to the pterygopalatine ganglion by joining the *nerve to the pterygoid canal.* The fibers do not synapse in the ganglion but pass directly through it into the branches (of CN V$_2$) arising from it. The postsynaptic parasympathetic and the sympathetic fibers pass to the lacrimal gland, the palatine glands, and the mucosal glands of the nasal cavity and superior pharynx.

Transantral Approach to the Pterygopalatine Fossa

Surgical access to the deeply placed pterygopalatine fossa is gained through the maxillary sinus. After elevating the upper lip, the maxillary gingiva and anterior wall of the sinus are transversed to enter the sinus. ▶

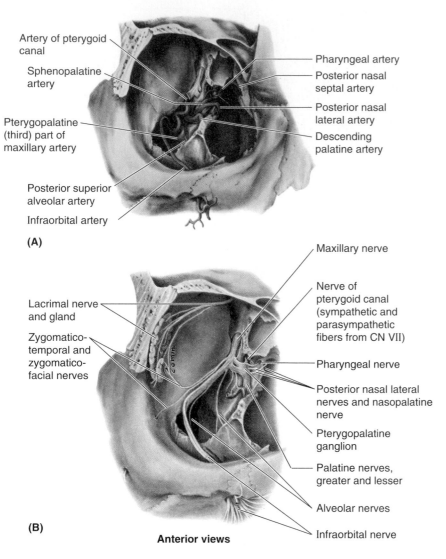

Artery of pterygoid canal

Sphenopalatine artery

Pterygopalatine (third) part of maxillary artery

Posterior superior alveolar artery

Infraorbital artery

Pharyngeal artery

Posterior nasal septal artery

Posterior nasal lateral artery

Descending palatine artery

(A)

Maxillary nerve

Lacrimal nerve and gland

Zygomatico-temporal and zygomatico-facial nerves

Nerve of pterygoid canal (sympathetic and parasympathetic fibers from CN VII)

Pharyngeal nerve

Posterior nasal lateral nerves and nasopalatine nerve

Pterygopalatine ganglion

Palatine nerves, greater and lesser

Alveolar nerves

Infraorbital nerve

(B)

Anterior views

Figure 7.62. Contents of pterygopalatine fossa. A. The pterygopalatine (third) part of the maxillary artery lies anterior to the lateral pterygoid muscle (Table 7.10). The branches of the third part arise just before and within the pterygopalatine fossa. **B.** The maxillary nerve (CN V_2) traverses the posterior wall of the pterygopalatine fossa via the foramen rotundum, sending two nerves (roots) to the pterygopalatine ganglion within the fossa. The branches arising from the ganglion are considered to be branches of CN V_2. **C.** Autonomic nerve fibers distributed by the maxillary nerve enter the nerve via the pterygopalatine ganglion. The greater petrosal nerve (carrying presynaptic parasympathetic fibers from the facial nerve) merges with the deep petrosal nerve (carrying postsynaptic sympathetic fibers conveyed from the superior cervical ganglion via the internal carotid plexus) to form the nerve of the pterygoid canal in the area of the foramen lacerum. The latter nerve thus brings both sympathetic and parasympathetic fibers to the pterygopalatine ganglion, where only the parasympathetic fibers synapse. The postsynaptic fibers of both divisions of the autonomic nervous system enter all the branches of the maxillary nerve that pass from the ganglion to the palatine, nasal, and uppermost pharyngeal mucosa. Some parasympathetic fibers pass retrograde, relative to the sensory fibers, through the pterygopalatine and maxillary nerves to reach the zygomatic nerve (CN V_2) for distribution to the lacrimal gland.

Greater petrosal nerve

Facial nerve (CN VII)

Geniculate ganglion

Internal carotid (sympathetic) plexus

Internal carotid artery

Deep petrosal nerve

Nerve of pterygoid canal

Foramen rotundum

Pterygopalatine nerves*

(C) Lateral view

Maxillary nerve*

Zygomatic nerve*

Lacrimal nerve (CN V_1)

Zygomaticotemporal nerve*

Zygomaticofacial nerve*

Infraorbital nerve*

Pterygopalatine ganglion

*CN V_2

The posterior wall is then chipped away as needed to open the anterior wall of the pterygopalatine fossa. In the case of chronic *epistaxis* (nosebleed), the third part of the maxillary artery may be ligated in the fossa to control the bleeding. ○

THE BOTTOM LINE: The pterygopalatine fossa is a major distributing center for branches of the maxillary nerve and the pterygopalatine (third) part of the maxillary artery. It is located between, and has communications with, the infratemporal fossa, nasal cavity, orbit, middle cranial fossa, pharyngeal vault, maxillary sinus, and oral cavity (palate). Its contents are the maxillary nerve (CN V_2), the parasympathetic pterygopalatine ganglion, the third part of the maxillary artery and accompanying veins, and a surrounding fatty matrix.

Nose

The **nose** is the part of the respiratory tract superior to the hard palate and contains the peripheral organ of smell. It includes the external nose and nasal cavity, which is divided into right and left cavities by the *nasal septum*. The functions of the nose are olfaction (smelling), respiration (breathing), filtration of dust, humidification of inspired air, and reception and elimination of secretions from the paranasal sinuses and nasolacrimal ducts.

External Nose

The external nose is the visible portion that projects from the face; its skeleton is mainly cartilaginous (Fig. 7.63). Noses vary considerably in size and shape, mainly because of differences in these cartilages. The **dorsum** of the nose extends from the **root** of the nose to the **apex** (**tip**) of the nose. The inferior surface of the nose is pierced by two piriform (L. pear-shaped) openings, the **nares** (nostrils, anterior nasal apertures), which are bound laterally by the **alae** (wings) of the nose. The superior bony part of the nose, including its root, is covered by thin skin. The skin over the cartilaginous part of the nose is covered with thicker skin, which contains many sebaceous glands. The skin extends into the **vestibule** of the nose (Fig. 7.64), where it has a variable number of stiff hairs (*vibrissae*). Because they are usually moist, these hairs filter dust particles from air entering the nasal cavity. The junction of the skin and mucous membrane is beyond the hair-bearing area.

Skeleton of the External Nose

The supporting skeleton of the nose is composed of bone and hyaline cartilage. The **bony part** of the nose (Figs. 7.63*B* and 7.64) consists of the nasal bones, frontal processes of the maxillae, the nasal part of the frontal bone and its nasal spine, and

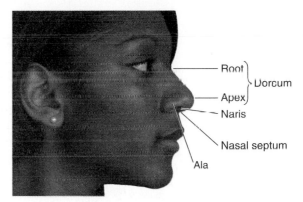

(A) Lateral view

- Root
- Dorsum
- Apex
- Naris
- Nasal septum
- Ala

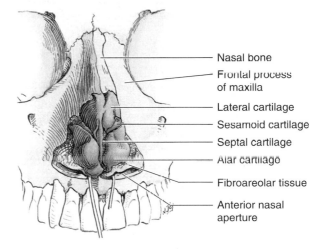

(B) Anterior view

- Nasal bone
- Frontal process of maxilla
- Lateral cartilage
- Sesamoid cartilage
- Septal cartilage
- Alar cartilage
- Fibroareolar tissue
- Anterior nasal aperture

Figure 7.63. External nose. A. The surface anatomy of the nose is shown. The nose is attached to the forehead by its root. The rounded border between the apex and the root is the dorsum. **B.** The cartilages of the nose are retracted inferiorly to expose the sesamoid cartilages. The lateral nasal cartilages are fixed by sutures to the nasal bones and are continuous with the septal cartilage.

the bony parts of the nasal septum. The **cartilaginous part** of the nose consists of five main cartilages: two lateral cartilages, two alar cartilages, and one septal cartilage. The U-shaped **alar cartilages** are free and movable; they dilate or constrict the nares when the muscles acting on the nose contract.

Nasal Septum

The *nasal septum* divides the chamber of the nose into two *nasal cavities* and has a bony part and a soft mobile cartilaginous part. The main components of the nasal septum are the perpendicular plate of the ethmoid, the vomer, and the septal cartilage. The thin **perpendicular plate of the ethmoid bone,** forming the superior part of the nasal septum, descends from the *cribriform plate* and is continued superior to this plate as the *crista galli.* The **vomer,** a thin flat bone, forms the posteroinferior part of the nasal septum, with some contribution from the nasal crests of the maxillary and palatine bones. The **septal cartilage** has a tongue-and-groove articulation with the edges of the bony septum.

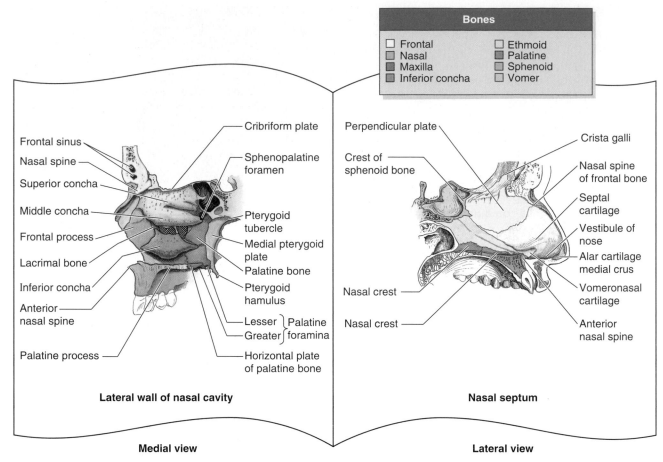

Bones

☐ Frontal   ☐ Ethmoid
☐ Nasal   ☐ Palatine
☐ Maxilla   ☐ Sphenoid
☐ Inferior concha ☐ Vomer

Lateral wall of nasal cavity

Frontal sinus
Nasal spine
Superior concha
Middle concha
Frontal process
Lacrimal bone
Inferior concha
Anterior nasal spine
Palatine process

Cribriform plate
Sphenopalatine foramen
Pterygoid tubercle
Medial pterygoid plate
Palatine bone
Pterygoid hamulus
Lesser ⎱ Palatine
Greater ⎰ foramina
Horizontal plate of palatine bone

Medial view

Nasal septum

Perpendicular plate
Crest of sphenoid bone
Nasal crest
Nasal crest

Crista galli
Nasal spine of frontal bone
Septal cartilage
Vestibule of nose
Alar cartilage medial crus
Vomeronasal cartilage
Anterior nasal spine

Lateral view

Figure 7.64. Lateral and medial (septal) walls of right side of nasal cavity. The walls are separated and shown as adjacent pages of a book. The medial view shows the right lateral wall of the nasal cavity, and the lateral view shows the nasal septum. The nasal septum has a hard (bony) part located deeply (posteriorly) where it is protected and a soft or mobile part located superficially (anteriorly) mostly in the more vulnerable external nose.

Nasal Fractures

Because of the prominence of the nose, fractures of the nasal bones are common facial fractures in automobile accidents and sports (unless face guards are worn). Fractures usually result in deformation of the nose, particularly when a lateral force is applied by someone's elbow, for example. *Epistaxis* (nosebleed) usually occurs. In severe fractures, disruption of the bones and cartilages results in displacement of the nose. When the injury results from a direct blow, the cribriform plate of the ethmoid bone may also fracture.

Deviation of the Nasal Septum

The nasal septum is usually deviated to one side or the other. This could be the result of a birth injury, but more often the deviation results during adolescence and adulthood from trauma (e.g., during a fist fight). Sometimes the deviation is so severe that the nasal septum is in contact with the lateral wall of the nasal cavity and often obstructs breathing or exacerbates snoring. The deviation can be corrected surgically. ✚

Nasal Cavity

The term *nasal cavity,* divided into right and left halves by the nasal septum, refers to either the entire cavity or one of its halves, depending on the context. The nasal cavity is entered anteriorly through the nares. It opens posteriorly into the nasopharynx through the *choanae.* Mucosa lines the nasal cavity, except for the *nasal vestibule,* which is lined with skin (Fig. 7.65*A*). The **nasal mucosa** is firmly bound to the periosteum and perichondrium of the supporting bones and cartilages of the nose. The mucosa is continuous with the lining of all the chambers with which the nasal cavities communicate: the nasopharynx posteriorly, the paranasal sinuses superiorly and laterally, and the lacrimal sac and conjunctiva superiorly. The inferior two thirds of the nasal mucosa is the respiratory area and the superior one third is the olfactory area. Air passing over the **respiratory area** is warmed and moistened before it passes through the rest of the upper respiratory tract to the lungs. The **olfactory area** contains the peripheral organ of smell; sniffing draws air to the area.

Boundaries of the Nasal Cavity

The nasal cavity has a roof, floor, and medial and lateral walls.

- The **roof** of the nasal cavity is curved and narrow, except at its posterior end; it is divided into three parts (frontonasal, ethmoidal, and sphenoidal) named from the bones forming each part (Fig. 7.64).

- The **floor** of the nasal cavity is wider than the roof and is formed by the palatine processes of the maxilla and the horizontal plates of the palatine bone.

- The **medial wall** of the nasal cavity is formed by the nasal septum.

- The **lateral walls** of the nasal cavity are irregular owing to three bony plates, the nasal conchae, which project inferiorly, somewhat like louvers (Figs. 7.64 and 7.65).

Features of the Nasal Cavity

The *nasal conchae* (superior, middle, and inferior) curve inferomedially, hanging like louvers or short curtains. The **conchae** (L. shells) or turbinates of many mammals (especially running mammals and those existing in extreme environments) are highly convoluted, scroll-like structures that offer a vast surface area for heat exchange. In both humans with simple nasal conchae and animals with complex turbinates, a recess or *meatus* (singular and plural; passage(s) in the nasal cavity) underlies each of the bony formations. The nasal cavity is thus divided into five passages: a posterosuperiorly placed *sphenoethmoidal recess,* three laterally located *nasal meatus* (superior, middle, and inferior), and a medially placed *common nasal meatus* into which the four lateral passages open. The **inferior concha** is the longest and broadest and is formed by an independent bone (of the same name, inferior concha) covered by a mucous membrane that contains large vascular spaces that can enlarge to control the caliber of the nasal cavity. When infected or irritated, the mucosa may swell rapidly, blocking the nasal passage(s) on that side.

The **sphenoethmoidal recess,** lying superoposterior to the superior concha, receives the opening of the *sphenoidal sinus,* an air-filled cavity in the body of the sphenoid. The **superior nasal meatus** is a narrow passage between the superior and the middle nasal conchae into which the posterior ethmoidal sinuses open by one or more orifices (Fig. 7.65*A*). The **middle nasal meatus** is longer and deeper than the superior one. The anterosuperior part of this passage leads into a funnel-shaped opening, the **ethmoidal infundibulum,** through which it communicates with the frontal sinus (Fig. 7.66). The passage that leads inferiorly from each frontal sinus to the infundibulum is the *frontonasal duct* (Fig. 7.65*B*). The **semilunar hiatus** (L. *hiatus semilunaris*) is a semicircular groove into which the frontal sinus opens. The **ethmoidal bulla** (L. bubble), a rounded elevation located superior to the hiatus, is visible when the middle concha is removed. The bulla is formed by middle ethmoidal cells that form the *ethmoidal sinuses.*

The **inferior nasal meatus** is a horizontal passage inferolateral to the inferior nasal concha. The *nasolacrimal duct,* which drains tears from the lacrimal sac, opens into the anterior part of this meatus. The **common nasal meatus** is the medial part of the nasal cavity between the conchae and the nasal septum, into which the lateral recesses and meatus open.

Vasculature and Innervation of the Nose

The **arterial supply of the medial and lateral walls** of the nasal cavity (Fig. 7.67) is from five sources:

1. *Anterior ethmoidal artery* (from the ophthalmic artery).

2. *Posterior ethmoidal artery* (from the ophthalmic artery).

3. *Sphenopalatine artery* (from the maxillary artery).

4. *Greater palatine artery* (from the maxillary artery).

5. *Septal branch of the superior labial artery* (from the facial artery).

The first three arteries divide into lateral and medial (septal) branches. The greater palatine artery reaches the septum via the incisive canal through the anterior hard palate. The anterior part of the nasal septum is the site (Kiesselbach area) of an anastomotic arterial plexus involving all five arteries supplying the septum. The external nose also receives blood from first and fifth arteries listed above plus nasal branches of the infraorbital artery and the lateral nasal branches of the facial artery.

(A) Medial view

Frontal sinus

Sphenoidal sinus

Respiratory area

Ethmoidal crest of maxilla

Atrium

Limen

Nasal vestibule

Vibrissae (nasal hairs)

Sphenoethmoidal recess

Superior nasal meatus

Middle nasal meatus

Inferior nasal meatus

Nasopharynx

Pharyngeal opening of pharyngotympanic tube

Medial surface of cerebral hemisphere

Corpus callosum

Third ventricle

Midbrain

Pons

Fourth ventricle

Medulla oblongata

Atlas (C1 vertebra)

Posterior cerebellomedullary cistern (cisterna magna)

Axis (C2 vertebra)

Spinal cord

Sup. concha

Mid. concha

Inf. concha

(B) Medial view

Frontal sinus

Rod passed from frontal sinus through frontonasal duct, and into ethmoidal infundibulum of middle meatus

Ethmoidal bulla

Nasal mucosa

Semilunar hiatus

Middle ethmoidal cells
Posterior ethmoidal cells
Form ethmoidal sinuses

Rod passed from sphenoidal sinus to sphenoethmoidal recess

Sphenoidal sinus

Nasopharynx

Pharyngeal opening of pharyngotympanic tube

Orifice of nasolacrimal duct

Rod passed from semilunar hiatus, through maxillary orifice, into maxillary sinus, and forced through wall of inferior meatus

Figure 7.65. Lateral wall of nasal cavity of right half of head. A. The inferior and middle conchae, curving medially and inferiorly from the lateral wall, divide the wall into three nearly equal parts and cover the inferior and middle meatus, respectively. The superior concha is small and anterior to the sphenoidal sinus and the middle concha has an angled inferior border and ends inferior to the sphenoidal sinus. The inferior concha has a slightly curved inferior border and ends inferior to the middle concha approximately 1 cm anterior to the orifice of the pharyngotympanic tube (approximately the width of the medial pterygoid plate). **B.** This dissection of the lateral wall of the nasal cavity shows the communications through the lateral wall of the nasal cavity. Parts of the superior, middle, and inferior conchae are cut away. The sphenoidal sinus occupies the body of the sphenoid bone; its orifice, superior to the middle of its anterior wall, opens into the sphenoethmoidal recess. The orifices of posterior, middle, and anterior ethmoidal cells open into the superior meatus, middle meatus, and semilunar hiatus, respectively.

Supraorbital artery and nerve

Frontal sinus

Superior oblique

Levator palpebrae
superioris
Superior rectus

Crista galli

Lacrimal gland
Check ligament

Ethmoidal
infundibulum

Eyeball

Lateral rectus

Ethmoidal cells

Air cell in middle concha

Semilunar hiatus

Middle meatus

Maxillary ostium

Common nasal meatus

Inferior nasal meatus
and concha

Nasal septum

Hard palate

Posterior view

Inferior oblique
Infraorbital vessels
and nerve

Maxillary sinus

Figure 7.66. Coronal section of right half of head. The orientation drawing illustrates the plane of the section. Observe the relationship of the orbit, nasal cavity, and paranasal sinuses. The orbital contents, including the four recti and the fascia uniting them, form a circle (a cone when viewed in three dimensions) around the posterior part (fundus) of the eyeball. *M. 1,* 1st molar; *R.I.,* rectus inferior, or inferior rectus; *R.M.,* rectus medius, or medial rectus.

A rich **submucosal venous plexus** deep to the nasal mucosa drains into the sphenopalatine, facial, and ophthalmic veins. This venous plexus is an important part of the body's thermoregulatory system, exchanging heat and warming air before it enters the lungs. Venous blood from the external nose drains mostly into the facial vein via the angular and lateral nasal veins. However, recall that it lies within the "danger area" of the face because of communications with the *cavernous (dural venous) sinus* (see clinical correlation [blue] box "Thrombophlebitis of the Facial Vein," earlier in this chapter).

Regarding its **nerve supply**, the nasal mucosa can be divided into posteroinferior and anterosuperior portions by an oblique line passing approximately through the apex of the nose and the sphenoethmoidal recess. The nerve supply of the posteroinferior portion of the nasal mucosa is chiefly from the *maxillary nerve*, by way of the *nasopalatine nerve* to the

nasal septum, and posterior superior lateral nasal and inferior lateral nasal branches of the *greater palatine nerve* to the lateral wall (Fig. 7.68). The nerve supply of the anterosuperior portion is from the ophthalmic nerve (CN V_1) by way of the **anterior** and **posterior ethmoidal nerves,** branches of the nasociliary nerve. Most of the external nose (dorsum and apex) is also supplied by CN V_1 (via the infratrochlear nerve and the external nasal branch of the anterior ethmoidal nerve), but the alae are supplied by the nasal branches of the infraorbital nerve (CN V_2).

The **olfactory nerves,** concerned with smell, arise from cells in the **olfactory epithelium** in the superior part of the lateral and septal walls of the nasal cavity. The central processes of these cells (forming the olfactory nerve) pass through the *cribriform plate* and end in the **olfactory bulb,** the rostral expansion of the **olfactory tract.**

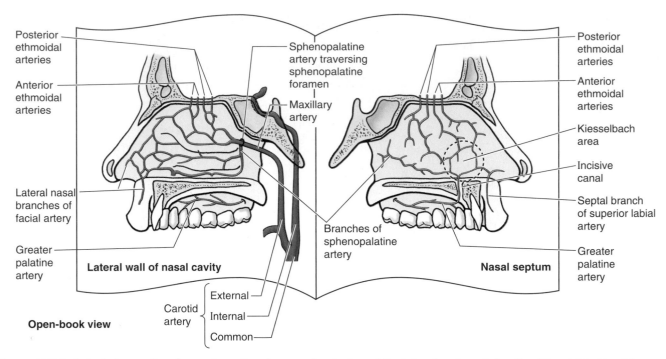

Figure 7.67. Arterial supply of nasal cavity. An open-book view of the lateral and medial walls of the right side of the nasal cavity is shown. The left "page" shows the lateral wall of the nasal cavity. The sphenopalatine artery (a branch of the maxillary) and the anterior ethmoidal artery (a branch of the ophthalmic) are the most important arteries to the nasal cavity. The right "page" shows the nasal septum. An anastomosis of four to five named arteries supplying the septum occurs in the anteroinferior portion of the nasal septum (Kiesselbach area, *dashed circle*), an area commonly involved in chronic epistaxis (nosebleeds).

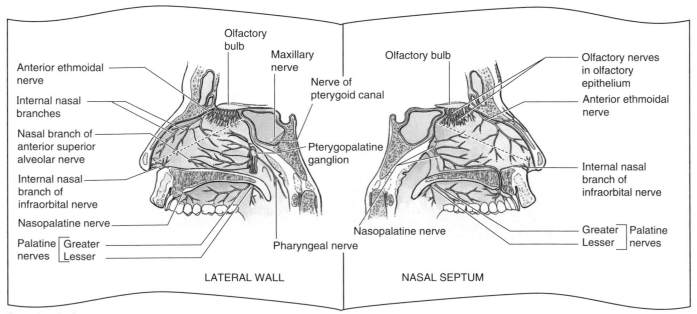

Figure 7.68. Innervation of nasal cavity. An open-book view of the lateral and medial (septal) walls of the right side of the nasal cavity is shown. A *dashed line* extrapolated approximately from the sphenoethmoidal recess to the apex of the nose demarcates the territories of the ophthalmic (CN V_1) and maxillary (CN V_2) nerves for supplying general sensation to both the lateral wall and the nasal septum. The olfactory nerve (CN I) is distributed to the olfactory mucosa superior to the level of the superior concha on both the lateral wall and the nasal septum.

Rhinitis

The nasal mucosa becomes swollen and inflamed (*rhinitis*) during severe upper respiratory infections and allergic reactions (e.g., hayfever). Swelling of the mucosa occurs readily because of its vascularity. Infections of the nasal cavities may spread to the:

- Anterior cranial fossa through the cribriform plate.
- Nasopharynx and retropharyngeal soft tissues.
- Middle ear through the *pharyngotympanic tube* (auditory tube), which connects the tympanic cavity and nasopharynx.
- Paranasal sinuses.
- Lacrimal apparatus and conjunctiva.

Epistaxis

Epistaxis (nosebleed) is relatively common because of the rich blood supply to the nasal mucosa. In most cases, the cause is trauma and the bleeding is from an area In the anterior third of the nose (Kiesselbach area). Epistaxis is also associated with infections and hypertension. Spurting of blood from the nose results from rupture of arteries. Mild epistaxis may also result from nose picking, which tears veins in the vestibule of the nose. ☉

Paranasal Sinuses

The **paranasal sinuses** are air-filled extensions of the respiratory part of the nasal cavity into the following cranial bones: frontal, ethmoid, sphenoid, and maxilla. They are named according to the bones in which they are located. The sinuses continue to invade the surrounding bone, and marked extensions are common in the crania of older individuals.

Sinusitis

Because the paranasal sinuses are continuous with the nasal cavities through apertures that open into them, infection may spread from the nasal cavities, producing inflammation and swelling of the mucosa of the sinuses (*sinusitis*) and local pain. Sometimes several sinuses are inflamed (*pansinusitis*), and the swelling of the mucosa may block one or more openings of the sinuses into the nasal cavities. ☉

Frontal Sinuses

The **frontal sinuses** are between the outer and the inner tables of the frontal bone, posterior to the superciliary arches and the root of the nose (Figs. 7.65, 7.66, and 7.69*A*).

Frontal sinuses are usually detectable in children by 7 years of age. Each sinus drains through a **frontonasal duct** into the *ethmoidal infundibulum*, which opens into the *semilunar hiatus* of the middle nasal meatus. The frontal sinuses are innervated by branches of the *supraorbital nerves* (CN V₁).

Variation of the Frontal Sinuses

The right and left frontal sinuses are rarely of equal size, and the septum between them is not usually situated entirely in the median plane. The frontal sinuses vary in size from approximately 5 mm to large spaces extending laterally into the greater wings of the sphenoid. Often a frontal sinus has two parts: a vertical part in the squamous part of the frontal bone and a horizontal part in the orbital part of the frontal bone. One or both parts may be large or small. When the supraorbital part is large, its roof forms the floor of the anterior cranial fossa and its floor forms the roof of the orbit. ☉

Ethmoidal Cells

The **ethmoidal cells** (**sinuses**) are small invaginations of the mucous membrane of the middle and superior nasal meatus into the ethmoid bone between the nasal cavity and the orbit (Figs. 7.66 and 7.69). The ethmoidal cells usually are not visible in plain radiographs before 2 years of age but are recognizable in CT scans. The **anterior ethmoidal cells** drain directly or indirectly into the middle nasal meatus through the ethmoidal infundibulum. The **middle ethmoidal cells** open directly into the middle meatus and are sometimes called "bullar cells" because they form the *ethmoidal bulla*, a swelling on the superior border of the semilunar hiatus (Fig. 7.65*B*). The **posterior ethmoidal cells** open directly into the superior meatus. The ethmoidal cells are supplied by the anterior and posterior ethmoidal branches of the *nasociliary nerves* (CN V₁) (Figs. 7.24 and 7.68).

Infection of the Ethmoidal Cells

If nasal drainage is blocked, infections of the ethmoidal cells may break through the fragile medial wall of the orbit. Severe infections from this source may cause blindness because some posterior ethmoidal cells lie close to the optic canal, which gives passage to the optic nerve and ophthalmic artery. Spread of infection from these cells could also affect the dural nerve sheath of the optic nerve, causing *optic neuritis*. ☉

Sphenoidal Sinuses

The **sphenoidal sinuses** are located in the body of the sphenoid and may extend into the wings of this bone (Figs. 7.65 and 7.69*A*). They are unevenly divided and separated by a bony

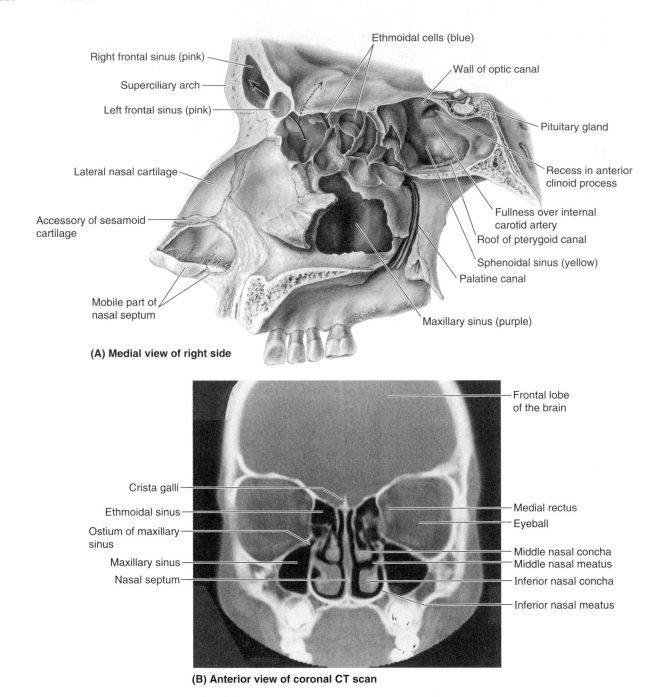

Figure 7.69. Paranasal sinuses. A. The paranasal sinuses of the right side have been opened from a nasal approach and color coded. An anterior ethmoidal cell (*pink*) is invading the diploë of the frontal bone to become a frontal sinus. An offshoot (*broken arrow*) invades the orbital plate of the frontal bone. The sphenoidal sinus in this specimen is extensive, extending (1) posteriorly, inferior to the pituitary gland, to the clivus; (2) laterally, inferior to the optic nerve (CN II), into the anterior clinoid process; and (3) inferior to the pterygoid process but leaving the pterygoid canal and rising as a ridge on the floor of the sinus. The maxillary sinus is pyramidal. **B.** A coronal CT scan is shown. (Courtesy of Dr. D. Armstrong, Associate Professor of Medical Imaging, University of Toronto, Toronto, Ontario, Canada.)

septum. Because of this extensive pneumatization (formation of air cells or sinuses), the body of the sphenoid is fragile. Only thin plates of bone separate the sinuses from several important structures: the optic nerves and optic chiasm, the pituitary gland, the internal carotid arteries, and the cavernous sinuses.

The sphenoidal sinuses are derived from a posterior ethmoidal cell that begins to invade the sphenoid at approximately 2 years of age. In some people, several posterior ethmoidal cells invade the sphenoid, giving rise to multiple sphenoidal sinuses that open separately into the *sphenoethmoidal recess*. The posterior

Skin
Subcutaneous tissue
Epicranial aponeurosis
Subaponeurotic space
Pericranium

Diploë

Superior sagittal sinus

Dura mater

Ethmoidal cells

Superior oblique

Auricularis anterior

Superior rectus

Levator palpebrae superioris

Optic nerve
Lateral rectus

Greater wing of sphenoid

Superior nasal concha
Middle nasal concha

Temporal fascia
Temporal muscle

Maxillary sinus

Infraorbital nerve
and artery

Zygomatic arch
Masseter

Inferior nasal concha
Inferior nasal meatus

Branches of palatine
artery and nerve

Intrinsic tongue muscles

Facial vein

Genioglossus
Sublingual gland

Vestibule of oral cavity

Buccinator

Geniohyoid
Mylohyoid

Inferior alveolar
nerve and artery
Digastric,
anterior belly

(C) Posterior view of anterior portion of head

Figure 7.69. *(Continued)* **C.** A coronal section of the head is shown. The orientation drawing shows the plane of the section shown in parts **B** and **C.** The ethmoid bone occupies a central position, with its horizontal component forming the central part of the anterior cranial fossa superiorly and the roof of the nasal cavity inferiorly. The ethmoidal cells give attachment to the superior and middle concha and form part of the medial wall of the orbit; the perpendicular plate of the ethmoid forms part of the nasal septum. The maxillary sinus forms the inferior part of the lateral wall of the nose and shares a common wall with the orbit. The middle concha shelters the hiatus semilunaris into which the maxillary ostium opens *(arrow)*.

ethmoidal arteries and posterior ethmoidal nerve supply the sphenoidal sinuses (Fig. 7.67).

Maxillary Sinuses

The **maxillary sinuses** are the largest of the paranasal sinuses. They occupy the bodies of the maxillae and communicate with the middle nasal meatus (Figs. 7.66 and 7.69).

- The **apex** of the maxillary sinus extends toward and often into the zygomatic bone.

- The **base** of the maxillary sinus forms the inferior part of the lateral wall of the nasal cavity.

- The **roof** of the maxillary sinus is formed by the floor of the orbit.

- The **floor** of the maxillary sinus is formed by the alveolar part of the maxilla. The roots of the maxillary teeth, particularly the first two molars, often produce conical elevations in the floor of the sinus.

Each maxillary sinus drains by one or more openings, the **maxillary ostium (ostia),** into the middle nasal meatus of the nasal cavity by way of the semilunar hiatus.

The **arterial supply of the maxillary sinus** is mainly from superior alveolar branches of the **maxillary artery** (Table 7.10); however, branches of the *descending* and *greater palatine arteries* supply the floor of the sinus (Figs. 7.62A and 7.67). **Innervation of the maxillary sinus** is from the anterior, middle, and posterior **superior alveolar nerves,** which are branches of the maxillary nerve (Fig. 7.42).

Infection of the Maxillary Sinuses

The maxillary sinuses are the most commonly infected, probably because their ostia are commonly small and are located high on their superomedial walls. When the mucous membrane of the sinus is congested, the maxillary ostia are often obstructed. Because of the high location of the ostia, when the head is erect it is impossible for the sinuses to drain until they are full. Because the ostia of the right and left sinuses lie on the medial sides (i.e., are directed toward each other), when lying on one's side only the upper sinus (e.g., the right sinus if lying on the left side) drains. A cold or allergy involving both sinuses can result in nights of rolling from side-to-side in an attempt to keep the sinuses drained. A maxillary sinus can be cannulated and drained by passing a cannula from the nares through the maxillary ostium into the sinus.

Relationship of the Teeth to the Maxillary Sinus

The close proximity of the three maxillary molar teeth to the floor of the maxillary sinus poses potentially serious problems. During removal of a molar tooth, a fracture of a root may occur. If proper retrieval methods are not used, a piece of the root may be driven superiorly into the maxillary sinus. A communication may be created between the oral cavity and the maxillary sinus as a result, and an infection may occur. Because the superior alveolar nerves (branches of the maxillary nerve) supply both the maxillary teeth and the mucous membrane of the maxillary sinuses, inflammation of the mucosa of the sinus is frequently accompanied by a sensation of toothache in the molar teeth.

Transillumination of the Sinuses

Transillumination of the maxillary sinuses is performed in a darkened room. A bright light is placed in the patient's mouth on one side of the hard palate. The light passes through the maxillary sinus and appears as a crescent-shaped, dull glow inferior to the orbit. If a sinus contains excess fluid, a mass, or a thickened mucosa, the glow is decreased. The frontal sinuses can also be transilluminated by directing the light superiorly under the medial aspect of the eyebrow, normally producing a glow superior to the orbit. Because of the great variation in the development of the sinuses, the pattern and extent of sinus illumination differs from person to person (Swartz, 2002). The ethmoidal and sphenoidal sinuses cannot be examined by transillumination. ✛

THE BOTTOM LINE: The nose is the ventilation system that traverses the head, enabling the flow of air between the external environment and the lower respiratory system (lungs). As the air is drawn in through the nose, its chemistry is sampled (smell and taste augmentation), and it is warmed, humidified, and filtered for the lungs. As it exits, heat and moisture are released with it. The nose also provides a drainage route for mucus and lacrimal fluid. Opening anteriorly via the nares, the nasal cavity is subdivided by a median nasal septum. The protruding external nose and anterior septum benefit from the flexibility provided by a cartilaginous skeleton, reducing the potential for nasal fractures. Except for the septum and floor, the walls of the nasal cavity are highly pneumatized by the paranasal sinuses and its lateral walls bear conchae. Both the sinuses and conchae increase the secretory surface area for exchange of moisture and heat.

Essentially, all surfaces are covered with thick, vascular, secretory mucosa, the anterosuperior portion of which (including that of most of the paranasal sinuses) is supplied by the ophthalmic artery and nerve (CN V_1), and the posteroinferior portion (including that of the maxillary sinus) by the maxillary artery and nerve (CN V_2). The mucosa of the roof and adjacent areas of walls and septum also receive special sensory innervation from the olfactory nerve (CN I).

Posteriorly, the nasal cavity is continuous with the nasopharynx via the choanae; the soft palate serves as a valve or gate controlling access to and from the nasal passageway. The bone and mucosa of the lateral walls of this passageway are perforated by openings of the nasolacrimal ducts, the paranasal sinuses and the pharyngotympanic tube. Only the bone is perforated by the pterygopalatine foramen, providing passage of neurovascular structures into the nasal mucosa. The paranasal sinuses are named for the bones they occupy. The maxillary sinus is the largest. Most open into the middle nasal meatus, but the sphenoidal sinuses enter the sphenoethmoidal recess.

Ear

The **ear** consists of external, middle, and internal parts (Fig. 7.70). The external and middle parts are mainly concerned with the transference of sound to the internal ear, which contains the organ for equilibrium (the condition of being evenly balanced) as well as for hearing. The *tympanic membrane* separates the external ear from the middle ear. The *pharyngotympanic tube* joins the middle ear to the nasopharynx.

External Ear

The **external ear** is composed of the shell-like *auricle* (*pinna*), which collects sound, and the *external acoustic meatus* (canal), which conducts sound to the tympanic membrane.

Auricle

The **auricle** (L. *auris,* an ear) is composed of an irregularly shaped plate of elastic cartilage that is covered by thin skin

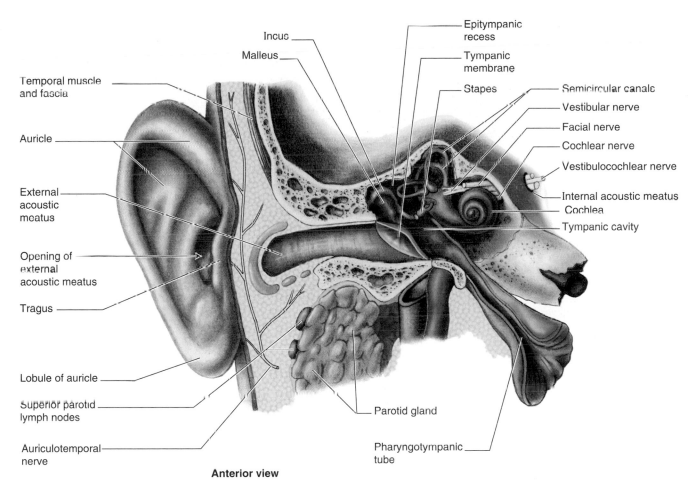

Incus

Malleus

Epitympanic recess

Tympanic membrane

Stapes

Semicircular canals

Vestibular nerve

Facial nerve

Cochlear nerve

Vestibulocochlear nerve

Internal acoustic meatus

Cochlea

Tympanic cavity

Temporal muscle and fascia

Auricle

External acoustic meatus

Opening of external acoustic meatus

Tragus

Lobule of auricle

Superior parotid lymph nodes

Auriculotemporal nerve

Parotid gland

Pharyngotympanic tube

Anterior view

Figure 7.70. Parts of ear. A coronal section of the ear is shown. The ear has three parts: external, middle, and internal. The external ear consists of the auricle and external acoustic meatus. The middle ear is an air space in which the auditory ossicles are located. The internal ear contains the membranous labyrinth; its chief divisions are the cochlear labyrinth and the vestibular labyrinth.

(Fig. 7.71). The auricle has several depressions and elevations. The **concha** is the deepest depression. The elevated margin of the auricle is the **helix**. The other depressions and elevations are identified in Figure 7.71. The non-cartilaginous **lobule** (earlobe) consists of fibrous tissue, fat, and blood vessels. It is easily pierced for taking small blood samples and inserting earrings. The **tragus** (G. *tragos,* goat; alluding to the hairs that tend to grow from this formation, like a goat's beard) is a tongue-like projection overlapping the opening of the external acoustic meatus.

The **arterial supply** to the auricle is derived mainly from the *posterior auricular* and *superficial temporal arteries* (Fig. 7.72*A*). The main **nerves to the skin of the auricle** are the great auricular and auriculotemporal nerves. The *great auricular nerve* supplies the cranial (medial) surface (commonly called the "back of the ear") and the posterior part (helix, antihelix, and lobule) of the lateral surface ("front"). The *auriculotemporal nerve,* a branch of CN V$_3$, supplies the skin of the auricle anterior to the external acoustic meatus. Minor contributions of embryological significance are made to the skin of the concha and its eminence by the vagus and facial nerves. The **lymphatic drainage** of the auricle is as follows: the lateral surface of the superior half of the auricle drains to

the *superficial parotid lymph nodes* (Fig. 7.72*B*); the cranial surface of the superior half of the auricle drains to the **mastoid nodes** and *deep cervical lymph nodes;* and the remainder of the auricle, including the lobule, drains into the **superficial cervical lymph nodes.**

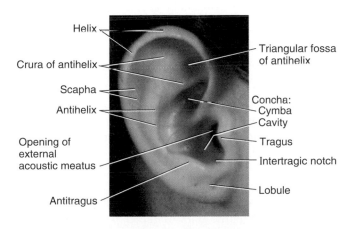

Helix

Crura of antihelix

Scapha

Antihelix

Opening of external acoustic meatus

Antitragus

Triangular fossa of antihelix

Concha:
Cymba
Cavity

Tragus

Intertragic notch

Lobule

Figure 7.71. External ear. The parts of the auricle commonly used in clinical descriptions are labeled. The external ear includes the auricle and external acoustic meatus.

(A) Lateral view

Lymph Node Groups

☐ Occipital	■ Submental
■ Mastoid	☐ Superficial cervical
■ Parotid	■ Deep cervical
■ Buccal	■ *Retropharyngeal
■ Submandibular	☐ *Jugulo-omohyoid

*Part of deep cervical group of lymph nodes

(B)

Figure 7.72. Dissection of face and lymphatic drainage of head. A. The posterior auricular and superficial temporal arteries and veins and the great auricular and auriculotemporal nerves provide the circulation and innervation of the external ear. **B.** Lymphatic drainage is to the parotid nodes and the mastoid and superficial cervical nodes, all which drain to the deep cervical nodes.

External Acoustic Meatus

The *external acoustic meatus* is a canal that leads inward through the tympanic part of the temporal bone from the auricle to the tympanic membrane, a distance of 2–3 cm in adults (Fig. 7.70). The lateral third of this slightly S-shaped canal is cartilaginous and lined with skin that is continuous with the auricular skin. Its medial two thirds is bony and lined with thin skin that is continuous with the external layer of the tympanic membrane. The ceruminous and sebaceous glands in the subcutaneous tissue of the cartilaginous part of the meatus produce *cerumen* (earwax).

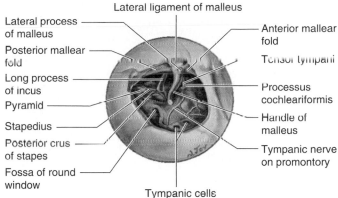

(A) Auriscopic view of right tympanic membrane

(B) Inferolateral view, right side

Figure 7.73. Tympanic membrane and lateral approach to tympanic cavity. A. An otoscopic view of the right tympanic membrane is demonstrated. The *cone of light* is a reflection of the light of the otoscope. **B.** The tympanic cavity after removal of the tympanic membrane is shown. The surface of the bulging promontory of the labyrinthine (medial) wall becomes grooved by the plexus of the tympanic nerve (a branch of CN IX).

The **tympanic membrane,** approximately 1 cm in diameter, is a thin, oval semitransparent membrane at the medial end of the external acoustic meatus (Figs. 7.70 and 7.73*A* & *B*). It forms a partition between the meatus and the *tympanic cavity* of the middle ear. The tympanic membrane is covered with thin skin externally and mucous membrane of the middle ear internally. Viewed through an otoscope, the tympanic membrane has a concavity toward the external acoustic meatus with a shallow, cone-like central depression, the peak of which is the **umbo** (Fig. 7.73*A*) (see clinical correlation [blue] box "Otoscopic Examination," on this page). The central axis of the tympanic membrane passes perpendicularly through the umbo like the handle of an umbrella, running anteriorly and inferiorly as it runs laterally. Thus the tympanic membrane is oriented like a mini radar or satellite dish positioned to receive signals coming from the ground in front and to the side of the head.

Superior to the lateral process of the *malleus* (one of the small ear bones, or *auditory ossicles,* of the middle ear), the membrane is thin and is called the **flaccid part** (L. *pars flaccida*). It lacks the radial and circular fibers present in the remainder of the membrane, called the **tense part** (L. *pars tensa*). The flaccid part forms the lateral wall of the superior recess of the tympanic cavity.

The tympanic membrane moves in response to air vibrations that pass to it through the external acoustic meatus. Movements of the membrane are transmitted by the auditory ossicles through the middle ear to the internal ear (Fig. 7.70). The external surface of the tympanic membrane is supplied mainly by the *auriculotemporal nerve* (Fig. 7.72*A*), a branch of CN V₃. Some innervation is supplied by a small *auricular branch of the vagus* (CN X). The internal surface of the tympanic membrane is supplied by the glossopharyngeal nerve (CN IX).

External Ear Injury

Bleeding within the auricle resulting from trauma may produce an *auricular hematoma.* A localized collection of blood forms between the perichondrium and the auricular cartilage, causing distortion of the contours of the auricle. As the hematoma enlarges, it compromises the blood supply to the cartilage. If untreated (e.g., by aspiration of blood), fibrosis (formation of fibrous tissue) develops in the overlying skin, forming a deformed auricle (e.g., the cauliflower or boxer's ear of some professional fighters).

Otoscopic Examination

Examination of the external acoustic meatus and tympanic membrane begins by straightening the meatus. In adults, the helix is grasped and pulled posterosuperiorly (up, out, and back). These movements reduce the curvature of the external acoustic meatus, facilitating insertion of the *otoscope* (Fig. B7.30*A*). The meatus is relatively short in infants; therefore, extra care must be exercised to prevent injury to the tympanic membrane. The meatus is straightened in infants by pulling the auricle inferoposteriorly (down and back). The examination also provides a clue to tenderness, which can indicate inflammation of the auricle and/or the meatus. The tympanic membrane is normally translucent and pearly gray (Fig. B7.30*B*). The handle of the malleus is usually visible near the center of the membrane (the umbo). From the inferior end of the handle, a bright *cone of light* is reflected from the otoscope's illuminator. This *light reflex* is visible radiating anteroinferiorly in the healthy ear. ▶

Figure B7.30. Otoscopic examination (A) and normal tympanic membrane (B).

Acute Otitis Externa

Otitis externa is an inflammation of the external acoustic meatus. The infection often develops in swimmers who do not dry their meatus after swimming and/or use ear drops, but it may also be the result of a bacterial infection of the skin lining the meatus. The affected individual complains of itching and pain in the external ear. Pulling the auricle or applying pressure on the tragus increases the pain. ✚

THE BOTTOM LINE: The ear is divided into external, middle, and internal parts. All three are concerned with the sense of hearing, but the internal ear also has a vestibular function. The external ear is a funnel-like conduit for airborne sound waves to reach the middle ear. The protruding auricle and lateral part of the external acoustic meatus have an elastic cartilage skeleton that allows flexibility. The primary sensory innervation of the external ear is provided by CN V and CN X.

Middle Ear

The **cavity of the middle ear** or **tympanic cavity** is the narrow air-filled chamber in the petrous part of the temporal bone (Fig. 7.70 and 7.74). The cavity has two parts: the **tympanic cavity proper**, the space directly internal to the tympanic membrane, and the **epitympanic recess**, the space superior to the membrane. The tympanic cavity is connected anteromedially with the nasopharynx by the *pharyngotympanic tube* and posterosuperiorly with the mastoid cells through the *mastoid antrum* (Fig. 7.75A). The tympanic cavity is lined with mucous membrane that is continuous with the lining of the pharyngotympanic tube, mastoid cells, and mastoid antrum. The contents of the middle ear are the:

- Auditory ossicles (malleus, incus, and stapes).

- Stapedius and tensor tympani muscles.

- Chorda tympani nerve, a branch of CN VII (Fig. 7.75).

- Tympanic plexus of nerves.

Walls of the Tympanic Cavity

The middle ear is shaped like a lozenge or narrow box with concave sides. It has six walls (Fig. 7.75*B*).

1. The **tegmental wall** (**tegmental roof**) is formed by a thin plate of bone, the *tegmen tympani,* which separates the tympanic cavity from the dura mater on the floor of the middle cranial fossa.

2. The **jugular wall** (**floor**) is formed by a layer of bone that separates the tympanic cavity from the superior bulb of the internal jugular vein.

3. The **membranous wall** (**lateral wall**) is formed almost entirely by the peaked convexity of the *tympanic membrane;* superiorly it is formed by the lateral bony wall of the *epitympanic recess.* The handle of the malleus is attached to the tympanic membrane, and its head extends into the epitympanic recess.

4. The **labyrinthine wall** (**medial wall**) separates the tympanic cavity from the internal ear. It also features the *promontory of the labyrinthine wall,* formed by the initial part (basal turn) of the cochlea, and the *oval* and *round windows,* which, in a dry cranium, communicate with the inner ear.

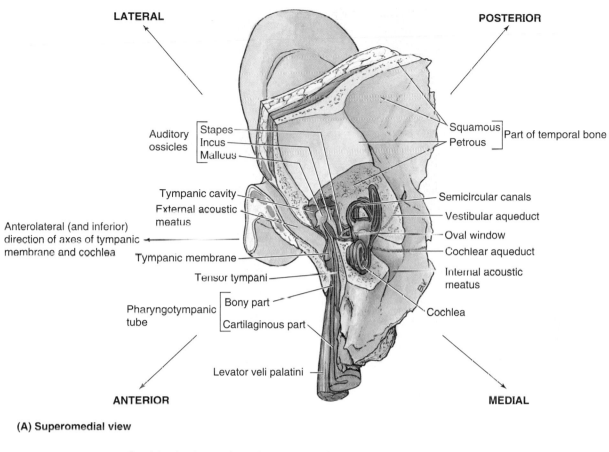

LATERAL

POSTERIOR

Auditory ossicles
- Stapes
- Incus
- Malleus

Squamous
Petrous
Part of temporal bone

Tympanic cavity

External acoustic meatus

Semicircular canals

Vestibular aqueduct

Anterolateral (and inferior) direction of axes of tympanic membrane and cochlea

Oval window

Cochlear aqueduct

Tympanic membrane

Tensor tympani

Internal acoustic meatus

Pharyngotympanic tube
- Bony part
- Cartilaginous part

Cochlea

Levator veli palatini

ANTERIOR

MEDIAL

(A) Superomedial view

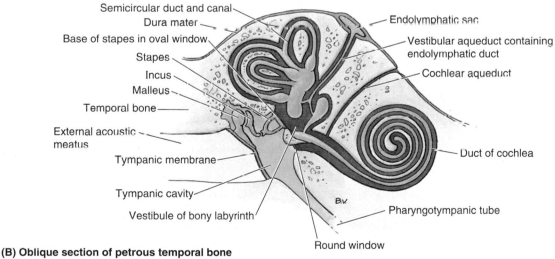

Semicircular duct and canal

Dura mater

Base of stapes in oval window

Stapes

Incus

Malleus

Temporal bone

External acoustic meatus

Tympanic membrane

Tympanic cavity

Vestibule of bony labyrinth

Endolymphatic sac

Vestibular aqueduct containing endolymphatic duct

Cochlear aqueduct

Duct of cochlea

Pharyngotympanic tube

Round window

(B) Oblique section of petrous temporal bone

Figure 7.74. General scheme of ear. A. The ear is shown in situ. The external acoustic meatus runs lateral to medial; the axis of the tympanic membrane and the axis about which the cochlea winds runs inferiorly and anteriorly as it proceeds laterally. The long axes of the bony and membranous labyrinths and of the pharyngotympanic tube and parallel tensor tympani and levator pala-tini muscles lie perpendicular to those of the tympanic membrane and cochlea (i.e., they run inferiorly and anteriorly as they proceed medially). **B.** The middle and internal parts of the ear are shown. The middle ear lies between the tympanic membrane and the internal ear. Three auditory ossicles stretch from the lateral to the medial wall of the tympanic cavity. The pharyngotympanic tube is a communication between the anterior wall of the tympanic cavity and the lateral wall of the nasopharynx. The internal ear is composed of a closed system of membranous tubes and bulbs, the membranous labyrinth, which is filled with a fluid called en-dolymph (*orange*) and bathed in surrounding fluid called perilymph (*purple*).

Chorda tympani nerve

Tensor tympani

Internal carotid artery

Anterior

Tympanic membrane forming
membranous (lateral) wall

(A) Superomedial view

Tegmen tympani [tegmental wall
(roof) of tympanic cavity]

Mastoid antrum

Opening of pharyngotympanic tube
in carotid (anterior) wall

Facial nerve

Jugular wall (floor)
of tympanic cavity

Posterior

Sigmoid sinus

Superior bulb of internal jugular vein

Epitympanic recess

Malleus
Incus
Stapes

Chorda tympani
nerve

Tensor tympani

Tympanic membrane

(B) Anterior view

Lesser petrosal nerve

Prominence of lateral
semicircular canal

Facial nerve

Aditus to mastoid antrum
(forming posterior wall)

Prominence of canal
for facial nerve

Tympanic plexus on promontory
of labyrinthine wall

Stapedius
Pyramidal eminence

Tympanic nerve (from CN IX)

1. Tegmental wall (roof)
2. Jugular wall (floor)
3. Membranous (lateral) wall
4. Labyrinthine (medial) wall
5. Mastoid (posterior) wall
   Carotid (anterior) wall was
   removed to provide this view

Figure 7.75. Walls of tympanic cavity. A. This specimen was dissected with a drill from the medial aspect. The tegmen tympani, forming the roof of the tympanic cavity and the mastoid antrum, is fairly thick in this specimen; usually it is extremely thin. The internal carotid artery is the main relation of the anterior wall, the internal jugular vein is the main relation of the floor, and the facial nerve (CN VII) is a main feature of the posterior wall. The chorda tympani nerve passes between the malleus and the incus. **B.** In this view of the middle ear, the carotid (anterior) wall of the tympanic cavity has been removed. The tympanic membrane forms most of the membranous (lateral) wall; superior to it is the epitympanic recess, in which are housed the larger parts of the malleus and incus. Branches of the tympanic plexus provide innervation to the mucosa of the middle ear and adjacent pharyngotympanic tube; but one branch, the lesser petrosal nerve, is conveying presynaptic parasympathetic fibers to the otic ganglion for secretomotor innervation of the parotid gland.

5. The anterior **carotid wall** separates the tympanic cavity from the carotid canal; superiorly, it has the **opening of the pharyngotympanic tube** and the **canal for the tensor tympani.**

6. The **mastoid wall (posterior wall)** features an opening in its superior part, the **aditus** (L. access) **to the mastoid antrum,** connecting the tympanic cavity to the mastoid cells; the canal for the facial nerve descends between the posterior wall and the antrum, medial to the aditus.

The **mastoid antrum** is a cavity in the mastoid process of the temporal bone (Fig. 7.75*A*). The antrum (L. from G., cave), like the tympanic cavity, is separated from the middle cranial fossa by a thin plate of the temporal bone, called the **tegmen tympani.** This structure forms the *tegmental wall* (roof) for the ear cavities and is also part of the floor of the lateral part of the middle cranial fossa. The antrum is the common cavity into which the mastoid cells open. The antrum and mastoid cells are lined by mucous membrane that is continuous with the lining of the middle ear. Anteroinferiorly, the antrum is related to the canal for the facial nerve.

Otitis Media

An earache and a bulging red tympanic membrane may indicate pus or fluid in the middle ear, a sign of *otitis media* (Fig. B7.31*A*). Infection of the middle ear is often secondary to upper respiratory infections. Inflammation and swelling of the mucous membrane lining the tympanic cavity may cause partial or complete *blockage of the pharyngotympanic tube.* The tympanic membrane becomes red and bulges, and the person may complain of "ear popping." An amber-colored bloody fluid may be observed through the tympanic membrane. If untreated, otitis media may produce impaired hearing as the result of scarring of the auditory ossicles, limiting their ability to move in response to sound.

Perforation of the Tympanic Membrane

Perforation of the tympanic membrane ("ruptured eardrum") may result from otitis media and is one of several causes of middle ear deafness. Perforation may also result from foreign bodies in the external acoustic meatus, trauma, or excessive pressure (e.g., during scuba diving). Minor ruptures of the tympanic membrane often heal spontaneously. Large ruptures usually require surgical repair. Because the superior half of the tympanic membrane is much more vascular than the inferior half, incisions to release pus from a middle ear abscess, for example, are made posteroinferiorly through the membrane. This incision also avoids injury to the chorda tympani nerve and auditory ossicles.

Mastoiditis

Infections of the mastoid antrum and mastoid cells *(mastoiditis)* result from a middle ear infection that causes inflammation of the mastoid process (Fig B7.31*B*). Infections may spread superiorly into the middle cranial fossa through the petrosquamous fissure in children and cause *osteomyelitis* (bone infection) of the tegmen tympani. Since the advent of antibiotics, mastoiditis is uncommon. During operations for mastoiditis, surgeons remain conscious of the course of the facial nerve to avoid injuring it. One point of access to the tympanic cavity is through the mastoid antrum. In children, only a thin plate of bone must be removed from the lateral wall of the antrum to expose the tympanic cavity. In adults, bone must be penetrated for 15 mm or more. At present, most mastoidectomies are endaural (i.e., performed through the posterior wall of the external acoustic meatus). ☉

(A)

(B)

Figure B7.31. Otitis media (A) and mastoiditis (ruptured retroauricular abscess) (B)

Pharyngotympanic Tube

The **pharyngotympanic tube** connects the tympanic cavity to the nasopharynx, where it opens posterior to the inferior nasal meatus (Fig. 7.74). The posterolateral third of the tube is bony and the remainder is cartilaginous. The pharyngotympanic tube is lined by mucous membrane that is continuous posteriorly with that of the tympanic cavity and anteriorly with that of the nasopharynx. The function of the pharyngotympanic tube is to equalize pressure in the middle ear with the atmospheric pressure, thereby allowing free movement of the tympanic membrane. By allowing air to enter and leave the tympanic cavity, this tube balances the pressure on both sides of the membrane. Because the walls (crura) of the cartilaginous part of the tube are normally in apposition, the tube must be actively opened. The tube is opened by the expanding girth of the belly of the *levator veli palatini* as it contracts longitudinally, pushing against one wall while the *tensor veli palatini* pulls on the other. Because these are muscles of the soft palate, equalizing pressure ("popping the eardrums") is commonly associated with activities such as yawning and swallowing.

The **arteries** of the pharyngotympanic tube are derived from the *ascending pharyngeal artery,* a branch of the external carotid artery, and the *middle meningeal artery* and *artery of the pterygoid canal,* branches of the maxillary artery (Fig. 7.76; Table 7.10). The **veins** of the pharyngotympanic tube drain into the pterygoid venous plexus. **Lymphatic drainage** of the pharyngotympanic tube is to the *deep cervical lymph nodes* (Fig. 7.72*B*). The **nerves** of the pharyngotympanic tube arise from the *tympanic plexus* (Fig. 7.75*B*), which is formed by fibers of the glossopharyngeal nerve (CN IX). Anteriorly, the tube also receives fibers from the *pterygopalatine ganglion* (Fig. 7.68).

Blockage of the Pharyngotympanic Tube

The pharyngotympanic tube forms a route for an infection to pass from the nasopharynx to the tympanic cavity. This tube is easily blocked by swelling of its mucous membrane, even as a result of mild infections (e.g., a cold), because the walls of its cartilaginous part are normally already in apposition. When the pharyngotympanic tube is occluded, residual air in the tympanic cavity is usually absorbed into the mucosal blood vessels, resulting in lower pressure in the tympanic cavity, retraction of the tympanic membrane, and interference with its free movement. Finally, hearing is affected. ✪

Auditory Ossicles

The **auditory ossicles** form a mobile chain of small bones across the tympanic cavity from the tympanic membrane to the **oval window** (L. *fenestra vestibuli*), an oval opening on the labyrinthine wall of the tympanic cavity leading to the *vestibule of the bony labyrinth* (Fig. 7.77*A*). The ossicles are the first bones to be fully ossified during development and are essentially mature at birth. The bone from which they are formed is exceptionally dense (hard). The ossicles are covered with the mucous membrane lining the tympanic cavity; but unlike other bones, they lack a surrounding layer of osteogenic periosteum.

Malleus. The **malleus** (L. a hammer) attaches to the tympanic membrane. The rounded superior **head** of the malleus lies in the epitympanic recess (Fig. 7.77*B*). The **neck** of the malleus lies against the flaccid part of the tympanic membrane, and the **handle** of the malleus is embedded in the tympanic membrane, with its tip at the umbo; thus the malleus moves with the membrane. The head of the malleus articulates with the incus; the tendon of the tensor tympani inserts into its handle near the neck. The *chorda tympani nerve* crosses the medial surface of the neck of the malleus. The malleus functions as a lever, with the longer of its two processes and its handle attached to the tympanic membrane.

Incus. The **incus** (L. an anvil) is located between the malleus and the stapes and articulates with them. It has a body and two limbs. Its large **body** lies in the epitympanic recess, where it articulates with the head of the malleus (Fig. 7.77*C*). The **long limb** lies parallel to the handle of the malleus, and its interior end articulates with the stapes by way of the **lenticular process,** a medially directed projection. The **short limb** is connected by a ligament to the posterior wall of the tympanic cavity.

Stapes. The **stapes** (L. a stirrup) is the smallest ossicle. It has a head, two limbs (crura), and a base (Fig. 7.77*D*). Its **head,** directed laterally, articulates with the incus. The **base** (footplate) of the stapes fits into the *oval window* on the medial wall of the tympanic cavity. The oval base is attached to the margins of the oval window. The base is considerably smaller than the tympanic membrane; as a result, the vibratory force of the stapes is increased approximately 10 times over that of the tympanic membrane. Consequently, the auditory ossicles increase the force but decrease the amplitude of the vibrations transmitted from the tympanic membrane.

Muscles Associated with the Auditory Ossicles. Two muscles dampen or resist movements of the auditory ossicles; one also dampens movements (vibration) of the tympanic membrane.

The **tensor tympani** is a short muscle that arises from the superior surface of the cartilaginous part of the pharyngotympanic tube, the greater wing of the sphenoid, and the petrous part of the temporal bone (Figs. 7.73*B* and 7.75). The muscle inserts into the handle of the malleus. The tensor tympani

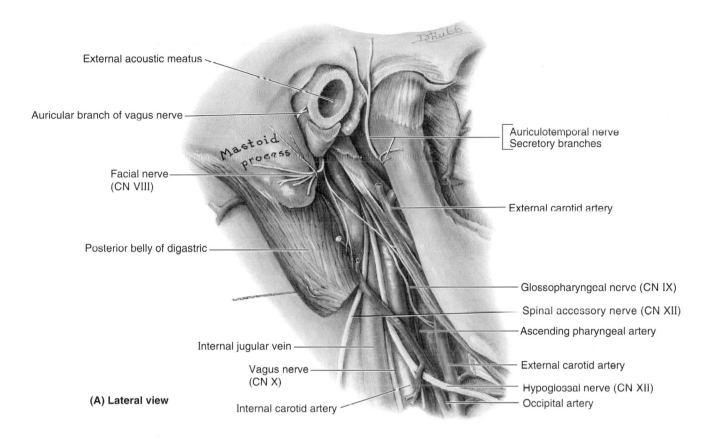

External acoustic meatus

Auricular branch of vagus nerve

Auriculotemporal nerve
Secretory branches

Facial nerve
(CN VIII)

Mastoid process

External carotid artery

Posterior belly of digastric

Glossopharyngeal nerve (CN IX)

Spinal accessory nerve (CN XII)

Ascending pharyngeal artery

Internal jugular vein

External carotid artery

Vagus nerve
(CN X)

Hypoglossal nerve (CN XII)

Occipital artery

Internal carotid artery

(A) Lateral view

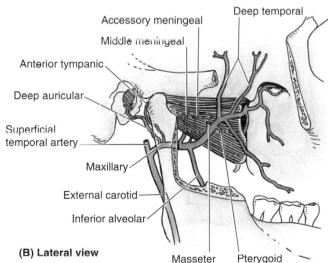

Deep temporal

Accessory meningeal

Middle meningeal

Anterior tympanic

Deep auricular

Superficial temporal artery

Maxillary

External carotid

Inferior alveolar

(B) Lateral view

Masseter   Pterygoid

Figure 7.76. Dissection of structures deep to parotid bed. A. The facial nerve (CN VII), the posterior belly of the digastric muscle, and the nerve to it are retracted. The deeply placed ascending pharyngeal artery is the only medial branch of the external carotid artery. It supplies the pharynx, palatine tonsil, pharyngotympanic tube, and the medial wall of the tympanic cavity before it terminates by sending meningeal branches to the cranial cavity. **B.** Maxillary artery and its branches. The branches of the first (mandibular) part supply the external acoustic meatus and tympanic membrane. The middle meningeal artery sends branches to the pharyngotympanic tube before entering the cranium through the foramen spinosum.

pulls the handle medially, tensing the tympanic membrane and reducing the amplitude of its oscillations. This action tends to prevent damage to the internal ear when one is exposed to loud sounds. The tensor tympani is supplied by the mandibular nerve (CN V$_3$).

The **stapedius** is a tiny muscle inside the **pyramidal eminence** (pyramid), a hollow, cone-shaped prominence on the posterior wall of the tympanic cavity (Figs. 7.73*B* and

7.75*B*). Its tendon enters the tympanic cavity by emerging from a pinpoint foramen in the apex of the eminence and inserts on the neck of the stapes. The stapedius pulls the stapes posteriorly and tilts its base in the *oval window*, thereby tightening the anular ligament and reducing the oscillatory range. It also prevents excessive movement of the stapes. The nerve to the stapedius arises from the facial nerve (CN VII).

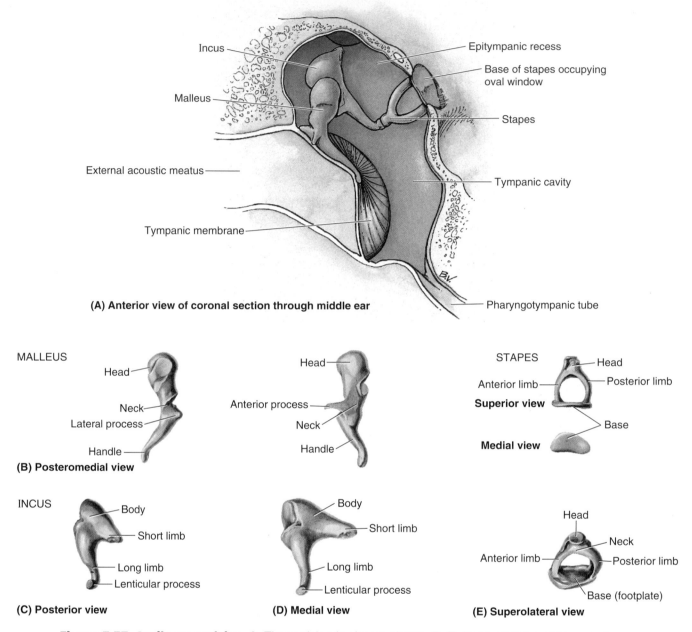

(A) Anterior view of coronal section through middle ear

MALLEUS

Head

Neck
Lateral process

Handle

(B) Posteromedial view

Head

Anterior process

Neck

Handle

STAPES — Head

Anterior limb — Posterior limb

Superior view

Base

Medial view

INCUS — Body

Short limb

Long limb
Lenticular process

(C) Posterior view

Body

Short limb

Long limb

Lenticular process

(D) Medial view

Head

Neck

Anterior limb — Posterior limb

Base (footplate)

(E) Superolateral view

Figure 7.77. Auditory ossicles. A. The ossicles *in situ* are shown. **B–E.** The isolated ossicles are shown.

Paralysis of the Stapedius

The tympanic muscles have a protective action in that they dampen large vibrations of the tympanic membrane resulting from loud noises. Paralysis of the stapedius (e.g., resulting from a lesion of the facial nerve) is associated with excessive acuteness of hearing called *hyperacusis* or *hyperacusia*. This condition results from uninhibited movements of the stapes. ✚

THE BOTTOM LINE: The tympanic membrane responds to airborne sound waves, converting them to vibrations transmitted by the solid medium of the ossicles of the middle ear. Because its entire lateral wall is formed by a thin membrane, the middle ear (tympanic cavity) is a pressure-sensitive space, ventilated by means of the pharyngotympanic tube. The mucosa lining both the cavity and the tube is innervated by CN IX. At the oval window, between the middle and internal ears, the solid medium vibrations of the ossicles are converted to fluidborne sonar waves.

Internal Ear

The **internal ear** contains the **vestibulocochlear organ** concerned with the reception of sound and the maintenance of balance. Buried in the petrous part of the temporal bone (Figs. 7.74 and 7.78A), the internal ear consists of the sacs and ducts of the membranous labyrinth. The *membranous labyrinth*, containing *endolymph*, is suspended within the perilymph-filled *bony labyrinth*, either by delicate filaments similar to the filaments of arachnoid mater that traverse the subarachnoid space or by the substantial spiral ligament. It does not float. These fluids are involved in stimulating the end organs for balance and hearing, respectively.

Bony Labyrinth

The **bony labyrinth** is a series of cavities (cochlea, vestibule, and semicircular canals) contained within the otic capsule of the petrous part of the temporal bone (Figs. 7.74A and 7.78B). The **otic capsule** is made of bone that is denser than the remainder of the petrous temporal bone and can be isolated (carved) from it using a dental drill. The otic capsule is often erroneously illustrated and identified as being the bony labyrinth. However, the bony labyrinth is the *fluid-filled space*, which is surrounded by the otic capsule, and is most accurately represented by a cast of the otic capsule after removal of the surrounding bone.

Cochlea. The **cochlea** is the shell-shaped part of the bony labyrinth that contains the **cochlear duct** (Fig. 7.78C), the part of the internal ear concerned with hearing. The **spiral canal** of the cochlea begins at the vestibule and makes 2.5 turns around a bony core, the *modiolus* (Fig. 7.79), the cone-shaped core of spongy bone about which the spiral canal of the cochlea turns. The modiolus contains canals for blood vessels and for distribution of the branches of the cochlear nerve. The apex of the cone-shaped modiolus, like the axis of the tympanic membrane, is directed laterally, anteriorly, and inferiorly. The large basal turn of the cochlea produces the *promontory of the labyrinthine wall* of the tympanic cavity (Fig. 7.75B). At the basal turn, the bony labyrinth communicates with the subarachnoid space superior to the jugular foramen through the **cochlear aqueduct** (Fig. 7.74B). It also features the **round window** (L. *fenestra cochleae*), closed by the **secondary tympanic membrane** (Fig. 7.78B & C).

Vestibule of the Bony Labyrinth. The **vestibule of the bony labyrinth** is a small oval chamber (approximately 5 mm long) that contains the **utricle** and **saccule** (Fig. 7.78C), and parts of the balancing apparatus (vestibular labyrinth). The vestibule features the *oval window* on its lateral wall, occupied by the base of the stapes. The vestibule is continuous with the bony cochlea anteriorly, the semicircular canals posteriorly, and the posterior cranial fossa by the **aqueduct of the vestibule** (Fig. 7.78A). The aqueduct extends to the posterior surface of the petrous part of the temporal bone, where it opens posterolateral to the *internal acoustic meatus* (Fig. 7.78A). The vestibular aqueduct transmits the **endolymphatic duct** (Fig. 7.78D) and two small blood vessels.

Semicircular Canals. The **semicircular canals** (anterior, posterior, and lateral) communicate with the vestibule of the bony labyrinth (Fig. 7.78B). The canals lie posterosuperior to the vestibule into which they open; they are set at right angles to each other. The canals occupy three planes in space. Each semicircular canal forms approximately two thirds of a circle and is approximately 1.5 mm in diameter, except at one end where there is a swelling, the **bony ampulla**. The canals have only five openings into the vestibule because the anterior and posterior canals have one limb common to both. Lodged within the canals are the *semicircular ducts* (Fig. 7.78C & D).

Membranous Labyrinth

The **membranous labyrinth** consists of a series of communicating sacs and ducts that are suspended in the bony labyrinth (Fig. 7.78C). It contains **endolymph**, a watery fluid similar in composition to intracellular fluid, thus differing in composition from the surrounding **perilymph** (which is like extracellular fluid) that fills the remainder of the bony labyrinth. The membranous labyrinth—composed of two divisions, the *vestibular labyrinth* and the *cochlear labyrinth*—consists of more parts than does the bony labyrinth:

- **Vestibular labyrinth:** utricle and saccule, two small communicating sacs in the vestibule of the bony labyrinth.

- Three semicircular ducts in the semicircular canals.

- **Cochlear labyrinth:** cochlear duct in the cochlea.

The **spiral ligament**, a spiral thickening of the periosteal lining of the cochlear canal, secures the *cochlear duct* to the spiral canal of the cochlea (Fig. 7.79). The remainder of the membranous labyrinth is suspended by delicate filaments that traverse the perilymph.

The **semicircular ducts** open into the *utricle* through five openings, reflective of the way the surrounding semicircular canals open into the vestibule. The utricle communicates with the saccule through the **utriculosaccular duct** from which the *endolymphatic duct* arises (Fig. 7.78D). The *saccule* is continuous with the cochlear duct through the **ductus reuniens**, a uniting duct. The utricle and saccule have specialized areas of sensory epithelium called *maculae*. The **macula of the utricle** (L. *macula utriculi*) is in the floor of the utricle, parallel with the base of the cranium, whereas the **macula of the saccule** (L. *macula sacculi*) is vertically placed on the medial wall of the saccule. The **hair cells in the maculae** are innervated by fibers of the vestibular division of the **vestibulocochlear nerve**. The primary sensory neurons are in the **vestibular ganglia** (Fig. 7.80), which are in the internal acoustic meatus.

The *endolymphatic duct* traverses the *vestibular aqueduct* (Fig. 7.74B) and emerges through the bone of the posterior cranial fossa, where it expands into a blind pouch called the **endolymphatic sac** (Figs. 7.78C and 7.80). The endolymphatic sac is located under the dura mater on the posterior surface of the petrous part of the temporal bone. The sac is a storage reservoir for excess endolymph, formed by the blood capillaries in the membranous labyrinth.

Direction of view for
parts B–D

Cochlea

Semicircular
canals {
Anterior
Lateral
Posterior

Vestibule

Aqueduct of vestibule

Squamous part
of temporal bone

Petrosquamous fissure

Petrous part }
Mastoid part } Of temporal
bone

Internal acoustic meatus

Foramen magnum

(A) Superior view of internal surface of cranial base

Anterior semicircular canal
and bony ampulla

Facial canal,
opened (canal
for facial nerve)

Cochlea {
Cupula
2nd turn
1st turn

Round window

Lateral semicircular
canal and bony ampulla

Posterior
semicircular
canal and
bony ampulla

Vestibule and oval window

(B) Anterolateral view of left otic capsule

Anterior semicircular duct
and membranous
ampulla

Cochlear duct

Saccule

Ductus reuniens

Lateral semicircular duct

Common crus

Posterior
semicircular
duct

Utricle

Secondary tympanic
membrane

Endolymphatic sac

**(C) Anterolateral view of left membranous labyrinth
(through transparent otic capsule)**

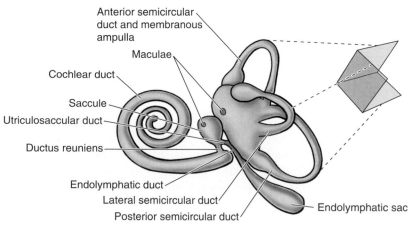

Anterior semicircular
duct and membranous
ampulla

Maculae

Cochlear duct

Saccule

Utriculosaccular duct

Ductus reuniens

Endolymphatic duct

Lateral semicircular duct

Posterior semicircular duct

Endolymphatic sac

(D) Anterolateral view of left membranous labyrinth

Figure 7.78. Bony and membranous labyrinths of internal ear. A. This view of the interior of the base of the cranium shows the temporal bone and the location of the bony labyrinth. **B.** The walls of the bony labyrinth have been carved out of the petrous temporal bone. **C.** A similar view of the bony labyrinth occupied by perilymph and the membranous labyrinth is shown. **D.** The membranous labyrinth, shown after removal from the bony labyrinth, is a closed system of ducts and chambers filled with endolymph and bathed by perilymph. It has three parts: the cochlear duct, which occupies the cochlea; the saccule and utricle, which occupy the vestibule; and the three semicircular ducts, which occupy the semicircular canals. The utricle communicates with the saccule through the utriculosaccular duct. The lateral semicircular duct lies in the horizontal plane and is more horizontal than it appears in this drawing.

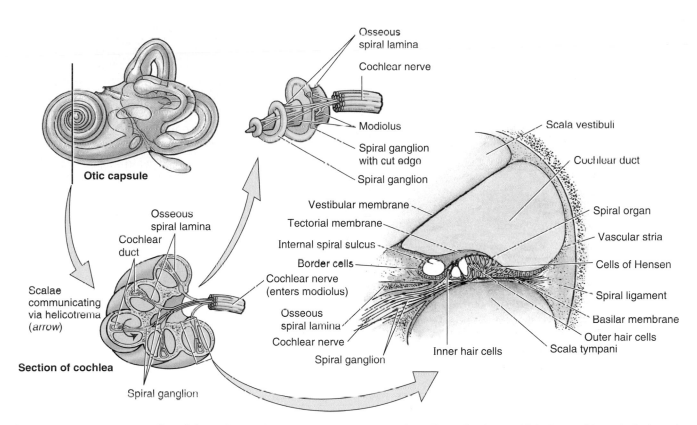

Figure 7.79. Structure of cochlea. The cochlea has been sectioned along the axis about which the cochlea winds (see the orientation figure in the upper left). An isolated, cone-like, bony core of the cochlea, the modiolus, is shown after the turns of the cochlea are removed, leaving only the spiral lamina winding around it like the thread of a screw. Details of the area enclosed in the rectangle are also shown.

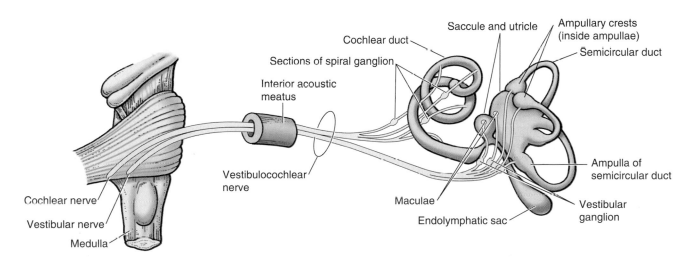

Figure 7.80. Vestibulocochlear nerve (CN VIII). CN VIII has two parts: the cochlear nerve (the nerve of hearing) and the vestibular nerve (the nerve of balance). The cell bodies of the sensory fibers (only) that make up the two parts of this nerve constitute the spiral and vestibular ganglia.

Motion Sickness

The maculae of the membranous labyrinth are primarily static organs, which have small dense particles (*otoliths*) embedded among hair cells. Under the influence of gravity, the otoliths cause bending of the hair cells, which stimulate the vestibular nerve and provide awareness of the position of the head in space; the hairs also respond to quick tilting movements and to linear acceleration and deceleration. *Motion sickness* results from discordance between vestibular and visual stimulation. ◑

Semicircular Ducts. Each semicircular duct has an **ampulla** at one end containing a sensory area, the **ampullary crest** (L. *crista ampullari*) (Fig. 7.80). The crests are sensors for recording movements of the endolymph in the ampulla resulting from rotation of the head in the plane of the duct. The hair cells of the crests, like those of the maculae, stimulate primary sensory neurons, whose cell bodies are in the *vestibular ganglia*.

Cochlear Duct. The cochlear duct is a spiral tube, closed at one end and triangular in cross section. The duct is firmly suspended across the cochlear canal between the *spiral ligament* on the external wall of the cochlear canal (Fig. 7.79) and the **osseous spiral lamina** of the modiolus. Spanning the spiral canal in this manner, the endolymph-filled cochlear duct divides the perilymph-filled spiral canal into two channels that are continuous at the apex of the cochlea at the **helicotrema,** a semilunar communication at the apex of the cochlea.

Waves of hydraulic pressure created in the perilymph of the vestibule by the vibrations of the base of the stapes ascend to the apex of the cochlea by one channel, the **scala vestibuli.** The pressure waves then pass through the helicotrema and then descend back to the basal turn of the cochlea by the other channel, the **scala tympani.** Here, the pressure waves again become vibrations, this time of the *secondary tympanic membrane* (Fig. 7.74*B*), and the energy initially received by the (primary) tympanic membrane is finally dissipated into the air of the tympanic cavity.

The roof of the cochlear duct is formed by the **vestibular membrane.** The floor of the duct is also formed by part of the duct, the **basilar membrane,** plus the outer edge of the osseous spiral lamina. The receptor of auditory stimuli is the **spiral organ** (of Corti), situated on the basilar membrane (Fig. 7.79). It is overlaid by the gelatinous **tectorial membrane.** The spiral organ contains hair cells, the tips of which are embedded in the tectorial membrane. The organ is stimulated to respond by deformation of the cochlear duct induced by the hydraulic pressure waves in the perilymph, which ascend and descend in the surrounding scalae vestibuli and tympani.

Dizziness and Hearing Loss

Injuries of the peripheral auditory system cause three major symptoms (Wazen, 2000): *hearing loss* (usually conductive hearing loss), *vertigo* (dizziness) when the injury involves the semicircular ducts, and *tinnitus* (buzzing or ringing) when the injury is localized in the cochlear duct. Tinnitus and hearing loss may result from lesions anywhere in the peripheral or central auditory pathways. The two types of hearing loss are as follows:

- *Conductive hearing loss:* resulting from anything in the external or middle ear that interferes with movement of the oval or round windows. People with this type of hearing loss often speak with a soft voice because, to them, their own voices sound louder than background sounds.

- *Sensorineural hearing loss:* resulting from defects in the cochlea, cochlear nerve, brainstem, or cortical connections.

Ménière Syndrome

Ménière syndrome is related to blockage of the cochlear aqueduct and is characterized by recurrent attacks of tinnitus, hearing loss, and vertigo. These symptoms are accompanied by a sense of pressure in the ear, distortion of sounds, and sensitivity to noises (Wazen, 2000). A characteristic sign is ballooning of the cochlear duct, utricle, and saccule caused by an increase in endolymphatic volume.

High Tone Deafness

Persistent exposure to excessively loud sounds causes degenerative changes in the spiral organ, resulting in high tone deafness. This type of hearing loss commonly occurs in workers who are exposed to loud noises and do not wear protective earmuffs (e.g., individuals working for long periods around jet engines).

Otic Barotrauma

Injury caused to the ear by an imbalance in pressure between ambient (surrounding) air and the air in the middle ear is called *otic barotrauma*. This type of injury usually occurs in fliers and divers. ◑

Internal Acoustic Meatus

The **internal acoustic meatus** is a narrow canal that runs laterally for approximately 1 cm within the petrous part of the temporal bone (Fig. 7.79*A*). The **internal acoustic opening** of the meatus is in the posteromedial part of this bone, in line with the external acoustic meatus. The internal acoustic meatus is closed laterally by a thin, perforated plate of bone that separates it from the internal ear. Through this plate pass the facial nerve (CN VII), the vestibulocochlear nerve (CN VIII) and its divisions, and blood vessels. The vestibulocochlear nerve divides near the lateral end of the internal acoustic meatus into two parts: a cochlear nerve and a vestibular nerve (Fig. 7.80).

THE BOTTOM LINE: The internal ear consists of a delicate and complex membranous labyrinth filled with intracellular fluid (endolymph), suspended within a bony cave otherwise occupied by extracellular fluid (perilymph). Although much larger and slightly less complex, the architecture of the bony labyrinth is a reflection of that of the membra-nous labyrinth. The posterior portion takes the form of three semicircular canals and ducts; the ampulla of each of the ducts contains an ampullary crest that is sensitive to motion of the head. The central bony vestibule contains a membranous utricle and saccule, each provided with a macula to monitor the position of the head relative to the line of gravitational pull. The neuroepithelial crests and maculae are innervated by the vestibular portion of CN VIII. The anterior portion of the internal ear contains a membranous cochlear duct suspended between two limbs of continuous pathway for the sonar waves that are conducted by the perilymph; the duct and perilymphatic channels spiral through the 2.5 turns of the bony cochlea. Deformation of the spiral organ within the cochlear duct by the sonar waves stimulates impulses conducted by the cochlear part of CN VIII for the sense of hearing.

Medical Imaging of the Head
Radiography

Although replaced by newer imaging modalities in many specific cases, radiography is often used for cranial examinations. The common radiographic projections used are lateral, posteroanterior (PA), anteroposterior (AP), and axial. Because crania vary considerably in shape, one must examine radiographs carefully for abnormalities. Several pathological conditions cause the head to enlarge (*hydrocephaly*) or remain small (*microcephaly*). Lateral radiographs are often made to examine the calvaria (Fig. 7.81), but they can also be useful for examining structures in the cranial base.

The facial skeleton in adults forms approximately half the cranium; in children, the facial area is proportionately smaller. The calvaria in adults varies from 3 to 8 mm in thickness, but the cranium is much thicker around the external occipital protuberance. In Figure 7.81, observe the hypophysial *fossa* for the pituitary gland and the grooves for the branches of the *middle meningeal vessels*. These vessels are often torn when someone is hit in the temporal fossa (e.g., with a stone). Also observe the frontal, ethmoidal, sphenoidal, and maxillary sinuses.

For examination of the orbits, nasal region, and certain paranasal sinuses, AP radiographs are also used (Fig. 7.82). In these views, the lateral masses of the atlas and the dens of the axis are superimposed on the facial skeleton. In Figure 7.82, observe that the right and left frontal sinuses are not the same size; this is normal. Also observe the lesser wing of the sphenoid, the superior orbital fissure, and the inferior and middle conchae on the lateral wall of the nose.

To visualize the arteries of the brain, a radiopaque contrast medium is injected into the carotid artery and radiographs are taken, producing *carotid arteriograms* (Fig. 7.83). This allows the four parts of the internal carotid artery—cervical, petrous, cavernous, and cerebral—to be visualized. This type of radiograph is used for detecting cerebral aneurysms and arteriovenous malformations.

Computed Tomography

CT is a premier imaging method in neurodiagnosis and is more informative than plain cranial radiographs (Fig. 7.84). For reasons of cost, speed, and availability, CT is widely used for evaluation of head injury. It is especially useful for people who are neurologically or medically unstable, uncooperative, or claustrophobic as well as for those with pacemakers or other metallic implants. The diagnosis of an *extradural* (*epidural*) *hematoma* can be made by CT (Fig. 7.85). When the injuries are more severe, the meninges and cerebral cortex are torn. Traumatic hemorrhages often produce hematomas in the cerebral hemispheres, basal ganglia, and brainstem.

Magnetic Resonance Imaging

MRI is slower and more expensive than CT but it shows more detail in the soft tissues than does CT (Fig. 7.86). MRI is the gold standard for detecting and delineating intracranial and spinal lesions (Delpaz and Chan, 2000) because it provides good soft tissue contrast of normal and pathologic structures. It also permits multiplanar capability, which provides three-dimensional information and relationships that are not so readily available with CT (Mohr and Delpaz, 2000). MRI can also demonstrate blood and CSF flow. Magnetic resonance angiography (MRA) is useful for determining the patency of vessels of the cerebral arterial circle. Acute occlusions of major vessels in this circle

Figure 7.81. Lateral radiograph of cranium. The paranasal sinuses are demonstrated: *E,* ethmoidal; *F,* frontal; *M,* maxillary; and *S,* sphenoidal. Also visible are the hypophysial fossa (*H*) for the pituitary gland, the great density of the petrous part of the temporal bone (*T*), and the mastoid cells (*Mc*). The right and left orbital parts of the frontal bone are not superimposed; thus the floor of the anterior cranial fossa appears as two lines (*L*). Observe the bony grooves for the branches of the middle meningeal vessels (*Mn*); the arch of the atlas (*A*), and the nasopharynx (*N*). (Courtesy of Dr. E. Becker, Associate Professor of Medical Imaging, University of Toronto, Toronto, Ontario, Canada.)

and the basilar artery are detectable, but occlusion of small branches is not easily observed (Delpaz and Chan, 2000).

Ultrasonography

Because of the nearly continuous layer of peripherally located bone, ultrasonography is not commonly used for evaluation of the head once ossification of the fontanelles has occurred. Ultrasonography is useful in evaluating subependymal and intraventricular hemorrhage in high-risk premature infants and in following them for possible later development of hydrocephalus. Ultrasonography requires minimal manipulation of critically ill infants.

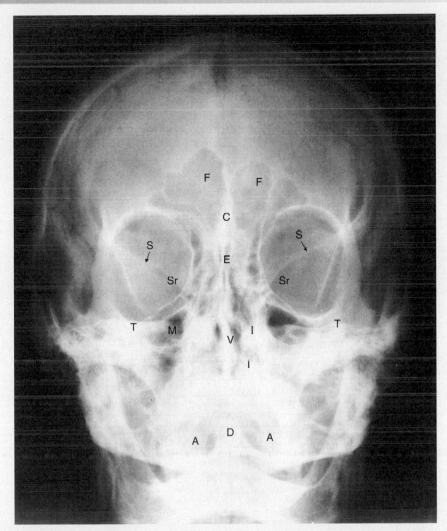

Anteroposterior view

Figure 7.82. Radiograph of cranium. The superior orbital fissure (*Sr*), the lesser wings of the sphenoid (*S*), and the superior surface of the petrous part of the temporal bone (*T*) are visible. The nasal septum is formed by the perpendicular plate of the ethmoid (*E*) and the vomer (*V*). The inferior and middle conchae (*I*) of the lateral wall of the nose, the crista galli (*C*), the frontal sinus (*F*), and the maxillary sinus (*M*) are also seen. Superimposed on the facial skeleton is the dens (*D*) and the lateral masses of the atlas (*A*). (Courtesy of Dr. E. Becker, Associate Professor of Medical Imaging, University of Toronto, Toronto, Ontario, Canada.)

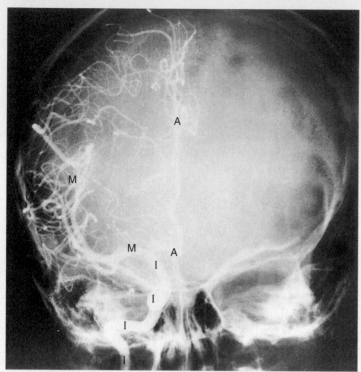

Posteroanterior view

Figure 7.83. Carotid arteriogram. The parts of the internal carotid artery—cervical, petrous, cavernous, and cerebral—are labeled with the letter *I*. The anterior cerebral artery and its branches (*A*), the middle cerebral artery and its branches (*M*) are demonstrated. (Courtesy of Dr. D. Armstrong, Associate Professor of Medical Imaging, University of Toronto, Toronto, Ontario, Canada.)

Calvaria

Grey matter

Lenticular nucleus

Choroid plexus of lateral ventricle

Cerebellum

Internal occipital protuberance

Longitudinal cerebral fissure

Anterior horn of lateral ventricle

Head of caudate nucleus

Thalamus

Quadrigeminal cistern (cistern of great cerebral vein)

Calcification in pineal body

Figure 7.84. Transverse (axial) CT image of brain. Observe the ventricles, various parts of the brain, and the choroid plexus of the lateral ventricle.

Figure 7.85. Extradural (epidural) hematoma. A. In this transverse (axial) CT image of the calvaria and brain, the large white area on the right indicates the site of extradural hemorrhage. **B.** This CT scan shows two adjacent fractures (*arrows*) of the calvaria; the anterior fracture is at the site of the groove for the middle meningeal artery.

Frontal lobe cortex

Frontal lobe
(white matter)

Head of caudate
nucleus

Thalamus

3rd ventricle

Splenium of
corpus callosum

Posterior horn of
lateral ventricle

Figure 7.86. Transverse MRI of brain. Various parts of the brain and ventricular system are shown.

References and Suggested Readings

Anderson MK, Hall SJ, Martin M: *Sports Injury Management,* 2nd ed. Baltimore, Lippincott Williams & Wilkins, 2000.

Behrman RE, Kliegman RM, Jensen HB (eds): *Nelson Textbook of Pediatrics,* 17th ed. Philadelphia, Saunders, 2004.

Bernardini GL: Focal infections. *In* Rowland LP (ed): *Merritt's Textbook of Neurology,* 10th ed. Baltimore, Lippincott Williams & Wilkins, 2000.

Brust JCM: Coma. *In* Rowland LP (ed): *Merritt's Textbook of Neurology,* 10th ed. Baltimore, Lippincott Williams & Wilkins, 2000.

Corbett JJ, Haines DE, Ard MD: The ventricles, choroid plexus, and cerebrospinal fluid. *In* Haines DE (ed): *Fundamental Neuroscience,* 2nd ed. New York, Churchill Livingstone, 2002.

Delpaz R, Chan S: CT and MRI. *In* Rowland LP (ed): *Merritt's Textbook of Neurology,* 10th ed. Baltimore, Lippincott Williams & Wilkins, 2000.

Fishman RA: Brain edema and disorders of intracranial pressure. *In* Rowland LP (ed): *Merritt's Textbook of Neurology,* 10th ed. Baltimore, Lippincott Williams & Wilkins, 2000b.

Fishman RA: Cerebral veins and sinuses. *In* Rowland LP (ed): *Merritt's Textbook of Neurology,* 10th ed. Baltimore, Lippincott Williams & Wilkins, 2000a.

Ger R, Abrahams P, Olson T: *Essentials of Clinical Anatomy,* 3rd ed. New York, Parthenon, 1996.

Haines DE (ed): *Fundamental Neuroscience,* 2nd ed. New York, Churchill Livingstone, 2002.

Haines DE: *Neuroanatomy: An Atlas of Structures, Sections, and Systems,* 6th ed. Baltimore, Lippincott Williams & Wilkins, 2003.

Haines DE, Harkey HL, Al-Mefty O: The "subdural" space: A new look at an outdated concept. *Neurosurgery* 32:111, 1993.

Kiernan JA: *Barr's The Human Nervous System: An Anatomical Viewpoint,* 7th ed. Baltimore, Lippincott Williams & Wilkins, 1998.

Lange DJ, Trojaborg W, Rowland LP: Peripheral and cranial nerve lesions. *In* Rowland LP (ed): *Merritt's Textbook of Neurology,* 10th ed. Baltimore, Lippincott Williams & Wilkins, 2000.

Miller JR, Jubelt B: Bacterial infections. *In* Rowland LP (ed): *Merritt's Textbook of Neurology,* 10th ed. Baltimore, Lippincott Williams & Wilkins, 2000.

Mohr JP, Delpaz R: Neurovascular imaging. *In* Rowland LP (ed): *Merritt's Textbook of Neurology,* 10th ed. Baltimore, Lippincott Williams & Wilkins, 2000.

Moore KL, Persaud TVN: *The Developing Human: Clinically Oriented Embryology,* 7th ed. Philadelphia, Saunders, 2003.

Prockop LD: Disorders of cerebrospinal and brain fluids. *In* Rowland LP (ed): *Merritt's Textbook of Neurology,* 10th ed. Baltimore, Lippincott Williams & Wilkins, 2000.

Raskin NH: Headache. *In* Rowland LP (ed): *Merritt's Textbook of Neurology,* 10th ed. Baltimore, Lippincott Williams & Wilkins, 2000.

Rowland LP (ed): *Merritt's Textbook of Neurology,* 10th ed. Baltimore, Lippincott Williams & Wilkins, 2000.

Sacco RL: Pathogenesis, classification, and epidemiology of cerebrovascular disease. *In* Rowland LP (ed): *Merritt's Textbook of Neurology,* 10th ed. Baltimore, Lippincott Williams & Wilkins, 2000.

Swartz MH: *Textbook of Physical Diagnosis, History and Examination,* 4th ed. Philadelphia, Saunders, 2002.

Wazen JJ: Ménière syndrome. *In* Rowland LP (ed): *Merritt's Textbook of Neurology,* 10th ed. Baltimore, Lippincott Williams & Wilkins, 2000.

Williams PL, Bannister LH, Berry MM, Collins P, Dyson M, Dussek JE, Fergusson MWJ (eds): *Gray's Anatomy,* 38th ed. Edinburgh, UK, Churchill Livingstone, 1995.

8 Neck

Overview

The **neck** (L. *collum, cervix*) is the transitional area between the cranium superiorly and the clavicles inferiorly that joins the head to the trunk and limbs.

It serves as a major conduit for structures passing between them. In addition, several important organs with unique functions are located here: the larynx and the thyroid and parathyroid glands, for example. The neck is relatively slender to allow the flexibility necessary to position the head to maximize the efficiency of its sensory organs (mainly the eyeballs but also the ears, mouth, and nose). Thus many important structures are crowded together in the neck, such as muscles, glands, arteries, veins, nerves, lymphatics, trachea, esophagus, and vertebrae.

The neck is a well-known region of vulnerability. Several vital structures, including the trachea, esophagus, and thyroid gland, lack the bony protection afforded other parts of the systems to which these structures belong. The main arterial blood flow to the head and neck (the *carotid arteries*) and the principal venous drainage (the *jugular veins*) lie anterolaterally in the neck (Fig. 8.1). Carotid/jugular blood vessels are the major structures commonly injured in penetrating wounds of the neck.

The *brachial plexuses of nerves* originate in the neck and pass inferolaterally to enter the axillae and continue into and supply the upper limbs. In the middle of the anterior aspect of the neck is the *thyroid cartilage,* the largest of the cartilages of the larynx, and the trachea. Lymph from structures in the head and neck drain into cervical lymph nodes. Lymph from all of the body except the superior right quadrant enters the venous system through the *thoracic duct* in the root of the neck.

Cervical Pain

Cervical pain (neck pain) has several causes, including inflamed lymph nodes, muscle strain, and protruding intervertebral (IV) discs. Enlarged cervical lymph nodes may indicate a malignant tumor in the head; however, the primary cancer may be in the thorax or abdomen because the neck connects the head to the trunk (e.g., lung cancer may metastasize through the neck to the cranium). Most chronic cervical pain is caused by ▶

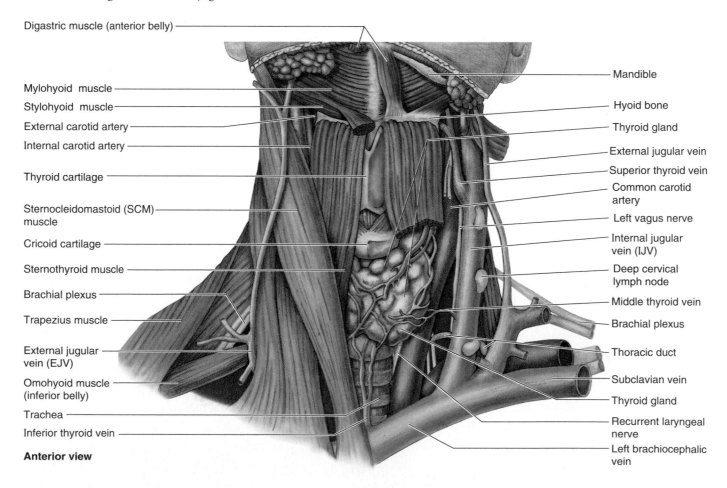

Digastric muscle (anterior belly)

Mylohyoid muscle
Stylohyoid muscle
External carotid artery
Internal carotid artery

Thyroid cartilage

Sternocleidomastoid (SCM) muscle

Cricoid cartilage

Sternothyroid muscle

Brachial plexus

Trapezius muscle

External jugular vein (EJV)

Omohyoid muscle (inferior belly)

Trachea

Inferior thyroid vein

Anterior view

Mandible
Hyoid bone
Thyroid gland
External jugular vein
Superior thyroid vein
Common carotid artery
Left vagus nerve
Internal jugular vein (IJV)
Deep cervical lymph node
Middle thyroid vein
Brachial plexus
Thoracic duct
Subclavian vein
Thyroid gland
Recurrent laryngeal nerve
Left brachiocephalic vein

Figure 8.1. Dissection of anterior neck. The fascia has been removed and the muscles on the left side have been reflected to show the hyoid bone, thyroid gland, and structures related to the carotid sheath: carotid artery, internal jugular vein (IJV), vagus nerve (CN X), and deep cervical lymph nodes.

bony abnormalities (e.g., cervical osteoarthritis) or by trauma (Rowland, 2000B). Cervical pain is usually affected by movement of the head and neck, and it may be exaggerated during coughing or sneezing, for example. ☉

Bones of the Neck

The skeleton of the neck is formed by the cervical vertebrae, hyoid bone, manubrium of the sternum, and clavicles (Figs. 8.2 and 8.3). These bones are parts of the axial skeleton except the clavicles, which are part of the superior appendicular skeleton.

Cervical Vertebrae

Seven **cervical vertebrae** form the cervical region of the vertebral column, which encloses the spinal cord and meninges (Fig. 8.2). The stacked, centrally placed vertebral bodies support the head, and the intervertebral (IV) articulations—especially the craniovertebral joints at its superior end—provide the flexibility necessary to allow positioning of the head. The cervical vertebrae, cervical IV joints, and movement of the cervical region of the vertebral column are described with the back (Chapter 4); therefore, only a brief review follows.

The four **typical cervical vertebrae** (3rd–6th) have the following characteristics:

- The vertebral body is small and longer from side to side than anteroposteriorly; the superior surface is concave, and the inferior surface is convex.

- The vertebral foramen is large and triangular.

- The transverse processes of all cervical vertebrae (typical or atypical) include **transverse foramina** (L. *foramina transversarium*) for the vertebral vessels (e.g., the vertebral vein and, except for C7, the vertebral artery).

- The superior facets of the articular processes are directed superoposteriorly, and the inferior facets are directed inferoposteriorly.

- Their spinous processes are short and bifid.

There are three **atypical cervical vertebrae:**

- The C1 vertebrae or **atlas:** a ring-like, kidney-shaped bone lacking a spinous process or body and consisting of two lateral masses connected by anterior and posterior arches. Its concave superior articular facets receive the occipital condyles.

- The C2 vertebrae or **axis:** a peg-like **dens** (odontoid process) projects superiorly from its body.

- The C7 vertebra or **vertebra prominens:** so-named because of its long spinous process, which is not bifid. Its transverse processes are large, but its transverse foramina are small.

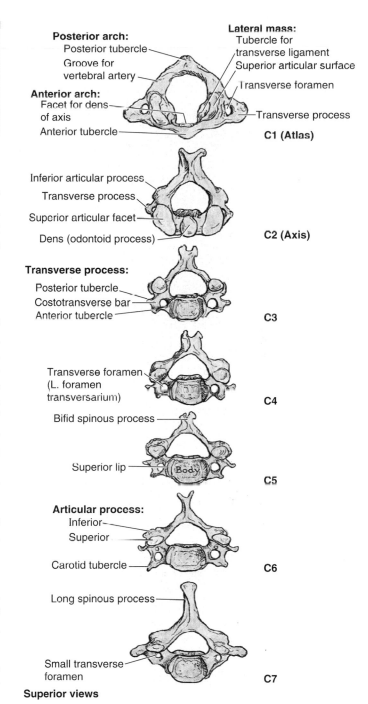

Figure 8.2. Cervical vertebrae. The 3rd–6th vertebrae "typical" cervical vertebrae; the 1st, 2nd, and 7th are "atypical." Typical vertebrae demonstrate rectangular bodies with articular uncinate processes on their lateral aspects, triangular vertebral foramina, bifid spinous processes, and transverse foramina.

Hyoid Bone

The mobile **hyoid bone** (referred to as the **hyoid** in common usage), lies in the anterior part of the neck at the level of the C3 vertebra in the angle between the mandible and the thyroid cartilage (Fig. 8.3). The hyoid is suspended by

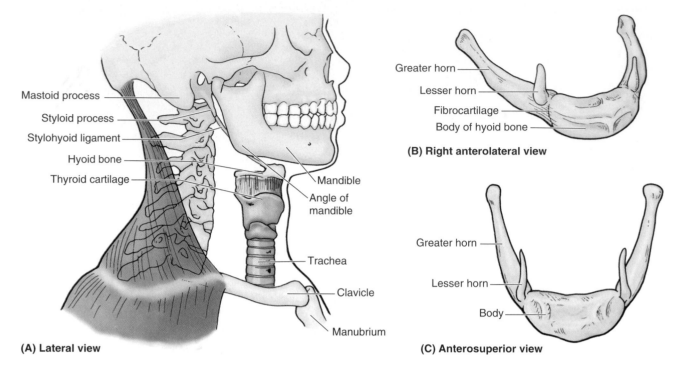

Figure 8.3. Bones and cartilages of neck. A. The bony and cartilaginous landmarks of the neck are the vertebrae, mastoid and styloid processes, angles of the mandible, hyoid bone, thyroid cartilage, clavicle, and manubrium of the sternum. **B and C.** The hyoid bone and its features are demonstrated.

muscles that connect it to the mandible, styloid processes, thyroid cartilage, manubrium, and scapulae. It is unique among bones for its isolation from the remainder of the skeleton. The U-shaped hyoid derives its name from the Greek word *hyoeidēs,* which means "shaped like the letter upsilon," the 20th letter in the Greek alphabet. The hyoid does not articulate with any other bone. It is suspended from the styloid processes of the temporal bones by the *stylohyoid ligaments* and is firmly bound to the thyroid cartilage. The hyoid consists of a body and greater and lesser horns (L. *cornua*). Functionally, the hyoid serves as an attachment for anterior neck muscles and a prop to keep the airway open.

The **body of the hyoid**, its middle part, faces anteriorly and is approximately 2.5 cm wide and 1 cm thick (Fig. 8.3*B* & *C*). Its anterior convex surface projects anterosuperiorly; its posterior concave surface projects posteroinferiorly. Each end of its body is united to a **greater horn** that projects posterosuperiorly and laterally from the body. In young people, the greater horns are united to the body by fibrocartilage. In older people, the horns are usually united by bone. Each **lesser horn** is a small bony projection from the superior part of the body of the hyoid near its union with the greater horn. It is connected to the body of the hyoid by fibrous tissue and sometimes to the greater horn by a synovial joint. The lesser horn projects superoposteriorly toward the styloid process; it may be partly or completely cartilaginous in some adults.

Fracture of the Hyoid

Fracture of the hyoid (or of the styloid processes of the temporal bone; see Chapter 7), occurs in people who are manually strangled by compression of the throat. This results in depression of the body of the bone onto the thyroid cartilage. Inability to elevate the hyoid and move it anteriorly beneath the tongue makes swallowing and maintenance of the separation of the alimentary and respiratory tracts difficult and may result in *aspiration pneumonia.* ⊘

THE BOTTOM LINE: The neck is a movable connecting stalk with a segmented, truly axial skeleton. The stacked, centrally placed vertebral bodies support the head, and the IV articulations—especially the craniovertebral joints at its superior end—provide the flexibility necessary to allow positioning of the head to maximize the use of its sensory organs. Multiple processes of the vertebrae provide both the attachments and the leverage necessary to move the head into and maintain those positions. The foramina of the cervical vertebrae provide protective passage for the spinal cord and the vertebral arteries that nourish the bones and are a major component of the brain's blood supply. However, the vertebrae provide surprisingly little protection for other structures of the neck.

Unique in terms of its isolation from the rest of the skeleton, the U-shaped hyoid is suspended between the U-shaped body of the mandible superiorly and the manubrium inferiorly. It provides a movable base for the tongue and attachment for the middle part of the pharynx. It also maintains the patency of the pharynx, required for swallowing and respiration.

Fascia of the Neck

Structures in the neck are surrounded by a layer of subcutaneous tissue (superficial fascia) and are compartmentalized by layers of deep cervical fascia. The fascial planes determine the direction in which an infection in the neck may spread.

Cervical Subcutaneous Tissue and the Platysma

The **subcutaneous tissue of the neck** (superficial cervical fascia) is a layer of fatty connective tissue that lies between the dermis of the skin and the investing layer of deep cervical fascia (Fig. 8.4A). It is usually thinner than in other regions, especially anteriorly. It contains cutaneous nerves, blood and lymphatic vessels, superficial lymph nodes, and variable amounts of fat. Anterolaterally it contains the platysma (Fig. 8.4B).

Platysma

The **platysma** (G. flat plate) is a broad, thin sheet of muscle in the subcutaneous tissue of the neck (Figs. 8.4B and 8.5; Table 8.1). Like other facial and scalp muscles, the platysma develops from a continuous sheet of musculature derived from mesenchyme in the 2nd pharyngeal arch of the embryo, supplied by branches of the facial nerve, CN VII (Moore and Persaud, 2003). The platysma is supplied by the cervical branch of CN VII. The external jugular vein (EJV), descending from the angle of the mandible to the middle of the clavicle (Fig. 8.1), and the main cutaneous nerves of the neck are deep to the platysma. The platysma covers the anterolateral aspect of the neck. Its fibers arise in the deep fascia covering the superior parts of the deltoid and pectoralis major muscles and sweep superomedially over the clavicle to the inferior border of the mandible. The anterior borders of the two muscles decussate over the chin and blend with the facial muscles. Inferiorly, the fibers diverge, leaving a gap anterior to the larynx and trachea (Fig. 8.5). Much variation exists in terms of the continuity (completeness) of this muscle sheet, which often occurs as isolated slips.

Acting from its superior attachment, the platysma tenses the skin, producing vertical skin ridges and releasing pressure on the superficial veins. Men commonly use this action of the platysma when shaving their necks and when easing tight collars. Acting from its inferior attachment, the platysma helps depress the mandible and draw the corners of the mouth inferiorly, as in a grimace. As a muscle of facial expression, the platysma serves to convey tension or stress.

Paralysis of the Platysma

Paralysis of the platysma, resulting from injury to the cervical branch of the facial nerve, causes the skin to fall away from the neck in slack folds. Consequently, during surgical dissections of the neck, extra care is necessary to preserve the cervical branch of the facial nerve. When suturing wounds of the neck, surgeons carefully suture the skin and edges of the platysma. If this is not done, the skin wound will be distracted (pulled in different directions) by the contracting platysma muscle fibers, and a broad ugly scar may develop. ✛

Deep Cervical Fascia

The **deep cervical fascia** consists of three fascial layers (sheaths): *investing, pretracheal,* and *prevertebral* (Fig. 8.4A & B). These layers support the viscera (e.g., the thyroid gland), muscles, vessels, and deep lymph nodes. The deep cervical fascia also condenses around the common carotid arteries, internal jugular veins (IJVs), and vagus nerves to form the *carotid sheath* (Fig. 8.4B & C). These fascial layers form natural cleavage planes through which tissues may be separated during surgery, and they limit the spread of abscesses (collections of pus) resulting from infections. The deep cervical fascial layers also afford the slipperiness that allows structures in the neck to move and pass over one another without difficulty, such as when swallowing and turning the head and neck.

Investing Layer of Deep Cervical Fascia

The **investing layer of deep cervical fascia,** the most superficial deep fascial layer, surrounds the entire neck deep to the skin and subcutaneous tissue. At the "four corners" of the neck, it splits into superficial and deep layers to enclose (invest) the *trapezius* and *sternocleidomastoid* (SCM) *muscles.* These muscles are derived from the same embryonic sheet of muscle and are innervated by the same nerve (CN XI). They have essentially continuous attachments to the cranial base superiorly and to the scapular spine and acromion and clavicle inferiorly (Fig. 8.4B & C). Superiorly, the investing layer of deep cervical fascia attaches to the:

- Superior nuchal line of the occipital bone.

- Mastoid processes of the temporal bones.

- Zygomatic arches.

- Inferior border of the mandible.

- Hyoid bone.

- Spinous processes of the cervical vertebrae.

Just inferior to its attachment to the mandible, the investing layer of fascia also splits to enclose the submandibular gland; posterior to the mandible, it splits to form the fibrous capsule of the parotid gland. The **stylomandibular ligament** is a

Figure 8.4. Sections of head and neck demonstrating cervical fascia. A. The right half of the head and neck have been sectioned in the median plane. The *detail* illustrates the fascia in the retropharyngeal region. **B.** This transverse section of the neck passes through the isthmus of the thyroid gland at the C7 vertebral level, as indicated in part **A**. The platysma is in the subcutaneous tissue. The outermost layer of deep cervical fascia, the investing layer, splits to enclose the trapezius and sternocleidomastoid (SCM) at the "four corners" of the neck. The investing layer and its embedded muscles surround two main fascial columns. The pretracheal (visceral) layer encloses muscles and viscera in the anterior neck; the prevertebral (musculoskeletal) layer encircles the vertebral column and associated muscles. The carotid sheaths are neurovascular conduits related to both fascial columns. **C.** The fascial compartments of the neck are shown to demonstrate an anterior midline approach to the thyroid gland. Although the larynx, trachea, and thyroid gland are nearly subcutaneous in the midline, two layers of deep cervical fascia (the investing and pretracheal layers) must also be incised to reach them.

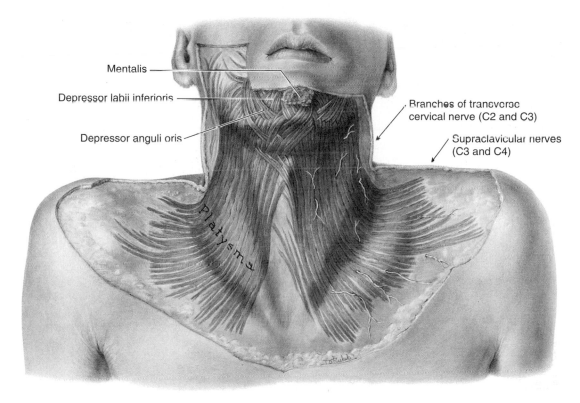

Figure 8.5. Platysma. The thin platysma muscle spreads subcutaneously like a sheet, passes over the clavicles, and is pierced by cutaneous nerves. Much variation is present in the continuity of this muscular sheet.

thickened modification of this layer. Inferiorly, the investing layer of deep cervical fascia attaches to the manubrium, clavicles, and acromions and spines of the scapulae. The investing layer of deep cervical fascia is continuous posteriorly with the periosteum covering the C7 spinous process, and with the **nuchal ligament** (L. *ligamentum nuchae*), a triangular membrane that forms a median fibrous septum between the muscles of the two sides of the neck (Fig. 8.4B). Inferiorly between the sternal heads of the SCMs and just superior to the manubrium, the investing layer of deep cervical fascia remains divided into two layers to enclose the SCM; one layer attaches to the anterior and the other to the posterior surface of the manubrium. A **suprasternal space** lies between these layers (Fig. 8.4A). It encloses the inferior ends of the anterior jugular veins, the jugular venous arch, fat, and a few deep lymph nodes.

Pretracheal Layer of Deep Cervical Fascia

The thin **pretracheal layer of deep cervical fascia** is limited to the anterior part of the neck (Fig. 8.4). It extends inferiorly from the hyoid into the thorax, where it blends with the fibrous pericardium covering the heart. The pretracheal layer of fascia includes a thin *muscular part,* which encloses the infrahyoid muscles, and a *visceral part,* which encloses the thyroid gland, trachea, and esophagus and is continuous posteriorly and superiorly with the *buccopharyngeal fascia* of the pharynx. The pretracheal fascia blends laterally with the *carotid sheaths.* In the region of the hyoid, a thickening of the pretracheal fascia forms a pulley or trochlea through which

the *intermediate tendon of the digastric muscle* passes, suspending the hyoid. By wrapping around its lateral border, the pretracheal layer also tethers the two-bellied *omohyoid muscle,* redirecting the course of the muscle between the bellies.

Prevertebral Layer of Deep Cervical Fascia

The **prevertebral layer of deep cervical fascia** forms a tubular sheath for the vertebral column and the muscles associated with it, such as the *longus colli* and *longus capitis* anteriorly, the *scalenes* laterally, and the *deep cervical muscles* posteriorly (Fig. 8.4). The prevertebral layer of fascia is fixed to the cranial base superiorly. Inferiorly, it blends with the *endothoracic fascia* peripherally and fuses with the *anterior longitudinal ligament* centrally at approximately the T3 vertebra (see Chapter 4) (Fig. 8.4A). The prevertebral fascia extends laterally as the *axillary sheath* (Chapter 6), which surrounds the axillary vessels and brachial plexus. The cervical parts of the sympathetic trunks are embedded in the prevertebral layer of deep cervical fascia.

The Carotid Sheath. The **carotid sheath** is a tubular fascial investment that extends from the cranial base to the root of the neck. This sheath blends anteriorly with the investing and pretracheal layers of fascia and posteriorly with the prevertebral layer of fascia (Fig. 8.4B & C). The carotid sheath contains (1) the common and internal carotid arteries, (2) the internal jugular vein, (3) the vagus nerve (CN X), (4) some deep cervical lymph nodes, (5) the carotid sinus nerve, and (6) sympathetic nerve fibers (carotid periarterial plexuses). The carotid sheath and pretracheal fascia communicate freely with

Table 8.1. Cutaneous and Superficial Muscles of the Neck

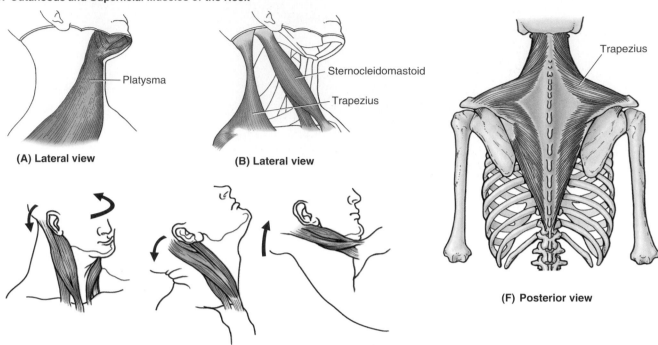

(A) Lateral view

(B) Lateral view

(F) Posterior view

(C) Anterolateral view:
Lateral flexion
with rotation

(D) Lateral view:
Extension at
atlanto-occipital
joints

(E) Lateral view: Flexion
of cervical vertebrae
(person is supine)

Muscle	Superior Attachment	Inferior Attachment	Innervation	Main Action(s)
Platysma	Inferior border of mandible, skin, and subcutaneous tissues of lower face	Fascia covering superior parts of pectoralis major and deltoid muscles	Cervical branch of facial nerve (CN VII)	Draws corners of mouth inferiorly and widens it as in expressions of sadness and fright; draws skin of neck superiorly when teeth are "clenched"
Sternocleidomastoid (SCM)	Lateral surface of mastoid process of temporal bone and lateral half of superior nuchal line	*Sternal head:* anterior surface of manubrium of sternum *Clavicular head:* superior surface of medial third of clavicle	Spinal accessory nerve (CN XI, motor); C2 and C3 nerves (pain and proprioception)	*Unilateral contraction:* tilts head to same side (i.e., laterally flexes neck) and rotates it so face is turned superiorly toward opposite side (fig. *C*) *Bilateral contraction:* (1) extends neck at atlanto-occipital joints (fig. *D*), (2) flexes cervical vertebrae so that chin approaches manubrium (fig. *E*), or (3) extends superior cervical vertebrae while flexing inferior vertebrae so chin is thrust forward with head kept level With cervical vertebrae fixed, may elevate manubrium and medial ends of clavicles, assisting pump-handle action of deep respiration (see Chapter 1)
Trapezius	Medial third of superior nuchal line, external occipital protuberance, nuchal ligament, spinous processes of C7–T12 vertebrae, and lumbar and sacral spinous processes	Lateral third of clavicle, acromion, and spine of scapula	Spinal accessory nerve (CN XI; motor); C2 and C3 nerves (pain and proprioception)	Elevates, retracts, and rotates scapula *Superior fibers:* elevate pectoral girdle, maintain level of shoulders against gravity or resistance *Middle fibers:* retract scapula *Inferior fibers:* depress shoulders *Superior and inferior fibers together:* rotate scapula upward With shoulders fixed, bilateral contraction extends neck; unilateral contraction produces lateral flexion to same side

the mediastinum of the thorax inferiorly and the cranial cavity superiorly. These communications represent potential pathways for the spread of infection and extravasated blood.

The Retropharyngeal Space. The retropharyngeal space is the largest and most important interfascial space in the neck (Fig. 8.4A & B). It is a potential space that consists of loose connective tissue between the visceral part of the prevertebral layer of deep cervical fascia and the buccopharyngeal fascia surrounding the pharynx superficially. Inferiorly, the buccopharyngeal fascia is continuous with the pretracheal layer of deep cervical fascia. The alar fascia forms a further subdivision of the retropharyngeal space. This thin layer is attached along the midline of the buccopharyngeal fascia from the cranium to the level of the C7 vertebra. From this attachment it extends laterally and terminates in the carotid sheath. The retropharyngeal space permits movement of the pharynx, esophagus, larynx, and trachea relative to the vertebral column during swallowing. This space is closed superiorly by the cranial base and on each side by the carotid sheath. It opens inferiorly into the superior mediastinum (see Chapter 1).

Spread of Infections in the Neck

The investing layer of deep cervical fascia helps prevent the spread of abscesses caused by tissue destruction. If an infection occurs between the investing layer of deep cervical fascia and the muscular part of the pretracheal fascia surrounding the infrahyoid muscles, the infection will usually not spread beyond the superior edge of the manubrium. If, however, the infection occurs between the investing fascia and the visceral part of pretracheal fascia, it can spread into the thoracic cavity anterior to the pericardium. Pus from an abscess posterior to the prevertebral layer of deep cervical fascia may extend laterally in the neck and form a swelling posterior to the SCM. The pus may perforate the prevertebral layer of deep cervical fascia and enter the retropharyngeal space, producing a bulge in the pharynx (*retropharyngeal abscess*). This abscess may cause difficulty in swallowing (*dysphagia*) and speaking (*dysarthria*). Infections in the head may also spread inferiorly posterior to the esophagus and enter the posterior mediastinum, or anterior to the trachea and enter the anterior mediastinum. Infections in the retropharyngeal space may also extend inferiorly into the superior mediastinum. Similarly, air from a ruptured trachea, bronchus, or esophagus (*pneumomediastinum*) can pass superiorly in the neck. ✪

THE BOTTOM LINE: The subcutaneous tissue is usually thinner in the neck than in other regions, especially anteriorly. It contains the platysma, a muscle of facial expression. Like deep fascia elsewhere, the function of the deep cervical fascia is: (1) to provide containment of muscles and viscera in

compartments with varying degrees of rigidity, (2) to provide the slipperiness that allows structures to slide over each other, and (3) to serve as a conduit for the passage of neurovascular structures. Two major fascial compartments of the neck are separated by the retropharyngeal space: Anteriorly, the pretracheal fascia surrounds the cervical viscera and the extrinsic musculature associated with it (suprahyoid and infrahyoid muscles). Posteriorly, the prevertebral fascia surrounds the musculoskeletal elements of the neck associated with and including the cervical vertebrae. These two fascial compartments are contained within the third and most superficial layer of deep cervical fascia, the investing layer, which includes the superficial muscles (trapezius and SCM). It attaches to the cranium superiorly and the pectoral girdle inferiorly. Lying anterolateral at the common junctions of these three layers are the major neurovascular conduits, the carotid sheaths. The superior and inferior boundaries and continuities of these fascial layers, compartments, and interfascial spaces establish pathways for the spread of infection, fluid, gas, or tumors.

Superficial Structures of the Neck: The Cervical Regions

To allow clear communications regarding the location of structures, injuries, or pathologies, the neck is divided into regions (Table 8.2). Between the cranium (mandible anteriorly and occipital bone posteriorly) and the clavicles, the neck is divided into four major regions based on the usually visible and/or palpable borders of the large and relatively superficial sternocleidomastoid and trapezius muscles, which are contained within the outermost (investing) layer of deep cervical fascia.

Sternocleidomastoid Region

The **sternocleidomastoid** is a key muscular landmark in the neck because it visibly divides each side of the neck into the *anterior* and *lateral cervical regions* (anterior and lateral triangles of the neck) (Tables 8.1 and 8.2). The region between these triangular regions, corresponding to the area of this broad, strap-like muscle, is the **sternocleidomastoid region of the neck**. The SCM has two heads: the rounded tendon of the **sternal head** attaches to the manubrium, and the thick fleshy **clavicular head** attaches to the superior surface of the medial third of the clavicle. The two heads are separated inferiorly by a space, visible superficially as a small triangular depression, the **lesser supraclavicular fossa**. The heads join superiorly as they pass obliquely upward toward the cranium. The superior attachment of the SCM is the mastoid process of the temporal bone and the superior nuchal line of the occipital bone. The investing layer of deep cervical fascia splits to form a sheath for the SCM (Fig. 8.4B).

The SCMs produce movement at the craniovertebral joints or the cervical intervertebral joints, or at both (Table 8.1). The cranial attachments of the SCMs lie posterior to

Table 8.2. Cervical Regions/Triangles and Contents[a]

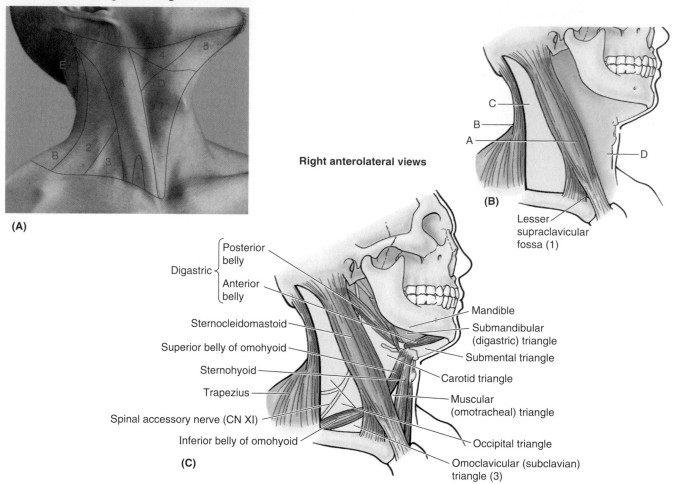

(A)

Right anterolateral views

(B)

Lesser supraclavicular fossa (1)

Digastric { Posterior belly / Anterior belly

Sternocleidomastoid

Superior belly of omohyoid

Sternohyoid

Trapezius

Spinal accessory nerve (CN XI)

Inferior belly of omohyoid

Mandible

Submandibular (digastric) triangle

Submental triangle

Carotid triangle

Muscular (omotracheal) triangle

Occipital triangle

Omoclavicular (subclavian) triangle (3)

(C)

Region[a]	Main Contents and Underlying Structures
Sternocleidomastoid region (A)	Sternocleidomastoid muscle; superior part of the external jugular vein; greater auricular nerve; transverse cervical nerve
Lesser supraclavicular fossa (1)	Inferior part of internal jugular vein
Posterior cervical region (B)	Trapezius muscle; cutaneous branches of posterior rami of cervical spinal nerves; suboccipital region or triangle (E) lies deep to superior part of this region
Lateral cervical region (posterior triangle of neck) (C)	
Occipital triangle (2)	Part of external jugular vein; posterior branches of cervical plexus of nerves; spinal accessory nerve (CN XI)[b]; trunks of brachial plexus; transverse cervical artery; cervical lymph node
Omoclavicular (subclavian) triangle (3)	Subclavian artery (third part); part of subclavian vein (sometimes); suprascapular artery; supraclavicular lymph nodes
Anterior cervical region (anterior triangle of neck) (D)	
Submandibular (digastric) triangle (4)	Submandibular gland almost fills triangle; submandibular lymph nodes; hypoglossal nerve; mylohyoid nerve; parts of facial artery and vein
Submental triangle (5)	Submental lymph nodes and small veins that unite to form anterior jugular vein
Carotid triangle (6)	Carotid sheath containing common carotid artery and its branches; internal jugular vein and its tributaries; vagus nerve; external carotid artery and some of its branches; hypoglossal nerve and superior root of ansa cervicalis; spinal accessory nerve (CN XI)[b]; thyroid gland, larynx, and pharynx; deep cervical lymph nodes; branches of cervical plexus
Muscular (omotracheal triangle) (7)	Sternothyroid and sternohyoid muscles; thyroid and parathyroid glands

[a]Letters and numbers in parentheses refer to figures (A) and (B).
[b]The spinal accessory nerve (CN XI) refers to the traditional "spinal root of CN XI." The traditional "cranial root" is now considered part of the vagus nerve (CN X) (Lachman et al., 2002).

the axis of the atlantooccipital (AO) joints. Starting from the anatomical position, with tonic contraction maintaining the position of the cervical vertebral column, bilateral contraction of the SCMs (especially their more posterior fibers) will cause extension of the head at the AO joints, elevating the chin (Table 8.1*D*). Acting bilaterally, the SCMs can also flex the neck. They can do this in two different ways:

1. If initially the head is flexed anteriorly at the AO joints by the prevertebral muscles (and/or the suprahyoid and infrahyoid muscles) against resistance, the SCMs (especially the anterior fibers) flex the entire cervical vertebral column so that the chin approaches the manubrium (Table 8.1*E*). However, gravity is usually the prime mover for this movement when standing erect.

2. Acting in conjunction with (against resistance provided by) the extensors of the neck (i.e., the deep cervical muscles), bilateral contraction of the SCMs can flex the lower neck while producing limited extension at the AO joint and upper neck, protruding the chin while keeping the head level. Such flexion movements also occur when lifting the head off the ground while lying supine (with gravity providing the resistance in place of the deep cervical muscles).

It is probable that most of the time smaller synergistic muscles and/or eccentric contraction (controlled relaxation of the muscle, gradually yielding to gravity; see the Introduction) are involved in initiating flexion or extension, with the SCMs providing the power and range of movement once initiated.

Acting unilaterally, the SCM laterally flexes the neck (bends the neck sideways) and rotates the head so the ear approaches the shoulder of the ipsilateral (same) side while rotating the head so that the chin is turned toward the contralateral (opposite) side and elevates.

If the head and neck are fixed, bilateral contraction of the SCMs elevates the clavicles and manubrium and thus the anterior ribs. In this way, the SCMs act as accessory muscles of respiration in assisting production of the pump-handle movement of the thoracic wall (see Chapter 1).

To test the SCM, the head is turned to the opposite side against resistance (hand against chin). If it is acting normally, the muscle can be seen and palpated.

Posterior Cervical Region

The region posterior to the anterior borders of (i.e., corresponding to the area of) the trapezius is the **posterior cervical region** (Fig. 8.6; Tables 8.1 and 8.2). The *suboccipital region* is deep to the superior part of this region (see Chapter 4). The **trapezius** is a large, flat triangular muscle that covers the posterolateral aspect of the neck and thorax. It is also a superficial muscle of the back (see Chapter 4), a muscle of the pectoral girdle (see Chapter 6), and a cervical muscle. The trapezius attaches the pectoral girdle to the cranium and the vertebral column and assists in suspending it. Its attachments, nerve supply, and main actions are described in Table 8.1. The skin of the posterior cervical region is innervated in a segmental pattern by the posterior rami of cervical spinal nerves.

To test the trapezius, the shoulder is shrugged against resistance. If the muscle is acting normally, its superior border can be seen and palpated. If the trapezius is paralyzed, the shoulder droops; however, the combined actions of the levator scapulae and superior fibers of the serratus anterior help support the shoulder and may compensate for the paralysis to some degree (see Chapter 6).

Congenital Torticollis

Torticollis (L. *tortus,* twisted + L. *collum,* neck) is a contraction of the cervical muscles that produces twisting of the neck and slanting of the head. The most common type of torticollis (wry neck) results from a *fibrous tissue tumor* (L. *fibromatosis colli*) that develops in the SCM before or shortly after birth. The lesion, like a normal unilateral SCM contraction, causes the head to tilt toward, and the face to turn away from, the affected side (Fig. B8.1*A*). When torticollis occurs prenatally, the position of the infant's head usually necessitates a breech delivery. Occasionally, the SCM is injured when an infant's head is pulled too much during a difficult birth, tearing its fibers (*muscular torticollis*) (Behrman et al., 2000). A *hematoma* occurs that may develop into a fibrotic mass that entraps a branch of the spinal accessory nerve (CN XI) and thus denervates part of the SCM. The stiffness and twisting of the neck results from fibrosis and shortening of the SCM. Surgical release of the SCM from its inferior attachments to the manubrium and clavicle inferior to the level of CN XI may be necessary to enable the person to hold and rotate the head normally.

Spasmodic Torticollis

Cervical dystonia (abnormal tonicity of the cervical muscles), commonly known as *spasmodic torticollis,* usually begins in adulthood. It may involve any bilateral combination of lateral neck muscles, especially the SCM and trapezius. Characteristics of this disorder are sustained turning, tilting, flexing, or extending of the neck (Fig. B8.1*B*). Shifting the head laterally or anteriorly can occur involuntarily (Fahn et al., 2000). The shoulder is usually elevated and displaced anteriorly on the side to which the chin turns. ▶

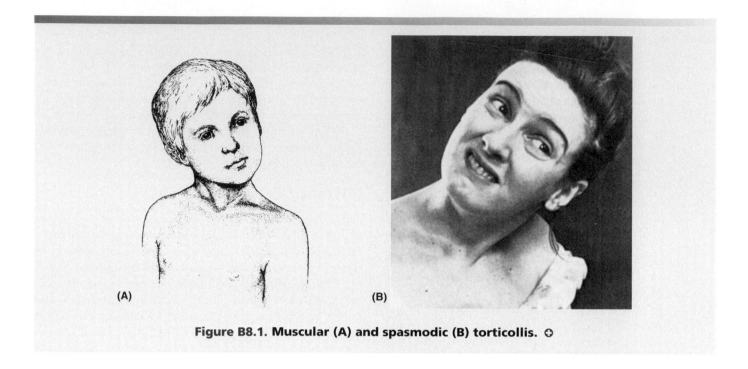

Figure B8.1. Muscular (A) and spasmodic (B) torticollis. ⊕

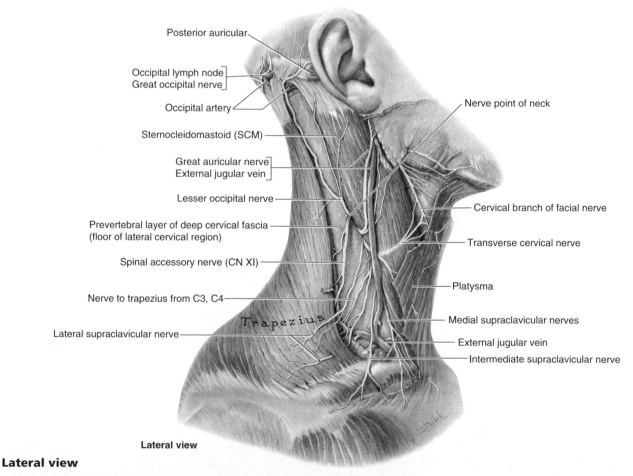

Posterior auricular

Occipital lymph node
Great occipital nerve

Occipital artery

Sternocleidomastoid (SCM)

Great auricular nerve
External jugular vein

Lesser occipital nerve

Prevertebral layer of deep cervical fascia
(floor of lateral cervical region)

Spinal accessory nerve (CN XI)

Nerve to trapezius from C3, C4

Lateral supraclavicular nerve

Nerve point of neck

Cervical branch of facial nerve

Transverse cervical nerve

Platysma

Medial supraclavicular nerves

External jugular vein

Intermediate supraclavicular nerve

Trapezius

Lateral view

Lateral view

Figure 8.6. Superficial dissection of lateral cervical region. The subcutaneous tissue and the investing layer of deep fascia have been removed, sparing most of the platysma and the cutaneous nerves. Between the trapezius (in the posterior cervical region) and the SCM, the prevertebral layer of deep cervical fascia forms the floor of the lateral cervical region. The spinal accessory nerve (CN XI) is the only motor nerve superficial to this fascia.

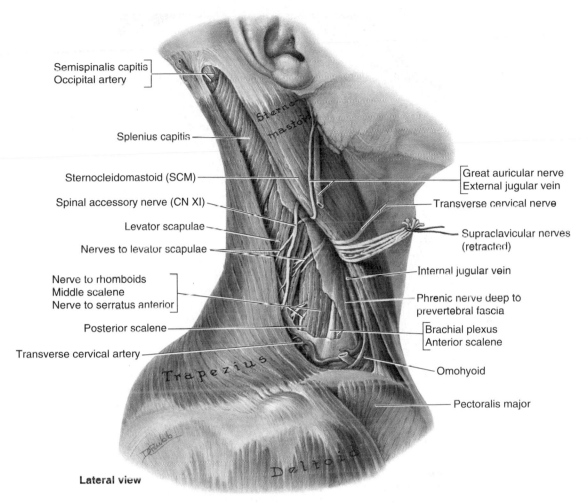

Semispinalis capitis
Occipital artery

Splenius capitis

Sternocleidomastoid (SCM)

Spinal accessory nerve (CN XI)

Levator scapulae

Nerves to levator scapulae

Nerve to rhomboids
Middle scalene
Nerve to serratus anterior

Posterior scalene

Transverse cervical artery

Trapezius

Deltoid

Lateral view

Great auricular nerve
External jugular vein

Transverse cervical nerve

Supraclavicular nerves
(retracted)

Internal jugular vein

Phrenic nerve deep to
prevertebral fascia

Brachial plexus
Anterior scalene

Omohyoid

Pectoralis major

Figure 8.7. Deep dissection of lateral cervical region. The investing layer of the deep cervical fascia has been removed. Although the spinal accessory nerve (CN XI) is superficial to it, the brachial plexus and motor nerves of the cervical plexus run deep to the prevertebral layer of deep cervical fascia that covers the floor of the triangle.

THE BOTTOM LINE: The SCM and trapezius muscles share their origins from a common embryologic source, innervation by the facial nerve (CN VII), enclosure by the investing layer of deep cervical fascia, a linear superior attachment to the cranial base, and an inferior attachment to the pectoral girdle. Their superficial masses and palpable borders provide the basis for describing the regions of the neck. The SCM produces multiple movements of the head and neck, and the trapezius causes multiple movements of the scapula, depending on whether the muscles act unilaterally or bilaterally and independently or in conjunction with concentric or eccentric contraction of other muscles.

Lateral Cervical Region

The **lateral cervical region** (posterior triangle of the neck) is bounded (Fig. 8.6; Table 8.2):

- Anteriorly by the posterior border of the SCM.

- Posteriorly by the anterior border of the trapezius.

- Inferiorly by the middle third of the clavicle between the trapezius and the SCM.

- By an *apex*, where the SCM and trapezius meet on the superior nuchal line of the occipital bone.

- By a *roof*, formed by the investing layer of deep cervical fascia.

- By a *floor*, formed by muscles covered by the prevertebral layer of deep cervical fascia.

The lateral cervical region wraps around the lateral surface of the neck like a spiral. The region is covered by skin and subcutaneous tissue containing the platysma.

Muscles in the Lateral Cervical Region

The floor of the lateral cervical region is usually formed by the prevertebral fascia overlying four muscles (Fig. 8.7): splenius capitis, levator scapulae, middle scalene (L. *scalenus medius*), and posterior scalene (L. *scalenus posterior*). Sometimes the inferior part of the anterior scalene (L. *scalenus anterior*) appears in the inferomedial angle of the lateral cervical region, where it is usually hidden by the SCM. An occasional offshoot of the anterior scalene, the smallest scalene (L. *scalenus minimus*), passes posterior to the subclavian artery to attach to the 1st rib (Agur and Dalley, 2004). For a more precise localization of structures, the lateral cervical region is divided into a large occipital triangle superiorly and a small omoclavicular triangle inferiorly by the *inferior belly of the omohyoid* (Table 8.2).

- The **occipital triangle** is so called because the *occipital artery* appears in its apex (Fig. 8.6). The most important nerve crossing the occipital triangle is the *spinal accessory nerve* (CN XI).

- The **omoclavicular** (subclavian) **triangle** is indicated on the surface of the neck by the *supraclavicular fossa.* The inferior part of the EJV crosses this triangle superficially (Fig. 8.6); the *subclavian artery* lies deep in it (Fig. 8.8). These vessels are separated by the investing layer of deep cervical fascia. Because the third part of the subclavian artery is located in this region, the omoclavicular triangle is often called the subclavian triangle.

Arteries in the Lateral Cervical Region

The **transverse cervical artery** originates from the *thyrocervical trunk,* a branch of the subclavian artery (Figs. 8.7–8.9).

The transverse cervical artery runs superficially and laterally across the phrenic nerve and anterior scalene muscle, 2–3 cm superior to the clavicle. It then crosses (passes through) the *trunks of the brachial plexus,* supplying branches to their *vasa nervorum* (blood vessels of nerves), and passing deep to the trapezius. The *superficial branch* of the transverse cervical artery accompanies the spinal accessory nerve (CN XI) along the anterior (deep) surface of the trapezius. The *deep branch* runs anterior to the rhomboid muscles as the *dorsal scapular artery,* accompanying the nerve of the same name. The dorsal scapular artery may arise independently, directly from the third (or, less often, the second) part of the subclavian artery.

The **suprascapular artery,** another branch of the thyrocervical trunk, passes inferolaterally across the anterior scalene muscle and phrenic nerve. It then crosses the third part of the subclavian artery and the cords of the brachial plexus. It then passes posterior to the clavicle to supply muscles on the posterior aspect of the scapula. Alternately, the suprascapular artery may arise directly from the third part of the subclavian artery.

The *occipital artery,* a branch of the external carotid artery, enters the lateral cervical region at its apex and ascends over the head to supply the posterior half of the scalp.

Trapezius — Sternocleidomastoid
Levator scapulae —
Branches of C5 — Phrenic nerve / Accessory phrenic nerve
Trunks of brachial plexus —
Posterior scalene / Transverse cervical artery — Anterior scalene
Branch of C6 — External jugular vein
Serratus anterior — Internal jugular vein / Jugular, subclavian, and bronchomediastinal lymph trunks / Brachiocephalic vein
Suprascapular nerve, artery, and vein — Subclavian vein
Subclavian artery —
Deltoid —
Axillary artery and vein — External intercostal muscle

Scalenus Medius · *Brachial Plexus* · *3rd* · *Subclavius* · *Pectoralis Minor* · *Pectoralis Major, sternal head*

Anterior view of right side

Figure 8.8. Deeper dissection of inferior part of lateral cervical region. All fascia, the omohyoid muscle, and the clavicular head of the pectoralis major have been removed to reveal the subclavian vein and third part of the subclavian artery. The internal jugular vein, deep to the SCM, is not in the lateral cervical region but is close to it. The brachial plexus of nerves and subclavian vessels pass to the upper limb, the name of the vessels changing to *axillary* inferior to the clavicle at the outer border of the 1st rib.

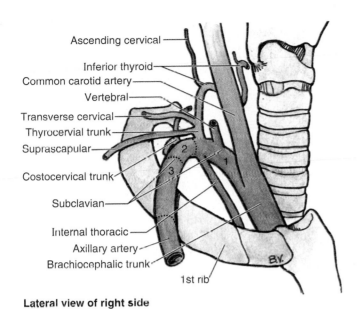

Lateral view of right side

Figure 8.9. Subclavian artery: its parts and branches.
There are three parts of the subclavian artery: medial (*1*), posterior (*2*), and lateral (*3*) to the anterior scalene muscle. The transverse cervical and suprascapular arteries occasionally arise directly (or via a common trunk) from the second or third parts of the subclavian artery instead of from the thyrocervical trunk, as shown here.

The **third part of the subclavian artery** supplies blood to the upper limb. It begins approximately a finger's breadth superior to the clavicle, opposite the lateral border of the anterior scalene muscle. It is hidden in the inferior part of the lateral cervical region, posterosuperior to the subclavian vein.

The third part of the artery is the longest and most superficial part. It lies on the 1st rib and its pulsations can be felt by applying deep pressure in the omoclavicular triangle. The artery is in contact with the 1st rib as it passes posterior to the anterior scalene muscle; consequently, compression of the subclavian artery against this rib can control bleeding in the upper limb. The inferior trunk of the brachial plexus lies directly posterior to the third part of the artery. The branches that occasionally arise from the third part (suprascapular artery, dorsal scapular artery) are aberrant forms of more typical patterns in which they arise elsewhere (from the thyrocervical trunk in particular).

Veins in the Lateral Cervical Region

The **external jugular vein** begins near the angle of the mandible (just inferior to the auricle) by the union of the posterior division of the *retromandibular vein* with the *posterior auricular vein* (Fig. 8.10). The EJV crosses the SCM obliquely, deep to the platysma, and enters the anteroinferior part of the lateral cervical region (Fig. 8.6). It then pierces the investing layer of deep cervical fascia, which forms the roof of this region, at the posterior border of the SCM. The EJV descends to the inferior part of the lateral cervical region and terminates in the subclavian vein (Figs. 8.8 and 8.10). It drains most of the scalp and side of the face.

The **subclavian vein,** the major venous channel draining the upper limb, curves through the inferior part of the lateral cervical region. It passes anterior to the anterior scalene muscle and phrenic nerve and unites at the medial border of the muscle with the IJV to form the **brachiocephalic vein,** posterior to the medial end of the clavicle. Just superior to the clavicle, the EJV receives the *transverse cervical, suprascapular,* and *anterior jugular veins.*

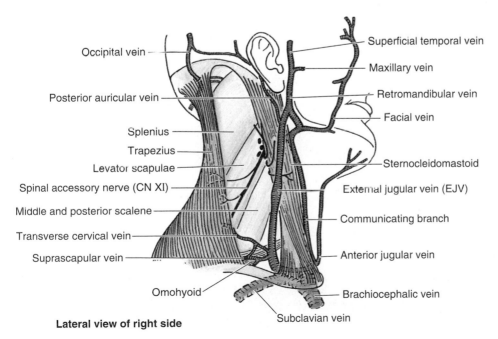

Lateral view of right side

Figure 8.10. Superficial veins of neck. The superficial temporal and maxillary veins merge, forming the retromandibular vein, the posterior division of which unites with the posterior auricular vein to form the EJV. The facial vein receives the anterior division of the retromandibular vein before emptying into the internal jugular vein, deep to the SCM. The anterior jugular veins may lie superficial or deep to the investing layer of the deep cervical fascia.

Subclavian Vein Puncture

The right or left subclavian vein is often the point of entry to the venous system for *central line placement,* such as a Swan-Ganz catheter. Central lines are inserted to administer parenteral (venous nutritional) fluids and medications and to measure central venous pressure. In an infraclavicular subclavian vein approach, the administrator places the thumb of one hand on the middle part of the clavicle and the index finger on the jugular notch in the manubrium (Ger et al., 1996) (Fig. B8.2). The needle punctures the skin inferior to the thumb (middle of the clavicle) and is advanced medially toward the tip of the index finger (jugular notch) until the tip enters the right venous angle, posterior to the sternoclavicular joint. Here the internal jugular and subclavian veins merge to form the brachiocephalic vein. If the needle is not inserted carefully, it may puncture the pleura and lung, resulting in *pneumothorax.* Furthermore, if the needle is inserted too far posteriorly, it may enter the subclavian artery. When the needle has been inserted correctly, a soft, flexible catheter is inserted into the subclavian vein, using the needle as a guide.

Right Cardiac Catheterization

For right cardiac catheterization (to take measurements of pressures in the right chambers of the heart), puncture of the IJV can be used to introduce a catheter through the right brachiocephalic vein into the superior vena cava (SVC) and the right side of the heart. Although the preferred route is through the IJV or the subclavian vein, it

may be necessary in some patients to use the EJV. This vein is not ideal for catheterization because its angle of junction with the subclavian vein makes passage of the catheter difficult (Ger et al., 1996).

Prominence of the External Jugular Vein

The EJV may serve as an "internal barometer." When venous pressure is in the normal range, the EJV is usually visible above the clavicle for only a short distance. However, when venous pressure rises (e.g., as in heart failure), the vein is prominent throughout its course along the side of the neck. Consequently, routine observation of the EJVs during physical examinations may give diagnostic signs of heart failure, SVC obstruction, enlarged supraclavicular lymph nodes, or increased intrathoracic pressure.

Severance of the External Jugular Vein

If the EJV is severed along the posterior border of the SCM where it pierces the roof of the lateral cervical region (e.g., by a knife slash), its lumen is held open by the tough investing layer of deep cervical fascia, and the negative intrathoracic pressure air will suck air into the vein. This action produces a churning noise in the thorax and **cyanosis** (a bluish discoloration of the skin and mucous membranes resulting from an excessive concentration of reduced hemoglobin in the blood). A *venous air* ▶

Sternocleidomastoid muscle (clavicular head)
Anterior scalene muscle
Clavicle
Right axillary vein
Right axillary artery
Right subclavian artery and vein

Sternocleidomastoid muscle (sternal head)
Index finger in jugular notch of manubrium
Superior vena cava

Figure B8.2

embolism produced in this way will fill the right side of the heart with froth, which nearly stops blood flow through it, resulting in *dyspnea*. The application of firm pressure to the severed jugular vein until it can be sutured will stop the bleeding and entry of air into the blood. ⊙

Nerves of the Lateral Cervical Region

The **spinal accessory nerve (CN XI)** passes deep to the SCM, supplying it before entering the lateral cervical region at or inferior to the junction of the superior and middle thirds of the posterior border of the SCM (Figs. 8.6 and 8.7). It passes posteroinferiorly, within or deep to the investing layer of deep cervical fascia, running on the levator scapulae from which it is separated by the prevertebral layer of fascia. CN XI then disappears deep to the anterior border of the trapezius at the junction of its superior two thirds with its inferior one third.

Lesions of the Spinal Accessory Nerve (CN XI)

Lesions of the spinal accessory nerve are uncommon. CN XI may be damaged by:

- Penetrating trauma, such as a stab or bullet wound.
- Surgical procedures in the lateral cervical region.
- Tumors at the cranial base or cancerous cervical lymph nodes.
- Fractures of the jugular foramen where CN XI leaves the cranium.

Although contraction of one SCM turns the head to one side, a unilateral lesion of CN XI usually does not produce an abnormal position of the head. However, people with CN XI damage usually have weakness in turning the head to the opposite side against resistance. Lesions of the CN XI produce weakness and atrophy of the trapezius, impairing neck movements. *Unilateral paralysis of the trapezius* is evident by the patient's inability to elevate and retract the shoulder and by difficulty in elevating the upper limb superior to the horizontal level. The normal prominence in the neck produced by the trapezius is also reduced. *Drooping of the shoulder* is an obvious sign of CN XI injury. During extensive surgical dissections in the lateral cervical region—for example, during removal of cancerous lymph nodes—the surgeon isolates CN XI to preserve it, if possible. An awareness of the superficial location of this nerve during superficial procedures in the lateral cervical region is important because CN XI is the most commonly iatrogenic nerve injury (G. *iatros,* physician or surgeon). ⊙

The **roots of the brachial plexus** (anterior rami of C5–C8 and T1) appear between the anterior and the middle scalene muscles (Fig. 8.8). The five rami unite to form the *three trunks of the brachial plexus,* which descend inferolaterally through the lateral cervical region. The plexus then passes between the 1st rib, clavicle, and superior border of the scapula (the *cervicoaxillary canal*) to enter the axilla, providing innervation for most of the upper limb (see Chapter 6).

The **suprascapular nerve,** which arises from the superior trunk of the *brachial plexus* (not cervical plexus), runs laterally across the lateral cervical region to supply the supraspinatus and infraspinatus muscles on the posterior aspect of the scapula. It also sends articular branches to the glenohumeral joint.

The anterior rami of C1–C4 make up the **roots** (limbs) **of the cervical plexus** (Fig. 8.11). The **cervical plexus** consists of an irregular series of nerve loops and the branches that arise from the loops. Each participating ramus, except the first, divides into ascending and descending branches that unite with the branches of the adjacent spinal nerve to form the loops. The cervical plexus lies anteromedial to the levator scapulae and middle scalene muscles and deep to the SCM. The superficial branches of the plexus that initially pass posteriorly are cutaneous branches. The deep branches passing anteromedially are motor branches, including the roots of the phrenic nerve (to the diaphragm) and the ansa cervicalis.

The superior root of the ansa briefly joins and then descends from the hypoglossal nerve (CN XII) as it traverses the lateral cervical region. The roots of the ansa cervicalis unite, forming a secondary loop, the **ansa cervicalis,** consisting of fibers from the C1–C3 spinal nerves, which branch from the loop to supply the infrahyoid muscles, including the omohyoid, sternothyroid, and sternohyoid (Figs. 8.11, 8.12A, and 8.13). The fourth infrahyoid muscle, the thyrohyoid, receives C1 and C2 fibers, which descend independently from the hypoglossal nerve, distal to the superior root of the ansa cervicalis.

Cutaneous branches of the cervical plexus emerge around the middle of the posterior border of the SCM, often called the **nerve point of the neck,** and supply the skin of the neck, superolateral thoracic wall, and scalp between the auricle and the external occipital protuberance (Figs. 8.11 and 8.12A). Close to their origin, the roots of the cervical plexus receive gray communicating branches (L. *rami communicantes*), most of which descend from the large *superior cervical ganglion* in the superior part of the neck.

Branches of cervical plexus arising from the nerve loop between the anterior rami of C2 and C3 are the (Fig. 8.11):

- **Lesser occipital nerve** (C2): supplies the skin of the neck and scalp posterosuperior to the auricle.
- **Great auricular nerve** (C2 and C3): ascends vertically across the oblique SCM to the inferior pole of the parotid gland, where it divides to supply the skin over—and the sheath surrounding—the gland, the mastoid process, and both surfaces of the auricle and an area of skin extending from the angle of the mandible to the mastoid process.

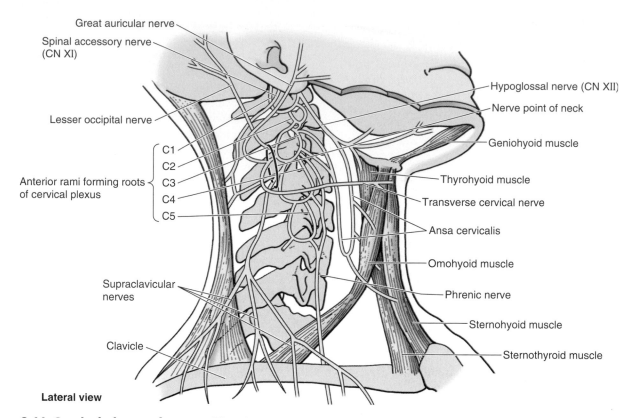

Great auricular nerve
Spinal accessory nerve (CN XI)
Lesser occipital nerve
Anterior rami forming roots of cervical plexus
C1
C2
C3
C4
C5
Supraclavicular nerves
Clavicle
Lateral view

Hypoglossal nerve (CN XII)
Nerve point of neck
Geniohyoid muscle
Thyrohyoid muscle
Transverse cervical nerve
Ansa cervicalis
Omohyoid muscle
Phrenic nerve
Sternohyoid muscle
Sternothyroid muscle

Figure 8.11. Cervical plexus of nerves. The plexus consists of nerve loops formed between the adjacent anterior rami of the first four cervical nerves and the receiving gray communicating branches from the superior cervical sympathetic ganglion (not shown) (Fig. 8.20*B*). The branches of the plexus arise from the loops. The ansa cervicalis is a second-level loop, the superior limb of which arises from the loop between the C1 (atlas) and the C2 (axis) vertebrae but travels initially with the hypoglossal nerve (CN XII), which is not part of the cervical plexus.

- **Transverse cervical nerve** (C2 and C3): supplies the skin covering the anterior cervical region. It curves around the middle of the posterior border of the SCM inferior to the great auricular nerve and passes anteriorly and horizontally across it deep to the EJV and platysma, dividing into superior and inferior branches.

The branches of the cervical plexus arising from the nerve loop formed between the anterior rami of C3–C4 are the:

- **Supraclavicular nerves** (C3 and C4): emerge as a common trunk under cover of the SCM, sending small branches to the skin of the neck that cross the clavicle and supply the skin over the shoulder.

In addition to the ansa cervicalis and phrenic nerves arising from the loops of the plexus, deep **motor branches of the cervical plexus** include branches arising from the roots that supply the rhomboids (dorsal scapular nerve; C4 and C5), serratus anterior (long thoracic nerve; C5–C7), and nearby prevertebral muscles.

The **phrenic nerves** originate chiefly from the C4 nerve but receive contributions from the C3 and C5 nerves (Figs. 8.7, 8.8, and 8.11). The phrenic nerves contain motor, sensory, and sympathetic nerve fibers. These nerves provide the sole motor supply to the diaphragm as well as sensation to its central part. In the thorax, each phrenic nerve supplies the mediastinal pleura and pericardium (see Chapter 1). Receiving variable communicating fibers in the neck from the cervical sympathetic ganglia or their branches, each phrenic nerve forms at the superior part of the lateral border of the anterior scalene muscle at the level of the superior border of the thyroid cartilage. The phrenic nerve descends obliquely with the IJV across the anterior scalene, deep to the prevertebral layer of deep cervical fascia and the transverse cervical and suprascapular arteries.

On the left, the phrenic nerve crosses anterior to the first part of the subclavian artery; *on the right,* it lies on the anterior scalene muscle and crosses anterior to the second part of the subclavian artery. On both sides, the phrenic nerve runs posterior to the subclavian vein and anterior to the internal thoracic artery as it enters the thorax.

The contribution of the C5 nerve to the phrenic nerve may be derived from an **accessory phrenic nerve** (Fig. 8.8). Frequently, it is a branch of the nerve to the subclavius and may contain a large number of phrenic nerve fibers. If present, the accessory phrenic nerve lies lateral to the main nerve and descends posterior and sometimes anterior to the subclavian vein. The accessory phrenic nerve joins the phrenic nerve either in the root of the neck or in the thorax.

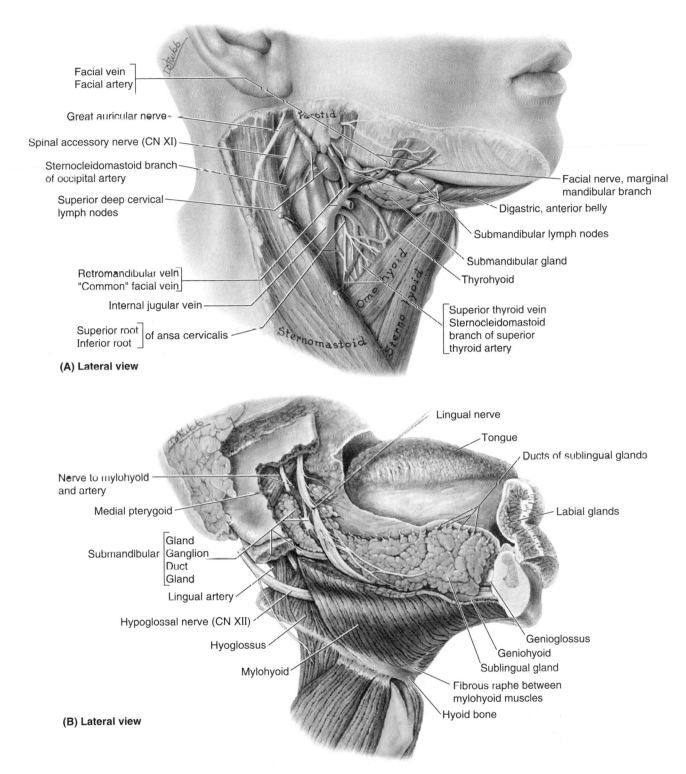

Facial vein
Facial artery

Great auricular nerve

Spinal accessory nerve (CN XI)

Sternocleidomastoid branch of occipital artery

Superior deep cervical lymph nodes

Parotid

Facial nerve, marginal mandibular branch

Digastric, anterior belly

Submandibular lymph nodes

Submandibular gland

Thyrohyoid

Retromandibular vein
"Common" facial vein

Internal jugular vein

Omohyoid

Superior root
Inferior root
of ansa cervicalis

Sternomastoid

Sternothyoid

Superior thyroid vein
Sternocleidomastoid branch of superior thyroid artery

(A) Lateral view

Lingual nerve

Tongue

Ducts of sublingual glands

Nerve to mylohyoid and artery

Medial pterygoid

Submandibular
Gland
Ganglion
Duct
Gland

Lingual artery

Hypoglossal nerve (CN XII)

Hyoglossus

Mylohyoid

Labial glands

Genioglossus
Geniohyoid
Sublingual gland
Fibrous raphe between mylohyoid muscles
Hyoid bone

(B) Lateral view

Figure 8.12. Dissections of anterior cervical and suprahyoid regions. A. This superficial dissection of the neck displays the submandibular gland and lymph nodes. **B.** In this dissection of the suprahyoid region, the right half of the mandible and the superior part of the mylohyoid muscle have been removed. The cut surface of the mylohyoid becomes progressively thinner as it is traced anteriorly.

Fascia investing submandibular gland
External carotid artery
Occipital artery
Hypoglossal nerve (CN XII)
Spinal accessory nerve (CN XI)
Superior root of ansa cervicalis
Sternocleidomastoid artery
Internal carotid artery
External carotid artery
Ansa cervicalis
Common carotid artery
Internal jugular vein
Sternocleidomastoid branch
Sternocleidomastoid (SCM)
Prevertebral layer of cervical fascia
("fascial carpet" of lateral
cervical region)
Transverse cervical vein
Muscular layer of pretracheal fascia
Sternocleidomastoid (SCM)

Common trunk of facial
and lingual arteries
Stylohyoid
Facial artery
Submental artery
Nerve to mylohyoid
Mylohyoid
Hyoid bone
Internal laryngeal nerve
Inferior constrictor
Thyrohyoid
External laryngeal nerve
Superior thyroid artery
Sternohyoid
Sternothyroid
Anterior jugular vein

Omohyoid
Clavicle
Clavicular head
Sternal head

Lateral view

Figure 8.13. Deep dissection of anterior cervical region. The common facial vein and its tributaries have been removed, revealing arteries and nerves, including the ansa cervicalis and its branches to the infrahyoid muscles. The facial and lingual arteries in this person arise by a common trunk that passes deep to the stylohyoid and digastric muscles to enter the submandibular triangle.

Severance of the Phrenic Nerve, Phrenic Nerve Block, and Phrenic Nerve Crush

Severance of a phrenic nerve results in paralysis of the corresponding half of the diaphragm (see clinical correlation [blue] box "Paralysis of the Diaphragm," in Chapter 1). A phrenic nerve block produces a short period of paralysis of the diaphragm on one side (e.g., for a lung operation). The anesthetic is injected around the nerve where it lies on the anterior surface of the middle third of the anterior scalene. A surgical phrenic nerve crush (e.g., compressing the nerve injuriously with forceps) produces a longer period of paralysis (sometimes for weeks after surgical repair of a diaphragmatic hernia). If an accessory phrenic nerve is present, it must also be crushed to produce complete paralysis of the hemidiaphragm.

Nerve Blocks in the Lateral Cervical Region

For regional anesthesia before neck surgery, a *cervical plexus block* inhibits nerve impulse conduction. The anesthetic agent is injected at several points along the posterior border of the SCM, mainly at the junction of its superior and middle thirds, the nerve point of the neck (Fig. 8.11). Because the phrenic nerve supplying half the diaphragm is usually paralyzed by a cervical nerve block, this procedure is not performed on persons with pulmonary or cardiac disease. For anesthesia of the upper limb, the anesthetic agent in a *supraclavicular brachial plexus block* is injected around the supraclavicular part of the brachial plexus. The main injection site is superior to the midpoint of the clavicle. ▶

Injury to the Suprascapular Nerve

The suprascapular nerve is vulnerable to injury in fractures of the middle third of the clavicle. Injury of this nerve results in loss of lateral rotation of the humerus at the glenohumeral joint. Consequently the relaxed limb rotates medially into the *waiter's tip position* (see Fig. B6.12*B*)). The ability to initiate abduction of the limb is also affected. ○

Lymph Nodes in the Lateral Cervical Region

Lymph from superficial tissues in the lateral cervical region enters the **superficial cervical lymph nodes** that lie along the EJV superficial to the SCM. Efferent vessels from these nodes drain into the **deep cervical lymph nodes**, which form a chain along the course of the IJV that is embedded in the fascia of the carotid sheath (Figs. 8.4*B* and 8.12*A*).

THE BOTTOM LINE: The lateral cervical region is bounded by the SCM, trapezius, and middle third of the clavicle, with a muscular floor formed by the lateral deep cervical muscles. It is subdivided by the diagonally placed inferior belly of the omohyoid. Most apparent within the superior occipital triangle is the lower half of the external jugular vein. Most important clinically is the superficially located spinal accessory nerve (CN XI). In the inferior and much smaller omoclavicular triangle, the brachial plexus emerges between the middle and the anterior scalene muscles, the latter of which is crossed anteriorly by the phrenic nerve. Superior to the brachial plexus and in the same plane, but deep to the SCM, is the cervical plexus. The cutaneous branches of this plexus emerge from the midpoint of the posterior border of the SCM and radiate toward the scalp, auricle, anterior neck, and shoulder.

Anterior Cervical Region

The **anterior cervical region** (anterior triangle of the neck) (Table 8.2) has:

- An *anterior boundary:* formed by the median line of the neck.

- A *posterior boundary:* formed by the anterior border of the SCM.

- A *superior boundary:* formed by the inferior border of the mandible.

- An *apex:* located at the jugular notch in the manubrium.

- A *roof:* formed by subcutaneous tissue containing the platysma.

- A *floor:* formed by the pharynx, larynx, and thyroid gland.

For more precise localization of structures, the anterior cervical region is subdivided into four smaller triangles (the unpaired submental triangle and three small paired triangles: submandibular, carotid, and muscular) by the digastric and omohyoid muscles.

The **submental triangle**, inferior to the chin, is an unpaired suprahyoid area bounded inferiorly by the body of the hyoid and laterally by the right and left anterior bellies of the digastric muscles. The floor of the submental triangle is formed by the two mylohyoid muscles, which meet in a median **fibrous raphe** (Fig. 8.12*B*). The apex of the submental triangle is at the **mandibular symphysis**, the site of union of the halves of the mandible during infancy. Its base is formed by the hyoid (Fig. 8.14). This triangle contains several small **submental lymph nodes** and small veins that unite to form the *anterior jugular vein* (Fig. 8.13).

The **submandibular triangle** is a glandular area between the inferior border of the mandible and the anterior and posterior bellies of the digastric muscle (Fig. 8.12*A*). The floor of the submandibular triangle is formed by the mylohyoid and hyoglossus muscles and the middle constrictor muscle of the pharynx. The **submandibular gland** nearly fills this triangle (Fig. 8.12*B*). (Because of its functional association with the mouth as well as its anatomical association with the floor of the mouth, the gland and its duct are discussed in Chapter 7.) **Submandibular lymph nodes** lie on each side of the submandibular gland and along the inferior border of the mandible. The *hypoglossal nerve* (CN XII) provides motor innervation to the intrinsic and extrinsic muscles of the tongue. It passes into the submandibular triangle, as do the *nerve to the mylohyoid muscle* (a branch of CN V₃, which also supplies the anterior belly of the digastric), parts of the *facial artery* and vein, and the *submental artery* (a branch of the facial artery) (Figs. 8.12 and 8.13).

The **carotid triangle** is a vascular area bounded by the superior belly of the omohyoid, the posterior belly of the digastric, and the anterior border of the SCM (Figs. 8.12*A* and 8.13). This triangle is important because the **common carotid artery** ascends into it. Its pulse can be auscultated or palpated by compressing it lightly against the transverse processes of the cervical vertebrae. At the level of the superior border of the thyroid cartilage, the common carotid artery divides into the *internal* and *external carotid arteries* (Figs. 8.13, 8.15, and 8.16). Located within the carotid triangle are the following:

- **Carotid sinus:** a slight dilation of the proximal part of the internal carotid artery, which may involve the common carotid artery (Figs. 8.15 and 8.16). Innervated principally by the glossopharyngeal nerve (CN IX) through the **carotid sinus nerve**, as well as by the vagus nerve (CN X), it is a *baroreceptor* (pressoreceptor) that reacts to changes in arterial blood pressure.

- **Carotid body:** a small, reddish brown ovoid mass of tissue in life that lies on the medial (deep) side of the bifurcation of the common carotid artery in close relation to the carotid sinus (Fig. 8.15). Supplied mainly by the carotid sinus

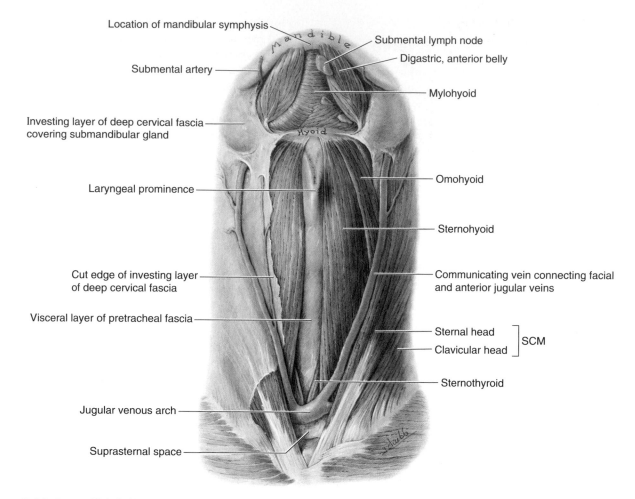

Location of mandibular symphysis

Submental artery

Investing layer of deep cervical fascia
covering submandibular gland

Laryngeal prominence

Cut edge of investing layer
of deep cervical fascia

Visceral layer of pretracheal fascia

Jugular venous arch

Suprasternal space

Submental lymph node

Digastric, anterior belly

Mylohyoid

Omohyoid

Sternohyoid

Communicating vein connecting facial
and anterior jugular veins

Sternal head ⎤
Clavicular head ⎦ SCM

Sternothyroid

Figure 8.14. Superficial dissection of anterior cervical region. The submental triangle is bounded inferiorly by the body of the hyoid and laterally by the right and left anterior bellies of the digastric muscles. The floor of this triangle is formed by the two mylohyoid muscles (the raphe common to the right and left mylohyoids is not distinct here) (Fig. 8.12B).

nerve (CN IX) and by CN X, it is a *chemoreceptor* that monitors the level of oxygen in the blood. It is stimulated by low levels of oxygen and initiates a reflex that increases the rate and depth of respiration, cardiac rate, and blood pressure.

The neurovascular structures of the carotid triangle are surrounded by the *carotid sheath:* the carotid arteries medially, the *IJV* laterally, and the *vagus nerve* posteriorly (Fig 8.4B). Superiorly, the common carotid is replaced by the internal carotid artery. The *ansa cervicalis* usually lies on (or is embedded in) the anterolateral aspect of the sheath. Many *deep cervical lymph nodes* lie along the carotid sheath and the IJV.

The **muscular triangle** is bounded by the superior belly of the omohyoid muscle, the anterior border of the SCM, and the median plane of the neck. This triangle contains the *infrahyoid muscles* and viscera (e.g., the thyroid and parathyroid glands).

Muscles in the Anterior Cervical Region

In the anterolateral part of the neck, the *hyoid* provides attachments for the suprahyoid muscles superior to it and the infrahyoid muscles inferior to it. These **hyoid muscles** steady or move the hyoid and larynx (Figs. 8.13 and 8.14). For

descriptive purposes, they are divided into suprahyoid and infrahyoid muscles, the attachments, innervation, and main actions of which are presented in Table 8.3.

The **suprahyoid muscles** are superior to the hyoid and connect it to the cranium (Figs. 8.12–8.14). The suprahyoid group of muscles includes the mylohyoid, geniohyoid, stylohyoid, and digastric muscles. As a group these muscles constitute the substance of the floor of the mouth, supporting the hyoid in providing a base from which the tongue functions, and elevating the hyoid and larynx in relation to swallowing and tone production.

Each **digastric muscle** has two bellies, joined by an **intermediate tendon,** that descends toward the hyoid. A **fibrous sling** derived from the pretracheal layer of deep cervical fascia allows the tendon to slide anteriorly and posteriorly as it connects this tendon to the body and greater horn of the hyoid. The difference in nerve supply between the anterior and posterior bellies of the digastric muscles results from their different embryological origin from the 1st and 2nd pharyngeal arches, respectively (Moore and Persaud, 2003). CN V supplies derivatives of the 1st arch, and CN VII supplies those of the 2nd arch.

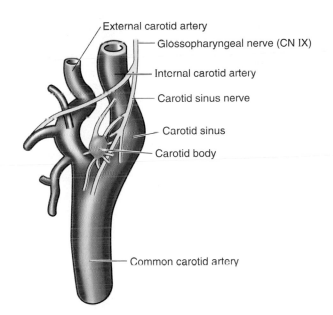

External carotid artery

Glossopharyngeal nerve (CN IX)

Internal carotid artery

Carotid sinus nerve

Carotid sinus

Carotid body

Common carotid artery

Medial view of right carotid artery

Figure 8.15. Carotid body and carotid sinus. This small epithelioid body lies within the bifurcation of the common carotid artery. The carotid sinus and the associated network of sensory fibers of the glossopharyngeal nerve (CN IX) are also shown. Some secondary innervation may be provided to the carotid body and/or sinus.

The **infrahyoid muscles**, often called *strap muscles* because of their ribbon-like appearance, are inferior to the hyoid (Fig. 8.14; Table 8.3). These four muscles anchor the hyoid, sternum, clavicle, and scapula and depress the hyoid and larynx during swallowing and speaking. They also work with the suprahyoid muscles to steady the hyoid, providing a firm base for the tongue. The infrahyoid group of muscles are arranged in two planes: a *superficial plane* made up of the sternohyoid and omohyoid, and a *deep plane* composed of the sternothyroid and thyrohyoid.

Like the digastric, the **omohyoid** has two bellies (superior and inferior) united by an *intermediate tendon*. The fascial sling for the intermediate tendon connects to the clavicle. The **sternothyroid** is wider than the **sternohyoid,** under which it lies. The sternothyroid covers the lateral lobe of the thyroid gland. Its attachment to the *oblique line* of the lamina of the thyroid cartilage immediately superior to the gland limits upward extension of an enlarged thyroid (see clinical correlation [blue] box "Enlargement of the Thyroid Gland," later in this chapter). The **thyrohyoid** appears to be the continuation of the sternothyroid muscle, running superiorly from the oblique line of the thyroid cartilage to the hyoid.

Arteries in the Anterior Cervical Region

The anterior cervical region contains the **carotid system of arteries,** consisting of the common carotid artery and its terminal branches, the internal and external carotid arteries. It also contains the IJV and its tributaries and the anterior

jugular veins (Figs. 8.16 and 8.17). The common carotid artery and one of its terminal branches, the *external carotid artery,* are the main arterial vessels in the carotid triangle. Branches of the external carotid (e.g., the superior thyroid artery) also originate in the carotid triangle. Each *common carotid artery* ascends within the *carotid sheath* with the IJV and vagus nerve to the level of the superior border of the thyroid cartilage. Here, each common carotid artery terminates by dividing into the internal and external carotid arteries (Fig. 8.18). The *internal carotid artery* has no branches in the neck; the external carotid has several.

The **right common carotid artery** begins at the bifurcation of the *brachiocephalic trunk* (Fig. 8.16). The right subclavian artery is the other branch of this trunk. From the arch of the aorta, the **left common carotid artery** ascends into the neck. Consequently, the left common carotid has a course of approximately 2 cm in the superior mediastinum before entering the neck.

The **internal carotid arteries** are direct continuations of the common carotids superior to the origin of the external carotid artery, at the level of the superior border of the thyroid cartilage. The proximal part of each internal carotid artery is the site of the *carotid sinus,* discussed earlier in this chapter (Figs. 8.15 and 8.16). The *carotid body* is located in the cleft between the internal and the external carotid arteries. The internal carotid arteries enter the cranium through the carotid canals in the petrous parts of the temporal bones and become the main arteries of the brain and structures in the orbits (see Chapter 7). No named branches arise from the internal carotid arteries in the neck.

The **external carotid arteries** supply most structures external to the cranium; the orbit and the part of the forehead and scalp supplied by the supraorbital artery are the major exceptions. There is some deep distribution as well (e.g., the middle meningeal artery). Each artery runs posterosuperiorly to the region between the neck of the mandible and the lobule of the auricle, where it is embedded in the parotid gland and terminates by dividing into two branches, the *maxillary artery* and the *superficial temporal artery* (Fig. 8.16). Before these terminal branches, six arteries arise from the external carotid artery:

1. **Ascending pharyngeal artery:** arises as the first or second branch of the external carotid artery and is its only medial branch. It ascends on the pharynx deep (medial) to the internal carotid artery and sends branches to the pharynx, prevertebral muscles, middle ear, and cranial meninges.

2. **Occipital artery:** arises from the posterior aspect of the external carotid artery, superior to the origin of the facial artery. It passes posteriorly, immediately medial and parallel to the attachment of the posterior belly of the digastric muscle, in the **occipital groove** in the temporal bone and ends by dividing into numerous branches in the posterior part of the scalp. During its course, it passes superficial to the internal carotid artery and CN IX–CN XI.

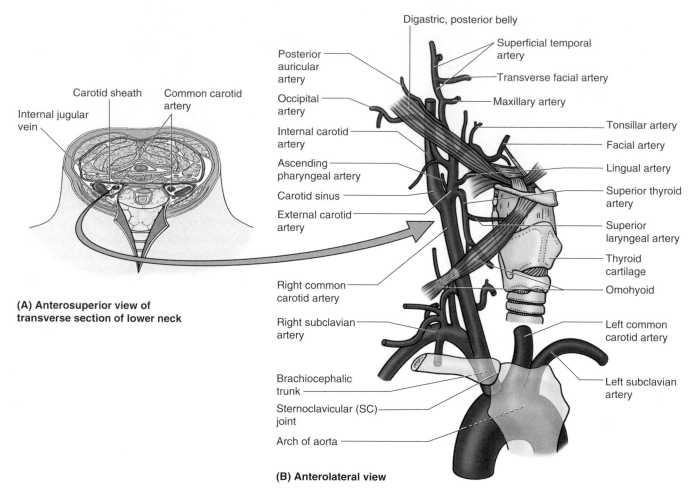

(A) Anterosuperior view of transverse section of lower neck

(B) Anterolateral view

Figure 8.16. Subclavian and carotid arteries and their branches. A. The position of the carotid sheath, the bilateral dense fibrous investment of the common carotid artery, the internal jugular vein, and the vagus nerve (CN X) are demonstrated. **B.** The muscles (posterior belly of the digastric and omohyoid muscles) indicate the superior and inferior boundaries of the carotid triangle.

3. **Posterior auricular artery:** is a small posterior branch of the external carotid artery, which is usually the last preterminal branch. It ascends posteriorly between the external acoustic meatus and the mastoid process to supply the adjacent muscles; parotid gland; facial nerve; and structures in the temporal bone, auricle, and scalp.

4. **Superior thyroid artery:** the most inferior of the three anterior branches of the external carotid artery, runs anteroinferiorly deep to the infrahyoid muscles to reach the thyroid gland. In addition to supplying this gland, it gives off branches to the infrahyoid muscles and the SCM and gives rise to the *superior laryngeal artery,* supplying the larynx.

5. **Lingual artery:** arises from the anterior aspect of the external carotid artery, where it lies on the middle constrictor muscle of the pharynx. It arches superoanteriorly and passes deep to the hypoglossal nerve (CN XII), the stylohyoid muscle, and the posterior belly of the digastric muscle. It disappears deep to the hyoglossus

muscle giving branches to the posterior tongue. It then turns superiorly at the anterior border of this muscle, bifurcating into the deep lingual and sublingual arteries.

6. **Facial artery:** arises anteriorly from the external carotid artery, either in common with the lingual artery or immediately superior to it (Figs. 8.13 and 8.16). After giving rise to the *ascending palatine artery* and a *tonsillar branch* (see Chapter 7), the facial artery passes superiorly under cover of the digastric and stylohyoid muscles and the angle of the mandible. It loops anteriorly and enters a deep groove in and supplies the submandibular gland. It then gives rise to the submental artery to the floor of the mouth and hooks around the middle of the inferior border of the mandible to enter the face.

Memory device for the six branches of the carotid artery: 1-2-3—one branch arises medially (ascending pharyngeal), two branches arise posteriorly (occipital and posterior auricular), and three branches arise anteriorly (superior thyroid, lingual, and facial).

Table 8.3. Muscles of the Anterior Cervical Region (Extrinsic Muscles of the Larynx)

Muscle	Origin	Insertion	Innervation	Main Action(s)
Suprahyoid muscles				
Mylohyoid	Mylohyoid line of mandible	Mylohyoid raphe and body of hyoid	Nerve to mylohyoid, a branch of inferior alveolar nerve (from mandibular nerve, CN V$_3$)	Elevates hyoid, floor of mouth, and tongue during swallowing and speaking
Geniohyoid	Inferior mental spine of mandible	Body of hyoid	C1 via hypoglossal nerve (CN XII)	Pulls hyoid anterosuperiorly; shortens floor of mouth; widens pharynx
Stylohyoid	Styloid process of temporal bone		Stylohyoid branch of (preparotid) facial nerve (CN VII)	Elevates and retracts hyoid, thus elongating floor of mouth
Digastric	*Anterior belly:* digastric fossa of mandible *Posterior belly:* mastoid notch of temporal bone	Intermediate tendon to body and greater horn of hyoid	*Anterior belly:* Nerve to mylohyoid, a branch of inferior alveolar nerve *Posterior belly:* Digastric branch of (preparotid) facial nerve (CN VII)	Working with infrahyoid muscles, depresses mandible against resistance; elevates and steadies hyoid during swallowing and speaking
Infrahyoid muscles				
Sternohyoid	Manubrium of sternum and medial end of clavicle	Body of hyoid	C1–C3 by a branch of ansa cervicalis	Depresses hyoid after elevation during swallowing
Omohyoid	Superior border of scapula near suprascapular notch	Inferior border of hyoid		Depresses, retracts, and steadies hyoid
Sternothyroid	Posterior surface of manubrium of sternum	Oblique line of thyroid cartilage	C2 and C3 by a branch of ansa cervicalis	Depresses hyoid and larynx
Thyrohyoid	Oblique line of thyroid cartilage	Inferior border of body and greater horn of hyoid	C1 via hypoglossal nerve (CN XII)	Depresses hyoid and elevates larynx

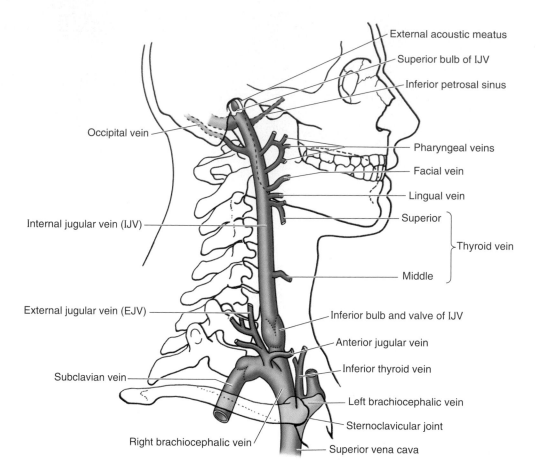

Figure 8.17. Internal jugular vein. The IJV is the main venous structure in the neck. It originates as a continuation of the S-shaped sigmoid (dural venous) sinus. As it descends in the neck, it is contained in the carotid sheath. It terminates at the T1 vertebral level, superior to the sternoclavicular joint, by uniting with the subclavian vein to form the brachiocephalic vein. A large valve near its termination prevents reflux of blood into the vein.

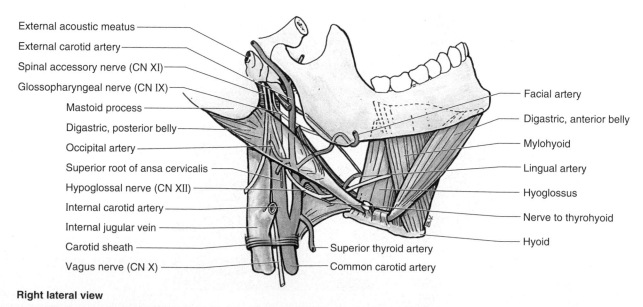

Right lateral view

Figure 8.18. Relationships of nerves and vessels to suprahyoid muscles of anterior cervical region. The posterior belly of the digastric muscle, running from the mastoid process to the hyoid, holds a superficial and key position in the neck. All vessels and nerves cross deep to this belly except for cervical branches of the facial nerve (CN VII), facial branches of the great auricular nerve, and the EJV and its connections, none of which is shown here.

Ligation of the External Carotid Artery

Ligation of an external carotid artery is sometimes necessary to control bleeding from one of its relatively inaccessible branches. This procedure decreases blood flow through the artery and its branches but does not eliminate it. Blood flows in a retrograde (backward) direction into the artery from the external carotid artery on the other side through communications between its branches (e.g., those in the face and scalp) and across the midline. When the external carotid or subclavian arteries are ligated, the descending branch of the occipital artery provides the main collateral circulation, anastomosing with the vertebral and deep cervical arteries.

Occlusion of carotid artery (Doppler color flow study)

Figure B8.3

Surgical Dissection of the Carotid Triangle

The carotid triangle provides an important surgical approach to the carotid system of arteries. It also provides access to the IJV, the vagus and hypoglossal nerves, and the cervical sympathetic trunk. Damage or compression of the vagus and/or recurrent laryngeal nerves during surgical dissection of the carotid triangle may produce an alteration in the voice because these nerves supply laryngeal muscles.

Carotid Occlusion and Endarterectomy

Atherosclerotic thickening of the intima (innermost coat) of the internal carotid artery may obstruct blood flow. Symptoms resulting from this obstruction depend on the degree of obstruction and the amount of collateral blood flow to the brain and structures in the orbit from other arteries. A partial occlusion of the internal carotid may cause a *transient ischemic attack* (TIA), a sudden focal loss of neurological function (e.g., dizziness and disorientation) that disappears within 24 hr. Arterial occlusion may also cause a *minor stroke,* a loss of neurological function such as weakness or sensory loss on one side of the body that exceeds 24 hr but disappears within 3 weeks (Sacco, 2000). Obstruction of blood flow can be observed in a *Doppler color study* (Fig. B8.3). A Doppler is a diagnostic instrument that emits an ultrasonic beam and detects its reflection from moving fluid (blood) in a manner that distinguishes the fluid from the static surrounding tissue, providing information about its pressure, velocity, and turbulence.

Carotid occlusion, causing stenosis (narrowing) in otherwise healthy persons can be relieved by opening the artery at its origin and stripping off the atherosclerotic plaque with the intima. This procedure is called *carotid*

endarterectomy. After the operation, drugs that inhibit clot formation are administered until the endothelium has regrown. Because of the relations of the internal carotid artery, there is risk of cranial nerve injury during the procedure involving one or more of the following nerves: CN IX, CN X (or its branch, the superior laryngeal nerve), CN XI, or CN XII (Fig. 8.18).

Carotid Pulse

The carotid pulse ("neck pulse") is easily felt by palpating the common carotid artery in the side of the neck, where it lies in a groove between the trachea and the infrahyoid muscles. It is usually easily palpated just deep to the anterior border of the SCM at the level of the superior border of the thyroid cartilage. It is routinely checked during *cardiopulmonary resuscitation* (CPR). Absence of a carotid pulse indicates cardiac arrest.

Carotid Sinus Hypersensitivity

In people with *carotid sinus hypersensitivity* (exceptional responsiveness of the carotid sinuses in various types of vascular disease), external pressure on the carotid artery may cause slowing of the heart rate, a fall in blood pressure, and cardiac ischemia resulting in fainting (syncope). In all forms of syncope, symptoms result from a sudden and critical decrease in cerebral perfusion (Pedley and Ziegler, 2000). Consequently, this method of checking the pulse is not recommended for people with cardiac or vascular disease. Alternate sites, such as the radial artery at the wrist, should be used to check pulse rate in people with carotid sinus hypersensitivity. ▶

Role of the Carotid Bodies

The carotid bodies are in an ideal position to monitor the oxygen content of the blood before it reaches the brain. A decrease in PO_2 (partial pressure of oxygen), as occurs at high altitudes or in pulmonary disease, activates the aortic and carotid chemoreceptors, increasing alveolar ventilation. The carotid bodies also respond to increased carbon dioxide (CO_2) tension or free hydrogen ions in the blood. The glossopharyngeal nerve (CN IX, perhaps with involvement of the vagus nerve) conducts the information centrally, resulting in reflexive stimulation of the respiratory centers of the brain that increase the depth and rate of breathing. The pulse rate and blood pressure also increase. With the increased ventilation and circulation, more oxygen is taken in and the concentration of CO_2 is reduced accordingly. ✛

Veins in the Anterior Cervical Region

Most veins in the anterior cervical region are tributaries of the IJV, typically the largest vein in the neck (Figs. 8.13 and 8.17). The IJV drains blood from the brain, anterior face, cervical viscera, and deep muscles of the neck. It commences at the jugular foramen in the posterior cranial fossa as the direct continuation of the sigmoid sinus (see Chapter 7). From a dilation at its origin, the **superior bulb of the IJV,** the vein descends in the *carotid sheath,* accompanying the internal carotid artery superior to the carotid bifurcation and the common carotid artery and vagus nerve inferiorly (Fig. 8.18). The vein lies laterally within the sheath, with the nerve located posteriorly. The *cervical sympathetic trunk* lies posterior to the carotid sheath. Although closely related, the trunk is not within the sheath; instead it is embedded in the prevertebral layer of deep cervical fascia. The IJV leaves the anterior cervical region by passing deep to the SCM. The inferior end of the vein passes deep to the gap between the sternal and the clavicular heads of this muscle.

Posterior to the sternal end of the clavicle, the IJV merges with the subclavian vein to form the *brachiocephalic vein* (Fig. 8.17). The inferior end of the IJV dilates to form the **inferior bulb of the IJV.** This bulb has a bicuspid valve that permits blood to flow toward the heart while preventing backflow into the vein, as might occur if inverted (e.g., standing on one's head or when intrathoracic pressure is increased). The tributaries of the IJV are the inferior petrosal sinus and the facial and lingual (often by a common trunk), pharyngeal, and superior and middle thyroid veins. The **occipital vein** usually drains into the *suboccipital venous plexus,* drained by the deep cervical vein and the vertebral vein, but it may drain into the IJV.

The **inferior petrosal sinus** leaves the cranium through the jugular foramen and enters the superior bulb of the IJV (Fig. 8.17). The *facial vein* empties into the IJV opposite or just inferior to the level of the hyoid. The facial vein may receive the superior thyroid, lingual, or sublingual veins. The *lingual veins* form a single vein from the tongue, which empties into the IJV at the level of origin of the lingual artery. The *pharyngeal veins* arise from the venous plexus on the pharyngeal wall and empty into the IJV at the level of the angle of the mandible. The superior and middle thyroid veins leave the thyroid gland and drain into the IJV.

Internal Jugular Pulse

Although pulsations are most commonly associated with arteries, pulsations of the internal jugular vein can provide information about heart activity corresponding to electrocardiogram (ECG) recordings and right atrial pressure. The IJV pulse is not palpable in the same manner as arterial pulses; however, the vein's pulsations are transmitted through the surrounding tissue and may be observed beneath the SCM superior to the medial end of the clavicle. Because there are no valves in the brachiocephalic vein or the superior vena cava, a wave of contraction passes up these vessels to the inferior bulb of the IJV. The pulsations are especially visible when the person's head is inferior to the lower limbs (the *Trendelenburg position*). The internal jugular pulse increases considerably in conditions such as mitral valve disease (see Chapter 1), which increases pressure in the pulmonary circulation and the right side of the heart. The right IJV runs a straighter, more direct course to the right atrium than does the left; thus it is the one that is examined (Swartz, 2001).

Internal Jugular Vein Puncture

A needle and catheter may be inserted into the IJV for diagnostic or therapeutic purposes. The right internal jugular is preferable because it is usually larger and straighter (Ger et al., 1996). During this procedure, the clinician palpates the common carotid artery and inserts the needle into the IJV just lateral to it at a 30° angle, aiming at the apex of the triangle between the sternal and the clavicular heads of the SCM, the lesser supraclavicular fossa (Fig. B8.4). The needle is then directed inferolaterally toward the ipsilateral nipple. ▶

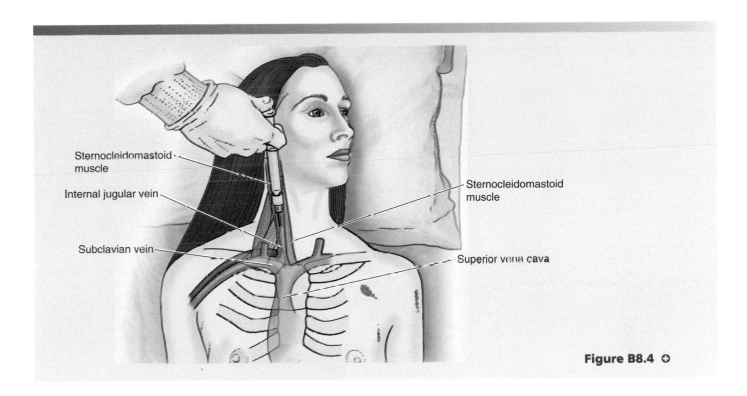

Sternocleidomastoid muscle

Internal jugular vein

Subclavian vein

Sternocleidomastoid muscle

Superior vena cava

Figure B8.4 ⊙

Nerves in the Anterior Cervical Region

Several nerves, including branches of cranial nerves, are located in the anterior cervical region.

- *Transverse cervical nerve* (C2 and C3). supplies the skin covering the anterior cervical region. This nerve was discussed with the cervical plexus earlier in this chapter (Figs. 8.6 and 8.11).

- **Hypoglossal nerve** (CN XII): the motor nerve of the tongue, enters the submandibular triangle deep to the posterior belly of the digastric muscle to supply the intrinsic and four of the five extrinsic muscles of the tongue (Figs. 8.11*B*, 8.13, and 8.18). The nerve passes between the external carotid and the jugular vessels and gives off the superior root of the ansa cervicalis and then a branch to the geniohyoid muscle (Fig. 8.11). In both cases, the branch conveys only fibers from the C1 spinal nerve, which joined its proximal part; no hypoglossal fibers are conveyed in these branches (see Chapter 9 for more details).

- Branches of the **glossopharyngeal** (CN IX) and **vagus** (CN X) **nerves:** in the submandibular and carotid triangles (Figs. 8.16 and 8.18). CN IX is primarily related to the tongue and pharynx. In the neck, CN X gives rise to pharyngeal, laryngeal, and cardiac branches.

THE BOTTOM LINE: The anterior cervical region is inferior to the body of the mandible, extending anteriorly from the SCM to the midline. The bellies of the digastric, the anterior belly of the omohyoid, and the hyoid subdivide the region into smaller triangles. The submental triangle is superficial to the floor of the mouth. The submandibular triangle, superior to the digastric bellies, is occupied by the submandibular salivary gland and submandibular lymph nodes. The facial artery, coursing within this triangle, is palpable as it emerges from it and crosses the body of the mandible. The carotid triangle, between the posterior digastric, inferior omohyoid, and SCM, includes much of the carotid sheath and related structures, including the bifurcation of the common carotid, the carotid sinus and body, and the initial branches of the external carotid artery. The muscular triangle is formed and occupied by the infrahyoid muscles.

Surface Anatomy of the Cervical Regions and Triangles of the Neck

The **skin of the neck** is thin and pliable. The subcutaneous tissue contains the **platysma**, a thin sheet of striated muscle that ascends to the face (Fig. SA8.1*A*). Its fibers can be observed, especially in thin people, by asking them to contract the platysma muscles by pretending to ease a tight collar.

The **SCM** is the key muscular landmark of the neck. It defines the **sternocleidomastoid region** ▶

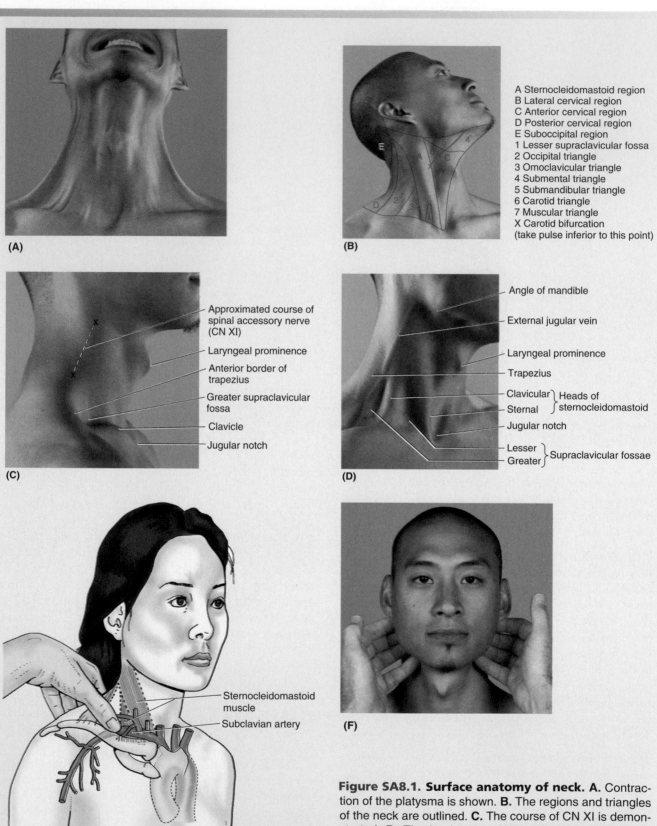

(A)

(B)

A Sternocleidomastoid region
B Lateral cervical region
C Anterior cervical region
D Posterior cervical region
E Suboccipital region
1 Lesser supraclavicular fossa
2 Occipital triangle
3 Omoclavicular triangle
4 Submental triangle
5 Submandibular triangle
6 Carotid triangle
7 Muscular triangle
X Carotid bifurcation
(take pulse inferior to this point)

(C)

Approximated course of spinal accessory nerve (CN XI)

Laryngeal prominence

Anterior border of trapezius

Greater supraclavicular fossa

Clavicle

Jugular notch

(D)

Angle of mandible

External jugular vein

Laryngeal prominence

Trapezius

Clavicular ⎫ Heads of
Sternal ⎭ sternocleidomastoid

Jugular notch

Lesser ⎫ Supraclavicular fossae
Greater ⎭

(E)

Sternocleidomastoid muscle

Subclavian artery

(F)

Figure SA8.1. Surface anatomy of neck. A. Contraction of the platysma is shown. **B.** The regions and triangles of the neck are outlined. **C.** The course of CN XI is demonstrated. **D.** The landmarks of the anterolateral neck are shown. **E.** Checking the subclavian artery pulse is demonstrated. **F.** Palpation of the submandibular lymph nodes is demonstrated. ▶

and divides the neck into anterior and lateral cervical regions (Fig. SA8.1*B;* Table 8.2). This broad bulging muscle is easy to observe and palpate throughout its length as it passes superolaterally from the **sternum** and **clavicle**. Its superior attachment to the **mastoid process** is palpable posterior to the lobule of the auricle. The SCM can be made to stand out by asking the person to rotate the face toward the contralateral side and elevate the chin. In this contracted state, the anterior and posterior borders of the muscle are clearly defined.

The **jugular notch** in the manubrium is the fossa between the sternal heads of the SCMs (Fig. SA8.1*C* & *D*). The **suprasternal space** and **jugular venous arch** are located superior to this notch (Fig. 8.14). The **lesser supraclavicular fossa**, between the sternal and the clavicular heads of the SCM, overlies the inferior end of the IJV (Fig. SA8.1*B* & *D*). It can be entered here by a needle or catheter (see clinical correlation [blue] box "Internal Jugular Vein Puncture," earlier in this chapter). The **EJV** runs vertically across the SCM toward the **angle of the mandible** (Fig. SA8.1*D*). It may be prominent, especially if distended by asking the person to take a deep breath and hold it, expiring against resistance (*Valsalva maneuver*), or by gentle pressure on the inferior part of the vein. These actions impede venous return to the right side of the heart. The EJV is less obvious in children and middle-aged women because their subcutaneous tissues tend to be thicker than those in men. The great auricular nerve parallels the vein, approximately a finger's breadth posterior to the vein. Deep to the superior half of the SCM is the cervical plexus, and deep to the inferior half of the SCM are the IJV, common carotid artery, and vagus nerve in the carotid sheath (Fig. 8.18).

The **trapezius**, which defines the **posterior cervical region**, can be observed and palpated by asking the person to shrug the shoulders against resistance (Fig. SA8.1*B–D*). Superiorly, where it attaches to the **external occipital protuberance**, the muscle overlies the **suboccipital region** (see Chapter 4). The inferior belly of the **omohyoid muscle** can just barely be seen and palpated as it passes superomedially across the inferior part of the **lateral cervical region**. Easiest to observe in thin people, the omohyoid muscle can often be seen contracting when they are speaking.

Just inferior to the inferior belly of the omohyoid is the **greater supraclavicular fossa**, the depression overlying the **omoclavicular triangle** (Fig. SA8.1*C* & *D*). The third part of the subclavian artery passes through this triangle before coursing posterior to the clavicle and across the 1st rib. The supraclavicular fossa is clinically important because **subclavian arterial pulsations** can be palpated here in most people. The course of the **subclavian artery** in the neck is represented by a curved line from the **sternoclavicular**

(SC) **joint** to the midpoint of the clavicle. To feel subclavian pulsations, press inferoposteriorly (down and back) immediately posterior to the junction of the medial and middle thirds of the clavicle (Fig. SA8.1*E*). This is the pressure point for the subclavian artery; firmer pressure, compressing the artery against the 1st rib, can occlude the artery when hemorrhage is occurring distally in the upper limb.

The chief contents of the larger **occipital triangle**, superior to the omohyoid muscle, are: the spinal accessory nerve (CN XI); cutaneous branches of cervical nerves C2, C3, and C4; and cervical lymph nodes. Because of its vulnerability and frequency of iatrogenic injury, it is important to be able to estimate the location of CN XI in the lateral cervical region. Its course can be approximated by a line that intersects the junction of the superior and middle thirds of the posterior border of the SCM and the junction of the middle and lower thirds of the anterior border of the trapezius (Fig. SA8.1*C*).

The cervical viscera and carotid arteries and their branches are approached surgically through the **anterior cervical region**, between the anterior border of the SCM and the midline (Fig. SA8.1*B;* Table 8.2). Of the four smaller triangles into which this region is subdivided, the submandibular and carotid triangles are especially important clinically. The **submandibular gland** nearly fills the **submandibular triangle**. It is palpable as a soft mass inferior to the body of the mandible, especially when the apex of the tongue is forced against the maxillary incisor teeth. The **submandibular lymph nodes** lie superficial to the gland (Fig. 8.12*A*). These nodes receive lymph from the face inferior to the eye and from the mouth. If enlarged, these nodes can be palpated by moving the fingertips from the angle of the mandible along its inferior border (Fig. SA8.1*D* & *F*). If continued until the fingers meet under the chin, enlarged **submental lymph nodes** could be palpated in the **submental triangle** (Fig. SA8.1*B*).

The carotid arterial system is located in the **carotid triangle**. This area is important for surgical approaches to the carotid sheath containing the common carotid artery, IJV, and vagus nerve (Fig. 8.18). The carotid triangle also contains the hypoglossal nerve (CN XII) and cervical sympathetic trunk. The **carotid sheath** can be marked out by a line joining the SC joint to a point midway between the mastoid process and the angle of the mandible. The **carotid pulse** can be palpated by placing the index and 3rd fingers on the thyroid cartilage and pointing them posterolaterally between the trachea and SCM. The pulse is palpable just medial to the SCM. The palpation is performed low in the neck to avoid pressure on the carotid sinus, which could cause a reflex drop in blood pressure and heart rate (Fig. SA8.1*B*). ☉

Deep Structures of the Neck

The **deep structures of the neck** are the prevertebral muscles, located posterior to the cervical viscera and anterolateral to the cervical vertebral column, and structures located on the cervical side of the superior thoracic aperture, the *root of the neck.*

Prevertebral Muscles

The anterior and lateral vertebral or **prevertebral muscles** are deep to prevertebral layer of deep cervical fascia. The **anterior vertebral muscles,** consisting of the longus colli and capitis, rectus capitis anterior, and anterior scalene muscles, lie directly posterior to the *retropharyngeal space* (Fig. 8.4) and medial to the neurovascular plane of the cervical and brachial plexuses and subclavian artery. The **lateral vertebral muscles,** consisting of the rectus capitis lateralis, splenius capitis, levator scapulae, and middle and posterior scalene muscles, lie posterior to this neurovascular plane and (except for the highly placed rectus capitis lateralis) form the floor of the lateral cervical region. These muscles are illustrated in Figure 8.19; their attachments, innervation, and main actions are presented in Table 8.4.

THE BOTTOM LINE: The prevertebral muscles, deep to the prevertebral layer of the deep cervical fascia, are divided into anterior and lateral vertebral muscles by the neurovascular plane of the cervical and brachial plexuses and subclavian artery. The anterior vertebral muscles flex the head and neck; however, this movement is normally produced by gravity in conjunction with eccentric contraction of the extensors of the neck. Thus the anterior vertebral muscles are called into action mainly when this movement is performed against resistance, probably initiating the movement while the strength of the movement is produced by the SCM. The lateral vertebral muscles laterally flex the neck, participate in rotation of the neck, and fix or elevate the superiormost ribs during forced inspiration.

Root of the Neck

The **root of the neck** is the junctional area between the thorax and the neck (Fig. 8.19). It is the cervical side of the superior thoracic aperture, through which pass all structures going from the thorax to the head or upper limb and vice versa (see Chapter 1). The inferior boundary of the root of the neck is the *superior thoracic aperture,* formed laterally by the 1st pair of ribs and their costal cartilages, anteriorly by the

Longus capitis
Middle scalene
Anterior scalene
Ascending cervical artery
Inferior thyroid artery
Longus colli
Vertebral artery
Suprascapular artery
Transverse cervical artery
Phrenic nerve
Right and left vagus nerves (CN X)
Right subclavian artery
Right common carotid artery
Right subclavian vein
Right recurrent laryngeal nerve
1st rib
Cervical pleura overlying lung
Right brachiocephalic vein

Esophagus
Carotid tubercle (C6)
Trachea
Left recurrent laryngeal nerve
Phrenic nerve
C5
C6
C7   Anterior rami
C8   forming roots of brachial plexus
T1
Left subclavian artery
Vertebral artery entering transverse foramen of C6
Thyrocervical trunk
Cervical pleura (cupula)
Left subclavian vein
Thoracic duct
Internal thoracic artery
Costal parietal pleura
Left common carotid artery
Left brachiocephalic vein

(A) Anterior view

Figure 8.19. Root of neck and prevertebral region. A. A dissection of the root of the neck is shown. The brachial plexus and the third part of the subclavian artery emerge between the anterior and the middle scalene muscles. The brachiocephalic veins, the first parts of the subclavian arteries, and the internal thoracic arteries arising from the subclavian arteries are closely related to the cervical pleura (cupula). The thoracic duct terminates in the root of the neck as it enters the left venous angle.

Cranial nerves
XII XI X and IX

Anterior tubercle of atlas
Jugular process
Rectus capitis lateralis
Nerve C1
Occipital artery
Digastric, posterior belly
Superior cervical sympathetic ganglion
Nerve C2
Gray rami communicantes to cervical spinal nerves
Nerve C3
Sympathetic trunk
Nerve C4
Longus colli
Phrenic nerve
Nerve C5
Cervicothoracic (stellate) sympathetic ganglion
Aberrant sympathetic ganglion
Ansa subclavia
Right recurrent laryngeal nerve
Subclavian artery
Brachiocephalic trunk
Manubrium

(B) Anterior view

Internal jugular vein
Facial nerve
**Rectus capitis anterior
Rectus capitis lateralis**
Mastoid process
Transverse process of atlas
Levator scapulae
Transverse process, C3 vertebra
Longus capitis
Middle scalene
Carotid tubercle of transverse process of C6 vertebra
Vertebral artery
Inferior thyroid artery
Ascending cervical artery
Transverse cervical artery
Costocervical trunk
Suprascapular artery
Thyrocervical trunk
Left recurrent laryngeal nerve
Internal thoracic artery
Subclavian artery
Common carotid artery

Figure 8.19. *(Continued)* **B.** In this dissection of the prevertebral region and root of the neck, the prevertebral layer of deep fascia has been removed, sparing the embedded sympathetic trunk; the longus capitis muscle has been excised on the left side. The cervical plexus of nerves, arising from the anterior rami of C1–C4, and the brachial plexus of nerves, arising from the anterior rami of C5–C8 and T1, are demonstrated on the right side.

manubrium of the sternum, and posteriorly by the body of T1 vertebra. The visceral structures in the root of the neck are described in "Viscera of the Neck," later in this chapter. Only the neurovascular elements of the root of the neck are described here.

Arteries in the Root of the Neck

The **brachiocephalic trunk** is covered anteriorly by the right sternohyoid and sternothyroid muscles; it is the largest branch of the arch of the aorta (Fig. 8.16). From 4 to 5 cm long, it arises in the midline from the beginning of the arch of the aorta, posterior to the manubrium. It passes superolaterally to the right where it divides into the right common carotid and right subclavian arteries posterior to the SC joint. The brachiocephalic trunk usually has no branches.

The **subclavian arteries** supply the upper limbs; they also send branches to the neck and brain (Fig. 8.19). The **right subclavian artery** arises from the brachiocephalic trunk. The **left subclavian artery** arises from the arch of the aorta, approximately 1 cm distal to the left common carotid artery. The left vagus nerve runs parallel to this part of the artery (Fig. 8.19A). Although the subclavian arteries of the two sides have different origins, their courses in the neck begin posterior to the respective SC joints as they ascend through the superior thoracic aperture and enter the root of the neck. The arteries arch superolaterally, reaching an apex as they pass posterior to the anterior scalene muscles. As they begin to descend, they disappear posterior to the middle of the clavicles. As the arteries cross the outer margin of the first ribs, their name changes; they become the axillary arteries.

Table 8.4. Prevertebral Muscles

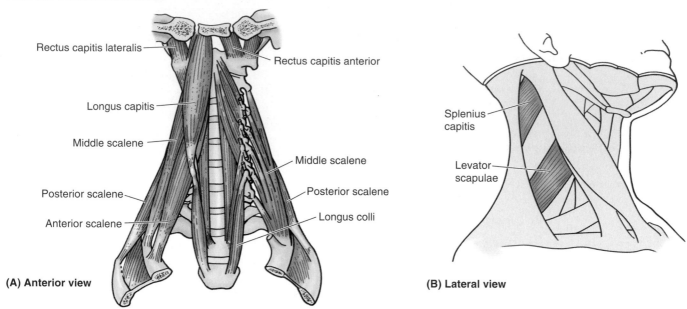

Rectus capitis lateralis

Rectus capitis anterior

Longus capitis

Middle scalene

Posterior scalene

Anterior scalene

Splenius capitis

Levator scapulae

Middle scalene

Posterior scalene

Longus colli

(A) Anterior view   **(B) Lateral view**

Muscle	Superior Attachment	Inferior Attachment	Innervation	Main Action(s)
Anterior vertebral muscles				
Longus colli	Anterior tubercle of C1 vertebra (atlas); bodies of C1–C3 and transverse processes of C3–C6 vertebrae	Bodies of C5–T3 vertebrae; transverse processes of C3–C5 vertebrae	Anterior rami of C2–C6 spinal nerves	Flexes neck with rotation (torsion) to opposite side if acting unilaterally[a]
Longus capitis	Basilar part of occipital bone	Anterior tubercles of C3–C6 transverse processes	Anterior rami of C1–C3 spinal nerves	Flex head[b]
Rectus capitis anterior	Base of skull, just anterior to occipital condyle	Anterior surface of lateral mass of atlas (C1 vertebra)	Branches from loop between C1 and C2 spinal nerves	
Anterior scalene	Transverse processes of C4–C6 vertebrae	1st rib	Cervical spinal nerves C4–C6	
Lateral vertebral muscles				
Rectus capitis lateralis	Jugular process of occipital bone	Transverse process of atlas (C1 vertebra)	Branches from loop between C1 and C2 spinal nerves	Flexes head and helps stabilize it[b]
Splenius capitis	Inferior half of nuchal ligament and spinous processes of superior six thoracic vertebrae	Lateral aspect of mastoid process and lateral third of superior nuchal line	Posterior rami of middle cervical spinal nerves	Laterally flexes and rotates head and neck to same side; acting bilaterally, extend head and neck[c]
Levator scapulae	Posterior tubercles of transverse processes C1–C4 vertebrae	Superior part of medial border of scapula	Dorsal scapular nerve C5 and cervical spinal nerves C3 and C4	Elevates scapula and tilts its glenoid cavity inferiorly by rotating scapula
Middle scalene	Posterior tubercles of transverse processes of C4–C6 vertebrae	Superior surface of 1st rib; posterior groove for subclavian artery	Anterior rami of cervical spinal nerves	Flexes neck laterally; elevates 1st rib during forced inspiration[a]
Posterior scalene		External border of 2nd rib	Anterior rami of cervical spinal nerves C7 and C8	Flexes neck laterally; elevates 2nd rib during forced inspiration[a]

[a]Flexion of neck = anterior (or lateral) bending of cervical vertebrae C2–C7.
[b]Flexion of head = anterior (or lateral) bending of the head relative to the vertebral column at the atlanto-occipital joints.
[c]Rotation of the head occurs at the atlantoaxial joints.

Three parts of each subclavian artery are described relative to the anterior scalene: the first part is medial to the muscle, the second part is posterior to it, and the third part is lateral to it (Figs. 8.9 and 8.19*B*). The cervical pleurae, apices of the lung, and sympathetic trunks lie posterior to the first part of the arteries. The third part of the subclavian artery was discussed previously in this chapter. The branches of the subclavian arteries are the:

- *Vertebral artery, internal thoracic artery,* and *thyrocervical trunk* from the first part of the subclavian artery.

- *Costocervical trunk* from the second part of the subclavian artery.

- *Dorsal scapular artery,* often arising from the third part of the subclavian artery.

The **cervical part of the vertebral artery** arises from the first part of the subclavian artery and ascends in the pyramidal space formed between the scalene and the longus muscles (Fig. 8.19). At the apex of this space, the artery passes deeply to course through the foramina of the transverse processes of vertebrae C1–C6. This is the **vertebral part of the vertebral artery.** Occasionally, the vertebral artery may enter a foramen more superior than vertebra C6. In approximately 5% of people, the left vertebral artery arises from the arch of the aorta. The **suboccipital part of the vertebral artery** courses in a groove on the posterior arch of the atlas before it enters the cranial cavity through the foramen magnum. The **cranial part of the vertebral artery** supplies branches to the medulla and spinal cord, parts of the cerebellum, and the dura of the posterior cranial fossa. At the inferior border of the pons of the brainstem, the vertebral arteries join to form the *basilar artery,* which participates in the formation of the cerebral arterial circle (see Chapter 7).

The **internal thoracic artery** arises from the anteroinferior aspect of the subclavian artery and passes inferomedially into the thorax. The cervical part of the internal thoracic artery has no branches; its thoracic distribution is described in Chapter 1.

The **thyrocervical trunk** arises from the anterosuperior aspect of the first part of the subclavian artery, near the medial border of the anterior scalene muscle. It has three branches, the largest and most important of which is the **inferior thyroid artery,** the primary visceral artery of the neck. Often arising from the thyrocervical trunk are the *suprascapular artery,* supplying muscles on the posterior scapula, and the *transverse cervical artery,* sending branches to muscles in the lateral cervical region, the trapezius and medial scapular muscles. These latter two arteries may arise via a common trunk from the thyrocervical trunk or may arise directly from the subclavian artery. The terminal branches of the thyrocervical trunk are the inferior thyroid and ascending cervical arteries. The latter artery supplies the lateral muscles of the upper neck.

The **costocervical trunk** arises from the posterior aspect of the second part of the subclavian artery (posterior to the anterior scalene on the right side and usually just medial to this muscle on the left side). The trunk passes posterosuperiorly and divides into the superior intercostal and deep cervical arteries, which supply the first two intercostal spaces and the posterior deep cervical muscles, respectively.

The **dorsal scapular artery** often arises as the deep descending branch of the transverse cervical artery, but it may be an independent branch of the second or third part of the subclavian artery (Fig. 8.19*A*). When it is a branch of the subclavian, the dorsal scapular artery passes laterally through the trunks of the brachial plexus, anterior to the middle scalene. It then runs deep to the levator scapulae and rhomboid muscles, supplying both and participating in the arterial anastomoses around the scapula (Chapter 6).

Veins in the Root of the Neck

Two large veins terminating in the root of the neck are the *EJV,* draining blood received mostly from the scalp and face, and the variable **anterior jugular vein** (AJV), usually the smallest of the jugular veins (Figs. 8.13 and 8.17). The AJV typically arises near the hyoid from the confluence of superficial submandibular veins. The AJV descends either in the subcutaneous tissue or deep to the investing layer of deep cervical fascia between the anterior median line and the anterior border of the SCM. At the root of the neck, the AJV turns laterally, posterior to the SCM, and opens into the termination of the EJV or into the subclavian vein. Superior to the manubrium, the right and left AJVs commonly unite across the midline to form the **jugular venous arch** in the suprasternal space (Fig. 8.14).

The *subclavian vein,* the continuation of the axillary vein, begins at the lateral border of the 1st rib and ends when it unites with the IJV (Fig. 8.19*A*). The subclavian vein passes over the 1st rib anterior to the scalene tubercle parallel to the subclavian artery, but it is separated from it by the anterior scalene muscle. It usually has only one named tributary, the *EJV* (Fig. 8.17). The IJV ends posterior to the medial end of the clavicle by uniting with the subclavian vein to form the brachiocephalic vein (Fig. 8.17). This union is commonly referred to as the **venous angle** and is the site where the *thoracic duct* (left side) and the *right lymphatic trunk* (right side) drain lymph collected throughout the body into the venous circulation (see Introduction). Throughout its course, the IJV is enclosed by the *carotid sheath* (Fig. 8.18).

Nerves in the Root of the Neck

There are three pairs of major nerves in the root of the neck: (1) the vagus nerves, (2) the phrenic nerves, and (3) the sympathetic trunks.

Vagus Nerves (CN X). Following its exit from the jugular foramen, each vagus nerve passes inferiorly in the neck within the posterior part of the carotid sheath in the angle between the IJV and the common carotid artery (Figs. 8.18–8.20). The **right vagus nerve** passes anterior to the first part of the subclavian artery and posterior to the brachiocephalic vein and SC joint to enter the thorax. The **left vagus nerve** descends between the left common carotid and the left subclavian arteries and posterior to the SC joint to enter the thorax.

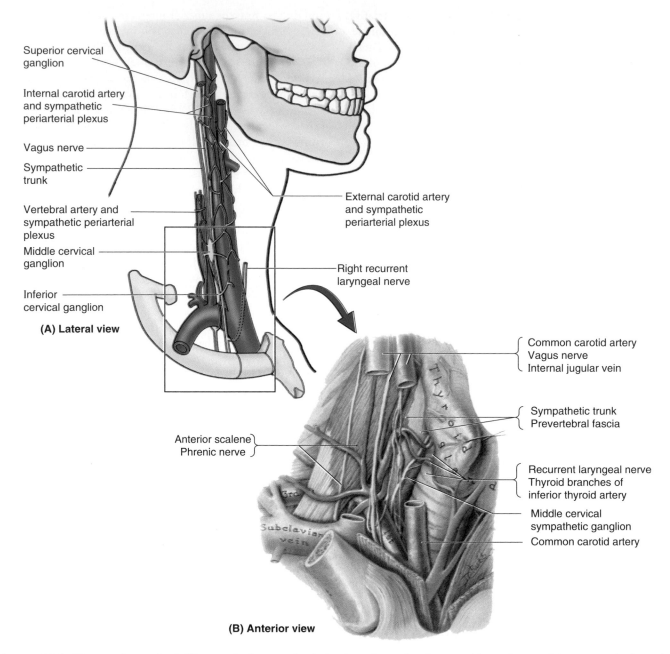

Figure 8.20. Nerves in neck. A. The cervical sympathetic trunk and ganglia, the carotid arteries, and the sympathetic periarterial plexuses surrounding them are shown. **B.** In this view of the root of the neck (right side), the clavicle is removed, sections are taken from the common carotid artery and IJV. The right lobe of the thyroid gland is retracted to reveal the nerves and middle cervical sympathetic ganglion.

The **recurrent laryngeal nerves** arise from the vagus nerves in the inferior part of the neck (Fig. 8.20). The nerves of the two sides have essentially the same distribution; however, they loop around different structures and at different levels on the two sides. The *right recurrent laryngeal nerve* loops inferior to the right subclavian artery at approximately the T1–T2 vertebral level, and the *left recurrent laryngeal nerve* loops inferior to the arch of the aorta at approximately the T4–T5 vertebral level. After looping, the recurrent laryngeal nerves

ascend superiorly to the posteromedial aspect of the thyroid gland (Figs. 8.20, 8.21*B,* and 8.22), where they ascend in the tracheoesophageal groove, supplying both trachea and esophagus and all the intrinsic muscles of the larynx except the cricothyroid.

The **cardiac branches of CN X** originate in the neck as well as in the thorax and convey presynpatic parasympathetic and visceral afferent fibers to the cardiac plexus of nerves (see Chapter 1).

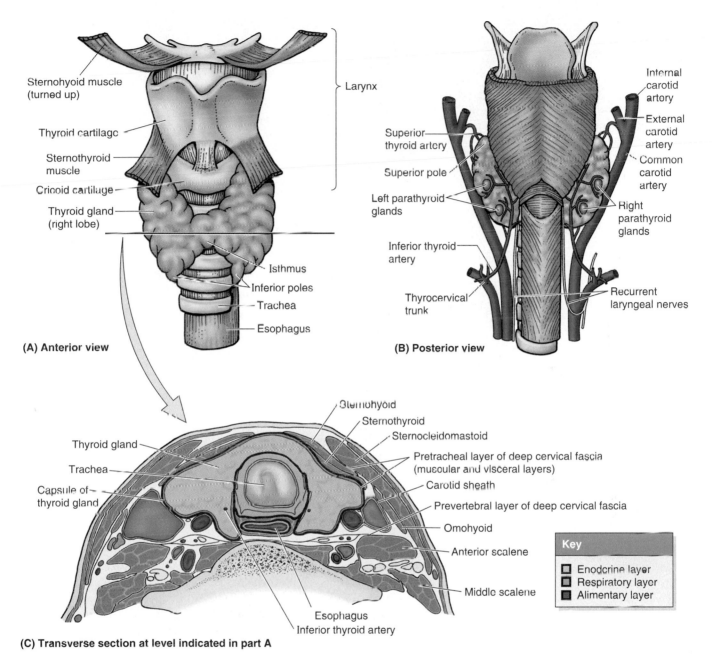

(A) Anterior view

Sternohyoid muscle (turned up)

Thyroid cartilage

Sternothyroid muscle

Cricoid cartilage

Thyroid gland (right lobe)

Larynx

Isthmus
Inferior poles
Trachea
Esophagus

(B) Posterior view

Internal carotid artery

External carotid artery

Common carotid artery

Superior thyroid artery

Superior pole

Left parathyroid glands

Inferior thyroid artery

Thyrocervical trunk

Right parathyroid glands

Recurrent laryngeal nerves

Sternohyoid
Sternothyroid
Sternocleidomastoid
Pretracheal layer of deep cervical fascia (muscular and visceral layers)
Carotid sheath
Prevertebral layer of deep cervical fascia
Omohyoid
Anterior scalene
Middle scalene

Thyroid gland
Trachea
Capsule of thyroid gland

Esophagus
Inferior thyroid artery

Key	
☐	Endocrine layer
☐	Respiratory layer
■	Alimentary layer

(C) Transverse section at level indicated in part A

Figure 8.21. Relationships of thyroid gland. A. The sternothyroid muscles have been cut to expose the lobes of the normal thyroid gland. The isthmus lies anterior to the second and third tracheal rings. **B.** The parathyroid glands are usually embedded in the fibrous capsule on the posterior surface of the thyroid gland. **C.** The functional layers of the cervical viscera are shown at the level noted in part **A.** The thyroid gland is asymmetrically enlarged in this specimen.

Phrenic Nerves. The phrenic nerves are formed at the lateral borders of the anterior scalene muscles (Figs. 8.19*A* and 8.20*B*), mainly from the C4 nerve with contributions from C3 and C5. The phrenic nerves descend anterior to the anterior scalene muscles under cover of the IJVs and the SCMs. They pass under the prevertebral layer of deep cervical fascia, between the subclavian arteries and veins, and proceed to the thorax to supply the diaphragm. The phrenic nerves are important because, in addition to their sensory distribution,

they provide the sole motor supply to their own half of the diaphragm (see Chapter 2 for details).

Sympathetic Trunks. The **cervical portion of the sympathetic trunks** lie anterolateral to the vertebral column, extending superiorly to the level of the C1 vertebra or cranial base (Figs. 8.19 and 8.20). The sympathetic trunks receive no white communicating branches (L. *rami communicantes*) in the neck (recall that none is associated with cervical spinal nerves). The cervical portion of the trunks includes three

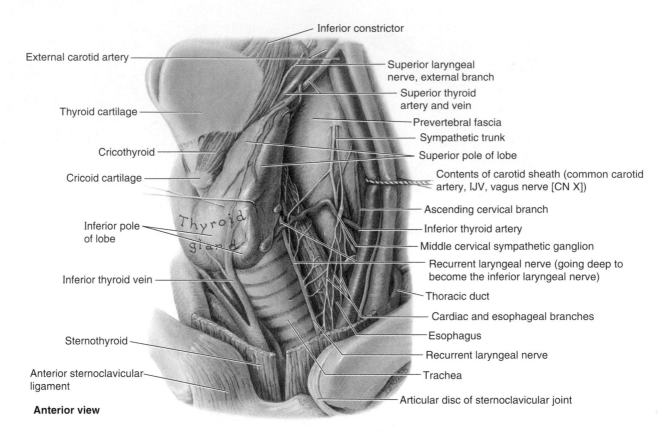

Inferior constrictor

External carotid artery

Thyroid cartilage

Cricothyroid

Cricoid cartilage

Inferior pole of lobe

Inferior thyroid vein

Sternothyroid

Anterior sternoclavicular ligament

Anterior view

Superior laryngeal nerve, external branch

Superior thyroid artery and vein

Prevertebral fascia

Sympathetic trunk

Superior pole of lobe

Contents of carotid sheath (common carotid artery, IJV, vagus nerve [CN X])

Ascending cervical branch

Inferior thyroid artery

Middle cervical sympathetic ganglion

Recurrent laryngeal nerve (going deep to become the inferior laryngeal nerve)

Thoracic duct

Cardiac and esophageal branches

Esophagus

Recurrent laryngeal nerve

Trachea

Articular disc of sternoclavicular joint

Thyroid gland

Figure 8.22. Dissection of left side of root of neck. The viscera (thyroid gland, trachea, and esophagus) are retracted to the right, and the contents of the left carotid sheath are retracted to the left. The middle thyroid vein, severed to allow such retraction, is not apparent. The recurrent laryngeal nerve ascends beside the trachea, in the angle between the trachea and the esophagus. The thoracic duct passes laterally, posterior to the contents of the carotid sheath as the thyrocervical trunk passes medially. Only the terminal branches of the thyrocervical trunk (the inferior thyroid and ascending cervical arteries) are seen here, emerging medial to the carotid sheath contents.

cervical sympathetic ganglia: superior, middle, and inferior. These ganglia receive presynaptic fibers conveyed to the trunk by the superior thoracic spinal nerves and their associated white communicating branches, which then ascend through the sympathetic trunk to the ganglia. After synapsing with the postsynaptic neuron in the cervical sympathetic ganglia, postsynaptic neurons send fibers to the:

1. Cervical spinal nerves via *gray communicating branches.*

2. Thoracic viscera via *cardiopulmonary splanchnic nerves.*

3. Head and viscera of the neck via *cephalic arterial branches* (rami).

The latter fibers accompany arteries as *sympathetic periarterial nerve plexuses,* especially the vertebral and internal and external carotid arteries (Fig. 8.20).

In approximately 80% of people, the **inferior cervical ganglion** fuses with the first thoracic ganglion to form the large **cervicothoracic ganglion (stellate ganglion).** This star-shaped (L. *stella,* a star) ganglion lies anterior to the transverse process of the C7 vertebra, just superior to the neck of the 1st rib on each side and posterior to the origin of the vertebral artery (Fig. 8.19B). Some postsynaptic fibers from

the ganglion pass via gray communicating branches to the anterior rami of the C7 and C8 spinal nerves (roots of the brachial plexus), and others pass to the heart via the *inferior cervical cardiac nerve* (a cardiopulmonary splanchnic nerve), which passes along the trachea to the deep *cardiac plexus.* Other fibers pass via arterial branches to contribute to the sympathetic periarterial nerve plexus around the vertebral artery running into the cranial cavity (Fig. 8.20A).

The **middle cervical ganglion,** the smallest of the three ganglia, is occasionally absent. When present, it lies on the anterior aspect of the inferior thyroid artery at the level of the cricoid cartilage and the transverse process of C6 vertebra, just anterior to the vertebral artery (Figs. 8.20 and 8.22). Postsynaptic fibers pass from the ganglion via gray communicating branches to the anterior rami of the C5 and C6 spinal nerves, via a middle cervical cardiac (cardiopulmonary splanchnic) nerve to the heart and via arterial branches to form the periarterial plexuses to the thyroid gland.

The **superior cervical ganglion** is at the level of the C1 and C2 vertebrae (Figs. 8.19B and 8.20A). Because of its large size, it forms a good landmark for locating the sympathetic trunk, but it may need to be distinguished from a large sensory (nodose) ganglion of the vagus (CN X) when present.

Postsynaptic fibers pass from it by means of cephalic arterial branches to form the internal carotid sympathetic plexus and enter the cranial cavity (Fig. 8.20). This ganglion also sends arterial branches to the external carotid artery and gray rami to the anterior rami of the superior four cervical spinal nerves. Other postsynaptic fibers pass from it to the cardiac plexus of nerves via a **superior cervical cardiac** (cardiopulmonary splanchnic) **nerve** (see Chapter 1).

Cervicothoracic Ganglion Block

Anesthetic injected around the large cervicothoracic ganglion blocks transmission of stimuli through the cervical and superior thoracic ganglia. This ganglion block may relieve vascular spasms involving the brain and upper limb. It is also useful when deciding if a surgical resection of the ganglion would be beneficial to a person with excess vasoconstriction in the ipsilateral limb.

Lesion of the Cervical Sympathetic Trunk

A lesion of a sympathetic trunk in the neck results in a sympathetic disturbance called *Horner syndrome*, which is characterized by:

- Contraction of the pupil (miosis), resulting from paralysis of the dilator pupillae muscle (see Chapter 7).

- Drooping of the superior eyelid (ptosis), resulting from paralysis of the smooth (tarsal) muscle intermingled with the striated muscle of the levator palpebrae superioris.

- Sinking in of the eye (enophthalmos), possibly caused by paralysis of the smooth (orbitalis) muscle in the floor of the orbit.

- Vasodilation and absence of sweating on the face and neck (anhydrosis), caused by lack of a sympathetic (vasoconstrictive) nerve supply to the blood vessels and sweat glands. ✚

THE BOTTOM LINE: The branches of the arch of the aorta bifurcate and/or traverse the root of the neck, with the branches of the subclavian artery arising here also. The internal jugular and subclavian veins converge at the root of the neck to form the brachiocephalic veins, with the major lymphatic trunks (right lymphatic duct and thoracic duct) entering the venous angles formed by the convergence of these veins. The phrenic and vagus nerves enter the thorax by passing anterior to the subclavian arteries and posterior to the brachiocephalic veins. The sympathetic trunks and

recurrent laryngeal nerves traverse the root of the neck posterior to the arteries, as do the visceral structures (trachea and esophagus). The cervical portion of the sympathetic trunks include three cervical sympathetic ganglia (inferior, middle, and superior) where presynaptic fibers from the superior thoracic spinal cord synapse with postsynaptic neurons. These neurons send fibers to the cervical spinal nerves, via gray communicating branches, to the head and viscera of the neck, via cephalic arterial branches and periarterial plexuses, and to the thoracic viscera, via cardiac (cardiopulmonary splanchnic) nerves.

Viscera of the Neck

The cervical viscera are disposed in three layers, named for their primary function (Fig. 8.21). Superficial to deep, they are the:

1. *Endocrine layer:* the thyroid and parathyroid glands.

2. *Respiratory layer:* the larynx and trachea.

3. *Alimentary layer:* the pharynx and esophagus.

Endocrine Layer of the Cervical Viscera

The cervical organs in the **endocrine layer** are part of the body's endocrine system of ductless, hormone-secreting glands. The thyroid gland is the body's largest endocrine gland. It produces *thyroid hormone*, which controls the rate of metabolism, and *calcitonin*, a hormone controlling calcium metabolism. The thyroid gland affects all areas of the body except itself and the spleen, testes, and uterus. The hormone produced by the *parathyroid glands, parathormone* (PTH), controls the metabolism of phosphorus and calcium in the blood. The parathyroid glands target the skeleton, kidneys, and intestine.

Thyroid Gland

The **thyroid gland** lies deep to the sternothyroid and sternohyoid muscles, located anteriorly in the neck at the level of the C5–T1 vertebrae (Fig. 8.21). It consists primarily of right and left **lobes**, anterolateral to the larynx and trachea. A relatively thin **isthmus** unites the lobes over the trachea, usually anterior to the second and third tracheal rings. The thyroid gland is surrounded by a thin **fibrous capsule**, which sends septa deeply into the gland. Dense connective tissue attaches the capsule to the cricoid cartilage and superior tracheal rings. External to the capsule is a loose sheath formed by the visceral portion of the pretracheal layer of deep cervical fascia.

Arteries of the Thyroid Gland. The highly vascular thyroid gland is supplied by the superior and inferior **thyroid arteries** (Figs. 8.21*B* and 8.22). These vessels lie between the fibrous capsule and the loose fascial sheath. Usually the first branches of the external carotid arteries, the *superior thyroid arteries*, descend to the superior poles of the gland, pierce the pretracheal layer of deep cervical fascia, and divide into anterior and posterior branches supplying mainly the antero-superior aspect of the gland. The *inferior thyroid arteries,* the largest branches of the thyrocervical trunks arising from the subclavian arteries, run superomedially posterior to the carotid sheaths to reach the posterior aspect of the thyroid gland. They divide into several branches that pierce the pre-tracheal layer of the deep cervical fascia and supply the pos-teroinferior aspect, including the **inferior poles** of the gland. The right and left superior and inferior thyroid arteries anas-tomose extensively within the gland, ensuring its supply while providing potential collateral circulation between the subcla-vian and external carotid arteries.

Thyroid Ima Artery

In approximately 10% of people, a small, unpaired **thy-roid ima artery** (L. *arteria thyroidea ima*) arises from the brachiocephalic trunk (Fig. B8.5); however, it may arise from the arch of the aorta or from the right common carotid, subclavian, or internal thoracic arteries. This small artery ascends on the anterior surface of the tra-chea, which it supplies, and continues to the isthmus of the thyroid gland, where it divides and supplies it. The possible presence of this artery must be considered when performing procedures in the midline of the neck inferior to the isthmus because it is a potential source of bleeding (see clinical correlation [blue] box "Tra-cheostomy," later in this chapter). ⊙

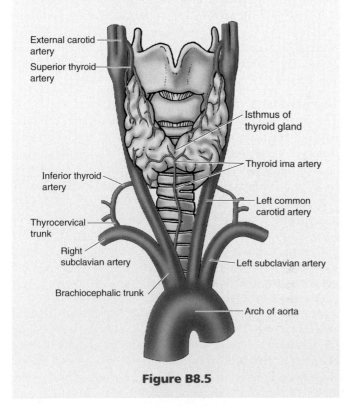

External carotid artery

Superior thyroid artery

Isthmus of thyroid gland

Inferior thyroid artery

Thyroid ima artery

Left common carotid artery

Thyrocervical trunk

Right subclavian artery

Left subclavian artery

Brachiocephalic trunk

Arch of aorta

Figure B8.5

Veins of the Thyroid Gland. Three pairs of thyroid veins usually form a **thyroid plexus of veins** on the anterior surface of the thyroid gland and anterior to the trachea (Figs. 8.22 and 8.23). The **superior thyroid veins** accompany the supe-rior thyroid arteries; they drain the **superior poles** of the thy-roid gland; the **middle thyroid veins** do not accompany but run essentially parallel courses with the inferior thyroid arter-ies; they drain the middle of the lobes. The usually indepen-dent **inferior thyroid veins** drain the inferior poles. The su-perior and middle thyroid veins drain into the IJVs; the inferior thyroid veins drain into the brachiocephalic veins posterior to the manubrium.

Lymphatic Drainage of the Thyroid Gland. The lym-phatic vessels of the thyroid gland run in the interlobular con-nective tissue, usually near the arteries; they communicate with a capsular network of lymphatic vessels. From here, the vessels pass initially to **prelaryngeal, pretracheal,** and **paratra-cheal lymph nodes,** which drain in turn to the **superior** (from the prelaryngeal nodes) and **inferior deep cervical nodes** (from the pretracheal and paratracheal nodes) (Fig. 8.24). Laterally, lymphatic vessels located along the superior thyroid veins pass directly to the inferior deep cervical lymph nodes. Some lymphatic vessels may drain into the *brachiocephalic lymph nodes* or the *thoracic duct* (Fig. 8.22).

Nerves of the Thyroid Gland. The nerves of the thyroid gland are derived from the superior, middle, and inferior *cer-vical sympathetic ganglia* (Figs. 8.20 and 8.22). They reach the gland through the *cardiac* and *superior* and *inferior thyroid pe-riarterial plexuses* that accompany the thyroid arteries. These fibers are vasomotor, not secretomotor. They cause constric-tion of blood vessels. Endocrine secretion from the thyroid gland is hormonally regulated by the pituitary gland.

Thyroglossal Duct Cysts

Development of the thyroid gland begins in the floor of the embryonic pharynx at the site indicated by a small pit, the **foramen cecum,** in the dorsum of the postnatal tongue. Subsequently, the developing gland descends from the tongue into the neck, passing anterior to the hyoid and thyroid cartilages to reach its final position anterolateral to the superior part of the trachea. During this descent, the thyroid gland is attached to the foramen cecum by the **thyroglossal duct** (Moore and Persaud, 2003). This duct normally disappears but remnants of epithelium may remain and form a *thyroglossal duct cyst* at any point along the path of its descent (Fig. B8.6). The cyst is usually near or within the body of the hyoid and forms a swelling in the anterior part of the neck.

Ectopic Thyroid Gland

Uncommonly, the thyroid gland fails to descend from its embryonic origin in the tongue, resulting in a ▶

Nerve to thyrohyoid

Superior laryngeal nerve, internal branch

External carotid artery

Superior laryngeal nerve, external branch
Superior thyroid artery

Sternocleidomastoid branch

Superior thyroid vein

Thyroid plexus of veins

Middle thyroid vein

Internal jugular vein
Vagus nerve
Common carotid artery

Subclavian artery

Inferior thyroid vein

Brachiocephalic trunk

Sternohyoid, reflected superiorly

Thyrohyoid

Accessory thyroid gland

Cricothyroid

Sternothyroid

Thyroid gland

Sternohyoid, reflected inferiorly

Anterior view

Figure 8.23. Thyroid gland. A dissection of the anterior aspect of the neck is shown. In this specimen, there is a small accessory thyroid gland on the right, lying on the thyrohyoid muscle, lateral to the thyroid cartilage. The superior thyroid artery is distributed primarily to the anterosuperior portion of the gland.

lingual thyroid gland. Incomplete descent results in the gland being located high in the neck, at or just inferior to the hyoid. As a rule, an ectopic thyroid gland in the median plane of the neck is the only thyroid tissue present. Occasionally, thyroid glandular tissue is associated with a thyroglossal duct cyst. Therefore, it is important to differentiate between an ectopic thyroid gland and a thyroglossal duct cyst when excising a cyst. Failure to do so may result in total thyroidectomy, leaving the person permanently dependent on thyroid medication (Leung et al., 1995).

Accessory Thyroid Glandular Tissue

Portions of the thyroglossal duct may persist to form thyroid tissue. Accessory thyroid glandular tissue may appear anywhere along the embryonic course of the thyroglossal duct (e.g., in the thymus inferior to the thyroid gland or in the thorax). Accessory thyroid tissue may develop in the neck lateral to the thyroid cartilage; it usually lies on the thyrohyoid muscle (Fig. 8.23). Although the accessory tis-

sue may be functional, it is often of insufficient size to maintain normal function if the thyroid gland is removed.

Pyramidal Lobe of the Thyroid Gland

Approximately 50% of thyroid glands have a pyramidal lobe. This lobe, which varies in size, extends superiorly from the isthmus of the thyroid gland, usually to the left of the median plane; the isthmus may be incomplete (Fig. B8.7). A band of connective tissue, often containing accessory thyroid tissue, may continue from the apex of the pyramidal lobe to the hyoid. The pyramidal lobe and the band develop from remnants of the epithelium and connective tissue of the thyroglossal duct.

Enlargement of the Thyroid Gland

A non-neoplastic and non-inflammatory enlargement of the thyroid gland, other than the variable enlargement that may occur during menstruation and pregnancy, is ▶

Key

■ Potential sites of aberrant thyroid glandular tissue or thyroglossal duct cysts

Figure B8.6

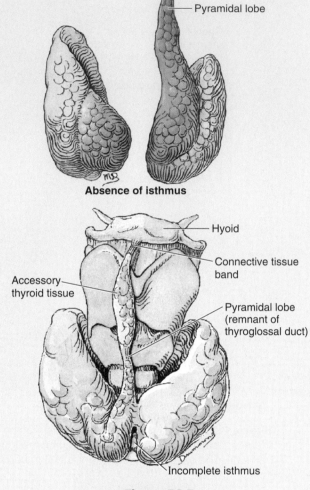

Figure B8.7

called a goiter. A *goiter* results from a lack of iodine. It is common in certain parts of the world where the soil and water are deficient in iodine. The enlarged gland causes a swelling in the neck that may compress the trachea, esophagus, and recurrent laryngeal nerves (Fig. B8.8). When the gland enlarges, it may do so anteriorly, posteriorly, inferiorly, or laterally. It cannot move superiorly because of the superior attachments of the sternothyroid and sternohyoid muscles (Table 8.3). Substernal extension of a goiter is also common.

Thyroidectomy

Excision of a malignant tumor of the thyroid gland or other surgical procedure sometimes necessitates removal of the gland *(thyroidectomy)*. In the surgical treatment of hyperthyroidism, the posterior part of each lobe of the enlarged thyroid is usually preserved, a procedure called *near-total thyroidectomy*, to protect the recurrent and superior laryngeal nerves and to spare the parathyroid glands. Postoperative hemorrhage after thyroid gland surgery may compress the trachea, making breathing difficult. The blood collects within the fibrous capsule of the gland.

Injury to the Recurrent Laryngeal Nerves

The risk of injury to the recurrent laryngeal nerves is ever present during neck surgery. Near the inferior pole of the thyroid gland, the right recurrent laryngeal nerve is ▶

Figure B8.8. Enlarged thyroid. A. A goiter is demonstrated.

(B)

Figure B8.8. *(Continued)* **B.** This scintigram shows a diffuse, enlarged thyroid gland.

intimately related to the inferior thyroid artery and its branches (Fig. B8.9). This nerve may cross anterior or posterior to branches of the artery, or it may pass between them. Because of this close relationship, the inferior thyroid artery is ligated some distance lateral to the thyroid gland, where it is not close to the nerve. Although the danger of injuring the left recurrent laryngeal nerve during surgery is not as great owing to its more vertical ascent from the superior mediastinum, the artery and nerve are also closely associated near the inferior pole of the thyroid gland (Fig. 8.22). Hoarseness is the usual sign of unilateral recurrent nerve injury; however, temporary aphonia or disturbance of phonation (voice production) and laryngeal spasm may occur. These signs usually result from bruising the recurrent laryngeal nerves during surgery or from the pressure of accumulated blood and serous exudate after the operation. ○

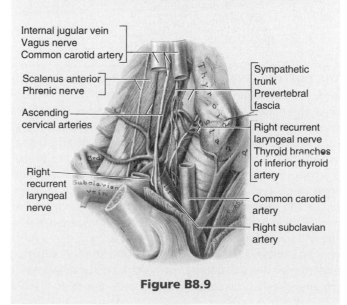

Figure B8.9

Labels:
- Internal jugular vein
- Vagus nerve
- Common carotid artery
- Scalenus anterior
- Phrenic nerve
- Ascending cervical arteries
- Right recurrent laryngeal nerve
- Sympathetic trunk
- Prevertebral fascia
- Right recurrent laryngeal nerve
- Thyroid branches of inferior thyroid artery
- Common carotid artery
- Right subclavian artery

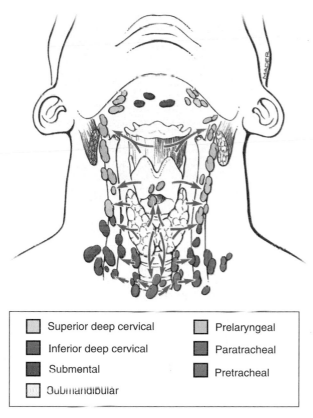

Legend:
- Superior deep cervical
- Inferior deep cervical
- Submental
- Submandibular
- Prelaryngeal
- Paratracheal
- Pretracheal

Figure 8.24. Lymphatic drainage of thyroid gland, larynx, and trachea. The *arrows* indicate the direction of lymph flow.

Parathyroid Glands

The small flattened, oval **parathyroid glands** usually lie external to the thyroid capsule on the medial half of the posterior surface of each lobe of the thyroid gland, inside its sheath (Fig. 8.25A). The **superior parathyroid glands** usually lie slightly more than 1 cm superior to the point of entry of the inferior thyroid arteries into the thyroid gland. The **inferior parathyroid glands** usually lie slightly more than 1 cm inferior to the arterial entry point (Skandalakis et al., 1995). Most people have four parathyroid glands. Approximately 5% of people have more; some have only two glands. The superior parathyroid glands, more constant in position than the inferior ones, are usually at the level of the inferior border of the cricoid cartilage. The inferior parathyroid glands are usually near the inferior poles of the thyroid gland, but they may lie in various positions (Fig. 8.25B). In 1–5% of people, an inferior parathyroid gland is deep in the superior mediastinum (Norton and Wells, 1994).

Vessels of the Parathyroid Glands. Because the *inferior thyroid arteries* provide the primary blood supply to the posterior aspect of the thyroid gland where the parathyroid glands are located, branches of these arteries usually supply the parathyroid glands (Fig. 8.25A). However, they may also be supplied by branches from the superior thyroid arteries; the thyroid ima artery; or the laryngeal, tracheal, and

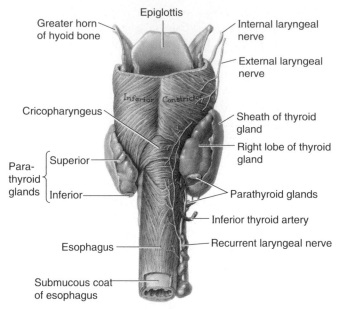

Epiglottis

Greater horn of hyoid bone

Internal laryngeal nerve

External laryngeal nerve

Cricopharyngeus

Inferior Constrictor

Sheath of thyroid gland

Right lobe of thyroid gland

Para-thyroid glands { Superior / Inferior

Parathyroid glands

Inferior thyroid artery

Esophagus

Recurrent laryngeal nerve

Submucous coat of esophagus

(A) Posterior view

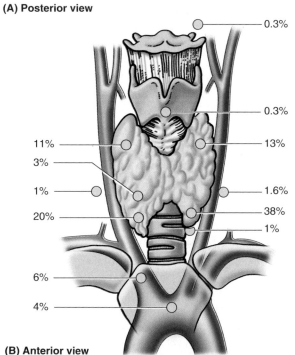

0.3%

0.3%

11%

13%

3%

1%

1.6%

20%

38%

1%

6%

4%

(B) Anterior view

Figure 8.25. Thyroid and parathyroid glands. A. The thyroid sheath has been dissected from the posterior surface of the thyroid gland to reveal the three embedded parathyroid glands. Both parathyroid glands on the right side are rather low, and the inferior gland is inferior to the thyroid gland. **B.** Sites and frequencies of aberrant parathyroid glandular tissue are shown.

esophageal arteries. **Parathyroid veins** drain into the *thyroid plexus of veins* of the thyroid gland and trachea (Fig. 8.23). *Lymphatic vessels* from the parathyroid glands drain with those from the thyroid gland into deep cervical lymph nodes and paratracheal lymph nodes (Fig. 8.24).

Nerves of the Parathyroid Glands. The nerve supply of the parathyroid glands is abundant; it is derived from thyroid branches of the cervical sympathetic ganglia (Fig. 8.20). Like the nerves to the thyroid, they are vasomotor rather than secretomotor because these glands are hormonally regulated.

Inadvertent Removal of the Parathyroid Glands

The variable position of the parathyroid glands, especially the inferior ones, puts them in danger of being damaged or removed during surgical procedures in the neck. The superior parathyroid glands may be as far superior as the thyroid cartilage, and the inferior ones may be as far inferior as the superior mediastinum. The aberrant sites of these glands are of concern when searching for abnormal parathyroid glands, as may be necessary in treating *parathyroid adenoma,* an ordinarily benign tumor of epithelial tissue associated with hyperparathyroidism.

Atrophy or inadvertent surgical removal of all the parathyroid glands results in *tetany,* a severe neurologic syndrome characterized by muscle twitches and cramps. The generalized spasms are caused by decreased serum calcium levels. Because laryngeal and respiratory muscles are involved, failure to respond immediately with appropriate therapy can result in death. To safeguard these glands during thyroidectomy, surgeons usually preserve the posterior part of the lobes of the thyroid gland. In cases in which it is necessary to remove all of the thyroid gland (e.g., because of malignant disease), the parathyroid glands are carefully isolated with their blood vessels intact before removal of the thyroid gland. Parathyroid tissue may also be transplanted, usually to the arm so it will not be damaged by subsequent surgery or radiation therapy. **☉**

THE BOTTOM LINE: Despite different developmental origins, the endocrine thyroid and parathyroid glands are intimately related. Typically the thyroid gland is roughly H-shaped, with right and left lobes linked by a thin central isthmus. The gland wraps around the anterior and lateral aspects of the trachea at the level of the second to fourth tracheal rings; the isthmus lies anterior to the second and third rings. Typically, there are four parathyroids (two superior and two inferior) within the capsule of the thyroid or in the gland itself. An abundant blood supply, essential to the endocrine function, is provided to the thyroid by a four-way anastomosis between the right and the left superior and inferior thyroid arteries, with the latter usually providing branches to the parathyroid glands. Superior thyroid veins accompany the arteries of the same name, draining the area they supply. However, unaccompanied middle and inferior thyroid veins drain the inferior part of the gland. The superior and middle thyroid veins drain to the IJV, whereas the usually singular inferior thyroid vein enters the left brachiocephalic vein. Vasomotor nerves course along the arteries, but the glands are regulated hormonally rather than by secretomotor nerve fibers. Lymphatic vessels pass directly to the deep cervical lymph nodes or via nodes associated with the larynx and trachea.

Respiratory Layer of the Cervical Viscera

The viscera of the **respiratory layer**, the larynx and trachea, contribute to the respiratory functions of the body. The main functions of the cervical respiratory viscera are as follows:

- Routing air and food into the respiratory tract and esophagus, respectively.

- Providing a patent airway and a means of sealing it off temporarily.

- Producing voice.

Larynx

The **larynx** is the complex organ of voice production (the "voice box") composed of nine cartilages connected by membranes and ligaments and containing the *vocal folds*. The larynx is located in the anterior neck at the level of the bodies of C3–C6 vertebrae. It connects the inferior part of the pharynx (oropharynx) with the trachea (Fig. 8.26). Although most commonly known for its role as the phonating mechanism for voice production, its most vital function is to guard the air passages, especially during swallowing when it serves as the "sphincter" or "valve" of the lower respiratory tract, thus maintaining a patent airway.

Laryngeal Skeleton. The laryngeal skeleton consists of nine cartilages: three are single (thyroid, cricoid, and epiglottic) and three are paired (arytenoid, corniculate, and cuneiform) (Fig. 8.27A & B).

The **thyroid cartilage** is the largest of the cartilages; its superior border lies opposite the C4 vertebra. The inferior two thirds of its two plate-like **laminae** fuse anteriorly in the median plane to form the **laryngeal prominence** (Fig. 8.27A & C). This projection is well marked in men but seldom visible in women. Superior to this prominence ("Adam's apple"), the laminae diverge to form a V-shaped **superior thyroid notch** (usually referred to as the thyroid notch). The small **inferior thyroid notch** is a shallow indentation in the middle of the inferior border of the cartilage. The posterior border of each lamina projects superiorly as the **superior horn** and inferiorly as the **inferior horn**. The superior border and superior horns attach to the hyoid by the **thyrohyoid membrane** (Fig. 8.27A & B). The thick median part of this membrane is the **median thyrohyoid ligament**; its lateral parts are the **lateral thyrohyoid ligaments**. The inferior horns articulate with the lateral surfaces of the cricoid cartilage at the **cricothyroid joints** (Fig. 8.27B). The main move-

Labels (left side, top to bottom): Pharyngeal tonsil (adenoids); Middle nasal concha; Inferior nasal concha; Palate — Soft / Hard; Mucosal surface of tongue; Tongue; Oropharynx; Mandible; Epiglottis; Larynx; Esophagus; Trachea

Labels (right side, top to bottom): Cerebellum; 4th ventricle; Pons; Medulla oblongata; Anterior arch of atl; Posterior arch of a; Dens of axis; Spinal cord; Body of C6 verteb; Intervertebral disc; Spinous process

Median section

Figure 8.26. Median MRI of head (viscerocranium) and neck. Because the air and food passages share the oropharynx, separation of food and air must occur to continue into the trachea (anterior) and esophagus (posterior). (Courtesy of Dr. W. Kucharczyk, Chair of Medical Imaging, University of Toronto, and Clinical Director, Tri-Hospital Resonance Centre, Toronto, Ontario, Canada.)

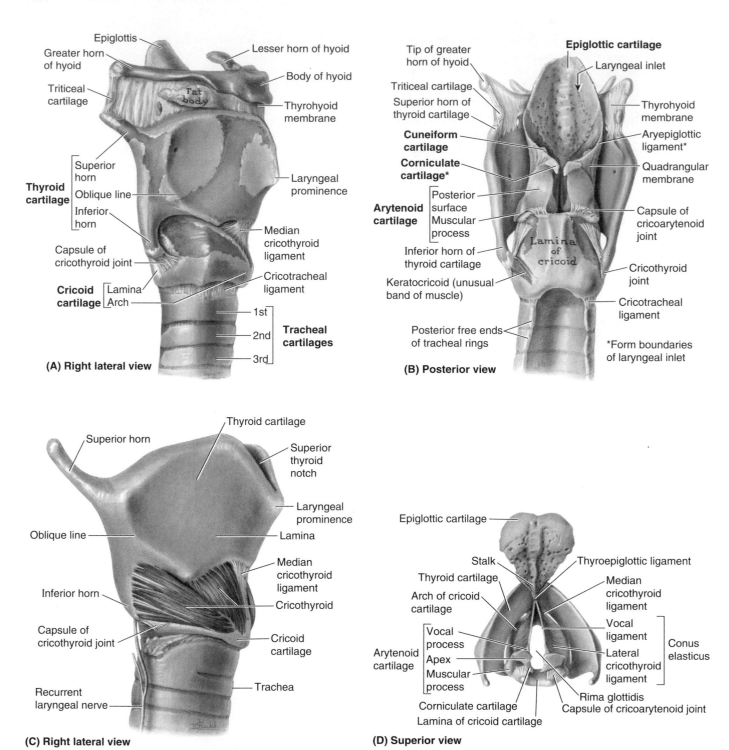

Epiglottis

Greater horn of hyoid

Triticeal cartilage

Thyroid cartilage
Superior horn
Oblique line
Inferior horn

Capsule of cricothyroid joint

Cricoid cartilage Lamina Arch

Lesser horn of hyoid

Body of hyoid

Thyrohyoid membrane

Laryngeal prominence

Median cricothyroid ligament

Cricotracheal ligament

1st
2nd **Tracheal cartilages**
3rd

(A) Right lateral view

Tip of greater horn of hyoid

Triticeal cartilage
Superior horn of thyroid cartilage

Cuneiform cartilage

Corniculate cartilage*

Arytenoid cartilage
Posterior surface
Muscular process

Inferior horn of thyroid cartilage

Keratocricoid (unusual band of muscle)

Posterior free ends of tracheal rings

Epiglottic cartilage
Laryngeal inlet

Thyrohyoid membrane

Aryepiglottic ligament*

Quadrangular membrane

Capsule of cricoarytenoid joint

Cricothyroid joint

Cricotracheal ligament

*Form boundaries of laryngeal inlet

(B) Posterior view

Thyroid cartilage

Superior horn

Superior thyroid notch

Laryngeal prominence

Oblique line

Lamina

Inferior horn

Median cricothyroid ligament

Cricothyroid

Capsule of cricothyroid joint

Cricoid cartilage

Recurrent laryngeal nerve

Trachea

(C) Right lateral view

Epiglottic cartilage

Stalk

Thyroid cartilage

Arch of cricoid cartilage

Arytenoid cartilage
Vocal process
Apex
Muscular process

Corniculate cartilage

Lamina of cricoid cartilage

Thyroepiglottic ligament

Median cricothyroid ligament

Vocal ligament

Lateral cricothyroid ligament

Conus elasticus

Rima glottidis

Capsule of cricoarytenoid joint

(D) Superior view

Figure 8.27. Skeleton of larynx. A. Although firmly connected to it, the hyoid is not part of the larynx. The larynx extends vertically from the tip of the heart-shaped epiglottis to the inferior border of the cricoid cartilage. **B.** The thyroid cartilage shields the smaller cartilages of the larynx, and the hyoid shields the superior part of the epiglottic cartilage. **C.** The thyroid cartilage and cricothyroid muscle are shown. This muscle produces movement at the cricothyroid joint. **D.** The epiglottic cartilage is pitted for mucous glands and its stalk is attached by the thyroepiglottic ligament to the angle of the thyroid cartilage superior to the vocal ligaments. The vocal ligament, which forms the skeleton of the vocal fold, extends from the vocal process to the "angle" of the thyroid cartilage, and there joins its fellow inferior to the thyroepiglottic ligament.

ments at these joints are rotation and gliding of the thyroid cartilage, which result in changes in the length of the vocal folds.

The **cricoid cartilage** is shaped like a signet ring with its band facing anteriorly. This ring-like opening of the carti lage fits an average finger. The posterior (signet) part of the cricoid is the *lamina,* and the anterior (band) part is the *arch* (Fig. 8.27*A*). Although much smaller than the thyroid carti lage, the cricoid cartilage is thicker and stronger and is the only complete ring of cartilage to encircle any part of the airway. It attaches to the interior margin of the thyroid car tilage by the **median cricothyroid ligament** and to the first tracheal ring by the **cricotracheal ligament.** Where the lar ynx is closest to the skin and most accessible, the median cricothyroid ligament may be felt as a soft spot during pal pation inferior to the thyroid cartilage.

The **arytenoid cartilages** are paired, three-sided pyramidal cartilages that articulate with the lateral parts of the superior border of the cricoid cartilage lamina (Fig. 8.27*B*). Each car tilage has an apex superiorly, a vocal process anteriorly, and a large muscular process that projects laterally from its base. The **apex** bears the corniculate cartilage and attaches to the aryepiglottic fold. The **vocal process** provides the posterior at tachment for the vocal ligament, and the muscular process serves as a lever to which the posterior and lateral cricoary tenoid muscles are attached.

The **cricoarytenoid joints,** located between the bases of the arytenoid cartilages and the superolateral surfaces of the lamina of the cricoid cartilage (Fig. 8.27*B*), permit the ary tenoid cartilages to slide toward or away from one to another, to tilt anteriorly and posteriorly, and to rotate. These move ments are important in approximating, tensing, and relaxing the vocal folds. The elastic **vocal ligaments** extend from the junction of the laminae of the thyroid cartilage anteriorly to the vocal process of the arytenoid cartilage posteriorly (Fig. 8.27*D*). The vocal ligaments make up the submucosal skele ton of the vocal folds. The vocal ligaments are the thickened, free superior border of the **conus elasticus** or **cricovocal membrane.** The parts of the membrane extending laterally between the vocal folds and the superior border of the cricoid are the **lateral cricothyroid ligaments.** The fibroelastic conus elasticus blends anteriorly with the *median cricothyroid liga ment.* The conus elasticus and overlying mucosa close the tracheal inlet except for the central **rima glottidis** (opening between the vocal folds).

The **epiglottic cartilage,** consisting of elastic cartilage, gives flexibility to the **epiglottis,** a heart-shaped cartilage cov ered with mucous membrane (Fig. 8.27*B*). Situated posterior to the root of the tongue and the hyoid and anterior to the **laryngeal inlet,** the epiglottic cartilage forms the superior part of the anterior wall and the superior margin of the inlet. Its broad superior end is free. Its tapered inferior end, the **stalk of the epiglottis,** is attached to the angle formed by the thy roid laminae by the **thyroepiglottic ligament** (Fig. 8.27*D*).

The **hyoepiglottic ligament** attaches the anterior surface

Body of hyoid

Lesser horn

Greater horn

Hyoepiglottic ligament

Median glossoepiglottic fold

Epiglottis

Superior view

Figure 8.28. Epiglottis and hyoepiglottic ligament. The epiglottis is a leaf-shaped plate of elastic fibrocartilage, which is covered with mucous membrane (*pink*) and is at tached anteriorly to the hyoid by the hyoepiglottic ligament (*blue*). The epiglottis serves as a diverter valve over the supe rior aperture of the larynx during swallowing.

of the epiglottic cartilage to the hyoid (Fig. 8.28). The **quadrangular membrane** (Fig. 8.27*B*) is a thin, submucosal sheet of connective tissue that extends between the lateral as pects of the arytenoid and epiglottic cartilages. Its free infe rior margin constitutes the **vestibular ligament,** which is covered loosely by mucosa to form the **vestibular fold** (Fig. 8.29). This fold lies superior to the vocal fold and extends from the thyroid cartilage to the arytenoid cartilage. The free superior margin of the quadrangular membrane forms the **aryepiglottic ligament,** which is covered with mucosa to form the **aryepiglottic fold.** The **corniculate** and **cuneiform cartilages** appear as small nodules in the posterior part of the aryepiglottic folds. The corniculate cartilages attach to the apices of the arytenoid cartilages; the cuneiform cartilages do not directly attach to other cartilages. The quadrangular membrane and conus elasticus are the superior and inferior parts of the submucosal **fibroelastic membrane of the larynx.**

Fractures of the Laryngeal Skeleton

Laryngeal fractures may result from blows received in sports such as kick boxing and hockey, or from com pression by a shoulder strap during an automobile accident. Because of the frequency of this type of injury, most goalies in ice hockey and catchers in baseball have protective guards hanging from their masks that cover their larynges. Laryngeal fractures produce sub mucous hemorrhage and edema, respiratory obstruc tion, hoarseness, and sometimes a temporary inability to speak. ✪

Left boundary of laryngeal inlet

Epiglottis
Aryepiglottic fold
Cuneiform tubercle
Corniculate tubercle

Epiglottic cartilage

Quadrangular membrane
Vestibular ligament

Cuneiform cartilage

Superior horn of thyroid cartilage

Corniculate cartilage

Arytenoid cartilage, medial surface

Posterior cricoarytenoid ligament

Vocal process of arytenoid cartilage

Lateral cricothyroid ligament
Vocal ligament
Conus elasticus

Arytenoid (cut surface)

Vestibular fold
Ventricle
Vocal fold

Lamina of cricoid cartilage

Mucous membrane

Surgical needle spreading halves of cricoid cartilage

Tracheal ring

Posterior view

Figure 8.29. Interior of larynx. The posterior wall of the larynx is split in the median plane, and the two sides are spread apart and held in place by a surgical needle. On the left side, the mucous membrane is intact. On the right side, the mucous and submucous coats are peeled off, and the skeletal coat—consisting of cartilages, ligaments, and the fibroelastic membrane—is uncovered.

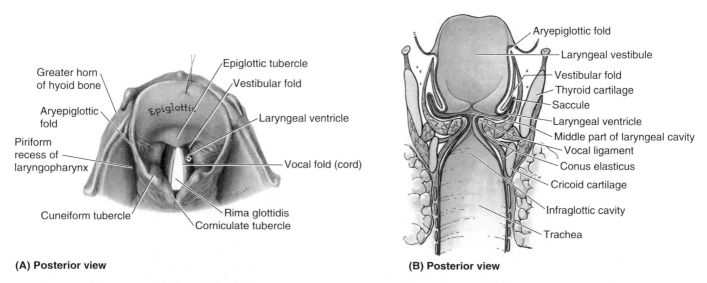

Greater horn of hyoid bone

Aryepiglottic fold

Piriform recess of laryngopharynx

Cuneiform tubercle

Epiglottic tubercle

Vestibular fold

Laryngeal ventricle

Vocal fold (cord)

Rima glottidis
Corniculate tubercle

(A) Posterior view

Aryepiglottic fold

Laryngeal vestibule

Vestibular fold
Thyroid cartilage
Saccule
Laryngeal ventricle
Middle part of laryngeal cavity
Vocal ligament
Conus elasticus
Cricoid cartilage
Infraglottic cavity
Trachea

(B) Posterior view

Figure 8.30. Folds and compartments of larynx. A. The rima glottidis (the space between the vocal folds) is visible through the laryngeal inlet and vestibule. The laryngeal inlet is bounded: (1) anteriorly by the free curved edge of the epiglottis; (2) posteriorly by the arytenoid cartilages, the corniculate cartilages that cap them, and the interarytenoid fold that unites them; and (3) on each side by the aryepiglottic fold that contains the superior end of the cuneiform cartilage. **B.** This coronal section shows the compartments of the larynx: the vestibule, middle compartment with left and right ventricles, and the infraglottic cavity.

Interior of the Larynx. The **laryngeal cavity** extends from the *laryngeal inlet,* through which it communicates with the *laryngopharynx,* to the level of the inferior border of the cricoid cartilage. Here the laryngeal cavity is continuous with the cavity of the trachea (Figs. 8.29 and 8.30). The laryngeal cavity includes the:

- **Laryngeal vestibule:** between the laryngeal inlet and the vestibular folds.

- **Middle part of the laryngeal cavity:** the central cavity (airway) between the vestibular and vocal folds.

- **Laryngeal ventricle:** recesses extending laterally from the middle part of the laryngeal cavity between vestibular and vocal folds. The **laryngeal saccule** is a blind pocket opening into each ventricle that is lined with mucosal glands.

- **Infraglottic cavity:** the inferior cavity of the larynx between the vocal folds and the inferior border of the cricoid cartilage, where it is continuous with the lumen of the trachea.

The **vocal folds** (true vocal cords) control sound production (Figs. 8.29–8.31). The apex of each wedge-shaped fold projects medially into the laryngeal cavity. Each vocal fold contains a:

- *Vocal ligament,* consisting of thickened elastic tissue that is the medial free edge of the conus elasticus.

- *Vocalis muscle,* composed of exceptionally fine muscle fibers immediately lateral to and terminating at intervals relative to the length of the vocal ligaments (Table 8.5).

The vocal folds are the source of the sounds (tone) that come from the larynx. These folds produce audible vibrations when their free margins are closely (but not tightly) apposed during phonation, and air is forcibly expired intermittently (Fig. 8.31B & C). The vocal folds also serve as the main inspiratory sphincter of the larynx when they are tightly closed. Complete adduction of the folds forms an effective sphincter that prevents entry of air.

The **glottis** (the vocal apparatus of the larynx) makes up the vocal folds and processes, together with the *rima glottidis,* the aperture between the vocal folds (Fig. 8.30A). The shape of the rima (L. slit) varies according to the position of the vocal folds (Fig. 8.31). During ordinary breathing, the rima is narrow and wedge shaped; during forced respiration it is wide and kite shaped. The rima glottidis is slit-like when the vocal folds are closely approximated during phonation. Variation in the tension and length of the vocal folds, in the width of the rima glottidis, and in the intensity of the expiratory effort produces changes in the pitch of the voice. The lower range of pitch of the voice of postpubertal males results from the greater length of the vocal folds.

The *vestibular folds* (false vocal cords), extending between the thyroid and the arytenoid cartilages (Figs. 8.29 and 8.30), play little or no part in voice production; they are protective in function. They consist of two thick folds of mucous membrane enclosing the *vestibular ligaments.* The space between these ligaments is the **rima vestibuli.** The lateral recesses between the vocal and the vestibular folds are the *laryngeal ventricles.*

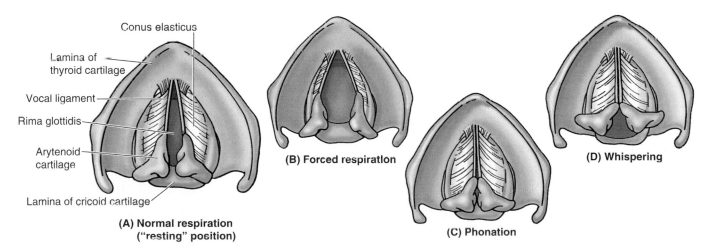

Conus elasticus

Lamina of thyroid cartilage

Vocal ligament

Rima glottidis

Arytenoid cartilage

Lamina of cricoid cartilage

(A) Normal respiration ("resting" position)

(B) Forced respiration

(C) Phonation

(D) Whispering

Figure 8.31. Variations in shape of rima glottidis. A. The shape of the rima glottidis, the aperture between the vocal folds, varies according to the position of the vocal folds. During normal respiration, the laryngeal muscles are relaxed and the rima glottidis assumes a narrow, slit-like position. **B.** During a deep inhalation, the vocal ligaments are abducted by contraction of the posterior cricoarytenoid muscles, opening the rima glottidis widely into an inverted kite shape. **C.** During phonation, the arytenoid muscles adduct the arytenoid cartilages at the same time that the lateral cricoarytenoid muscles moderately adduct. Air forced between the adducted vocal ligaments produces tone. Stronger contraction of the same muscles seals the rima glottidis (Valsalva maneuver). **C.** During whispering, the vocal ligaments are strongly adducted by the lateral cricoarytenoid muscles, but the relaxed arytenoid muscles allow air to pass between the arytenoid cartilages (intercartilaginous part of rima glottidis), which is modified into toneless speech. No tone is produced.

Table 8.5. Muscles of the Larynx

Lateral view
Cricothyroid

Superior view
Posterior cricoarytenoid

Superior view
Transverse arytenoid

Superior view
Thyroarytenoid

Superior view
Lateral cricoarytenoid

Superior view
Oblique arytenoid

Muscle	Origin	Insertion	Innervation	Main Action(s)
Cricothyroid	Anterolateral part of cricoid cartilage	Inferior margin and inferior horn of thyroid cartilage	External laryngeal nerve (from CN X)	Stretches and tenses vocal ligament
Thyroarytenoid[a]	Lower half of posterior aspect of angle of thyroid laminae and cricothyroid ligament	Anterolateral arytenoid surface	Inferior laryngeal nerve (terminal part of recurrent laryngeal nerve, from CN X)	Relaxes vocal ligament
Posterior cricoarytenoid	Posterior surface of lamina of cricoid cartilage	Vocal process of arytenoid cartilage		Abducts vocal folds
Lateral cricoarytenoid	Arch of cricoid cartilage			Adducts vocal folds (interligamentous portion)
Transverse and oblique arytenoids[b]	One arytenoid cartilage	Contralateral arytenoid cartilage		Adduct arytenoid cartilages (adducting intercartilaginous portion of vocal folds, closing posterior rima glottidis)
Vocalis[c]	Lateral surface of vocal process of arytenoid cartilage	Ipsilateral vocal ligament		Relaxes posterior vocal ligament while maintaining (or increasing) tension of anterior part

[a]Superior fibers of the thyroarytenoid muscles pass into the aryepiglottic fold, and some of them reach the epiglottic cartilage; These fibers constitute the thyroepiglottic muscle, which widens the laryngeal inlet.
[b]Some fibers of the oblique arytenoids muscles continue as aryepiglottic muscles (Fig. 8.33).
[c]This slender muscle slip lies medial to and is composed of fibers finer than those of the thyroarytenoid muscle.

Laryngoscopy

Laryngoscopy is the procedure used to examine the interior of the larynx. The larynx may be examined visually by *indirect laryngoscopy* using a laryngeal mirror (Fig. B8.10*A*). The anterior part of the tongue is gently pulled from the oral cavity to minimize the extent to which the posterior part of the tongue covers the epiglottis and laryngeal inlet. Because the rima vestibuli is larger than the rima glottidis during normal respiration, the vestibular folds and vocal folds are visible during a laryngoscopic examination (Fig. B8.10*B*). The larynx can also be viewed by *direct laryngoscopy,* using a tubular endoscopic instrument, a laryngoscope. A laryngoscope is a tube or flexible fiber optic endoscope equipped with electrical lighting for examining or operating on the interior of the larynx through the mouth. The vestibular folds normally appear pink, whereas the vocal folds are usually pearly white.

Valsalva Maneuver

The sphincteric actions of the vestibular and vocal folds are important during the Valsalva maneuver, any forced expiratory effort against a closed airway, such as a cough, sneeze, or strain during a bowel movement or weight lifting. The vestibular and vocal folds abduct widely as the lungs inflate during deep inspiration. In the Valsalva maneuver, both the vestibular and vocal folds are tightly adducted at the end of deep inspiration. The anterolateral abdominal muscles then contract strongly to increase the intrathoracic and intra-abdominal pressures. The relaxed diaphragm passively transmits the increased abdominopelvic pressure to the thoracic cavity. Because high intrathoracic pressure impedes venous return to the right atrium, researchers use the Valsalva maneuver to study cardiovascular effects of raised peripheral venous pressure and decreased cardiac filling and cardiac output.

Aspiration of Foreign Bodies and the Heimlich Maneuver

A foreign object, such as a piece of steak, may accidentally *aspirate* through the laryngeal inlet into the vestibule of the larynx, where it becomes trapped superior to the vestibular folds. When a foreign object enters the vestibule of the larynx, the laryngeal muscles go into spasm, tensing the vocal folds. The rima glottidis closes and no air enters the trachea. The resulting blockage may completely seal off the larynx (laryngeal obstruction) and choke the person, leaving the individual speechless because the larynx is blocked. Asphyxiation occurs, and the person will die in approximately 5 min from lack of oxygen if the obstruction is not removed.

A person who is choking will cough in an attempt to dislodge the object. The vestibular folds are part of the protective mechanism that closes the larynx. The mucosa of the vestibule is sensitive to foreign objects such as food. When an object passes through the laryngeal inlet and contacts the vestibular epithelium, violent coughing occurs. Emergency therapy must be given to open the airway. The procedure used depends on the condition of the person, the facilities available, and the experience of the person giving first aid.

Because the lungs still contain air, sudden compression of the abdomen (Heimlich maneuver) causes the ▶

Laryngeal mirror

(A) Indirect laryngoscopy

Posterior wall of laryngopharynx

Piriform fossa (recess)
To esophagus
Mucosa over cricoid cartilage
Interarytenoid notch
Site of corniculate cartilages
Site of cuneiform cartilages
Aryepiglottic fold
Trachea
Vocal folds
Lateral walls of laryngeal vestibule (mucosa over quadrangular membrane)
Vestibular folds (medial edge)
Epiglottis
Median glossoepiglottic fold
Right and left valleculae

(B)   Dorsum of tongue

Figure B8.10

diaphragm to elevate and compress the lungs, expelling air from the trachea into the larynx. This maneuver usually dislodges the food or other material from the larynx. To perform the Heimlich maneuver, the person giving first aid uses subdiaphragmatic abdominal thrusts to expel the foreign object from the larynx. First, the closed fist, with the base of the palm facing inward, is placed on the victim's abdomen between the umbilicus and the xiphoid process of the sternum (Fig. B8.11). The fist is grasped by the other hand and forcefully thrust inward and superiorly, forcing the diaphragm superiorly. This action forces air from the lungs and creates an artificial cough that usually expels the foreign object. Several abdominal thrusts may be necessary to remove the obstruction in the larynx.

In extreme cases, experienced persons (e.g., physicians) insert a large-bore needle through the cricothyroid ligament *(needle cricothyrotomy,* or "coniotomy") to permit fast entry of air. Later, a *surgical cricothyrotomy* may be performed, which involves an incision through the skin and cricothyroid ligament and insertion of a small *tracheostomy tube* into the trachea (see clinical correlation [blue] box "Tracheostomy," later in this chapter). ○

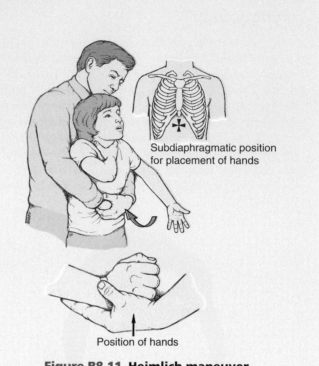

Subdiaphragmatic position for placement of hands

Position of hands

Figure B8.11. Heimlich maneuver.

Laryngeal Muscles. The laryngeal muscles are divided into extrinsic and intrinsic groups.

- **Extrinsic laryngeal muscles** (discussed earlier in this chapter) move the larynx as a whole (Table 8.3). The *infrahyoid muscles* are depressors of the hyoid and larynx, whereas the *suprahyoid muscles* (and the *stylopharyngeus,* a pharyngeal muscle, discussed later in this chapter) are elevators of the hyoid and larynx.

- **Intrinsic laryngeal muscles** move the laryngeal parts, altering the length and tension of the vocal folds and the size and shape of the rima glottidis (Fig. 8.31). All but one of the intrinsic muscles of the larynx are supplied by the *recurrent laryngeal nerve* (Figs. 8.32–8.34), a branch of CN X. The cricothyroid is supplied by the external laryngeal nerve, one of the two terminal branches of the *superior laryngeal nerve.*

The actions of the intrinsic laryngeal muscles are easiest to understand when they are considered as functional groups: adductors and abductors, sphincters, and tensors and relaxers. The intrinsic muscles are illustrated in situ in Figures 8.30 and 8.32; their attachments, innervation, and main actions are summarized in Table 8.5.

- *Adductors and abductors:* These muscles move the vocal folds to open and close the rima glottidis. The principal adductors are the **lateral cricoarytenoid muscles,** which

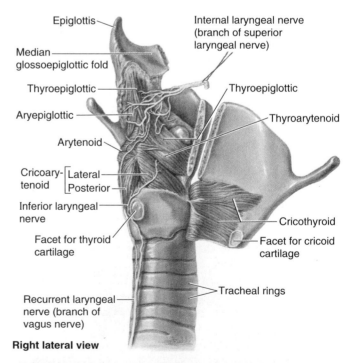

Epiglottis

Median glossoepiglottic fold

Thyroepiglottic

Aryepiglottic

Arytenoid

Cricoary-[Lateral
tenoid [Posterior

Inferior laryngeal nerve

Facet for thyroid cartilage

Internal laryngeal nerve (branch of superior laryngeal nerve)

Thyroepiglottic

Thyroarytenoid

Cricothyroid

Facet for cricoid cartilage

Tracheal rings

Recurrent laryngeal nerve (branch of vagus nerve)

Right lateral view

Figure 8.32. Muscles and nerves of larynx and cricothyroid joint. The thyroid cartilage is sawn through to the right of the median plane. The cricothyroid joint is disarticulated and the right lamina of the thyroid cartilage is turned anteriorly (like opening a book), stripping the cricothyroid muscles off the arch of the cricoid cartilage.

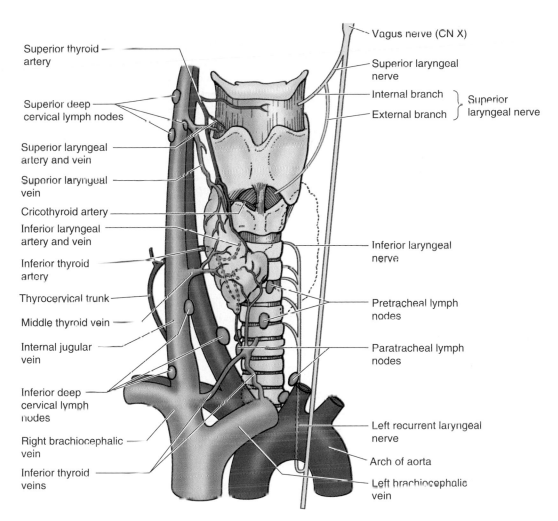

Figure 8.33. Vessels, nerves, and lymph nodes of larynx. The superior and inferior thyroid arteries give rise to the superior and inferior laryngeal arteries, respectively; they anastomose with each other. The laryngeal nerves are derived from the vagus (CN X) through the internal and external branches of the superior laryngeal nerve and the inferior laryngeal nerve from the recurrent laryngeal nerve. The left recurrent laryngeal nerve passes inferior to the arch of the aorta.

pull the muscular processes anteriorly, rotating the arytenoid cartilages so that their vocal processes swing medially. When this action is combined with that of the **transverse** and **oblique arytenoid muscles**, which pull the arytenoid cartilages together, air pushed through the rima glottidis causes vibrations of the vocal ligaments (phonation). When the vocal ligaments are adducted but the transverse arytenoid muscles do not act, the arytenoid cartilages remain apart and air may bypass the ligaments. This is the position of whispering, when the breath is modified into voice in the absence of tone. The sole abductors are the **posterior cricoarytenoid muscles**, which pull the muscular processes posteriorly, rotating the vocal processes laterally and thus widening the rima glottidis.

- *Sphincters:* The combined actions of most of the muscles of the laryngeal inlet result in a sphincteric action that closes the laryngeal inlet as a protective mechanism during swallowing. Contraction of the *lateral cricoarytenoids,*

transverse and *oblique arytenoids,* and *aryepiglottic muscles* brings the aryepiglottic folds together and pulls the arytenoid cartilages toward the epiglottis. This action occurs reflexively in response to the presence of liquid or particles approaching or within the laryngeal vestibule. It is perhaps our strongest reflex, diminishing only after loss of consciousness, as in drowning.

- *Tensors:* The principal tensors are the **cricothyroid muscles,** which tilt or pull the prominence or angle of the thyroid cartilage anteriorly and inferiorly toward the arch of the cricoid cartilage. This increases the distance between the thyroid prominence and the arytenoid cartilages. Because the anterior ends of the vocal ligaments attach to the posterior aspect of the prominence, the vocal ligaments elongate and tighten, raising the pitch of the voice.

- *Relaxers:* The principal muscles in this group are the **thyroarytenoid muscles,** which pull the arytenoid

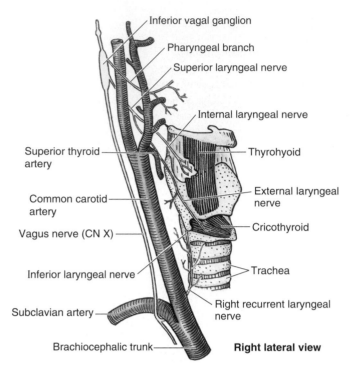

Inferior vagal ganglion
Pharyngeal branch
Superior laryngeal nerve
Internal laryngeal nerve
Superior thyroid artery
Thyrohyoid
Common carotid artery
External laryngeal nerve
Vagus nerve (CN X)
Cricothyroid
Inferior laryngeal nerve
Trachea
Subclavian artery
Right recurrent laryngeal nerve
Brachiocephalic trunk
Right lateral view

Figure 8.34. Laryngeal branches of right vagus nerve (CN X). The nerves of the larynx are the internal and external branches of the superior laryngeal nerve and the inferior laryngeal nerve from the recurrent laryngeal nerve. The right recurrent laryngeal nerve passes inferior to the right subclavian artery.

cartilages anteriorly, toward the thyroid angle (prominence), thereby relaxing the vocal ligaments to lower the pitch of the voice. The **vocalis muscles** lie medial to the thyroarytenoid muscles and lateral to the vocal ligaments within the vocal folds. Some authors consider them as the medial part of the thyroarytenoid muscles, but they are distinct in being formed of shorter, finer muscles fibers and extending only part of the length of the vocal ligaments. The vocalis muscles produce minute adjustments of the vocal ligaments, selectively tensing and relaxing the anterior and posterior parts, respectively, of the vocal folds during animated speech and singing.

Arteries of the Larynx. The laryngeal arteries, branches of the superior and inferior thyroid arteries, supply the larynx (Fig. 8.33). The **superior laryngeal artery** accompanies the internal branch of the superior laryngeal nerve through the thyrohyoid membrane and branches to supply the internal surface of the larynx. The **cricothyroid artery,** a small branch of the superior thyroid artery, supplies the cricothyroid muscle. The **inferior laryngeal artery,** a branch of the inferior thyroid artery, accompanies the *inferior laryngeal nerve* (terminal part of the recurrent laryngeal nerve) and supplies the mucous membrane and muscles in the inferior part of the larynx.

Veins of the Larynx. The laryngeal veins accompany the laryngeal arteries. The **superior laryngeal vein** usually joins the superior thyroid vein and through it drains into the IJV (Fig. 8.33). The **inferior laryngeal vein** joins the inferior thyroid vein or the venous plexus of veins on the anterior aspect of the trachea, which empties into the left brachiocephalic vein.

Lymphatics of the Larynx. The laryngeal lymphatic vessels superior to the vocal folds accompany the superior laryngeal artery through the thyrohyoid membrane and drain into the **superior deep cervical lymph nodes.** The lymphatic vessels inferior to the vocal folds drain into the *pretracheal* or *paratracheal lymph nodes,* which drain into the **inferior deep cervical lymph nodes.**

Nerves of the Larynx. The nerves of the larynx are the superior and inferior laryngeal branches of the vagus nerves (CN X). The **superior laryngeal nerve** arises from the **inferior vagal ganglion** at the superior end of the carotid triangle (Fig. 8.34). The nerve divides into two terminal branches within the carotid sheath: the internal laryngeal nerve (sensory and autonomic) and the external laryngeal nerve (motor). The **internal laryngeal nerve,** the larger of the terminal branches of the superior laryngeal nerve, pierces the thyrohyoid membrane with the superior laryngeal artery, supplying sensory fibers to the laryngeal mucous membrane of the laryngeal vestibule and middle laryngeal cavity, including the superior surface of the vocal folds. The **external laryngeal nerve,** the smaller terminal branch of the superior laryngeal nerve, descends posterior to the sternothyroid muscle in company with the superior thyroid artery. At first, the external laryngeal nerve lies on the inferior constrictor muscle of the pharynx; it then pierces the muscle, contributing to its innervation (with the pharyngeal plexus), and continues to supply the cricothyroid muscle.

The **inferior laryngeal nerve,** the continuation of the recurrent laryngeal nerve (a branch of the vagus nerve) enters the larynx by passing deep to the inferior border of the inferior constrictor muscle of the pharynx and medial to the lamina of the thyroid cartilage (Fig. 8.34). It divides into anterior and posterior branches, which accompany the inferior laryngeal artery into the larynx. The anterior branch supplies the lateral cricothyroid, thyroarytenoid, vocalis, aryepiglottic, and thyroepiglottic muscles. The posterior branch supplies the posterior cricoarytenoid and transverse and oblique arytenoid muscles. Because it supplies all the intrinsic muscles except the cricothyroid, it is the primary motor nerve of the larynx. However, it also provides sensory fibers to the mucosa of the infraglottic cavity.

Injury to the Laryngeal Nerves

Because the inferior laryngeal nerve, the continuation of the recurrent laryngeal nerve, innervates the muscles moving the vocal fold, paralysis of the vocal fold results when the nerve (or its parent nerve) is injured. The voice is poor initially because the paralyzed vocal fold cannot adduct to meet the normal vocal fold. ▶

Within weeks, the contralateral fold crosses the midline when its muscles act to compensate. When bilateral paralysis of the vocal folds occurs, the voice is almost absent because the vocal folds are motionless in a position that is slightly narrower than the usually neutral respiratory position. They cannot be adducted for phonation, nor can they be abducted for increased respiration, resulting in *stridor* (high pitched, noisy respiration) often accompanied by anxiety similar to that accompanying an asthmatic episode.

In progressive lesions of the recurrent laryngeal nerve, abduction of the vocal ligaments is lost before adduction; conversely, during recovery, adduction returns before abduction (Williams et al., 1995). Hoarseness is the common symptom of serious disorders of the larynx, such as carcinoma of the vocal folds. Paralysis of the superior laryngeal nerve causes anesthesia of the superior laryngeal mucosa. As a result, the protective mechanism designed to keep foreign bodies out of the larynx is inactive, and foreign bodies can easily enter the larynx.

Injury to the external branch of the superior laryngeal nerve results in a voice that is monotonous in character because the paralyzed cricothyroid muscle supplied by it is unable to vary the length and tension of the vocal fold (Table 8.5). Such an injury may be unnoticed in individuals who don't usually employ a wide range of tone in their speech, but it may be critical to singers or public speakers. To avoid injury to the external branch of the superior laryngeal nerve (e.g., during thyroidectomy), the superior thyroid artery is ligated and sectioned more superior to the gland, where it is not as closely related to the nerve. Because an enlarged thyroid gland (goiter) may itself cause impaired innervation of the larynx by compressing the laryngeal nerves, the vocal folds are examined by laryngoscopy before an operation in this area. In this way, damage to the larynx or its nerves resulting from a surgical mishap may be distinguished from a pre-existing injury resulting from nerve compression.

Superior Laryngeal Nerve Block

A superior laryngeal nerve block is often administered with endotracheal intubation in the conscious patient. This technique is used for peroral endoscopy, transesophageal echocardiography, and laryngeal and esophageal instru-mentation. The needle is inserted midway between the thyroid cartilage and the hyoid, 1–5 cm anterior to the greater horn of the hyoid. The needle passes through the thyrohyoid membrane, and the anesthetic agent bathes the internal laryngeal nerve, the larger terminal branch of the superior laryngeal nerve. Anesthesia of the laryngeal mucosa occurs superior to the vocal folds and includes the superior surface of these folds.

Cancer of the Larynx

The incidence of cancer of the larynx is high in individuals who smoke cigarettes or chew tobacco. Most persons present with persistent hoarseness (Scher and Richtsmeier, 1994), often associated with *otalgia* (earache) and dysphagia. Enlarged pretracheal or paratracheal lymph nodes may indicate the presence of laryngeal cancer. *Laryngectomy* (removal of the larynx) may be performed in severe cases of laryngeal cancer. Vocal rehabilitation can be accomplished by the use of an electrolarynx, a tracheoesophageal prosthesis, or esophageal speech (regurgitation of ingested air).

Age Changes in the Larynx

The larynx grows steadily until approximately 3 years of age, after which time little growth occurs until approximately 12 years of age. Before puberty, no major laryngeal sex differences exist. Owing to the presence of testosterone at puberty in males, the walls of the larynx strengthen and the laryngeal cavity enlarges. There is only a slight increase in the size of the larynx of most girls. In boys, all of the laryngeal cartilages enlarge, and the laryngeal prominence becomes conspicuous in most males. The anteroposterior diameter of the rima glottidis almost doubles its prepubescent measurement in males, the vocal folds lengthening and thickening proportionately and abruptly. This growth accounts for the voice changes that occur in males: The pitch typically becomes an octave lower. The pitch of the voice of *eunuchs*, males whose testes have not developed (agonadal males), does not become lower without administration of male hormones. The thyroid, cricoid, and most of the arytenoid cartilages often ossify as age advances, commencing at approximately 25 years of age in the thyroid cartilage. By 65 years of age, the cartilages are frequently visible in radiographs. ☉

Trachea

The **trachea**, extending from the larynx into the thorax, terminates inferiorly as it divides into right and left main bronchi. It transports air to and from the lungs, and its epithelium propels debris-laden mucus toward the pharynx for expulsion from the mouth. The trachea is a fibrocartilaginous tube, supported by incomplete cartilaginous **tracheal rings,** that occupies a median position in the neck (Fig. 8.32). The tracheal rings keep the trachea patent; they are deficient posteriorly where the trachea is adjacent to the esophagus. The posterior gap in the tracheal rings is spanned by the involuntary **trachealis muscle,** smooth muscle connecting the ends of the rings (Fig. 8.35). Hence the posterior wall of the trachea is flat.

In adults, the trachea is approximately 2.5 cm in diameter, whereas in infants it has the diameter of a pencil. The trachea

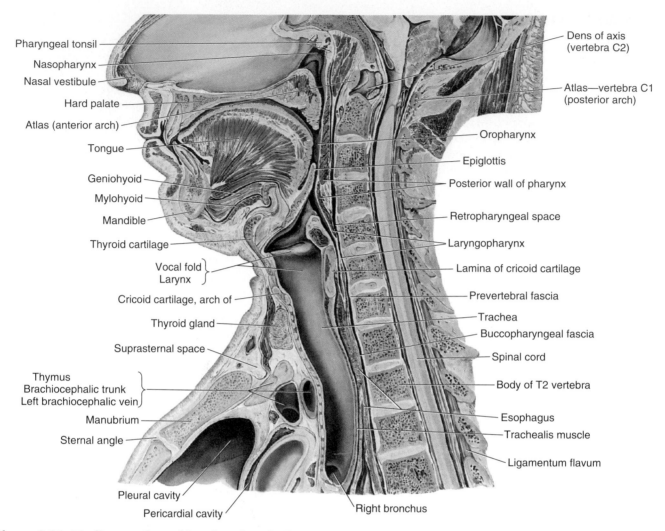

Pharyngeal tonsil

Nasopharynx

Nasal vestibule

Hard palate

Atlas (anterior arch)

Tongue

Geniohyoid

Mylohyoid

Mandible

Thyroid cartilage

Vocal fold
Larynx

Cricoid cartilage, arch of

Thyroid gland

Suprasternal space

Thymus
Brachiocephalic trunk
Left brachiocephalic vein

Manubrium

Sternal angle

Pleural cavity

Pericardial cavity

Dens of axis
(vertebra C2)

Atlas—vertebra C1
(posterior arch)

Oropharynx

Epiglottis

Posterior wall of pharynx

Retropharyngeal space

Laryngopharynx

Lamina of cricoid cartilage

Prevertebral fascia

Trachea

Buccopharyngeal fascia

Spinal cord

Body of T2 vertebra

Esophagus

Trachealis muscle

Ligamentum flavum

Right bronchus

Figure 8.35. Median section of head and neck. The pharynx extends from the cranial base to the level of the cricoid carti-lage (body of C6 vertebra or the C6–C7 IV disc, as shown here), where it is continuous with the esophagus.

extends from the inferior end of the larynx at the level of the C6 vertebra. It ends at the level of the sternal angle or the T4–T5 IV disc, where it divides into the right and left main bronchi (see Chapter 1). Lateral to the trachea are the common carotid arteries and the thyroid lobes (Fig. 8.23). Inferior to the isthmus of the thyroid gland are the jugular venous arch and the inferior thyroid veins. The brachiocephalic trunk is related to the right side of the trachea in the root of the neck. Deviation of the trachea from the midline, apparent superficially or radiographically, often signals the presence of a pathological process. Tracheal trauma often affects the closely adherent esophagus.

Tracheostomy

A transverse incision through the skin of the neck and anterior wall of the trachea (*tracheostomy*) establishes an airway in patients with upper airway obstruction or respiratory failure (Fig. B8.12). The infrahyoid muscles are retracted laterally, and the isthmus of the thyroid gland is either divided or retracted superiorly. An opening is made in the trachea between the first and second tracheal rings or through the second through fourth tracheal rings. A *tracheostomy tube* is then inserted into the trachea and secured. To avoid complications during a tracheostomy, the following anatomical relationships are important:

• The *inferior thyroid veins* arise from a venous plexus on the thyroid gland and descend anterior to the trachea.

• A small *thyroid ima artery* is present in approximately 10% of people; it ascends from the brachiocephalic ▶

Deep cervical fascia

Tracheostomy tube

Pretracheal fascia

Esophagus

Incision in trachea after retracting infrahyoid muscles and incising isthmus of thyroid

2nd and 4th tracheal rings

Figure B8.12

trunk or the arch of the aorta to the isthmus of the thyroid gland.

- The *left brachiocephalic vein,* jugular venous arch, and pleurae may be encountered, particularly in infants and children.

- The *thymus* covers the inferior part of the trachea in infants and children.

- The trachea is small, mobile, and soft in infants, making it easy to cut through its posterior wall and damage the esophagus. ✪

THE BOTTOM LINE: The larynx is the superior end of the lower respiratory tract, modified to regulate entry into or close off the lower respiratory tract. The larynx also modifies the exit of air from the tract to produce tone for vocalization. With the diaphragm, it regulates intra-abdominal pressure through air retention and the force and suddenness by which air exits the tract (e.g., exhaling verses coughing or sneezing). The larynx consists of a cartilaginous articulating skeleton joined by ligaments, membranes, and muscles, lined with mucous membrane. All the laryngeal muscles except one (posterior cricoarytenoid) participate in closure of the rima glottidis. Active opening of the rima is required only during deep inspiration. Otherwise, opening occurs passively by the tidal flow of air, with the other muscles controlling the amount and nature of resistance provided at the rima glottidis to produce tone and to control its pitch. In addition to intrinsically produced movements between its components, extrinsic musculature (the hyoid muscles) can move the entire larynx for swallowing and to modify pitch further.

The internal laryngeal nerve, a branch of the superior laryngeal nerve, is the sensory nerve of the larynx. The recurrent laryngeal nerve (via its terminal branch, the inferior laryngeal nerve) is the motor nerve, which supplies all muscles of the larynx, with one exception. The external laryngeal nerve, a smaller branch of the superior laryngeal nerve, supplies the cricothyroid muscle.

The trachea is the median fibrocartilaginous tube extending between the cricoid cartilage at the C6 vertebral level and its bifurcation into main bronchi at the T4–T5 IV disc level (level of sternal angle).

Alimentary Layer of the Cervical Viscera

In the **alimentary layer,** cervical viscera take part in the digestive functions of the body. Although the pharynx conducts air to the larynx, trachea, and lungs, its constrictor muscles direct (and the *epiglottis* deflects) food to the esophagus. The esophagus, also involved in food propulsion, is the beginning of the *alimentary canal* (digestive tract).

Pharynx

The **pharynx** is the superior expanded part of the alimentary system posterior to the nasal and oral cavities, extending

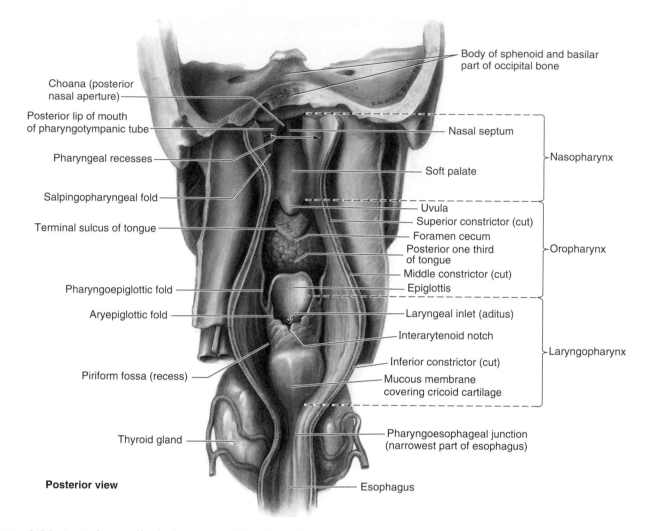

Figure 8.36. Anterior wall of pharynx. In this dissection, the posterior wall has been incised along the midline and spread apart. Openings in the anterior wall communicate with the nasal, oral, and laryngeal cavities. On each side of the laryngeal inlet, separated from it by the aryepiglottic fold, a piriform fossa (recess) is formed by the invagination of the larynx into the anterior wall of the laryngopharynx.

inferiorly past the larynx (Figs. 8.35 and 8.36). The pharynx extends from the cranial base to the inferior border of the cricoid cartilage anteriorly and the inferior border of the C6 vertebra posteriorly. The pharynx is widest (approximately 5 cm) opposite the hyoid and narrowest (approximately 1.5 cm) at its inferior end, where it is continuous with the esophagus. The flat posterior wall of the pharynx lies against the prevertebral layer of deep cervical fascia.

Interior of the Pharynx. The pharynx is divided into three parts (Figs. 8.35 and 8.36):

* *Nasopharynx:* posterior to the nose and superior to the soft palate.

* *Oropharynx:* posterior to the mouth.

* *Laryngopharynx:* posterior to the larynx.

The **nasopharynx** has a respiratory function. It lies superior to the *soft palate* and is the posterior extension of the nasal cavities (Figs. 8.35–8.37). The nose opens into the nasopharynx through two **choanae** (paired openings between the nasal cavity and nasopharynx). The roof and posterior wall of the nasopharynx form a continuous surface that lies inferior to the body of the sphenoid bone and the basilar part of the occipital bone (Fig. 8.36).

The abundant lymphoid tissue in the pharynx forms an incomplete *tonsillar ring* around the superior part of the pharynx (discussed later in this chapter). The lymphoid tissue is aggregated in certain regions to form masses called *tonsils.* The **pharyngeal tonsil** (commonly called the adenoids when enlarged) is in the mucous membrane of the roof and posterior wall of the nasopharynx (Figs. 8.35 and 8.37). Extending inferiorly from the medial end of the pharyngotympanic tube is a vertical fold of mucous membrane, the **salpingopharyngeal fold** (Figs. 8.36 and 8.37). It covers the salpingopharyngeus muscle, which opens the pharyngeal orifice of the pharyngotympanic tube during swallowing. The collection of

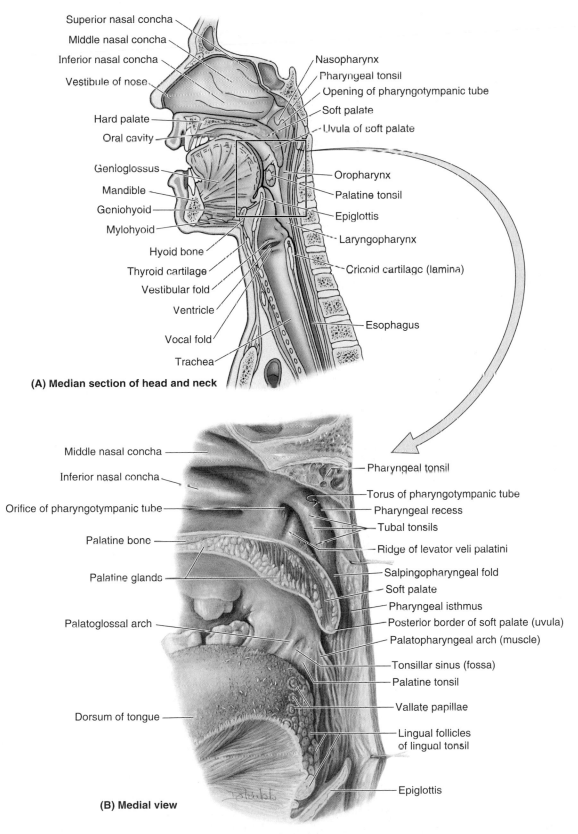

Superior nasal concha
Middle nasal concha
Inferior nasal concha
Vestibule of nose
Hard palate
Oral cavity
Genioglossus
Mandible
Geniohyoid
Mylohyoid
Hyoid bone
Thyroid cartilage
Vestibular fold
Ventricle
Vocal fold
Trachea

Nasopharynx
Pharyngeal tonsil
Opening of pharyngotympanic tube
Soft palate
Uvula of soft palate
Oropharynx
Palatine tonsil
Epiglottis
Laryngopharynx
Cricoid cartilage (lamina)
Esophagus

(A) Median section of head and neck

Middle nasal concha
Inferior nasal concha
Orifice of pharyngotympanic tube
Palatine bone
Palatine glands
Palatoglossal arch
Dorsum of tongue

Pharyngeal tonsil
Torus of pharyngotympanic tube
Pharyngeal recess
Tubal tonsils
Ridge of levator veli palatini
Salpingopharyngeal fold
Soft palate
Pharyngeal isthmus
Posterior border of soft palate (uvula)
Palatopharyngeal arch (muscle)
Tonsillar sinus (fossa)
Palatine tonsil
Vallate papillae
Lingual follicles of lingual tonsil
Epiglottis

(B) Medial view

Figure 8.37. Internal aspect of lateral wall of pharynx. A. The upper respiratory passages and alimentary canal in the right half of a bisected head and neck are shown. The *square* indicates the location of the section shown in part **B. B.** A closer view of the nasopharynx and oropharynx, which are separated anteriorly by the soft palate, is provided. The posterior border of the soft palate forms the anterior margin of the pharyngeal isthmus through which the two spaces communicate posteriorly.

lymphoid tissue in the submucosa of the pharynx near the pharyngeal orifice of the pharyngotympanic tube is the **tubal tonsil** (Fig. 8.37). Posterior to the **torus of the pharyngotympanic tube** and the salpingopharyngeal fold is a slit-like lateral projection of the pharynx, the **pharyngeal recess**, which extends laterally and posteriorly.

The **oropharynx** has a digestive function. It is bounded by the soft palate superiorly, the base of the tongue inferiorly, and the palatoglossal and palatopharyngeal arches laterally (Figs. 8.37 and 8.38*A*). It extends from the soft palate to the superior border of the epiglottis. **Deglutition** (swallowing) is the complex process that transfers a food bolus from the mouth through the pharynx and esophagus into the stomach. Solid food is masticated (chewed) and mixed with saliva to form a soft bolus that is easier to swallow. Deglutition occurs in three stages:

- **Stage 1:** voluntary; the bolus is compressed against the palate and pushed from the mouth into the oropharynx, mainly by movements of the muscles of the tongue and soft palate (Fig. 8.39*A* & *B*).

- **Stage 2:** involuntary and rapid; the soft palate is elevated, sealing off the nasopharynx from the oropharynx and laryngopharynx (Fig. 8.39*C*). The pharynx widens and shortens to receive the bolus of food as the suprahyoid muscles and longitudinal pharyngeal muscles contract, elevating the larynx.

- **Stage 3:** involuntary; sequential contraction of all three constrictor muscles forces the food bolus inferiorly into the esophagus (Fig. 8.39*D*).

The **palatine tonsils** are collections of lymphoid tissue on each side of the oropharynx in the interval between the palatine arches (Figs. 8.37 and 8.38*A*). The tonsil does not fill the **tonsillar sinus** between the palatoglossal and palatopharyngeal arches in adults. The **tonsillar bed,** in which the palatine tonsil lies, is between these arches (Fig. 8.38*B*). The ton-

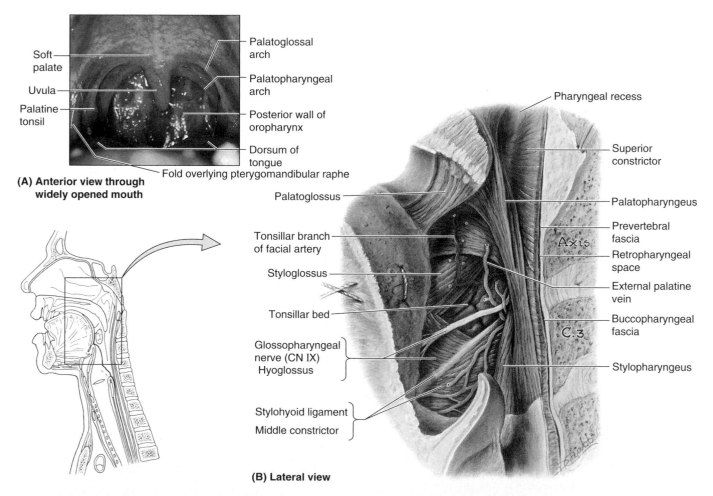

(A) Anterior view through widely opened mouth

Soft palate
Uvula
Palatine tonsil
Palatoglossal arch
Palatopharyngeal arch
Posterior wall of oropharynx
Dorsum of tongue
Fold overlying pterygomandibular raphe

(B) Lateral view

Palatoglossus
Tonsillar branch of facial artery
Styloglossus
Tonsillar bed
Glossopharyngeal nerve (CN IX)
Hyoglossus
Stylohyoid ligament
Middle constrictor

Pharyngeal recess
Superior constrictor
Palatopharyngeus
Prevertebral fascia
Retropharyngeal space
External palatine vein
Buccopharyngeal fascia
Stylopharyngeus
Axis
C.3

Figure 8.38. Oral cavity and tonsillar bed. A. The oral cavity and palatine tonsils with the mouth wide open and the tongue protruding as far as possible. The uvula is a muscular projection from the posterior edge of the soft palate. (Courtesy of Dr. B. Liebgott, Professor, Division of Anatomy, Department of Surgery, University of Toronto, Ontario, Canada.) **B.** In this deep dissection of the tonsillar bed, the palatine tonsil has been removed. The tongue is pulled anteriorly, and the inferior (lingual) attachment of the superior constrictor muscle is cut away.

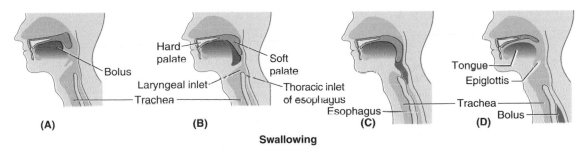

Swallowing

Figure 8.39. Swallowing. A. The bolus of food is squeezed to the back of the mouth by pushing the tongue against the palate. **B.** The nasopharynx is sealed off and the larynx is elevated, enlarging the pharynx to receive food. **C.** The pharyngeal sphincters contract sequentially, squeezing food into the esophagus. The epiglottis deflects the bolus from but does not close the inlet to the larynx and trachea. **D.** The bolus of food moves down the esophagus by peristaltic contractions.

sillar bed is formed by the superior constrictor of the pharynx and the thin, fibrous sheet of **pharyngobasilar fascia** (Fig. 8.40). This fascia blends with the periosteum of the cranial base and defines the limits of the pharyngeal wall in its superior part.

The **laryngopharynx** (hypopharynx) lies posterior to the larynx (Figs. 8.35 and 8.37), extending from the superior border of the epiglottis and the pharyngoepiglottic folds to the inferior border of the cricoid cartilage, where it narrows and becomes continuous with the esophagus. Posteriorly,

(A) Posterior view

Figure 8.40. Pharynx and cranial nerves. A. This dissection shows the posterior aspect of the pharynx and associated structures. The buccopharyngeal fascia has been removed. Of the three pharyngeal constrictor muscles, the inferior muscle overlaps the middle one and the middle one overlaps the superior one. All three muscles form a common median pharyngeal raphe posteriorly.

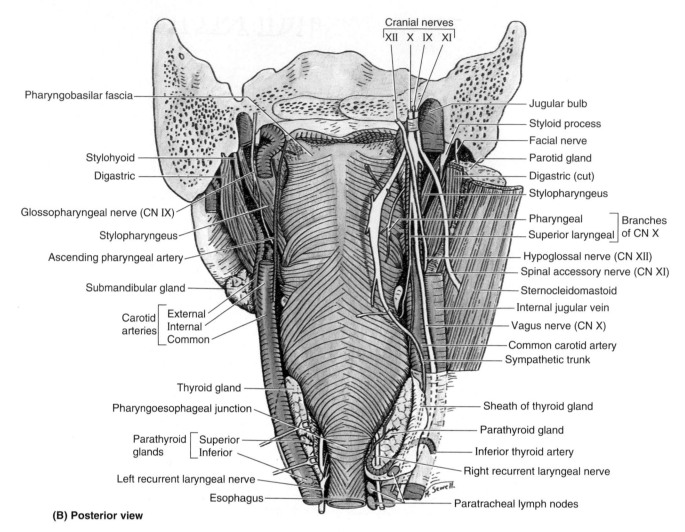

Cranial nerves
XII X IX XI

Pharyngobasilar fascia

Stylohyoid

Digastric

Glossopharyngeal nerve (CN IX)

Stylopharyngeus

Ascending pharyngeal artery

Submandibular gland

Carotid arteries — External
Internal
Common

Thyroid gland

Pharyngoesophageal junction

Parathyroid glands — Superior
Inferior

Left recurrent laryngeal nerve

Esophagus

Jugular bulb

Styloid process

Facial nerve

Parotid gland

Digastric (cut)

Stylopharyngeus

Pharyngeal — Branches
Superior laryngeal — of CN X

Hypoglossal nerve (CN XII)

Spinal accessory nerve (CN XI)

Sternocleidomastoid

Internal jugular vein

Vagus nerve (CN X)

Common carotid artery

Sympathetic trunk

Sheath of thyroid gland

Parathyroid gland

Inferior thyroid artery

Right recurrent laryngeal nerve

Paratracheal lymph nodes

(B) Posterior view

Figure 8.40. *(Continued)* **B.** The narrowest and least distensible part of the alimentary tract is the pharyngoesophageal junction, where the laryngopharynx becomes the esophagus.

the laryngopharynx is related to the bodies of the C4–C6 vertebrae. Its posterior and lateral walls are formed by the **middle** and **inferior constrictor muscles** (Fig. 8.40*A*). Internally the wall is formed by the *palatopharyngeus* and *stylopharyngeus muscles*. The laryngopharynx communicates with the larynx through the *laryngeal inlet* on its anterior wall (Fig. 8.36).

The **piriform fossa** (**recess**) is a small depression of the laryngopharyngeal cavity on either side of the laryngeal inlet. This mucosa-lined recess is separated from the laryngeal inlet by the *aryepiglottic fold*. Laterally, the piriform fossa is bounded by the medial surfaces of the thyroid cartilage and the *thyrohyoid membrane*. Branches of the internal laryngeal and recurrent laryngeal nerves lie deep to the mucous membrane of the piriform fossa and are vulnerable to injury when a foreign body lodges in the recess.

Pharyngeal Muscles. The wall of the pharynx is exceptional for the **alimentary canal,** having a muscular layer composed entirely of voluntary muscle arranged mainly into an external circular and an internal longitudinal layer of muscles.

In most of the canal, the muscular layer consists of smooth muscle opposite in its arrangement. The external circular layer of pharyngeal muscles consists of three **pharyngeal constrictors: superior, middle,** and **inferior** (Figs. 8.38 and 8.40). The internal, mainly longitudinal layer of muscles consists of the **palatopharyngeus, stylopharyngeus,** and **salpingopharyngeus.** These muscles elevate the larynx and shorten the pharynx during swallowing and speaking. The attachments, nerve supply, and actions of the pharyngeal muscles are described in Table 8.6.

The pharyngeal constrictors have a strong internal fascial lining, the *pharyngobasilar fascia* (Fig. 8.40*B*), and a thin external fascial lining, the *buccopharyngeal fascia.* Inferiorly, the buccopharyngeal fascia blends with the pretracheal layer of the *deep cervical fascia.* The pharyngeal constrictors contract involuntarily so that contraction takes place sequentially from the superior to the inferior end of the pharynx, propelling food into the esophagus. All three constrictors are supplied by the pharyngeal plexus of nerves that is formed by pharyngeal branches of the vagus and glossopharyngeal nerves and by

Table 8.6. Muscles of the Pharynx

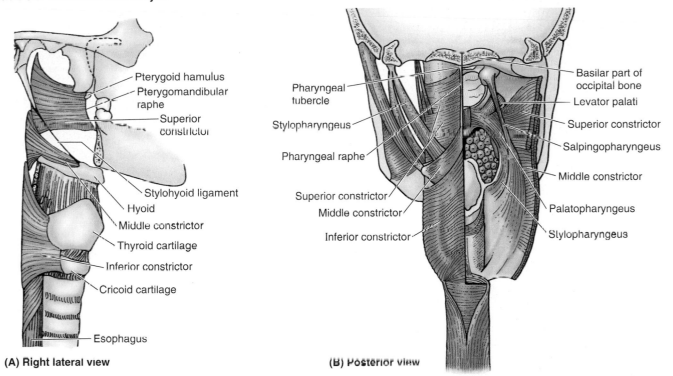

(A) Right lateral view

(B) Posterior view

Muscle	Origin	Insertion	Innervation	Main Action(s)
External layer				
Superior constrictor	Pterygoid hamulus, pterygomandibular raphe; posterior end of mylohyoid line of mandible and side of tongue	Pharyngeal tubercle on basilar part of occipital bone	Pharyngeal branch of vagus (CN X) and pharyngeal plexus	Constrict walls of pharynx during swallowing
Middle constrictor	Stylohyoid ligament and greater and lesser horns of hyoid	Pharyngeal raphe	Pharyngeal branch of vagus (CN X) and pharyngeal plexus, plus branches of external and recurrent laryngeal nerves of vagus	
Inferior constrictor	Oblique line of thyroid cartilage and side of cricoid cartilage	Cricopharyngeal part encircles pharyngo-esophageal junction without forming a raphe		
Internal layer				
Palatopharyngeus	Hard palate and palatine aponeurosis	Posterior border of lamina of thyroid cartilage and side of pharynx and esophagus	Pharyngeal branch of vagus (CN X) and pharyngeal plexus	Elevate (shorten and widen) pharynx and larynx during swallowing and speaking
Salpingopharyngeus	Cartilaginous part of pharyngotympanic tube	Blends with palatopharyngeus		
Stylopharyngeus	Styloid process of temporal bone	Posterior and superior borders of thyroid cartilage with palatopharyngeus	Glossopharyngeal nerve (CN IX)	

(A)

(B)

(C)

Key

- ☐ Occipital
- ☐ Retroauricular (mastoid)
- ☐ Parotid
- ☐ Buccal
- ■ Submental
- ☐ Submandibular
- ☐ Jugulo-omohyoid
- ☐ Superficial cervical
- ☐ Deep cervical
- ■ Retropharyngeal
- ☐ Jugulodigastric
- ☐ Infrahyoid
- **A** Pharyngeal tonsil
- **P** Palatine tonsil

Thyroid gland

Right internal jugular vein

Left internal jugular vein

Jugular lymphatic trunk

Right lymphatic duct

Right venous angle

Thoracic duct

Left venous angle

Left brachiocephalic vein

Key

- ☐ Superior deep cervical
- ■ Inferior deep cervical
- ☐ Prelaryngeal
- ■ Paratracheal
- ■ Pretracheal

Figure 8.41. Lymphatic drainage of head and neck. The pathways of the superficial (**A**) and deep (**B**) lymphatic drainages are shown. **C.** The lymph nodes, lymphatic trunks, and thoracic duct are shown.

sympathetic branches from the superior cervical ganglion (Fig. 8.40*A;* Table 8.6). The pharyngeal plexus lies on the lateral wall of the pharynx, mainly on the middle constrictor. The overlapping of the constrictor muscles leaves four gaps in the musculature for structures to enter or leave the pharynx:

1. Superior to the superior constrictor, the levator veli palatini, pharyngotympanic tube, and ascending palatine artery pass through a *gap between the superior constrictor and the cranium.* It is here that the pharyngobasilar fascia blends with the buccopharyngeal fascia to form, with the mucous membrane, the thin wall of the pharyngeal recess (Fig. 8.36).

2. A *gap between the superior and middle constrictors* forms a passageway that allows the stylopharyngeus, glossopharyngeal nerve, and stylohyoid ligament to pass to the internal aspect of the pharyngeal wall.

3. A *gap between the middle and inferior constrictors* allows the internal laryngeal nerve and superior laryngeal artery and vein to pass to the larynx.

4. A *gap inferior to the inferior constrictor* allows the recurrent laryngeal nerve and inferior laryngeal artery to pass superiorly into the larynx.

Vessels of the Pharynx. A branch of the facial artery, the **tonsillar artery** (Fig. 8.38*B*) passes through the superior constrictor muscle and enters the inferior pole of the tonsil. The tonsil also receives arterial twigs from the ascending palatine, lingual, descending palatine, and ascending pharyngeal arteries. The large **external palatine vein** (paratonsillar vein) descends from the soft palate and passes close to the lateral surface of the tonsil before it enters the pharyngeal venous plexus.

The **tonsillar lymphatic vessels** pass laterally and inferiorly to the lymph nodes near the angle of the mandible and the **jugulodigastric node,** referred to as the *tonsillar node* because of its frequent enlargement when the tonsil is inflamed (*tonsillitis*) (Fig. 8.41). The palatine, lingual, and pharyngeal tonsils form the pharyngeal **tonsillar ring** (of Waldeyer), an incomplete circular band of lymphoid tissue around the superior part of the pharynx (Fig. 8.42). The anteroinferior part of the ring is formed by the *lingual tonsil* in the posterior part of the tongue. Lateral parts of the ring are formed by the palatine and tubal tonsils, and posterior and superior parts are formed by the pharyngeal tonsil.

Pharyngeal Nerves. The nerve supply to the pharynx (motor and most of sensory) derives from the **pharyngeal plexus of nerves** (Fig. 8.40). Motor fibers in the plexus are derived from the vagus nerve (CN X) via its pharyngeal branch or branches. They supply all muscles of the pharynx and soft palate, except the stylopharyngeus (supplied by CN IX) and the tensor veli palatini (supplied by CN V$_3$). The inferior pharyngeal constrictor also receives some motor fibers from the external and recurrent laryngeal branches of the vagus. Sensory fibers in the plexus are derived from the glossopharyngeal nerve. They supply most of the mucosa of all three

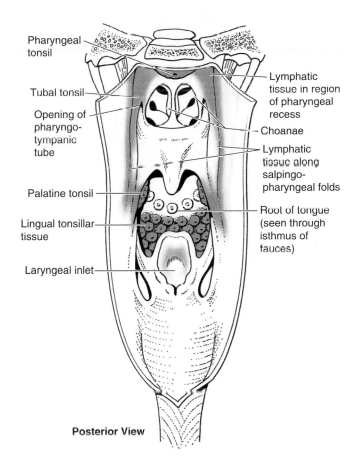

Figure 8.42. Lymphoid tissue in tongue and pharynx. The tonsillar ring (*pink*) around the superior pharynx is formed of the pharyngeal, tubal, palatine, and lingual tonsils.

parts of the pharynx. The sensory nerve supply of the mucous membrane of the anterior and superior nasopharynx is mainly from the maxillary nerve (CN V$_2$). The **tonsillar nerves** are derived from the *tonsillar plexus of nerves* formed by branches of the glossopharyngeal and vagus nerves. Other branches are derived from the pharyngeal plexus of nerves (Fig. 8.40*B*).

Foreign Bodies in the Laryngopharynx

When food passes through the laryngopharynx during swallowing, some of it enters the piriform fossae. Foreign bodies (e.g., a chicken bone or fishbone) entering the pharynx may lodge in this recess. If the object is sharp, it may pierce the mucous membrane and injure the internal laryngeal nerve. The superior laryngeal nerve and its internal laryngeal branch are also vulnerable to injury during removal of the object if the instrument used to remove the foreign body accidentally pierces the mucous membrane. Injury to these nerves may result in anesthesia of the laryngeal mucous ▶

membrane as far inferiorly as the vocal folds. Young children swallow a variety of objects, most of which reach the stomach and pass through the alimentary tract without difficulty. In some cases, the foreign body stops at the inferior end of the laryngopharynx, its narrowest part. A medical image such as a radiograph or a CT scan will reveal the presence of a radiopaque foreign body. Foreign bodies in the pharynx are often removed under direct vision through a pharyngoscope.

Sinus Tract from the Piriform Recess

Although uncommon, a sinus tract may pass from the piriform fossa to the thyroid gland, becoming a potential site for recurring thyroiditis (inflammation of the thyroid gland). This sinus tract apparently develops from a remnant of the thyroglossal duct that adheres to the developing laryngopharynx. Removal of this sinus tract essentially involves a partial thyroidectomy because the piriform fossa lies deep to the superior pole of the gland (Scher and Richtsmeier, 1994).

Tonsillectomy

Tonsillectomy (removal of the tonsils) is performed by dissecting the palatine tonsil from the tonsillar bed or by a guillotine or snare operation. Each procedure involves removal of the tonsil and the fascial sheet covering the tonsillar bed (Fig. B8.13). Because of the rich blood supply of the tonsil, bleeding commonly arises from the large *external palatine vein* (Fig. 8.38B) or, less commonly, from the tonsillar artery or other arterial twigs. The glossopharyngeal nerve (CN IX) accompanies the tonsillar artery on the lateral wall of the pharynx. Because this wall is thin, the nerve is vulnerable to injury. The internal carotid artery is especially vulnerable when it is tortuous and lies directly lateral to the tonsil.

Adenoiditis

Inflammation of the pharyngeal tonsils (adenoids) is called *adenoiditis.* This condition can obstruct the passage of air from the nasal cavities through the choanae into the nasopharynx, making mouth breathing necessary. Infection from the enlarged pharyngeal tonsils may spread to the tubal tonsils, causing swelling and closure of the pharyngotympanic tubes. Impairment of hearing may result from nasal obstruction and blockage of the pharyngotympanic tubes. Infection spreading from the nasopharynx to the middle ear causes *otitis media* (middle ear infection), which may produce temporary or permanent hearing loss. Sometimes the palatine and pharyngeal tonsils are removed during the same operation (tonsillectomy and adenoidectomy; T & A).

Membranous lateral wall of pharyngotympanic tube

Tensor veli palatini

Cartilage of pharyngotympanic tube

Levator veli palatini

Salpingopharyngeus

Tonsillar branch of ascending palatine artery

Tonsillar branch of facial artery

Ligature retracting palatine tonsil

Figure B8.13

Branchial Fistula

A branchial fistula is an abnormal canal that opens internally into the tonsillar cleft and externally on the side of the neck (Fig. B8.14A). This uncommon cervical canal results from persistence of remnants of the 2nd pharyngeal pouch and 2nd pharyngeal groove (Moore and Persaud, 2003). The fistula ascends from its cervical opening, ▶

Figure B8.14

usually along the anterior border of the SCM in the inferior third of the neck, through the subcutaneous tissue, platysma, and fascia of the neck to enter the carotid sheath. It then passes between the internal and the external carotid arteries on its way to its opening in the tonsillar cleft. Its course can be demonstrated by radiography (Fig. B8.14*B*).

Branchial Sinuses and Cysts

When the embryonic cervical sinus fails to disappear, it may retain its connection with the lateral surface of the neck by a *branchial sinus,* a narrow canal. The opening of the sinus may be anywhere along the anterior border of the SCM (Fig. B8.15). If the remnant of the cervical sinus is not connected with the surface, it may form a branchial cyst (lateral cervical cyst), usually located just inferior to the angle of the mandible. Although these cysts may be present in infants and children, they may not enlarge and become visible until early adulthood. The sinus and cyst are usually excised. ⊕

Figure B8.15

Esophagus

The **esophagus** is a muscular tube that is continuous with the laryngopharynx at the **pharyngoesophageal junction** (Figs. 8.35 and 8.40). The esophagus consists of striated (voluntary) muscle in its upper third, smooth (involuntary) muscle in its lower third, and a mixture of striated and smooth muscle in between. Its first part, the **cervical esophagus,** is part of the voluntary upper third. It begins immediately posterior to, and at

the level of, the inferior border of the cricoid cartilage in the median plane. This is the level of the C6 vertebra. Externally, the pharyngoesophageal junction appears as a constriction produced by the **cricopharyngeal part of the inferior constrictor muscle** (the superior esophageal sphincter) and is the narrowest part of the esophagus (Figs. 8.36 and 8.40). The cervical esophagus inclines slightly to the left as it descends and enters the superior mediastinum, becoming the thoracic esophagus.

When the esophagus is empty, it has a slit-like lumen. When a food bolus descends in it, the lumen expands, eliciting reflex peristalsis in the inferior two thirds of the esophagus. The cervical esophagus lies between the trachea and the cervical vertebral column (Figs. 8.35 and 8.37*A*). The *recurrent laryngeal nerve* lies in the tracheoesophageal groove on each side of the esophagus (Fig. 8.40). On the right of the esophagus is the right lobe of the *thyroid gland* and the right *carotid sheath* and its contents. The esophagus is in contact with the cervical pleura at the root of the neck. On the left is the left lobe of the thyroid gland and the left carotid sheath. The thoracic duct adheres to the left side of the esophagus and lies between the pleura and the esophagus. For details concerning the thoracic and abdominal regions of the esophagus, see Chapters 1 and 2.

Vessels of the Cervical Esophagus. The arteries to the cervical esophagus are branches of the *inferior thyroid arteries.* Each artery gives off ascending and descending branches that anastomose with each other and across the midline. Veins from the cervical esophagus are tributaries of the *inferior thyroid veins.* Lymphatic vessels of the cervical part of the esophagus drain into the *paratracheal lymph nodes* and *inferior deep cervical lymph nodes* (Fig. 8.41).

Nerves of the Cervical Esophagus. The nerve supply to the esophagus is somatic motor and sensory to the upper half and parasympathetic (vagal) sympathetic and visceral sensory to the lower half. The cervical esophagus receives somatic fibers via branches from the *recurrent laryngeal nerves* and vasomotor fibers from the *cervical sympathetic trunks* through the plexus around the inferior thyroid artery (Fig. 8.40).

Esophageal Injuries

Esophageal injuries are the rarest kinds of penetrating neck trauma, but they cause most complications following a surgical procedure or other treatment. Most esophageal injuries occur in conjunction with an airway injury because the airway lies anterior to the esophagus and provides some protection to it. Esophageal injuries are often occult (hidden), which makes the injury difficult to detect, especially when it is isolated. Unrecognized esophageal perforation causes death in nearly all patients who do not have surgery and in approximately 50% of those who do (Sinkinson, 1991).

Tracheoesophageal Fistula

The most common congenital anomaly of the esophagus is *tracheoesophageal fistula* (TEF). Usually, it is combined with some form of esophageal atresia. In the most common type of TEF (approximately 90% of cases), the superior part of the esophagus ends in a blind pouch and the inferior part communicates with the trachea (Fig. B8.16*A*). In these cases, the pouch fills with mucus, which the infant aspirates. In some cases, the superior esophagus communicates with the trachea and the inferior esophagus joins the stomach (Fig. B8.16*B*), but sometimes it does not, ▶

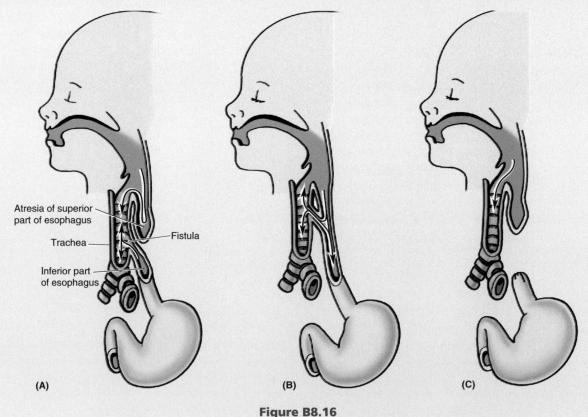

Atresia of superior part of esophagus

Trachea — Fistula

Inferior part of esophagus

(A)   (B)   (C)

Figure B8.16

producing TEF with esophageal atresia (Fig B8.16C). TEFs result from abnormalities in partitioning of the esophagus and trachea by the tracheoesophageal septum.

Esophageal Cancer

The most common presenting complaint of cancer of the esophagus is dysphagia, which is not usually recognized until the lumen is reduced by 30–50%. *Esophagoscopy* is a common diagnostic tool for observing these cancers. Painful swallowing in some patients suggests extension of the tumor to periesophageal tissues. Enlargement of the inferior deep cervical lymph nodes also suggests esophageal cancer. Compression of the recurrent laryngeal nerves by an esophageal tumor produces hoarseness.

Zones of Penetrating Neck Trauma

Three zones are common clinical guides to the seriousness of neck trauma (Fig. B8.17). The zones give physicians an understanding of the structures that are at risk with penetrating neck injuries.

- **Zone I:** includes the root of the neck and extends from the clavicles and the manubrium to the level of the inferior border of the cricoid cartilage. Structures at risk are the cervical pleurae, apices of lungs, thyroid and parathyroid glands, trachea, esophagus, common carotid arteries, jugular veins, and the cervical region of the vertebral column.

- **Zone II:** extends from the cricoid cartilage to the level of the angles of the mandible. Structures at risk are the superior poles of the thyroid gland, thyroid and cricoid cartilages, larynx, laryngopharynx, carotid arteries, jugular veins, esophagus, and cervical region of the vertebral column.

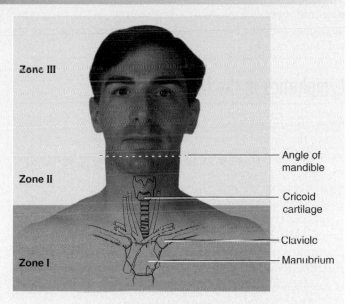

Figure B8.17

- **Zone III:** occurs at the angles of the mandibles superiorly. Structures at risk are the salivary glands, oral and nasal cavities, oropharynx, and nasopharynx.

Injuries in zones I and III obstruct the airway and have the greatest risk for **morbidity** (complications following surgical procedures and other treatments) and **mortality** (a fatal outcome) because the injured structures are difficult to visualize and repair and vascular damage is difficult to control. Injuries in zone II are most common; however, morbidity and mortality are lower because physicians can control vascular damage by direct pressure and surgeons can visualize and treat injured structures more easily than they can in zones I and III. ⊕

THE BOTTOM LINE: Although generally considered part of the alimentary tract, the pharynx is shared with the respiratory system. The superior, non-collapsible nasopharynx is exclusively respiratory, and the air and food pathways cross within the oropharynx and laryngopharynx. The contractile pharynx is unique within the alimentary tract in being constructed of voluntary muscle with the circular layer (pharyngeal constrictors) external to the longitudinal layer. Its flat posterior wall, abutting the musculoskeletal neck at the retropharyngeal space, is without openings; however, its anterior wall includes openings to the nose, mouth, and larynx. These openings determine the three segments of the pharynx. The soft palate serves as a flap valve regulating access to or from the nasopharynx and oropharynx, whereas the larynx is the "valve" ultimately separating food and air before they enter the esophagus and trachea, respectively

The superior two openings of the pharynx, which connect to the external environment, are encircled by a ring of lymphoid (tonsillar) tissue. Gaps in the submucosal lateral wall, between attachments of the constrictor muscles, permit the passage of slip-like longitudinal muscles and neurovascular elements. Innervation is from the pharyngeal nerve plexus, with the vagus providing motor fibers and the glossopharyngeal providing sensory fibers.

At the level of the cricoid cartilage (C6 vertebral level), a relatively abrupt change is made to the muscular pattern more typical of the alimentary tract. The cricopharyngeal part of the inferior pharyngeal constrictor, the most inferior part of the external circular layer, forms the superior esophageal sphincter. Immediately inferior, as the outer muscular layer becomes longitudinal, the esophagus begins. Also at approximately this point, sensory and motor innervation is transferred to the recurrent laryngeal nerves. The cervical esophagus is composed of voluntary muscle.

Lymphatics in the Neck

Most superficial tissues in the neck are drained by lymphatic vessels that enter the *superficial cervical lymph nodes,* which are located along the course of the EJV. Lymph from these nodes, like lymph from all of the head and neck, drains into *inferior deep cervical lymph nodes* (Figs. 8.41 and 8.43). The specific group of inferior deep cervical nodes involved here descends across the lateral cervical region with the spinal accessory nerve. Most lymph from the six to eight lymph nodes then drains into the *supraclavicular group of nodes,* which accompany the transverse cervical artery. The main group of deep cervical nodes forms a chain along the IJV, mostly under

cover of the SCM. Other deep cervical nodes include the prelaryngeal, pretracheal, paratracheal, and retropharyngeal nodes. Efferent lymphatic vessels from the deep cervical nodes join to form the **jugular lymphatic trunks,** which usually join the thoracic duct on the left side and enter the junction of the internal jugular and subclavian veins (right venous angle) directly or via a short right lymphatic duct on the right.

The *thoracic duct* passes superiorly through the superior thoracic aperture along the left border of the esophagus. It arches laterally in the root of the neck, posterior to the carotid sheath and anterior to the sympathetic trunk and vertebral and subclavian arteries (Fig. 8.43*A*). The thoracic duct enters the left brachiocephalic vein at the junction of the subclavian and IJVs (*left venous angle*). When the right jugular, subclavian, and bronchomediastinal lymphatic trunks unite to form a *right lymphatic duct,* it enters the right venous angle as the thoracic duct does on the left (Fig. 8.43*B*). Often, however, these lymphatic trunks enter the venous system independently in the region of the right venous angle.

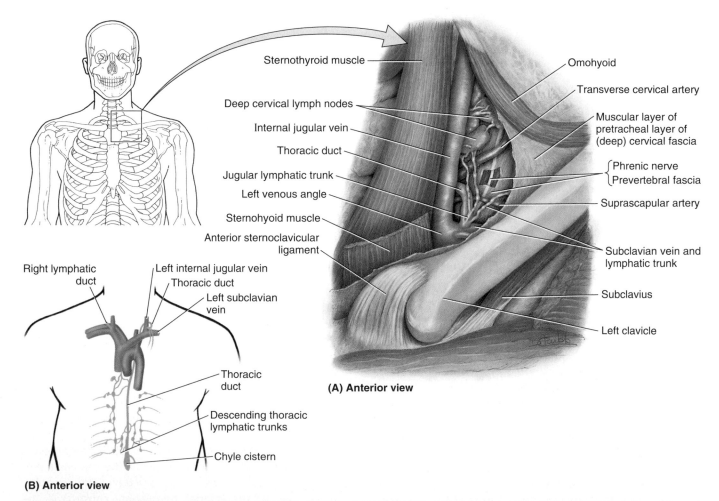

(A) Anterior view

(B) Anterior view

Figure 8.43. Lymphatic vessels in root of neck. A. This dissection of the left side shows the deep cervical lymph nodes and the termination of the thoracic duct at the junction of the subclavian and internal jugular veins (left venous angle). **B.** This overview demonstrates the course of the thoracic duct and site of the termination of the thoracic and right lymphatic ducts.

Radical Neck Dissections

Radical neck dissections are performed when cancer invades the lymphatics. During the procedure, the deep cervical lymph nodes and tissues around them are removed as completely as possible. The major arteries, brachial plexus, CN X, and phrenic nerve are preserved; however, most cutaneous branches of the cervical plexus are removed. The aim of the dissection is to remove all tissue that bears lymph nodes in one piece. The deep cervical lymph nodes, particularly those located along the transverse cervical artery, may be involved in the spread of cancer from the thorax and abdomen. As their enlargement may give the first clue to cancer in these regions, they are often referred to as the *cervical sentinel lymph nodes.* ●

Surface Anatomy of the Endocrine and Respiratory Layers of the Cervical Viscera

The neck of an infant is short; therefore the cervical viscera are located more superiorly in infants than in adults. The cervical viscera do not reach their final levels until after the 7th year. The elongation of the neck is accompanied by growth changes in the skin. Consequently, a midline incision in the inferior neck of an infant results in a scar that will lie over the superior sternum as a child.

The U-shaped **hyoid bone** lies in the anterior part of the neck in the deep angle between the mandible and the thyroid cartilage at the level of the C3 vertebra (Fig. SA8.2). Swallow and the hyoid will move under your fingers when they are placed at the angle between the chin and anterior neck. The greater horn of one side of the hyoid is palpable only when the greater horn on the opposite side is steadied. The **laryngeal prominence** is produced by the meeting of the laminae of the thyroid cartilage at an acute angle in the anterior midline. This thyroid angle, most acute in postpubertal males, forms the laryngeal prominence ("Adam's apple"), which is palpable and frequently visible. During palpation of the prominence, it can be felt to recede on swallowing. The vocal folds are at the level of the middle of the laryngeal prominence.

The **cricoid cartilage** can be felt inferior to the laryngeal prominence at the level of the C6 vertebra. Extend your neck as far as possible and run your finger over the laryngeal prominence. As your finger passes inferiorly from the prominence, feel the **cricothyroid ligament,** the site for a *needle cricothyrotomy* or coniotomy (see clinical correlation [blue] box "Aspiration of Foreign Bodies and the Heimlich Maneuver," earlier in this chapter). After your finger passes over the arch of the cricoid cartilage, note that your fingertip sinks in because the arch of the cartilage projects farther anteriorly than the rings of the trachea. The cricoid cartilage, a key landmark in the neck, indicates the:

- Level of the C6 vertebra.

- Site where the carotid artery can be compressed against the transverse process of the C6 vertebra.

- Junction of the larynx and trachea.

- Joining of the pharynx and esophagus.

- Point where the recurrent laryngeal nerve enters the larynx.

- Site that is approximately 3 cm superior to the isthmus of the thyroid gland.

The **tracheal rings** are palpable in the inferior part of the neck. The second through fourth cartilaginous rings cannot be felt because the isthmus connecting the right and left thyroid lobes covers them. The first tracheal ring is just superior to the isthmus of the thyroid gland.

The **thyroid gland** may be palpated by anterior or posterior approaches (i.e., standing in front of or behind the person); place the fingertips anterior (for the isthmus) or immediately lateral (for the lobes) to the trachea and then direct the person to swallow (see Bickley and Szilayi, 2003 for details). Although both approaches are typically performed (the posterior approach usually allows better palpation, whereas the anterior approach is combined with ▶

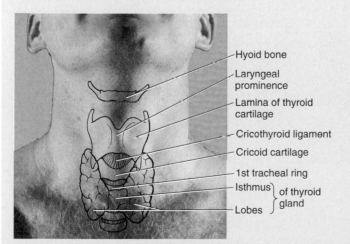

— Hyoid bone
— Laryngeal prominence
— Lamina of thyroid cartilage
— Cricothyroid ligament
— Cricoid cartilage
— 1st tracheal ring
— Isthmus } of thyroid gland
— Lobes }

Figure SA8.2

observation), a perfectly normal thyroid gland may not be visible or distinctly palpable in some females except during menstruation or pregnancy. The normal gland has the consistency of muscle tissue.

The **isthmus of the thyroid gland** lies immediately inferior to the cricoid cartilage; it extends approximately 1.25 cm on either side of the midline. It can usually be felt by placing the fingertips of one hand on the midline below the cricoid arch and then having the person swallow. The isthmus will be felt moving up and then down. The apex of each **lobe of the thyroid gland** is at the middle of the lamina of the thyroid cartilage.

The surface anatomy of the posterior aspect of the neck is described in Chapter 4. Key points are the following:

- The **spinous processes of the C6 and C7 vertebrae** are palpable and visible, especially when the neck is flexed.
- The **transverse processes of the C1, C6, and C7 vertebrae** are palpable.
- The **tubercles of the C1 vertebra** can be palpated by deep pressure posteroinferior to the tips of the mastoid processes. ☉

Medical Imaging of the Neck

Radiography

Standard radiographic examinations of the cervical vertebral column include anteroposterior (AP), lateral, and oblique projections. In a routine AP projection of the cer-

vical vertebral column, the mandible usually obscures the first two cervical vertebrae (Fig. 8.44). To visualize these bones, the neck is extended so that the occiput and maxillary teeth are in the same plane. The central X-ray beam aims through the open mouth, perpendicular to the X-ray detector or film cassette (Fig. 8.45). This radiograph shows the relationship of the atlas to the axis. The ligaments of

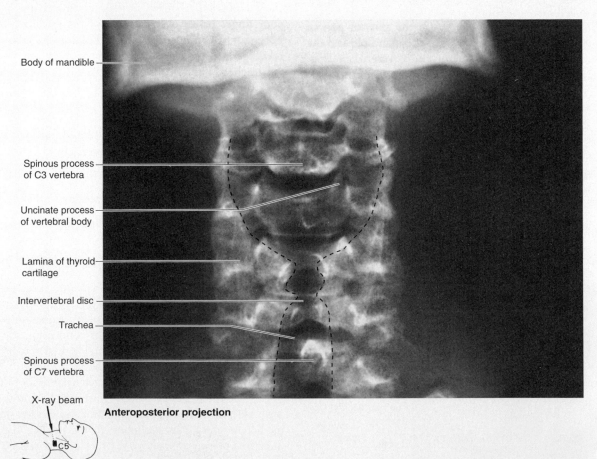

Body of mandible

Spinous process of C3 vertebra

Uncinate process of vertebral body

Lamina of thyroid cartilage

Intervertebral disc

Trachea

Spinous process of C7 vertebra

X-ray beam

C5

X-ray film

Anteroposterior projection

Figure 8.44. Radiograph of middle and lower cervical region of vertebral column. The shadows of the pharynx and trachea (*dashed line*) are superimposed.

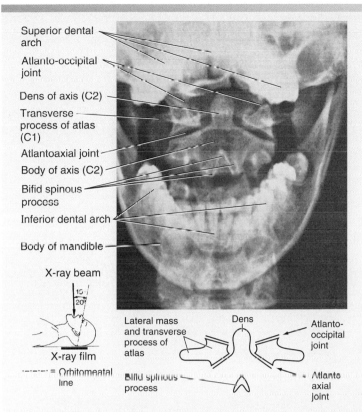

Superior dental arch
Atlanto-occipital joint
Dens of axis (C2)
Transverse process of atlas (C1)
Atlantoaxial joint
Body of axis (C2)
Bifid spinous process
Inferior dental arch
Body of mandible

X-ray beam

X-ray film
------- = Orbitomeatal line

Lateral mass and transverse process of atlas
Dens
Atlanto-occipital joint
Bifid spinous process
Atlanto axial joint

Figure 8.45. Open-mouth radiograph of dens. The dens projects superiorly from the body of the axis (C2 vertebra), around which the atlas (C1 vertebra) rotates.

the atlantoaxial joint are radiolucent and therefore do not cast a shadow. The lateral masses of the atlas are triangular or wedge shaped and are easy to recognize. Laterally, the long transverse processes of the atlas are clearly visible. Between the lateral masses of the atlas, the dens of the axis is also readily discernible.

When taking a lateral projection of the cervical vertebral column, the person is usually sitting erect, with the neck slightly extended (Fig. 8.46). The central X-ray beam aims perpendicular to the X-ray detector or film cassette at the level of the thyroid cartilage. Lateral projections are common for evaluating severe neck injuries. When a fracture is suspected, the lateral projection is examined before the person is moved for other projections. Observe the anterior and posterior margins of the vertebral bodies. Any deviation from the smooth curvature of these margins suggests a fracture and tearing of the associated ligaments. Observe that the IV disc spaces are wider anteriorly than posteriorly, indicating that the IV discs are wedge shaped. As the discs degenerate, the vertical height of the disc spaces decreases. Also observe the long, prominent spinous process of vertebra C7. The posterior margins of the bodies of cervical vertebra form the anterior aspect of the vertebral canal containing the spinal cord.

Oblique radiographs of the neck may be required in some cases for a complete study of the cervical vertebral column. The standard 45° oblique projection shows the IV foramina as well as the uncovertebral joints (see Chapter 5).

Bony outgrowths, such as *osteophytes* from the joints of the vertebral column, can be detected in oblique projections.

Contrast visualization of the esophagus is achieved by having the patient swallow a mixture of barium sulfate and water (Fig. 8.47). The first of four constrictions in the esophagus occurs at the pharyngoesophageal junction. The commencement of the esophagus is its narrowest part.

Computed Tomography

Transverse CT scans through the thyroid gland show sections of the neck (Fig. 8.48A). They are oriented to show how a horizontal section of the person's neck appears to the physician standing at the foot of the bed. The superior edge of the CT image represents the anterior surface of the neck, and the right lateral edge of the image represents the left lateral surface. CT is used mainly as a diagnostic adjunct to conventional radiography. CT scans are superior to radiographs because they reveal radiodensity differences among and within soft tissues (e.g., the thyroid gland).

Magnetic Resonance Imaging

MRI systems construct images of transverse, sagittal, and coronal sections of the neck and have the advantage of using no radiation. MRI studies of the neck are superior to CT studies for showing detail in the soft tissues, but they provide little information about bones (Figs. 8.26 and 8.48–8.51).

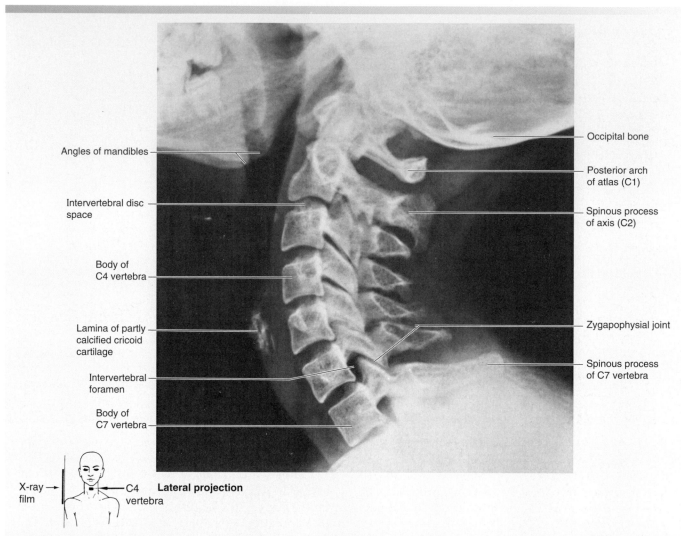

Angles of mandibles

Intervertebral disc space

Body of C4 vertebra

Lamina of partly calcified cricoid cartilage

Intervertebral foramen

Body of C7 vertebra

Occipital bone

Posterior arch of atlas (C1)

Spinous process of axis (C2)

Zygapophysial joint

Spinous process of C7 vertebra

X-ray film

C4 vertebra

Lateral projection

Figure 8.46. Radiograph of cervical vertebral column. The long spinous process of vertebra C7 is typically the most prominent superficially. Zygapophysial (facet) joints are also visible.

Cervical part of esophagus

Necklace

Narrowing of the thoracic part of the esophagus (caused by aorta and left primary bronchus)

Diaphragm

Esophagus, abdominal part

(A)

(B)

Figure 8.47. Radiograph of esophagus. This radiograph was taken after barium was swallowed. Necklaces should be removed before radiographs are taken.

Figure 8.48. Transverse scans of neck through thyroid gland. A. A CT study through the lobes of the thyroid gland is shown. (Courtesy of Dr. M. Keller, Assistant Professor of Medical Imaging, University of Toronto, Toronto, Ontario, Canada.) **B.** An MRI study through the thyroid isthmus is shown. (Courtesy of Dr. W. Kucharczyk, Clinical Director, Tri-Hospital Resonance Centre, Toronto, Ontario, Canada.) *1,* esophagus; *2,* trachea; *3,* lobes of the thyroid gland; *4,* thyroid isthmus; *5,* SCM; *6,* sternohyoid muscles; *7,* common carotid artery; *8,* IJV; *9,* vertebral artery; *10,* vertebral body; *11,* spinal cord surrounded by cerebrospinal fluid in the subarachnoid space; *12,* deep muscles of the back; *13,* retropharyngeal space.

(A)   **(B)**

Figure 8.49. Transverse MRI studies of larynx. A. This scan is through the thyroid cartilage. **B.** This scan is through the cricoid cartilage. *1,* esophagus; *2,* thyroid cartilage; *3,* lamina of the cricoid cartilage; *4,* sternothyroid and sternohyoid muscles; *5,* common carotid artery; *6,* IJV; *7,* anterior root; *8,* SCM; *9,* inferior constrictor; *10,* vertebral body; *11,* spinal cord; *12,* vertebral artery. (Courtesy of Dr. W. Kucharczyk, Chair of Medical Imaging, University of Toronto, and Clinical Director, Tri-Hospital Resonance Centre, Toronto, Ontario, Canada.)

Figure 8.50. Median MRI study of floor of mouth and neck. The tongue, oropharynx, hyoid, thyroid and cricoid cartilages, vocal fold, and trachea are visible. (Courtesy of Dr. W. Kucharczyk, Chair of Medical Imaging, University of Toronto, and Clinical Director, Tri-Hospital Resonance Centre, Toronto, Ontario, Canada.)

Tongue

Mandible

Epiglottis

Vestibule

Vestibular fold

Ventricle

Vocal folds
(opposed)

Trachea

Aryepiglottic fold

Piriform fossa (recess)

Thyroid cartilage

Cricoid cartilage

Figure 8.51. Coronal MRI study of larynx. The valleculae of the oropharynx, piriform fossae of the laryngopharynx, and vestibular and vocal folds of the larynx are visible. (Courtesy of Dr. W. Kucharczyk, Chair of Medical Imaging, University of Toronto, and Clinical Director, Tri-Hospital Resonance Centre, Toronto, Ontario, Canada.)

Ultrasonography

Ultrasonography is also a useful diagnostic imaging technique for studying the soft tissues of the neck. Ultrasound provides images of many abnormal conditions of the neck non-invasively, at relatively low cost, and with minimal discomfort. Ultrasound is useful for distinguishing solid from cystic masses, for example, which may be difficult to determine during physical examinations. Vascular imaging of arteries and veins of the neck is possible using intravascular ultrasonography. The images are produced by placing a transducer within a blood vessel. Doppler ultrasound techniques help evaluate blood flow through a vessel (Fig. 8.52), for detecting stenosis of a carotid artery, for example. ○

Figure 8.52. Doppler color flow study of internal carotid artery. The study reveals normal blood flow.

References and Suggested Readings

Agur AMR, Dalley AF: *Grant's Atlas of Anatomy,* 11th ed. Baltimore, Lippincott Williams & Wilkins, 2004.

Behrman RE, Kliegman RM, Arvin AM (eds): *Nelson Textbook of Pediatrics,* 16th ed. Philadelphia, Saunders, 2000.

Bickley LS, Szilagyi: *Bate's Guide to Physical Examination and History Taking,* 8th ed. Baltimore, Lippincott Williams & Wilkins, 2003.

Fahn S, Bressman SB: Dystonia. *In* Rowland LP (ed): *Merritt's Textbook of Neurology,* 10th ed. Baltimore, Lippincott Williams & Wilkins, 2000.

Ger R, Abrahams P, Olson TR: *Essentials of Clinical Anatomy,* 2nd ed. New York, Parthenon, 1996.

Lachman N, Acland RD, Rosse C: Anatomical evidence for the absence of a morphologically distinct cranial root of the accessory nerve in man. *Clin Anat* 15:4–10 2002.

Leung AKC, Wong AL, Robson WLLM: Ectopic thyroid gland simulating a thyroglossal duct cyst: A case report. *Can J Surg* 38:87, 1995.

Moore KL, Persaud TVN: *The Developing Human: Clinically Oriented Embryology,* 7th ed. Philadelphia, Saunders, 2003.

Norton JA, Wells SA Jr: The parathyroid glands. *In* Sabiston DC Jr, Lyerly HK (eds): *Sabiston Essentials of Surgery,* 2nd ed. Philadelphia, Saunders, 1994.

Pedley TA, Ziegler DK: Syncope and seizure. *In* Rowland LP (ed): *Merritt's Textbook of Neurology,* 10th ed. Baltimore, Lippincott Williams & Wilkins, 2000.

Rowland LP (ed): *Merritt's Textbook of Neurology,* 10th ed. Baltimore: Lippincott Williams & Wilkins, 2000A.

Rowland LP: Diagnosis of pain and paresthesias. *In* Rowland LP (ed): *Merritt's Textbook of Neurology,* 10th ed. Baltimore, Lippincott Williams & Wilkins, 2000B.

Sabiston DC Jr, Lyerly H: *Sabiston Essentials of Surgery,* 2nd ed. Philadelphia, Saunders, 1994.

Sacco RL: Pathogenesis, classification, and epidemiology of cerebrovascular disease. *In* Rowland LP (ed): *Merritt's Textbook of Neurology,* 10th ed. Baltimore, Lippincott Williams & Wilkins, 2000.

Scher RL, Richtsmeier WJ: Otolaryngology: head and neck surgery. *In* Sabiston DC Jr, Lyerly HK (eds): *Sabiston Essentials of Surgery,* 2nd ed. Philadelphia, Saunders, 1994.

Sinkinson CA: The continuing saga of penetrating neck injuries. *Emerg Med* 12:135, 1991.

Skandalakis JE, Skandalakis PN, Skandalakis LJ: *Surgical Anatomy and Technique. A Pocket Manual.* New York, Springer-Verlag, 1995.

Swartz MH: *Textbook of Physical Diagnosis: History and Examination,* 2nd ed. Philadelphia, Saunders, 2001.

Williams PH, Bannister LH, Berry MM, Collins P, Dyson M, Dussek JE, Ferguson MWJ: *Gray's Anatomy,* 38th ed. New York, Churchill Livingstone, 1995.

9 Summary of Cranial Nerves

The regional aspects of the cranial nerves are described in the preceding chapters, especially those for the head and neck.

This chapter summarizes all of the cranial nerves, largely in figures and tables. Tables 9.1 and 9.2 summarize specific cranial nerves. Table 9.3 summarizes some common cranial nerve injuries, indicating the type or site of lesion and the abnormal findings that result.

Overview

Like spinal nerves, **cranial nerves** are bundles of sensory or motor fibers that innervate muscles or glands; carry impulses from sensory receptors, or show a combination of these fiber types. They are called cranial nerves because they emerge through foramina or fissures in the cranium and are covered by tubular sheaths derived from the cranial meninges. There are twelve pairs of cranial nerves, which are numbered I to XII, from rostral to caudal, according to their attachment to the brain and penetration of the cranial dura (Fig. 9.1). Their names reflect their general distribution or function.

Cranial nerves carry one or more of the following five main functional components.

- Motor (efferent) fibers.

  1. *Motor fibers to voluntary* (striated) *muscle.* Two subtypes are distinguished, based on the embryologic origin of the specific muscles:

     a. *Somatic motor* (general somatic efferent) axons innervate the striated muscles in the orbit (e.g., ocular muscles), tongue, and external muscles of the neck (sternocleidomastoid and trapezius[1]) derived from sources other than the embryonic pharyngeal arches.

     b. *Branchial motor* (special visceral efferent) axons innervate striated muscles (e.g., muscles of mastication, or chewing muscles) derived from the pharyngeal arches (face, palate, pharynx, and larynx).

  2. *Motor fibers involved in innervating involuntary* (smooth) *muscles or glands.* These include visceral motor (general visceral efferent) axons that constitute the cranial outflow of the parasympathetic division of the autonomic nervous system (ANS). The presynaptic (preganglionic) fibers that emerge from the brain synapse outside the central nervous system (CNS) in a parasympathetic ganglion. The postsynapatic (postganglionic) fibers continue to innervate smooth muscles and glands (e.g., the sphincter pupillae and lacrimal gland).

- Sensory (afferent) fibers.

  3. *Fibers conveying sensation from the viscera.* These include visceral sensory (general visceral afferent) fibers conveying information from the carotid body and sinus, pharynx, larynx, trachea, bronchi, lungs, heart, and gastrointestinal tract.

  4. *Fibers transmitting general sensation* (e.g., touch, pressure, heat, cold, etc.) from the skin and mucous membranes. These include general sensory (general somatic afferent) fibers, mainly carried by CN V but also by CN VII, CN IX, and CN X.

  5. *Fibers transmitting unique sensations.* These include special sensory fibers conveying taste and smell (special visceral afferent fibers) and those serving the special senses of vision, hearing, and balance (special somatic afferent fibers).

Somatic cranial nerves are wholly sensory, others are considered "purely" motor, and several are mixed. CN III, CN IV, CN VI, CN XI, CN XII and the motor root of CN V are considered to be "pure" motor nerves that appear to have evolved from primordial anterior roots. However, a small number of sensory fibers for proprioception (non-visual perception of movement and position) are also present in these nerves, the cell bodies of which are probably located in the mesencephalic nucleus of CN V. Four cranial nerves (CN III, CN VII, CN IX, and CN X) contain presynaptic parasympathetic (visceral motor) axons as they emerge from the brainstem. CN V, CN VII, CN IX, and CN X are mixed nerves with both motor and sensory components, and each nerve supplies derivatives of a different pharyngeal arch.

The fibers of cranial nerves connect centrally to **cranial nerve nuclei**—groups of neurons in which sensory or afferent fibers terminate and from which motor or efferent fibers originate (Fig. 9.2). Except for CN I and CN II, which involve extensions of the forebrain, the nuclei of the cranial nerves are located in the brainstem. Nuclei of similar functional components (e.g., general somatic or visceral motor, or general somatic or visceral sensory) are generally aligned into functional columns in the brainstem.

Cranial Nerve Injuries

Injury to the cranial nerves is a frequent complication of a fracture in the base of the cranium (Table 9.3). Furthermore, excessive movement of the brain within the cranium may tear or bruise cranial nerve fibers, especially those of CN I. Paralysis of cranial nerves as a result of trauma can usually be detected as soon as the patient's state of consciousness permits (Lange et al., 2000); however, in some people, the paralysis may not be evident for several days. ▶

(*cont'd on page 1129*)

---

[1]Historically, the sternocleidomastoid and trapezius have been classified as branchiomeric muscles; students may see them classified as such in other references.

Table 9.1. Summary of Cranial Nerves

Oculomotor—CN III

Motor: ciliary muscles, sphincter of pupil, all extrinsic muscles of eye except those listed for CN IV and VI

Motor: superior oblique muscle of eye

Abducent—CN VI

Motor: lateral rectus muscle of eye

Key

- - - Spinal nerve fibers
—— Efferent (motor) fibers
—— Afferent (sensory) fibers

Optic—CN II

Sensory: vision

Olfactory—CN I

Sensory: smell

Facial—CN VII Primary root

Motor: muscles of facial expression

Trigeminal—CN V Sensory root

Sensory: face, sinuses, teeth

Facial—CN VII Intermediate nerve

Motor: submandibular, sublingual, lacrimal glands
Sensory: taste to anterior two thirds of tongue, soft palate

Trigeminal—CN V Motor root

Motor: muscles of mastication

Vestibulocochlear—CN VIII

Vestibular nerve, sensory: orientation, motion
Cochlear nerve, sensory: hearing

Hypoglossal—CN XII

Motor: all intrinsic and extrinsic muscles of tongue (excluding palatoglossus—a palatine muscle)

* **Spinal accessory— CN XI**

Motor: sternocleido-mastoid and trapezius

* **Vagus—CN X**

Motor: palate, pharynx, larynx, trachea, bronchial tree, heart, GI tract to left colic flexure
Sensory: pharynx, larynx; reflex sensory from trachio-bronchial tree, lungs, heart, GI tract to left colic flexure

Glossopharyngeal—CN IX

Motor: stylopharyngeus, parotid gland
Sensory: taste: posterior third of tongue; general sensation: pharynx, tonsillar sinus, pharyngotympanic tube, middle ear cavity

CN III   CN II   CN I

CN IV

CN VI

CN V

CN V   CN XII   CN XI   CN X   CN IX

CN VII

CN VII

CN VIII

(continues)

Table 9.1. Summary of Cranial Nerves (*continued*)

Nerve	Components	Location of Nerve Cell Bodies	Cranial Exit	Main Action(s)
Olfactory (CN I)	Special sensory	Olfactory epithelium (olfactory cells)	Foramina in cribriform plate of ethmoid bone	Smell from nasal mucosa of roof of each nasal cavity and superior sides of nasal septum and superior concha
Optic (CN II)	Special sensory	Retina (ganglion cells)	Optic canal	Vision from retina
Oculomotor (CN III)	Somatic motor	Midbrain	Superior orbital fissure	Motor to superior rectus, inferior rectus, medial rectus, inferior oblique, and levator palpebrae superioris muscles; raises superior eyelid; turns eyeball superiorly, inferiorly, and medially
	Visceral motor	Presynaptic: midbrain Postsynaptic: ciliary ganglion		Parasympathetic innervation to sphincter of pupil and ciliary muscle; constricts pupil and accommodates lens of eye
Trochlear (CN IV)	Somatic motor	Midbrain		Motor to superior oblique that assists in turning eye infero-laterally (or inferiorly when adducted)
Trigeminal (CN V)				
Ophthalmic (CN V₁)	General sensory	Trigeminal ganglion	Superior orbital fissure	Sensation from cornea, skin of forehead, scalp, eyelids, nose, and mucosa of nasal cavity and paranasal sinuses
Maxillary (CN V₂)			Foramen rotundum	Sensation from skin of face over maxilla, including upper lip, maxillary teeth, mucosa of nose, maxillary sinuses, and palate
Mandibular (CN V₃)			Foramen ovale	Sensation from skin and over side of head mandible including lower lip, mandibular teeth, temporomandibular joint, mucosa of mouth and anterior two thirds of tongue
	Branchial motor	Pons		Motor to muscles of mastication, mylohyoid, anterior belly of digastric, tensor veli palatini, and tensor tympani
Abducent (CN VI)	Somatic motor	Pons	Superior orbital fissure	Motor to lateral rectus that turns eye laterally
Facial (CN VII)	Branchial motor	Pons	Internal acoustic meatus; facial canal; stylomastoid foramen	Motor to muscles of facial expression and scalp; also supplies stapedius of middle ear, stylohyoid, and posterior belly of digastric
	Special sensory	Geniculate ganglion		Taste from anterior two thirds of tongue and the palate
	Visceral motor	Presynaptic: pons Postsynaptic: pterygopalatine ganglion; submandibular ganglion		Parasympathetic innervation to submandibular and sublingual salivary glands, lacrimal gland, and glands of nose and palate

(continues)

Table 9.1. Summary of Cranial Nerves (*continued*)

Nerve	Components	Location of Nerve Cell Bodies	Cranial Exit	Main Action(s)
Vestibulocochlear (CN VIII)				
Vestibular	Special sensory	Vestibular ganglion	Internal acoustic meatus	Vestibular sensation from semicircular ducts, utricle, and saccule related to position and movement of head
Cochlear	Special sensory	Spiral ganglion		Hearing from spiral organ
Glossopharyngeal (CN IX)	Branchial motor	Medulla	Jugular foramen	Motor to stylopharyngeus to assist with swallowing
	Visceral motor	Presynaptic: medulla Postsynaptic: otic ganglion		Parasympathetic innervation to parotid gland
	Visceral sensory	Superior ganglion		Visceral sensation from parotid gland, carotid body and sinus, pharynx, and middle ear
	Special sensory	Inferior ganglion		Taste from posterior third of tongue
	General sensory	Inferior ganglion		Cutaneous sensation from external ear
Vagus (CN X)	Branchial motor	Medulla		Motor to constrictor muscles of pharynx (except stylopharyngeus), intrinsic muscles of larynx, muscles of palate (except tensor veli palatini), and striated muscle in superior two thirds of esophagus
	Visceral motor	Presynaptic: medulla Postsynaptic: neurons in, on, or near viscera		Parasympathetic innervation to smooth muscle of trachea, bronchi, digestive tract, and cardiac muscle of heart
	Visceral sensory	Superior ganglion		Visceral sensation from base of tongue, pharynx, larynx, trachea, bronchi, heart, esophagus, stomach, and intestine to left colic flexure
	Special sensory	Inferior ganglion		Taste from epiglottis and palate
	General sensory	Superior ganglion		Sensation from auricle, external acoustic meatus, and dura mater of posterior cranial fossa
Spinal accessory (CN XI)	Somatic motor	Spinal cord		Motor to sternocleidomastoid and trapezius
Hypoglossal (CN XII)	Somatic motor	Medulla	Hypoglossal canal	Motor to intrinsic and extrinsic muscles of tongue (except palatoglossus)

*The traditional "cranial root of the accessory nerve" is considered here as part of the vagus nerve (CN X); the spinal accessory nerve (CN XI) as listed here refers only to the traditional "spinal root of the accessory nerve."

Table 9.2. Cranial Nerves: Attachment to Central Nervous System, General Functions, and Distribution[a]

Inferior (ventral) view

Cranial Nerves		Part of Central Nervous System Nerve(s) Enter(s) or Emerge(s) From		General Functional Types of Fibers[b]	General Distribution
Number	Name				
I	Olfactory	Forebrain (prosencephalon)	Telencephalon	Special sensory only	Olfactory mucosa of nose
II	Optic		Diencephalon		Retina of eye
III	Oculomotor	Midbrain (mesencephalon)		Motor only	Intraocular and four extraocular muscles;
					One extraocular muscle

(continues)

Table 9.2. Cranial Nerves: Attachment to Central Nervous System, General Functions, and Distributiona (*continued*)

Cranial Nerves Number	Cranial Nerves Name	Part of Central Nervous System Nerve(s) Enter(s) or Emerge(s) From		General Functional Types of Fibersb		General Distribution
V	Trigeminal	Brainstem	Pons (mesencephalon)	Mixed	Motor root	Derivative of fronto-nasal process and 1st pharyngeal arch
					Sensory root	
VI	Abducent		Junction between pons and medulla	Motor only		One extraocular muscle
VII	Facial			Mixed	Motor root	Derivatives of 2nd pharyngeal arch
					Intermediate nerve	
VIII	Vestibulocochlear			Special sensory only		Internal (inner) ear
IX	Glossopharyngeal		Medulla (myelencephalon)	Mixed		Derivatives of 3rd pharyngeal arch
X	Vagusc					Derivatives of 4th pharyngeal arch
XII	Hypoglossal					Muscles of tongue
XI	Spinal accessoryd	Superior spinal cord		Motor only		Superficial layer of neck

aThe superficial origins of the cranial nerves from the central nervous system (except for CN IV, which arises from the posterior aspect of the midbrain).
bNote that the colors in this column match those of the nerves in the figure.
cThe traditional "cranial root of the accessory nerve" is considered here as part of the vagus nerve.
dThe spinal accessory nerve as listed here refers to only the traditional "spinal root of the accessory nerve."

Because of their location within the confined cranial cavity, relatively fixed positions, and sometimes close relationships to bony or vascular formations, the intracranial portions of certain cranial nerves are also susceptible to compression owing to a tumor or aneurysm. In such cases, the onset of symptoms usually occurs gradually, and the effects depend on the extent of the pressure exerted. Because of their close relationship to the cavernous sinus, CN III, CN IV, CN V_1 and especially CN VI are susceptible to compression or injury related to pathologies (infections, thrombophlebitis) affecting the sinus. ○

Olfactory Nerve (CN I)

Function: Special sensory (special visceral afferent)—that is, the special sense of smell. "*Olfaction* is the sensation of odors that results from the detection of odorous substances aerosolized in the environment" (Sweazey, 2002).

The cell bodies of **olfactory receptor neurons** are located in the **olfactory organ** (the olfactory part of the nasal mucosa or olfactory area), which is located in the roof of the nasal cavity and along the nasal septum and medial wall of the superior nasal concha. Olfactory receptor neurons are both receptors and conductors (Fig. 9.3). The apical surfaces of the neurons possess fine **olfactory cilia**, bathed by a film of watery

Table 9.3. Summary of Cranial Nerve Lesions

Nerve	Type(s) and/or Site(s) of Lesion	Abnormal Findings
CN I	Fracture of cribiform plate	Anosmia (loss of smell); cerebrospinal fluid rhinorrhea
CN II	Direct trauma to orbit or eyeball; fracture involving optic canal	Loss of pupillary constriction
	Pressure on optic pathway; laceration or intracerebral clot in the temporal, parietal, or occipital lobes of brain	Visual field defects
CN III	Pressure from herniating uncus on nerve; fracture involving cavernous sinus; aneurysms	Dilated pupil; ptosis; eye turns down and out; pupillary reflex on the side of the lesion will be lost
CN IV	Stretching of nerve during its course around brainstem; fracture of orbit	Inability to look down when eye is adducted
CN V	Injury to terminal branches (particularly CN V$_2$) in roof of maxillary sinus; pathological processes affecting trigeminal ganglion	Loss of pain and touch sensations; paraesthesia; masseter and temporalis muscles do not contract; deviation of mandible to side of lesion when mouth is opened
CN VI	Base of brain or fracture involving cavernous sinus or orbit	Eye falls to move laterally; diplopia on lateral gaze
CN VII	Laceration or contusion in parotid region	Paralysis of facial muscles; eye remains open; angle of mouth droops; forehead does not wrinkle
	Fracture of temporal bone	As above, plus associated involvement of cochlear nerve and chorda tympani; dry cornea; loss of taste on anterior two thirds of tongue
	Intracranial hematoma ("stroke")	Forehead wrinkles because of bilateral innervation of the frontalis muscle; otherwise paralysis of contralateral facial muscles
CN VIII	Tumor of nerve (acoustic neuroma)	Progressive unilateral hearing loss; tinnitus (noises in ear)
CN IX	Brainstem lesion or deep laceration of neck	Loss of taste on posterior third of tongue; loss of sensation on affected side of soft palate
CN X	Brainstem lesion or deep laceration of neck	Sagging of soft palate; deviation of uvula to normal side; hoarseness owing to paralysis of vocal fold
CN XI	Laceration of neck	Paralysis of sternocleidomastoid and superior fibers of trapezius; drooping of shoulder
CN XII	Neck laceration; basal skull fractures	Protruded tongue deviates toward affected side; moderate dysarthria (disturbance of articulation)

mucus secreted by the **olfactory glands** of the epithelium. The cilia are stimulated by molecules of an odiferous gas dissolved in the fluid.

The basal surfaces of the bipolar olfactory receptor neurons of the nasal cavity of one side give rise to central processes that are collected into approximately 20 **olfactory nerves** (L. *fila olfactoria*), constituting the right or left **olfactory nerve (CN I)**. They pass through tiny foramina in the **cribriform plate** of the ethmoid bone, surrounded by sleeves of dura and arachnoid, and enter the **olfactory bulb** in the anterior cranial fossa (Fig. 9.1). The olfactory bulb lies in contact with the inferior or orbital surface of the frontal lobe of the cerebral hemisphere. The olfactory nerve fibers synapse with **mitral cells** in the olfactory bulb. The axons of these secondary neurons form the **olfactory tract**. The olfactory bulbs and tracts are technically anterior extensions of the forebrain.

Each olfactory tract divides into lateral and medial **olfactory striae** (distinct fiber bands). The lateral olfactory stria terminates in the piriform cortex of the anterior part of the temporal lobe, and the medial olfactory stria projects through the anterior commissure to contralateral olfactory structures. The olfactory nerves are the only cranial nerves to enter the cerebrum directly.

Anosmia—Loss of Smell

Loss of olfactory fibers usually occurs with aging. Consequently, elderly people often have reduced acuity of the sensation of smell, resulting from progressive reduction in the number of olfactory receptor neurons in the olfactory epithelium. The chief complaint of most people with anosmia is the loss or alteration of taste; however, clinical studies reveal that in all but a few people, the dysfunction is in the olfactory system (Sweazey, 2002). The reason is that most people confuse taste with flavor. Transitory olfactory impairment occurs as ▶

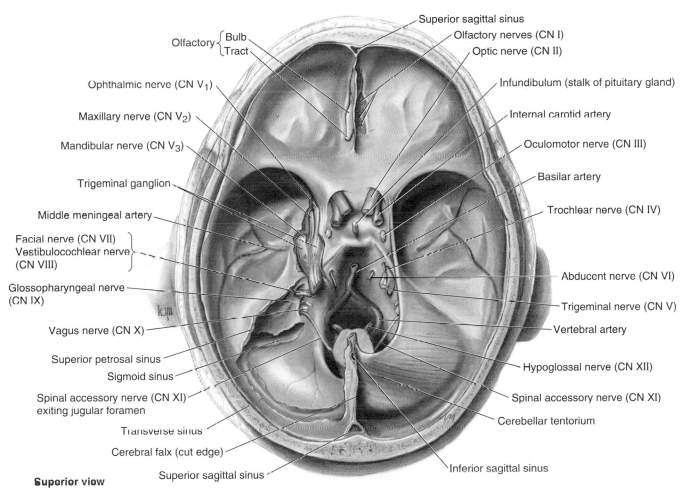

Olfactory {Bulb, Tract}
Ophthalmic nerve (CN V₁)
Maxillary nerve (CN V₂)
Mandibular nerve (CN V₃)
Trigeminal ganglion
Middle meningeal artery
Facial nerve (CN VII)
Vestibulocochlear nerve (CN VIII)
Glossopharyngeal nerve (CN IX)
Vagus nerve (CN X)
Superior petrosal sinus
Sigmoid sinus
Spinal accessory nerve (CN XI) exiting jugular foramen
Transverse sinus
Cerebral falx (cut edge)
Superior sagittal sinus

Superior sagittal sinus
Olfactory nerves (CN I)
Optic nerve (CN II)
Infundibulum (stalk of pituitary gland)
Internal carotid artery
Oculomotor nerve (CN III)
Basilar artery
Trochlear nerve (CN IV)
Abducent nerve (CN VI)
Trigeminal nerve (CN V)
Vertebral artery
Hypoglossal nerve (CN XII)
Spinal accessory nerve (CN XI)
Cerebellar tentorium
Inferior sagittal sinus

Superior view

Figure 9.1. Internal surface of cranial base. This view shows the cranial nerves, dura, and blood vessels. On the left side, the dura is cut away to expose the trigeminal cave housing the trigeminal ganglion and its roots and the nerves arising from it: CN V₁, CN V₂, and CN V₃. The cerebellar tentorium is also removed on the left side to show the nerves exiting the internal acoustic meatus (CN VII and CN VIII) and jugular foramen (CN IX, CN X, and CN XI).

a result of viral or allergic rhinitis—inflammation of the nasal mucous membrane.

To test the sense of smell, the person is blindfolded and asked to identify common odors, such as freshly ground coffee placed near the external nares (nostrils). One naris is occluded and the eyes are closed. Because anosmia is usually unilateral, each naris is tested separately. If the loss of smell is unilateral, the person may not be aware of it without clinical testing.

Injury to the nasal mucosa, olfactory nerve fibers, olfactory bulbs, or olfactory tracts may also impair smell. In severe head injuries, the olfactory bulbs may be torn away from the olfactory nerves, or some olfactory nerve fibers may be torn as they pass through a *fractured cribriform plate.* If all the nerve bundles on one side are torn, a complete loss of smell will occur on that side; consequently, anosmia may be

a clue to a fracture of the cranial base and cerebrospinal fluid rhinorrhea (leakage of the fluid through the nose). A tumor and/or abscess (collection of pus) in the frontal lobe of the brain or a tumor of the meninges (meningioma) in the anterior cranial fossa may also cause anosmia by compressing the olfactory bulb and/or tract (Bruce and Fetell, 2000).

Olfactory Hallucinations

Occasionally *olfactory hallucinations* (false perceptions of smell) may accompany lesions in the temporal lobe of the cerebral hemisphere. A lesion that irritates the lateral olfactory area (deep to the uncus) may cause *temporal lobe epilepsy* or "uncinate fits," which are characterized by imaginary disagreeable odors and involuntary movements of the lips and tongue (Table 9.2). ☉

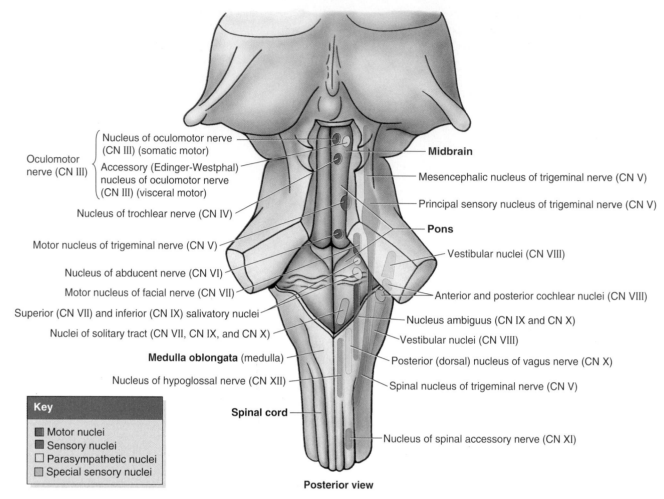

Oculomotor nerve (CN III)
{
Nucleus of oculomotor nerve (CN III) (somatic motor)

Accessory (Edinger-Westphal) nucleus of oculomotor nerve (CN III) (visceral motor)
}

Nucleus of trochlear nerve (CN IV)

Motor nucleus of trigeminal nerve (CN V)

Nucleus of abducent nerve (CN VI)

Motor nucleus of facial nerve (CN VII)

Superior (CN VII) and inferior (CN IX) salivatory nuclei

Nuclei of solitary tract (CN VII, CN IX, and CN X)

Medulla oblongata (medulla)

Nucleus of hypoglossal nerve (CN XII)

Spinal cord

Midbrain

Mesencephalic nucleus of trigeminal nerve (CN V)

Principal sensory nucleus of trigeminal nerve (CN V)

Pons

Vestibular nuclei (CN VIII)

Anterior and posterior cochlear nuclei (CN VIII)

Nucleus ambiguus (CN IX and CN X)

Vestibular nuclei (CN VIII)

Posterior (dorsal) nucleus of vagus nerve (CN X)

Spinal nucleus of trigeminal nerve (CN V)

Nucleus of spinal accessory nerve (CN XI)

Key
- Motor nuclei
- Sensory nuclei
- Parasympathetic nuclei
- Special sensory nuclei

Posterior view

Figure 9.2. Cranial nerve nuclei. Observe the location of the motor, sensory, parasympathetic, and special sensory nuclei.

THE BOTTOM LINE: The olfactory nerves (CN I) have sensory fibers concerned with the special sense of smell. The olfactory receptor neurons are in the olfactory epithelium (olfactory mucosa) in the roof of the nasal cavity. The central processes of the olfactory receptor neurons ascend through foramina in the cribriform plate of the ethmoid to reach the olfactory bulbs in the anterior cranial fossa. These nerves synapse on neurons in the bulbs, and the processes of these neurons follow the olfactory tracts to the primary and associated areas of the cerebral cortex. Fracture of the cranial base can injure the olfactory nerve fibers, resulting in anosmia (loss of smell), tearing of the meninges, and/or cerebrospinal fluid rhinorrhea.

Optic Nerve (CN II)

Function: Special sensory (special somatic afferent)—that is, the special sense of vision.

Although they are officially nerves by convention, the **optic nerves** (CN II) develop in a completely different manner

from the other cranial nerves. The structures involved in receiving and transmitting optical stimuli (the optical fibers and neural retina, together with the pigmented epithelium of the eyeball) develop as evaginations of the diencephalon (Moore and Persaud, 2003). The optic nerves are paired, anterior extensions of the forebrain (diencephalon) and are, therefore, actually CNS fiber tracts formed by axons of **retinal ganglion cells**. In other words, they are third-order neurons, with their cell bodies located in the retina (Fig. 9.4).

The optic nerves are surrounded by extensions of the cranial meninges and subarachnoid space, which is filled with cerebrospinal fluid (CSF). The meninges extend all the way to the eyeball. The central artery and vein of the retina traverse the meningeal layers and course in the anterior part of the optic nerve. CN II begins where the unmyelinated axons of retinal ganglion cells pierce the sclera (the opaque part of the external fibrous coat of the eyeball) and become myelinated, deep to the **optic disc.**

The nerve passes posteromedially in the orbit, exiting through the **optic canal** to enter the middle cranial fossa, where it forms the **optic chiasm** (L. *chiasma opticum*). Here, fibers from the nasal (medial) half of each retina decussate in the chiasm and join uncrossed fibers from the temporal (lateral) half of the retina to form the **optic tract.** The partial crossing of optic nerve fibers in the chiasm is a requirement for binocular vision, allowing depth-of-field perception (three-dimensional vision). Thus fibers from the right halves of both retinas form the left optic tract. The decussation of nerve fibers in the chiasm results in the right optic tract conveying impulses from the left visual field and vice versa. The **visual field** is what is seen by a person who has both eyes wide open and who is looking straight ahead (Hutchins and Corbett, 2002). Most fibers in the optic tracts terminate in the **lateral geniculate bodies** of the thalamus. From these nuclei, axons are relayed to the visual cortices of the occipital lobes of the brain.

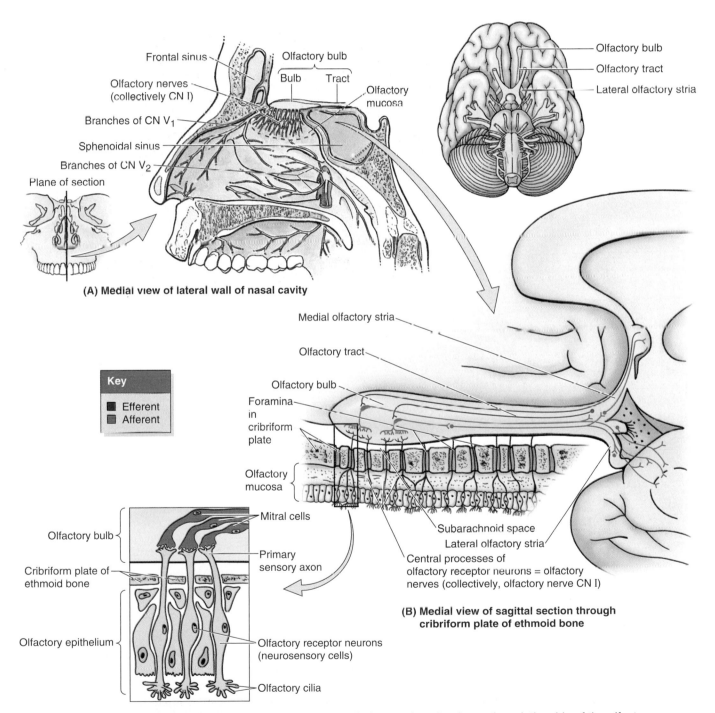

Figure 9.3. Olfactory system A. This sagittal section through the nasal cavity shows the relationship of the olfactory mucosa to the olfactory bulb. **B.** The bodies of the olfactory receptor neurons are in the olfactory epithelium. These bundles of axons are collectively called the olfactory nerve (CN I).

Temporal (T) Nasal (N) Nasal (N) Temporal (T)

Left visual field

Right visual field

Retina

Optic nerve (CN II)

Optic chiasm

Right optic tract

Lateral geniculate body

Midbrain (diencephalon)

(A)

Visual cortices of occipital lobes

Optic disc

Axons of retinal ganglion cells

Ganglion cell layer

Bipolar cell layer

Layer of rods and cores

Sclera

Optic nerve

(B)

Figure 9.4. Visual system. A. The origin, course, and distribution of the visual pathway are shown. The axons of retinal ganglionic neurons convey visual information to the lateral geniculate body of the thalamus through the optic nerve (CN II) and optic tract. Fibers from the lateral geniculate body project to the visual cortices of the occipital lobes. The axons of ganglion cells of the nasal halves of the retinas cross in the optic chiasm; those from the temporal halves do not cross. **B.** The visual pathway begins with photoreceptor cells (rods and cones) in the retina. The responses of the photoreceptors are transmitted by bipolar cells (neurons having two processes) to ganglion cells in the ganglion cell layer of the retina. The central processes of this third-order neuron are the fibers conducted by the optic nerves.

Demyelinating Diseases and the Optic Nerve

Because the optic nerves are actually CNS tracts, the myelin sheath that surrounds the sensory fibers from the point at which the fibers penetrate the sclera is formed by oligodendrocytes (glial cells) rather than by neurolemma (Schwann) cells, as in other cranial or spinal nerves of the parasympathetic nervous system (PNS). Consequently, the optic nerves are susceptible to the effects of demyelinating diseases of the CNS, such as *multiple sclerosis* (MS), which usually do not affect other nerves of the PNS.

Optic Neuritis

Optic neuritis refers to lesions of the optic nerve that cause diminution of visual acuity, with or without changes in peripheral fields of vision (Lange et al., 2000). Optic neuritis may be caused by inflammatory, degenerative, demyelinating, or toxic disorders. The optic disc appears pale and smaller than usual on ophthalmoscopic examination. Many toxic substances (e.g., methyl and ethyl alcohol, tobacco, lead, and mercury) may also injure the optic nerve.

Visual Field Defects

Visual field defects result from lesions that affect different parts of the visual pathway. The type of defect depends on where the pathway is interrupted (Fig. B9.1):

- Complete section of an optic nerve results in blindness in the temporal (*T*) and nasal (*N*) visual fields of the ipsilateral eye (depicted in *black*).

- Complete section of the optic chiasm reduces peripheral vision and results in *bitemporal hemianopsia*, the loss of vision of one half of the visual field of both eyes.

- Complete section of the right optic tract at the midline eliminates vision from the left temporal and right nasal visual fields. A lesion of the right or left optic tract causes a contralateral homonymous hemianopsia, indicating that visual loss is in similar fields. This defect is the most common form of visual field loss and is often observed in patients with strokes (Swartz, 2002).

Defects of vision caused by compression of the optic pathway, as may result from tumors of the pituitary gland or berry aneurysms of the internal carotid or the precommissural part of the anterior cerebral arteries (see Chapter 7), may produce only part of the visual losses described here for complete section of the pathway. Patients may not be aware of changes in their visual fields until late in the course of disease, because lesions affecting the visual pathway often develop insidiously. ⊙

Right monocular blindness

Visual fields

Bitemporal hemianopsia

Visual fields

Left homonymous hemianopsia

Visual fields

Section of right optic nerve

Section of optic chiasm

Section of right optic tract

Figure B9.1

THE BOTTOM LINE: The optic nerves (CN II) have sensory fibers concerned with the special sense of vision. The nerve fibers arise from ganglion cells in the retina. They exit the orbit via the optic canals; fibers from the nasal half of the retina cross to the contralateral side at the optic chiasm. The fibers then pass via the optic tracts to the geniculate bodies of the thalamus, where they synapse on neurons whose processes form the optic radiations to the primary visual cortex of the occipital lobe. Pressure on the optic pathway or laceration or intracerebral thrombus in the temporal, parietal, or occipital lobes of the brain can result in visual field defects.

Oculomotor Nerve (CN III)

Functions: Somatic motor (general somatic efferent) and visceral motor (general visceral efferent–parasympathetic).

Nuclei: There are two oculomotor nuclei, each serving one of the functional components of the nerve. The somatic motor nucleus of the oculomotor nerve is in the midbrain (Fig. 9.2). The visceral motor (parasympathetic) accessory (Edinger-Westphal) nucleus of the oculomotor nerve lies dorsal to the rostral two thirds of the somatic motor nucleus (Haines, 2002).

The **oculomotor nerve** (CN III) provides the following (Fig. 9.5):

- Motor to the striated muscle of four of the six extraocular muscles (*superior, medial,* and *inferior recti* and *inferior oblique*) and superior eyelid (L. *levator palpebrae superioris*); hence the nerve's name.

- Proprioceptive to the muscles listed above.

- Parasympathetic through the ciliary ganglion to the smooth muscle of the sphincter of the pupil (L. *sphincter pupillae*), which causes constriction of the pupil and ciliary body, which produces accommodation (allowing the lens to become more rounded) for near vision.

CN III is the chief motor nerve to the ocular and extraocular muscles. It emerges from the midbrain, pierces the dura lateral to the sellar diaphragm roofing over the hypophysis, and then runs through the roof and lateral wall of the *cavernous*

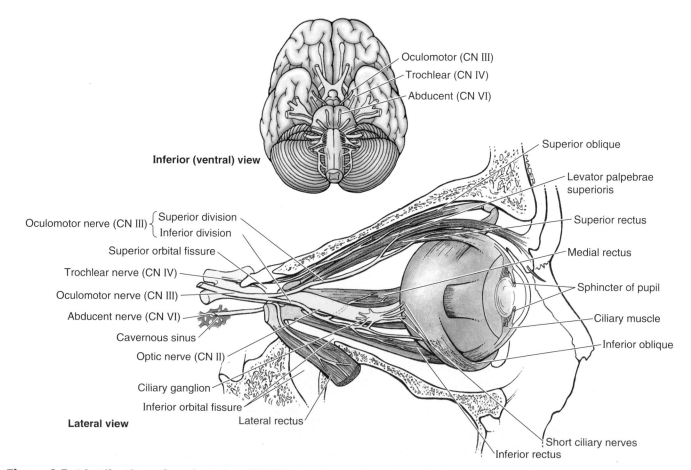

Figure 9.5. Distribution of oculomotor (CN III), trochlear (CN IV), and abducent (CN VI) nerves. CN IV supplies the superior oblique, CN VI supplies the lateral rectus, and CN III supplies five striated extraocular muscles (levator palpebrae superioris, superior rectus, medial rectus, inferior rectus, and inferior oblique) and two intraocular muscles (ciliary muscle and sphincter of pupil).

sinus. CN III leaves the cranial cavity and enters the orbit through the *superior orbital fissure.* Within this fissure, CN III divides into a **superior division** (which supplies the superior rectus and levator palpebrae superioris) and an **inferior division** (which supplies the inferior and medial rectus and inferior oblique). The inferior division also carries presynaptic parasympathetic (visceral efferent) fibers to the **ciliary ganglion,** where they synapse (Table 9.4). Postsynaptic fibers from this ganglion pass to the eyeball in the *short ciliary nerves* to innervate the ciliary body and sphincter of the pupil.

Injury to the Oculomotor Nerve

A lesion of CN III results in *ipsilateral oculomotor palsy,* summarized in Table 9.3 and discussed in detail in Chapter 7.

Compression of the Oculomotor Nerve

Rapidly increasing intracranial pressure (e.g., resulting from an extradural hematoma) often compresses CN III against the crest of the petrous part of the temporal bone. Because autonomic fibers in CN III are superficial, they are affected first. As a result, the pupil dilates progressively on the injured side. Consequently, the first sign of CN III compression is ipsilateral slowness of the pupillary response to light.

Aneurysm of the Posterior Cerebral or Superior Cerebellar Artery

An aneurysm of a posterior cerebral or superior cerebellar artery may also exert pressure on CN III as it passes between these vessels. The effects of this pressure depend on its severity. Because CN III lies in the lateral wall of the cavernous sinus, injuries or infections of the sinus may also affect this nerve. ⊙

THE BOTTOM LINE: The oculomotor nerves (CN III) send somatic motor fibers to all extraocular muscles, except the superior oblique and lateral rectus. They also send presynaptic parasympathetic fibers to the ciliary ganglion for innervation of the ciliary body and sphincter pupillae. These nerves originate from the brainstem, emerging medial to the cerebral peduncles, and run in the lateral wall of the cavernous sinus. They enter the orbit through the superior orbital fissures and divide into superior and inferior branches. Pressure on CN III from a herniating uncus, injury from a fracture involving the cavernous sinus, or an aneurysm can result in a dilated pupil, ptosis, turning of the eyeball down and out, and loss of the pupillary reflex on the side of the lesion.

Trochlear Nerve (CN IV)

Functions: Somatic motor (general somatic efferent) and proprioceptive to one extraocular muscle (superior oblique).

Nucleus: The nucleus of the trochlear nerve is located in the midbrain, immediately caudal to the oculomotor nucleus (Fig. 9.2).

The **trochlear nerve** (CN IV) is the smallest cranial nerve. It emerges from the posterior surface of the midbrain (the only cranial nerve to do so), passing anteriorly around the brainstem, running the longest intracranial (subarachnoid) course of the cranial nerves. It pierces the dura mater at the margin of the cerebellar tentorium (L. *tentorium cerebelli*) and passes anteriorly in the lateral wall of the cavernous sinus (Fig. 9.5). CN IV continues past the sinus to pass through the superior orbital fissure into the orbit, where it supplies the superior oblique—the only extraocular muscle that uses a pulley, or trochlea, to redirect its line of action (hence the nerve's name).

Injury to the Trochlear Nerve

CN IV is rarely paralyzed alone. Lesions of this nerve or its nucleus cause paralysis of the superior oblique and impair the ability to turn the affected eyeball inferomedially. CN IV may be torn when there are severe head injuries because of its long intracranial course. The characteristic sign of trochlear nerve injury is *diplopia* (double vision) when looking down (e.g., when going down stairs). Diplopia occurs because the superior oblique normally assists the inferior rectus in depressing the pupil (directing the gaze downward) and is the only muscle to do so when the pupil is adducted. In addition, because the superior oblique is the primary muscle producing intorsion of the eyeball, the primary muscle producing extorsion (the inferior oblique) is unopposed when the superior oblique is paralyzed. Thus the direction of gaze and rotation of the eyeball about its anteroposterior axis is different for the two eyes when an attempt is made to look downward, and especially when looking downward and medially. The person can compensate for the diplopia by inclining the head anteriorly and laterally toward the side of the normal eye. ⊙

THE BOTTOM LINE: The trochlear nerves (CN IV) supply somatic motor fibers to the superior oblique muscles and send proprioceptive fibers to this muscle, which abducts, depresses, and medially rotates the eyeball. The nerves emerge from the posterior aspect of the brainstem. They run a long intracranial course, passing around the brainstem to enter the dura mater in the free edge of the

Table 9.4.   Summary of Cranial Parasympathetic Ganglia

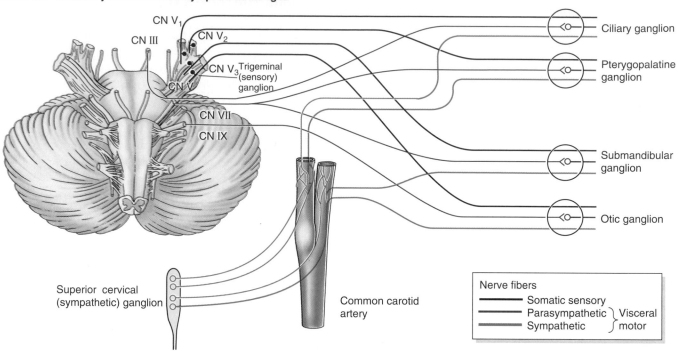

Ganglion	Location	Parasympathetic Root	Sympathetic Root	Main Distribution
Ciliary	Between optic nerve and lateral rectus, close to apex of orbit	Inferior branch of oculomotor nerve (CN III)	Branches from internal carotid plexus in cavernous sinus	Parasympathetic postsynaptic fibers from ciliary ganglion pass to ciliary muscle and sphincter pupillae of iris; sympathetic postganglionic fibers from superior cervical ganglion pass to dilator of pupil and blood vessels of eye
Pterygopalatine	In pterygopalatine fossa, where it is suspended by ganglionic branches of maxillary nerve (sensory roots of pterygopalatine ganglion); just anterior to opening of pterygoid canal and inferior to CN V_2	Greater petrosal nerve from facial nerve (CN VII) via nerve of pterygoid canal	Deep petrosal nerve, a branch of internal carotid plexus that is a continuation of postsynaptic fibers of cervical sympathetic trunk; fibers from superior cervical ganglion pass through pterygopalatine ganglion and enter branches of CN V_2	Parasympathetic postganglionic (secretomotor) fibers from pterygopalatine ganglion innervate lacrimal gland via zygomatic branch of CN V_2; sympathetic postsynaptic fibers from superior cervical ganglion accompany branches of pterygopalatine nerve that are distributed to blood vessels of nasal cavity, palate, and superior parts of pharynx
Otic	Between tensor veli palatini and mandibular nerve (CN V_3); lies inferior to foramen ovale of sphenoid bone	Tympanic nerve from glossopharyngeal nerve (CN IX); continues from the tympanic plexus as the lesser petrosal nerve	Fibers from superior cervical ganglion come from plexus on middle meningeal artery	Parasympathetic postsynaptic fibers from otic ganglion are distributed to parotid gland via auriculotemporal nerve (branch of CN V_3); sympathetic postsynaptic fibers from superior cervical ganglion pass to parotid gland and supply its blood vessels
Submandibular	Suspended from lingual nerve by two ganglionic branches (sensory roots); lies on surface of hyoglossus muscle inferior to submandibular duct	Parasympathetic fibers join facial nerve (CN VII) and leave it in its chorda tympani branch, which unites with lingual nerve	Sympathetic fibers from superior cervical ganglion via plexus on facial artery	Parasympathetic postsynaptic (secretomotor) fibers from submandibular ganglion are distributed to sublingual and submandibular glands; sympathetic fibers supply sublingual and submandibular glands

cerebellar tentorium close to the posterior clinoid process. They then run in the lateral wall of the cavernous sinus, entering the orbit via the superior orbital fissures. Stretching of CN IV during its course around the brainstem, or fracture of the orbit can result in an inability to look down (depress the pupil) when the eyeball is adducted.

Trigeminal Nerve (CN V)

Functions: General sensory (general somatic afferent) and branchial motor (special visceral efferent) to derivatives of the 1st pharyngeal arch.

Nuclei: There are four trigeminal nuclei—one motor and three sensory (Fig. 9.2).

The **trigeminal nerve** (CN V) is the largest cranial nerve (if the atypical optic nerve is excluded). It emerges from the lateral aspect of the pons by a large sensory root and a small motor root. The roots of CN V are comparable to the posterior and anterior roots of spinal nerves. CN V is the principal general sensory nerve for the head (face, teeth, mouth, nasal cavity, and dura of the cranial cavity). The large **sensory root of CN V** is composed mainly of the central processes of the pseudounipolar neurons that make up the trigeminal ganglion (Fig. 9.6B). The trigeminal ganglion is flattened and crescent shaped (hence its unofficial name, semilunar ganglion) and is housed within a dural recess (**trigeminal cave**) lateral to the cavernous sinus. The peripheral processes of the ganglionic neurons form three nerves or divisions: **ophthalmic nerve** (CN V₁), **maxillary nerve** (CN V₂), and sensory component of the **mandibular nerve** (CN V₃). Maps of the zones of cutaneous innervation by the three divisions resemble the dermatome maps for cutaneous innervation by spinal nerves (Fig. 9.6A). Unlike dermatomes, however, there is little overlap in innervation by the divisions; lesions of a single nerve result in clearly demarcated areas of numbness.

The fibers of the **motor root of CN V** pass inferior to the trigeminal ganglion along the floor of the trigeminal cave, bypassing the ganglion just as the anterior roots of spinal nerves bypass the spinal sensory ganglia. They are distributed exclusively via the mandibular nerve (CN V₃), blending with the sensory fibers as the nerve traverses the foramen ovale in the cranium; entering branches pass to the muscles of mastication, mylohyoid, anterior belly of the digastric, tensor veli palatini, and tensor tympani, which are derived from the 1st pharyngeal arch.

Although CN V conveys no presynaptic parasympathetic (visceral efferent) fibers from the CNS, all four parasympathetic ganglia are associated with the divisions of CN V. Postsynaptic parasympathetic fibers from the ganglia join branches of CN V and are carried to their destinations along with the CN V sensory and motor fibers (Fig. 9.5; Table 9.4).

The three divisions of the trigeminal nerve are discussed in the following sections.

Ophthalmic Nerve (CN V₁)

In contrast to the other two CN V divisions, CN V₁ is not a "branchial" nerve (i.e., it does not supply pharyngeal arch derivatives). It serves structures derived from the paraxial mesoderm of the embryonic frontonasal process. The ophthalmic nerve's association with the other CN V divisions is a secondary occurrence. The sensory (somatic afferent) fibers of CN V₁ are distributed to skin and mucous membranes and conjunctiva of the front of the head and nose (Table 9.1).

Testing CN V₁: The integrity of this division is tested by checking the corneal reflex—touching the cornea, which is also supplied by CN V₁, with a wisp of cotton will evoke a reflexive blink if the nerve is functional (Table 9.4).

Maxillary Nerve (CN V₂)

CN V₂ innervates derivatives of the maxillary prominence of the 1st pharyngeal arch. Exiting the cranial cavity via the foramen rotundum, its sensory (somatic afferent) fibers are generally distributed to skin and mucous membranes associated with the upper jaw. The pterygopalatine (parasympathetic) ganglion is associated with this division of CN V, involved in innervating the lacrimal and mucus glands.

Mandibular Nerve (CN V₃)

CN V₃ innervates derivatives of the mandibular prominence of the 1st pharyngeal arch. CN V₃ is the only division of CN V to convey motor (branchial efferent) fibers, distributed to the striated muscle derived from mandibular prominence mesoderm, primarily the muscles of mastication. Two parasympathetic ganglia, the otic and submandibular, are associated with this division of CN V; both are concerned with the innervation of salivary glands.

Tables 9.1 and 9.2 provide a general summary of CN V; Table 9.5 summarizes the branches of the three divisions.

Injury to the Trigeminal Nerve

CN V may be injured by trauma, tumors, aneurysms, or meningeal infections (Lange et al., 2000). It may be involved occasionally in poliomyelitis and generalized polyneuropathy, a disease process involving several nerves. The sensory and motor nuclei in the pons and medulla may be destroyed by intramedullary tumors or vascular lesions. An isolated lesion of the spinal trigeminal tract also may occur with multiple sclerosis (MS). Injury to the CN V causes the following:

- Paralysis of the muscles of mastication with deviation of the mandible toward the side of the lesion (Table 9.3). ▶

(A) Lateral view

(B) Lateral view

Key
- Ophthalmic nerve (CN V₁)
- Maxillary nerve (CN V₂)
- Mandibular nerve (CN V₃)

(C) Open-book view

Figure 9.6. Distribution of trigeminal nerve (CN V). A. Cutaneous (sensory) zones are innervated by the three divisions of the trigeminal nerve. **B.** Each cranial nerve division supplies skin and mucous membranes and sends a branch to the dura. Each division is associated with one or two parasympathetic ganglia and delivers the postsynaptic parasympathetic fibers from that ganglion: CN V₁ for the ciliary ganglion, CN V₂ for the pterygopalatine ganglion, and CN V₃ for the submandibular and otic ganglia. CN V₃ is also motor to the muscles of mastication and other striated muscles derived from the 1st pharyngeal arch. **C.** This open-book view shows the innervation of the lateral wall and septum of the nasal cavity and palate. CN V₁ supplies the anterosuperior portions of the cavity, and CN V₂ the posteroinferior portions and the palate.

Table 9.5. Summary of Divisions of Trigeminal Nerve (CN V)

Divisions/Distributions	Branches

Ophthalmic nerve (CN V₁)
Sensory only
Passes through superior orbital fissure
Supplies cornea, upper conjunctiva, mucosa of anterosuperior nasal cavity, frontal and ethmoidal sinuses, anterior and supratentorial dura mater, skin of dorsum of external nose, superior eyelid, forehead, and scalp
	Tentorial nerve (a meningeal branch)
	Lacrimal nerve
	   Communicating branch from zygomatic nerve
	Frontal nerve
	   Supraorbital nerve
	   Supratrochlear nerve
	Nasociliary nerve
	   Sensory root of ciliary ganglion
	   Short ciliary nerves
	   Long ciliary nerves
	   Infratrochlear nerves
	   Anterior and posterior ethmoidal nerves

Maxillary nerve (CN V₂)
Sensory only
Passes through foramen rotundum
Supplies dura mater of anterior part of middle cranial fossa; conjunctiva of inferior eyelid; mucosa of posteroinferior nasal cavity, maxillary sinus, palate and anterior part of superior oral vestibule; maxillary teeth; and skin of lateral external nose, inferior eyelid, anterior cheek, and upper lip
	Meningeal branch
	Zygomatic nerve
	   Zygomaticofacial branch
	   Zygomaticotemporal branch
	   Communicating branch to lacrimal nerve
	Ganglionic branches to (sensory root of) pterygopalatine ganglion
	Posterior superior alveolar branches
	   Infraorbital nerve
	   Anterior and middle superior alveolar branches
	   Superior labial branches
	   Inferior palpebral branches
	   External nasal branches
	Greater palatine nerves
	   Posterior inferior lateral nasal nerves
	Lesser palatine nerves
	Posterior superior lateral nasal branches
	Nasopalatine nerve
	Pharyngeal nerve

Mandibular nerve (CN V₃)
Sensory and motor
Passes through foramen ovale
Supplies sensory innervation to mucosa of anterior two thirds of tongue, floor of mouth, and posterior and anterior inferior oral vestibule; mandibular teeth; and skin of lower lip, buccal, parotid, and temporal regions of face; and external ear (auricle, upper external auditory meatus, and tympanic membrane)
	General sensory branches
	   Meningeal branch (nervus spinosum)
	   Buccal nerve
	   Auriculotemporal nerve
	   Lingual nerve
	   Inferior alveolar nerve
	      Nerve to mylohyoid
	      Inferior dental plexus
	      Mental nerve
	Branchiomotor branches
	   Masseter
	   Temporal
	   Medial and lateral pterygoids
	   Mylohyoid
	   Anterior belly of digastric
	   Tensor tympani

- Loss of the ability to appreciate soft tactile, thermal, or painful sensations in the face.

- Loss of corneal reflex (blinking in response to the cornea being touched) and the sneezing reflex (stimulated by irritants to clear the respiratory tract).

Common causes of facial numbness are dental trauma, herpes zoster (infection caused by a herpes virus), cranial trauma, head and neck tumors, intracranial tumors, and idiopathic trigeminal neuropathy (a nerve disease of unknown cause).

Trigeminal neuralgia (tic douloureux), the principal disease affecting the sensory root of CN V, produces excruciating, episodic pain that is usually restricted to the areas supplied by the maxillary and/or mandibular divisions of this nerve. This condition is discussed in detail in Chapter 7.

Dental Anesthesia

Anesthetic agents are commonly administered by injection to block pain during dental procedures. CN V is of great ▶

importance in the practice of dentistry because it is the sensory nerve of the head, serving teeth and mucosa of the oral cavity. Because the superior alveolar nerves (branches of CN V_2) are not accessible, the maxillary teeth are locally anesthetized by injecting the agent into the tissues surrounding the roots of the teeth and allowing the solution to infiltrate the tissue to reach the terminal (dental) nerve branches that enter the roots. By contrast, the inferior alveolar nerve (CN V_3) is readily accessible and is probably anesthetized more frequently than any other nerve. This procedure is discussed in clinical correlation (blue) box "Inferior Alveolar Nerve Block," in Chapter 7. ⊙

THE BOTTOM LINE: The trigeminal nerves (CN V) supply somatic motor fibers to the muscles of mastication, mylohyoid, anterior belly of the digastric, tensor tympani, and tensor veli palatini muscles. They also distribute postsynaptic parasympathetic fibers of the head to their destinations. CN V is sensory to the dura of the anterior and middle cranial fossae, skin of the face, teeth, gingiva, mucous membrane of the nasal cavity, paranasal sinuses, and mouth. CN V originates from the lateral surface of the pons by two roots: motor and sensory. These roots cross the medial part of the crest of the petrous part of the temporal bone. They enter the trigeminal cave of the dura lateral to the body of the sphenoid and cavernous sinus. The sensory root leads to the trigeminal ganglion; the motor root runs parallel to the sensory root, then bypasses the ganglion and becomes part of the mandibular nerve (CN V_3). Injury to the terminal branches and pathologic processes (tumors, aneurysms, infections) affecting CN V can result in loss of pain and touch sensations/paresthesia on the face, loss of corneal reflex, paralysis of the muscles of mastication, and deviation of the mandible on the side of the lesion when the mouth is opened.

Abducent Nerve (CN VI)

Functions: Somatic motor (general somatic efferent and proprioceptive) to one extraocular muscle (lateral rectus).

Nucleus: The abducent (*L. abducens*) nucleus is in the pons near the median plane (Fig. 9.2).

The **abducent nerves** (CN VI) emerge from the brainstem between the pons and the medulla and traverse the pontine cistern of the subarachnoid space, straddling the basilar artery (Fig. 9.5). Each abducent nerve then pierces the dura to run the longest intradural course within the cranial cavity of the cranial nerves—that is, its point of entry into the dura covering the clivus is the most distant from its exit from the cranium via the superior orbital fissure. During its intradural course, it bends

sharply over the crest of the petrous part of the temporal bone and then courses through the cavernous sinus, surrounded by the venous blood in the same manner as the internal carotid artery, which it parallels in the sinus. CN VI traverses the common tendinous ring (*L. anulus tendineus communis*) as it enters the orbit (see Chapter 7), running on and penetrating the medial surface of the lateral rectus, which abducts the eye (this function being the basis for the name of the nerve).

Injury to the Abducent Nerve

Because CN VI has a long intracranial course, it is often stretched when intracranial pressure rises, partly because of the sharp bend it makes over the crest of the petrous part of the temporal bone after entering the dura. A space-occupying lesion, such as a brain tumor, may compress CN VI, causing paralysis of the lateral rectus. Complete paralysis of CN VI causes medial deviation of the affected eye—that is, it is fully adducted owing to the unopposed action of the medial rectus, leaving the person unable to abduct the eye (Fig. B9.2). *Diplopia* is present in all ranges of movement of the eyeball, except on gazing to the side opposite the lesion. Paralysis of CN VI may also result from:

- An aneurysm of the cerebral arterial circle (at the base of the brain) (see Chapter 7).

- Pressure from an atherosclerotic internal carotid artery in the cavernous sinus, where CN VI is closely related to this artery.

- Septic thrombosis of the sinus subsequent to infection in the nasal cavities and/or paranasal sinuses. ⊙

Figure B9.2. Injury to abducent nerve.

THE BOTTOM LINE: The abducent nerves (CN VI) supply somatic motor fibers to the lateral rectus muscles of the eyeballs and proprioceptive fibers to these muscles. The nerves originate from the pons, pierce the dura on the clivis, traverse the cavernous sinus and superior orbital fissures, and enter the orbits. Injury to the base of the brain or a fracture of the cranial base involving the cavernous sinus or orbit can result in inability to move the eye laterally, and diplopia occurs on lateral gaze.

Facial Nerve (CN VII)

Functions: Sensory (special visceral afferent and general somatic afferent), motor (branchial motor or special visceral efferent), and parasympathetic (general visceral efferent). It also carries proprioceptive fibers from the muscles it innervates.

Nuclei: The motor nucleus of the facial nerve is a branchiomotor nucleus in the ventrolateral part of the pons (Fig. 9.2). The cell bodies of the primary sensory neurons are in the geniculate ganglion (Fig. 9.7). The central processes of those concerned with taste end in the nuclei of the solitary tract in the medulla. The processes of those concerned with general sensations (pain, touch, and thermal) from around the external ear end in the *spinal nucleus of the trigeminal nerve.*

The **facial nerve** (CN VII) emerges from the junction of the pons and medulla as two divisions, the motor root and the intermediate nerve. The larger **motor root** (facial nerve proper) innervates the muscles of facial expression, and the smaller **intermediate nerve** (L. *nervus intermedius*) carries taste, parasympathetic, and somatic sensory fibers. During its course, CN VII traverses the posterior cranial fossa, internal acoustic meatus, facial canal, stylomastoid foramen of the temporal bone, and parotid gland. After traversing the internal acoustic meatus, the nerve proceeds a short distance anteriorly within the temporal bone and then turns abruptly posteriorly to course along the medial wall of the tympanic cavity. The sharp bend is the **geniculum of the facial nerve** (L. *genu,* knee), sometimes called the external genu of CN VII, the site of the **geniculate ganglion** (sensory ganglion of CN VII). While traversing the temporal bone within the facial canal, CN VII gives rise to the:

- Greater petrosal nerve.
- Nerve to the stapedius.
- Chorda tympani nerve.

Then, after running the longest intraosseous course of any cranial nerve, CN VII emerges from the cranium via the *stylomastoid foramen;* gives off the posterior auricular branch; enters the parotid gland; and forms the **parotid plexus,** which gives rise to the following five terminal motor branches: temporal, zygomatic, buccal, marginal mandibular, and cervical.

Branchial Motor

As the nerve of the 2nd pharyngeal arch, the facial nerve supplies striated muscles derived from its mesoderm, mainly the muscles of facial expression and auricular muscles. It also supplies the posterior bellies of the digastric, stylohyoid, and stapedius muscles.

Presynaptic Parasympathetic

The parasympathetic (general visceral efferent) distribution of the facial nerve is presented in Figure 9.8. CN VII provides presynaptic parasympathetic fibers to the **pterygopalatine ganglion** for innervation of the lacrimal mucous glands and to the **submandibular ganglion** for innervation of the sublingual and submandibular salivary glands. The pterygopalatine ganglion is associated with the maxillary nerve (CN V_2), which distributes its postsynaptic fibers, whereas the submandibular ganglion is associated with the mandibular nerve (CN V_3). The main features of parasympathetic ganglia supplied by the facial nerve and other cranial nerves are summarized in Table 9.4. Parasympathetic fibers synapse in these ganglia, whereas sympathetic and other fibers pass through them.

General Sensory

Some fibers from the geniculate ganglion supply a small area of the skin of the concha of the auricle, close to external acoustic meatus.

Taste (Special Sensory)

Fibers carried by the chorda tympani join the **lingual nerve** to convey taste sensation from the anterior two thirds of the tongue and soft palate.

Injury to the Facial Nerve

Among motor nerves, CN VII is the most frequently paralyzed of all the cranial nerves. Depending on the part of the nerve involved, injury to CN VII may cause paralysis of facial muscles without loss of taste on the anterior two thirds of the tongue, or altered secretion of the lacrimal and salivary glands.

A *lesion of CN VII near its origin* or near the geniculate ganglion is accompanied by loss of motor, gustatory (taste), and autonomic functions. The motor paralysis of facial muscles involves superior and inferior parts of the face on the ipsilateral side.

A *central lesion of CN VII* (lesion of the CNS) results in paralysis of muscles in the inferior face on the contralateral side; consequently, forehead wrinkling is not visibly impaired because it is innervated bilaterally. Lesions between the geniculate ganglion and ▶

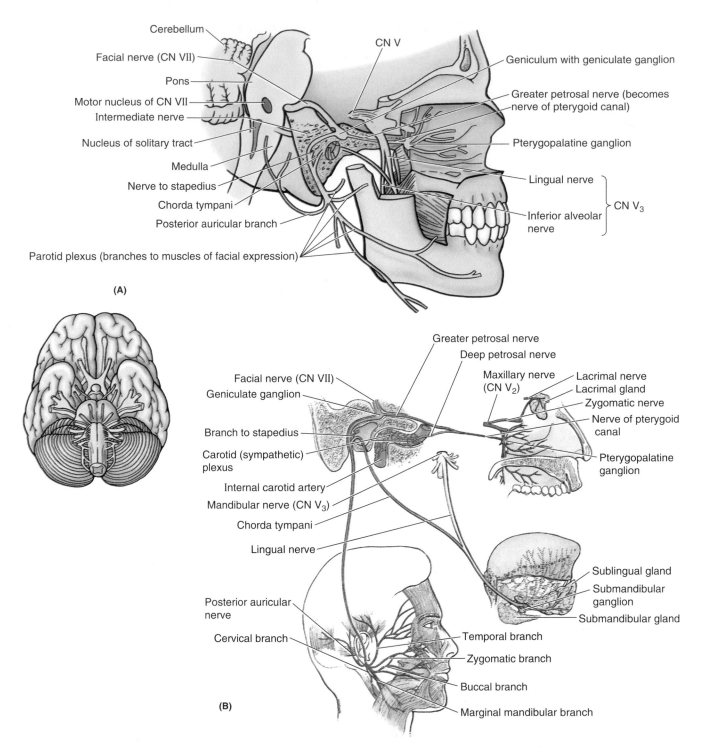

Figure 9.7. Distribution of facial nerve (CN VII). A. The facial nerve in situ demonstrates its intraosseous course and branches. **B.** The distribution of the facial nerve fibers is shown. Observe that CN VII supplies (1) branchial motor innervation (*blue*) to derivatives of the 2nd pharyngeal arch (muscles of facial expression, including the auricular and occipitofrontalis muscles plus the stapedius and posterior bellies of the digastric and stylohyoid); (2) special sensory (taste) and presynaptic parasympathetic (secretomotor) fibers (*green*) to the anterior tongue and submandibular ganglion via the chorda tympani; and (3) presynaptic parasympathetic (secretomotor) fibers (*purple*) to the pterygopalatine ganglion via the greater petrosal nerve.

(A) Parasympathetic (visceral motor) to lacrimal gland

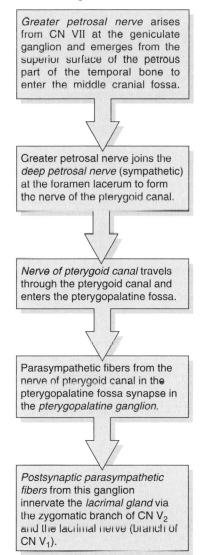

Greater petrosal nerve arises from CN VII at the geniculate ganglion and emerges from the superior surface of the petrous part of the temporal bone to enter the middle cranial fossa.

↓

Greater petrosal nerve joins the *deep petrosal nerve* (sympathetic) at the foramen lacerum to form the nerve of the pterygoid canal.

↓

Nerve of pterygoid canal travels through the pterygoid canal and enters the pterygopalatine fossa.

↓

Parasympathetic fibers from the nerve of pterygoid canal in the pterygopalatine fossa synapse in the *pterygopalatine ganglion*.

↓

Postsynaptic parasympathetic fibers from this ganglion innervate the *lacrimal gland* via the zygomatic branch of CN V$_2$ and the lacrimal nerve (branch of CN V$_1$).

(B) Parasympathetic (visceral motor) to submandibular and sublingual glands

The chorda tympani branch arises from CN VII just superior to stylomastoid foramen.

↓

The chorda tympani crosses the tympanic cavity medial to handle of malleus.

↓

The chorda tympani passes through the petrotympanic fissure between the tympanic and the petrous parts of the temporal bone to join the lingual nerve (CN V$_3$) in the infratemporal fossa.

↓

Parasympathetic fibers of the chorda tympani synapse in the submandibular ganglion; postsynaptic fibers follow arteries to glands

Figure 9.8. Parasympathetic innervation involving CN VII. A. Innervation of the lacrimal gland is outlined. **B.** Innervation of the submandibular and sublingual glands is outlined.

the origin of the chorda tympani produce the same effects as that resulting from injury near the ganglion, except that lacrimal secretion is not affected. Because it passes through the facial canal in the temporal bone, CN VII is vulnerable to compression when a viral infection produces inflammation (viral neuritis) and swelling of the nerve just before it emerges from the stylomastoid foramen.

Because the branches of CN VII are superficial, they are subject to injury from knife and gunshot wounds, cuts, and birth injury. Damage to CN VII is common with fracture of the temporal bone and is usually detectable immediately after the injury. CN VII may also

be affected by tumors of the brain and cranium, aneurysms, meningeal infections, and herpes viruses. Although injuries to CN VII cause paralysis of facial muscles, sensory loss in the small area of skin on the posteromedial surface of the auricle and around the opening of the external acoustic meatus is rare. Similarly, hearing is not usually impaired, but the ear may become more sensitive to low tones when the stapedius (supplied by CN VII) is paralyzed; this muscle dampens vibration of the stapes (see Chapter 7).

Bell palsy is a unilateral facial paralysis of sudden onset resulting from a lesion of CN VII. This syndrome is illustrated and discussed in detail in Chapter 7. ◐

THE BOTTOM LINE: The facial nerves (CN VII) supply motor fibers to the stapedius, posterior belly of the digastric, stylohyoid, facial, and scalp muscles. They also supply presynaptic parasympathetic fibers via the intermediate nerve (smaller root of CN VII) destined for the pterygopalatine and submandibular ganglia via the greater petrosal nerve and chorda tympani, respectively. CN VII is sensory to some skin of the external acoustic meatus and, via the intermediate nerve, is sensory to taste from the anterior two thirds of the tongue and the soft palate. CN VII originates from the posterior border of the pons and runs through the internal acoustic meatus and facial canal in the petrous part of the temporal bone. CN VII exits via the stylomastoid foramen; its main trunk forms the intraparotid nerve plexus. Laceration or contusion of CN VII in the parotid region results in paralysis of the facial muscles—the eye remains open, the angle of the mouth droops, and the forehead does not wrinkle. Fracture of the temporal bone can result in the abnormalities just described plus increased sensitivity to noise, a dry mouth and cornea, and loss of taste on the anterior two thirds of the tongue.

Vestibulocochlear Nerve (CN VIII)

Functions: Special sensory (special somatic afferent)—that is, special sensations of hearing and equilibrium.

Nuclei: Four vestibular nuclei are located at the junction of the pons and medulla in the lateral part of the floor of the 4th ventricle; two cochlear nuclei are in the medulla (Fig. 9.2).

The **vestibulocochlear nerve** (CN VIII) emerges from the junction of the pons and medulla and enters the **internal acoustic meatus** (Fig. 9.9). Here it separates into the vestibular and cochlear nerves.

- The **vestibular nerve** is concerned with equilibrium. It is composed of the central processes of bipolar neurons in the **vestibular ganglion;** the peripheral processes of the neurons extend to the maculae of the utricle and saccule (sensitive to the line of linear acceleration relative to the position of the head) and to the ampullae of the semicircular ducts (sensitive to rotational acceleration).

- The **cochlear nerve** is concerned with hearing. It is composed of the central processes of bipolar neurons in the **spinal ganglion;** the peripheral processes of the neurons extend to the spiral organ.

Within the internal acoustic meatus, the two divisions of CN VIII are accompanied by the motor root and intermediate nerve of CN VII and the labyrinthine artery (see Chapter 7).

Injuries of the Vestibulocochlear Nerve

Although the vestibular and cochlear nerves are essentially independent, peripheral lesions often produce concurrent clinical effects because of their close relationship. Hence lesions of CN VIII may cause *tinnitus* (ringing or buzzing in ears), *vertigo* (dizziness, loss of balance), and impairment or loss of hearing. Central lesions may involve either the cochlear or vestibular divisions of CN VIII.

Deafness

There are two kinds of deafness: conductive deafness, involving the external or middle ear (e.g., otitis media, inflammation in the middle ear), and sensorineural deafness, which results from disease in the cochlea or in the pathway from the cochlea to the brain.

Acoustic Neuroma

An *acoustic neuroma* (neurofibroma) is a slow-growing benign tumor of the neurolemma (Schwann) cells. The tumor begins in the vestibular nerve while it is in the internal acoustic meatus, but the early symptom of an acoustic neuroma is usually loss of hearing. Dysequilibrium (derangement of the sense of equilibrium) and tinnitus occur in approximately 70% of patients (Bruce and Fetell, 2000).

Trauma and Vertigo

People with head trauma often experience headache, dizziness, vertigo, and other features of posttraumatic injury. *Vertigo* is a hallucination of movement involving the person or the environment (Wazen, 2000). It often involves a spinning sensation but may be felt as a swaying back and forth or falling. These symptoms, often accompanied by nausea and vomiting, are usually related to a peripheral vestibular nerve lesion. ⊕

THE BOTTOM LINE: The vestibulocochlear nerves (CN VIII) carry fibers concerned with the special senses of hearing and balance. The nerves originate from the grooves between the pons and the medulla. They run through the internal acoustic meatus and divide into the cochlear and vestibular nerves. The cochlear nerve is sensory to the spiral organ (for the sense of hearing). The vestibular nerve is sensory to the cristae of the ampullae of the semicircular ducts and the maculae of the saccule and utricle (for the sense of equilibration). A tumor of CN VIII can result in progressive, unilateral hearing loss, tinnitus (noises in the ear), and vertigo (loss of balance).

Figure 9.9. Vestibulocochlear nerve (CN VIII). A. The internal surface of the cranial base shows the location of the bony labyrinth of the internal ear within the temporal bone. **B.** This depiction of the bony and membranous labyrinths shows (1) innervation of the cochlea by the cochlear nerve of CN VIII for the sense of hearing and (2) innervation of the vestibular apparatus by the vestibular nerve of CN VIII for balance and equilibrium.

Inferior view

(A) Superior view

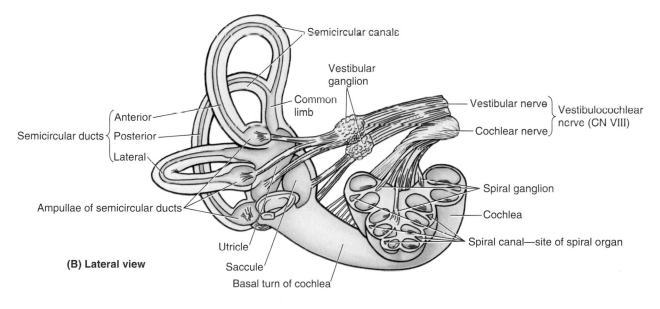

(B) Lateral view

Glossopharyngeal Nerve (CN IX)

Functions: Sensory (general somatic afferent, special visceral afferent, general visceral afferent), motor (special visceral efferent), and parasympathetic (general visceral efferent) for derivatives of the 3rd pharyngeal arch.

Nuclei: Four nuclei in the medulla send or receive fibers via CN IX: two motor and two sensory. Three of these nuclei are shared with CN X (Fig. 9.2).

The **glossopharyngeal nerve** (CN IX) emerges from the lateral aspect of the medulla and passes anterolaterally to leave the cranium through the anterior aspect of the *jugular foramen* (Figs. 9.10 and 9.11). At this foramen are **superior** and **inferior** (sensory) **ganglia,** which contain the pseudounipolar cell bodies for the afferent components of the nerve. CN IX follows the stylopharyngeus, the only muscle the nerve supplies, and passes between the superior and the middle constrictor muscles of the pharynx to reach the oropharynx and tongue. It contributes sensory fibers to the *pharyngeal plexus* of nerves. CN IX is afferent from the tongue and pharynx (hence its name) and efferent to the stylopharyngeus and parotid gland.

Branchial Motor

Motor fibers pass to one muscle, the stylopharyngeus, derived from the 3rd pharyngeal arch.

Parasympathetic (Visceral Motor)

Following a circuitous route initially involving the tympanic nerve, presynaptic parasympathetic fibers are provided to the otic ganglion for innervation of the parotid gland. The otic

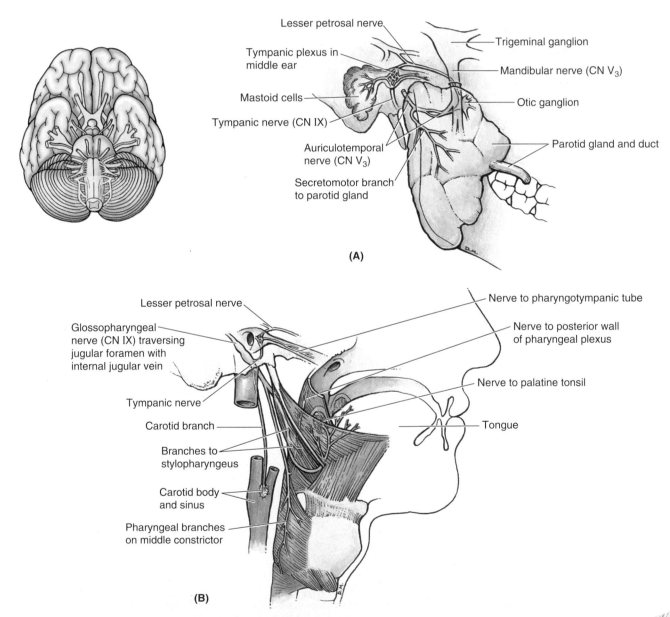

Figure 9.10. Distribution of glossopharyngeal nerve (CN IX). A. CN IX is motor to one striated pharyngeal muscle, the stylopharyngeus. It also carries sensory fibers from the carotid body and sinus, conveying information about blood pressure and gas levels as well as general sensation from the internal ear, pharynx, and fauces and taste from the posterior tongue. **B.** The parasympathetic compartment of CN IX supplies presynaptic secretory fibers to the otic ganglion; postsynaptic fibers pass to the parotid gland via the auriculotemporal nerve (CN V$_3$).

Figure 9.11. Relationship of structures traversing jugular foramen. CN IX, CN X, and CN XI are, in numerical order, anterior to the internal jugular vein as they traverse the foramen. They are immediately posterior to the internal carotid artery as they emerge from it. The superior and inferior sensory ganglia of CN IX and CN X are seen as thickenings of those nerves immediately inferior to their exit from the cranium.

ganglion is associated with the mandibular nerve (CN V₃), branches of which convey the postsynaptic parasympathetic fibers to the parotid gland (Fig. 9.12).

Sensory (General Sensory)

The general sensory branches of CN IX are as follows (Fig. 9.10):

- The *tympanic nerve.*
- The *carotid sinus nerve* to the carotid sinus, a baro- (presso) receptor sensitive to changes in blood pressure, and the carotid body, a chemoreceptor sensitive to blood gas (oxygen and carbon dioxide levels).

- The *pharyngeal, tonsillar,* and *lingual nerves* to the mucosa of the oropharynx and isthmus of the fauces (L. throat), including palatine tonsil, soft palate, and posterior third of the tongue. In addition to general sensation (touch, pain, temperature), tactile (actual or threatened) stimuli determined to be unusual or unpleasant here may evoke the gag reflex or even vomiting.

Taste (Special Sensory)

Taste fibers are conveyed from the posterior third of the tongue to the sensory ganglia. Details of the distribution of CN IX are outlined in Figure 9.12.

Lesions of the Glossopharyngeal Nerve

Isolated lesions of CN IX or its nuclei are uncommon and are not associated with perceptible disability (Lange et al., 2000). Taste is absent on the posterior third of the tongue, and the gag reflex is absent on the side of the lesion. Ipsilateral weakness may produce a noticeable change in swallowing. Injuries of CN IX resulting from infection or tumors are usually accompanied by signs of involvement of adjacent nerves. Because CN IX, CN X, and CN XI pass through the jugular foramen, tumors in this region produce multiple cranial nerve palsies, called

the *jugular foramen syndrome.* Pain in the distribution of CN IX may be associated with involvement of the nerve in a tumor in the neck.

Glossopharyngeal Neuralgia

Glossopharyngeal neuralgia (glossopharyngeal tic) is uncommon and its cause is unknown. The sudden intensification of pain is of a burning or stabbing nature. These paroxysms of pain are often initiated by swallowing, protruding the tongue, talking, or touching the palatine tonsil (Lange et al., 2000). Pain paroxysms occur during eating when trigger areas are stimulated. ○

Parasympathetic (visceral motor)

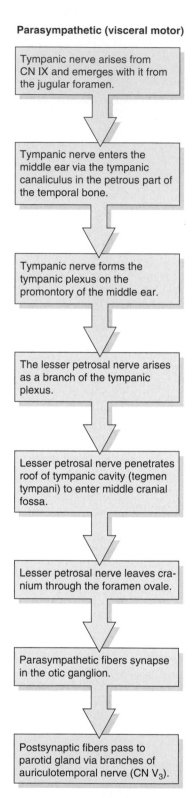

Figure 9.12. Parasympathetic innervation involving the glossopharyngeal nerve (CN IX). CN IX sends presynaptic parasympathetic (secretomotor) fibers to the otic ganglion via a convoluted route; postsynaptic fibers pass from the ganglion to the parotid gland via the auriculotemporal nerve (Fig. 9.10*B*).

THE BOTTOM LINE: The glossopharyngeal nerves (CN IX) send somatic motor fibers to the stylopharyngeus and visceral motor (presynaptic parasympathetic) fibers to the otic ganglion for innervation of the parotid gland. They also send sensory fibers to the posterior third of the tongue (including taste), pharynx, tympanic cavity, pharyngotympanic cavity, carotid body, and sinus. The nerves originate from the rostral end of the medulla and exit from the cranium via the jugular foramina. They pass between the superior and the middle constrictors of the pharynx to the tonsillar sinus and enter the posterior third of the tongue. A brainstem lesion or deep laceration of the neck can result in loss of taste on the posterior third of the tongue, loss of sensation on the affected side of the soft palate, and loss of the gag reflex on the affected side.

Vagus Nerve (CN X)

Functions: Sensory (general somatic afferent, special visceral afferent, general visceral afferent), motor (special visceral efferent), and parasympathetic (general visceral efferent).

- Sensory from the inferior pharynx, larynx, and thoracic and abdominal organs.
- Sense of taste from the root of the tongue and taste buds on the epiglottis. Branches of the internal laryngeal nerve (a branch of CN X) supply a small area, mostly general but some special sensation; most general and special sensation to the root is supplied by CN IX.
- Motor to the soft palate; pharynx; intrinsic laryngeal muscles (phonation); and a nominal extrinsic tongue muscle, the palatoglossus, which is actually a palatine muscle based on its derivation and innervation.
- Proprioceptive to the muscles listed above.
- Parasympathetic to thoracic and abdominal viscera.

Nuclei: Four nuclei of CN X in the medulla send or receive fibers via CN IX—two motor and two sensory (Fig. 9.2). Three of these nuclei are shared with CN IX.

The **vagus nerve** (CN X) has the longest course and most extensive distribution of all the cranial nerves, most of which is outside of (inferior to) the head. The term *vagus* is derived from the Latin word *vagari* meaning "wandering." CN X was so called because of its extensive distribution (Table 9.6). It arises by a series of rootlets from the lateral aspect of the medulla that merge and leave the cranium through the *jugular foramen* positioned between CN IX and CN XI (Figs. 9.11 and 9.13).

Table 9.6. Summary of Vagus Nerve (CN X)

Divisions (Parts)	Branches
Cranial Vagi arise by a series of rootlets from medulla (includes traditional cranial root of CN XI)	Meningeal branch to dura mater (sensory; actually fibers of C2 spinal ganglion neurons that hitch a ride with vagus nerve) Auricular branch
Cervical Exit cranium/enter neck through jugular foramen; right and left vagus nerves enter carotid sheaths and continue to root of neck	Pharyngeal branches to pharyngeal plexus (motor) Cervical cardiac branches (parasympathetic, visceral afferent) Superior laryngeal nerve (mixed) internal (sensory) and external (motor) branches Right recurrent laryngeal nerve (mixed)
Thoracic Vagi enter thorax through superior thoracic aperture; left vagus contributes to anterior esophageal plexus; right vagus to posterior plexus; form anterior and posterior trunks	Left recurrent laryngeal nerve (mixed; all distal branches convey parasympathetic and visceral afferent fibers for reflex stimuli) Thoracic cardiac branches Pulmonary branches Esophageal plexus
Abdominal Anterior and posterior vagal trunks enter abdomen through esophageal hiatus in diaphragm; distribute asymmetrically	Esophageal branches Gastric branches Hepatic branches Celiac branches (from posterior trunk) Pyloric branch (from anterior trunk) Renal branches Intestinal branches (to left colic flexure)

What was formerly called the "cranial root of the accessory nerve" is actually a part of CN X (Fig. 9.14). CN X has a *superior ganglion* in the jugular foramen that is mainly concerned with the general sensory component of the nerve. Inferior to the foramen is an *inferior ganglion* (nodose ganglion) concerned with the visceral sensory components of the nerve. In the region of the superior ganglion are connections to CN IX and the superior cervical (sympathetic) ganglion. CN X continues inferiorly in the *carotid sheath* to the root of the neck (see Chapter 8), supplying branches to the palate, pharynx, and larynx (Fig. 9.13; Table 9.6).

The course of CN X in the thorax differs on the two sides, a consequence of rotation of the midgut during development (see Chapters 1 and 2). CN X supplies branches to the heart, bronchi, and lungs. The vagi join the *esophageal plexus* surrounding the esophagus, which is formed by branches of the vagi and sympathetic trunks. This plexus follows the esophagus through the diaphragm into the abdomen, where the **anterior** and **posterior vagal trunks** break up into branches that innervate the esophagus, stomach, and intestinal tract as far as the left colic flexure.

Lesions of the Vagus Nerve

Isolated lesions of CN X are uncommon. Injury to pharyngeal branches of CN X results in *dysphagia* (difficulty in swallowing). Lesions of the superior laryngeal nerve produce anesthesia of the superior part of the larynx and paralysis of the cricothyroid muscle (see Chapter 8). The voice is weak and tires easily. Injury of a recurrent laryngeal nerve may be caused by aneurysms of the arch of the aorta and may occur during neck operations. Injury of the recurrent laryngeal nerve causes hoarseness and *dysphonia* (difficulty in speaking) because of paralysis of the vocal folds (cords). Paralysis of both recurrent laryngeal nerves causes *aphonia* (loss of voice) and *inspiratory stridor* (a harsh, high pitched respiratory sound). Paralysis of recurrent laryngeal nerves usually results from cancer of the larynx and thyroid gland and/or from injury during surgery on the thyroid gland, neck, esophagus, heart, and lungs. Because of its longer course, lesions of the left recurrent laryngeal nerve are more common than those of the right. Proximal lesions of CN X also affect the pharyngeal and superior laryngeal nerves, causing difficulty in swallowing and speaking. ⊕

THE BOTTOM LINE: The vagus nerves (CN X) supply motor fibers to the voluntary muscles of the larynx and superior esophagus. They also send visceral motor (presynaptic parasympathetic) fibers to (1) involuntary muscles and glands of the tracheobronchial tree and esophagus via the pulmonary and esophageal plexuses, (2) to the heart via the cardiac plexus, and (3) to the alimentary tract as far as the left colic flexure. The nerves also send sensory fibers to the pharynx, larynx, and reflex afferents from these same areas. They originate via 8–10 rootlets from the lateral sides of the medulla of the brainstem. They enter the superior mediastinum posterior to the sternoclavicular joints and brachiocephalic veins. The nerves give rise to right and left recurrent nerves and then, from the esophageal plexus, reform as anterior and posterior vagal trunks that continue into the abdomen. A brainstem lesion or a deep laceration of the neck can result in sagging of the soft palate, deviation of the uvula to the unaffected side, hoarseness owing to paralysis of the vocal fold, and difficulty in swallowing and speaking.

Spinal Accessory Nerve (CN XI)

Functions: Motor to the striated sternocleidomastoid and trapezius muscles.

Nuclei: The spinal accessory nerve arises from the nucleus of the accessory nerve, a column of anterior horn motor neurons

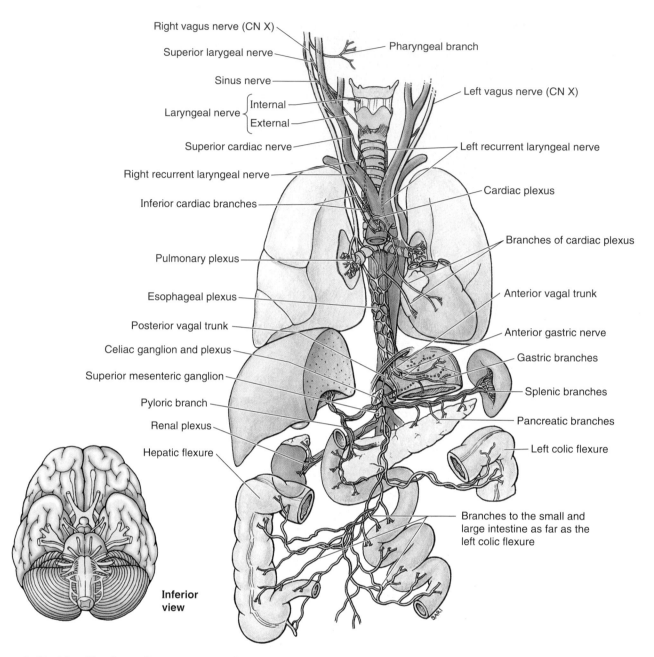

Right vagus nerve (CN X)
Superior larygeal nerve
Sinus nerve
Laryngeal nerve { Internal / External }
Superior cardiac nerve
Right recurrent laryngeal nerve
Inferior cardiac branches
Pulmonary plexus
Esophageal plexus
Posterior vagal trunk
Celiac ganglion and plexus
Superior mesenteric ganglion
Pyloric branch
Renal plexus
Hepatic flexure

Pharyngeal branch
Left vagus nerve (CN X)
Left recurrent laryngeal nerve
Cardiac plexus
Branches of cardiac plexus
Anterior vagal trunk
Anterior gastric nerve
Gastric branches
Splenic branches
Pancreatic branches
Left colic flexure
Branches to the small and large intestine as far as the left colic flexure

Inferior view

Figure 9.13. Distribution of vagus nerve (CN X). After supplying the palatine, pharyngeal, and laryngeal branches, CN X descends into the thorax. The recurrent laryngeal nerves ascend to the larynx, the left from a more inferior (thoracic) level. In the abdomen, the anterior and posterior vagal trunks demonstrate further asymmetry as they supply the terminal esophagus, stomach, and intestinal tract as far distally as the left colic flexure.

in the superior five or six cervical segments of the spinal cord (Fig. 9.2).

The traditional "cranial root" of CN XI is actually a part of CN X (Lachman et al., 2002). It is united for a short distance with the **spinal accessory nerve** (CN XI) (Fig. 9.14). CN XI emerges as a series of rootlets from the first five or six cervical segments of the spinal cord. It joins the CN X temporarily as they pass through the *jugular foramen,* separating again as they exit. CN XI descends along the internal carotid

artery, penetrates and innervates the sternocleidomastoid, and emerges from the muscle near the middle of its posterior border. It crosses the posterior cervical region and passes deep to the superior border of the trapezius to descend on its deep surface, providing multiple branches to the muscle as it does so. Branches of the cervical plexus conveying sensory fibers from spinal nerves C2–C4 join the spinal accessory nerve in the posterior cervical region, providing these muscles with pain and proprioceptive fibers.

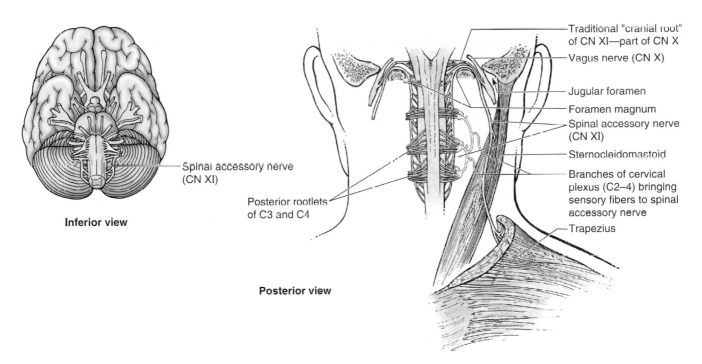

Inferior view

Spinal accessory nerve
(CN XI)

Posterior rootlets
of C3 and C4

Posterior view

Traditional "cranial root"
of CN XI—part of CN X

Vagus nerve (CN X)

Jugular foramen

Foramen magnum

Spinal accessory nerve
(CN XI)

Sternocleidomastoid

Branches of cervical
plexus (C2–4) bringing
sensory fibers to spinal
accessory nerve

Trapezius

Figure 9.14. Distribution of spinal accessory nerve (CN XI). The traditional cranial root consists of vagal fibers that arise via four or five rootlets from the lateral part of the medulla, join CN XI, and then leave it to join and be distributed by the vagus (CN X). CN XI (the traditional spinal root) arises from the cervical region of the spinal cord and supplies the sternocleidomastoid and trapezius muscles. CN XI is now called the spinal accessory nerve.

Injury to the Spinal Accessory Nerve

Because of its nearly subcutaneous passage through the posterior cervical region, CN XI is susceptible to injury during surgical procedures such as lymph node biopsy, cannulation of the internal jugular vein, and carotid endarterectomy (see Chapter 8). ✪

THE BOTTOM LINE: The spinal accessory nerves (CN XI) supply motor fibers to the striated sternocleidomastoid and trapezius muscles. The nerves arise as rootlets from the sides of the spinal cord in the superior five or six cervical segments. They ascend into the cranial cavity via the foramen magnum and exit through the jugular foramina, crossing the lateral cervical region. A laceration of the neck can cause paralysis of the sternocleidomastoid and superior fibers of the trapezius, which results in drooping of the shoulder.

Hypoglossal Nerve (CN XII)

Functions: Motor (general somatic efferent) to the intrinsic and extrinsic muscles of the tongue (G. *glossa*)—styloglossus, hyoglossus, and genioglossus.

The **hypoglossal nerve** (CN XII) arises as a purely motor nerve by several rootlets from the medulla and leaves the cranium through the *hypoglossal canal.* After exiting the

cranial cavity, CN XII is joined by a branch or branches of the cervical plexus conveying general somatic motor fibers from C1 and C2 spinal nerves and general somatic sensory fibers from the spinal ganglion of C2. These spinal nerve fibers "hitch a ride" with CN XII to reach the hyoid muscles, with some of the sensory fibers passing retrograde along it to reach the dura mater of the posterior cranial fossa. CN XII passes inferiorly medial to the angle of the mandible and then curves anteriorly to enter the tongue (Fig. 9.15).

CN XII ends in many branches that supply all the extrinsic muscles of the tongue, except the palatoglossus (which is actually a palatine muscle). CN XII has the following branches:

- A **meningeal branch** returns to the cranium through the hypoglossal canal and innervates the dura mater on the floor and posterior wall of the posterior cranial fossa. The nerve fibers conveyed are from the sensory spinal ganglion of spinal nerve C2 and are not hypoglossal fibers.

- The **superior root of the ansa cervicalis** branches from CN XII to supply the infrahyoid muscles (sternohyoid, sternothyroid, and omohyoid). This branch actually conveys only fibers from the cervical plexus (the loop between the anterior rami of C1 and C2) that joined the nerve outside the cranial cavity, not hypoglossal fibers. Some fibers continue past the descending branch to reach the thyrohyoid muscle.

- Terminal **lingual branches** supply the styloglossus, hyoglossus, genioglossus, and intrinsic muscles of the tongue.

Inferior view

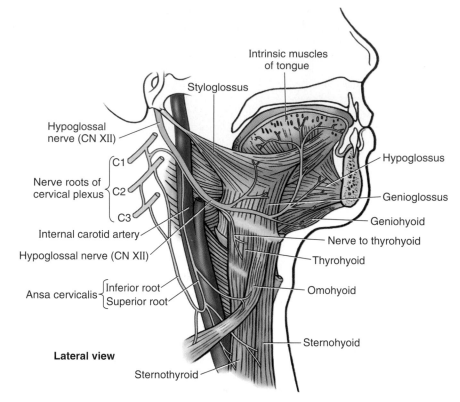

Intrinsic muscles of tongue

Styloglossus

Hypoglossal nerve (CN XII)

Nerve roots of cervical plexus { C1 C2 C3

Internal carotid artery

Hypoglossal nerve (CN XII)

Ansa cervicalis { Inferior root / Superior root

Hypoglossus

Genioglossus

Geniohyoid

Nerve to thyrohyoid

Thyrohyoid

Omohyoid

Sternohyoid

Sternothyroid

Lateral view

Figure 9.15. Distribution of hypoglossal nerve (CN XII). CN XII leaves the cranium through the hypoglossal canal and passes deep to the mandible to enter the tongue, where it supplies all intrinsic and extrinsic lingual muscles, except the palatoglossus. CN XII is joined immediately distal to the hypoglossal canal by a branch conveying fibers from the C1 and C2 loop of the cervical plexus. These fibers hitch a ride with CN XII, leaving it as the superior root of the ansa cervicalis and the nerve to the thyrohyoid muscle. Cervical spinal nerves, not CN XII, supply the infrahyoid muscles.

Injury to the Hypoglossal Nerve

Injury to CN XII paralyzes the ipsilateral half of the tongue. After some time, the tongue atrophies, making it appear shrunken and wrinkled. When the tongue is protruded, its apex deviates toward the paralyzed side because of the unopposed action of the genioglossus muscle on the normal side of the tongue. ✚

THE BOTTOM LINE: The hypoglossal nerves (CN XII) supply somatic motor fibers to the intrinsic and extrinsic muscles of the tongue, except the palatoglossus (actually a palatine muscle). They arise by several rootlets between the pyramids and the olives of the medulla. They pass through the hypoglossal canals and run inferiorly and anteriorly, passing medial to the angles of the mandible and between the mylohyoid and the hypoglossus to reach the muscles of the tongue. A neck laceration or a fracture of the cranial base can result in deviation of a protruded tongue toward the affected side and moderate dysarthria (disturbance of articulation).

References and Suggested Readings

Agur, AMR, Dalley AF: *Grant's Atlas of Anatomy,* 11th ed. Baltimore, Lippincott Williams & Wilkins, 2005.

Bruce JN, Balmaceda CM, Fetell MR: Tumors of the skull and cranial nerves. *In* Rowland LP (ed): *Merritt's Textbook of Neurology,* 10th ed. Baltimore, Lippincott Williams & Wilkins, 2000.

Fetell MR: General considerations. *In* Rowland LP (ed) *Merritt's Textbook of Neurology,* 10th ed. Baltimore, Lippincott Williams & Wilkins, 2000.

Haines DE: *Fundamental Neuroscience,* 2nd ed. New York, Churchill Livingstone, 2002.

Haines DE: *Neuroanatomy: An Atlas of Structures, Sections, and Systems,* 6th ed. Baltimore, Lippincott Williams & Wilkins, 2000.

Haines DE, Mihailoff GA: An overview of the brainstem. *In* Haines DE (ed): *Fundamental Neuroscience,* 2nd ed. New York, Churchill Livingstone, 2002.

Hutchins JB, Corbett JJ: The visual system. *In* Haines DE (ed): *Fundamental Neuroscience,* 2nd ed. New York, Churchill Livingstone, 2002.

Kiernan JA: *Barr's the Human Nervous System: An Anatomical Viewpoint,* 7th ed. Baltimore, Lippincott Williams & Wilkins, 1998.

Lachman N, Acland RD, Rosse C: Anatomical evidence for the absence of a morphologically distinct cranial root of the accessory nerve in man. Clin Anat 15:4, 2002.

Lange DL, Trojaborg W, Rowland LP: Peripheral and cranial nerve lesions. *In* Rowland LP (ed): *Merritt's Textbook of Neurology*, 10th ed. Baltimore, Lippincott Williams & Wilkins, 2000.

Moore KL, Persaud TVN: *The Developing Human. Clinically Oriented Embryology*, 7th ed. Philadelphia, Saunders, 2003

Rowland LP (ed): *Merritt's Textbook of Neurology*, 10th ed. Baltimore, Lippincott Williams & Wilkins, 2000.

Sacco RL: Pathogenesis, classification, and epidemiology of cerebrovascular disease. *In* Rowland LP (ed): *Merritt's Textbook of Neurology*, 10th ed. Baltimore, Lippincott Williams & Wilkins, 2000.

Swartz MH: *Textbook of Physical Diagnosis: History and Diagnosis*, 4th ed. Philadelphia, Saunders, 2002.

Sweazey RD: Olfaction and taste. *In* Haines DE (ed): *Fundamental Neuroscience*, 2nd ed. New York, Churchill Livingstone, 2002.

Wazen JJ: Dizziness and hearing loss. *In* Rowland LP (ed): *Merritt's Textbook of Neurology*, 10th ed. Baltimore, Lippincott Williams & Wilkins, 2000.

Wilson-Pauwels L, Akesson EJ, Stewart PA: *Cranial Nerves: Anatomy and Clinical Comments*. Toronto, Decker, 1988.

Index

Page numbers in *italics* denote figures; those followed by "t" denote tables

A

Abbreviations, 12
Abdomen
  acute, 206, *276*
  description of, 193
  computed tomography of, 347, *352*
  fat accumulation on, 205
  functions of, 193
  hernias of, 205
  magnetic resonance imaging of,
      347, *350*
  medical imaging of, 343–353
  paracentesis of, *233*
  protuberance of, 205
  radiographs of, 343–344, *344*
  regions of, 194, *195*
  ultrasound of, *71*, 347, *348–349*
  viscera of
    description of, 194, 241–244
    innervation of, 321–325
    parasympathetic innervation of,
        324–325
    physiology of, 243–244
    sympathetic innervation of, 321–324
  walls of (*see* Abdominal wall)
Abdominal wall
  anterolateral
    blood vessels of, 210–213
    description of, 194, 196
    elements of, 196, *197*
    fascia of, 196–198
    incisions of
      description of, 208
      gridiron (muscle-splitting), 209
      longitudinal, 208–209
      McBurney, 209
      median, 208–209
      midline, 208–209
      oblique, 209
      paramedian, 208–209
      pararectus, 209
      Pfannenstiel, 209
      suprapubic, 209
      transverse, 209
    internal surface of, 213–214
    lymphatic system for, *210*
    muscles of, 198–206
    nerves of, 206–207t
    palpation of, 206
    physical examination of, 196
    structure of, *200*
    surface anatomy of, 230–231
  description of, 194
  inferior, *202*
  posterior
    anatomy of, 331, *332–333*
    arteries of, 337–343
    autonomic nerves of, *322*
    blood vessels of, 337–343
    fascia of, 331–333, *332*
    lymphatic system of, *342*, *342*
    muscles of, 333–334, *336*
    nerves of, 335–336, *336*
  subdivisions of, *196*
Abduction, *9–10*, 11
Abscess
  ischioanal, 449–450
  parotid gland, 955
  pelvirectal, 450
  perianal, 450
  perinephric, 308
  peritoneal, 238
  popliteal, 636
  psoas, 333, 596
  retroauricular, 1029, *1029*
  retropharyngeal, 1053
  seminal gland, 406
  subphrenic, 292
  tooth, 995
Acetabulum
  anatomy of, *28*, *359*, *558–560*, 562, 675
  fracture of, *364*
  lunate surface of, *675*
Acetylcholine, 59
Acoustic neuroma, 1146
Acromion
  anatomy of, *28*, 753
  of scapula, *728*, 731, *731*
  surface anatomy of, 781, *783*
Acute abdomen, 206, 275
Acute arterial occlusion, 671
Acute respiratory distress, 131
Adduction, *9–10*, 11
Adenocarcinoma, ductular, 288
Adenoiditis, 1110
Adenoma, parathyroid, 1088
Adhesions
  definition of, 233
  diaphragmatic, *251*
  peritoneal, 233
  splenic, *251*
Adhesiotomy, 233

Adhesive capsulitis, 859
Aging
  of costal cartilage, 81
  of vertebrae, 495–496
Ala
  of ilium, *613*
  of sacrum, *468*
Alimentary system, 4
Alveolar bone resorption, 892
Alveolus, *127*
  pulmonary, 125
Amastia, 111
Ampulla
  bony, 1033
  of ductus deferens, 376, *378*, *404*,
      405, *407*
  duodenum, 259, *344*
  hepatopancreatic, 260, 287, *296*
  rectal, *397*, *429*, 430, *430*, 445
  of semicircular canals, *1147*
  of uterine tube, 424
Anastomoses (*see also* Arteries; Vein(s))
  arterial, 29
    around scapula, 767, *767–768*
    of elbow joint, 863
    of elbow region, 792, *792*
  arteriolovenular, 44
  arteriovenous, 448
  of cerebral arteries, 930
  cruciate, 604, 605t
    of thigh, 624
  definition of, 29, 41
  of gastro-omental arteries, *240*, *249*
  genicular, *635*, 695
  of intercostal arteries, *770*
  of knee, *695*
  periarticular arterial, 29
  portocaval/porto-systemic, 306, 307,
      390, 431
  splenorenal, 307
  venous, 42
Anatomical planes, 5–6, *6*
Anatomical position, 5
Anatomical snuff box, 741, 812, *812*,
      838, *846*
Anatomical variations, 12
Anatomicomedical terminology, 4–12
  abbreviation of, 12
  anatomical planes, 5–6, *6*
  anatomical position, 5
  description of, 4–5
  laterality terms, 7
  movement terms, 7–11, *9–10*

Macula lutea, 966
Magnetic resonance imaging
  of back, 548–549, *552*